Handbook of Sexual Assault and Sexual Assault Prevention

William T. O'Donohue
Paul A. Schewe
Editors

Handbook of Sexual Assault and Sexual Assault Prevention

Springer

Editors
William T. O'Donohue
Department of Psychology
University of Nevada
Reno, NV, USA

Paul A. Schewe
Department of Criminology, Law, and Justice
University of Illinois at Chicago
Chicago, IL, USA

ISBN 978-3-030-23644-1 ISBN 978-3-030-23645-8 (eBook)
https://doi.org/10.1007/978-3-030-23645-8

This Springer imprint is published by the registered company Springer Nature Switzerland AG
The registered company address is: Gewerbestrasse 11, 6330 Cham, Switzerland

Introduction

Controversies, a Path Forward for Prevention, and Summary of this Volume

Major Controversies in Sexual Assault

Any field of science is not without its controversies and the field of sexual assault research is no exception. This section will provide an overview of eight important but controversial issues in the contemporary sexual assault field. Further research that provides a basis for increased understanding and perhaps resolving these controversies represents an important path forward for advancing the science around sexual assault and sexual assault prevention.

The Incidence of Sexual Assault: "One in Four"?

Epidemiology is the scientific study of the incidence and prevalence of health problems. Incidence is defined as the frequency of new cases of the phenomenon and is usually given with respect to both a specific time-period, e.g., the incidence of sexual assault in a one-year period would be the rate of new cases of sexual assault in that time-period; as well as by the size of the population, e.g., the incidence of sexual assault is x within a year for the y million female undergraduate students in the United States. Prevalence, on the other hand, is the number of cases that are current, which is a combination of new cases plus previous cases. Prevalence in some sense is a cumulative number—with lifetime prevalence providing just that—the frequency of sexual assault occurring sometime in an individual's life.

Obviously, within the epidemiology of sexual assault there are a number of complex issues that need to handled well to derive accurate numbers: (a) how sexual assault is defined—e.g., does any sort of unwanted sexual contact count, e.g., does an unwanted kiss on a date count just as does forced vaginal penetration, or does an inappropriate touching of a chest when 5 by a 4-year-older sibling count as a case of sexual assault (or should it count as child sexual abuse, a different phenomenon, or as problematic sex play?) Sexual assault can be a vague term and it is useful to be more specific and clear about how this term is operationalized—e.g., is penetration involved in the statistic or simply any unwanted touching? One reason so many incidences are not reported as assault is that the recipient does not label them as such. Others indicate that the incidents are not significant enough to be reported (e.g., an unwanted kiss on a date). Perhaps other distinctions between sexual assault and unwanted sexual touching are needed —something like unwanted minor sexual advances during a date. The latter are in no way being excused or condoned—just distinguished from something that is more serious. Second, should every self-report of sexual assault count as a true incidence or should some sort of screen or some sort of additional burden of proof be met, i.e., only "founded" cases that involve some sort of positive finding from some sort of reasonable investigation are included in the statistic? Should reported cases be used, or should self-report data of unreported cases also be used; or both? If formal reports of sexual assault are used, how does one deal with the fact that many self-reported instances of unwanted sexual contact are never formally reported at all: does one include in these epidemiological numbers only reported cases (assuming all are true), or does one take some sort of estimate of the number of unreported cases (e.g., only one in 16 cases is reported; therefore, every reported case is multiplied by 16) and use this estimate to calculate incidence or prevalence? A further nuance to this issue is that Koss and colleagues (1987) in a classic study found that the report of sexual assault is subject to a number of important methodological variables such as the wording of questions (use of the word "rape" vs. use of something like "unwanted sexual contact") as well as assessment strategy (face to face interviews vs. questionnaires) and thus these methodological characteristics can influence the epidemiological numbers reported.

Here are just a few examples of these sorts of problematic epidemiological statistics that are commonly reported:

- An American Association of University survey indicated that 1 in 4 women will be victims of sexual assault or misconduct—which can be taken as evidence of this commonly reported prevalence rate. However, those reporting penetration was 10.8%—and thus if penetration is taken to be a definitional criterion of rape—this rate decreases from 1 in 4 to 1 in 9.
- One in five women and one in 71 men will be raped at some point in their lives (a) (National Sexual Violence Center (nsvc.org). This organization also states on the same website: "One in 5 women and one in 16 men are sexually assaulted while in college (i)," which would problematically imply given the first statistic no woman will be raped after she graduates from college or that the rate of sexual assault in college is substantially greater than the general population).
- However, in a study of college-age females between the years of 1995 and 2014 Sinozich and Langton (2014) found that the incidence of rape and sexual assault was 7.6 per 1000 for nonstudents and for students 6.1 per 1000—a rate of about 1 in 164. This is obviously quite different than 1 in 4.

It is not the purpose of this section to clear up the numerous and complex controversies concerning the epidemiology of sexual assault. It is to say, however, that in science as well as any rational debate, accuracy and clarity are desirable characteristics. Perhaps the function of the phrase "1 in 4" women will be raped is to have an important and desirable rhetorical function: individuals ought not to minimize this problem; it is a problem that ought to be taken seriously: sexual assault clearly occurs all too frequently. However, the persuasive and informative function ought to be achieved with accurate numbers with clearly defined terms. Moreover, there does not seem to be any cutoff that sexual assault advocates ought to be worried about, e.g., no one has argued that if "only" 1 in 200 individuals are sexually assaulted the problem is then unimportant. Scholars in the field are encouraged to use accurate numbers and precise terms regarding the incidence and prevalence of sexual assault, communicate assumptions or problems with these numbers, so that only clear accurate information is being disseminated.

False Allegations

Relatedly, there is also a controversial issue of the existence of false allegations of sexual assault. This is a multidimensional issue involving a moral dimension, a pragmatic dimension, and a scientific dimension. The moral dimension may currently be predominating and involves at least two interrelated issues: calling a true report of sexual report false is often seen as a moral failing as it further harms the sexual assault victim (and possibly even allows the perpetrator to abuse other individuals). This error arguably seems to be a legitimate moral failing—however, the only nuance to consider is that if the erroneous judgment is made in good faith (e.g., without bias toward women or toward victims, and after a reasonably thorough—but obviously faulty—examination of all evidence, and so on) or it is made more problematically—e.g., due to sexism. This moral problem of course can be rectified by simply believing all allegations of sexual assault—a course that at times seems to be advocated by some. However, the opposing moral consideration then comes into play: alleging that an individual committed a sexual assault when this individual did not also causes moral harm against that individual. It would seem that the best moral position would be to try to minimize both sorts of error and harm.

However, there seems to be a problematic meta-moral position taken and that is that merely asserting that false allegations exist is itself a moral failing. For some, it is a matter of morality that ethically one must always "believe the victim" (which of course is question begging) or in a less question begging form, "believe all women." This position takes any rational scrutiny of the claim, or its evidence (or lack thereof) or any recognition of due process rights of the accused as in and of itself morally problematic. It also fails to recognize that false claims have been made in the past (see O'Donohue, Chap. 32, this volume); as well as the practical consideration that it is not a law of nature—i.e., an impossibility—that a person cannot falsely claim that sexual assault has occurred. These false allegations may be due to a complex array of factors including mental disorders, lying, intoxication, or suggestibility (see Engle & O'Donohue, 2012). Of course, part of the rationale for the ethical condemnation of a belief in false allegations may be well-intentioned: it is certainly the case that historically and even currently in some situations, women's true accounts of sexual assault are not believed. However, this can be a problem that can be more precisely stated: *The field needs to develop methods to distinguish between true and false allegations with a high degree of accuracy and in a way that is not further traumatizing to the victim.* This is an important and urgent problem and is better formed than the simplistic and problematic "believe all victims or "believe all women."

The pragmatic dimension is centered on how does one (and this can vary across contexts—e.g., a research context would be different than a legal context) rationally determine whether an allegation is true or false? This leads to the scientific dimension and a complex research agenda. This is not an easy task but too little research is currently being reported that is oriented toward making progress on this problem. What standard of proof ought to be used? What evidence is relevant and how should it be analyzed? What evidence is most important? What ought to be done with missing evidence, especially if the claimant does not want to cooperate with the investigation? What should a procedure look like to come to some accurate judgment—should it involve cross-examination? Should it involve subpoena power? Should a recantation always be considered as sufficient evidence of a false report (even though a true allegation can be recanted)? What is relevant from either the alleged victim's or alleged perpetrator's past (e.g., a history of other allegations, a history of lying, or continued amicable relationships after the alleged assault?). Are current protocols for investigation sufficient or how can they be improved? Do current protocols involve any biases such as sexism or confirmation bias? These are critical questions that need to be addressed.

Existence of a "*Rape Culture*"?

Some advocates in the sexual assault field have suggested that there is a *rape culture*. Rape culture typically is taken to mean ideologies that normalize or promote sexual assault. For example, Keller, Mendes and Ringrose (2018) stated:

> According to feminists then, rape culture is manifested in a number of ways. While rape culture inevitably involves rape and sexual assault, it is also defined by a number of other harmful practices, including rape jokes, sexual harassment, cat-calling, sexualized 'banter'; the routine policing of women's bodies, dress, appearance, and code of conduct; the re-direction of blame from the perpetrator in an assault to the victim; and impunity for perpetrators, despite their conduct or crimes (Mendes, 2015). We thus employ the term 'rape culture' to describe a multitude of practices that range in terms of legality, prevalence, and cultural acceptance (p. 24).

Phipps, Ringrose, Renold and Jackson (2018), on the other hand, provided a somewhat different definition of rape culture:

> …refers to a set of general cultural beliefs supporting men's violence against women, including the idea that this violence is a fact of life, that there is an association between violence and sexuality, that men are active while women are passive, and that men have a right to sexual intercourse. These also produce prevalent 'rape myths' such as that women enjoy being raped, and give credence to the idea that there are 'blurred' lines around consent, which has generated widespread disbelief of rape victims and low conviction rates of perpetrators (p. 1).

We can see at least one problem immediately: the construct of rape culture has a good deal of variability in its definition. However, both definitions (and there are other definitions) agree that the construct is complex: it has multiple dimensions and is linked to other more general problematic beliefs such as sexism. Secondly, there is a lack of scientific evidence for the existence of a rape culture. There are no measurement procedures to measure the presence, absence, or degree of "rape culture." The definition also fails to acknowledge the true complexity of this construct in that it fails to acknowledge that all may not buy in or adhere to rape culture—one would hypothesize that feminists certainly would create environments and safe spaces that would be inconsistent with this; but it also is the case that not all males would endorse such a culture. Some may not endorse the rape culture for reasons similar to feminists although some males may not endorse a rape culture as there are females that they care about and do not want to be sexually assaulted—wives, daughters, sisters, mothers, friends, and so on. The construct of rape culture paints indirectly a very negative and false view of males and such extraordinary claims need extraordinary evidence, which is lacking. This is not to say that there are problematic attitudes in cultures that may interfere with preventing sexual assault; however, it is to say that such a poorly defined, not currently measurable construct, may paint with too broad a brush. More careful and nuanced work is needed.

The Funding of Sexual Assault Research, Prevention, and Therapy

Efforts designed to positively impact sexual assault are grossly underfunded. There is too little money in local, state, and federal justice agencies to support victims and to prosecute sexual assault perpetrators; too little federal or private grant money to research key issues in sexual assault; too little money on college campuses for prevention efforts (it is useful to compute a ratio of amount spent on college football vs. the amount spent on sexual assault—from a behavioral economics point of view it would seem that college campuses value touchdowns more than safe campuses); and too little money spent in trying to rehabilitate perpetrators (e.g., there is no DSMV category of "rapist" in the paraphilias and therefore cannot receive third-party payments for therapy delivered to these individuals). It would be useful to deal with this practical issue and determine what constitutes a fair and reasonable amount of funds to support all dimensions of the sexual assault field. This would seem to be a priority for sexual assault advocates.

Evidence-Based Practice

Evidence-based practice is a useful construct that has positive effects on the quality of services in health care in general. Basically, the idea is that interventions (including assessments) ought to be continually evaluated by scientific study such as randomly controlled trials and only those that produce the best results (including effectiveness and safety) be disseminated. In addition, there is a notion of evidence-based assessment, where any purported measurement procedure is examined for its error rate by understanding its psychometric properties such as reliability and validity. However, too often in the field of sexual assault, fads, anecdotes, or extra-scientific concerns like politics have influenced practice and thus too few have received the best evidence-based sexual assault prevention programming. More needs to be done to make the data relevant to key practical decisions in this field clearer, available, and transparent.

DSM Diagnosis and Rape Perpetrators

As stated previously there is no diagnostic category for a rapist. This needs to change. In general, mental disorders in the DSM5 (American Psychiatric Association, 2013) are defined as:

1. A behavioral or psychological syndrome or pattern that occurs in an individual
2. The consequences of which are clinically significant distress (e.g., a painful symptom) or disability (i.e., impairment in one or more important areas of functioning)
3. Must not be merely an expectable response to common stressors and losses (e.g., the loss of a loved one) or a culturally sanctioned response to a particular event (e.g., trance states in religious rituals)
4. That reflects an underlying psychobiological dysfunction
5. That is not solely a result of social deviance or conflicts with society
6. That has diagnostic validity using one or more sets of diagnostic validators (e.g., prognostic significance, psychobiological disruption, response to treatment) that has clinical utility (e.g., contributes to better conceptualization of diagnoses, or to better assessment and treatment)

These definitional criteria of mental disorder have received a lot of criticism: including whether existing diagnostic conditions currently included in the DSM5 actually meet these—e.g., given how little is known about the "psychobiological dysfunction" underlying most mental disorders (criterion 4). However, it seems like if a paraphilia like pedophilia meets these criteria then some sort of "willingness to rape or arousal to rape" ought to also. Rape ought to be seen as a paraphilia and treated by mental health professionals.

Memory Wars

There are unresolved issues in the science of remembering trauma (see McNally's (2003) classic book). Key questions include: are memories of sexual assault trauma recalled with significant detail—at least for the central components such as what was done—or is trauma remembered poorly so that a rape victim's account will typically contain significant gaps or inconsistent statements? Or even more strongly, can trauma be completely repressed so that the victim even comes to believe for at time that he or she was never assaulted—but after some sort of memory trigger has detailed memories rushing back? These issues are battles in what is known as "the memory wars" and have received a lot of attention in recent years. In some ways this also pits factions in the field—those more influenced by science against those more associated with practice and what the APA problematically calls "professional knowledge."

This issue is related to the general notion of evidence-based practice above. Again, the field needs to orient more toward science and less away from mere political advocacy.

Low Reporting Rates and Low Rates of Successful Prosecution

This is an important pragmatic problem in the field that needs attention. How can more victims report their assaults in a way that is effective, supportive, and non-traumatic? How can these victims feel comfortable about pursuing further adjudication, particularly criminal prosecution so that hopefully they can feel some sense of justice and closure and perpetrators can be justly punished and prevented from victimizing others? Cummings and O'Donohue (2019) have developed a barrier screen as well as an interview protocol for use with sexual assault victims that have some preliminary data on its acceptability. However, more efforts are needed so that sexual assault perpetrators end up being punished instead of having a low probability of detection, prosecution, and sentencing.

Understanding and Preventing Sexual Assault: A Path Forward

A Developmental Socio-Ecological Approach to Preventing Sexual Assault Across the Lifespan

Sexual assault does not exist within the bodies of individual perpetrators or victims like some rare disease. The problem of sexual assault does not occur in a vacuum. There are a host of individual, relationship, community, societal, and environmental factors that all serve as either risk factors or protective factors. Of course, for sexual assault to occur at least two individuals need to be involved; hence, there also is an interaction between perpetrator variables and victim variables. These risk factors, the data and theories that attempt to explain and expose them, are the focus of several chapters in this volume. Certainly, sexual assault shares characteristics and risk factors with other forms of interpersonal violence such as child abuse, bullying, dating violence, and spouse abuse. The problem of preventing violence in relationships has drawn attention from investigators from diverse fields including Psychology, Sociology, Public Health, Social Work, Psychiatry, Medicine, Neuroscience, Criminology, Gender Studies, Nursing, and Education. Almost without fail, journal articles addressing relationship violence include a section describing the implications of research results for prevention. Until recently, however, most violence prevention efforts have focused on reducing the incidence of assaults by strangers, despite long-standing evidence that people are twice as likely to be victimized by an acquaintance/friend, relative, or intimate partner (Catalano, 2007). As is typical with many efforts to address important social problems, sexual assault prevention efforts have been largely spearheaded by advocates, and research has generally followed their lead. Early efforts to prevent sexual assault focused on preventing violent assaults by strangers (Schewe & O'Donohue, 1993). College freshmen were given rape whistles, women were taught to use their keys to defend themselves against an attack, and emergency call boxes and increased lighting were installed on college campuses. Increased understanding that sexual assault often occurs within relationships has led to efforts to prevent men from assaulting or abusing their partners, efforts to teach young people healthy relationship skills, and efforts to teach bystanders how to safely intervene to prevent sexual assault among their friends and acquaintances.

The focus of this handbook is the integration of theory, research, and practice, guided by a vision of developing policies and programs to facilitate healing, promote healthy relationships and prevent sexual violence within society. One of the core questions that drive prevention research is, "What can be done from the start and throughout the lifecourse to maximize the probability of children developing in wholesome ways?" Anyone who works with survivors of sexual assault quickly realizes that the only humane way to address sexual assault is to prevent it in the first place. In the early 1990s, Schewe and O'Donohue worked to develop educational interventions directed towards college males intended to instill knowledge, attitudes, beliefs, and skills that would prevent them from committing rape (Schewe & O'Donohue, 1993a, 1993b, 1996). From those projects, they learned that educational interventions with college males are entirely insufficient, and that if we are to be successful in preventing rape we must intervene at all developmental stages and address all levels of the social ecology (individual attitudes, beliefs and behaviors; relationship skills; community values, policies and norms; and societal/cultural values, policies, and laws). To further complicate this socio-ecological lifespan approach, programs, treatment, and policies are needed to address primary, secondary, and tertiary prevention. At the *primary* level, programs and policies are designed to prevent first instances of sexual assault, focusing both on potential perpetrators and victims. At the *secondary* level, programs, treatment, and policies are directed at increasing early detection of victims, or identifying and intervening with individuals at higher risk for either perpetration or victimization (i.e., delinquent individuals, run-aways, substance users, etc.). *Tertiary* interventions are aimed at restoring functioning for survivors of sexual violence, or preventing recidivism among perpetrators.

Clearly, the focus and methods of sexual assault prevention will vary widely depending upon the developmental stage of the target audience. Interventions directed at the **Individual and Relationship** level often focus on educational efforts at various developmental stages. The following examples of interventions are not intended to be exhaustive, but rather are intended to spark ideas regarding potential areas of intervention using developmental stages, levels of prevention, and the social-ecological model as a guide.

Young Children. **Primary**—Promote social emotional skills and emotional intelligence. **Secondary**—Provide resources and treatment for children in families that are exposed to domestic violence. **Tertiary**—Provide referrals for child victims of sexual violence and their families. As mandated reporters, teachers need to report suspicions of child abuse to their state's child protection agency. Since the tertiary level of prevention is really intervention after sexual abuse has occurred, it will not be covered in detail here but is addressed elsewhere in this Handbook.

Early Elementary. **Primary**—Continue to teach social-emotional skills, build language for respect, teach respect, sharing, and equality. Instill ethical principles of autonomy, justice, beneficence, and non-maleficence. **Secondary**—Child victims may respond with either internalizing or externalizing behaviors. Be sensitive to children who suddenly begin acting out, or who may become overly compliant or shy and withdrawn.

Elementary. **Primary**—Work to prevent bullying. Implement bullying prevention programs. Teach healthy communication skills. **Secondary**—Directly intervene in bully–victim relationships. Provide education and support to all parties.

Middle School. **Primary**—Begin to address dating violence and healthy relationship skills. **Secondary**—Identify aggressive or sexually aggressive students, as well as overly shy or withdrawn students. Provide them with additional mentoring. Engage them in conversations and encourage them to share their experiences. Encourage participation in supervised afterschool activities.

High School. **Primary**—Begin to address sexual assault more directly, continue teaching healthy relationships skills and begin to incorporate rape myths, consent, healthy sexuality, and bystander intervention concepts. **Secondary**—Address the use of pornography. Develop specialized interventions for youth identified as sexually aggressive or those who abuse substances.

Parenting. **Primary**—Parents need to be taught how to adequately supervise their children, and to understand that children are often victimized by individuals who are known and trusted by the family. Parents can teach children body autonomy and respect, and should practice nonviolent forms of discipline. **Secondary**—Parents should teach their children proper labels for body parts (e.g., penis and vagina) and let them know that they can safely talk to their parents or other trusted adults (e.g., teachers, doctors, police) about sex. Parents can talk to young children about secrets, and that it is okay to disclose secrets to a trusted adult. As children grow, talk to them about bullying, about dating, and about sex. Make expectations clear, and keep lines of communication open. **Tertiary**—Parents are often the first ones to discover or suspect sexual victimization. This is often difficult because the perpetrator is often someone loved or trusted by the parent. Parents should express support and belief to their child, and enlist the help of professionals from medical centers, rape crisis centers, child advocacy centers, or law enforcement to help navigate a path forward.

Community-Level Interventions: While many individual and relationship risk factors can be addressed through education, Community and Societal level responses require a different approach. At the **Community Level**, resources, community norms, policies, training, alcohol-related policies, etc. need to be addressed. For instance, what if alcohol were allowed at college Sororities, but banned from college Fraternities? This change in community-level policies could have a significant impact on sexual assault on college campuses. Other community-level interventions could involve training bartenders and bouncers in sexual assault and bystander intervention.

Societal-Level Interventions: Of course, all of the levels of the social ecology and developmental stages exist with societies. Again, the ethical principles of autonomy, justice, beneficence, and non-maleficence can be applied here. Constructs to be addressed here include patriarchy/equality between genders, fair judicial proceedings, respect for each person's autonomy/right to self-determination. Societal interventions generally entail the creation of laws and policies. The movie rating system that restricts access or warns of sexually explicit or violent material is one set of policies intended to protect children from exposure to potentially harmful material. Title IX policies, statutes of limitations for prosecuting sex offenses, rape shield laws, orders of protection, efforts to remove guns from domestic violence offenders, zoning laws that separate bars from schools, and sex offender registration are all examples of laws and policies that have attempted to address sexual assault.

Special Populations: Within each of the levels of the social ecology and developmental stages, of course, are special populations that warrant specialized attention. Developmentally delayed individuals, individuals with disabilities, LGBTQIA individuals, and prisoners are just a few examples of special populations where sexual assault is a particular concern and where specialized interventions are warranted. Race, religion, nationality might also warrant special attention, as well as those affiliated with specific institutions (i.e., military).

The goal of this handbook is to compile much of what research has taught us about sexual assault, as well as to identify a path forward in the understanding and prevention of sexual assault. The prevention of sexual assault is an amazingly complex problem to solve, and it will take the combined efforts of advocates and professionals from diverse fields to accomplish this goal.

Summary of the Book

This handbook is divided into 7 major sections that explore prevention, intervention, risk factors, and other topics related to sexual assault victimization and perpetration.

The first section, Theories of Sexual Assault, includes two chapters that conceptualize sexual assault using separate theoretical frameworks. Sasha and Levand (*this volume*) present literature on the emergence of feminism and its intersection with sexual assault. Second, Huppin, Malamuth and Linz (*this volume*) discuss how evolutionary psychology might explain the presence of sexual violence and elucidate methods of reducing the prevalence rate of victimization and perpetration.

The second section, Culture and Society, is dedicated to chapters focused on how culture as well as societal issues and policies explain sexual assault. McMahon (*this volume*) explains the evolution of the anti-rape movement, spanning back to the founding years of the United States. Benuto, Gonzalez, Casas, Newlands, and Leany (*this volume*) discuss the extant literature on sexual victimization of ethnic minority individuals, as well as provide perspectives on culturally sensitive practices to utilize when interviewing and treating these populations. McMahon (*this volume*) discusses social and legal policies (e.g., Clery Act; Title IX; Violence Against Women Act) developed to target sexual assault and provides recommendations for future social policy development. McDonald (*this volume*) highlights the historic impact of the #MeToo movement and the role of social media to create, reflect, and reinforce public perception around sexual assault on an increasingly politicized platform. Both Bridges (*this volume*) and Foubert, Blanchard, Houston and Williams, Jr. (*this volume*) provide perspectives of the effects of pornography use on the prevalence of sexual assault, as well as how additional factors (e.g., age, culture) moderate these associations. Ryan (*this volume*) provides a review of rape myths, how these reframe societies' attitudes and beliefs of sexual victimization, and recommendations for how to intervene to change these misbeliefs.

Next, the third section, Risk Factors of Sexual Victimization and Perpetration, presents literature on multiple risk factors related to the perpetration of sexual assault, as well as risk of victimization. Yucel, Cantor, Joppa, and Angelone (*this volume*) provide a review of commonly studied risk factors, including demographic, individual, behavioral, and environmental risk factors, as these pertain to sexual victimization. Mouilso and Wilson (*this volume*) discuss the underlying mechanisms by which alcohol is associated with increased risk of both sexual assault victimization and perpetration. Messman-Moore and Salim (*this volume*) present literature on risk recognition, how this influences the likelihood of victimization, as well as factors that affect individuals' perceived risk. Marshall and Marshall (*this volume*) provide a critical review of the extant literature on empathy deficits in perpetrators of sexual assault and discuss the limitations of using this construct as a primary target of sexual offender treatment. Wojcik and Fisher (*this volume*) discuss typologies (i.e., patterns of characteristics) of four major categories of sexual offenders: adult rapists, child abusers, female offenders, and cyber sexual offenders. Vechiu (*this volume*) reviews the theoretical framework of hypermasculinity as it pertains to sexual assault perpetration, including sociocultural factors that influence the development of hypermasculinity.

The fourth section, Victimology, discusses the after effects victims of sexual assault often suffer from post-assault. Arditte Hall, Healy, and Galovski (*this volume*) examine literature regarding short-term and long-term negative outcomes commonly experienced by sexual assault victims, including mental, physiological, physical, and functional health concerns. Dworkin and colleagues (*this volume*) then provide a comprehensive review of theories explaining the development of posttraumatic stress disorder after being a victim of sexual violence, including symptoms and risk factors, as well as treatments to address the psychological sequela. Bhuptani and Messman-Moore (*this volume*) discuss the effects of blame and shame on outcomes in victims of child sexual abuse and adult sexual assault, as well as how these can be targeted in treatment for victims. Mann and Naugle (*this volume*) discuss the evolution of our understanding of how recovered memories occur in the context of child sexual assault cases, specifically. Zoellner and colleagues (*this *volume*) provide an in-depth review of how memory encoding of a sexual assault occurs (including physiological processes) and is often subject to biases. Vechiu (*this volume*) presents literature on the effects of sexual victimization on sexual functioning, with an emphasis on sexual dysfunction disorders, and calls for an exploration of this in treatment for victims. Holcomb, Mahoney, and Lawyer (*this volume*) argue how impulsive decision-making is both a risk factor for sexual assault perpetration, as well as a negative outcome in victims of sexual assault, through an examination of underlying mechanisms linking impulsivity to cognitions and behaviors of both populations.

The fifth section, Prevention and Intervention, is an expansive section presenting literature and recommendations on effective methods of both preventing and intervening in crimes of sexual violence. McMahon, Wood, and Cusano (*this volume*) provide a review of multiple theories (e.g., ecological theory, social learning theory) of sexual assault that explain prevention from micro- to macro-level systems approaches. Wood, Rikkonen, and Davis (*this volume*) provide a critical review of variability in definitions of consent and sexual assault, including those specific to the legal, academic, and military contexts, and how consent is both interpreted and conveyed. Mazar (*this volume*) discusses the existing interventions targeted at reducing the rate at which witnesses of a sexual crime avoid intervening (i.e., bystander), including education about possible methods of intervening, as well as the limitations of such intervention efforts. Bell, Coker, and Clear (*this volume*) provide a review of both in-person and technology-based bystander interventions commonly utilized in educational settings to prevent sexual violence. Stern (*this volume*) presents a novel mechanism for speakers to utilize when attempting to effectively deliver sexual assault prevention education: humor. Szoke and Hazlett-Stevens (*this volume*) examine the translation of the underlying mechanisms of change in mindfulness-based interventions, an evidence-based psychological treatment, into sexual assault treatment programs for both victims and sexual assault victim advocates. Leach and Orchowski (*this volume*) present a thorough review of both psychological interventions and medical treatments that victims often benefit from immediately post-assault to prevent and/or assuage the various long-term effects of sexual victimization. Vechiu and Zimmermann (*this volume*) provide an overview of the efficacy of various brief-focused and psychoeducational interventions available to victims to help overcome the barriers to obtaining psychological treatment this population is often subject to experiencing. Heffernan and Ward (*this volume*) explain how Ward's "Good Lives Model" can be utilized to improve sexual assault offender treatment and reduce rates of recidivism, through the inclusion of additional risk targets and taking a more individualized approach toward designating treatment.

The sixth section, Sexual Assault and Law, is composed of chapters focused on how sexual violence is examined at various levels of the legal system. O'Donohue (Chap. 32, *this volume*) provides a literature review examining the rates of false allegations and discusses limitations in the measurement of false rates of sexual violence. Rerick, Livingston, and Davis (*this volume*) discuss individual, societal, and other related factors that influence how jurors make decisions in cases of sexual violence. Tellis and Spohn (*this volume*) present their data on decision-making in the criminal justice system, including that of officers' decision to arrest and prosecutors' decision to charge the perpetrator, and the effects of these two decision-making processes on the later stages of sexual assault cases. O'Donohue (Chap. 35, *this volume*) reviews extant literature pertaining to the steps victims take when reporting sexual violence to various entities (e.g., police; Title IX office) and barriers victims endorse that reduce their likelihood of reporting sexual violence. Caruso (*this volume*) discusses the process of a forensic sexual assault medical legal examination, including the role of a Sexual Assault Nurse Examiner and considerations in conducting the exam, given the acuity often experienced by victims post-assault combined with time restraints in completing the exam in a legally and medically appropriate manner. Beauregard and Reale (*this volume*) discuss both victim and perpetrator characteristics associated with an increased risk of a sexually violent crime ending in a homicide, and urge for literature to continue examining this and, importantly, address the current limitations in the measurement of these correlates.

The final section, Special Populations, explore themes addressed in other sections but provide considerations about how these factors and processes differentially occur across specific populations. Messinger and Koon-Magnin (*this volume*) present literature on sexual violence in LGBTQ communities, including risk factors and, especially, how this affects reporting and help-seeking in victims who self-identify as a sexual minority. Lopez, Yeater, Ross, and Vitek (this volume) focus on the intersectionality between sexual, ethnic, and gender minority status and how these variables influence the experience of sexual violence, as well as considerations in treating victims from these demographic backgrounds. Tyler and Wright (*this volume*) focus on sexual violence occurring in homeless populations, from a lifespan approach, and explore outcomes occurring at high rates within this population. Bourgeois and Marx (*this volume*) discuss the multiple forms of sexual violence that occur in the military-context, as well as outcomes and treatments utilized for victims of sexual violence in the military. Potter and Tewksbury (*this volume*) discuss the evolution of prison rape and both societal and political views toward the violence, culminating in the development of the Prison Rape Elimination Act, and how policies have affected the prevention of this particular sexual crime. McCray (*this volume*) discuss how rape culture and hypermasculinity are often fostered in college athletic departments resulting in increased rates of sexual violence perpetration by athletes, as well as methods of preventing and identifying those athletic-contexts that require further resolution. Kaylor and Jeglic (*this volume*) focus on exhibitionism, describing the prevalence of this sexual crime and ways of rehabilitating offenders of this specific form of sexual violence. McDonald (*this volume*) explains how gang involvement is correlated with child sexual abuse in females, with an emphasis on the importance of addressing sexual abuse history in interventions aimed at reducing female gang involvement and sexual revictimization. Salfati (*this volume*) presents literature on how crime analysis may yield further identification of patterns of behavior that serial sexual offenders follow, thereby noting specific targets of individualized rehabilitation for high-risk repeat offenders. Nguyen and Naugle (*this volume*) explore gender symmetry in the study of intimate partner sexual violence and methods of preventing an asymmetric approach towards investigating this form of sexual violence that occurs at high rates across all genders. Harper (*this volume*) explains how coercive control is a mechanism utilized by perpetrators of intimate partner sexual violence resulting in negative emotional, physical health, and behavioral outcomes that limit victims' ability to depart from the relationship.

References

American Psychiatric Association. (2013). *The diagnostic and statistical manual, 5*. Washington, DC: American Psychiatric Association Press.

Catalano, S. (2007). *Intimate partner violence in the United States*. U.S Department of Justice, Bureau of Justice Statistics.

Cummings, C., & O'Donohue, W. (2019). *A forensic interview protocol for adult sexual assault: Content validity and consumer acceptability*. Unpublished manuscript.

Engle, J., & O'Donohue, W. (2012). Pathways to false allegations of sexual abuse. *Journal of Forensic Practice,* 97–123.

Keller, J., Mendes, K., & Ringrose, J. (2018). Speaking 'unspeakable things': Documenting digital feminist responses to rape culture. *Journal of Gender Studies, 27*(1), 22–36.

Koss, M. P., Gidycz, C. A., & Wisniewski, N. (1987). The scope of rape: Incidence and prevalence of sexual aggression and victimization in a national sample of higher education students. *Journal of Consulting and Clinical Psychology, 55*(2), 162–170.

McNally, R. (2003). *Remembering trauma*. Cambridge, MA: Harvard University Press.

Phipps, A., Ringrose, J., Renold, E., & Jackson, C. (2018). Rape culture, lad culture and everyday sexism: Researching, conceptualizing and politicizing new mediations of gender and sexual violence, *Journal of Gender Studies, 27*(1), 1–8.

Schewe, P. A., & O'Donohue, W. T. (1996). Rape prevention with high risk males: Short-term outcome of two interventions. *Archives of Sexual Behavior, 25*(5), 455–471.

Schewe, P. A., & O'Donohue, W. T. (1993a). Rape prevention: Methodological problems and new directions. *Clinical Psychology Review, 13*, 667–682.

Schewe, P. A., & O'Donohue, W. T. (1993b). Sexual abuse prevention with high risk males: The roles of victim empathy and rape myths. *Violence and Victims, 8*(4), 339–351.

Sinozich, S., & Langton, L. (2014). Rape and sexual assault among college-age females, 1995–2013. *Bureau of Justice Statistics.*

Contents

Part III Risk Factors of Sexual Victimization and Perpetration

Part IV Victimology

Part I

Theories of Sexual Assault

A Feminist Perspective on Sexual Assault

1

Sasha N. Canan and Mark A. Levand

The word *feminism* is derived from the French term *féminisme* and is defined by Merriam-Webster (2018), who chose it as their 2017 Word of the Year, as "the theory of the political, economic, and social equality of the sexes." There are many different types of feminism that have developed throughout history and from a variety of theoretical perspectives. Within this chapter, we find feminist activist bell hooks' conceptualization of feminism most useful when discussing sexual assault. She describes feminism as "a movement to end sexism, sexist exploitation, and oppression" (Hooks, 2000, p. 1). We choose this framing of feminism because it demands action in its use of the phrase "to end," the ultimate goal of feminist work regarding sexual assault. Also, we choose it because with this definition, hooks asserts sexual assault is predicated on the concept of sexism, not simply a struggle between men (perpetrators) and women (victims). She goes on further to say that "…sexist thinking and action is the problem, whether those who perpetuate it are female or male, child or adult" (Hooks, 2000, p. 1).

The terms *sexual assault*, *sexual violence*, and *rape* all overlap with and diverge from each other in important ways. Definitions of each of these terms have changed over time, and currently, definitions may differ within and between researchers, activist, journalists, and the community at large (Kelly, Burton, & Regan, 1996). Beyond definitional incongruences, use of the terminology is further complicated because we may choose to use certain terms over others due to varying connotations and linguistic powers associated with each term. For example, due to its more intense emotional connotation presently, it is not uncommon for individuals to avoid using the term *rape* and, instead, substitute it for the less jarring term *sexual assault*. Due to the array of definitions and uses of these terms, when reviewing previous work in this chapter, we will retain the original wording used by the original speakers as to not distort their voice.

Nevertheless, when we use these terms ourselves, we describe *sexual violence* as the broadest of the terms and *rape* as the most specific of the terms. That is, sexual violence encompasses both behaviors that involve attempted or completed bodily contact (e.g., sexual assault) and behaviors that may not include bodily contact (e.g., sexual harassment). Sexual assault only includes attempted or completed bodily contact, yet this contact can be either penetrative (rape) or nonpenetrative (e.g., grabbing genitals). Rape only describes attempted or completed bodily contact that is penetrative. Therefore, all rape is sexual violence, but not all sexual violence is

S. N. Canan (✉)
Monmouth University, West Long Branch, NJ, USA
e-mail: scanan@monmouth.edu

M. A. Levand
Widener University, Chester, PA, USA
e-mail: malevand1@widener.edu

W. T. O'Donohue and P. A. Schewe (eds.), *Handbook of Sexual Assault and Sexual Assault Prevention*,
https://doi.org/10.1007/978-3-030-23645-8_1

rape. The core commonality of all these terms is that they involve sexual or sexualized behaviors that occur without at least one involved person's consent.

Western Historical Ideas of Sexual Assault Pre-1960s

During the Colonial Era and into parts of the nineteenth century, rape was treated like property crime wherein women were the property of their fathers until they became the property of their husbands (Burgess-Jackson, 1999). If an unmarried, virgin woman was raped, the crime committed was considered a crime against her father to whom the woman may now remain an economic liability if she could not marry (Donat & D'Emilio, 1992). Similarly, if someone raped a married woman, the rape was considered a property crime against her husband. Remnants of this view of rape existed within US law as late as 1993 when marital rape became a crime in all 50 states (Bennice & Resick, 2003). Prior to this time, husbands could rape their wives without committing the crime of rape because, as women had previously been the property of their husbands, the husband could not commit a property crime against himself.

Donat and D'Emilio (1992) discuss in their review of the historical foundations of sexual assault that, during this time, women were viewed as naturally sexually "pure" while men were assumed to have an innate sexual lust. It was women's responsibility to use their purity to manage men's lust. If a woman was sexually attacked she "needed to comply with male standards of her behavior by proving her nonconsent through physical and verbal resistance, and through immediate disclosure of the attack..." (Donat & D'Emilio, 1992, p. 10). However, any woman who defied these ideas of purity, either via consensual sex or rape, was considered to be corrupted (Donat & D'Emilio, 1992).

In the early twentieth century, perhaps coinciding with the increasing popularity of the field of psychology, perpetrators were increasingly viewed as mentally unwell, "sick," or having a diagnosable character disorder (Donat & D'Emilio, 1992). At this time, these views served to reduce the perceived control a perpetrator had over his actions, and therefore reduce his responsibility of those actions. For example, Donat and D'Emilio (1992) review historical "sexual psychopath laws" that allowed for men, particularly white men, to be sent to state hospitals instead of receiving jail sentences. This created public discourse which focuses conversations of sexual violence around the perpetrator's experiences, not the victim's experiences—"her victimization was simply a by-product of his pathology" (Donat & D'Emilio, 1992, p. 12). Again, when victims—who were exclusively considered women during this period—were brought into the conversation it was to either to note their now "fallen" or flawed status or to assert how their behavior contributed to their victimization (Rennison, 2014).

Prior to the 1960s, theoretical explanations of sexual assault and, more often, rape, specifically, centered around the Androcentric Theoretical Tradition. This model often described sexual assault in a biologically imperative manner (Marcus, 1992). Rennison (2014) notes that

> …when these traditional perspectives discussed "gender difference," it was done in a way to highlight differences and to deny the presences of gender inequality. For instance, disparities in strength and in aggression (in general) between males and females and the greater innate nurturing and care giving behaviors (in general) found among females compared to males were seen as reflecting the natural order of things… (p. 1619)

Because of this, few people advocated for social change as a means to curb sexual assault.

Western Historical Ideas of Sexual Assault During and Post 1960s: Introduction of the Feminist Movement

It was not until feminist discourse began to enter the mainstream conversation about sexual assault in the 1960s that social change was demanded in order to address the issue (Donat & D'Emilio,

1992; Rennison, 2014). The feminist movement greatly concerned itself with addressing sexual assault (Donat & D'Emilio, 1992), and therefore, had a profound impact on the issue's framing (McPhail, 2016). For example, in the first steps of the movement, feminists advocated that gender socialization, not merely biological sex, needed to be considered within criminological behavior research (Marcus, 1992; Rennison, 2014). In other words, feminists claimed that criminal behavior was affected by learned gender assumptions like the endorsement of adversarial sexual scripts—where sex is viewed as a conquest by men whose job it is to "get" sex from women—instead of being affected by an inherent, unchangeable biological trait of men or women. Feminists also focused conversations toward the actual experiences of the women who were assaulted (Marcus, 1992; Whisnant, 2017) when the conversations had previously centered around either the perpetrator's experiences or the women's father's/husband's experience (Donat & D'Emilio, 1992).

Leading up to and during the 1960s, rape was primarily thought of as an act of sex rather than an act of violence (Donat & D'Emilio, 1992). Because rape was sexually motivated, the victim's sexual history was deemed relevant and could be included in legal procedures (Hegeman & Meikle, 1980). As female desire for sexuality began to be legitimated during the Sexual Revolution, this could serve to further blame her for her own sexual assault or rape—she must have "asked for it" (Donat & D'Emilio, 1992). Because of this, some scholars argued that rape was sometimes viewed as a punishment for deviance from the traditional feminine gender norms of purity (Donat & D'Emilio, 1992; Marcus, 1992). Feminists worked to reform policies that institutionalized the discussion of disproportionate gender violence suffered by women in order to better serve these women (e.g., Violence Against Women Act of 1994; Burt, Newmark, Norris, Dyer, & Harrell, 1996). These changes included Rape Shield Laws, which excluded some victim characteristics—like the victim's sexual history—from court proceedings (Burt et al., 1996).

Additionally, as perpetrators were more often conceptualized as mentally "sick," two distinct approaches to dealing with perpetrators arose: extreme penal sentences and rehabilitation through mental health systems (Donat & D'Emilio, 1992; Freedman, 1987). Neither approach provided practical justice or resolution to the affected women because, with both approaches, perpetrators were less likely to be convicted for their crimes (Donat & D'Emilio, 1992). Feminists lobbied to include laws with several levels of sexual assault types that carried a wider range of penalties—some with mild penalties and others with more serious penalties. This was necessary because few perpetrators were ever convicted with the harsh "all or nothing" penalties in state statutes at this time; knowing that a perpetrator would be sentenced to life in prison, juries would be less likely to convict unless the rape was particularly violent or heinous (Donat & D'Emilio, 1992). Simultaneously, feminists worked to dispel previous beliefs that perpetrators were helplessly controlled by their overwhelming sexual impulses and therefore were less accountable for their actions (Donat & D'Emilio, 1992).

Through these efforts, rape began to be recognized as an act of violence, not sex (Donat & D'Emilio, 1992). Perhaps most famously, Brownmiller (1975) shaped the conversation with her work *Against Our Will: Men, Women, and Rape*, which suggested, among many things, that rape was about power and a form of male domination over women. Her work and others broadened the view of sexual assault from a micro lens at the interpersonal level to a macro lens that discussed how sexual assault is situated within the broader patriarchal culture and is cultivated and substantiated by systems within that culture (e.g., Sanday, 1981). Feminist researchers have commented on this by saying, "in a feminist analysis, sexual assault is understood to be intrinsic to a system of male supremacy" (Herman, 1990, p. 177) and "rape was no longer viewed as an outcome of an individual deviant, but a product of a larger rape culture that condoned and excused male violence" (McPhail, 2016, p. 2).

These ideas helped to launch the sexual assault conversation into the political realm.

The authors of the *New York Radical Feminists Manifesto of Shared Rape* (1971) were credited with declaring that "when more than two people have suffered the same oppression the problem is no longer personal but political—and rape is a political matter" (Manhart & Rush, 1971, p. 1). Many scholars and activists describe that this "same oppression" not only includes acts of rape but also a ubiquitous fear of rape among women. Marcus (1992) reviews and critiques some of these ideas that women are "always either already raped or already rapable" (p. 386) and never not rapable. Because this fear of rape is so common for women, the constant threat limits their ability to be active participants in the public arena, including in politics (Donat & D'Emilio, 1992). In fact, Brownmiller (1975) specifically discusses rape as a political function that preserves a system of male dominance, which benefits all men regardless of if they have ever committed rape.

Types of Feminist Theory

Over the years, the broad spectrum of feminist ideologies have been conceptualized as historic waves (Genz & Brabon, 2009), as a spectrum (Whisnant, 2017), and as varied by discipline and purpose (Kelly et al., 1996). Some disciplines (e.g., law and criminology) have been particularly impacted by feminism, especially around views of sexual assault. For example, in trying to define feminist theories for a criminological lens of sexual violence, Rennison (2014) says:

> As such, the phrase "feminist theories" refers to a decentered and diverse collection of perspectives and methodologies based on various ideas about the basic assumptions regarding inequality, the role of gender and gender relations, the issues and problems requiring attention, and the methods needed to address these issues and problems (p. 1618).

Below, we briefly examine a few different paradigms of feminist theory, conceptualizations of feminist identities, and an overall feminist perspective of sexual assault. Due to the ebb and flow of feminist thought and leadership, the following feminist theory paradigms are listed loosely in chronological order of their broad influential debut.

Liberal Feminist Theory

Liberal Feminist Theory is often concerned with policy and legal changes that foster equal economic and social opportunities for women. Through structurally equal treatment of the law, symptoms of women's oppression, which can include sexual assault, will be resolved. Rennison (2014) argues that although this theory is not directly related to sexual violence (because it addresses legal/economic issues broadly), it laid a foundation for the emergence of contemporary feminist theories that do. However, some feminists criticize Liberal Feminist Theory for "playing by the rules" of a governing system that is inherently unequal because it was built on patriarchal values. For example, liberal feminist efforts to put forth new legislation and judicial policies that were still decided on by a heavily male-dominated legislative and judicial branch in the US; therefore, largely men still got to decide what opportunities and protections were permissible for women.

Additionally, some modern feminists have moved beyond the liberal feminist's push for equality in law and policy. Today, many feminists advocate moving toward equitability rather than equality because "a focus on equal treatment uses males as the yardstick by which females are treated," which does not fix the underlying issues of women's oppression in a patriarchy as it still holds a male standard (Rennison, 2014, p. 1620). For example, within prosecution of sexual assault, it is common to provide evidence that the victim "fought back" against her perpetrator in order to be certain that it was not a consensual experience (Donat & D'Emilio, 1992). Although some women do fight against their perpetrators, many women are not socialized to resort to physical violence in order to resolve conflict. Holding women to this "equal standard" of physically violent resistance may hinder women's likelihood of receiving justice in the judicial process.

Radical Feminist Theory

Radical Feminist Theory finds that patriarchy is the key cause of gender inequality and sexual violence (Whisnant, 2017). Broadly defined, patriarchy is a social system that values traditional masculine social norms (e.g., strong, powerful, stoic, sexually aggressive, protective) and where men disproportionately occupy positions of power. The radical feminist perspective frames sexual violence as not merely random acts of aggression but a means of social domination over women (Rennison, 2014). This social domination occurs because the continual threat of sexual violence perpetuates continual fear in women (Rennison, 2014). This theory helped to expand conceptualizations of sexual violence beyond stranger rape to include other types of rape (e.g., acquaintance rape) given that "…every man is a potential rapist and all women are potential victims" (Donat & D'Emilio, 1992, p. 17). Radical Feminist Theory has perhaps had the largest influence in framing sexual assault as an act of violence instead of an act of sex (e.g., Brownmiller, 1975).

Radical feminists and women of color feminists criticized the liberal feminist sexual violence agenda both for not addressing racism, classism, poverty, etc. (McPhail, 2016) and also for reinforcing the patriarchy by working within the preexisting patriarchal confines. Marcus (1992) argues this by stating.

> Attempts to stop rape through legal deterrence fundamentally choose to *persuade men* not to rape… they do not envision strategies which will enable women to sabotage men's power to rape, which will empower women to take the ability to rape completely out of men's hands. (p. 388)

Nevertheless, criticisms of Radical Feminist Theory also exist. Some, particularly intersectional and transnational feminists, find the idea of a universal patriarchy and timelessness of sexual victimization narrow in scope because patriarchy and sexual victimization exist in varying degrees across culture and time (Donat & D'Emilio, 1992). Others criticize Radical Feminist Theory because they credit it with focusing the women's movement solely around negative issues, like rape (Donat & D'Emilio, 1992).

Marxist Feminist Theory

Marxist Feminist Theory finds that the primary basis of sexual violence is class inequality; gender is a secondary concern (Rennison, 2014). In traditional marriage where husbands are lone income earners and wives perform unpaid domestic work, class forms the base for female disadvantage because of an economic master–slave relationship between husbands and wives (Rennison, 2014). Schwendinger and Schwendinger (1983) state that "inequality bred by a capitalist society enhances the conditions for female subordination and sexual violence…. In noncapitalist societies, rape is rare, and egalitarianism between males and females is high" (Rennison, 2014, p. 1621). Although this lens brings in important issues of the relatedness of gender and poverty, it stops short of examining the intersections of gender and poverty with race, citizenship, sexual orientation, and other important social strata.

Intersectional Feminist Theory

Intersectionality focuses on the idea that people occupy multiple social identities simultaneously, and each of these identities intersect with one another to form a person's unique experience of the world, particularly as it relates to their experiences of oppression. For example, a person can have the identities: indigenous, Mexican, immigrant, transwoman of low socioeconomic status. Each one of these identities has social implications alone and creates a distinct identity when layered together—the whole (person) is more than the sum of their parts (identities). Intersectional Feminist Theory notes the shortcomings of other theories focused on one identity, which can distort and misrepresent people's holistic experiences (Bright, Malinsky, & Thompson, 2016). By grouping all women together, singular identity theories assume that, for example, a woman who is trans, indigenous, Mexican, teenager, and low socioeconomic status has a similar experience of sexual assault compared to a woman who holds other identities (e.g., cisgender, of American citizenship, White, middle-aged, and high socioeconomic status).

Kimberlé Crenshaw (1989), coined the term "intersectionality" first within discussions of employment discrimination and quickly applied Intersectionality to violence literature (Crenshaw, 1991). Crenshaw (1991) discusses how both race and gender identities simultaneously and uniquely affect women of color's experiences of violence. For example, Black women are more likely to experience sexual assault compared to both White women or Black men (Black et al., 2011). The layering of both racial and gender oppression creates higher risk for victimization for these women. If sexual assault is situated on ideas of power and control, Mustaine and Tewksbury (2002) argue that this increased victimization makes sense because White men "may especially need to control minority women whose increasing status is particularly threatening" (p. 96).

Intersectional considerations also exist for perpetrators. Donat and D'Emilio (1992) discuss the racial myth of the "animalistic," sexually uncontrollable Black man as it relates to sexual assault perpetration. This myth, born out of slave imagery, was used as a threat to all White women while simultaneously used as an excuse for White men's violence toward Black men via lynching. Angela Davis (1981) uses Intersectional Feminist Theory to add classism to the discussion by addressing these intersections within the historical context of slavery—a form of both economic and racial domination. Further theorists have also addressed how these identities intersect with ableism, heterosexism, colonialism, as well as other identities.

Emerging as a blend between Intersectional Feminist Theory and Decolonial Theory—a theory based on the concept of deconstructing the ways colonization has negatively impacted indigenous societies (Salem, 2014)—Transnational Feminism focuses on women's issues on a global perspective where feminism is not solely defined by Western standards, particularly White Western women's standards. Transnational Feminism seeks to address global women's issues that affect different cultures, nationalities, and races in varying degrees without trying to westernize women across the globe. Transnational Feminism also critiques the idea of patriarchy as it often contains problems of unidimensionality and universality while also failing to address cross-border gender relations and identities (Patil, 2013).

"Doing" Gender Theory: Masculinities

Some gender theorists conceptualize gender as a performance, rather than an innate quality that a person holds. Similar to an actor performing on a stage, people perform their gender on the stage of life. Judith Butler (1988) explains that "gender is an act that has been rehearsed, much as a script survives the particular actors who make use of it, but which requires individual actors in order to be actualized" (p. 526). People learn how to perform these actions (gender expression) through learned gender scripts. That is, how to perform masculinity and femininity is both actively learned (e.g., a father explicitly telling his son "a real man takes what he wants") and/or passively learned (e.g., watching media that rewards male violence with "getting the girl") within a culture. Feminist theory of masculinities finds that some cultures or subcultures may endorse and, subsequently, teach men to perform different types of masculinity or perform traditional masculinity to varying degrees.

Messerschmidt (1993) argues that, because masculinity is not an inherent or fixed characteristic, it must be continually accomplished by men. Because dominance and aggression are characteristics associated with traditional masculinity, sexual violence against women is one way to accomplish this type of masculinity (Mustaine & Tewksbury, 2002; Rennison, 2014). This can especially be seen in revenge rape cases where, in an effort to restore threatened masculinity, some men engage in sexual violence against romantic partners that have been unfaithful or have attempted to end the relationship (Rennison, 2014; Schwartz, DeKeseredy, Tait, & Alvi, 2001). Godenzi, Schwartz, and Dekeseredy (2001) assert that performing masculinity is why men who are associated with hypermasculine peer groups (e.g., college athletic teams) are more likely to commit sexual violence against women.

Performing masculinity combines with Marxist Feminist Theory to create the Left Realist Gendered Subcultural Theory. This related theory addresses the Marxist shortcomings of deemphasizing gender. Left Realist Gendered Subcultural Theory discusses how destructive economic policies (e.g., weak labor laws, deregulation of predatory money lending practices) make men's attempts to accomplish masculinity more difficult, at least masculinity that values financial success as a means to attain power and control (Rennison, 2014). When it is difficult to accomplish masculinity through these means, men can turn to rape as a way of accomplishing masculinity because rape can afford them a different type of power and control (Rennison, 2014). Additionally, Schwartz et al. (2001) describe that men rape women especially when they have other men's complacency, or even encouragement, for doing so.

Feminist Framework Plus

A newer feminist theory that aims to understand sexual assault via "knitting" together several preexisting theories is Beverly McPhail's (2016) Feminist Framework Plus. Each theory partially explains motivations for sexual assault, but no one theory fully explains it alone. She argues the need for a more comprehensive theory because the idea that sexual assault is motivated by power and control, not sex, "while very important and groundbreaking in its time, does not wholly account for the etiology of sexual assault" (p. 1). To look at sexual assault through a broader lens, she brings together five core ideas while noting the strengths and weaknesses of each.

The first, Patriarchal Power and Control, describes the key theme born of Radical Feminist Theory; sexual assault is about power and control. Sexual assault is a result of a male supremacy and patriarchy, and, therefore, is political. Although McPhail critiques that this idea cannot fully explain sexual assault, she finds that it is one piece of the overall phenomenon. The second idea, Normative Heterosexuality Perspective, is similar to the first but acknowledges that sexual violence is both sex and violence at the same time. It frames rape as an inherent part of normative heterosexuality due to rape's frequency of occurrence and the sexual pleasure those with more power (men) sometimes report receiving from aggressing against those with less power (women).

The third core idea of the Feminist Framework Plus holds that Intersectional Feminist Theory also possesses important explanatory power for understanding sexual assault. She explicitly notes that the intersection of oppressed identities "results in less credibility for women of color survivors as well as longer prison terms for rapists of color" (McPhail, 2016, p. 6). The fourth core idea reflects the concepts of "doing" gender and masculinity where rape, rather than being a deviant sexual practice, is related to normative masculine practices (e.g., Malamuth, 1981). The fifth and final idea knitted into the theory is the Embodied Sexual Practice Perspective. This perspective brings discussions of rape inward focusing on how it is experienced by the victim in order to, in part, acknowledge that rape does not carry the same experience for all women. It also finds that "rape is a sexually specific act with sexual consequences for the victim…" (McPhail, 2016, p. 7).

Overall, these five core ideas blend together to assert five key concepts. One, rape is a sexual act that can create sexual consequences for the survivor. Two, there are multiple motives for rape, not only power and control. Three, it is imperative to understand rape at both a political level while also addressing that it occurs at the individual bodily level. Four, there should always be an emphasis on the intersectional experience of rape which highlights oppressed identities. Five, rape can do great harm to a survivor. Lastly, the "Plus" part of this theory aims to add developmental, biological, environmental, situational, and psychological causal explanations for rape, which McPhail (2016) argues are often left out of many feminist theories.

Even with bringing together these varied feminist explanations of sexual assault and rape to create a broader model with more explanatory power, the Feminist Framework Plus still has limitations. McPhail (2016) notes that it does not provide a theoretical explanation for female sexual offenders, an area of research that, though historically neglected, is included in more contemporary sexual violence research. For example, in a recent national sample of lesbian, bisexual, and heterosexual women, 9% of women who experienced sexual assault indicated that their perpetrators were other women (Canan, 2017), giving evidence to an undertheorized topic in previous feminist perspectives of sexual assault: women as perpetrators.

Feminist Identities Related to Sexual Assault

While people use different theories and paradigms to *understand* sexual assault, feminists have also applied these theories to the modes in which they *interact* with sexual assault. Kelly et al. (1996) describe various "feminist identities" or different modes of feminism as distinctions to make sense of feminist activity, particularly in western countries. These authors describe four distinct feminist identities that, despite being conceptualized over 20 years ago, are still culturally relevant to the ways many feminists interact with sexual assault today. These are: academic feminist, activist feminists, commercialized feminists, and "power" and "victimhood" feminists.

Academic feminists aim to create knowledge about sexual assault from the perspective of women. However, theory has become increasingly disconnected from action to create change around the issue or, at least, to create change outside of the institutions in which these academics work (Kelly et al., 1996). On the contrary, activist feminists predominantly aim to challenge the current social order through grassroots organizing of media awareness campaigns, policy creation, lobbying, etc. Activist feminists are often doing the community work "on the ground." Many feminists, activist feminists in particular, criticize academic feminists and the knowledge they create because much of the information is inaccessible to the community at large.

Commercialized feminists are concerned with making feminism marketable and profitable. This occurs in both media and therapeutic services (e.g., films marketing as feminist blockbusters and feminist self-help books; Kelly et al., 1996). Kelly et al. (1996) credit this type of feminism with creating the concept of "survival" after experiencing sexual assault. The shift in terminology was developed within the self-help movements to move away from the stigma associated with the word "victim." They also note that the increased divergence between academic feminist and activist feminist helps to create commercialized feminists. More specifically, they state that "it is the lack of connection between the first two which, in our view, adds power to the latter" (Kelly et al., 1996, p 96).

"Power" and "Victimhood" feminists conceptualize a dichotomy that Kelly et al. (1996) heavily criticize as unhelpful to the overall cause. In this dichotomy, "power" feminists advocate to move away from victimhood framings of sexual assault as they find them to be disempowering to women. "Victimhood" feminists frame sexual assault within experiences of victimization in order to politicize the issue, and they, conversely, criticize the self-help movement's depoliticization of the issue. Both "power" and "victimhood" feminists overlap in that they both emphasize the importance of telling women's stories in order to make private pain into public discourse. Kelly et al. (1996) describe how both power and victimization exist for people who have endured sexual assault in that

> all sexual violence involves an experience of victimization, and if individuals do not die as a consequence they have physically survived... being victimized is what was done—a statement of

historical fact; survival is what individuals who are victimized achieve in relation to, and often in spite of, that historical reality (Kelly et al., 1996, p. 91–92).

A Feminist Perspective of Sexual Assault

The plethora of feminist theories, some of which are identified above, allows for much philosophical and theoretical debate on what feminism entails. We have identified theoretical paradigms identifying the gendered experience on personal and systemic levels, in political and economic spheres, and from generalized, specific, and intersectional identities. With McPhail's knitting together of several feminist theories regarding rape and sexual assault, we get closer to an understanding of the complexities of sexual assault as an individual and personal act that carries implications both for that person and for society more broadly. Even McPhail, however, identifies that the expertly knitted theories still have some shortcomings—namely, not having a frame for understanding female perpetration of rape and sexual assault. Therefore, although the above theories offer bits and pieces of rhetoric to understand the phenomenon of rape and sexual assault, we must expand our scope to gain an overall feminist perspective of rape and sexual assault.

An Intersectional Imperative

Although women of color feminists have been doing intersectional feminism for decades, due to racial biases inherent within White western feminism, Intersectional Feminist Theory has only recently begun to gain mainstream traction in sexual assault discussions. Its increasing acceptance is exemplified in McPhail's inclusion of intersectionality in the Feminist Framework Plus. However, we argue a need to make Intersectional Feminist Theory *the central* component to an overall feminist perspective of sexual assault. When feminist theory lacks an intersectional grounding to reality, theories become increasingly disconnected from the lived experience of individuals. When lacking an anchor to intersectional experiences, concepts of gender, economics, power, and socialization—though exhaustively discoursed upon—offer little in the way of how sexual assault exists in our world and how we must address these issues. In other words, all other theoretical framings or feminist identities related to sexual assault lack holistic efficacy without Intersectional Feminist Theory.

With the joining of the various modes of feminism discussed above, we see where academic feminism leaves gaps and activist feminism offers insight. This is exemplified in Friedman and Valenti's (2008) book *Yes Means Yes: Visions of Female Sexual Power & a World Without Rape*—a book with an activist-focus on positively affecting rape culture and female sexual pleasure. The editors and contributors compile a view of female sexuality, pleasure, and sexual violence from a variety of lived experiences focusing on the nuances of identity in the sexual experience. They move toward a more intersectional understanding of female sexuality by starting with the lived experience and supplying a space to articulate differences, difficulties, and disparities with the intent to affect rape culture. They discuss body size, immigration, citizenship, race, pregnancy, and sex work among other identity factors. These examinations make clear the need for an intersectional feminist perspective by highlighting the possible oversight of various types of oppression by a single-dimension feminist analysis.

In a more contextual example, the way Black women are subject to a sexual racism identifies how a simple gendered examination is not enough. Collins (1990) famously breaks down the racialization of female sexuality and White and Black womanhood. She says,

> In this context of a gender-specific, White, heterosexual normality, the jezebel or hoochie becomes a racialized, gendered symbol of deviant female sexuality. Normal female heterosexuality is expressed via the cult of true White womanhood, whereas deviant female heterosexuality is typified by the "hot mommas" of Black womanhood (p. 83)

Collins identifies how female sexuality and womanhood is seen differently based on race. This examination stemming from the experience of Black, female sexuality—the source for discussing intersectionality (Crenshaw, 1989) and Patricia Hill Collins' (1990) subsequent interrogation of the theory, embedding it further into the dialogue of sexuality—is another example of how this discussion benefits from more than just a monolithic gendered critique.

With the dawn of intersectional and transnational feminism, we have a broader scope through which to view sexual assault. We see that feminism offers an examination of gender, sex, age, power, economic situation, political context, etc. As such, a feminist perspective of sexual assault is critical of the many dynamics that exist within the experience of sexual assault—both as it occurs on an individual basis and as society interacts with the concept and consequences on a macro level. Here, we briefly examine how four major components influence sexual assault through a more intersectional lens.

Gender/Sex

As an activist and author, bell hooks (1984) first identified feminism as a movement to end sexist oppression in the mid-1980s. Several years later, hooks expounded on the idea, offering insight into the complexities of how feminism can move the discussion on sexual assault forward. For hooks, feminism is much more than the social schema that pitted women against men. When considering sexual assault in a patriarchal system, many of the theorists above made gendered assumptions—that victims are always women and perpetrators are always men. While some authors identified this assumption, they did little to address the complexities of how sexual assault is portrayed beyond a unidirectional, binary gendered experience. More recently, hooks elaborated:

> When I boldly affirmed that I advocate feminist politics, folks wanted to know just what I meant by that. Their questions, their interrogations gave me the opportunity to challenge notions of feminism as being about women against men. It gave me the opportunity to share the definition of feminism that was for me clear and simple: "Feminism is a movement to end sexism, sexist exploitation, and oppression." Feminist politics aims to challenge and change patriarchy. (Hooks, 2015, para. 6)

As McPhail (2016) mentioned, the previous gendered scope has been insufficiently useful in addressing female perpetrators. When men are raped by women, oppression may exist in the patriarchal system preventing men from seeking emotional or legal support. When the gender identity of a sexual assault survivor—transgender or gender nonconforming, for example—may be dangerous to discuss, report, or identify in a narrative, what is needed to offer consolation and justice when their gendered experience is contributing to the stigma of sexual assault? Activist campaigns such as the 1 in 6 drive (1in6, 2018), or studies on male survivors of sexual assault exemplify the usefulness of identifying oppression in ways that have brought about awareness moving toward social change. In the edited book *Queering Sexual Violence*, genderqueer author River Willow Fagan notes "people of all genders experience sexual violence and have valid needs for support and access to healing spaces" (Fagan, 2016, p. 18). An intersectional feminist perspective of sexual assault includes the reality that sexual assault happens across all genders and is equally as intersectional in its support of these individuals.

Race

The race of sexual assailants and sexual assault survivors cannot be overlooked in a feminist perspective that aims to end oppression. Sexual assaults do not exist outside of a racial context. When race is ignored, implicit bias and racist thoughts influence how we discuss and address individuals involved in sexual assaults. An intersectional feminist perspective identifies how race plays a role in a given assault and the ways in which racial oppression may contribute to perceived harm to individuals or groups. Collins (1990) discusses in *Black Feminist Thought* the complexities of addressing rape within racial boundaries:

> ...to talk of White racist constructions of Black women's sexuality is acceptable. But developing analyses of sexuality that implicate Black men is not —it violates norms of racial solidarity that counsel Black women always to put our own needs second. Even within these racial boundaries, some topics are more acceptable than others—White men's rape of Black women during slavery can be discussed whereas Black men's rape of Black women today cannot (p. 124)

Collins gives voice to the nature of how discourse on sexual assault can be influenced by race—in this excerpt, by identifying what is acceptable or unacceptable. She identities the difficulty in discussing race and sexual assault by illustrating how the current gendered/racial dynamics affect what is more or less acceptable to discuss in a given social context at a given time. The historic oppression of the sexualities of people of color—from the rape of slaves discussed by Collins to forced sterilization noted by Angela Davis (1982)—has influenced how we discuss the existence of sexual assault in our world. A feminist perspective of sexual assault recognizes racial dynamics as inseparable from conversation of how oppression relates to sexual assault.

Class/Economics

When sexual assault occurs in a heteropatriarchy, there is much to say about who had the economic power that gave them access to commit sexual assault or the economic power to avoid consequences for sexual assault. For example, cases like Harvey Weinstein, Bill O'Reilly, and many other wealthy men in film and television have recently been exposed for sexually harassing and assaulting women in the industry for decades. Of the individuals who came forward against these men, several cited that Weinstein, O'Reilly, and others held key positions of power in the industry which kept the assaulted individuals from reporting their experiences lest they forfeit their own careers. These men held positions of economic power over their victims that both helped foster the sexual assaults as well as allowed these men to postpone or entirely avoid negative fallout of their actions. Therefore, there are economic circumstances for perpetrators, victims, and victims relative to their perpetrators that intersect with further identities (e.g., gender) to shape the context of sexual assault.

Sexual assault in the context of sex work is another intersectional economic consideration. The radical feminist view of sex work often equates all sex work or prostitution to sexual assault (e.g., Jeffreys, 1997). Intersectional, transnational, and global feminist authors advocate for examining sex work as beyond the view that all sex work is sexual slavery or violence against women (Jeffreys, 1997). Kamala Kempadoo (2001) notes that when sex work is reduced to "a violence inflicted upon women due to notions of a universality of patriarchy and masculinist ideologies and structures...[it] dismisses the great variety of historical and socio-economic conditions, as well as cultural histories, that produce sexual relations and desire" (p. 38). Neglecting to identify the economic impact of sex work undermines the reality that it can be a form of income and survival for some individuals. When sexual assault occurs in the context of sex work, there may be laws preventing sex workers from reporting rape (New York Consolidated Laws, n.d.; Anderson, 2002); also some police themselves perpetuate sexual assault on sex workers (Deering et al., 2014). These realities contribute to the oppression and stigmatization experienced by sex workers.

Political

In Friedman and Valenti's (2008) book, Miriam Zoila Pérez (2008) writes a chapter about immigrant women and their experience of sexual violence. She discusses the way that sexual violence assumes an added layer of intersectional complexity when considering structures of citizenship, poverty, and racism. More specifically, immigration laws and policies can create and sustain opportunities for perpetrators to sexually assault others, especially noncitizens, who hold less political power. When rape or sexual assault occurs in the context of immigration, a simple awareness of gender and patriarchy offers an incomplete rhetoric to how we can move toward the end of this kind of oppression.

We must be clear in identifying the oppression in political power that impacts survivors and influences perpetrators' decisions to move toward sexual violation. An intersectional approach to sexual assault understands that political climate will shape a survivor's experience of sexual assault (e.g., political decisions to insufficiently fund rape crisis centers, victim blaming comments made by political officials). Furthermore, additional political intersections exist when it comes to police abuse of sexual power or the military's use of sexual assault as weapon. While McPhail stated the importance of recognizing the many motives of individual perpetrators of sexual assault, we must also identify the political motivations as part of a system, not simply an individual's relation to power, sexual pleasure, or socialization.

Recommendations

We offer two key recommendations to address the problem of sexual assault. These recommendations are broad as to include things that everyone can do, not just people of one particular gender, one particular race, one particular class, etc. For example, although their help is essential to solving this issue, we cannot only recommend men to act. Men exist in all forms in the sexual assault process—as perpetrators, as victims, as bystanders, as advocates, and as the uninformed public that upholds rape culture. Therefore, in keeping with the need for an intersectional approach to this problem we offer general recommendations which, we hope, can be adapted in culturally appropriate ways to fit calls to action for a variety of groups.

Our first and foremost recommendation is that it is imperative to see sexual assault as intersectional. These above feminist theories imply that we need a more holistic understanding of this phenomenon in order to most effectively address sexual assault in our world. Perpetuating a belief about where or how sexual assaults happen while overlooking evidence contrary to this belief, holding a single group of people responsible for perpetration while ignoring other types of perpetrators, or believing that sex and power are the only dynamics that exist in a sexual assault are all examples of nonintersectional ways of working around sexual assault. We must first break free of the narratives ruling the sexual assault discourse that prevent us from seeing oppression in all forms caused by sexual assault—oppression of all genders, racial oppression, economic disparities, oppression of victims through legal channels, overlooking perpetrators, false accusations, or allowing sexual assault to be tolerated in society. We start by seeking an education about sexual assault that is trauma-informed and aware of the many facets present in sexual assault.

Our second recommendation is that it is important to understand the role we play as individuals in perpetuating an atmosphere that upholds sexual assault as permissible or, at the very least, inconsequential. In what ways do we partake in a society that allows a nonchalance about sexual assault, often called rape culture? These theories above carry the implications that we must identify our own biases and learned beliefs that prevent us from speaking out about injustices that happen around sexual assault. The simplest form of not perpetuating this atmosphere is to avoid sexually assaulting people. This is, however, an incredibly low bar as a moral imperative for what these theories advocate. We must also analyze how we speak about sexual assault, to what extent we employ rape myths in our speech and beliefs, how our lived experience makes us responsible bystanders, or why we do or do not disclose our own sexually coercive experiences. We need to seek out how we can best work against the oppression of sexual assault in our life—talk to friends about it, ask teachers, counselors, or trained professionals about how we as individuals can work against these injustices.

Conclusion

With a seemingly endless matrix of intersectional identities, a feminist perspective of sexual assault encompasses more than the individual identities of a person. It includes an understanding of feminism that offers insight about sexual assault that brings about freedom from oppression in a multidimensional way. When we understand sexual assault to be a form of oppression, we might start from the lived experience and extrapolate the oppressive components.

Because individuals all have identities that may experience oppression in some way, we must consider the effects of sexual assault in the context of each of those identities. Though perhaps incredibly obvious, these components are not mutually exclusive. The four components above are also not the only components to consider—the list of identities is practically endless.

Whether a survivor is oppressed in a single-dimensional way or has a multifaceted oppressive experience, a feminist perspective of sexual assault—rooted in the experience of the patriarchy as an oppressive system in a symbiotic relationship with other systems—identifies the oppression that uniquely exists as a result of sexual assault. Because sexual assault happens to people of all kinds, a feminist response is equally varied and complex. A feminist perspective of sexual assault is intersectional. It is intersectional not only in its consideration of identity components and oppressive factors therein but also in its ontological, teleological, and epistemological approaches.

References

1in6. (2018). *About us*. Retrieved from https://1in6.org/about-1in6/

Anderson, M.J. (2002). From chastity requirement to sexuality license: sexual consent and a new rape shield law. George Washington Law Review, Forthcoming. Retrieved from https://papers.ssrn.com/sol3/papers.cfm?abstract_id=326260

Bennice, J. A., & Resick, P. A. (2003). Marital rape: History, research, and practice. *Trauma, Violence & Abuse, 4*(3), 228–246. https://doi.org/10.1177/1524838003004003003

Black, M. C., Basile, K. C., Breiding, M. J., Smith, S. G., Walters, M. L., Merrick, M. T., & Stevens, M. R. (2011). *National intimate partner and sexual violence survey: 2010 summary report* (Vol. 75). Atlanta, GA: Centers for Disease Control and Prevention. Retrieved from http://vawnet.org/Assoc_Files_VAWnet/NRCWebinar_NISVSBriefingHandout.pdf

Bright, L. K., Malinsky, D., & Thompson, M. (2016). Causally interpreting intersectionality theory. *Philosophy of Science, 83*(1), 60–81. https://doi.org/10.1086/684173

Brownmiller, S. (1975). *Against our will: men, women and rape*. New York: Bantam Books.

Burgess-Jackson, K. (Ed.). (1999). *A most detestable crime: New philosophical essays on rape*. New York: Oxford University Press.

Burt, M., Newmark, L., Norris, M., Dyer, D., & Harrell, A. (1996). *The Violence Against Women Act of 1994: Evaluation of the STOP block grants to combat violence against women: (721332011-001) [Data set]*. American Psychological Association. https://doi.org/10.1037/e721332011-001

Butler, J. (1988). Performative acts and gender constitution: An essay in phenomenology and feminist theory. *Theatre Journal, 40*(4), 519–531.

Canan, S. N. (2017). *A mixed-methods study of sexual assault in lesbian, gay, and bisexual adults in the US* (Doctoral dissertation). Retrieved from University of Arkansas ScholarWorks (2464).

Collins, P. H. (1990). *Black feminist thought: Knowledge, consciousness, and the politics of empowerment.* Boston, MA: Unwin Hyman.

Crenshaw, K. (1991). Mapping the margins: Intersectionality, identity politics, and violence against women of color. *Stanford Law Review, 43*(6), 1241. https://doi.org/10.2307/1229039

Crenshaw, K.W. (1989). *Demarginalizing the intersection of race and sex: A black feminist critique of antidiscrimination doctrine, feminist theory and antiracist politics* (pp. 139–167). University of Chicago Legal Forum.

Davis, A. (1982). Racism, birth control and reproductive rights. In A. Davis (Ed.), *Women, race and class* (pp. 202–271). New York, NY: Random House.

Davis, A. Y. (1981). *Women, race & class*. New York: Vintage Books. Retrieved from http://search.ebscohost.com/login.aspx?direct=true&scope=site&db=nlebk&db=nlabk&AN=738888

Deering, K. N., Nesbitt, A., Shoveller, J., Amin, A., García-Moreno, C., & Shannon, K. (2014). A systematic review of the correlates of violence against sex workers. *American Journal of Public Health, 104*(5), e42–e54. https://doi.org/10.2105/AJPH.2014.301909

Donat, P. L. N., & D'Emilio, J. (1992). A feminist redefinition of rape and sexual assault: Historical foundations and change. *Journal of Social Issues, 48*(1), 9–22. https://doi.org/10.1111/j.1540-4560.1992.tb01154.x

Fagan, R. W. (2016). Fluctuations in voice: A genderqueer response to traumatic violence. In J. Patterson (Ed.), *Queering sexual violence: Radical voices from within the anti-violence movement* (pp. 17–21). Riverdale, NY: Magnus.

Freedman, E. B. (1987). "Uncontrolled desires": The response to the sexual psychopath, 1920–1960. *Journal of American History (Bloomington, Ind.), 74*(1), 83–106.

Friedman, J., & Valenti, J. (Eds.). (2008). *Yes means yes: Visions of female sexual power & a world without rape*. Berkley, CA: Seal Press.

Genz, S., & Brabon, B. A. (2009). *Postfeminism: Cultural texts and theories*. Edinburgh: Edinburgh University Press.

Godenzi, A., Schwartz, M. D., & Dekeseredy, W. S. (2001). Toward a gendered social bond/male peer support theory of university woman abuse. *Critical Criminology, 10*(1), 1–16. https://doi.org/10.1023/A:1013105118592

Hegeman, N., & Meikle, S. (1980). Motives and attitudes of rapists. *Canadian Journal of Behavioural Science/Revue Canadienne Des Sciences Du Comportement, 12*(4), 359–372. https://doi.org/10.1037/h0081079

Herman, J. L. (1990). Sex offenders: A feminist perspective. In *Handbook of sexual assault: issues, theories, and treatment of the offender* (pp. 177–193). Boston, MA: Springer. https://doi.org/10.1007/978-1-4899-0915-2_11

Hooks, B. (1984). *Feminist theory: From margin to center*. Cambridge, MA: South End Press.

Hooks, B. (2000). *Feminism is for everybody: Passionate politics*. Cambridge, MA: South End Press.

Hooks, B. (2015). *Feminism is fun! By bell hooks*. Retrieved from http://www.bellhooksinstitute.com/blog/2015/12/12/feminism-is-fun-by-bell-hooks

Jeffreys, S. (1997). *The idea of prostitution*. North Melbourne, AU: Spinifex.

Kelly, L., Burton, S., & Regan, L. (1996). Beyond victim or survivor: Sexual violence, identity and feminist theory and practice. In *Sexualizing the social* (pp. 77–101). London: Palgrave Macmillan. https://doi.org/10.1007/978-1-349-24549-9_5

Kempadoo, K. (2001). Women of color and the global sex trade: Transnational feminist perspectives. *Meridians: Feminism, Race, Transnationalism (Project Muse), 1*(2), 28–51.

Manhart, M. A., & Rush, F. (1971). *New York radical feminists manifesto of shared rape*. Retrieved May 15, 2018, from https://web.viu.ca/davies/H323Vietnam/Manifesto.SharedRape.1971.htm

Marcus, S. (1992). Fighting bodies, fighting words: A theory and politics of rape prevention. In *Feminists theorize the political* (pp. 385–403).

McPhail, B. A. (2016). Feminist Framework Plus: Knitting feminist theories of rape etiology into a comprehensive model. *Trauma, Violence, & Abuse, 17*(3), 314–329. https://doi.org/10.1177/1524838015584367

Messerschmidt, J. W. (1993). *Masculinities and crime: critique and reconceptualization of theory*. Lanham, MD: Rowman & Littlefield.

Miriam-Webster. (2018). *Definition of feminism*. Retrieved May 15, 2018, from https://www.merriam-webster.com/dictionary/feminism.

Mustaine, E. E., & Tewksbury, R. (2002). Sexual assault of college women: A feminist interpretation of a routine activities analysis. *Criminal Justice Review, 27*(1), 89–123. https://doi.org/10.1177/073401680202700106

New York Consolidated Laws (n.d.). Criminal Procedure Law—CPL §60.42. *Rules of evidence: Admissibility of evidence of victim's sexual conduct in sex offense cases*. Retrieved from https://codes.findlaw.com/ny/criminal-procedure-law/cpl-sect-60-42.html

Patil, V. (2013). From patriarchy to intersectionality: A transnational feminist assessment of how far we've really come. *Signs: Journal of Women in Culture and Society, 38*(4), 847–867. https://doi.org/10.1086/669560

Rennison, C. M. (2014). Feminist theory in the context of sexual violence. In G. Bruinsma & D. Weisburd (Eds.), *Encyclopedia of criminology and criminal justice* (pp. 1617–1627). New York, NY: Springer New York. https://doi.org/10.1007/978-1-4614-5690-2_70

Salem, S. (2014, April). *Decolonial intersectionality and a transnational feminist movement*. Retrieved May 22, 2018, from http://www.thefeministwire.com/2014/04/decolonial-intersectionality/.

Sanday, P. R. (1981). The socio-cultural context of rape: A cross-cultural study. *Journal of Social Issues, 37*(4), 5–27. https://doi.org/10.1111/j.1540-4560.1981.tb01068.x

Schwartz, M., DeKeseredy, W., Tait, D., & Alvi, S. (2001). Male peer support and feminist routine activities theory: Understanding sexual assault on the college campus. *Justice Quarterly, 18*(3), 623–649.

Schwendinger, J. R., & Schwendinger, H. (1983). *Rape and inequality*. Thousand Oaks, CA: Sage Publications, Inc.

Whisnant, R. (2017). Feminist perspectives on rape. In E. N. Zalta (Ed.), *The Stanford encyclopedia of philosophy* (Fall 2017). Metaphysics Research Lab, Stanford University. Retrieved from https://plato.stanford.edu/archives/fall2017/entries/feminism-rape/

Zoila Pérez, M. (2008). When sexual autonomy isn't enough: Sexual violence against immigrant women in the United States. In J. Friedman & J. Valenti (Eds.), *Yes means yes: Visions of female sexual power & a world without rape* (pp. 141–150). Berkley, CA: Seal Press.

An Evolutionary Perspective on Sexual Assault and Implications for Interventions

2

Mark Huppin, Neil M. Malamuth, and Daniel Linz

Although acts of sexual aggression have been reported throughout human history, recently this topic has garnered much public awareness and concern. Many countries have publicly reckoned with the problem of sexual assault in recent years (Sengupta, 2017). In 2015, the World Health Organization and United Nations Office on Drugs and Crime launched a toolkit to help countries respond to sexual violence (WHO & UNODC, 2015). *Time* magazine named "The Silence Breakers," denoting the voices that launched the #MeToo movement, as its Person of the Year 2017 (Zacharek, Dockterman, & Edwards, 2017).

In this chapter, we use an evolutionary psychological (EP) perspective to discuss sexual assault and what might be done to reduce it. There has often been the misperception that evolutionary psychological perspectives and feminist ideology and goals conflict with each other, particularly on the topic of sexual assault. Although a discussion of such misconceptions is beyond the scope of this chapter, we note that over many years, researchers have attempted to dispel such beliefs (see, e.g., Buss & Malamuth, 1996, and more recently https://blog.oup.com/2014/02/evolutionary-psychology-affront-feminism/ and https://quillette.com/2017/10/29/human-behaviour-feminism/).

We use terms such as sexual aggression and sexual assault interchangeably herein, defined as acts that involve sexual contact whereby one of the individuals does not fully consent to the acts. These can include some use of physical force, threat, deception, or some other form of coercion. Rape is an extreme form of sexual assault.

EP perspectives seek to identify ultimate causes of behavior, complementing the focus on proximate causes characteristic of other psychological theorizing. In addressing ultimate causation, evolutionary psychologists have often asked whether the ability to inflict sexual aggression or to avoid it contributed to reproductive success in our species' ancestral history, possibly giving rise to dedicated psychological mechanisms pertaining to coercive sex. Although addressing such questions is standard in EP theorizing, some critics have raised concerns that this might imply that sexual aggression is "natural" in the sense of inevitable or morally neutral (i.e., "biology is destiny"), an implication we clearly wish to avoid. This is not an implication of the EP theorizing discussed here (for a discussion of the error committed by critics by mistakenly inferring this about the logic of evolutionary psychology, see, e.g., Confer et al., 2010).

Much EP theorizing on sexual aggression has focused on models that implicate condition-dependent psychological mechanisms affecting

M. Huppin (✉) · N. M. Malamuth
University of California, Los Angeles, CA, USA
e-mail: huppin@ucla.edu

D. Linz
University of California, Santa Barbara, CA, USA

W. T. O'Donohue and P. A. Schewe (eds.), *Handbook of Sexual Assault and Sexual Assault Prevention*,
https://doi.org/10.1007/978-3-030-23645-8_2

an individual's propensity to coerce. As Buss and Greiling (1999) explain, such information-processing devices are "designed to take in certain classes of input, operate on that input with a set of decision rules, and transform it into output in the form of decision rules" (p. 212). Environmental experiences, particularly in critical early stages, are said to result in the *calibration* of mechanisms at relatively fixed values, which can lead to lifelong differences in thresholds for evoking sexual coercion. In contrast, EP theorizing typically has not stressed any direct links between genetic differences and sexual coercion. However, there has been some consideration of the possibility that some genetic differences underlie certain personality and other characteristics that indirectly affect the propensity to sexually coerce (Ellis, 1989; Malamuth, 1998). Lending support to the potential usefulness of considering genetic factors is evidence of the ability to genetically breed mice that are either more or less sexually aggressive (Canastar & Maxson, 2003). Also suggestive is research showing strong evidence of familial clustering of sexual offending, primarily accounted for by genes rather than shared environmental influences (see, e.g., Barnes, TenEyck, Boutwell, & Beaver, 2013, finding that genetic factors accounted for 51% of the variance in forcing sexual activity on one's domestic or intimate partner; see also Längström, Babchishin, Fazel, Lichtenstein, & Friesel, 2015).

Sexual Aggression in Humans

In applying the EP paradigm, we begin by considering clues to motivational differences between men and women that may have a bearing on the potential occurrence of sexual coercion. Differences in minimal parental investment (Trivers, 1972) contribute to a greater likelihood that a man will be motivated to have sex with certain women than vice versa and that, for men, sex may be more easily separated from emotions associated with long-term mating (Buss & Schmitt, 1993). Such differences create conflicts that can result in some men using coercion to overcome female reluctance and resistance (Gorelik, Shackelford, & Weeks-Shackelford, 2012). Consistent with the predictions derived from parental investment theory is the finding that across various societies and recorded human history, as well as across virtually all species where sexual coercion occurs, there are large sex differences in the use of sexual coercion. Males are typically the perpetrators and females are disproportionately the victims. According to the CDC's Division of Violence Prevention, an estimated 19.3% of women have been raped during their lifetime versus an estimated 1.7% of men (Breiding et al., 2014). For female rape victims, an estimated 99% had only male perpetrators; 79% of male victims also had only male perpetrators, although for some other forms of sexual violence such as being made to penetrate, a majority of male victims had only female perpetrators (Breiding et al., 2014). Data from ten European countries revealed self-reported sexual aggression in a total of 16.3% of men compared to 5.0% of women (Längström et al., 2015). Perpetration rates were significantly higher among men than women for each of the four coercive strategies measured: (1) the use or threat of physical force, (2) the exploitation of the other person's incapacity, (3) the use of verbal pressure, and (4) the exploitation of authority. The sex difference in reported victimization rates was much smaller, however.

Although there are cultural differences in the frequency of sexual aggression, large sex differences can be found even in the most egalitarian and low general violence nations. For example, a review of datasets of youth sexual aggression in Europe (Krahé, Tomaszewska, Kuyper, & Vanwesenbeeck, 2014) found that among Danish youth, the rates of female sexual victimization were 63.5% compared to a male victimization rate of 40%. From the perpetrator perspective, Danish males reported far higher rates of lifetime sexual aggression than did females, 46.4% as against 9.3%. While recognizing the importance of a gender inclusive conception of sexual violence (Turchik, Hebenstreit, & Judson, 2016), our focus in this chapter is on the majority of adulthood sexual violence involving a male perpetrator and a female victim and implications for effective interventions.

Another issue relevant to an evolutionary-based model of sexual coercion is its frequency in human history, because regularly occurring events are more likely to have a "… logic embedded in the dynamics of natural selection for reproductive success" (Wrangham & Peterson, 1996, p. 138). Sexual coercion does appear to have occurred throughout human history (e.g., Chagnon, 1994), and cross-cultural surveys reveal that it occurs in most societies today (Basile, 2002; Broude & Greene, 1978; Fulu, Jewkes, Roselli, & Garcia-Moreno, 2013; Levinson, 1989; Monson & Langhinrichsen-Rohling, 2002). Moreover, even relatively rape-free societies described in such surveys (e.g., Sanday, 1981) have social rules intended to counter male sexual aggression, suggesting that there is universal risk for such behavior.

Particularly when fear of punishment is reduced, signaling conditions in which the costs of sexual coercion are low or the perpetrator has anonymity, many men do rape. This is most evident in times of war (see Allen, 1996; Stiglmayer, 1994). Even though the extent of sexual violence varies considerably between wars, sexual violence occurs in all wars (Wood, 2006). In surveys of undergraduate men, about one-third report some likelihood that they personally would rape a woman if they could be assured that they would not suffer negative consequences (e.g., Malamuth, 1989).

Sexual Aggression in Other Species

Also relevant to EP theories of sexual coercion is evidence of sexual aggression in other species. In fact, physical force, harassment, and other intimidation to obtain sex have been reported in many species. Based on a review of the literature on forced copulation among nonhumans, Lalumière, Harris, Quinsey, and Rice (2005) identified specific characteristics in those species that exhibit sexual coercion. Across all nonhuman species, forced copulation is always perpetrated by males on females. Despite the tendency of females in some species to be assertive in the mating process, the authors could not find one instance of a female forcing sex on a male. Further, males are more likely to target fertile than infertile females for forced copulation, and forced copulation does occasionally result in insemination, fertilization, and offspring. Also, males of most species tend not to engage solely in coercive sexual behaviors. Most males that engage in forced copulation at other times court females. Finally, Lalumière et al. (2005) recognized the role of individual differences in sexual coercion. Certain males are more likely than others to engage in forced copulation, and some males are more successful at sexual coercion than others. They conclude that sexual coercion (particularly in the form of forced copulation) "… is a tactic used by some males under some conditions to increase reproduction" (p. 59).

A particularly interesting species to consider is the orangutan, one of the few nonhuman primates for which sexual coercion is common. There is evidence for two distinct classes of orangutan males: large or flanged males, who develop secondary sexual characteristics such as cheek pads and large throat sacs, and small or unflanged males. Both types are sexually mature, though the onset of sexual maturity can be highly variable. Large males typically weigh over 80 kg in the wild, about twice the size of the small males (Knott, 2009; Knott & Kahlenberg, 2007). Although both types resort to forced copulations, they are significantly more often used strategically by small males, who force more than 80% of their total copulations at some orangutan sites (although only about half or fewer of their copulations are forced at other sites, suggesting the role of environmental contingencies such as population density and sex ratio in the incidence of sexual aggression) (Knott, 2009; Knott & Kahlenberg, 2007).

In a study of chimpanzees, our closest genetic relatives, sexual coercion as long-term intimidation was positively associated with paternity, particularly among high-ranking males, suggesting that it is a strategy used to increase reproductive fitness (Feldman et al., 2014). Sexually coercive tactics toward a female also provide delayed mating benefits in chacma baboons, due in part to the fact that male aggression preferentially targets fertile females (Baniel, Cowlishaw, & Huchard, 2017). As the authors explain, "By repeatedly attacking females in the weeks preceding ovulation, males appear to increase their chances of monopolizing sexual access to females around ovulation, which in turn increases their probability of successful reproduction" (p. 2166). The authors were able to rule out several competing hypotheses for male sexual violence perpetration (e.g., cycling females are more aggressive than noncycling females; females prefer to mate with aggressive males).

Generalist vs. Specialist Models

Historically, investigations focusing on convicted rapists had been guided by the following somewhat simplistic question: Are sexually aggressive individuals those who commit a wide range of antisocial acts, including sexual coercion (e.g., generic antisocial offenders), or are they individuals with characteristics that make them prone uniquely to commit acts of coercion against women? Although there isn't a single profile, there are considerable data regarding convicted rapists showing that many are antisocial generally. Among criminal men convicted of rape, it is clear that a majority also have a history of nonsexual offenses (Harris, Mazerolle, & Knight, 2009; Harris, Smallbone, Dennison, & Knight, 2009; Kingston, Seto, Firestone, & Bradford, 2010), and on most measures of antisocial traits and behaviors they are comparable to other types of violent criminals (Lalumière et al., 2005). These men typically differ from other men not necessarily on some specific mechanism for sexual coercion but on mechanisms underlying general antisocial behaviors. They may be more likely to steal or to use coercion for obtaining any desired goal. In keeping with this evidence, there may be a common genetic factor influencing both antisocial behavior and sexual coercion (Johansson et al., 2008).

Nevertheless, although associations between sexual and nonsexual offenders are substantial, generalist explanations of male sexual aggression fail to fully account for the data. Fanniff, Schubert, Mulvey, Iselin, and Piquero (2016) found that whereas juvenile sexual and nonsexual offenders showed equivalent general recidivism rates over a 7-year follow-up, juvenile sex offenders showed higher sexual recidivism rates. A meta-analysis of 59 studies comparing male adolescent sex and nonsex offenders also did not support the notion that adolescent sexual offending can be parsimoniously explained by generalist theories of sexual aggression (Seto & Lalumière, 2010). A more recent meta-analysis of 68 datasets that included behavioral measures of the perpetration of sexual and nonsexual aggression similarly lends support to specialist explanations of sexual aggression, concluding that the generalist explanation is insufficient (Wilson, Mouilso, Gentile, Calhoun, & Zeichner, 2015).

Findings such as these suggest the need to consider specialist models of sexual aggression, or to supplement contributors to general delinquency (e.g., lack of inhibitory self-control, high impulsivity, low empathy, and/or callousness) with risk factors specific to sexual aggression (e.g., hostile masculinity, impersonal sexual attitudes) in a combined model (Lussier & Cale, 2016). In the literature on convicted rapists, there has been the development of a complex and sophisticated classification system known as MTC: R3 (Knight & Prentky, 1990; Knight & Sims-Knight, 2016), consisting of eight subtypes, which has sought to integrate "general" and "specific" characteristics for some rapists, and indeed a small minority of these criminal men do show such a mixture.

EP theorizing on sexual aggression includes models that vary along the dimension of specialized to general explanations for the behavior. Symons (1979) first discussed extensively whether adaptations or by-products of adaptations produce rape. Adaptations are naturally selected (i.e., they resulted in increased ancestral reproductive success). Criteria for establishing adaptation within evolutionary science include attributes of economy, efficiency, complexity, precision, reliability of development, and functionality in solving a specific problem (Buss, Haselton, Shackelford, Bleske, & Wakefield, 1998; see also Tooby & Cosmides, 1992). By-products are incidental characteristics that did not evolve because they solved adaptive problems. For example, male nipples, which have no design functionality, are by-products of the adaptive value of nipples in women (Symons, 1979).

Symons (1979) concluded that the available data were insufficient to conclude that rape is a facultative adaptation in humans. Rather, rape may be a by-product of male adaptations that produce sexual arousal and adaptations that motivate coercion to secure desired goods. This model, in that it places the propensity to sexually coerce within a larger framework of aggressive tendencies that describes a propensity for antisocial behavior in general, is an example of a generalist model. Other EP models of rape have extended Symons's proposal to include rape as a by-product of both sexual desire and a generalized possessiveness or desire to control others (Ellis, 1989).

Representative of specialist theories of sexual aggression is the work of Thornhill and Palmer (2000). They proposed a set of possible specialized adaptive mechanisms designed to address fundamental problems of sexual access, including mechanisms designed specifically to: (a) evaluate female vulnerability to rape; (b) identify cues associated with fertility (e.g., age, ovulation status); (c) optimize sperm counts produced during rape; (d) motivate rape under conditions of sperm competition; (e) motivate rape in men who lack sexual access to females (the "mate deprivation" hypothesis); or (f) produce sexual arousal specific to opportunities of rape. What distinguishes this type of EP theorizing on specialized mechanisms from the typology research not informed by an evolutionary perspective is the idea that the potential for such mechanisms is part of an "adaptively functional" alternative strategy of reproduction. In other words, EP theorizing seeks to explain why such specialized mechanisms may have evolved, but in no way suggests that they are desirable, inevitable, or that they are "functional" in current environments.

Many of these hypotheses have been evaluated in more detail elsewhere (see, e.g., Camilleri & Stiver, 2014). In this chapter, we will evaluate the adaptation hypothesis in the context of theory and data specially pertaining to sexual arousal specific to forced sex. Although our primary focus in this chapter is on the male perpetrator's psychology, we first consider potential female adaptations to avoid being sexually assaulted. In the past decade, this has been an area of emphasis of EP rape research.

Female Adaptations to Avoid Sexual Assault

Considering the specific adaptive problems faced by our ancestors, it is actually more likely that specialized mechanisms for avoiding sexual assault evolved in women than that specialized mechanisms for engaging in sexual aggression evolved in men. Underlying this assertion is the notion that the reproductive costs to ancestral women of losing the ability to choose among mating partners due to sexual coercion would have been greater than the reproductive benefits to men of, at times, using coercive sex. As one group of authors recently noted, "It would be astonishing if selection had not produced any defenses against [the huge costs of rape and sexual coercion] on female choice" (Al-Shawaf, Lewis, & Buss, 2018, p. 152).

On this point, it may well be that females' trauma in today's modern environments is to some degree still particularly affected by human psychological mechanisms "designed" in the evolutionary landscape, where even one brief act of forced sex may have had truly devastating consequences for a lifetime (e.g., beyond the possibility of injury and the circumvention of mate choice, there was no contraception, no pills that could prevent pregnancy after the attack, no way of determining who the father of the offspring was), even to a greater degree than other types of physical assault. While it is, of course, very difficult to study this issue with well-designed research, there is some support for the possibility that as compared to nonsexual traumatic events, sexual assault of females may result in greater posttraumatic stress disorder consequences generally and sexual problems specifically (e.g., DiMauro, Renshaw, & Blais, 2018; see also Thornhill & Thornhill, 1990, finding that reproductive-aged victims of rape are more psychologically traumatized by rape than are nonreproductive aged victims).

Researchers have observed a number of female behaviors that may suggest anti-rape adaptations, although most hypotheses and accompanying data in support have been tentatively asserted. Wilson and Mesnick (1997) suggest that women's preference for mating with physically and socially dominant men may indicate anti-rape adaptation. In indirect support, married women at all ages are significantly less likely to experience sexual aggression than unmarried women (Wilson & Mesnick, 1997). Their "bodyguard hypothesis" of female mate choice is also supported by field studies and by research across a diverse range of species indicating that attraction to dominant males varies positively with risk of sexual aggression, such that attraction increases in proportion to conditions of risk (Wilson & Mesnick, 1997; see also Mesnick, 1997; but see, e.g., Ryder, Maltby, Rai, Jones, & Flowe, 2016, finding that although women's preferences for physically dominant and formidable males is positively associated with fear of crime, the relationship does not vary according to risk situation, perpetrator gender, or crime type, suggesting that the underlying psychological mechanisms are general in nature). Similarly, Smuts (1992) explains patterns of women's social alliances by looking to the benefits of protection against potential rapists. Future research should continue to attempt to disentangle whether the psychological mechanisms underlying these relationship preferences are specialized to protect against sexual aggression or designed to counter the risk of aggressive behavior in general, including nonsexual aggression untethered to issues of sexual access (for a discussion, see McKibbin & Shackelford, 2012).

Studies on the effects of ovulatory cycle status on women's risk-related behaviors provide some further support for female anti-rape adaptations. This line of research starts from the assumption that rape is most costly when pregnancy is most likely, i.e., during the ovulatory phase of the menstrual cycle. Consistent with a model of specialization, Bröder and Hohmann (2003) found that during the ovulatory phase naturally cycling women reduced risky behaviors (e.g., "come home alone late," "get dressed sexily when going out") and increased nonrisky behaviors (e.g., "watch TV at home," "visit relatives"), whereas women using hormonally based contraceptives suppressing ovulation did not show either effect. Given that motor activity, sexual activities, and sexual desire increase during the ovulatory phase of the cycle, these results cannot be accounted for by theorizing a sum total reduction in women's activity around the time of ovulation (Bröder & Hohmann, 2003). This research replicates and extends earlier work on reduced risk-taking behavior during the fertile phase of the cycle (Chavanne & Gallup, 1998). Both of these studies, however, relied upon potentially unreliable self-reporting methods for identifying the fertile phase of the cycle.

Related research has found that naturally cycling women evidence greater handgrip strength in response to imagined sexual assault (compared to a baseline measure of handgrip strength), but only when in the fertile phase (Petralia & Gallup, 2002). In contrast, women using hormonally based contraceptives do not show any evidence of this. Moreover, this same effect did not occur at any time for either group when they were presented a neutral scenario. This study used not only the forward cycle self-reporting method but also a self-administered ovulation test that identified luteinizing hormone in urine to assess menstrual cycle phase. These results suggest the existence of female adaptation designed to mobilize resources aimed to resist sexual assault when the risks to a woman's reproductive success are especially high.

Garver-Apgar, Gangestad, and Simpson (2007) discovered that fertile-phase women who had viewed taped short interviews of men rated them as more sexually coercive than did similarly situated nonfertile women. Fertility status failed to influence women's ratings regarding other male traits such as kindness, commitment, and faithfulness, suggesting to the researchers that women may possess dedicated perceptual mechanisms specifically designed to limit the incidence of male sexual coercion. On the other hand, Ryder et al. (2016) found that fertility status did not predict perceived risk of being raped by a man in either crime hotspots or safe spots, although no exposure to a male occurred during this experiment.

Navarrete, Fessler, Fleischman, and Geyer (2009) found that white women demonstrated greater out-group bias against black men when in the fertile phase, which the authors interpreted as consistent with the "coercion avoidance perspective" (p. 664). This assumes that group membership is a feature relevant to assessing risk of sexual coercion, given that out-group members are not subject to in-group social norms and controls. Drawing on this perspective, McDonald, Donnellan, Cesario, and Navarette (2015) found that undergraduate women self-identified as vulnerable to sexual coercion were significantly less likely to agree to dating requests from an out-group member but not an in-group member when conception risk was elevated.

Other investigators have examined the influence on coercion avoidance of individual difference factors such as a woman's physical attractiveness, age, relationship status, and proximity to kin. McKibbin, Shackelford, Miner, Bates, and Liddle (2011) suggest how these factors could be related to psychological mechanisms designed to reduce the risk of rape. First, a woman's attractiveness should correlate positively with her frequency of rape avoidance behavior. This prediction is based on research suggesting that would-be rapists prefer and target more attractive women (see, e.g., McKibbin, Shackelford, Goetz, & Starratt, 2008; Thornhill & Palmer, 2000). Second, given that a woman's fertility peaks in the early 20s and declines thereafter, a woman's age should correlate negatively with the frequency of rape avoidance behavior. Third, because mated women have more to lose than unmated women from rape, including the risk of partner abandonment, they should engage in higher frequencies of rape avoidance behavior. Finally, in view of the fact that if a female is raped then genetic relatives may also incur fitness costs, it follows from inclusive fitness theory that a woman's rape avoidance behavior should increase with the number of family members living in close proximity, who can be expected to monitor and influence her sexual behavior. In their own investigations, with the exception of the age-related factor, these researchers found some measure of support for each of these predictions (McKibbin et al., 2011). For example, total scores on a rape avoidance inventory correlated significantly and positively with the other three predictor variables. In multiple regression analyses, however, in most cases only a woman's relationship status uniquely predicted her rape avoidance. Additionally, other researchers have questioned the necessity of resorting to an EP explanation for these results when other narratives may more parsimoniously account for them (for a discussion see Snyder & Fessler, 2012; for a response see McKibbin & Shackelford, 2013).

In sum, while some promising avenues of exploration into the area of female anti-rape adaptation do exist, supporting a model of psychological mechanisms solving specialized design problems, more research is needed.

The Adaptation Hypothesis

The adaptation hypothesis suggests that in ancestral environments, being sexually coercive under some circumstances (and, particularly for women, having the capacity to avoid being sexually coerced) contributed to reproductive success sufficiently frequently to have resulted in some change in the evolved psychological architecture that would not have occurred without the recurring fitness consequences of sexual coercion. Accordingly, this hypothesis posits specific psychological mechanisms pertaining to sexual assault. Such specialized mechanisms might include reactions such as emotions or arousal patterns that, in the proximate environment, mediate between relevant environmental cues and behaviors.

From an EP perspective, the question is not whether sexual assault is a better strategy for males than engaging in consensual sex but whether for some ancestral males, under some circumstances, it may have been reproductively effective to use sexual coercion as compared to not using it. In other words, did recurrent ancestral conditions exist under which for some men, some of the time, an overall fitness increase resulted from sexual coercion? Although the hypothesis that sexually assaultive behavior contributed to reproductive success has been criticized on grounds that rape rarely leads to conception, evidence suggests otherwise. Gottschall and Gottschall (2003) estimated pregnancy rates resulting from an incident of penile–vaginal rape among women of reproductive age to be twice that of consensual per-incident rates (6.4% to 3.1%). Controlling for age, rape pregnancy rates per incident remained 2% higher than consensual rates. A national sample of adult American women of reproductive age found a rape-related pregnancy rate of 5.0% per rape or 6.0% per victim (Holmes, Resnick, Kilpatrick, & Best, 1996). Among a representative sample of women in the Netherlands, 7% reported that they got pregnant as the result of a rape (de Haas, van Berlo, Bakker, & Vanwesenbeeck, 2012). There is some indirect corroboration of sexual assault as a strategy for increasing reproductive success in a study by Beirne, Hall, Grills, and Moore (2011). In a sample of 105 normally ovulating sexual assault victims, they identified "a trend and a distinct rise in the number of assaults when the victims were in the middle of their cycle," that is to say at peak fertility (p. 315).

Another factor to think about when considering the potential fitness outcomes of sexual coercion is the fact that a substantial minority of women continue to have sex with the men who sexually assault them (Koss, 1988). This is particularly true of completed sexual assault, pointing to the use of sexual coercion as a tactic to secure subsequent copulations. From a comparative EP perspective, this shares in common with the intimidation tactics of chimpanzees and baboons discussed above, in which the reproductive benefits of sexual coercion are long-term but not immediate.

Ellis, Widmayer, and Palmer (2009) identified more than two thousand North American undergraduate women who reported having been sexually assaulted sometime in their lives, dividing victims into two groups: assault blocked (59.4%) and assault completed (40.6%; i.e., sexual intercourse occurred). 19.4% of women in the assault-blocked and 27.2% in the assault-completed group reported future intercourse at least one time with their assaulter. According to the authors, these results suggest that, "at least a minority of men may have evolved tendencies to use assaultive tactics to secure mating opportunities beyond those obtained by men who only employ 'voluntary' tactics" (p. 461).

In earlier related work, other researchers found that 39% of rape victims compared to 12% of victims of attempted rape dated their attackers again (Wilson & Durrenberger, 1982). Ellis et al. (2009) suggest that completed sexual assault may be more likely to secure subsequent copulations than attempted assault because it leads to greater experienced female trauma or to a need for support in the event of pregnancy. In accord, Perilloux, Duntley, and Buss (2012) found that victims of a completed rape experienced significantly more negative outcomes than did victims of an attempted sexual assault, including with respect to effects on self-esteem, sexual reputation, and self-perceived mate value.

Sexual Arousal to Force

One hypothesized candidate for a specialized psychological mechanism motivating sexual assault that has received the most focused attention is sexual arousal specific to forced sex, referred to here as *sexual arousal to force* ("SAF"). Such arousal may be a manifestation of a broader category of sexual arousal generated by controlling or dominating women, which can be accomplished by the use of force.

Using an adaptation model, R. Thornhill and N. Thornhill (Thornhill & Thornhill, 1992) discussed SAF and argued that higher sexual arousal to coercive sex among men should be associated with greater success with coercive sexual tactics, thereby contributing to ancestral reproductive fitness under some circumstances. They noted that given the costs of forced mating in ancestral environments, including possible loss of status or life, men might be expected *not* to have evolved preferences for forced sex and, therefore, *not* to evidence SAF. If, however, under some recurrent ancestral conditions, the reproductive benefits of forced mating outweighed the costs, then psychological mechanisms enabling sexual arousal despite a woman's lack of consent may have evolved. Harris, Rice, Hilton, Lalumière, and Quinsey's (2007) selectionist hypothesis of psychopathy provides an example of a model suggesting that SAF could reflect a design feature of a rape adaptation. This hypothesis asks: "Do psychopaths respond more to sexual stimuli depicting violence, coercion, and rape simply because they are indifferent to the suffering of others, or does psychopathy entail a mechanism promoting coercive sex?" (p. 20). In their work, these researchers have found psychopathy to be strongly associated with the factor of coercive and precocious sexuality, which factor analyses confirmed to be a core component of psychopathy. They also reported a marginally positive association between psychopathy score and number of biological offspring. In view of this they conclude that psychopathy may exist today because it was part of a successful reproductive strategy for some of our ancestors.

Buss (2003) suggests that the model pertaining to SAF and the data presented by Thornhill and Palmer (2000) do not enable differentiating among alternative hypotheses. Hagen (2004) argues that specialized mechanisms pertaining to rape would not be expected unless the problems involved in "successfully" committing such an act in ancestral environments were not the same problems as with the use of aggression in other contexts. The occurrence of sexual arousal in the context of coercive acts may be an important distinguishing characteristic. For most aggressive acts, sexual arousal would be irrelevant or even detrimental. Because the preferred sexual strategy for most men in most circumstances is to pursue consensual sex, the most common calibration of sexual arousal mechanisms should be to become sexually inhibited by indications of lack of sexual receptivity by women. However, if an individual were to effectively rape in ancestral environments, such aggression may have required reversing of the default arousal pattern. This may be hypothesized as a unique adaptive problem associated with sexual coercion as contrasted with the use of coercion in nonsexual contexts.

Proposed Evolved Function of Sexual Arousal to Force

Within some ancestral circumstances, the inhibition or activation of sexual arousal in response to cues associated with using force might have affected the likelihood of successfully exerting sexual control over an unwilling woman. Some emotions motivate avoidance of particular stimuli, whereas others motivate approaching or pursuing particular stimuli (for an overview see Elliot, 2008). Just as fear of snakes or spiders motivates avoidance of specific threats, sexual arousal cued to the use of force may motivate sexual coercion. This hypothesis is supported by the meta-analysis of Allen, D'Alessio, and Emmers-Sommer (2000), which documented that sexual arousal is associated with positive psychological affect, a precursor of approach or pursuit.

An evolutionary-based model suggests that, due to calibrating mechanisms grounded in the consequences in ancestral environments, a substantial minority of men in the general population may evidence the sexual arousal pattern that facilitates sexual assault. In support of this assumption, in a study of college students, Malamuth, Check, and Briere (1986) identified about 30% of the students as more at risk for sexual aggression. For these men, they were more sexually aroused by depictions including forced sex than by nearly identical depictions without sexual coercion.

Such arousal to forced sex may be part of a constellation of "hostile masculinity" characteristics (Russell, 2018) "designed" to engage in sexually coercive acts in ancestral environments. Indeed, many studies focusing on the *confluence model of sexual aggression*, which suggests that hostile masculinity and an impersonal orientation to sex interact to predict sexual aggression, have found a strong connection between measures of individual differences in men's hostility toward women and their SAF or similar constructs such as dominance as a motive for sex and rape fantasies (Malamuth & Hald, 2017). With rape fantasies, analysis of their impact suggests that they become closely associated with sexual arousal and orgasm, influencing expectancies about the rewards of coercive activity (Greendlinger & Byrne, 1987). Such fantasies are correlated with past coercive sexual behavior and predict sexual aggression (Dean & Malamuth, 1997; Knight, 2010; Seto & Kuban, 1996). In a sample of community men, 33% reported fantasizing about a scene "where you rape a woman" (Crèpault & Couture, 1980). Rape fantasies may reveal important information about evolved mental mechanisms (Ellis & Symons, 1989; Kenrick & Sheets, 1993). EP theorizing may be unique in offering an explanation as to why such characteristics as hostility towards women, fantasizing about rape, attitudes supporting violence against women, and SAF become part of a constellation of factors that are highly inter-correlated.

How might calibration of increased SAF occur? In keeping with the proposition that humans share a common evolved psychology that enables relevant developmental experiences to "set" mechanisms at different levels (Belsky, Steinberg, & Draper, 1991; Draper & Harpending, 1982; Trivers, 1972), the model we outline here emphasizes some relevant perceived negative experiences with women that may set the sexual arousal versus sexual inhibition to force mechanism more in one direction or the other. Although full testing of such a process would require a longitudinal study that would be difficult to conduct, it may be possible to prime similar processes to create a *state condition* related to the *trait condition.* Yates, Marshall, and Barbaree (1984) found that college men who were insulted by a woman were more sexually aroused by rape portrayals as compared to portrayals of consensual sex. Creating general arousal by physiological exercise instead of an insult by a woman did not result in a similar increase.

Other relevant findings pertain to the trait rather than the state of anger and hostility toward women. These studies, including many focusing on the confluence model, indicate that men who are hostile to women, typically on measures that include items referring to perceived rejection from women, show relatively high SAF as contrasted with men who are relatively low on such measures of hostility toward women (e.g., Check, Malamuth, Elias, & Barton, 1985; Malamuth & Hald, 2017). Other studies examining differences between behaviorally sexually nonaggressive men and sexual aggressors (some of whom are likely to have the relevant calibration of increased SAF) have found similar results (e.g., Murnen, Wright, & Kaluzny, 2002). Several priming studies have revealed that sexually aggressive men may be more prone to automatically associate women with hostility, sex, and power (Bargh, Raymond, Pryor, & Strack, 1995; Leibold & McConnell, 2004). Barbaree (1990) reported a study with a rapist who was asked to imagine raping women for whom he held different emotional feelings. He found that the greater the hostility to the woman, the greater the sexual arousal to rape cues. Forbes, Adams-Curtis, and White (2004) showed that the key component linking various measures of male dominance ideology (e.g., attitudes supporting aggression or sexism) to aggression against women is hostility toward women. Seto (2017) identifies hostile masculinity as a key trait facilitation factor in his motivation-facilitation model of sexual offending.

Men who are high in hostile masculinity and generally insensitive to women's distress (i.e., low in empathy) are the most likely candidates to have the relevant calibration of increased SAF or to be disinhibited in the presence of an unwilling partner. Bernat, Calhoun, and Adams (1999) found that the penile tumescence of self-identified sexually aggressive men who also held callous sexual beliefs (e.g., "Prick teasers should be raped") increased when force was introduced into a sexual scenario. Lawing, Frick, and Cruise (2010) reported that adolescent sexual offenders high in callous/unemotional traits showed more sexualized aggression and had a greater number of victims than other adolescents with a sex offense. Studies examining the differentiating characteristics of sex offenders have shown that rapists score higher on the callousness-unemotionality component scale of psychopathy than nonsex offenders, including violent nonsex offenders (e.g., Harris et al., 2007; Knight & Sims-Knight, 2011). In a study of college men, high-risk males with low empathy reported higher rates of sexual aggression than all other men, but high-risk males with high dispositional empathy were comparable to lower-risk males (Wheeler, George, & Dahl, 2002).

In sum, although sexual arousal to force may be viewed as potentially the most likely to be a specialized evolved mechanism promoting sexual assault, the other risk factors identified in the literature such as those encompassed in the confluence model may be conceptualized along somewhat similar lines, potentially "designed" in concert to facilitate a sexually coercive strategy. Not being turned off but actually being turned on by the use of force may be important for committing an act of sexual assault, but if, for example, a person feels little hostility and high empathy for the potential victim, it is difficult to imagine how such a person could "effectively" carry out a coercive sexual act.

Fixed or Flexible

The evolutionary functional model that we have outlined here suggests that sexually aggressive men possess psychological mechanisms calibrated to motivate sexual assault in response to perceived blocked access to desired females. Importantly, however, evolutionary approaches also allow for developmental variability, depending on heritable genetic variation and exposure to environmental inputs that can help shape lifelong patterns of behavior. The degree of "fixing" of evolved mechanisms depends on the role and influence on a particular life history trajectory of these factors (Camilleri & Stiver, 2014), which can contribute to differences in the stability over time of the decision rules or algorithms underlying an individual's sexual strategies. This is consistent with research by Swartout and colleagues, who found that the rape trajectories of sexually aggressive young men across high school and college showed three distinct trajectories: time-limited, decreasing, and increasing (Swartout et al., 2015).

An example of a relatively fixed path is psychopathy (Camilleri & Stiver, 2014), in which substantial genetic contributions are associated with an individual's developmental trajectory and sexual aggression appears to be a core factor of the male's sexual strategy (for a discussion of genetic contributions to psychopathy, see, e.g., Ferguson, 2010). From a comparative EP perspective, psychopathy can be considered a psychological phenotype most closely resembling the fixed morphological phenotype of the small male orangutans. Other men's persistent sexual aggression is influenced to a greater extent by early environmental conditions such as violent and abusive home conditions and parent–child interactions that lead to adolescent delinquency, sexual promiscuity, and adversarial or hostile schema related to male–female relationships (Malamuth, Heavey, & Linz, 1996). Early neural adversity due to poor environmental conditions, resulting in a competitive mating disadvantage, can also contribute to life-persistent offending based on what may be termed a developmentally fixed path (Lalumière et al., 2005). Early social and neural adversity may interact to increase the risk of expression of sexual aggression (Camilleri & Stiver, 2014).

High-risk men falling into relatively fixed life-course categories comprise the minority of sexual offenders, however (Camilleri & Stiver, 2014). More often, sexually aggressive men are unlikely to persist with sexual offending as they age. For example, Moffitt and colleagues have identified a substantial group of adolescent-limited sexual aggressors (Moffitt, Caspi, Harrington, & Milne, 2002). Many of these men may have experienced early environmental conditions that are less severe or pervasive than those of life-course-persistent offenders. As a result, they would be considered to have developmentally flexible psychological mechanisms.

Summary and Recommendations for Sexual Assault Interventions

How might an evolutionary psychological (EP) approach help inform the structure of sexual assault interventions? The following is a summary based on the discussion above of the EP perspective with regard to understanding sexual violence. Next, we apply each of the main points in the summary to arrive at a set of specific recommendations and cautions about sexual violence interventions.

An EP perspective seeks to identify ultimate causes of behavior. This perspective is best seen as complementing the focus on more proximate causes of behavior characteristic of other psychological theorizing. EP suggests that the propensity to be sexually coercive might be profitably located within a larger framework of aggressive tendencies or propensities for antisocial behavior in general. This is an example of a generalist model. However, this is only one possible approach. There is also a specialist explanation which stresses adaptive mechanisms designed to address fundamental problems of sexual access. One possible candidate for a specialized psychological mechanism motivating sexual coercion in men is sexual arousal specific to forced sex ("SAF"). Such arousal to force may be a manifestation of a broader category of sexual arousal generated by controlling or dominating women, which can be accomplished by the use of force. An evolutionary-based model uniquely suggests that, due to calibrating mechanisms grounded in the consequences of ancestral environments, a substantial percentage of men today may evidence the sexual arousal pattern that facilitates sexual assault. Other risk factors shown to predict sexual aggression may be conceptualized in similar ways.

Even relatively rape-free societies have social rules intended to counter male sexual aggression, suggesting that there is universal risk for such behavior. When fear of punishment is reduced, signaling conditions in which the costs of sexual coercion are low or the perpetrator has anonymity, many men do rape.

Sexual selection has undoubtedly produced defenses against the huge costs of rape and sexual assault on female choice. There is therefore an emphasis in EP on the idea of a coevolutionary "arms race" between men and women in which women have evolved adaptive strategies designed to reduce female vulnerability to sexual assault and increase control over their reproductive choices. We have discussed how these adaptations can operate both at the individual level and on an interpersonal level in the form of strategic social alliances.

Finally, men can vary on how fixed or flexible their sexual strategies are, depending on the role and influence of genetic and environmental factors on the life history trajectory of each individual.

These EP precepts form the foundation for several observations about what techniques or methods may or may not be effective when designing sexual assault prevention programs. We note that although similar recommendations may be made by others not informed by an evolutionary model, it may not be clear what theoretical framework, if any, has led to these recommendations.

An EP perspective suggests that to effectively modify the mechanisms to engage in sexual assault that are in place for some men requires prevention programs that recognize several points of importance. (1) Although much of the focus has been on intervention programs on college campuses, early calibration of hostile masculinity psychological mechanisms suggests that interventions are first needed at relatively early ages such as in middle school. (2) One-shot or other brief interventions are unlikely to achieve lasting behavior change. More comprehensive programs are required. (3) An emphasis on female control and empowerment is likely to be an effective intervention strategy. (4) Clear laws and policies, and the corresponding fear of punishment if caught violating these rules, are needed to inhibit the expression of sexual aggression. (5) An emphasis on changing certain social-environmental inputs is important, such as peer support for sexual violence. (6) Sexual assault prevention programs must include a focus on changing the behavior of the 30% or so of men who are at higher risk of committing sexual assault, in part by identifying and addressing factors attenuating the relationship between psychological risk factors and sexual aggression. (7) Because many commonly used programs have not highlighted this population, there is a real possibility that current interventions may be interacting with high-risk men's psychological makeup (e.g., hostile masculinity characteristics) to cause the opposite of the intended effects, or boomerang reactance effects. To avoid these effects, prevention programs should consider introducing exercises likely to reduce the possibility of hostile/reactive aggression. (8) To effectively modify sexually aggressive mechanisms requires intervention emphasis at emotional levels, not only cognitive levels. Therefore, empathy-based interventions may be particularly important for high-risk males.

1. Early calibration of hostile masculinity psychological mechanisms suggests that interventions are first needed at relatively early ages.

Individual differences in life history, especially at certain critical periods early in life, play a role in organizing later behavior. The theory is that variation in ecological factors leads to tradeoffs in an individual's "optimal" energy allocation (Del Guidice, Gangestad, & Kaplan, 2015). Increased risk taking and shorter time preferences are favored for those individuals exposed to harsh, insensitive, early environments (Del Guidice et al., 2015). This has been referred to by EP theorists as taking a fast life track into account.

For example, Nettle, Dickens, Coall, and de Mornay Davies (2013) found that patterns of physical and psychological development in young girls predicted the likelihood of teenage childbearing. Future young mothers weighed significantly less than their peers at birth and experienced increased levels of behavioral and emotional disturbance by age 7, among other differences between groups. In this perspective, teenage childbearing can be seen as the outcome of a coherent reproductive strategy in which the optimal behavioral approach—increased early allocation of effort to mating and reproduction—differs from those individuals in more stable life circumstances.

Using survey data from the National Longitudinal Study of Adolescent Health, Brumbach, Figueredo, and Ellis (2009) found that exposure during adolescence to violence and unpredictability (defined as frequent changes or ongoing inconsistency in childhood environments) was associated with several life history traits, including social deviance. Specifically, there was a positive association between environmental unpredictability experienced in adolescence and social deviance expressed in young adulthood. Unpredictability was also related to the development of a fast life track. Collectively, these studies demonstrate the relevance of life history to human behavior (Reynolds & McCrea, 2016).

Because life history factors can also have profound effects on the development and expression of sexual aggression as a sexual strategy (Camilleri & Stiver, 2014), EP theorizing suggests that interventions regarding sexual behavior should begin as early as possible in the life course. This implication is no different from recommendations in other health areas (e.g., depression screening) that also highlight the value of early intervention.

Thus, although institutions of higher education are required by law to offer sexual violence prevention programs to all incoming undergraduate and graduate students (see https://www.congress.gov/bill/113th-congress/senate-bill/47), additional programs and tools at the middle and high school levels are highly recommended. Consistent with this idea, a 2014 report prepared for the *White House Task Force to Protect Students from Sexual Assault*, using rigorous evaluation criteria, found that the only two primary prevention programs to date that had shown significant reductions in sexual violence behaviors had both been developed for and implemented with middle school students (Centers for Disease Control and Prevention, 2014). As the authors of one of these projects discussed,

"Long-term effects may have been realized [e.g., a reduction in sexual violence perpetration and victimization in the treatment group compared to controls at 4-year follow-up] because Safe Dates [the intervention program] was offered at the beginning of the adolescents' dating careers (8th grade) and included information and skills that could be incorporated into individual dating practices that continued through the high school years" (Foshee et al., 2004, p. 619).

2. One-shot or other brief interventions are unlikely to achieve lasting behavior change.

An EP perspective suggests that the ultimate causes of behavior must be taken into account and recognized as stable (but certainly not immutable) background variables. This implies that one-shot or time-limited interventions will not achieve any lasting behavior change. More comprehensive programs are required. Indeed, one of the basic principles associated with effective prevention programs is that participants need to be exposed to enough of the intervention to have an effect, as measured by the quality and quantity of contact hours (Nation et al., 2003). In accord, the effective implementation of the middle school Safe Dates program included a curriculum of sexual violence literacy comprising ten 45-minute sessions (Foshee et al., 2004). Among sexual violence prevention researchers there has been a growing recognition for the need for such a comprehensive framework, underscored similarly by the Social-Ecological Model used by the Centers for Disease Control and Prevention, which incorporates the dynamic interplay between individual, relationship, community, and societal factors (Dahlberg & Krug, 2002).

Recent examples to provide more comprehensive sexual health instruction in our own state include the California Healthy Youth Act, which requires instruction to middle school and high school students on healthy relationships and communication (California Legislative Information, 2016). A related California law, also effective as of 2016, requires that "all school districts that have health education as a graduation requirement must include instruction on California's affirmative consent standard" (California Department of Education, 2018).

An instructive example of a more comprehensive program within the collegiate setting is the Sexual Violence Prevention Project announced in January 2015 at Dartmouth University. The goal is to reduce sexual assault, dating violence, stalking, and harassment on Dartmouth's campus. What makes this program unique is its intensive focus on sexual assault prevention throughout the entire four-year educational experience. The program eschews a more limited intervention approach by fundamentally addressing over time the norms and behaviors that perpetuate sexual violence on campus. The program emphasizes that sexual violence is a problem that negatively affects all campus community members, preventing them from thriving intellectually, socially, emotionally, spiritually, and physically.

To significantly reduce, and ideally eliminate sexual violence, the Dartmouth program aims to influence multiple behavioral outcomes (e.g., communication and interactions between individuals, bystander intervention). Because the program aims to fundamentally change campus cultural norms regarding sexual violence, we would argue that it is congruent with an EP perspective by realistically considering that stable background variables motivating sexual behavior must be taken into account and addressed using a multi-pronged, intensive approach.

3. An emphasis on female control and empowerment is likely to be an effective strategy.

EP theorists contend that sexual selection has undoubtedly produced defenses against the huge costs of rape and sexual assault on females. Sexual assault prevention programs should therefore include interventions specifically designed for women that account for these adaptive algorithms and motivational systems.

This suggests that self-defense and risk recognition programming for women should be a critical component of prevention programs. Recent research supports this view. Senn et al. (2017) assigned first-year female undergraduate students either to receive a 12-hour resistance program that teaches risk-recognition skills and effective responding or to a control group. The treatment group was significantly less likely than the group of control women to have been victimized by completed or attempted rape, attempted coercion, or nonconsensual sexual contact over a 2-year follow-up period. So, too, women in the treatment group reported significant increases in self-defense self-efficacy and knowledge of verbal and physical resistance strategies over the entire follow-up period. Other studies confirm that women who participate in self-defense training are less likely to experience sexual assault (see, e.g., Hollander, 2014). A recent review of research indicates that, "The vast majority of programs [for women] where effectiveness has been demonstrated include a feminist or empowerment self-defense program" (Gidycz, 2018). The benefits of participation in these programs include increases in (1) feelings of self-efficacy to avoid an assault, (2) confidence that they could defend themselves if attacked, (3) assertive communication, and (4) the use of defensive strategies.

An EP perspective also suggests that an emphasis on female control via creating or simulating strategic alliances can be particularly beneficial to women (Smuts, 1992; Wilson & Mesnick, 1997). One implication of this is that the goal of increasing bystander intervention is highly congruent with an EP approach. Research on programs designed to short-circuit sexual violence by increasing bystander intervention show that this is indeed a promising method. For example, encouraging female and male college students who see someone trying to isolate a heavily intoxicated woman to ask the women if she needs help or to create a distraction has been shown to be an effective strategy (Banyard, Moynihan, & Plante, 2007). Observational research in the related domain of bullying behaviors has found that intervening bystanders "successfully abate victimization more than 50% of the time" (Polanin, Esplanage, & Pigott, 2012).

Such research suggests that bystander intervention programs can achieve some success. However, because bystander intervention training is relatively new, research into its efficacy is still developing. Moreover, as described below, although these interventions undoubtedly can have beneficial indirect effects by changing the surrounding environment, the impact of these programs on the attitudes and behaviors of sexually aggressive men is likely to be minimal.

4. Clear laws and policies, and the corresponding fear of punishment if caught violating these rules, are needed to inhibit the expression of sexual aggression.

As EP researchers have reported, even relatively rape-free societies have social rules intended to counter male sexual aggression, suggesting that there is universal risk for such behavior (Sanday, 1981). Conditions of anonymity and lack of accountability increase the risk of sexual aggression (Allen, 1996; Stiglmayer, 1994). Compounding the problem, sexual assault often goes unreported to police (Truman & Morgan, 2016). The EP perspective is highly congruent with the idea that explicit limitations on unacceptable behavior through laws and policies are required on college campuses.

Colleges and universities are now subject to a number of state laws meant to address the problem of sexual misconduct on campus. An essential part of this legal and regulatory approach, consistent with an EP approach, is an increasing emphasis on the right of women to be free of all forms of unwanted sexual contact. The legal regulation in this area is expanding to become increasingly protective of victims' rights.

Examples of this include victim-centered institutional responses to campus peer sexual violence (Banyard, Moynihan, Cares, & Warner, 2014). At the state level, in 2014 California became the first state to pass legislation (see https://leginfo.legislature.ca.gov/faces/billNavClient.xhtml?bill_id=201320140SB967) requiring consent on college campuses to be "affirmative, conscious, and voluntary" (see consent chapter this volume). A handful of states have since followed California's model, and affirmative consent laws are presently under consideration in other states as well.

California's affirmative consent law provides explicit standards for appropriate sexual conduct. It states: "Lack of protest or resistance does not mean consent, nor does silence mean consent. Affirmative consent must be ongoing throughout a sexual activity and can be revoked at any time."

The existence of a dating or past sexual relationship between the persons involved is not assumed to be an indicator of consent. The law also clearly states instances in which someone cannot give affirmative consent, including being asleep, unconscious, or incapacitated due to the influence of drugs.

Whether such new initiatives will actually result in increased accountability remains to be seen, but their effectiveness seems likely given an EP analysis. Suggestive in this regard, in her ethnographic research of an Indonesian "rape-free" society, Sanday's interview subjects reported that "rape was impossible in their society because custom, law, and religion forbade it and punished it severely" (Sanday, 1996, p. 202). In the same article, she suggests that studying naturally occurring relatively rape-free environments on college campuses and their sociocultural correlates may be useful in finding solutions to the problem of campus sexual assault (Sanday, 1996).

5. An emphasis on changing certain social-environmental inputs is important, such as peer support for sexual violence.

Social factors may be important moderating influences on sexual aggression. EP theory as applied to sexual aggression contends that while sexually aggressive men possess psychological mechanisms calibrated to motivate sexual assault, these mechanisms have a higher or lower probability of being enacted depending on environmental conditions. Group and social support may be important moderators of aggressive psychological mechanisms.

Young men look to their peers for information, especially concerning women, dating, and sex (Sim & Koh, 2003). Research suggests that individuals take peer attitudes toward sexual aggression into account when making the decision to intervene in a sexually aggressive situation (Brown & Messman-Moore, 2010). A recent study found that men high in hostile sexism ("HS") who received peer supportive feedback showed higher rape proclivity than did high HS men in a low HS peer-group condition (Durán, Megías, & Moya, 2018). Other studies have revealed that perceived peer rape justification predicts hostility toward women and sexual violence, whereas the diversity of men's social networks protects them against perpetrating sexual assault (Kaczkowski, Brennan, & Swartout, 2017; see also Swartout, 2013, for a general discussion of this line of research). Related research indicates that men with an external locus of control are more likely to inflict injury on their intimate partners if they report a negative peer group climate (e.g., "The group of people I hang out with tell jokes about girls or women"; "The group of people I hang out with hit someone they are seeing or going out with") (Schmidt, Lisco, Parrot, & Tharp, 2016).

A recent somewhat encouraging pilot prevention program for college men with a norms and group-based component focused on 20 men who engage in heavy drinking (Orchowski et al., 2018). About half of the sample had reported engaging in some form of sexual coercion since the age of 14. Facilitators delivered a three-session sexual assault and alcohol feedback and education program to these men. This included personalized normative feedback regarding alcohol use, sexual activity, alcohol-related sexual consequences, understanding of consent, and engagement in bystander intervention, delivered individually in a motivational interviewing style. A group-based sexual assault prevention workshop focusing on social norms, empathy, masculinity, consent, and bystander intervention was then undertaken. Finally, a booster group session was administered. The authors reported positive effects on some measures of alcohol intentions and sexual assault-related outcomes, e.g., greater recognition of peer engagement in sexual coercion. The program also increased bystander intervention intentions and confidence to intervene to help strangers. No effects were seen on men's actual drinking behavior (i.e., heavy drinking days in past month, number of reported drinks per week), however, and 25% of the sample (5/20) reported engaging in sexual coercion during the two-month follow-up period.

From an EP perspective, it is important to recognize the influence of environmental factors such as peer groups. Men who hold highly hostile attitudes toward women tend to associate with peers who share these attitudes and to be motivated to engage in within-group status seeking. Participation in a sexual assault prevention program needs to address these peer influences—there will be sustained social pressure on these men to embody their peer group's sexual norms. Social norms campaigns designed to reduce negative peer influences and to expose men to more diverse points of view—similar to those that have been developed to reduce alcohol use on college campuses—might therefore be combined into a coherent strategy, e.g., with bystander intervention programs, to reduce sexual violence.

6. Interventions must include a focus on high-risk males.

High-risk males in the general population are likely to possess a combination of general antisocial tendencies (e.g., a narcissistic personality, a high sense of entitlement, a tendency towards psychopathy) as well as specific characteristics pertaining to sexual violence (e.g., hostility toward women, attitudes accepting of violence against women, an impersonal sexual orientation). Studies indicate that men who are hostile to women, typically on measures that include items referring to perceived rejection from women (e.g., Check et al., 1985), show relatively high sexual arousal to force ("SAF") as contrasted with men who are relatively low on such measures of hostility toward women. There is also a strong connection between measures of individual differences in men's hostility toward women and similar constructs such as dominance as a motive for sex and rape fantasies (Malamuth et al., 1996; Malamuth & Hald, 2017). Such psychological characteristics can make these men especially resistant to attitudinal, emotional, or behavioral changes.

A recent study for example shows that reproductive strategies are directly influenced by hostility towards women (Wegner et al., 2017). This study measured men's intentions to use coercive condom use resistance ("CUR") to obtain unprotected but "consensual" sex. Coercive CUR tactics include the use of lies, manipulation, threats, and physical force to have sex without a condom with a partner who wants to use one. The experiment also randomly assigned participants to an alcohol administration or a control condition. After receiving a condom request from a hypothetical partner, men with greater hostility toward women reported stronger intentions to use coercive CUR tactics. Men high in hostility toward women were at particularly high risk for the use of coercion around condom negotiation when intoxicated. The authors concluded that men high in hostility toward women pose a threat to women's sexual safety.

The implication from an EP perspective is that high-risk males must be a focus of sustained attention on college campuses and elsewhere. Recent revelations about the violent tendencies of high-hostility men who feel they have been unjustly deprived of sex with women, known as the INCEL movement, should alert us to the extreme lengths certain males will go, to act upon their hostility toward women who they believe have denied them of deserved sexual contact. Because sexual predation may be a successful strategy for gaining sexual access, these males will be resistant to change. Not only this, but also attempts to change these men may actually backfire if not approached comprehensively.

7. Interventions that are effective for women and most men may show "boomerang" effects with high-risk males. In order to effectively change the behavior of these men, prevention programs should consider introducing exercises likely to reduce the possibility of hostile/reactive aggression.

To the extent that recurrent ancestral conditions existed such that for some men sexual coercion contributed to overall reproductive success, the psychological architecture of men today who have experienced relevant developmental adversity may be calibrated in a way that helps motivate sexual assault to obtain sex from an unwilling partner. What's more, there is a real possibility that many current sexual assault prevention programs may be interacting with the psychological makeup of these high-risk males to create boomerang reactance effects.

Many high-risk men may experience current programs on college campuses as both manipulative and provocative. To these young men such intervention efforts are directed at supporting more positive treatment for a group, undergraduate women, who seem to them to already "get all the breaks." These programs may therefore threaten these men's self-concept and perceived freedoms. Especially if they see intervention messages as condescending and therefore insulting, they may respond in anger and with greater support for aggression. From an EP perspective, if we conceive of sexual strategies within the framework of a coevolutionary "arms race" between men and women, it is unsurprising that messages suggesting or dictating to sexually coercive young men how they should behave toward women will be ineffective, especially if these men feel that they have something to lose from this (Mealey, 2003).

The evaluations of current sexual assault programs generally have not examined the impact on sexually aggressive men. If currently effective programs work at all for such men, they may do so only indirectly. For example, bystander intervention programs may reduce the ability of high-risk men to carry out an assault by changing the responses of the low-risk, less violent people around them. Any net positive effect, however, is most likely due to a change in the environment in which some assaults occur rather than by having an effect on the high-risk male himself.

An extensive critical review of the scientific literature on prevention efforts on U.S. college campuses was recently published by Newlands and O'Donohue (2016). In order to facilitate improvement, the authors made some recommendations for developing more rigorous research programs. Among them is the idea that attending to "differences between participants can elucidate what factors influence or moderate treatment success or failure" (p. 10). In light of growing evidence of boomerang reactance effects described below, whereby interventions may result in an increased probability that relatively high-risk males will endorse sexually violent attitudes and be willing to behave more aggressively after the intervention compared to before, attending specifically to men's individual risk profiles appears highly important.

For many years, based on repeated findings in various areas (e.g., alcohol consumption, home energy use), reviewers of public health campaigns have called attention to the possibility of adverse boomerang effects. As some reviewers have noted, "An obvious implication is that boomerang effects should be taken into account as one of the potential costs of launching a mass communication campaign" (Ringold, 2012, p. 27). Most relevant to the current focus, boomerang effects have been well documented in areas of interventions designed to change antisocial behaviors, including sexual and nonsexual violence (see, e.g., Byrne & Hart, 2016; Wilson, Linz, Donnerstein, & Stipp, 1992). For example, an analysis of the consequences of a domestic violence campaign that included multiple television and newspaper advertisements demonstrated such unintended effects (Keller, Wilkinson, & Otjen, 2010). One of the stated goals of the program was to change the attitudes and behaviors of potential perpetrators. Only women's perception of the severity of domestic violence (e.g., "Domestic violence is a serious issue that requires government or police involvement") increased after the campaign, however. Perceptions of the severity of domestic violence actually substantially decreased for the men in the study.

Cardaba, Brinol, Brandle, and Ruiz-SanRoman (2016) conducted research on the effects of anti-violence campaigns in different countries with different age populations. In one study, they found that individuals with relatively higher scores in trait aggressiveness showed a boomerang effect of anti-violence messages since they actually increased their favorability of attitudes toward violence. In contrast, the anti-violence campaigns were effective for those with relatively lower trait aggressiveness. In a second study, the intervention campaign again worked for the low trait-aggressive individuals but not for the high trait-aggressive participants. Another study reporting boomerang effects in the area of violence was conducted by Rivera, Santos, Brandle, and Cardaba (2016). The authors randomly assigned a large number of Italian students to participate in an intervention campaign designed to reduce participants' acceptance of violent video games. Participants were classified according to their relational lifestyle, consisting of four groups: e.g., "communicative" adolescents were more highly engaged in "civic values duties" in their communities than other groups; "meta-reflexive" adolescents had the lowest probability of seeking parents' support; whereas "fractured" adolescents had a higher probability of taking drugs than other groups and of engaging in other relatively delinquent behaviors. The group with a "fractured" or problematic lifestyle showed a boomerang effect, increasing their intent to play violent video games, whereas the other participants reduced their desire as a result of the intervention or there was a null effect. This finding is noteworthy as it is consistent with the idea in EP that sexually aggressive men can be "generalists" or "specialists," with implications for how different men might be expected to respond differently to the same sexual assault prevention program based on group membership.

We could not find any studies that specifically examined the impact of any elaborate interventions on high-risk males. The studies we did find all involved some form of intervention of less than one or two hours. One of these was a systematic experiment using a well-validated laboratory analogue of sexual aggression. In a community sample of American men, Bosson, Parrott, Swan, Kuchynka, and Schramm (2015) found that men low in sexism showed less aggressive tendencies following exposure to messages emphasizing norms of gender equality (e.g., most men approve of "men doing half of the housework and childcare"). Conversely, men high in hostile sexist attitudes showed a boomerang effect of increased sexually aggressive tendencies.

In a study of undergraduate men, Stephens and George (2009) examined the impact of a rape prevention intervention on low- vs. high-risk men. Risk level was determined by whether individuals had reported previously engaging in sexually aggressive behavior. The researchers found that men in general showed reductions in rape myth acceptance and an increase in victim empathy at a 5-week follow-up. Subgroup analyses, however, indicated that low-risk men were responsible for these findings. High-risk men showed no reliable attitudinal changes from the intervention. More alarmingly, high-risk men in the intervention group were more likely at follow-up to report higher sexually coercive behaviors than were high-risk men in a control group, although the sample size was small.

In another study that presented men a bystander sexual violence prevention program consisting of multifaceted training and skills development, outcome measures of rape myth acceptance and sexually coercive behavioral intentions were reduced among low-risk men (Elias-Lambert & Black, 2016). The program was relatively ineffective with high-risk men, however, leading the authors to conclude that "high-risk males may require a different type of prevention program that can help change the stubborn attitudes and habits they have developed" (p. 3229).

In order to avoid the possibility of boomerang effects, prevention programs should consider introducing exercises likely to reduce the perception of women as out-group threat. Using techniques such as self-affirmation and identity verification may be effective in this regard. These could be incorporated as part of a more comprehensive program for high-risk males, prior to the introduction of specific educational interventions. By moderating perceptions of out-group threat, these experiences can serve to mitigate hostile reactance.

According to self-affirmation theory (Steele, 1988), individuals have a fundamental motivation to protect their personal image. Self-threatening information is likely to elicit defensive responses such as rejecting the information, presenting counterarguments, or expressing resistance to change in order to restore one's self-integrity. When one's self-integrity is supported via self-affirmation, however, one can more carefully consider views and information that otherwise would be too threatening to accept (Cohen & Sherman, 2014; Sherman, 2013).

Self-affirmations have been found to increase positive other-directed feelings (Crocker, Niiya, & Mischkowski, 2008). They have been shown to have physiological bases for their desired effects by buffering neuroendocrine and psychological stress responses (Creswell et al., 2005) and by activating relevant brain-reward systems (Dutcher et al., 2016). By reducing defensive information processing, self-affirmations can increase the effectiveness of educational campaigns (Cohen, Aronson, & Steele, 2000) via how campaigns are framed and embodied. To our knowledge, existing efforts to educate undergraduate students, and high-risk men specifically, about sexual violence prevention have not included these self-image maintenance processes. Because of this, these programs are more likely to have unintended, counterproductive consequences.

Similarly, research on identity verification has found that when the set of meanings in a situation does not match people's internal standards, and someone else does not confirm or verify their identities, they can experience negative emotional arousal such as hostility (Cast & Burke, 2002). If the lack of verification persists, an individual ultimately may resort to tactics of physical or sexual aggression over others in order to reassert control over the environment (Stets, 1992). Many current sexual assault prevention programs contain admonishments that may create hostility and lead to a diminished sense of control for high-risk men, such that a resort to sexual violence to compensate for this loss is possible.

Identity-verification can serve to reduce or eliminate such backlash responses by creating feelings of positive arousal including high self-esteem and mastery (Burke & Stets, 1999; Cast & Burke, 2002), setting the stage, e.g., for approach behaviors to programmatic information such as increased perspective taking. Research from identity theory suggests that verifying high-risk men in areas affiliated with their aggressive personality, such as masculinity, athletics, or a personal identity related to the degree to which they see themselves as more or less controlling may be most likely to create the conditions for attitudinal and behavioral change (Stets & Burke, 1994), as part of a comprehensive educational program for change.

8. Empathy-based interventions may be particularly important for high-risk males.

To effectively modify sexually aggressive mechanisms requires an intervention emphasis at emotional levels, not only a cognitive level. Focusing on remedying empathy and sympathy deficits may be useful as one component of an effective strategy with high-risk males, although the results of studies emphasizing these variables are tentative and inconsistent. Frans de Waal has conjectured that emotional contagion and empathy, compassion and sympathy, or automatic and deliberate empathy are all connected emotions that have been developed in humans through evolutionary processes. Most EP theorists agree that these constructs are the result of evolution although there is disagreement about the precise development of each component. However, there is a serious drawback to relying too heavily on the cultivation of empathy in high-risk males. As de Waal (2012) and others have noted, psychopaths may be capable of perspective-taking that superficially looks like empathy but given their lack of emotional investment, they cannot truly be called empathetic (Mullins-Nelson, Salekin, & Leistico, 2006). For high-risk males who have tendencies toward psychopathic personality characteristics, i.e., those men on the far end of the spectrum with relatively fixed calibration of decision rules, attempts to increase empathy and victim sympathy therefore may be ineffective at best and lead to unintended boomerang reactance effects at worst. As we describe above, however, the prior use of self-affirmation and identity verification techniques might help to avoid boomerang effects with these men. Further, for those high-risk males who have developmentally flexible psychological mechanisms, empathy interventions are more likely to produce positive outcomes.

One line of research has shown some positive, albeit mixed effects, of a short-term intervention on measures of empathy for men classified as high risk. In one of the studies, high-risk males, based on scores on a modified version of Malamuth's Likelihood of Raping scale (Malamuth, 1981), were randomly assigned to one of three conditions: (1) a no-treatment control group, (2) viewing videos intended to induce greater empathy, or (3) viewing videos designed to counter rape myths by presenting rape facts (Schewe & O'Donohue, 1993). The condition presenting rape facts failed to show any significant effects and indeed the high-risk men scored more negatively on rape-related variables than the control group. However, the rape empathy condition, which showed a presentation depicting victims of rape, child sexual abuse, and sexual harassment and their subsequent pain and suffering, did result in improvements in rape empathy and a decrease in attitudes supporting aggression against women. In a second study using similar procedures, a condition designed to facilitate empathy towards victims of sexual abuse and to increase awareness of the destructive consequences of rape for the male aggressor lowered the scores of high-risk males at two-week follow-up on measures of attraction to sexual aggression and acceptance of interpersonal violence, although not on rape myth acceptance and adversarial sexual beliefs (Schewe & O'Donohue, 1996).

A promising new avenue for change is virtual reality simulations. As a leading creator of virtual reality experiences describes, "I sometimes call virtual reality an empathy generator. It's astonishing to me. People all of a sudden connect to the characters in a way that they don't when they've read about it in the newspaper or watched it on TV" (Delahoussaye, 2015). Virtual experiences involve using new technologies to enable more intensive and immersive experiences that permit a radical change in perspective. Embodied virtual experiences lead to greater feelings of connectedness to a target than traditional perspective-taking, even for people low in interpersonal reactivity (i.e., low in empathic concern, perspective taking, fantasy, and personal distress) (Ahn, Le, & Bailenson, 2013).

Recent research on immersion in virtual reality, including work by Abbey, Pegram, Woerner, and Wegner (2018), who have developed a virtual dating simulation of sexual aggression, Brewster (2017), who has suggested that VR is especially suited to tapping into our emotions to produce a sense of "real feelings," and other researchers who have shown the value of VR for helping offenders with emotion recognition (Seinfeld et al., 2018), suggests promising opportunities for sexual assault risk reduction. Seinfeld et al. (2018), for example, had a group of male domestic violence offenders experience a virtual scene of abuse in first-person perspective. The virtual encounter improved deficits in these men's emotion recognition skills by improving their ability to recognize fear in female faces compared to baseline and reducing a bias toward classifying fearful faces as happy. These effects occurred in offenders and not in a control group of men. In view of the fact that men who are violent toward their female partners are poorer at recognizing fear in female faces than are nonviolent men (Seinfeld et al., 2018), these results are suggestive of the potential of virtual reality perspective-taking for changing real-world behavior. Although more research is needed on how best to fine-tune VR experiences to increase perspective-taking, the use of VR simulations holds promise as an empathy generator for sexually aggressive men.

It is also significant that other research on the effects of perspective taking has shown that increased perspective-taking can in some cases diminish out-group stereotypes (Galinsky & Ku, 2004; Galinsky & Moskowitz, 2000) and combat automatic expressions of biases, denial of discrimination, and stereotype maintenance processes (e.g., Todd, Bodenhausen, Richeson, & Galinsky, 2011; Todd & Galinsky, 2014). To the extent that sexually aggressive men can be seen as "prejudiced" against women, there is therefore reason to expect positive benefits of empathy-focused interventions when these men are not too fixed in their path. Encouragingly, for undergraduate men in general, research shows that as they engage with new people, experiences, and ideas in the college environment, empathy is amenable to change (Hudson-Flege & Thompson, 2017). For college men who possess important risk factors (hostile masculinity, impersonal sexual attitudes), empathy has been found to moderate these risk factors in predicting sexual aggression, such that men high on these constructs but who are also high in empathy have been found to behave comparably to low-risk men (Wheeler et al., 2002).

Schewe and O'Donohue (1993) provide tentative evidence that an empathy-based intervention can have short-term positive effects on high-risk men, at least at the attitudinal level. Involvement in organizations that tend to promote a strong sense of in-group identity, such as fraternities, may inhibit positive growth, however (Hudson-Flege & Thompson, 2017), highlighting the need for interventions that also target group-level factors, such as peer groups supportive of sexual aggression (Swartout, 2013).

Final Observations

In a recent interview with former President Clinton, Comedy Central's Trevor Noah asked him about the #MeToo movement: "Honest question: Has it been hard for you to reprogram your brain? Has it been difficult for you to go, 'I have to relearn something that is happening now as to how I have always seen the world?... As a man, the instinct is to go to a defensive place... What would you recommend to other men out there to begin the journey of understanding and self-reflection?" To which President Clinton responded, "To become first other-directed. That is look at what's happening in people's lives. Then you have to ask yourself how do I think, how do I feel, how do I act. And, both try to make sure you're doing better, even if you think you're a really good person and you're not aware of ever having done anything wrong, and then... asking the women in your life..." (*The Daily Show with Trevor Noah*, June 26, 2018). From an evolutionary psychological perspective, there is much to recommend in this exchange. Moving sexually aggressive men to better engage with others' perspectives, such as by incorporating the use of affirming and immersive strategies that can help function to recalibrate previous decision rules and subsequent choices, may be essential to yield better preventative policies.

References

Abbey, A., Pegram, S. E., Woerner, J., & Wegner, R. (2018). Men's responses to women's sexual refusals: Development and construct validity of a virtual dating simulation of sexual aggression. *Psychology of Violence, 8*, 87–99.

Ahn, S. J., Le, A. M. T., & Bailenson, J. N. (2013). The effect of embodied experiences on self-other merging, attitude, and helping behavior. *Media Psychology, 16*, 7–38.

Allen, B. (1996). *Rape warfare: The hidden genocide in Bosnia-Herzegovina and Croatia*. Minneapolis: University of Minnesota Press.

Allen, M., D'Alessio, D., & Emmers-Sommer, T. M. (2000). Reactions of criminal sexual offenders to pornography: A meta-analytic summary. In M. Roloff (Ed.), *Communication yearbook 22* (pp. 139–169). Thousand Oaks, CA: Sage.

Al-Shawaf, L., Lewis, D. M. G., & Buss, D. M. (2018). Sex differences in disgust: Why are women more easily disgusted than men? *Emotion Review, 10*(2), 149–160.

Baniel, A., Cowlishaw, G., & Huchard, E. (2017). Male violence and sexual intimidation in a wild primate society. *Current Biology, 27*(14), 2163–2168.

Banyard, V. L., Moynihan, M. M., Cares, A. C., & Warner, R. (2014). How do we know if it works? Measuring outcomes in bystander-focused abuse prevention on campus. *Psychology of Violence, 4*, 101–114.

Banyard, V. L., Moynihan, M. M., & Plante, E. G. (2007). Sexual violence prevention through bystander education: An experimental evaluation. *Journal of Community Psychology, 35*, 463–466.

Barbaree, H. E. (1990). Stimulus control of sexual arousal: Its role in sexual assault. In W. L. Marshall, D. Laws, & H. E. Barbaree (Eds.), *Handbook of sexual assault: Issues, theories, and treatment of the offender* (pp. 115–142). New York, NY: Plenum Press.

Bargh, J. A., Raymond, P., Pryor, J. B., & Strack, F. (1995). Attractiveness of the underling: An automatic power → sex association and its consequences for sexual harassment and aggression. *Journal of Personality and Social Psychology, 68*, 768–781.

Barnes, J. C., TenEyck, M., Boutwell, B. B., & Beaver, K. M. (2013). Indicators of domestic/intimate partner violence are structured by genetic and nonshared environmental influences. *Journal of Psychiatric Research, 47*(3), 371–376.

Basile, K. C. (2002). Prevalence of wife rape and other intimate partner sexual coercion in a nationally representative sample of women. *Violence and Victims, 17*, 511–524.

Beirne, P., Hall, J., Grills, C., & Moore, T. (2011). Female hormone influences on sexual assaults in Northern Ireland from 2002 to 2009. *Journal of Forensic and Legal Medicine, 18*, 313–316.

Belsky, J., Steinberg, L., & Draper, P. (1991). Childhood experience, interpersonal development, and reproductive strategy: An evolutionary theory of socialization. *Child Development, 62*, 647–670.

Bernat, J. A., Calhoun, K. S., & Adams, H. E. (1999). Sexually aggressive and nonaggressive men: Sexual arousal and judgments in response to acquaintance rape and consensual analogues. *Journal of Abnormal Psychology, 108*, 662–673.

Bosson, J. K., Parrott, D. J., Swan, S. C., Kuchynka, S. L., & Schramm, A. T. (2015). A dangerous boomerang: Injunctive norms, hostile sexist attitudes, and male-to-female sexual aggression. *Aggressive Behavior, 41*, 580–593.

Breiding, M. J., Smith, S. G., Basile, K. C., Walters, M. L., Chen, J., & Merrick, M. T. (2014). Prevalence and characteristics of sexual violence, stalking, and intimate partner violence victimization—National intimate partner and sexual violence survey, United States, 2011. *MMWR, 63*(SS-8), 1–18.

Brewster, S. (2017). *Designing for real feelings in a virtual reality*. Retrieved from https://medium.com/s/designing-for-virtual-reality/designing-for-real-feelings-in-a-virtual-reality-41f2a2c7046

Bröder, A., & Hohmann, N. (2003). Variations in risk taking behavior over the menstrual cycle: An improved replication. *Evolution and Human Behavior, 24*, 391–398.

Broude, G. J., & Greene, S. J. (1978). Cross-cultural codes on 20 sexual attitudes and practices. *Ethnology, 15*, 409–430.

Brown, A. L., & Messman-Moore, T. L. (2010). Personal and perceived peer attitudes supporting sexual aggression as predictors of male college students' willingness to intervene against sexual aggression. *Journal of Interpersonal Violence, 25*(3), 503–517.

Brumbach, B. H., Figueredo, A. J., & Ellis, B. J. (2009). Effects of harsh and unpredictable environments in adolescence on development of life history strategies. *Human Nature, 20*(1), 25–51.

Burke, P. J., & Stets, J. E. (1999). Trust and commitment through self-verification. *Social Psychology Quarterly, 62*, 347–360.

Buss, D., & Malamuth, N. (Eds.). (1996). *Sex, power, conflict: Evolutionary and feminist perspectives*. New York: Oxford University Press.

Buss, D. M. (2003). *The evolution of desire: Strategies of human mating*. New York, NY: Basic Books. (Original work published 1994).

Buss, D. M., & Greiling, H. (1999). Adaptive individual differences. *Journal of Personality, 67*(2), 209–243.

Buss, D. M., Haselton, M. G., Shackelford, T. K., Bleske, A. L., & Wakefield, J. C. (1998). Adaptations, exaptations, and spandrels. *American Psychologist, 53*, 533–548.

Buss, D. M., & Schmitt, D. P. (1993). Sexual strategy theory: An evolutionary perspective on human mating. *Psychological Review, 100*, 204–232.

Byrne, S., & Hart, P. S. (2016). The Boomerang Effect A synthesis of findings and a preliminary theoretical framework. *Annals of the International Communication Association, 33*, 3–37. https://doi.org/10.1080/23808985.2009.11679083

California Department of Education (2018). *Questions and answers regarding comprehensive sexual health education, HIV/AIDS and STD instruction*. Retrieved from https://www.cde.ca.gov/ls/he/se/faq.asp

California Legislative Information. (2016). *California education code sections 51930-51939*. Retrieved from https://leginfo.legislature.ca.gov/faces/billNavClient.xhtml?bill_id=201520160AB329

Camilleri, J. A., & Stiver, K. A. (2014). Adaptation and sexual offending. In V. A. Weekes-Shackelford & T. K. Shackelford (Eds.), *Evolutionary perspectives on human sexual psychology and behavior* (pp. 43–67). New York, NY: Springer.

Canastar, A., & Maxson, S. (2003). Sexual aggression in mice: Effects of male strain and of female estrous state. *Behavior Genetics, 33*, 521–528.

Cardaba, M. G., Brinol, P., Brandle, G., & Ruiz-SanRoman, J. A. (2016). The moderating role of aggressiveness to campaigns and interventions promoting anti-violence attitudes. *Aggressive Behavior, 99*, 1–12.

Cast, A. D., & Burke, P. J. (2002). A theory of self-esteem. *Social Forces, 80*, 1041–1068.

Centers for Disease Control and Prevention. (2014). *Preventing sexual violence on college campuses: Lessons from research and practice*. Retrieved from https://www.notalone.gov/schools/

Chagnon, N. A. (1994, August). How important was "marriage by capture" as a mating strategy in the EEA? *Human Behavior and Evolution Society Newsletter, 3*, 1–2.

Chavanne, T. J., & Gallup, G. G. (1998). Variation in risk taking behavior among female college students as a function of the menstrual cycle. *Evolution and Human Behavior, 19*, 27–32.

Check, M. V. P., Malamuth, N., Elias, B., & Barton, S. (1985). On hostile ground. *Psychology Today, 19*, 56–61.

Cohen, G. L., Aronson, J., & Steele, C. M. (2000). When beliefs yield to evidence: Reducing biased evaluation by affirming the self. *Personality and Social Psychology Bulletin, 26*, 1151–1164.

Cohen, G. L., & Sherman, D. K. (2014). The psychology of change: Self-affirmation and social psychological intervention. *Annual Review of Psychology, 65*, 333–371.

Confer, J. C., Easton, J. A., Fleischman, D. S., Goetz, C. D., Lewis, D. M. G., Perilloux, C., & Buss, D. M. (2010). Evolutionary psychology: Controversies, questions, prospects, and limitations. *The American Psychologist, 65*, 110–126.

Creswell, J. D., Welch, W., Taylor, S. E., Sherman, D. K., Gruenewald, T., & Mann, T. (2005). Affirmation of personal values buffers neuroendocrine and psychological stress responses. *Psychological Science, 16*, 846–851.

Crèpault, C., & Couture, M. (1980). Men's erotic fantasies. *Archives of Sexual Behavior, 9*(6), 565–581.

Crocker, J., Niiya, Y., & Mischkowski, D. (2008). Why does writing about important values reduce defensiveness? Self-affirmation and the role of positive other-directed feelings. *Psychological Science, 19*(7), 740–747.

Dahlberg, L. L., & Krug, E. G. (2002). Violence: A global health public program. In E. G. Krug, L. L. Dahlberg, J. A. Mercy, A. B. Zwi, & R. Lozano (Eds.), *World report on violence and health* (pp. 1–56). Geneva: World Health Organization.

de Haas, S., van Berlo, W., Bakker, F., & Vanwesenbeeck, I. (2012). Prevalence and characteristics of sexual violence in the Netherlands, the risk of revictimization and pregnancy: Results from a national population survey. *Violence and Victims, 27*(4), 592–608.

de Waal, F. B. (2012). Empathy in primates and other mammals. In J. Decety (Ed.), *Empathy: From bench to bedside* (pp. 87–106). Cambridge, MA: MIT Press.

Dean, K., & Malamuth, N. (1997). Characteristics of men who aggress sexually and of men who imagine aggressing: Risk and moderating variables. *Journal of Personality and Social Psychology, 72*, 449–455.

Del Guidice, M., Gangestad, S. W., & Kaplan, H. S. (2015). Life history theory and evolutionary psychology. In D. M. Buss (Ed.), *The handbook of evolutionary psychology—Vol. 1: Foundations* (2nd ed., pp. 88–114). New York: Wiley.

Delahoussaye, J. (2015, February 2). *Virtual games try to generate real empathy for faraway conflict (quoting Nonny de la Peña)*. Retrieved from www.npr.org/sections/alltechconsidered/2015/01/25/379417927/virtual-games-try-to-generate-real-empathy-for-far-away-conflict

DiMauro, J., Renshaw, K. D., & Blais, R. K. (2018). Sexual vs. non-sexual trauma, sexual satisfaction and function, and mental health in female veterans. *Journal of Trauma & Dissociation, 19*, 403–416.

Draper, P., & Harpending, H. (1982). Father absence and reproductive strategy: An evolutionary perspective. *Journal of Anthropological Research, 38*, 255–273.

Durán, M., Megías, J. L., & Moya, M. (2018). Male peer support to hostile sexist attitudes influences rape proclivity. *Journal of Interpersonal Violence, 33*(14), 2180–2196.

Dutcher, J. M., Creswell, J. D., Pacilio, L. E., Harris, P. R., Klein, W. M. P., Levine, J. M., … Eisenberger, N. I. (2016). Self-affirmation activates the ventral striatum: A possible reward-related mechanism for self-affirmation. *Psychological Science, 27*, 455–666.

Elias-Lambert, N., & Black, B. M. (2016). Bystander sexual violence prevention program: Outcomes for high- and low-risk university men. *Journal of Interpersonal Violence, 31*, 3211–3235. https://doi.org/10.1177/0886260515584346

Elliot, A. J. (2008). Approach and avoidance motivation. In A. Elliot (Ed.), *Handbook of approach and avoidance motivation* (pp. 3–14). New York, NY: Psychology Press.

Ellis, B., & Symons, D. (1989). Sex differences in sexual fantasy. *Journal of Sex Research, 27*, 527–555.

Ellis, L. (1989). *Theories of rape: Inquiries into the causes of sexual aggression*. New York, NY: Hemisphere.

Ellis, L., Widmayer, A., & Palmer, C. T. (2009). Perpetrators of sexual assault continuing to have sex with their victims following the initial assault: Evidence for evolved reproductive strategies. *International Journal of Offender Therapy and Comparative Criminology, 53*(4), 454–463.

Fanniff, A. M., Schubert, C. A., Mulvey, E. P., Iselin, A.-M. R., & Piquero, A. (2016). Risk and outcomes: Are adolescents charged with sex offenses different from other adolescent offenders? *Journal of Youth and Adolescence, 46*, 1394. https://doi.org/10.1007/s10964-016-0536-9

Feldman, J. T., Wroblewski, E. E., Rudicell, R. S., Hahn, B. H., Paiva, T., Cetinkaya-Rundel, M., … Gilby, I. C. (2014). Sexually coercive male chimpanzees sire more offspring. *Current Biology, 24*(23), 2855–2860.

Ferguson, C. J. (2010). Genetic contributions to antisocial personality and behavior: A meta-analytic review from an evolutionary psychological perspective. *The Journal of Social Psychology, 150*, 160–180.

Forbes, G. B., Adams-Curtis, L. E., & White, K. B. (2004). First- and second-generation measures of sexism, rape myths and related beliefs, and hostility toward women. *Violence Against Women, 10*, 236–261.

Foshee, V. A., Bauman, K. E., Ennett, S. T., Linder, G. F., Benefield, T., & Suchindran, C. (2004). Assessing the long-term effects of the Safe Dates program and a booster in preventing and reducing adolescent dating violence victimization and perpetration. *American Journal of Public Health, 94*(4), 619–624.

Fulu, E., Jewkes, R., Roselli, T., & Garcia-Moreno, C. (2013). Prevalence of and factors associated with non-partner rape perpetration: Findings from the UN multi-country cross-sectional study on men and violence in Asia and the Pacific. *The Lancet Global Health, 1*, e208–e218.

Galinsky, A. D., & Ku, G. (2004). The effects of perspective-taking on prejudice: The moderating role of self-evaluation. *Personality and Social Psychology Bulletin, 30*(5), 594–604.

Galinsky, A. D., & Moskowitz, G. B. (2000). Perspective-taking: Decreasing stereotype expression, stereotype accessibility, and in-group favoritism. *Journal of Personality and Social Psychology, 78*(4), 708–724.

Garver-Apgar, C. E., Gangestad, S. W., & Simpson, J. A. (2007). Women's perceptions of men's sexual coerciveness change across the menstrual cycle. *Acta Psychologica Sinica, 39*, 536–540.

Gidycz, C. A. (2018). Sexual assault risk reduction: Current state and historical underpinnings. In L. M. Orchowski & C. A. Gidycz (Eds.), *Sexual assault risk reduction and resistance: Theory, research, and practice* (pp. 3–14). San Diego: Academic Press, an imprint of Elsevier.

Gorelik, G., Shackelford, T. K., & Weeks-Shackelford, V. A. (2012). Human violence and evolutionary consciousness. *Review of General Psychology, 16*, 343–356.

Gottschall, J., & Gottschall, T. (2003). Are per-incident rape-pregnancy rates higher than per-incident consensual pregnancy rates? *Human Nature, 14*, 1–20.

Greendlinger, V., & Byrne, D. (1987). Coercive sexual fantasies of college men as predictors of self-reported likelihood to rape and overt sexual aggression. *Journal of Sex Research, 23*, 1–11.

Hagen, E. H. (2004). Is rape an adaptation? *The Evolutionary Psychology FAQ*. Retrieved from www.anth.ucsb.edu/projects/human/evpsychfaq.html

Harris, D. A., Mazerolle, P., & Knight, R. A. (2009). Understanding male sexual offending: A comparison of general and specialist theories. *Criminal Justice and Behavior, 36*(10), 1051–1069.

Harris, D. A., Smallbone, S., Dennison, S., & Knight, R. A. (2009). Specialization and versatility of sexual offenders referred for civil commitment. *Journal of Criminal Justice, 37*, 37–44.

Harris, G. T., Rice, M. E., Hilton, N. Z., Lalumière, M. L., & Quinsey, V. L. (2007). Coercive and precocious sexuality as a fundamental aspect of psychopathy. *Journal of Personality Disorders, 21*(1), 1–27.

Hollander, J. A. (2014). Does self-defense training prevent sexual violence against women? *Violence Against Women, 20*(3), 252–269.

Holmes, M. M., Resnick, H. S., Kilpatrick, D. G., & Best, C. L. (1996). Rape-related pregnancy: Estimates and descriptive characteristics from a national sample of women. *American Journal of Obstetrics and Gynecology, 175*(2), 320–324.

Hudson-Flege, M., & Thompson, M. P. (2017). Empathy and extracurricular involvement in emerging adulthood: Findings from a longitudinal study of undergraduate college males. *Journal of College Student Development, 58*(5), 674–684.

Johansson, A., Santtila, P., Harlaar, N., von der Pahlen, B., Witting, K., Algars, M., … Sandnabba, N. K. (2008). Genetic effects on male sexual coercion. *Aggressive Behavior, 34*, 190–202.

Kaczkowski, W., Brennan, C. L., & Swartout, K. M. (2017). In good company: Social network diversity may protect men against perpetrating sexual violence. *Psychology of Violence, 7*(2), 276–285.

Keller, S. N., Wilkinson, T., & Otjen, A. J. (2010). Unintended effects of a domestic violence campaign. *Journal of Advertising, 39*, 53–68.

Kenrick, D. T., & Sheets, V. (1993). Homicidal fantasies. *Ethology and Sociobiology, 14*, 231–246.

Kingston, D. A., Seto, M. C., Firestone, P., & Bradford, J. M. (2010). Comparing indicators of sexual sadism as predictors of recidivism among adult male sexual offenders. *Journal of Consulting and Clinical Psychology, 78*(4), 574–584.

Knight, R. A. (2010). Is a diagnostic category for paraphilic coercive disorder defensible? *Archives of Sexual Behavior, 39*(2), 419–426.

Knight, R. A., & Prentky, R. A. (1990). Classifying sexual offenders: The development and corroboration of taxonomic models. In W. L. Marshall, D. R. Laws, & H. E. Barbaree (Eds.), *Handbook of sexual assault: issues, theories, and treatment of the offender* (pp. 23–52). New York: Plenum Press.

Knight, R. A., & Sims-Knight, J. E. (2011). Risk factors for sexual violence. In J. W. White, M. P. Koss, & A. E. Kadzin (Eds.), *Violence against women and children: Mapping the terrain* (Vol. 1, pp. 125–150). Washington, DC: American Psychological Association.

Knight, R. A., & Sims-Knight, J. E. (2016). A theoretical integration of etiological and typological models of rape. In A. R. Beech & T. Ward (Eds.), *The Wiley handbook on the theories, assessment and treatment of sexual offending* (Vol. Vol. 1, pp. 73–102). Hoboken, NJ: Wiley.

Knott, C. D. (2009). Orangutans: Sexual coercion without sexual violence. In M. N. Muller & R. W. Wrangham (Eds.), *Sexual coercion in primates: An evolutionary perspective on male aggression against females* (pp. 81–111). Cambridge, MA: Harvard University Press.

Knott, C. D., & Kahlenberg, S. (2007). Orangutans in perspective: Forced copulations and female mating resistance. In S. Bearder, C. J. Campbell, A. Fuentes, K. C. MacKinnon, & M. Panger (Eds.), *Primates in perspective* (pp. 290–305). Oxford, England: Oxford University Press.

Koss, M. (1988). Hidden rape: Sexual aggression and victimization in a national sample of students in higher education. In A. W. Burgess (Ed.), *Rape and sexual assault* (pp. 3–25). New York, NY: Garland Press.

Krahé, B., Tomaszewska, P., Kuyper, L., & Vanwesenbeeck, I. (2014). Prevalence of sexual aggression among young people in Europe: A review of the evidence from 27 EU countries. *Aggression and Violent Behavior, 19*, 545–558.

Lalumière, M. L., Harris, G. T., Quinsey, V. L., & Rice, M. E. (2005). *The nature of rape: Understanding male propensity for sexual aggression*. Washington, DC: American Psychological Association.

Längström, N., Babchishin, K. M., Fazel, S., Lichtenstein, P., & Friesel, T. (2015). Sexual offending runs in families: A 37-year nationwide study. *International Journal of Epidemiology, 44*(2), 713–720.

Lawing, K., Frick, P. J., & Cruise, K. R. (2010). Differences in offending patterns between adolescent sex offenders high or low in callous-unemotional traits. *Psychological Assessment, 22*(2), 298–305.

Leibold, J. M., & McConnell, A. R. (2004). Women, sex, hostility, power, and suspicion: Sexually aggressive men's cognitive associations. *Journal of Experimental Social Psychology, 40*, 256–263.

Levinson, D. (1989). *Family violence in cross-cultural perspective*. Thousand Oaks, CA: Sage.

Lussier, P., & Cale, J. (2016). Understanding the origins and the development of rape and sexual aggression against women: Four generations of research and theorizing. *Aggression and Violent Behavior, 31*, 66–81.

Malamuth, N. (1981). Rape proclivity among males. *Journal of Social Issues, 37*, 138–157.

Malamuth, N. (1989). The attraction to sexual aggression scale: Part one. *Journal of Sex Research, 26*, 26–49.

Malamuth, N., Check, J., & Briere, J. (1986). Sexual arousal in response to aggression: Ideological, aggressive and sexual correlates. *Journal of Personality and Social Psychology, 50*, 330–340.

Malamuth, N., & Hald, G. M. (2017). The confluence mediational model of sexual aggression. In A. R. Beech & T. Ward (Eds.), *The Wiley handbook on the theories, assessment and treatment of sexual offending* (Vol. 1, pp. 53–72). Hoboken, NJ: Wiley.

Malamuth, N. M. (1998). An evolutionary-based model integrating research on the characteristics of sexually aggressive men. In J. G. Adair & D. Belanger (Eds.), *Advances in psychological science. Vol. 1: Social, personal, and cultural aspects* (pp. 151–184). Hove, England: Psychology Press/Erlbaum.

Malamuth, N. M., Heavey, C. L., & Linz, D. (1996). The confluence model of sexual aggression. *Journal of Offender Rehabilitation, 23*, 13–37.

McDonald, M. M., Donnellan, M. B., Cesario, J., & Navarette, C. D. (2015). Mate choice preferences in an intergroup context: Evidence for a sexual coercion threat-management system among women. *Evolution and Human Behavior, 36*(6), 438–445.

McKibbin, W. F., & Shackelford, T. K. (2012). Women's avoidance of rape: An evolutionary psychological perspective. In K. M. Beaver & A. Walsh (Eds.), *The Ashgate research companion to biosocial theories of crime*. Farnham, UK: Ashgate.

McKibbin, W. F., & Shackelford, T. K. (2013). Comment on "Reexamining individual differences in rape avoidance" by Snyder and Fessler (2012). *Archives of Sexual Behavior, 42*, 1–4.

McKibbin, W. F., Shackelford, T. K., Goetz, A. T., & Starratt, V. G. (2008). Why do men rape? An evolutionary psychological perspective. *Review of General Psychology, 12*(1), 86–97.

McKibbin, W. F., Shackelford, T. K., Miner, E. J., Bates, V. M., & Liddle, J. R. (2011). Individual differences in women's rape avoidance behaviors. *Archives of Sexual Behavior, 40*, 343–349.

Mealey, L. (2003). Combating rape: Views of an evolutionary psychologist. In R. W. Bloom & N. Dess (Eds.), *Evolutionary psychology and violence: A primer for policymakers and public policy advocates* (pp. 83–114). Westport, CT: Praeger Publishers.

Mesnick, S. L. (1997). Sexual alliances: Evidence and evolutionary implications. In P. A. Gowaty (Ed.), *Feminism and evolutionary biology: Boundaries, intersections and frontiers* (pp. 207–260). New York, NY: Chapman and Hall.

Moffitt, T. E., Caspi, A., Harrington, H., & Milne, B. J. (2002). Males on the life-course-persistent and adolescence-limited antisocial pathways: Follow-up at age 26 years. *Development and Psychopathology, 14*, 179–207.

Monson, C. M., & Langhinrichsen-Rohling, J. (2002). Sexual and nonsexual dating violence perpetration: Testing an integrated perpetrator typology. *Violence and Victims, 17*, 403–428.

Mullins-Nelson, J. L., Salekin, R. T., & Leistico, A.-M. R. (2006). Psychopathy, empathy, and perspective-taking ability in a community sample: Implications for the successful psychopathy concept. *International Journal of Forensic Mental Health, 5*(2), 133–149.

Murnen, S., Wright, C., & Kaluzny, G. (2002). If "boys will be boys," then girls will be victims? A meta-analytic review of the research that relates masculine ideology to sexual aggression. *Sex Roles, 46*, 359–375.

Nation, M., Crusto, C., Wandersman, A., Kumpfer, K. L., Seybolt, D., Morrissey-Kane, E., & Davino, K. (2003). Applying the principles of prevention: What do prevention practitioners need to know about what works. *American Psychologist, 58*, 449–456.

Navarrete, C. D., Fessler, D. M. T., Fleischman, D. S., & Geyer, J. (2009). Race bias tracks conception risk across the menstrual cycle. *Psychological Science, 20*(6), 661–665.

Nettle, D., Dickens, T. E., Coall, D. A., & de Mornay Davies, P. (2013). Patterns of physical and psychological development in future teenage mothers. *Evolution, Medicine, and Public Health, 2013*(1), 187–196.

Newlands, R., & O'Donohue, W. (2016). A critical review of sexual violence prevention on college campuses. *Acta Psychopathologica*, 2–14. https://doi.org/10.4172/2469-6676.100040

Orchowski, L. M., Barnett, N. P., Berkowitz, A., Borsari, B., Oesterle, D., & Zlotnick, C. (2018). Sexual assault prevention for heavy drinking college men: Development and feasibility of an integrated approach. *Violence Against Women, 24*(11), 1369–1396.

Perilloux, C., Duntley, J. D., & Buss, D. M. (2012). The costs of rape. *Archives of Sexual Behavior, 41*(5), 1099–1106.

Petralia, S. M., & Gallup, G. G. (2002). Effects of a sexual assault scenario on handgrip strength across the menstrual cycle. *Evolution and Human Behavior, 23*, 3–10.

Polanin, J. R., Esplanage, D. L., & Pigott, T. D. (2012). A meta-analysis of school-based bullying prevention programs' effects on bystander prevention behavior. *School Psychology Review, 41*(1), 47–65.

Reynolds, J. J., & McCrea, S. M. (2016). Life history theory and exploitative strategies. *Evolutionary Psychology, 14*(3), 1–16.

Ringold, D. R. (2012). Boomerang effects in response to public health interventions: Some unintended consequences in the alcoholic beverages market. *Journal of Consumer Policy, 25*(1), 27–63.

Rivera, R., Santos, D., Brandle, G., & Cardaba, M. A. M. (2016). Design effectiveness analysis of a media literacy intervention to reduce violent video games consumption among adolescents: The relevance of lifestyles segmentation. *Evaluation Review, 40*, 142–161. https://doi.org/10.1177/0193841X16666196

Russell, T. D. (2018). Hostile masculinity. In T. K. Shackelford & V. A. Weekes-Shackelford (Eds.), *Encyclopedia of evolutionary psychological science*. Cham: Springer.

Ryder, H., Maltby, J., Rai, L., Jones, P., & Flowe, H. D. (2016). Women's fear of crime and preference for formidable mates: How specific are the underlying psychological mechanisms? *Evolution and Human Behavior, 37*(4), 293–302.

Sanday, P. R. (1981). The sociocultural context of rape: A cross-cultural study. *Journal of Social Issues, 37*, 5–27.

Sanday, P. R. (1996). Rape-free versus rape-prone campus cultures. *Violence Against Women, 2*(2), 191–208.

Schewe, P. A., & O'Donohue, W. (1993). Sexual abuse prevention with high-risk males: The roles of victim empathy and rape myths. *Violence and Victims, 8*, 339–351.

Schewe, P. A., & O'Donohue, W. (1996). Rape prevention with high-risk males: Short-term outcome of two interventions. *Archives of Sexual Behavior, 5*, 455–471.

Schmidt, M. R., Lisco, C. G., Parrot, D. J., & Tharp, A. T. (2016). Moderating effect of negative peer group climate on the relation between men's locus of control and aggression toward intimate partners. *Journal of Interpersonal Violence, 31*(5), 755–773.

Seinfeld, S., Arroyo-Palacios, J., Iruretagoyena, G., Hortensius, R., Zapata, L. E., Borland, D., … Sanchez-Vives, M. V. (2018). Offenders become the victim in virtual reality: Impact of changing perspective in domestic violence. *Scientific Reports, 8*(1), 2692. https://doi.org/10.1038/s41598-018-19987-7

Sengupta, S. (2017, December 22). The #MeToo moment: what happened after women broke their silence elsewhere. *New York Times*. Retrieved from https://www.nytimes.com/2017/12/22/us/the-metoo-moment-what-happened-after-women-broke-the-silence-elsewhere.html

Senn, C. Y., Eliasziw, M., Hobden, K. L., Newby-Clark, I. R., Barata, P. C., Radtke, H. L., & Thurston, W. E. (2017). Secondary and 2-year outcomes of a sexual assault resistance program for university women. *Psychology of Women Quarterly, 41*(2), 147–162.

Seto, M. C. (2017). The motivation-facilitation model of sexual offending. *Sexual Abuse: A Journal of Research and Treatment*, 1–22. https://doi.org/10.1177/1079063217720919

Seto, M. C., & Kuban, M. (1996). Criterion-related validity of a phallometric test for paraphilic rape and sadism. *Behaviour Research and Therapy, 34*, 175–183.

Seto, M. C., & Lalumière, M. L. (2010). What is so special about male adolescent sexual offending? A review and test of explanations through meta-analysis. *Psychological Bulletin, 136*(4), 526–575.

Sherman, D. K. (2013). Self-affirmation: Understanding the effects. *Social and Personality Psychology Compass, 7*, 834–845.

Sim, T. N., & Koh, S. F. (2003). A domain conceptualization of adolescent susceptibility to peer pressure. *Journal of Research on Adolescence, 13*(1), 57–80.

Smuts, B. (1992). Male aggression against women: An evolutionary perspective. *Human Nature, 3*(1), 1–44.

Snyder, J. K., & Fessler, D. M. T. (2012). Reexamining individual differences in women's rape avoidance behaviors. *Archives of Sexual Behavior, 42*(4), 543–551.

Steele, C. M. (1988). The psychology of self-affirmation: Sustaining the integrity of the self. In L. Berkowitz (Ed.), *Advances in experimental social psychology* (Vol. 21, pp. 261–302). New York: Academic Press.

Stephens, K. A., & George, W. H. (2009). Rape prevention with college men: Evaluating risk status. *Journal of Interpersonal Violence, 24*, 996–1013.

Stets, J. E. (1992). Interactive processes in dating aggression: A national study. *Journal of Marriage and the Family, 54*, 165–177.

Stets, J. E., & Burke, P. J. (1994). Inconsistent self-views in the identity control model. *Social Science Research, 23*, 236–262.

Stiglmayer, A. (Ed.). (1994). *Mass rape*. Lincoln: University of Nebraska Press.

Swartout, K. M. (2013). The company they keep: How peer networks influence male sexual aggression. *Psychology of Violence, 3*(2), 157–171.

Swartout, K. M., Koss, M. P., White, J. W., Thompson, M. P., Abbey, A., & Bellis, A. L. (2015). Trajectory analysis of the campus serial rapist assumption. *JAMA Pediatrics, 169*(12), 1148–1154.

Symons, D. (1979). *The evolution of human sexuality*. New York, NY: Oxford University Press.

The Daily Show with Trevor Noah. (2018, June 26). *Comedy Central*. Retrieved from http://www.cc.com/video-clips/b037d1/the-daily-show-with-trevor-noah-bill-clinton%2D%2D-james-patterson%2D%2D%2D%2Dthe-president-is-missing%2D%2D%2D%2Dextended-interview

Thornhill, N. W., & Thornhill, R. (1990). An evolutionary analysis of psychological pain following rape. III: Effects of force and violence. *Aggressive Behavior, 16*, 297–320.

Thornhill, R., & Palmer, C. T. (2000). *A natural history of rape: Biological bases of sexual coercion*. Cambridge, MA: MIT Press.

Thornhill, R., & Thornhill, N. (1992). The evolutionary psychology of men's coercive sexuality. *Behavioral and Brain Sciences, 15*, 363–421.

Todd, A. R., Bodenhausen, G. V., Richeson, J. A., & Galinsky, A. D. (2011). Perspective taking combats automatic expression of racial bias. *Journal of Personality and Social Psychology, 100*(6), 1027–1042.

Todd, A. R., & Galinsky, A. D. (2014). Perspective-taking as a strategy for improving intergroup relations: Evidence, mechanisms, and qualifications. *Social and Personality Psychology Compass, 8*(7), 374–387.

Tooby, J., & Cosmides, L. (1992). Psychological foundations of culture. In J. Barkow, L. Cosmides, & J. Tooby (Eds.), *The adapted mind* (pp. 19–136). Chicago, IL: Aldine.

Trivers, R. (1972). Parental investment and sexual selection. In B. Campbell (Ed.), *Sexual selection and the descent of man, 1871–1971* (pp. 136–179). Chicago, IL: Aldine.

Truman, J. L., & Morgan, R. E. (2016). *Criminal victimization, 2015 (NCJ 250180)* (pp. 1–23). U.S. Department of Justice, Office of Justice Programs, Bureau of Justice Statistics.

Turchik, J. A., Hebenstreit, C. L., & Judson, S. S. (2016). An exanimation of the gender inclusiveness of current theories of sexual violence in adulthood: Recognizing male victims, female perpetrators, and same-sex violence. *Trauma, Violence & Abuse, 17*(2), 133–148.

Wegner, R., Davis, K., Stappenbeck, C. A., Kajumulo, K. F., Norris, J., & George, W. H. (2017). The effects of men's hostility toward women, acute alcohol intoxication, and women's condom request style on men's condom use resistance tactics. *Psychology of Violence, 7*(4), 593–601.

Wheeler, J. G., George, W. H., & Dahl, B. J. (2002). Sexually aggressive college males: Empathy as a moderator in the "confluence model" of sexual aggression. *Personality and Individual Differences, 33*, 759–775.

WHO & UNODC. (2015). *Strengthening the medico-legal response to sexual violence*. Geneva: WHO. Retrieved from https://www.who.int/reproductivehealth/publications/violence/medico-legal-response/en/

Wilson, A. P., & Durrenberger, R. (1982). Comparison of rape and attempted rape victims. *Psychological Reports, 50*, 198–199.

Wilson, B. J., Linz, D., Donnerstein, E., & Stipp, H. (1992). The impact of social issue television programming on attitudes toward rape. *Human Communication Research, 19*, 179–208.

Wilson, L., Mouilso, E., Gentile, B., Calhoun, K., & Zeichner, A. (2015). How is sexual aggression related to nonsexual aggression? A meta-analytic review. *Aggression and Violent Behavior, 24*, 199–213.

Wilson, M., & Mesnick, S. L. (1997). An empirical test of the bodyguard hypothesis. In P. A. Gowaty (Ed.), *Feminism and evolutionary biology: Boundaries, intersections and frontiers* (pp. 505–511). New York, NY: Chapman and Hall.

Wood, E. J. (2006). Variation in sexual violence during war. *Politics and Society, 34*(3), 307–341.

Wrangham, R. W., & Peterson, D. (1996). *Demonic males: Apes and the origins of human violence*. Boston, MA: Houghton Mifflon.

Yates, E., Marshall, W. L., & Barbaree, H. E. (1984). Anger and deviant sexual arousal. *Behavior Therapy, 15*(3), 287–294.

Zacharek, S., Dockterman, E., & Edwards, H. S. (2017, December 18). TIME person of the year: The Silence Breakers. *Time*. Retrieved from http://time.com/time-person-of-the-year-2017-silence-breakers/

Part II

Culture and Society

History of the Anti-Rape Movement

3

Sheila M. McMahon

What Is Sexual Assault?

"Sexual assault" is a term that was introduced in the 1980s to replace the term "rape" in many states, because the term "sexual assault" is considered gender neutral i.e. includes male victims and covers a broader range of sexually violent acts, including but not necessarily limited to rape, which is often defined as vaginal penetration using a penis or other object, by some use of force (Campbell & Townsend, 2011; Reddington & Kreisel, 2005). According to the Centers for Disease Control (CDC), an estimated 1.7% of men and 19.3% of women in the US have been raped during their lifetimes (Breideg, Smith, Basile, et al., 2014). At least 50% of individuals who identify as transgender, 43.9% of women, and 23.4% of men have experienced other forms of sexual violence in their lifetimes, such as sexual coercion and unwanted sexual contact (Breideg, Smith, Basile, et al., 2014; Stotzer, 2009).

Early US History and Sexual Assault

Beginning with the Puritans and the founding of the United States, much of the legal system and thinking with regard to the rights of women has been based on the tenets of English Common Law. English Common Law defined rape as "carnal knowledge of a woman by force and against her will" (Reddington & Kreisel, 2005, p. 319). At that historical moment, rape was considered a crime because it damaged a man's property (e.g., the woman, who was considered an object owned by her spouse or father). Consequently, the focus of laws about sexual assault and other forms of sexual violence was a question of the impact of this crime on the male head of household, not on the actual victims. Husbands could not be punished for forcing sex on their wives under this system. Consent was assumed as a continuous aspect of the marital contract. In addition, women who were raped were viewed as responsible for the crime. Victim-blaming was prevalent, as women were considered unreliable and prone to lying, particularly when "scorned" by a male lover (Bernat, 2002). Hence, sexual assault wasn't viewed as a problem requiring widespread intervention, but as an issue to be addressed on a case-by-case basis.

Sexual Assault in the US: Nineteenth Century

Sexual assault was first recognized as a social problem in the United States in the late nineteenth century, when Ida B. Wells, whose career was largely focused on anti-lynching campaigns,

S. M. McMahon (✉)
Barry University School of Social Work,
Miami Shores, FL, USA
e-mail: smcmahon@barry.edu

W. T. O'Donohue and P. A. Schewe (eds.), *Handbook of Sexual Assault and Sexual Assault Prevention*,
https://doi.org/10.1007/978-3-030-23645-8_3

pointed out publicly the connection between lynching and rape (Bevacqua, 2000). She spoke openly about the stereotypical image of the black man as a rapist, and the black woman as sexually promiscuous. She pointed out the consequences of these sinister images: namely, that while Black women raped by White men were often overlooked, charges of rape by Black men (even if false) were routinely used to justify lynching (Bevacqua, 2000). Unfortunately, at that time, Wells' insights about the problem of sexual assault were not taken up more broadly in the public consciousness.

Sexual Assault in the US: Twentieth Century

Sexual Assault in the Context of Marriage: 1920s

Even as courts began to hear cases in the 1920s regarding incidents of domestic violence, sexual assault by spouses was not recognized as a violation of the law. Rather, these rulings were often focused on family reconciliation. The assumption was that husbands were permitted to abuse their wives when they were considered disobedient (Pleck, 1987) and wives were often blamed for marital difficulties that resulted in violence in the home. Moreover, stereotypical gender roles were often enforced, with men as aggressive heads of household, women as passive caregivers, and a code of silence that enshrouded violence against women in the home. Sexual assault within the context of marriage was still *not* considered a crime in some states as recently as 1993 (Basile, 2002), only a year before the first passage of the Violence Against Women Act.

Sexual Assault: 1940s

In the 1940s, the decade leading up to the landmark Civil Rights case, *Brown vs. Board of Education* (a landmark US Supreme Court case that declared racially separated schools unconstitutional), African American women in the US courageously spoke to the press and mobilized their communities in response to sexual assaults against Black women perpetrated by White men as part of the larger campaign of racialized segregation in the US (McGuire, 2010). For example, Rosa Parks, well known for her pivotal role in the Civil Rights movement Montgomery bus boycott, interviewed women of color who were sexually assaulted as part of her role as secretary of the NAACP (National Association for the Advancement of Colored Persons) Chapter. In that capacity, she coordinated support for Recy Taylor, an African American woman who was abducted and gang raped by a group of White men in Alabama in 1944. The case, while not successful in court, led to a national campaign that drew attention to the unjust and systematic violation of Black women's bodies (McGuire, 2010). The widespread use of rape as a tool of segregationists was recognized by Daisy Bates and her husband, L.C. Bates, owner of the *Arkansas State Press*, who focused media attention on these rapes (McGuire, 2010). However, the ire among White segregationists raised by *Brown*, which led to increased death threats and attacks on African Americans, also resulted in increased silence about racially motivated crimes of sexual violence in the following decade (McGuire, 2010).

Sexual Assault: 1950s

In 1955, the American Law Institute, a legal think tank, was charged with developing the Model Penal Code (MPC) for rape, which they finalized in 1962 and revised in 1980. Much like the executive branch's approach, the MPC made some improvements over US Common Law, but still retained key features of anti-victim laws, such as maintaining corroboration requirements in rape cases (Bevacqua, 2000). This meant that the state had to "corroborate the identity of the accused, the fact of penetration, and the victim's nonconsent before proceeding with prosecution" (Bevacqua, 2000). The MPC also retained the common law emphasis on the victim's resistance juxtaposed against the perpetrator's use of force; in cases in which the victim's level of resistance is considered questionable, the outcome may be less favorable for the victim (Bernat, 2002).

Sexual Assault and the Civil Rights Era: 1960s

It would take decades and the rise of the Civil Rights Movement, and the subsequent rise of the women's liberation movement, for public recognition of sexual assault as a social problem in the US. According to Bevacqua (2000), social movements arise when there is "an organizational base, a network of communication among potential organizers, shared consciousness of a common oppression, and a critical mobilizing event or events" (p. 26). By the time the issue of rape came to the fore within the Women's Liberation Movement, there was already an established base of supporters, established through the organizing that was done during the Civil Rights Movement.

The Women's Liberation Movement vs. Sexual Assault: 1970s

Because of work on the Equal Rights Amendment and Roe vs. Wade, the anti-rape movement, a movement within the broader women's liberation movement, also had the benefit of a network of communication. Grassroots activists were already mobilized through work on these other issues, which made them easier to reach for anti-rape activism.

Liberal Feminists vs. Radical Feminists

The anti-rape movement, like the broader women's liberation movement, emerged with two primary ideological camps, liberal and radical feminists. The anti-rape movement that emerged as a result of work by both groups can be viewed as a movement within a movement, which accounts for at least some of the success of the anti-rape movement; women working to raise awareness about rape and to change rape laws had had significant, relevant previous political organizing experience in other parts of the women's movement.

Liberal Feminists

Liberal feminists tended to operate within the norms of the prevailing political system, and often used the language of equal rights to frame their causes. Modeled after the structure of the National Association of Colored People (NAACP), liberal feminists borrowed from this organization's well-run operation to develop the National Organization for Women (NOW) (Bevacqua, 2000). They were able to use political and legal channels to fight for women's rights. In 1972, they founded *Ms. Magazine* in order to disseminate and share movement ideas with a broader audience (Bevacqua, 2000). They organized women in support of the Equal Rights Amendment and the Roe vs. Wade Supreme Court ruling legalizing abortion, so by the mid-1970s, they had become seasoned activists. With this training and a significant infrastructure (largely visible in the form of NOW), liberal feminists began looking at rape laws in the US after a 1973 national meeting of NOW where this issue came to the fore. However, this was after the other main camp of feminists, radical feminists, brought the question of sexual assault to public consciousness (Bevacqua, 2000).

Radical Feminists

Radical feminists relied on unorthodox and often bold strategies to creatively challenge the prevailing rape culture of the late 1960s and early 1970s. Led by radical feminists, consciousness-raising (C-R) groups provided a safe space in which women could articulate the gender-specific challenges they were facing. The purpose of these gatherings was to make a public statement that would counter prevalent rape myths (i.e. the myth that women can't be raped against their will; the myth that women really want to be raped; and the myth that women make false accusations of rape) (Bevacqua, 2000). In her memoir *In Our Time,* feminist activist Susan Brownmiller writes poignantly about attending her first C-R group where she found herself among women who shared openly, often for the first time, about their experiences of back alley abortions and unwanted sexual experiences (Brownmiller, 1999). It was among these women that the phrase "the personal is political" became a rallying cry, and resulted in women organized in cities including New York, Boston, Washington, DC, Berkeley, Los Angeles, Seattle and Chicago to create rape crisis centers in the early 1970s as a result of their collective experiences in C-R groups (Bevacqua, 2000).

Consciousness-Raising Groups

Through the Consciousness-Raising groups, anti-rape activists had developed a shared consciousness about the broader culture in which they were living and a shared critique of patriarchy was developed. There were ample critical events to drive the movement, both through the broader debate about women's bodies due to the Roe vs. Wade abortion case, and also through planned activism led by the groups of radical feminists in urban centers such as New York, Boston, Washington, DC, and Seattle. In fact, in 1971, the New York Radical Feminists held a speak-out and conference about rape, both of which were seen as pivotal events that launched the anti-rape movement (Bevacqua, 2000).

Establishment of Rape Crisis Centers

One of the most tangible and lasting legacies of the anti-rape movement's efforts is visible in the formation and continued existence of rape crisis centers throughout the United States. With training and established networks created during the Civil Rights Movement and subsequent work on the Equal Rights Amendment and Roe vs. Wade, feminist leaders brought forth concerns about violence against women, establishing women's shelters for victims of domestic violence as well as rape crisis centers to support victims of sexual assault (Bevacqua, 2000).

Rape crisis centers are significant not only because of the services they provide, and the empowerment model in which they operate, but also because they symbolize the ongoing struggle feminist activists have faced since the beginning of the anti-rape movement: how to remain at the forefront of the women's liberation movement, a movement for societal transformation, while at the same time cooperating with the institutions they wanted to transform in order to accomplish their work (Bevacqua, 2000). For example, the Washington DC rape crisis center was the first in the nation. When it opened its doors in 1972, it operated as a collective of dedicated volunteers (Bevacqua, 2000). The center took a neutral stance on whether or not women should report rapes because they recognized that the people and institutions (i.e. hospitals, police, and prosecutors) that were supposed to help rape survivors could blame them instead.

Because of their suspicion of existing institutions, rape crisis centers often operated based on private funding in order to avoid state control of their work philosophy and operating style (Bevacqua, 2000). Not unlike the spontaneous rise of soup kitchens in response to hunger in a community, rape crisis centers arose in response to the needs identified by activists who became dedicated volunteers (Smith & Lipsky, 1993). However, as the demand for rape crisis center services expanded and rape came to be viewed more broadly as a social problem, tensions arose among feminist activists regarding the aims and sources of funding for the work of rape crisis centers. This conflict is embodied in the emergence of competing national organizations of rape crisis centers.

By 1974, with rape crisis centers in 43 states, national coordination of centers made sense. The first national clearinghouse for rape crisis centers, the Feminist Alliance Against Rape (FAAR), was established in 1974. In 1978, the National Coalition Against Sexual Assault (NCASA) was founded. The two groups' philosophies differed greatly on the question of staffing and scope. FAAR members tended to view sexual assault as endemic of a larger societal dynamic of male dominance, while NCASA was both interested in the professionalization of the field and in addressing immediate client needs rather than an analysis of the larger systems of interlocking forms of oppression, of which sexual assault was a symptom (Bevacqua, 2000). FAAR is no longer in existence, but NCASA was open to accepting government funding, which meant that they became publicly accountable in ways that were sometimes in conflict with radical feminists' original vision for rape crisis centers, but they also became more stable and viable organizations

(Smith & Lipsky, 1993). Public funding for rape crisis centers came from the Law Enforcement Assistance Administration (LEAA). LEAA was a branch of the Department of Justice established by President Johnson to "end crime." The funding from this government agency often went toward research and rape crisis programs headed by professionals instead of activists. Support for these programs sometimes required victims to report to the police (Bevacqua, 2000). This was a major move away from the radical feminists' vision of neutral support for sexual assault survivors. As rape crisis centers were locked in battle with government funders about the purpose and direction of their work, women's liberation movement activists were also embroiled in legal fights with law enforcement and "tough on crime" politicians about the future of rape crisis laws.

It is important to note that, even as the broader public grappled with issues of racism and white supremacy, there were many challenges within the women's movement regarding issues of race. Black women activists often worked successfully with their male counterparts in the black liberation movement. However, they were often excluded from liberal feminists' agenda, as liberal feminists were often concerned about the needs of middle-class white women. There were also instances in which radical white women's consciousness-raising ("C-R ") groups excluded black women (Bevacqua, 2000). This type of exclusion sometimes resulted in women of color founding their own feminist organizations, such as the Combahee River Collective, which was established in 1975 (Bevacqua, 2000).

Legal Battles

Increased focus on rape as a social problem was also evident in Congress, but with outcomes sometimes emblematic of the larger fight anti-rape activists were waging against the patronizing nature of rape culture. For example, in 1975, Senator Mathias pursued the Rape Prevention and Control Bill using a 'protect our women' approach (Bevacqua, 2000). It is important to note that Mathias did indeed seek information from the Prince Georges County Rape Task Force as well as the Public Safety Committee Task Force in Washington, DC. Both groups included members who were feminist anti-rape activists. Nonetheless, when Mathias introduced the bill, he argued that it was necessary legislation because, "We fight no war, adopt no program, create no law that is not ultimately and unselfishly aimed at making life better for our women" (US Congress, Bevacqua, 2000, 29,830; quoted in Bevacqua, 2000, p. 144). This commentary suggests a haunting refrain that goes back to the days of lynching, when "our women" may have signified white women, the property of white men. Nonetheless, the bill was enacted by Congress and resulted in the creation of the National Center for the Prevention and Control of Rape (NCPCR) within the National Institute of Mental Health, as well as the LEAA's Office of Community Anti-Crime Programs, which gave money to community-based organizations, such as rape crisis centers, as long as these agencies had full-time directors and boards (Bevacqua, 2000). Following Mathias's bill, Representative Elizabeth Holtzman introduced the Rape Victims Privacy Act, which amended federal law regarding the disclosure of information about a victim's past. Considered a pro-victim piece of legislation, it was signed into law by President Carter in 1978 (Bevacqua, 2000).

Although feminist activists were successful in getting rape on the public agenda in the 1970s, their understanding of rape [i.e. victims are not at fault; rapists are not crazed sociopaths; rape is an act of power and violence rather than sexual desire] did not gain support on the public agenda (Bevacqua, 2000). The tensions between feminists and policy makers regarding the understanding of what constitutes rape is critical because it explains the broader policy agenda that formed and directed expert understanding of rape.

Regarding policy changes that affect how sexual assault is understood as a social problem in the US, Underwood and Edmunds (2003) write,

> The demands for rights tend to be more evolutionary than revolutionary. As victims' rights become established through formal policies, victims and advocacy groups press for the next level of services and practices. But public policy is a process that is lethargic to change. It is also a process that often involves a compromise of competing interests or values. (p. 230)

Despite anti-rape activists' best efforts to shape public understanding of rape, the public debate often went in directions antithetical to anti-rape activists' efforts. For example, beginning in the 1980s, it actually became more common for rapes to be placed into categories, especially by the media. While this categorization reflected the reality of what rape crisis centers were seeing (i.e. the vast majority of victims were raped by someone known to them), it also created a sense in the public that certain categories of rapes (i.e. date or acquaintance) were viewed as less serious (Bevacqua, 2000).

1980s: Recognition of Acquaintance Rape

By 1982, *Ms. Magazine* had gotten data that suggested that "date rape" or acquaintance rape was much more common than people realized. As a result, the magazine approached the National Institute of Mental Health and the Center for Prevention and Control of Rape to discuss a possible follow-up study. Because researcher Mary P. Koss was already working in the field on this topic, they identified her as the lead researcher for the study, for which they collected data from 6159 college students on 32 college campuses across the nation (Warshaw, 1994). Completed in 1985, the study showed staggering rates of acquaintance rape among college students. In fact, the college years quickly became identified as the time in life of highest sexual assault victimization rates among US females (Koss, 1994).

And yet, because of the categorization of rape into categories in which acquaintance rape was considered less serious, it was difficult to gain legal ground to make pro-victim changes. Caringella (2009) argues that this ranking has very real consequences in the legal system, "So, it winds up that only the strongest cases, with the most evidence, with characteristics that meet old requirements, that fit the stereotype of stranger-out-of-the-bushes ("real") ambush (and yet infrequent) rape, that most often end up in conviction (p. 61)." Moreover, most rape reforms tend to focus on "real" or aggravated rape, and because courts enjoy discretionary decision-making, the extent to which reform provisions are implemented varies and this explains the failure and dismissal of acquaintance rape cases (Caringella, 2009).

1990s

Federal Legislation to Address Sexual Assault

In 1994, then Senator Joseph Biden sponsored the Violence Against Women Act (VAWA). The purpose of VAWA was to criminalize acts of violence against women, including acquaintance rape, domestic violence, and stalking; to provide better support to victim-survivors of these crimes; and to prevent violence against women, who were disproportionately victims of sexual assault (Boba & Lilley, 2009). Because of its focus on deterrence and crime, VAWA included greater punishment for repeat offenders, criminal and civil court restitution for victims, protection of victim's identity, reimbursement to victims for financial losses, and funding, education, and training for rape crisis center staff (Caringella, 2009). The passage of VAWA included the establishment of two streams of funding for VAWA initiatives: one through the Department of Health and Human Services (HHS) and the other through the Department of Justice (DOJ). The efficacy of the legislation would take years to measure, but VAWA's passage with bipartisan support suggested the possibility of a future in which there would be fewer sexual assault victims and less stigma attached to survivors.

2000s

Sexual Assault and Social Media

As cell phones have become ubiquitous in the US, sexual assault has been both captured on social media and also challenged on social media.

Steubenville rape case. The infamous Steubenville rape case of 2012, in which two high school football players used their cellphones and social media apps to document their sexual assault of an incapacitated peer, provides a disturbing example of the pervasiveness of rape culture in our communities, including the active collusion or apathy of bystanders, the use of social media to shame and silence victims, and the reluctance to hold offenders accountable when they hold significant social capital (Pennington & Birthisel, 2016). The case also illustrated the value of family support for survivors and the increasing visibility of survivors, who are speaking out about crimes that in past decades would have been rendered victims silent and alone (Szalavitz, 2013).

#MeToo Movement. In 2006, Civil Rights activist Tarana Burke created a nonprofit organization to support sexual assault survivors in response to a disclosure she received from a young girl who had experienced sexual assault years before (Garcia, 2017). She created the hashtag in 2007 to invite survivors to give voice to their experiences via social media. The campaign went viral in 2017 after actress Alyssa Milano and others used the hashtag to share their experiences of sexual assault in Hollywood (Ohlheiser, 2017)

Conclusion

The history of sexual assault in the US is inextricably linked to the nation's complex history of misogyny and racism. Women of color, who were often on the forefront of speaking out against sexual assault, were frequently ignored. The women's liberation movement, which was credited with creating social change regarding sexual assault largely due to the passage of VAWA, failed to include women of color in significant leadership roles and simultaneously lost control of the narrative about sexual assault to White, male policymakers who were focused on preservation of the status quo through a narrow criminal justice approach to sexual assault. The result has been that the root causes of sexual assault are rarely addressed in a holistic way.

References

Basile, K. C. (2002). Prevalence of wife rape and other intimate partner sexual coercion in a nationally representative sample of women. Violence and victims, 17(5), 511.

Basile, K. C., Smith, S. G., Breiding, M., Black, M. C., & Mahendra, R. R. (2014). Sexual violence surveillance: Uniform definitions and recommended data elements. Version 2.0.

Bernat, F. P. (2002). Rape law reform. In J. F. Hodgson & D. S. Kelley (Eds.), *Sexual violence: Policies, practices, and challenges in the United States and Canada* (pp. 85–100). Westport, CT: Praeger.

Bevacqua, M. (2000). *Rape on the public agenda: Feminism and the politics of sexual assault*. Boston: Northeastern University Press.

Boba, R., & Lilley, D. (2009). Violence against women act (VAWA) funding: A nationwide assessment of effects on rape and assault. *Violence Against Women, 15*(2), 168–185.

Brownmiller, S. (1999). *In our time: Memoir of a revolution*. New York: Random House.

Campbell, R., & Townsend, S. (2011). *Defining the scope of sexual violence against women. Sourcebook on violence against women, second edition*. Thousand Oaks, CA: Sage Publications.

Caringella, S. (2009). *Addressing rape reform in law and practice*. New York: Columbia University Press.

Garcia, S. E. (2017, October 20). The woman who created #MeToo long before hashtags. *The New York Times*. Retrieved from https://www.nytimes.com/2017/10/20/us/me-too-movement-tarana-burke.html

Koss, M. P. (1994). Afterword. In *I never called it rape* (pp. 189–210). New York: HarperCollins.

McGuire, D. L. (2010). At the dark end of the street: Black women, rape, and resistance--A new history of the civil rights movement from Rosa Parks to the rise of black power. Vintage.

Ohlheiser, A. (2017, 19 October). The woman behind 'Me Too' knew the power of the phrase when she created it—10 years ago. *Washington Post*.

Pennington, R., & Birthisel, J. (2016). When new media make news: Framing technology and sexual assault in the Steubenville rape case. *New Media and Society, 18*, 1–17.

Pleck, E. H. (1987). *Domestic tyranny: The making of social policy against family violence from colonial times to the present*. New York: Oxford University Press.

Reddington, F. P., & Kreisel, B. W. (2005). *Sexual assault: The victims, the perpetrators, and the criminal justice system*. Durham, NC: Academic Press.

Smith, S. R., & Lipsky, M. (1993). *Nonprofits for hire: The welfare state in the age of contracting*. Cambridge, MA: Harvard University Press.

Stotzer, R. L. (2009). Violence against transgender people: A review of United States data. Aggression and Violent Behavior, 14(3), 170–179.

Szalavitz, Maia. (March 20, 2013). What About the Victim: The Steubenville Rape Victim's Recovery. Time. Retrieved from http://healthland.time.com/2013/03/20/what-about-the-victim-the-steubenville-rape-victims-recovery/

Underwood, T. L., & Edmunds, C. (2003). *Victim assistance: Exploring individual practice, organizational policy, and societal responses*. Springer Publishing Company.

Warshaw, R. (1994). *I never called it rape*. New York: HarperCollins.

Cultural Considerations in Sexual Assault

4

Lorraine T. Benuto, Frances Gonzalez, Jena Casas, Rory Newlands, and Brian D. Leany

What Is Sexual Assault?

Sexual assault is a broad term, encompassing a myriad of acts and experiences. Sexual assault (depending on the definition being employed) ranges from inappropriate sexual behaviors, such as unwanted groping or fondling, to forcible rape (Muehlenhard, Humphreys, Jozkowski, & Peterson, 2016). While the inclusiveness of the term allows law makers, enforcers, and adjudicators to categorize a wide variety of unwanted sexual experiences, its lack of specificity makes it difficult for researchers and clinicians to operationalize and measure accurately, and thereby permits flexibility in how the legal system interprets events. For instance, the United States Department of Justice defines sexual assault as "any nonconsensual sexual act proscribed by Federal, tribal, or State law, including when the victim lacks capacity to consent." (Sexual Assault, 2018). However, what exactly constitutes "consent" is never articulated, providing leeway in how this mandate is interpreted. Further complicating the issue, states vary in how they define sexual assault, meaning what constitutes as sexual assault in one state or jurisdiction may not in another (Eileraas, 2011; Palmer, 2011).

L. T. Benuto (✉) · F. Gonzalez · J. Casas
R. Newlands · B. D. Leany
Department of Psychology, University of Nevada
Reno, Reno, NV, USA

The National Institute of Justice provides a drastically different definition of sexual assault, stating:

> Sexual assault covers a wide range of unwanted behaviors—up to but not including penetration—that are attempted or completed against a victim's will or when a victim cannot consent because of age, disability, or the influence of alcohol or drugs. Sexual assault may involve actual or threatened physical force, use of weapons, coercion, intimidation, or pressure. (Rape and Sexual Violence, 2017)

Further they explain that sexual assault can include: "intentional touching of the victim's genitals, anus, groin, or breasts, voyeurism, exposure to exhibitionism, undesired exposure to pornography, and public display of images that were taken in a private context or when the victim was unaware" (Rape and Sexual Violence, 2017).

While the United States Center for Disease Control (CDC) does not use the term sexual assault, opting for the term sexual violence, their definition provides a more comprehensive description. The CDC states that sexual violence (sexual assault) includes: completed or attempted penetration via force, threats, incapacitation (due to drugs or alcohol intoxication), or verbal coercion (i.e. manipulation, sexual pressure by an authority, or nonphysical threats); completed or attempted efforts to make a victim penetrate someone via, force, threats, or incapacitation (but interestingly not verbal coercion); unwanted

W. T. O'Donohue and P. A. Schewe (eds.), *Handbook of Sexual Assault and Sexual Assault Prevention*,
https://doi.org/10.1007/978-3-030-23645-8_4

sexual contact intentional touching "of the genitalia, anus, groin, breast, inner thigh, or buttocks of any person without his or her consent, or of a person who is unable to consent. Unwanted sexual contact also includes making a victim touch the perpetrator"; and noncontact unwanted sexual experiences, such as being made to watch pornography or inappropriate sexual comments (Violence Prevention, 2018).

Give the inconsistencies in how sexual assault is defined within official government agencies, it is not surprising that researchers also struggle to employ a consistent definition across studies (Muehlenhard et al., 2016). For example, some studies operationalize sexual assault as any unwanted sexual experience, including rape (Conley, Overstret, Hawn, Dick & Amstader, 2017), where as others specific that sexual assault requires force or intoxication (Hines, Armstrong, Reed, & Cameron, 2012). However, we opine that the CDC's definition of sexual violence represents a useful way to conceptualize sexual assault, attending to both the acts themselves and the strategies used by perpetrators. This definition may be useful to researchers and mental health care providers, but is not necessarily representative of how individuals, societies, and cultural groups conceptualize sexual assault. Cultural groups vary in what they consider normative gender roles (Padilla & Baird, 1991; Rice & Coates, 1995; Upchurch et al., 2001), rape scripts (Littleton, Carmen, & Berenson, 2007), attitudes towards rape (Jacques-Tiura, Tkatch, Abbey, & Wegner, 2010; Jimenez & Abreu, 2003; Price, Davidson, Ruggiero, Acierno, & Resnick, 2014), and the acceptance of violence (Covington, 2003; Miller & Peterson, 2008; Vandello, Cohen, & Ransom, 2008). Research has found that male and female African Americans, Latinos, and Asian Americans are more likely to endorse rape myths than White-Americans, even if they had been sexually victimized themselves (Carmody & Washington, 2001; Jimenez & Abreu, 2003). The authors posit that various culturally bound stereotypes increase the likelihood that certain ethnic groups will endorse such myths (Carmody & Washington, 2001). For example, Latino populations have been found to adhere to values such as *simpatia* (valuing pleasant, conflict free, social relationships [Fraga, 2008]), *personalismo* (connectedness with others founded on trust [Fraga, 2008]), *marianismo* (defined as women who "aspire to be like Virgin Mary by acquiring the characteristics of humbleness, self-sacrifice, and other-centeredness" [Fraga, 2008, p. 1196]), and machismo (hypermasculinity [Fraga, 2008]). These values, and the degree to which they are held, likely influence how individuals conceptualize their experiences as well as their willingness to report their experiences and seek treatment. Thus, when working with victims of sexual assault the clinicians should consider the cultural background of the victim as it may play a fundamental role in the case conceptualization.

Prevalence Rates of Sexual Assault

On average, there are 321,500 victims (age 12 and older) of rape or sexual assault each year in the United States (U.S. Department of Justice, 2015). Rates of sexual assault vary across different ethnic groups. Women who identify as American Indian or Alaskan are twice as likely to experience a sexual assault compared to other ethnicities with one out of two American Indian or Alaskan women (56%) experiencing sexual assault in their lifetime (Rosay, 2016). Over 41% of sexual assaults among American Indian and Alaskan women are committed by a stranger with sexual violence without penetration (e.g., unwanted sexual contact, sexual coercion) being the most prevalent form of sexual assault (52%; Rosay, 2016).

Sexual assault is also prevalent among Latinas and African American women. A systematic review of the literature on rates of interpersonal violence among Latinas (Gonzalez, Benuto, & Casas, 2018) found that that prevalence rates of sexual abuse among Latinas ranged from 1% to 38%. This wide range of prevalence rates was attributable to the manner in which interpersonal violence was defined, the lumping together of sub-ethnicities, and the methods used to collect data.

Specific to sexual assault the systematic review of the literature indicated that 1% (Benson, Gohm, & Gross, 2007) to 38% (Cavanaugh et al., 2014) of Latinos experience sexual assault. According to West and Johnson (2013), one in five (20%) African American women will experience a form of sexual assault in their lifetime. Data on the rates of sexual assault among Asian Americans and Pacific Islanders are less available; one resource indicated that 31.9% of Asian and Pacific Islander women experienced sexual violence other than rape during their lifetime, with 23% reporting some form of contact sexual violence, 10% reporting completed or attempted rape, and 21% had noncontact unwanted sexual experiences during their lifetime (Center for Disease Control and Prevention, 2017). Another report indicated the lifetime prevalence rate of sexual assault among Asian Americans to be 53% (KAN-WIN, 2017). The above literature makes it evident that rates of sexual assault are high among ethnic minorities.

Reporting Sexual Assault

Cultural and societal factors may influence reporting incidents of sexual assault among various ethnic groups which in turn can influence prevalence rates of sexual assault and may explain the large variation observed across prevalence rates. As with other forms of interpersonal violence, incidents of sexual assault remain underreported even with minority cultures. For example, only about one in fifteen African American women who have experienced rape will report the rape (Hart & Rennison, 2003). The following barriers have been identified among African American women in not reporting incidents of sexual assault: (1) fear of being stereotyped and/or victim-blaming response to victims who had been using drugs and/or alcohol; (2) experiences of racism by police officers; and (3) reluctance to report sexual crimes of African American males (Weist et al., 2014).

Among Asian Americans, and Pacific Islanders, disclosing personal or familial information, even in a confidential setting, is contrary to traditional values. In Asian American and Pacific Islander culture, bringing attention to negative situations is shameful, especially if it is a family matter (Kercher & Kuo, 2008). In an unpublished study by the KAN-WIN (2017), a nonprofit organization in Chicago that provided sexual assault and domestic violence services to the Asian community, survivors of sexual assault reported that they were worried about being blamed after disclosing sexual assault. Worries about victim-shaming by their community, guilt, and shame arose when considering reporting incidents of sexual assault (KAN-WIN, 2017). In addition, survivors were worried about the consequences of reporting their sexual abuse with 45% of survivors of sexual assault indicating that they were afraid of the prejudice and stigma they may face by their community (KAN-WIN, 2017). Among Latinas similar barriers were reported regarding feeling shame and guilt after reporting incidents of sexual assault (Ahrens, Rios-Mandel, Isas, & Lopez, 2010; Benuto & Bennett, 2015). Latinas reported additional barriers to reporting sexual assault such as: (1) having traditional beliefs about marriage (being a virgin until married); (2) familismo; (3) taboos against talking about sex; (4) respect of authority; and (5) lack of community resources (Ahrens et al., 2010).

Immigration status may also impact the experience of sexual assault. Language barriers are a common barrier to reporting crimes in addition to seeking psychological help (Benuto & Bennett, 2015; Kercher & Kuo, 2008). Moreover, being an unauthorized immigrant can lead to low reporting of incidents of sexual assault due to the fear of authority and deportation (Messing, Becerra, Ward-Lasher, & Androff, 2015; Rizo & Macy, 2011). One study asked Latinas in the community why would Latinas not report domestic violence or sexual crimes to the police ("No More" Report, 2015). Forty-one percent of Latinas believed the primary reason Latina victims may not come forward is fear of deportation; 39% of Latinas say the primary reason Latina victims may not come forward is fear of more violence for themselves and their family; and 39% of Latinas say the primary reason Latina victims may not come forward is fear of their children being taken away ("No More" Report, 2015). This fear could possibly explain why immigrant Latinas are less likely to seek help than U.S. born Latinas (Sabina, Cuevas, & Schally, 2015).

Cultural Considerations in Forensic Interviews

When there is an accusation of sexual abuse, a forensic interview can be used to investigate what occurred (Laney & Loftus, 2016). The functions of these interviews are to objectively gather facts and details about the alleged abuse from the victim (Krueger, 2016) and to use this information in legal actions: establishing jurisdiction over the person and the matter, determining venue, determining when the crime allegedly occurred, figuring out which crimes to charge, and identifying the defendant among other factors (Daly, 2016). Although forensic interviews often produce true and accurate reports of events, they can also produce erroneous or false reports. In general, poor interviewer techniques (e.g. using fear, anticipation of a reward, coaching, suggestive or leading questions, and so forth) are thought to be especially harmful in seeking the truth as these techniques can produce false memories, be wrongfully influential, and can ultimately undermine an investigation (Laney & Loftus, 2016).

There are many factors that require cultural considerations in the context of a forensic interview. Problematically, research on forensic assessment practices with cultural minorities is lacking (Benuto & Garrick, 2016). Forensic evaluations should include evidence-based assessments that have been researched with the population of interest because evaluations that fail to consider cultural factors and use culturally sensitive assessment measures can have deleterious consequences. Although limited and at times conflicting, research has suggested that sociodemographic factors (e.g. SES, gender, ethnicity) can influence suggestibility, memory, and disclosure in forensic interviews in many ways (Benuto & Garrick, 2016). For instance, it is suggested that a child's disclosure of abuse can be influenced by race, ethnicity, culture, and gender differences between the interviewer and interviewee (Fontes & Faller, 2006; Lovett, 2004). Thus, being culturally sensitive and using culturally appropriate assessments during a forensic interview is thought to be integral to the success of the interview. Benuto and Garrick (2016) made the following recommendations for forensic interviews: assessing for the interviewee's language preference and proficiency level and conducting the interview in their native language (using translated protocols and a translator who has been trained in forensic interviewing (never using family or friends to fill this role) only as necessary); aiming for ethnic matching and racial/ethnic concordance, and if absent, ensuring rapport is sufficient before proceeding with the interview; and considering the interviewees environment and any specific sociocultural factors (e.g., shame, guilt, immigration status, ethnic identity, acculturation, racism) in the context of the interview (Chapman, DeLapp, & Richards, 2015).

Assessment of the Sequelae after Sexual Assault

A person who experiences sexual assault can experience a host of behavioral health issues as a consequence of the trauma. The common sequelae of sexual assault include depression and anxiety disorders, particularly Posttraumatic Stress Disorder (Briere & Elliott, 2003) among other psychological problems, and forensic interviews often incorporate assessments for these disorders to facilitate treatment (Breland-Noble, Sotomayor, & Burriss, 2015).

Major Depressive Disorder. Major Depressive Disorder is an affective disorder marked by depressed mood or anhedonia, where five or more symptoms (e.g., fatigue, change in appetite, change in sleep, psychomotor agitation or retardation, feelings of worthlessness or inappropriate guilt, inability to concentrate, suicidal ideation) have been present during the same 2-week period (APA, 2013). There are several assessments used to assess for the presence of depression in a forensic interview that have been validated for use with African American, Asian American, and Latino cultural minorities

(Breland-Noble et al., 2015; Kalibatseva, Wu, & Leong, 2014; Wiebe, Sauceda, & Lara, 2013). These assessments are primarily self-report, have good psychometric properties (i.e., in terms of being standardized using diverse samples, and demonstrating high internal consistency, criterion validity, and construct validity in validation studies), and are available in different languages (e.g., Spanish, Chinese, Japanese, Korean, Thai, Hmong, Taiwanese, Mandarin, Cantonese, and Vietnamese) depending on the measure: the Beck Depression Inventory (BDI: Beck, Ward, Mendelson, Mock, & Erbaugh, 1961), the Beck Depression Inventory-II ((BDI-II: Beck, Steer, & Brown, 1996), the Patient Health Questionnaire-9 (PHQ-9: Kronke, Spitzer, & Williams, 2001), the Hospital Anxiety and Depression Scale (HADS: Zigmond & Snaith, 1983), the Center for Epidemiologic Studies Depression Scale (CESD: Radloff, 1977), the Geriatric Depression Scale (GDS: Strauss, Sherman, & Spreen, 2006), the Hamilton Rating Scale of Depression (HDRS: Hamilton, 1960), and the Zung Self-Rating Depression Scale (SDS: Zung, Richards, & Short, 1965) (Benuto, 2012; Benuto & Leany, 2015; Benuto, Thaler, & Leany, 2014). In general, these assessments are used to identify the presence of a depressive disorder, to monitor depressive symptomology, or to differentiate between depressive or anxiety disorders and the decision to use one measure over another measure depends on the referral question of the assessment as well as the client (Benuto & Leany, 2015).

Anxiety Disorders. The DSM-V categorizes several disorders under the umbrella term "anxiety disorder": Posttraumatic Stress Disorder, Generalized Anxiety Disorder, Social Anxiety Disorder, Obsessive Compulsive Disorder, and Panic Disorder (APA, 2013). In a forensic interview, there is some variation in the measures used to assess for specific anxiety disorders. In general, these assessments are primarily self-report, have good to excellent validity and reliability among cultural minority populations in the United States, and are available in different languages depending on the measure (e.g. Spanish, Japanese, Chinese, and Korean) (Benuto, 2012; Benuto et al., 2014; Benuto & Leany, 2015). Researchers caution interviewers to be aware of culture-specific syndromes in anxiety presentations that may affect a client's understanding and reporting of anxiety symptoms (e.g., Koreans experiencing *hwabyung*, or fire disease or anger disease: Lee, 2014).

Posttraumatic Stress Disorder (PTSD). Posttraumatic Stress Disorder is an anxiety disorder marked by the exposure to a stressor, and the subsequent presence of intrusive and avoidant symptoms, and alterations in cognitions, mood, arousal, and reactivity, that have been present for at least 1 month (APA, 2013). Common assessments used to screen for the presence of PTSD are: The Clinician Administered PTSD Scale (CAPS: Weathers, Keane, & Davidson, 2001 [available in Spanish: Benuto, Olmo-Terasa, & Reyes-Rabanillo, 2011]); the Traumatic Life Events Questionnaire (TLEF: Kubany et al., 2000); the Distressing Event Questionnaire (DEQ: Kubany, Leisen, Kaplan, & Kelly, 2000); the Impact of Events Scale-Revised (IES-R: Weiss & Marmar, 1997); the Los Angeles Symptom Checklist (LASC: King, King, Leskin, & Foy, 1995); the Penn Inventory for Posttraumatic Stress Disorder (Penn Inventory: Hammarberg, 1992); the Posttraumatic Diagnostic Scale (PDS: Foa, Cashman, Jaycox, & Perry, 1997); the PTSD Severity Scale-Interview Version (PSS-I: Foa, Riggs, Dancu, & Rothbaum, 1993); the Screen for Posttraumatic Stress Symptoms (SPTSS: Carlson, 2001); the Davidson Trauma Scale (DTS: Davidson et al., 1997); the Posttraumatic Stress Disorder Checklist (PCL: Weathers, Litz, Herman, Huska, & Keane, 1993); the Structured Clinical Interview for DSM (SCID: First, Williams, Karg, & Spitzer, 2015); and the Anxiety Disorder Interview Scale (ADIS-IV: Brown, Barlow, & DiNardo, 1994).

Lee (2014) summarized the research on the assessment of anxiety with Asian Americans and noted these assessments to have excellent psychometric properties in terms of validity and reliability for Asian Americans as well as to have been validated in different Asian languages (Benuto et al., 2014). Similarly, Snipes (2013) summarized the research on the assessment of anxiety with Latinos and noted these assessments to have sound psychometric properties (i.e. the CAPS and the PCL have been specifically researched with this population, are available in English and Spanish, and both language versions were deemed equivalent, suggesting these measures to be acceptable for use with this population) and to be recommended for use with Latinos. Finally, Williams, Malcoun, and Bahojb Nouri (2015) summarized the research on the assessment of PTSD with African Americans and while in general they found these measures to have acceptable psychometric properties (i.e. 3 out of 14 measures were validated in studies using a predominantly African American sample, while the psychometric properties, primarily internal consistency, of only 8 out of the 14 measures have been examined for African Americans), they also noted that many measures lack validation research with African Americans and their appropriateness for use with African Americans remain largely unknown (e.g. DEQ, LASC, SPTSS).

Generalized Anxiety Disorder (GAD). Generalized Anxiety Disorder is an anxiety disorder marked by excessive uncontrollable anxiety or worry, where three or more symptoms (e.g., restlessness, fatigue, difficulty concentrating, irritability, muscle tension, and sleep disturbances), have been present for more days than not over a six-month period (APA, 2013). Common assessments used to screen for the presence of GAD include: the Generalized Anxiety Disorder Questionnaire-IV (GAD-Q-IV: Newman et al., 2002); the Penn State Worry Questionnaires (PSWQ: Meyer, Miller, Metzger, & Borkovec, 1990), the Hamilton Rating Scale (HARS: Hamilton, 1959); the Worry Domains Questionnaire (WDQ: Tallis, Eysenck, & Mathews, 1992); the State-Trait Anxiety Inventory (STAI: Spielberger, Gorsuch, Lushene, Vagg, & Jacobs, 1983); the Beck Anxiety Inventory (BWAI: Beck, Epstein, Brown, & Steer, 1988); the Anxiety Severity Index (ASI: Reiss, Peterson, Gursky, & McNally, 1986; Taylor, Koch, & Crockett, 1991; Telch, Shermis, & Lucas, 1989), the Structured Clinical Interview for DSM (SCID: First et al., 2015), and the Anxiety Disorder Interview Scale (ADIS-IV: Brown et al., 1994) (Benuto, 2012; Benuto et al., 2014; Benuto & Leany, 2015). Prior research suggests that these assessments have good sensitivity in terms of being able to distinguish between GAD and other anxiety disorders and good to strong psychometric properties (i.e., having available standardization research that determined good inter-rater reliability, internal reliability, and test-retest reliability: See Chapman et al. (2015), Lee (2014), Snipes (2013), and Benuto et al. (2014) for a review of the psychometric properties of specific assessments). As a consideration for Latinos, the ADIS-IV and the GAD-Q-IV are not available in Spanish (Snipes, 2013), and thus would not be appropriate for limited English proficient Latinos. As a consideration for African Americans, the WDQ covers a limited number of life events and may overlook culturally specific worries (Chapman et al., 2015).

Panic Disorder. Panic Disorder is an anxiety disorder marked by intense fear or physical discomfort (at least four of the following symptoms are present: palpitations, sweating, trembling, shortness of breath, chest pain, choking sensations, nausea, dizziness, derealization, fear of dying, numbness, chills) and recurring, unexpected panic attacks, where at least one attack is followed by a 1-month period, where the person worries about having additional attacks (APA, 2013). Common assessments used to identify the presence of Panic Disorder in a forensic interview are: the Beck Anxiety Inventory (BAI: Beck et al., 1988), the Panic Disorder Severity Scale (PDSS: Shear et al., 1997), the Anxiety Sensitivity Index (ASI: Reiss et al., 1986; the Brief Panic Disorder Screen (BPDS: Apfeldorf, Shear, Leon, & Portera, 1994); the Albany Panic and Phobia Questionnaire (APPQ: Rapee, Craske, & Barlow, 1995); the Structured Clinical Interview for DSM (SCID: First et al., 2015), and the Anxiety Disorder Interview Scale (ADIS-IV: Brown, Di Nardo, & Barlow, 1994) (Benuto, 2012; Benuto et al., 2014; Benuto & Leany, 2015). Lee (2014) noted these assessments to have excellent psychometric properties for Asian Americans (i.e. as many have been standardized for use with this population) as well as to have been validated in different Asian languages (Benuto et al., 2014), while Snipes (2013) and Chapman et al. (2015) noted that although many of these assessments have not been exclusively researched with Latinos or African Americans, they are still being recommended for use with the population. Thus, because the psychometric properties and clinical utility of these measures has not been examined in predominantly Latino or African American samples, caution should be exercised (Chapman et al., 2015) as their acceptability specifically for these populations is not well known.

Social Anxiety Disorder. Social Anxiety Disorder is an anxiety disorder marked by a fear of social or performance situations where the person may be exposed to scrutiny by others, where the individual recognizes the fear to be unreasonable or excessive, and where the situations are avoided or endured with extreme anxiety and distress (APA, 2013). Common assessments used to identify the presence of Social Anxiety Disorder in a forensic interview are: the Social Phobia and Anxiety Inventory (SPAI: Beidel, Turner, Dancu, & Stanley, 1989); the Liebowitz Social Anxiety Scale (LSAS: Liebowitz, 1987); the Fear of Negative Evaluation Scale and Social Avoidance Distress Scale (FNES; SADS: Watson & Friend, 1969); Positive Affect and Negative Affect Scale (PANAS: Watson, Clark, & Carey, 1988); the Social Avoidance and Distress Scale (SADS: Watson & Friend, 1969), the Social Interaction Anxiety Scale (SIAS: Mattick & Clarke, 1998); the Structured Clinical Interview for DSM (SCID: First et al., 2015); and the Anxiety Disorder Interview Scale (ADIS-IV: Brown et al., 1994; Benuto et al., 2014). Overall, Lee (2014), Chapman et al. (2015), and Snipes (2013) noted these assessments to have excellent psychometric properties for cultural minorities, to be fairly easy to administer, to control for underreporting of cognitive symptoms, and to have been validated in many different languages (Benuto et al., 2014).

Best Practices for Treatment

The most common reactions to sexual assault include Acute Stress Disorder (which may or may not evolve into Posttraumatic Stress Disorder [PTSD]), PTSD, Major Depressive Disorder, Generalized Anxiety Disorder, and Panic Disorder. There has been controversy regarding whether intervention in the early aftermath of trauma are effective (Koucky, Galovski, & Nixon, 2012) and there is a small body of literature that suggests that utilizing trauma-focused CBT for clients who present with Acute Stress Disorder meet the possibly efficacious category (Ponniah & Hollon, 2009).

PTSD represents the most common sequalae to sexual assault. The gold standard treatment for PTSD is Prolonged Exposure Therapy (Powers, Halpern, Ferenschack, Gillihan, & Foa, 2010). Prolonged Exposure Therapy is delivered in approximately 12 individual sessions and consists of psychoeducation about common reactions to trauma and breathing retraining; in-vivo exposure where the client engages in in-vivo exposure to objectively safe situations, places, or people that s/he is avoiding because the these objectively safe situations, places, or people serve as reminders to the trauma; and imaginal exposure where the client describes what occurred directly before, during, and after the traumatic event. The extant literature on Prolonged Exposure Therapy and ethnic minorities is minimal. Benuto, Bennett, Casas, Norton, and Massey (2019) systematically reviewed the randomized controlled trial literature on Prolonged Exposure Therapy and found that ethnic minorities were substantially underrepresented in the treatment outcome literature. A single randomized controlled trial conducted in Japan with Japanese patients who had PTSD indicated that Prolonged Exposure Therapy is an efficacious treatment for PTSD even in non-Western settings. Per the results from the systematic review of the literature (Benuto et al., 2019) randomized controlled trials of Prolonged Exposure Therapy that have included samples with more than 50% African American (adolescents) have indicated strong support for Prolonged Exposure Therapy.

While randomized controlled trials on Prolonged Exposure Therapy with ethnic minorities are few and far between, an effectiveness study has indicated that at least for Latinos Prolonged Exposure appears to be a reasonable treatment option that produces substantial treatment gains even when free of cultural adaptations (Benuto, O'Donohue, Bennett, & Casas, 2019). This conclusion is further supported via case study research which has indicated that Prolonged exposure therapy represents an effective treatment option for Latina victims of sexual assault (Benuto & Bennett, 2015). With regard African Americans Williams, Chapman, Buckner, and Durrett (2016) noted that there is evidence that CBT can be effectively used with African Americans that in many ways for it is suitable for African American families and youth because of its empowering nature and because it focuses on building strengths and achieving goals. A review of the extant literature did not yield much research on the use of CBT with Asian participants but of the literature that does exist shows promising effects with this population (Tang, Li, Rodgers, & Ballou, 2016; Wong & Sun, 2006).

The evidence-based treatments for other common sequalae of sexual assault (including Major Depressive Disorder and other anxiety disorders) all include iterations of Cognitive Behavioral Therapy (CBT). Benuto and O'Donohue (2015) reviewed the literature on CBT and Latinos and found evidence that CBT can be used to generally effectively with this group. Additional research on other related interventions for (i.e., Behavioral Activation) also indicate positive results for Latinos (Benson-Flórez, Santiago-Rivera, & Nagy, 2017) and for both younger (Jacob, Keeley, Ritschel, & Craighead, 2013) and older African Americans (Gitlin, Harris, McCoy, Hess, & Hauck, 2016). Thus the extant literature supports the use of evidence-based interventions (most notably CBT) for use with ethnic minority clients. It is worth noting that much has been written about cultural adaptations with the central premise of these works being based on the notion that empirically supported treatments can be enhanced for ethnic minority clients if they are culturally adapted. Benuto and O'Donohue (2015) concluded that there was evidence that standard (nonculturally adapted interventions) were effective for use with Latinos.

Legal and Cultural Intersections

To reduce the fear of immigrants reporting crimes, the United States has created the U nonimmigrant status visa (U-Visa). Yearly, 10,000 visas are awarded to victims of certain crimes who have suffered mental or physical abuse and are helpful to law enforcement or government officials in the investigation or prosecution of criminal activity (U.S. Citizenship and Immigration Services [USCIS], 2018a, 2018b). This visa is intended to investigate and prosecute cases of domestic violence, sexual assault, and other crimes, while protecting victims of crime (USCIS, 2018a, 2018b). Applicants must provide proof that they have suffered mental or physical abuse using police reports, police photos, court documents, affidavits from medical personal, school officials, behavioral health providers, or family members. Family members of the victim may also qualify for a U-visa application. Individuals who have had a U-visa for a minimum of 3 years may apply for green card (USCIS, 2018a, 2018b). Family members of U-visa applicants may also apply for a green card. During the 2017 fiscal year, 36,531 victim applications had been submitted while 110, 511 were pending from previous years (USCIS, 2018a, 2018b). For family members, 25,155 applications were submitted in the 2017 fiscal year while 79, 850 were pending from previous years (USCIS, 2018a, 2018b). Those who work with victims of sexual assault should have an awareness of the U-Visa policies so that victims can be referred to legal services when needed.

Best Practices for Prevention Programming

Despite numerous efforts to prevent sexual assault, effective prevention programs are lacking (Mikton, Maguire, & Shakespeare, 2014; Newlands & O'Donohue, 2016). While some risk reduction programs have shown promise, such as those that target alcohol use, those that incorporate self-defense training (Lonsway et al., 2009), or bystander approaches (Katz & Moore, 2013), cultural factors are rarely considered. One particular intervention "Sexual Assault Resistance Education (SARE)" has demonstrated impressive initial results with Canadian college women (Senn et al., 2015). This intervention focuses on (1) improving women's assessment of possible dangerous situations and developing problem-solving strategies; (2) teaching women to recognize when situations have become dangerous and providing skills to overcome any emotional barriers that may prevent them from escaping or resisting the situation; (3) teaching resistance skills appropriate to a the situation (including self-defense and addressing barriers that may contribute to women's reluctance to implement self-defense); (4) enabling women to talk more openly about sexuality, identification of one's sexual wants and boundaries, and communicating this in an effective manner (Senn et al., 2013). Although some interventions have demonstrated success, it is important to note that they have primarily been conducted with Caucasian college students.

Research is needed to examine how cultural factors intersect with these prevention approaches. Some cultural backgrounds may be better suited for certain prevention approaches (e.g. African American women may do well with self-defense and bystander-oriented prevention programs, as research indicates this population tends to be more assertive [Lineberger & Calhoun, 1983]) and other populations may need additional tailoring, as this approaches may be inconsistent or in direct conflict with their cultural values (e.g. Asian cultures tend to promote passivity and hyperfemininity in Asian women [Pyke & Johnson, 2003]). Additionally, researchers need to consider how issues of intersectionality factor into prevention efforts. In other words, should prevention programs consider and attend to the multiple facets of culture, such as sexual orientation, gender identify, ethnicity, socioeconomic status, or disability, are the mechanisms that culminate in sexual assault (e.g. binge drinking) the same for all groups? Examining the efficacy of such interventions with more diverse population is sorely needed.

Summary and Conclusions

The extant literature indicates variations in how sexual assault is defined. This in part has resulted in wide ranges in reported prevalence rates of sexual assault for ethnic minorities. Despite these wide ranges, it is evident that sexual assault prevalence rates among ethnic minorities are high. While the research on forensic interviews with ethnic minorities is limited, at a minimum forensic interviewers assess for the interviewee's language preference and proficiency level and conduct the interview in their native language; attempt ethnic matching and racial/ethnic concordance between the interviewer and interviewee; where ethnic matching is not possible, interviewers should ensure that rapport is sufficient before proceeding with the interview; and finally interviewers considering specific cultural factors (e.g. shame, guilt, immigration status) in the context of the interview. The extant literature does indicate that there are assessment measures that can be used effectively with ethnic minority clients to assess for the common sequelae after sexual assault and that evidence-based interventions (iterations of CBT) can be used to effectively treat the common sequalae of sexual assault. When using evidence-based interventions clinicians should ensure they are aware of the possible intersections between the law and the cultural characteristics of their clients (i.e., being aware of immigration status and the existence of the U-Visa).

References

Ahrens, C., Rios-Mandel, L., Isas, L., & Lopez, M. (2010). Talking about interpersonal violence: Cultural influences on Latinas' identification and disclosure of sexual assault and intimate partner violence. *Psychological Trauma-Theory Research Practice and Policy, 2*(4), 284–295. https://doi.org/10.1037/a0018605

American Psychiatric Association (APA). (2013). *Diagnostic and statistical manual of mental disorders* (5th ed.). Arlington, VA: American Psychiatric Publishing.

Apfeldorf, W., Shear, M. K., Leon, A. C., & Portera, L. (1994). A brief screen for panic disorder. *Journal of Anxiety Disorders, 8*, 71–78. https://doi.org/10.1016/0887-6185(94)90024-8

Beck, A. T., Epstein, N., Brown, G., & Steer, R. A. (1988). An inventory for measuring clinical anxiety: Psychometric properties. *Journal of Consulting and Clinical Psychology, 56*(6), 893. https://doi.org/10.1037/0022-006X.56.6.893

Beck, A. T., Steer, R. A., & Brown, G. K. (1996). *Manual for the Beck depression inventory-II*. San Antonio, TX: Psychological Corporation.

Beck, A. T., Ward, C. H., Mendelson, M., Mock, J., & Erbaugh, J. (1961). An inventory for measuring depression. *Archives of General Psychiatry, 4*, 561–571. https://doi.org/10.1001/archpsyc.1961.01710120031004

Beidel, D. C., Turner, S. M., Stanley, M. A., & Dancu, C. V. (1989). The social phobia and anxiety inventory: Concurrent and external validity. *Behavior Therapy, 20*, 417–427. https://doi.org/10.1016/S0005-7894(89)80060-7

Benson, B. J., Gohm, C. L., & Gross, A. M. (2007). College women and sexual assault: The role of sex-related alcohol expectancies. *Journal of Family Violence, 22*(6), 341–351. https://doi.org/10.1007/s10896-007-9085-z

Benson-Flórez, G., Santiago-Rivera, A., & Nagy, G. (2017). Culturally adapted behavioral activation: A treatment approach for a Latino family. *Clinical Case Studies, 16*(1), 9–24. https://doi.org/10.1177/1534650116668630

Benuto, L., Olmo-Terasa, A., & Reyes-Rabanillo, M. (2011). Exploring the factor structure and psychometric properties of a Spanish translation of the clinician-administered PTSD scale. *The International Journal of Educational and Psychological Assessment, 9*(1), 14.

Benuto, L., & O'Donohue, W. (2015). Is culturally sensitive cognitive behavioral therapy an empirically supported treatment?: The case for hispanics. *International Journal of Psychology and Psychological Therapy, 15*(3), 405.

Benuto, L. T. (Ed.). (2012). *Guide to psychological assessment with Hispanics*. New York: Springer Science & Business Media.

Benuto, L. T., & Bennett, N. (2015). Using prolonged exposure therapy to treat post-traumatic stress disorder a Latina female with a complex trauma history. *International Journal of Psychology and Psychological Therapy, 15*(1), 143–153.

Benuto, L. T., & Garrick, J. (2016). Cultural considerations in forensic interviewing of children. In W. O'Donohue & M. Fanetti (Eds.), *Forensic interviews regarding child sexual abuse*. Cham: Springer. https://doi.org/10.1007/978-3-319-21097-1_20

Benuto, L. T., & Leany, B. D. (Eds.). (2015). *Guide to psychological assessment with African Americans*. New York: Springer.

Benuto, L. T., Thaler, N. S., & Leany, B. D. (Eds.). (2014). *Guide to psychological assessment with Asians*. New York: Springer.

Benuto, L.T., Bennett, N.M., & Casas, J.B., (2019). Minority participation in randomized controlled trials for prolonged exposure therapy: A systematic review of the literature. Manuscript submitted for publication.

Benuto, L., O'Donohue, W., Bennett, N., & Casas, J. (2019). Treatment outcomes for Latinos and non-Hispanic white victims of crime: An effectiveness study. *Hispanic Journal of the Behavioral Sciences*.

Breland-Noble, A., Sotomayor, J., & Burriss, F. (2015). Assessing mood disorders and suicidality in African Americans. In L. Benuto & B. Leany (Eds.), *Guide to psychological assessment with African Americans*. New York, NY: Springer.

Briere, J., & Elliott, D. M. (2003). Prevalence and psychological sequelae of self-reported childhood physical and sexual abuse in a general population sample of men and women. *Child Abuse & Neglect, 27*(10), 1205–1222. https://doi.org/10.1016/j.chiabu.2003.09.008

Brown, T. A., Barlow, D. H., & DiNardo, P. A. (1994). *Anxiety Disorders Interview Schedule for DSM-IV (ADIS-IV): Client Interview Schedule*. New York: Graywind Publications Incorporated/Cambridge University Press.

Brown, T. A., Di Nardo, P. A., & Barlow, D. H. (1994). *Anxiety disorders interview schedule for DSM-IV (ADIS-IV).: Clinician's manual*. Graywind Publications.

Carlson, E. B. (2001). Psychometric study of a brief screen for PTSD: Assessing the impact of multiple traumatic events. *Assessment, 8*, 431–441. https://doi.org/10.1177/107319110100800408

Carmody, D. C., & Washington, L. M. (2001). Rape myth acceptance among college women: The impact of race and prior victimization. *Journal of Interpersonal Violence, 16*(5), 424–436. https://doi.org/10.1177/088626001016005003

Cavanaugh, C. E., Messing, J. T., Amanor-Boadu, Y., O'Sullivan, C. S., Webster, D., & Campbell, J. (2014). Intimate partner sexual violence: A comparison of foreign- versus US-born physically abused Latinas. *Journal of Urban Health, 91*(1), 122–135. https://doi.org/10.1007/s11524-013-9817-8

Center for Disease Control and Prevention. (2017). *The National Intimate Partner and sexual violence survey: 2010–2012 state report*. Retrieved September 4, 2018, from https://www.cdc.gov/violenceprevention/pdf/NISVS-StateReportBook.pdf

Chapman, L., DeLapp, R., & Richards, A. (2015). Assessment of generalized anxiety disorder, panic, and phobias with African Americans. In L. Benuto & B. Leany (Eds.), *Guide to psychological assessment with African Americans*. New York, NY: Springer.

Conley, A. H., Overstreet, C. M., Hawn, S. E., Kendler, K. S., Dick, D. M., & Amstadter, A. B. (2017). Prevalence and predictors of sexual assault among a college sample. *Journal of American College Health, 65*(1), 41–49. https://doi.org/10.1080/07448481.2016.1235578

Covington, J. (2003). *The violent black male: Conceptions of race in criminological theories*. Cambridge: Cambridge University Press.

Daly, K. (2016). The purpose of the forensic interview: A Lawyer's perspective. In W. O'Donohue & M. Fanetti (Eds.), *Forensic interviews regarding child sexual abuse*. Cham: Springer. https://doi.org/10.1007/978-3-319-21097-1_2

Davidson, J. R. T., Book, S. W., Colket, J. T., Tupler, L. A., Roth, S., David, D., … Feldman, M. (1997).

Assessment of a new self-rating scale for post-traumatic stress disorder. *Psychological Medicine, 27*, 153–160.

Department of Justice. (2015). *Office of Justice Programs, Bureau of Justice Statistics, National Crime Victimization Survey, 2010–2014*. Retrieved September 4, 2018, from https://www.bjs.gov/content/pub/pdf/cv15.pdf

Eileraas, K. (2011). Rape, legal definitions of. In M. Stange & C. Oyster (Eds.), *The multimedia encyclopedia of women in today's world*. Thousand Oaks, CA: Sage Publications. Retrieved from https://search.credoreference.com/content/topic/rape

First, M. B., Williams, J. B. W., Karg, R. S., & Spitzer, R. L. (2015). *Structured clinical interview for DSM-5—Research version (SCID-5 for DSM-5, research version; SCID-5-RV)*. Arlington, VA: American Psychiatric Association.

Foa, E., Riggs, D. S., Dancu, C. V., & Rothbaum, B. O. (1993). Reliability and validity of a brief instrument for assessing post-traumatic stress disorder. *Journal of Traumatic Stress, 6*, 459–473. https://doi.org/10.1002/jts.2490060405

Foa, E. B., Cashman, L., Jaycox, L., & Perry, K. (1997). The validation of a self-report measure of PTSD: The Posttraumatic Diagnostic Scale. *Psychological Assessment, 9*, 445–451. https://doi.org/10.1037/1040-3590.9.4.445

Fontes, L. A., & Faller, K. C. (2006). Conducting culturally competent sexual abuse interviews with children from diverse racial, cultural, and socioeconomic backgrounds. In K. C. Faller (Ed.), *Interviewing children about sexual abuse: Controversies and best practice* (p. 164). New York, NY: Oxford University Press.

Fraga, E. (2008). *Latinos. In cross-cultural counseling*. Thousand Oaks, CA: Sage.

Gitlin, L. N., Harris, L. F., McCoy, M. C., Hess, E., & Hauck, W. W. (2016). Delivery characteristics, acceptability, and depression outcomes of a home-based depression intervention for older African Americans: The Get Busy Get Better program. *The Gerontologist, 56*(5), 956–965. https://doi.org/10.1093/geront/gnv117

Gonzalez, F. R., Benuto, L. T., & Casas, J. (2018). Prevalence of interpersonal violence among Latinas: A systematic review. *Trauma, Violence, Abuse*. https://doi.org/10.1177/1524838018806507

Hamilton, M. (1959). The assessment of anxiety states by rating. *British Journal of Medical Psychology, 32*, 50–55. https://doi.org/10.1111/j.2044-8341.1959.tb00467.x

Hamilton, M. (1960). A rating scale for depression. *Journal of Neurology, Neurosurgery, and Psychiatry, 23*(1), 56. https://doi.org/10.1136/jnnp.23.1.56

Hammarberg, M. (1992). Penn inventory for post-traumatic stress disorder: Psychometric properties. *Psychological Assessment, 4*, 67–76.

Hart, T. C., & Rennison, C. (2003). *Bureau of Justice Statistics Special Report, reporting crime to the police, 1992–2000*. Retrieved September 4, 2018, from http://www.icasa.org/docs/reporting_to_police_1992-2000.pdf

Hines, D., Armstrong, J., Reed, K., & Cameron, A. (2012). Gender differences in sexual assault victimization among college students. *Violence and Victims, 27*(6), 922–940. https://doi.org/10.1891/0886-6708.27.6.922

Jacob, M., Keeley, M. L., Ritschel, L., & Craighead, W. E. (2013). Behavioural activation for the treatment of low-income, African American adolescents with major depressive disorder: A case series. *Clinical Psychology & Psychotherapy, 20*(1), 87–96. https://doi.org/10.1002/cpp.774

Jacques-Tiura, A. J., Tkatch, R., Abbey, A., & Wegner, R. (2010). Disclosure of sexual assault: Characteristics and implications for posttraumatic stress symptoms among African American and Caucasian survivors. *Journal of Trauma and Dissociation, 11*(2), 174–192. https://doi.org/10.1080/15299730903502938

Jimenez, J. A., & Abreu, J. M. (2003). Race and sex effects on attitudinal perceptions of acquaintance rape. *Journal of Counseling Psychology, 50*(2), 252–256. https://doi.org/10.1037/0022-0167.50.2.252

Kalibatseva, Z., Wu, I. H., & Leong, F. T. (2014). Assessing depression and suicidality in Asian-Americans. In *Guide to psychological assessment with Asians* (pp. 181–198). New York, NY: Springer.

Katz, J., & Moore, J. (2013). Bystander education training for campus sexual assault prevention: An initial meta-analysis. *Violence and Victims, 28*(6), 1054–1067. https://doi.org/10.1891/0886-6708.VV-D-12-00113

KAN-WIN. (2017). Community survey report on sexual violence in Asian American/immigrant community.. Retrieved September 4, 2018, from https://www.api-gbv.org/resources/sexual-violence-community-survey-bykanwin/

Kercher, G., & Kuo, C. (2008). *Victimization of immigrants*. Retrieved September 4, 2018, from http://www.crimevictimsinstitute.org/documents/ImmigrantVictimizationfinalcorrected.pdf

King, L. A., King, D. W., Leskin, G., & Foy, D. W. (1995). The Los Angeles Symptom Checklist: A self-report measure of posttraumatic stress disorder. *Assessment, 2*(1), 1–17. https://doi.org/10.1177/1073191195002001001

Koucky, E. M., Galovski, T. E., & Nixon, R. V. (2012). Acute stress disorder: Conceptual issues and treatment outcomes. *Cognitive and Behavioral Practice, 19*(3), 437–450. https://doi.org/10.1016/j.cbpra.2011.07.002

Krueger, M. (2016). Forensic interviewing and charging: A prosecutor's perspective. In W. O'Donohue & M. Fanetti (Eds.), *Forensic interviews regarding child sexual abuse*. Cham: Springer. https://doi.org/10.1007/978-3-319-21097-1_4

Kubany, E. S., Haynes, S. N., Leisen, M. B., Owens, J. A., Kaplan, A. S., & Watson, S. B. (2000). Development and preliminary validation of a brief broad-spectrum measure of trauma exposure: The Traumatic Life Events Questionnaire. *Psychological Assessment, 12*(2), 210–224.

Kubany, E. S., Leisen, M. B., Kaplan, A. S., & Kelly, M. P. (2000). Validation of a brief measure of posttraumatic stress disorder: The distressing event questionnaire (DEQ). *Psychological Assessment, 12*(2), 197–209.

Laney, C., & Loftus, E. F. (2016). History of forensic interviewing. In W. O'Donohue & M. Fanetti (Eds.), *Forensic interviews regarding child sexual abuse*. Cham: Springer. https://doi.org/10.1007/978-3-319-21097-1_1

Lee, J. (2014). Assessment of anxiety with Asians. In L. Benuto, N. Thaler, & B. Leany (Eds.), *Guide to psychological assessment with Asians*. New York, NY: Springer.

Liebowitz, M. R. (1987). Social phobia. *Modern Problems in Pharmacopsychiatry, 22*, 141–173.

Lineberger, M. H., & Calhoun, K. S. (1983). Assertive behavior in black and white American undergraduates. *The Journal of Psychology, 113*(1), 139–148. https://doi.org/10.1080/00223980.1983.9923568

Littleton, H., Carmen, R. B., & Berenson, A. B. (2007). Rape scripts of low-income European American and Latina women. *Sex Roles, 56*(7–8), 509–516. https://doi.org/10.1007/s11199-007-9189-1

Lonsway, K. A., Banyard, V. L., Berkowitz, A. D., Gidycz, C. A., Katz, J. T., Ross, M. P., … Edwards, D. (2009). *Rape prevention and risk reduction: Review of the research literature for practitioners*. VAWnet.

Lovett, B. B. (2004). Child sexual abuse disclosure: Maternal response and other variables impacting the victim. *Child and Adolescent Social Work Journal, 21*(4), 355–371. https://doi.org/10.1023/B:CASW.0000035221.78729.d6

Mattick, R. P., & Clarke, J. C. (1998). Development and validation of measures of social phobia scrutiny fear and social interaction anxiety. *Behaviour Research and Therapy, 36*, 455–470. https://doi.org/10.1016/S0005-7967(97)

Messing, J. T., Becerra, D., Ward-Lasher, A., & Androff, D. K. (2015). Latinas' perceptions of law enforcement: Fear of deportation, crime reporting, and trust in the system. *Affilia, 30*(3), 328–340. https://doi.org/10.1177/0886109915576520

Meyer, T. J., Miller, M. L., Metzger, R. L., & Borkovec, T. D. (1990). Development and validation of the penn state worry questionnaire. *Behaviour Research and Therapy, 28*(6), 487–495. https://doi.org/10.1016/0005-7967(90)90135-6

Mikton, C., Maguire, H., & Shakespeare, T. (2014). A systematic review of the effectiveness of interventions to prevent and respond to violence against persons with disabilities. *Journal of Interpersonal Violence, 29*(17), 3207–3226. https://doi.org/10.1177/0886260514534530

Miller, J., & Peterson, R. D. (2008). *Getting played: African American girls, urban inequality, and gendered violence*. New York: New York University Press.

Muehlenhard, C. L., Humphreys, T. P., Jozkowski, K. N., & Peterson, Z. D. (2016). The complexities of sexual consent among college students: A conceptual and empirical review. *The Journal of Sex Research, 53*(4–5), 457–487. https://doi.org/10.1080/00224499.2016.1146651

Newlands, R., & O'Donohue, W. (2016). A critical review of sexual violence prevention on college campuses. *Acta Psychopathologica, 2*(2), 14), 1–14),13. https://doi.org/10.4172/2469-6676.100040

Newman, M. G., Zuellig, A. R., Kachin, K. E., Constantino, M. J., Przeworski, A., Erickson, T., & Cashman-McGrath, L. (2002). Preliminary reliability and validity of the Generalized Anxiety Disorder Questionnaire-IV: A revised self-report diagnostic measure of generalized anxiety disorder. *Behavior Therapy, 33*, 215–233. https://doi.org/10.1016/S0005-7894(02)80026-0

No More. (2015). *THE NO MÁS STUDY: Domestic Violence and Sexual Assault in the Latin@ Community*. Retrieved September 4, 2018, from https://nomore.org/wp-content/uploads/2015/04/NO-MAS-STUDY-Embargoed-Until-4.21.15.pdf

Padilla, A. M., & Baird, T. L. (1991). Mexican-American adolescent sexuality and sexual knowledge: An exploratory study. *Hispanic Journal of Behavioral Sciences, 13*, 83–104. https://doi.org/10.1177/07399863910131007

Palmer, B. (2011, Feburary). What's the difference between "Rape" and "Sexual Assault"? Slate. Retrieved from https://slate.com/news-and-politics/2011/02/cbscorrespondent-lara-logan-was-a-victim-of-sexual-assault-is-that-the-same-as-rape.html

Ponniah, K., & Hollon, S. D. (2009). Empirically supported psychological treatments for adult acute stress disorder and posttraumatic stress disorder: A review. *Depression and Anxiety, 26*(12), 1086–1109. https://doi.org/10.1002/da.20635

Powers, M. B., Halpern, J. M., Ferenschak, M. P., Gillihan, S. J., & Foa, E. B. (2010). A meta-analytic review of prolonged exposure for posttraumatic stress disorder. *Clinical Psychology Review, 30*(6), 635–641. https://doi.org/10.1016/j.cpr.2010.04.007.

Price, M., Davidson, T. M., Ruggiero, K. J., Acierno, R., & Resnick, H. S. (2014). Predictors of using mental health services after sexual assault. *Journal of Traumatic Stress, 27*(3), 331–337. https://doi.org/10.1002/jts.21915

Pyke, K. D., & Johnson, D. L. (2003). Asian American women and Racialized femininities: "Doing" gender across cultural worlds. *Gender & Society, 17*(1), 33–53. https://doi.org/10.1177/0891243202238977

Radloff, L. S. (1977). The CES-D scale a self-report depression scale for research in the general population. *Applied Psychological Measurement, 1*(3), 385–401. https://doi.org/10.1177/014662167700100306

Rape and sexual violence. (2017, March 21). Retrieved September 5, 2018, from https://www.nij.gov/topics/crime/rape-sexual-violence/Pages/welcome.aspx

Rapee, R. M., Craske, M. G., & Barlow, D. H. (1995). Assessment instrument for panic disorder that includes fear of sensation-producing activities: The Albany Panic and Phobia Questionnaire. *Anxiety, 1*, 114–122. https://doi.org/10.1002/anxi.3070010303

Reiss, S., Peterson, R. A., Gursky, D. M., & McNally, R. (1986). Anxiety sensitivity, anxiety frequency and the prediction of fearfulness. *Behaviour*

Research and Therapy, 24, 1–8. https://doi.org/10.1016/0005-7967(86)90143-9
Rice, T., & Coates, D. (1995). Gender role attitudes in the southern United States. *Gender and Society, 9*(6), 744–756. https://doi.org/10.1177/089124395009006007
Rizo, C. F., & Macy, R. J. (2011). Help seeking and barriers of Hispanic partner violence survivors: A systematic review of the literature. *Aggression and Violent Behavior, 16*, 250–264. https://doi.org/10.1016/j.avb.2011.03.004
Rosay, A. B. (2016). *National Institute of Justice Research Report: Violence against American Indian and Alaska Native Women and Men 2010 findings from the National Intimate Partner and Sexual Violence Survey*. Retrieved September 4, 2018, from https://www.ncjrs.gov/pdffiles1/nij/249736.pdf
Sabina, C., Cuevas, C., & Schally, J. (2015). The influence of ethnic group variation on victimization and help seeking among Latino women. *Cultural Diversity & Ethnic Minority Psychology, 21*(1), 19–30. https://doi.org/10.1037/a0036526
Senn, C., Eliasziw, M., Barata, P., Thurston, W., Newby-Clark, I., & Radtke, H.. SARE Study Team(2013). Sexual assault resistance education for university women: Study protocol for a randomized controlled trial (SARE trial). *BMC Womens Health, 13*(1), 25–25. https://doi.org/10.1186/1472-6874-13-25
Senn, C., Eliasziw, M., Barata, P., Thurston, W., Newby-Clark, I., Radtke, H., & Hobden, K. (2015). Efficacy of a sexual assault resistance program for university women. *New England Journal of Medicine, 372*(24), 2326–2335. https://doi.org/10.1056/NEJMsa1411131
Sexual assault. (2018, August 27). Retrieved September 5, 2018, from https://www.justice.gov/ovw/sexual-assault#sa
Shear, M. K., Brown, T. A., Barlow, D. H., Money, R., Sholomskas, D. E., Woods, S. W., … Papp, L. A. (1997). Multicenter collaborative panic disorder severity scale. *American Journal of Psychiatry, 154*(11), 1571–1575. https://doi.org/10.1176/ajp.154.11.1571
Snipes, C. (2013). Assessment of anxiety with Hispanics. In L.B (Ed.), *Guide to psychological assessment with Hispanics* (pp. 153–162). Boston, MA: Springer.
Spielberger, C. D., Gorsuch, R. L., Lushene, R., Vagg, P. R., & Jacobs, G. A. (1983). *Manual for the state-trait anxiety inventory*. Palo Alto, CA: Consulting Psychologists Press.
Tallis, F., Eysenck, M., & Mathews, A. (1992). A questionnaire for the measurement of non-pathological worry. *Personality and Individual Differences, 13*(2), 161–168. https://doi.org/10.1016/0191-8869(92)90038-Q
Tang, J. Y., Li, C., Rodgers, R. F., & Ballou, M. (2016). Ethnic differences in the effectiveness of cognitive behavioral therapy combined with medication: Comparing Asian American and white psychiatric patients. *Asian Journal of Psychiatry, 24*, 2446–2450. https://doi.org/10.1016/j.ajp.2016.08.012
Taylor, S., Koch, W. J., & Crockett, D. J. (1991). Anxiety sensitivity, trait anxiety, and the anxiety disorders. *J Anxiety Disorders, 5*, 293–311. https://doi.org/10.1016/0887-6185(91)90030-W
Telch, M. J., Shermis, M. D., & Lucas, J. A. (1989). Anxiety sensitivity: Unitary personality trait or domain-specific appraisals? *J Anxiety Disorders, 3*, 25–32. https://doi.org/10.1016/0887-6185(89)90026-1
U.S. Citizenship and Immigration Services. (2018a). *Number of Form I-918, petition for U nonimmigrant status, by fiscal year, quarter, and case status 2009–2017*. Retrieved September 4, 2018, from https://www.uscis.gov/sites/default/files/USCIS/Resources/Reports%20and%20Studies/Immigration%20Forms%20Data/Victims/I918u_visastatistics_fy2017_qtr4.pdf
U.S. Citizenship and Immigration Services. (2018b). *Victims of Criminal Activity: U Nonimmigrant Status*. Retrieved September 4, 2018, from https://www.uscis.gov/humanitarian/victims-human-trafficking-other-crimes/victims-criminal-activity-u-nonimmigrant-status/victims-criminal-activity-u-nonimmigrant-status
Upchurch, D., et al. (2001). Sociocultural contexts of time to first sex among Hispanic adolescents. *Journal of Marriage and Family, 63*(4), 1158–1169. https://doi.org/10.1111/j.1741-3737.2001.01158.x
Vandello, J. A., Cohen, D., & Ransom, S. (2008). US Southern and Northern differences in perceptions of norms about aggression: Mechanisms for the perpetuation of a culture of honor. *Journal of Cross-Cultural Psychology, 39*(2), 162–177. https://doi.org/10.1177/0022022107313862
Violence Prevention. (2018, April 10). Retrieved September 5, 2018, from https://www.cdc.gov/violenceprevention/sexualviolence/definitions.html
Watson, D., Clark, L. A., & Carey, G. (1988). Development and validation of brief measures of positive and negative affect: The PANAS scales. *Journal of Personality and Social Psychology, 54*, 1063–1070.
Watson, D., & Friend, R. (1969). Measurement of social-evaluation anxiety. *Journal of Consulting and Clinical Psychology, 33*, 448–457. https://doi.org/10.1037/h0027806
Weathers, F. W., Keane, T. M., & Davidson, M. D. (2001). Clinician-Administered PTSD Scale: A review of the first ten years of research. *Depression and Anxiety, 13*(2001), 132–156.
Weathers, F. W., Litz, B. T., Herman, D. S., Huska, J. A., Keane, T. M. (eds). (1993). The PTSD checklist: Reliability, validity, and diagnostic utility. In *Annual meeting of the International Society for Traumatic Stress Studies; San Antonio, CA*.
Weiss, D. S., & Marmar, C. R. (1997). The Impact of Event Scale—Revised. In J. P. Wilson & T. M. Keane (Eds.), *Assessing psychological trauma and PTSD* (pp. 399–411). New York, NY, US: Guilford Press.
Weist, M. D., Kinney, L., Taylor, L. K., Pollitt-Hill, J., Bryant, Y., Anthony, L., & Wilkerson, J. (2014).

African American and white women's experience of sexual assault and services for sexual assault. *Journal of Aggression, Maltreatment & Trauma, 23*(9), 901–916. https://doi.org/10.1080/10926771.2014.953715

West, C. M. M & Johnson, K. (2013. *Sexual violence in the lives of African American women.* National Online Resource Center on Violence Against Women. Retrieved September 4, 2018, from https://vawnet.org/sites/default/files/materials/files/2016-09/AR_SVAAWomenRevised.pdf

Wiebe, J. S., Sauceda, J. A., & Lara, C. (2013). Assessing mood disorders and suicidality in hispanics. In L. Benuto (Ed.), *Guide to psychological assessment with hispanics*. Boston, MA: Springer. https://doi.org/10.1007/978-1-4614-4412-1_8

Williams, M., Malcoun, E., & Bahojb Nouri, L. (2015). Assessment of posttraumatic stress disorder with African Americans. In L. Benuto & B. Leany (Eds.), *Guide to psychological assessment with African Americans*. New York, NY: Springer.

Williams, M. T., Chapman, L. K., Buckner, E. V., & Durrett, E. L. (2016). Cognitive behavioral therapies. In A. Breland-Noble, C. S. Al-Mateen, & N. N. Singh (Eds.), *Handbook of mental health in African American youth* (pp. 63–77). Cham: Springer International Publishing. https://doi.org/10.1007/978-3-319-25501-9_4

Wong, D. K., & Sun, S. K. (2006). A preliminary study of the efficacy of group cognitive-behavioural therapy for people with social anxiety in Hong Kong. *Hong Kong Journal of Psychiatry, 16*(2), 50–56.

Zigmond, A., & Snaith, R. (1983). The hospital anxiety and depression scale. *Acta Psychiatrica Scandinavica, 67*, 361–370. https://doi.org/10.1111/j.1600-0447.1983.tb09716.x

Zung, W. W., Richards, C. B., & Short, M. J. (1965). Self-rating depression scale in an outpatient clinic: Further validation of the SDS. *Archives of General Psychiatry, 13*(6), 508–515. https://doi.org/10.1001/archpsyc.1965.01730060026004

Social Policy and Sexual Assault 5

Sheila M. McMahon

Social policy is a term that is used to denote government action to meet human needs; because these needs may be in conflict (on the basis of class, race, sex, and so on), it is critical to consider whose values and biases guide any given social policy implementation (Titmuss, 1974). Within the context of social policy, sexual assault can be defined as "any type of sexual contact or behavior that occurs without the explicit consent of the recipient" (U.S. Department of Justice, 2016) including forced intercourse, incest, child molestation, and attempted rape. According to the Centers for Disease Control (CDC), an estimated 1.7% of men and 19.3% of women in the US have been raped during their lifetimes (Breideg, Smith, Basile, et al., 2014). At least 50% of individuals who identify as transgender, 43.9% of women, and 23.4% of men have experienced other forms of sexual violence in their lifetimes, such as sexual coercion and unwanted sexual contact (Breideg et al., 2014; Stotzer, 2009). These national estimates suggest that sexual violence is an issue that affects many in the US and generates a great deal of need. Social policy to address sexual assault in the US has been shaped by competing values, needs, and concepts of sexual assault victimization, perpetration, and prevention.

S. M. McMahon (✉)
Barry University School of Social Work,
Miami Shores, FL, USA
e-mail: smcmahon@barry.edu

The US legal system, with its legacy of preserving traditional gender roles, particularly within the family, has included state laws that were very uneven regarding protections for victims of domestic violence and sexual assault. Many anti-rape activists' early battles for social policy solutions to sexual assault in the US were in state legislatures because states exercised much control over their local rape laws (Valente, Hart, Zeya, & Malefyt, 2001). Traditionally, state laws relied on myths about rape to drive legal processes (Caringella, 2009); this meant that the rules of evidence included the victim/survivor's sexual history, survivors had to show that they had clearly resisted, and hence the burden of proof was on the survivor. Similarly, victims' orders of protection were often not recognized across state lines, leaving survivors vulnerable. Michigan was the first state to pass a revised anti-rape law, and in doing so, became the first in the nation to expand the definition of rape to include broader acts of sexual violence, to provide a "staircase" of penalties (penalties ranging from misdemeanors to felony crimes based on the severity of harm and the statutory age of the victim), to institute rape shield laws, and to end resistance requirements (e.g. requirements that the survivor show proof that they physically resisted the attack) (Bevacqua, 2000). While these changes in Michigan state law were profound and did have a ripple effect in other states, feminist criminologist Susan Caringella (2009) points out that it is important to trace not only the changes to laws on the

W. T. O'Donohue and P. A. Schewe (eds.), *Handbook of Sexual Assault and Sexual Assault Prevention*,
https://doi.org/10.1007/978-3-030-23645-8_5

books, but to examine closely whether corrective action was taken in court proceedings to be more fair to survivors. Unfortunately, sexual assault cases often used assumptions about victims' abilities to consent and victims' personal sexual history in trials, signs that reforms did not result in more fair outcomes for survivors of sexual assault (Caringella, 2009).

Beginning in the early 1970s, survivor advocates increasingly turned to the federal government for support and change. These efforts to nationalize the issue of violence against women led to passage of the Victims of Crime Act in 1984, which included grant support for victims of child abuse, domestic violence, and sexual assault (Brooks, 1997). However, it was not until 1990 when the first version of VAWA was put forth in Congress by then Senator Joseph Biden that there was a legislative effort in the US to pass comprehensive legislation addressing issues of violence against women. This legislative work combined advocates' concerns about domestic violence, sexual assault, and stalking under a single legislative umbrella that culminated in the 1994 passage of the Violence Against Women Act (VAWA, "Title IV" of the Violent Crime Control and Law Enforcement Act, 1994) (Valente et al., 2001).

VAWA

The passage of VAWA marked a significant shift in policymakers' understanding of sexual assault because VAWA specifically attempted to address attitudes that suggest rape is less serious than other violent crimes, and also to refocus attention on the perpetrator's conduct instead of that of the victim (Caringella, 2009). Perhaps most importantly, VAWA represented a shift in public opinion and policy maker's views of rape, replacing protectionist language with a discourse about justice. Authored by then Senator Joe Biden with assistance from NCASA (National Coalition Against Sexual Assault) and the National Organization for Women (NOW) Legal Defense Fund, this piece of legislation included greater punishment for repeat offenders, criminal and civil court restitution for victims, reimbursement to victims for financial losses, protection of victim's identity, and funding, education, and training for rape crisis centers, shelters, and so on (Caringella, 2009). Because it incorporated civil rights language, the Act actually inspired the ire of the (American Civil Liberties Union) ACLU and U.S. Judicial Conference. Opponents of the bill said it would be impossible to establish legally whether a woman was sexually assaulted specifically because of her gender (hence, allowing for additional civil rights protections). As Caringella observes, "According to Biden, if women have to change their lives to accommodate the fear of rape, while men don't, that's not equality" (Caringella, 2009).

Moreover, VAWA's passage also reflected a significant change in public policy regarding violence against women, from policymakers viewing violence against women as a private matter involving quarreling family members to a matter of public concern about violent crimes against women (Boba & Lilley, 2009). This shift was considered a victory among liberal feminists, who had been working through legal and judicial channels for over two decades toward greater gender equality for women in the US. Yet, this landmark violence against women legislation was also characterized by fundamental compromises by feminist activists to get the bill passed, including the inclusion of VAWA in a larger crime bill, and the relinquishing of a critically conscious view of violence against women in our society.

While a discussion of the nuances between radical and liberal feminists regarding approaches to policymaking are beyond the scope of this paper, it is important to understand that, overall, feminist approaches to policy design, implementation, and analysis differ significantly from traditional policymakers because of feminists' ideological and practical commitments to understanding social policy from a gendered perspective. This feminist approach requires policymakers to carefully analyze and challenge the more common androcentric approaches to policymaking that are used in the mainstream (Bevacqua, 2000; Hyde, 2009).

Notably, the social context leading up to the passage of VAWA included several high-profile cases involving violence against women, including the Anita Hill/Clarence Thomas sexual harassment case in 1991 and the Nicole Brown Simpson/O.J. Simpson domestic violence murder case in 1994 (Bevacqua, 2000). Additionally, there were violence against women cases such as the slashing of a female model by a stranger in 1991, which raised media attention on issues of violence against women (Brooks, 1997). As Congress hosted hearings featuring testimony from lawmakers, anti-rape advocates, domestic violence advocates, and survivors, these media-featured crimes stood out as palpable reminders of the national statistics showing rates of violence against women increasing at twice the rate of violence against men (Biden, 2000). The confluence of these very public instances of sexual violence against women, ranging from harassment to stalking and death, and VAWA's placement in a crime bill are important indicators of the thinking that guided the development and passage of the legislation. Namely, this legislation aimed to take violence against women seriously.

And yet, as Meyer-Emerick (2001) points out, unlike subtle forms of violence against women covered in workplace sexual harassment legislation (Title VII of the 1964 Civil Rights Act), VAWA emphasizes the criminal aspects after overt violent crimes against women have been committed. VAWA doesn't address subtler forms of intimidation or other threats of violence against women. The law is meant to assist individual victims and potential victims, as well as to punish perpetrators, rather than directly addressing the conditions that allow violence to occur through a primary prevention approach (Meyer-Emerick, 2001). Nonetheless, VAWA is the primary federal law concerned with addressing sexual assault in the US.

VAWA I: Purpose and Funding

The purpose of VAWA was threefold: (1) to criminalize acts of violence against women, including acquaintance rape, domestic violence, and stalking, (2) to provide better support to survivors of these crimes, and (3) to prevent violence against women (Boba & Lilley, 2009). VAWA-I included greater punishment for repeat offenders, criminal and civil court restitution for victims, protection of victims' identity, reimbursement to victims for financial losses, and funding, education, training for rape crisis centers, and shelters for victims (Caringella, 2009).

The passage of VAWA resulted in the establishment of two funding streams for VAWA initiatives: one through the Department of Health and Human Services (HHS) and the other through the Department of Justice (DOJ). HHS grants were provided to fund a national domestic abuse hotline, shelters, rape prevention programs, and programs to prevent sexual abuse of street youth (Boba & Lilley, 2009). DOJ grants included funding for prosecution and related law enforcement activities for sexual assault crisis response, domestic violence, and child abuse. Funding was also provided for research on violence against women (Parmley, 2004).

In 1995, the Office on Violence Against Women (OVW) was established under the auspices of the Department of Justice to provide financial and technical support to VAWA-funded programs. Currently, the OVW oversees 18 discretionary grant programs and three formula-based programs (e.g. where the funds will be spent is stipulated in the grant). The three formula-based programs are Services, Training, Officers, Prosecutors (STOP); Sexual Assault Services Program (SASP); and State Coalitions. The purpose of the 18 discretionary programs is to provide support for community-based responses which support victims and hold perpetrators accountable. These funds are provided to community-based organizations, nonprofits, universities, courts, schools, and tribal coalitions that provide services to victims and their families, crisis intervention, housing assistance, and support for special victim populations including the elderly, teenagers, or persons with disabilities (http://www.ovw.usdoj.gov/overview.htm).

VAWA 2000 (GovTrack.us. 2019a)

When VAWA-I expired at the end of fiscal year 2000, President Clinton reauthorized VAWA as "Division B" of the Victims of Trafficking and Violence Protection Act of 2000. This reauthorized preexisting programs and funding under VAWA, added requirements to evaluate program effectiveness, and also made it easier for battered immigrant women to leave abusers who were also their sponsors for US citizenship while remaining in the US. At this time, STOP (Services, Training, Officers, and Prosecutors) and Arrest Grants were added. The purpose of these grants was to fund training efforts for law enforcement officials focusing on the arrest and prosecution of perpetrators.

VAWA 2005 (GovTrack.us. 2019b)

Signed into law by President Bush, VAWA 2005 was primarily concerned with providing additional funding for closer monitoring of program performance, often in the form of more stringent program evaluation. VAWA 2005 also added provisions to encourage collaboration among law enforcement, hospitals, judicial officials, and social service providers to improve victim services for special populations (Laney, 2010). Funding for broader research efforts on relevant issues of violence against women were largely removed from this version of the bill, consistent with this presidential administration's cuts for research work in many disciplines.

VAWA 2013 (GovTrack.us. 2019c)

In 2011, VAWA, which enjoyed bipartisan support when it was enacted, faced a significant delay in reauthorization due to Republican opposition to the bill's expanded protections for undocumented immigrants in domestic violence situations seeking temporary visas, greater support for tribal communities to internally prosecute domestic violence and sexual assault crimes committed against Native American women, and a broader definition of domestic violence that would include same-sex couples (Culp-Ressler, 2013; Weisman, 2012). After a protracted political battle, the bill passed the Senate and the House; it was signed into law by President Obama in March of 2013 (Henderson, 2013), but did not include additional protections for undocumented survivors of intimate partner violence (Modi, Palmer, & Armstrong, 2014). While VAWA 2013 provides fewer appropriations than previous versions of the law, it also added a nondiscrimination provision, improved the privacy protections regarding victims' personal information, and increased the certification requirements for grantees providing legal assistance to survivors. VAWA 2013 also aimed to address human trafficking through increased grant funding (Sacco, 2015).

Attention to vulnerable populations. While all victims of sexual assault experience vulnerabilities, social factors can increase the likelihood of victimization. For example, rates of sexual assault against American Indian and Alaskan Native women are extremely high; 56.1% of American Indian and Alaskan Native women and 27.5% of American Indian and Alaskan Native men have experienced some form of sexual assault in their lifetime (Rosay, 2016). Similarly, sexual assault victimization rates of individuals with disabilities in the US are very high and often ignored (Shapiro, 2018). VAWA attempts to mitigate some of these effects through the following program allocations: (1) Services for survivors with disabilities equip domestic violence shelters to meet the needs of individuals with disabilities. (2) Services and training to prevent elder abuse. (3) Grant funding for tribal communities. (4) Grant funding for communities of color and diverse communities with distinct needs that are not addressed by the dominant social policy and practice paradigm in the US. (5) Funding for coordinated community responses to prevent and address sexual assault within LGBT communities and in immigrant communities (APA, n.d.) (Table 5.1).

Colleges & Universities: VAWA 2013 reporting and prevention education requirements. The Campus Sexual Violence Elimination Act of 2013, often referred to as the "Campus SaVE Act," VAWA 2013, Section 304 added significant

Table 5.1 Chart of VAWA provisions

Year of (Re) Authorization	Provisions
1994	Department of Justice (DOJ):
	• Established the Office on Violence Against Women
	• Established the following DOJ grants:
	– STOP (Services∗Training∗Officers∗ Prosecutors) Violence Against Women Formula Grant Program
	– STOP Violence Against Indian Women Discretionary Program
	– Grants to Encourage Arrest Policies Program
	– Rural Domestic Violence and Child Abuse Assistance Grant Program
	Department of Health & Human Services (HHS):
	• Established and funded the National Domestic Violence Hotline
	• Provided support for battered women's shelters
	• Provided support for development of rape prevention education programs
	• Provided support for coordinated community responses to domestic violence, sexual assault, and stalking
2000	Provided new programs to support the following:
	• Legal assistance for victims
	• Grants to state coalitions and tribal coalitions
	• Grants for law enforcement training; training for prosecutors and courts on elder abuse; training on violence against individuals with disabilities
	• Grants to provide services that are accessible to victims with disabilities
	Added definition of "dating violence" to the four VAWA grant programs
	Encouraged the enforcement of protection orders
	Required grantee agencies to show that survivors do not have to pay for services
	Allowed STOP funds to be used to train sexual assault nurse examiners
	Expanded interstate stalking laws
	Added Indian territory to the list of jurisdictions under interstate domestic violence and stalking crimes
	Expanded battered immigrants' access to immigration services
2005	Authorized new programs with the following foci:
	• Native American women
	• Sexual assault
	• Youth victims
2013	Imposed new accountability requirements on VAWA grantees
	Increased auditing requirements for rape kit backlogs through grant funds for DNA analysis
	Provided funding for trafficked persons through amendments to the Trafficking Victims Protection Act of 2000 (Division A of P.L. 106-386)
	Granted authority to American Indian Tribes to exercise civil and criminal jurisdiction over crimes of domestic violence
	Included stalking in the definition of the nonimmigrant U visa
	Provided funding to address the needs of underserved populations
	Included a provision that survivors of domestic violence, dating violence, sexual assault or stalking could not be denied public housing assistance nor expected to undergo unnecessary background checks in order to gain entry to such housing
	Established new mandatory guidelines for institutions of higher education regarding programs to prevent sexual assault, dating violence, domestic violence and stalking through amendments to the Higher Education Act of 1965
	Mandated that federal detention facilities adopt national standards through the Prison Rape Elimination act of 2003

prevention education and response requirements for colleges and universities. Under this reauthorization, college and universities were required to add dating violence, domestic violence, and stalking to the reportable offenses in the Annual Security Report (ASR) that must be issued annually. Schools' policies must include information for sexual assault victims on options to notify or not notify law enforcement, and victims' rights/universities' responsibilities to provide no contact orders and information about where to obtain protective orders. Institutional representatives who conduct campus-based hearings on sexual assault must receive appropriate training to do so in order to promote offender accountability and victim safety. The accuser and accused must be simultaneously notified of the outcomes of campus-based adjudication proceedings, with the option for each to appeal. All new students and faculty must receive sexual assault prevention and education training that includes the definitions of sexual assault, dating violence, domestic violence, and stalking in the relevant jurisdiction; the definition of consent; a statement that the institution prohibits sexual misconduct offenses; options for bystander intervention; training on the signs of abusive relationships; as well as ongoing prevention and awareness campaigns (American Council on Education, 2014). These educational requirements represent an important shift in thinking about sexual assault in the US because they include a broad-based focus on prevention that includes the whole campus community rather than focusing on the victim alone.

To accomplish the additional educational and campus-based crime reporting requirements for colleges and universities, VAWA 2013 made important changes to the Higher Education Act of 1965 statute Jeanne Clery Disclosure of Campus Security Policy and Campus Crime Statistics Act, commonly known as "the Clery Act."

The Clery Act

The Clery Act was signed into law in 1990 as an amendment to the Higher Education Act of 1965 ("History of the Clery Act," 2014). Named in honor of Jeanne Clery, a college student who was raped and murdered in her university residence hall dormitory room in 1986, the Clery Act established crime reporting requirements for colleges and universities (Clery Center, n.d.). The Act required US colleges and universities to publicly report crimes that occurred on or near their campuses, including sexual assault. In 1992, the Clery Act was amended to include a "Sexual Assault Victims' Bill of Rights," requiring colleges and universities to have policies in place to address sexual assault on campus (Clery Center, n.d.). This Act has been instrumental in increasing public awareness about the rates of reported sexual assaults on US college campuses and providing a framework for campus safety efforts to address sexual assault. Changes to VAWA pertaining to colleges and universities in the 2013 reauthorization coincided with increased enforcement of Title IX requirements that colleges and universities maintain environments free of sexual assault, and an outpouring of anti-sexual violence activism by students.

Title IX

Enacted in 1972, education amendment Title IX stated simply, "No person in the United States shall, on the basis of sex, be excluded from participation in, be denied the benefits of, or be subjected to discrimination under any education program or activity receiving Federal financial assistance" (Office for Civil Rights, 2015). Typically, Title IX has been synonymous with gender equity in school sports programs. However, in the 1990s, there were two important Supreme Court cases that clearly reflected the importance of addressing sexual assault in schools under the auspices of Title IX. In *Franklin* vs. *Gwinnett County Public Schools*, Christine Franklin, a high school student in Gwinnett County, was sexually harassed by her teacher and coach. When she reported the incidents to the school, she was discouraged from filing criminal charges and ultimately the case went to the Supreme Court, which affirmed her right to seek monetary damages from the school under Title IX (*Oyez*, 2018). In 1999, under Title IX, a mother sued her daughter's school district for failure to address ongoing peer-on-peer harassment by the daughter's fifth grade classmate in *Davis* vs. *Monroe County Board of Education*, the Supreme Court held the school responsible for failing to intervene in this known harassment. Title IX was applied in this case because the harassment interfered with Miss Davis's ability to engage in the benefits of her education (*Oyez*, 2018).

In 2011, the Department of Education Office for Civil Rights, which administers Title IX, issued guidance to schools (K-12 and postsecondary education) that underscored the importance of taking steps to address incidents of sexual misconduct promptly, protecting the safety of the complainant, and the need to use a preponderance of the evidence standard in disciplinary procedures (Ali, 2011). The letter underscored the need for schools receiving federal funds to publish their grievance proceedings, ensure that their procedures were fair, and designate a school official to coordinate Title IX compliance activities (Grassgreen, 2011). The guidance, which was supported by enforcement efforts and widespread activism by college student survivors and their allies, was met with criticism by men's rights groups, and was repealed in 2017 by the Trump administration (U.S. Department of Education, 2017).

Social Policy, Sexual Assault, and Vulnerable Populations

As previously noted, social policy is intended to address human needs. In the context of sexual assault, individuals and groups may more vulnerable to victimization on the basis of gender identity or expression, race, age, ability, or other factors. Victims are not to blame for these differences; yet it is important to be aware of them so that future social policy can be crafted to prevent sexual assault among all, especially those who are most vulnerable, and in order to provide appropriate and necessary support to survivors. To date, the only additional federal legislation to specifically address the needs of a vulnerable population outside of VAWA was the Prison Rape Elimination Act.

Sexual Assault and Individuals Who Are Incarcerated

The Prison Rape Elimination Act (PREA) was the first US federal law aimed at eliminating sexual violence against prisoners. Signed into law in 2003 by President Bush, PREA established the National Prison Rape Elimination Commission to examine the prevalence rates of sexual victimization in prisons and to create national standards to curb this violence (Just Detention International, 2009). Rape in prison is believed to be widespread but it has been very difficult to get accurate estimates of this violence; because PREA sunset in 2009, it is unclear when these estimates and remedies will be addressed (Moster & Jeglic, 2009).

Conclusion

It is difficult to measure the effectiveness of social policies to ameliorate sexual assault. VAWA, as the only comprehensive national legislation to address sexual assault, was created in a social context in which policymakers were often focused on the criminal nature of sexual violence. While sexual assault is a crime, a "tough on crime" perspective fails to consider root causes and conditions that lay the ground for sexual assault to occur, such as rigid gender roles, racism, gender-based entitlement and misogyny, and so on. As well, the focus of social policy is often centered on response rather than prevention of harm. Moreover, from a research perspective, it is difficult to attribute changes in sexual assault to specific social policies, as it is nearly impossible to rule out other temporal, social, cultural, and developmental factors that may influence the complex social problem of sexual assault. Thus, the success of future social policies to prevent sexual assault will require bridging significant ideological perspectives, eradicating social inequalities, and prioritizing funding for evidence-based victim services and prevention programming.

References

Ali, R. (2011, April 4). *Dear colleague letter*. Washington, DC: U.S. Department of Education, Office for Civil Rights. Retrieved from https://www2.ed.gov/about/offices/list/ocr/letters/colleague-201104.pdf

American Council on Education. (2014, April 1). *New requirements imposed by the violence against women reauthorization act*. Retrieved from http://www.acenet.edu/news-room/Documents/VAWA-Summary.pdf

American Psychological Association (APA). (n.d.) *The Violence Against Women Act*. Retrieved from http://www.apa.org/advocacy/interpersonal-violence/violence-against-women-act.pdf

Bevacqua, M. (2000). Rape on the public agenda: Feminism and the politics of sexual assault.

Biden, J. R., Jr. (2000). The civil rights remedy of the violence against women act: A defense. Harvard Journal on Legislation, 37(1), 1–43.

Boba, R., & Lilley, D. (2009). Violence against women act (VAWA) funding: A nationwide assessment of effects on rape and assault. *Violence Against Women, 15*(2), 168–185.

Breiding, M. J., Smith, S. G., Basile, K. C., Walters, M. L., Chen, J., Merrick, M. T. (2014). Prevalence and characteristics of sexual violence, stalking, and intimate partner violence victimization—National Intimate Partner and Sexual Violence Survey, United States, 2011. *MMWR, 63*(8).

Brooks, R. (1997). Feminists Negotiate the Legislative Branch: The Violence Against Women Act. In Cynthia R. Daniels (Ed.), Feminists Negotiate the State, pp.1–5. New York: University Press of America.

Caringella, S. (2009). *Addressing rape reform in law and practice*. New York: Columbia University Press.

Clery Center. (n.d.). Retrieved from https://clerycenter.org/policy-resources/

Culp-Ressler, T. (2013, January 3). Violence against women act debacle: Why congress should be more diverse. *The Atlantic*. Retrieved from https://www.theatlantic.com/sexes/archive/2013/01/violence-against-women-act-debacle-why-congress-should-be-more-diverse/266784/

Davis v. Monroe County Board of Education. (2018). *Oyez*. Retrieved May 1, 2018, from https://www.oyez.org/cases/1998/97-843

Fisher, B., Cullen, F. T., Turner, M. G., & National Institute of Justice. (2000). *The sexual victimization of college women*. Washington, DC: U.S. Dept. of Justice, Office of Justice Programs, National Institute of Justice.

Fisher, B., Daigle, L. E., & Cullen, F. T. (2010). *Unsafe in the ivory tower: The sexual victimization of college women*. Los Angeles: Sage Publications.

"Franklin v. Gwinnett County Public Schools." (2018, 1 May). *Oyez*. Retrieved from www.oyez.org/cases/1991/90-918

GovTrack.us. (2019a). S. 2787—106th Congress: Violence against women act of 2000. Retrieved from https://www.govtrack.us/congress/bills/106/s2787

GovTrack.us. (2019b). S. 1197—109th Congress: Violence against women act of 2005. Retrieved from https://www.govtrack.us/congress/bills/109/s1197

GovTrack.us. (2019c). S. 47—113th Congress: Violence against women reauthorization act of 2013. Retrieved from https://www.govtrack.us/congress/bills/113/s47

Grassgreen, A. (2011, April 4). Call to action on sexual harassment. *Insider Higher Ed*. Retrieved from https://www.insidehighered.com/news/2011/04/04/education_department_civil_rights_office_clarifies_colleges_sexual_harassment_obligations_title_ix

Henderson, N.-M. (2013, March 7). Obama signs a strengthened violence against women act. *The Washington Post*. Retrieved from https://www.washingtonpost.com/politics/obama-signs-a-strengthened-violence-against-women-act/2013/03/07/e50d585e-8740-11e2-98a3-b3db6b9ac586_story.html?utm_term=.c0a4824f2013

Hyde, C. (2009). "Feminist Approaches to Social Policy". In The Handbook of Social Policy. Los Angeles: SAGE Publications, Inc.

Just Detention International. (2009, February). *The prison rape elimination act. Fact sheet*. Retrieved from https://justdetention.org/publication/

Laney, G. P. (2010). Violence against women act: History and federal funding. Washington, DC: Congressional Research Service. Retrieved from http://digitalcommons.ilr.cornell.edu/key_workplace/711

Meyer-Emerick, N. (2001). Policymakers, Practitioners, Citizens: Perceptions of the Violence Against Women Act of 1994. Administration & Society, Vol. 33: 629–663.

Modi, M. N., Palmer, S., & Armstrong, A. (2014). The role of violence against women act in addressing intimate partner violence: A public health issue. *Journal of Women's Health, 23*(3), 253–259. https://doi.org/10.1089/jwh.2013.4387

Moster, A. N., & Jeglic, E. L. (2009). Prison warden attitudes toward prison rape and sexual assault: Findings since the Prison Rape Elimination Act (PREA). *The Prison Journal, 89*(1), 65–78. https://doi.org/10.1177/0032885508329981

Office for Civil Rights. (2015, April 29). *Title IX and sex discrimination*. Retrieved from https://www2.ed.gov/about/offices/list/ocr/docs/tix_dis.html

Parmley, A. M. (2004). Violence against women research post VAWA: Where have we been, where are we going? Violence Against Women, 10(12), 1417–1430.

Rosay, A. B. (2016). *Violence against American Indian and Alaska Native women and men: 2010 findings from the National Intimate Partner and Sexual Violence Survey (NCJ # 249736)*. Washington, DC: National Institute of Justice, Office of Justice Program, U.S. Department of Justice.

Sacco, L. N. (2015). *The violence against women act: Overview, legislation, and Federal Funding*. Washington, DC: Congressional Research Service.

Shapiro, J. (2018, January 8). The sexual assault epidemic no one talks about. *All Things Considered*. Retrieved from https://www.npr.org/2018/01/08/570224090/the-sexual-assault-epidemic-no-one-talks-about

Stotzer, R. L. (2009). Violence against transgender people: A review of United States data. *Aggression and Violent Behavior, 14*(3), 170–179. https://doi.org/10.1016/j.avb.2009.01.006

Titmuss, R. M. (1974). *Social policy* (pp. 1–2). London: Allen & Unwin.

U.S. Department of Education. (2017, September 22). *Department of Education Issues new Interim Guidance on campus sexual misconduct*. Retrieved from https://www.ed.gov/news/press-releases/department-education-issues-new-interim-guidance-campus-sexual-misconduct

U.S. Department of Justice. (2016). *Sexual assault*. Retrieved from https://www.justice.gov/ovw/sexual-assault

Valente, R., Hart, B., Zeya, S., & Malefyt, M. (2001). The violence against women act of 1994: The Federal Commitment to ending domestic violence, sexual assault, stalking, and gender-based crimes of violence. In C. Renzetti, J. Edleson, & R. Bergen (Eds.), *Sourcebook on violence against women* (pp. 279–302). Thousand Oaks: Sage Publications.

Violence Against Women Act (VAWA). (1994). Title IV of the violent crime control and law enforcement act, H.R. 3355, Pub.L. 103–322.

Weisman, J. (2012, March 15). Women figure anew in Senate's latest Battle. The New York Times , p. A1.

Framing #MeToo: Assessing the Power and Unintended Consequences of a Social Media Movement to Address Sexual Assault

6

Aubri F. McDonald

Introduction

Social media has become a predominant way for people to express themselves, interact with others, and learn what is going on in the world. In the Fall of 2017 millions of social media users affixed the phrase #MeToo to their experiences of being sexually assaulted and harassed. The collection of responses spurred a cultural movement that has illuminated the universality of sexual assault and harassment. The #MeToo movement has encouraged victims to break their silence by emphasizing the credibility of women and victims and by highlighting the impunity that many powerful white men have experienced. Social media grants individuals a voice and the ability to control their message, wherein past social movement actors often did not have control over how media represented their claims (Gamson & Modigliani, 1989).

In this chapter, framing concepts are applied to the #MeToo movement to better understand the influence of the #MeToo frame on certain beliefs and actions regarding the issue of sexual assault. The #MeToo movement is examined with regard to its impact on politics, identity, policy, and gender relations. Social media is discussed in terms of its potential advantages and risks as a justice-seeking tool.

A. F. McDonald (✉)
Criminal Justice Department, University of Wisconsin-Parkside, Kenosha, WI, USA

Social Media and #MeToo

Social media serves a catch-all term for internet platforms—websites ("sites"), or applications ("apps") for mobile devices—where users create and share content and interact with each other. Platforms across social media emerged in the early 2000s and are used for social networking (i.e., Facebook), professional networking (e.g., LinkedIn), video sharing (e.g., YouTube), and sharing videos, photos, and typed content (e.g., Twitter, Instagram, Snapchat, Reddit).[1] In 2017 there were an estimated 209 million social media users in the US and 2.46 billon worldwide (*Statista*, 2018a). By 2022, social media use is projected to increase to about 221 million US users and around 3 billon users globally (*Statista*, 2018b).

The #MeToo movement gained widespread recognition on social media after the #MeToo "hashtag," a keyword or phrase preceded by a pound sign, "went viral" or was circulated rapidly and extensively, on the social media platform Twitter. Twitter allows users to broadcast short messages called "tweets" limited to 140 characters. When users include a hashtag in a tweet, Twitter converts the keyword or phrase into a clickable link allowing users to track

[1]Other social media platforms are for photo messaging (e.g., Snapchat); video calling (e.g., Skype); gaming in a multiplayer virtual world (e.g., Fortnite) or dating (e.g., Match, Tinder, Bumble).

W. T. O'Donohue and P. A. Schewe (eds.), *Handbook of Sexual Assault and Sexual Assault Prevention*,
https://doi.org/10.1007/978-3-030-23645-8_6

discussions of certain topics.[2,3] Users can also "follow" each other to receive updates in real time about what others are creating, sharing, and their reactions to content. Twitter users set up virtual identities or profiles consisting of a short bio and image.

The notion of "MeToo" as an initiative to support survivors of sexual violence predates social media. In 1997, Tarana Burke came up with the phrase "me too" while working at a youth camp after a 13-year-old sexual abuse survivor shared her story. Burke recalls on her website, "[I]n the middle of her sharing her pain with me, I cut her off and immediately directed her to another female counselor who could 'help her better…' I couldn't even bring myself to whisper…me too" (JustBeInc, 2013a). In 2006 Burke founded the nonprofit organization Just Be Inc. which serves survivors of sexual harassment and abuse (JustBeInc, 2013b).[4]

The #MeToo movement caught fire in October 2017 in the wake of sexual assault and harassment allegations against media mogul Harvey Weinstein by female celebrities and numerous other women in the entertainment industry. Weinstein was exposed by Kantor and Twohey (2017) writing for the *New York Times* and Rowan Farrow in the *New Yorker*. The Weinstein company, the production company Weinstein ran with his brother, was forced into bankruptcy. Kantor and Twohey along with others who brought awareness to sexual violence were named *TIME* magazine's "Person of the Year" for Farrow, 2017 as "Silence Breakers." Farrow won a Pulitzer Prize for his Weinstein story.

In response to the allegations against Weinstein actress Alyssa Milano, known for her television roles on *Who's The Boss?* and *Charmed,* sent a tweet encouraging her three million Twitter followers to reply to her tweet and write "me too" if they've been sexually harassed or assaulted. The #MeToo hashtag circulated rapidly and extensively or "went viral" on Twitter. Milano's tweet prompted millions of people worldwide to post their #MeToo experiences. Women in different countries have translated the hashtag or created a new one. In the Arab world "#Ana_kaman," translated as "me too," has been used millions of times. In France "#BalanceTonPorc" meaning "rat out your pig," went viral (Nicolaou, 2018).

The #MeToo hashtag was used roughly 19 million times on Twitter in the year after it went viral (Anderson & Toor, 2018). Though hashtags originated as a feature on Twitter, they have become part of the language on other social media platforms. #MeToo spawned other hashtags which have become political statements aimed at challenging society's skepticism toward victims of sexual assault and harassment and a long history of women's voices being dismissed or ignored (Hodge, 2018). #BelieveWomen or #BelieveVictims, and #TimesUp encapsulate the ideas that women should be taken seriously when they allege they have been victims of sexual misconduct and the time has come for abusive men to be held accountable for their behavior.

Social media movements or "hashtag" movements such as #MeToo facilitate social movement participation. In the vast social media landscape, hashtags make it easy to find related posts, spread messages, and unite with allies. The elasticity of the #MeToo hashtag contributes to its broad appeal. #MeToo ties together experiences from all ages and different backgrounds into a broader whole to illustrate the scale of the sexual assault problem.

Framing and Frames

The framing approach derives from literatures in sociology (Goffman, 1974) and communication (Entman, 1993). Framing theory explains that the way information about a particular issue is presented influences how that issue is understood. Framing has been applied to social movements

[2]A twitter "handle" is the users identifying name. Using the @ symbol and the Twitter user's name sends messages directly to that user's Twitter feed (or collection of messages).

[3]Reddit content is organized within areas of interest called "subreddits" or "subs" for short. Users vote on content which then moves it toward the top or bottom of a subreddit feed.

[4]To learn more about JustBeInc see: https://justbeinc.wixsite.com/justbeinc/purpose-mission-and-vision

(Benford, 1997; Snow & Benford, 1992), media (see Scheufele, 1999 for an overview) and political communication (e.g., Edelman, 1964). From a sociological perspective a frame provides "a central organizing idea or story line that provides meaning to an unfolding strip of events, weaving a connection among them. The frame suggests what the controversy is about, the essence of the issue" (Gamson & Modigliani, 1987, p. 143). The social movements literature defines a frame as "an interpretive schemata that simplifies and condenses the 'world out there' by selectively punctuating and encoding objects, situations, events, experiences, and sequences of actions within one's present or past environment" (Snow & Benford, 1992, p. 137). Framing is characterized by selection, emphasis, salience, and exclusion. While some facts are selected and emphasized to make them more salient, other facts are downplayed or excluded (Entman, 1993).

#MeToo represents a collective action frame, an "action-oriented sets of beliefs that inspire meaning and legitimate social movement activities and campaigns" (Benford, 1997, p. 416). Collective action frames "underscore and embellish the seriousness and injustice of a particular social condition," amplify the suffering of victims, and cast moral judgements upon those who represent the cause of the problem (Snow & Benford, 1992, p. 137). Simplifying and crafting information to promote a certain set of beliefs can be very effective for getting people on board to support a particular cause, though it may also limit a movement's ability to address issues in an effective way and lead to other injustices or unintended consequences.

The Power of the #MeToo Frame: Credibility and Salience

The phrase and hashtag #MeToo is one of the most viral and powerful occurrences in social media history. The #MeToo frame characterizes a "Superframe," a highly recognizable and resonant frame that serves as an "interpretive medium" for evaluating the issues and assigning blame for problems (Benford & Hunt, 1992; Minsky, 1974, p. 237). Superframes like #MeToo are easily activated and retrieved from memory (Minsky, 1974). Why is #MeToo so powerful? Why do some framings seem to be effective or "resonate" while others do not? The strength of a frame depends on its credibility and salience (Snow & Benford, 1988).

The credibility of any framing depends on its *empirical credibility* or its apparent fit between framings and events in the world. The greater the number of slices of evidence for the frame, the more credible the framing and the broader its appeal (Benford & Snow, 2000). The volume of #MeToo-related posts, news items, and discussions on social media and off-line actions prompted by #MeToo serve as "slices of evidence" for legitimizing the #MeToo frame. A frame's credibility also has to do with the credibility of the frame articulators, the greater their status, the more plausible and resonant the frame (Benford & Snow, 2000). #MeToo gained recognition amid sexual misconduct allegations by celebrities against Hollywood producer Harvey Weinstein. Famous actresses like Alyssa Milano, Gwenyth Paltrow, Ashley Judd, and Angelina Jolie and countless other celebrities validated the claims against Weinstein. The interest in celebrity culture lends to the resonance of the #MeToo frame.

Social media plays an important role in the salience of the #MeToo frame. The accessibility of social media and its extensive reach increases the visibility of #MeToo-related content. Pew Research found that since #MeToo went viral, 65% of adult social media users in the US reported regularly seeing posts about sexual harassment-related content online with 29% reporting it comprised a great deal of content they saw on social networking sites (Anderson & Toor, 2018).[5] #MeToo has been linked to a substantial increase in internet searches related to

[5]The study noted that usage surged around news events with the most posts in September 9, 2018, when CBS CEO Leslie Moonves resigned after allegations of sexual assault followed by Harvey Weinstein's resignation from the board of his entertainment company on October 17, 2017 (Anderson & Toor, 2018).

reporting sexual harassment and assault (Caputi, Nobles, & Ayers, 2018).

News media in particular influences beliefs about a variety of topics, including sexual assault (Ardovini-Brooker & Caringella-MacDonald, 2002). As of 2018 68% of adults in the US were getting their news from social media (Matsa & Shearer, 2018). Traditional news outlets such as broadcast news and newspapers report on social media activity and vice versa, creating a feedback loop. The content of news feeds vary depending on the social media platform, but they consist mainly of the posts, articles, and images from other people whom the user has chosen to "follow." People tend to search for, interpret, favor, and recall information in a way that confirms how they see the world (Plous, 1993, p. 233).

Interactions over social media serve as important identity signals that help people navigate the networked social world. As social movements play out online, social media interactions play an important role in identity construction, transformation, and validation (Benford, 1997; Donath & Boyd, 2004). "Identity discourse in social movements helps to concretize activists' perceptions of social movement dramas, demonstrate personal identities, reconstruct biographies, impute group identities and align personal and collective identities in movement groups" (Benford, 1997, p. 421).

How Do Frames Influence Thinking?

Framing refers to both the "frames" people use in communication and mental "frames" or schemas that people use to interpret information. Frames, in communication and in the mind, are never constructed from scratch, but always draw on already existing schemas (Gamson & Modigliani, 1989; Snow & Benford, 1988). Concepts from social cognition offer insight into how frames influence thinking. The "schema" concept (Bartlett, 1932) refers to "internal structures of the mind" (Goffman, 1974; Kinder & Sanders, 1990, p. 74). Research finds that our brains set up mental schemas, or stereotyped categories to make sense of the world (Allport, 1954; Bartlett, 1932; Fiske & Taylor, 1991; Tajfel, 1974).[6] Much like how user content on Twitter is organized by hashtags, our brains catalog vast amounts of incoming information by taking "cognitive shortcuts" and by setting up schemas to streamline the meaning making process (Fiske & Taylor, 1991; Lippmann, 1946). Walter Lippmann (1946) explains that "we are not equipped to deal with so much subtlety, so much variety, so many permutations and combinations" and must reconstruct information to a "simpler model" in order to manage it (p. 16).

Schemas are shaped by experience and reflect our beliefs, values, and worldview. Through "priming," certain frames can unconsciously activate an associated mental schema, which then influences how new information is perceived and evaluated (Bartlett, 1932; Fiske & Taylor, 1991; Winter, 2005). For instance, attaching the #MeToo hashtag to a post on social media links it to the broader #MeToo frame. The #MeToo frame activates the reader's mental schema with their beliefs and values regarding the #MeToo movement and influences how the reader evaluates the content of the post and the person who posted it.

Simplifying operations or heuristics that function to conserve mental effort often reduce the complexity of thinking and renders individuals ill-equipped to deal with complex social matters in a critical way and can lead to errors in judgement and illogical thinking (Nelson, Clawson, & Oxley, 1997; Shah & Oppenheimer, 2008). While we cannot avoid automatic, cognitive processes that often operate without our knowledge, we can certainly acknowledge that a better understanding of #MeToo and the frames embedded in discussions around #MeToo is critical given its salience and potential to affect real change.

[6] Related ideas can be found in Bartlett's (1932) research on the schematic nature of perception and Tajfel's (1969) cognitive determinants of social interaction.

Setting the Stage for the #MeToo Movement

Frames are influential when they resonate with a certain schema. The likelihood that a frame will activate a schema increases if information in that schema is activated frequently or has been recently activated (Graber, 1988). While sexually abusive behavior toward women has been a problem for a very long time, in the year leading up to #MeToo going viral, glimpses of the activities that characterize the #MeToo movement "primed" the public's schemas to be activated and to resonate once #MeToo went viral.

Twelve months before #MeToo went viral in October 2016, during the presidential election between Donald Trump and Hilary Clinton, the *Washington Post* publicized a recording of Trump from 2005 talking about his treatment toward women and that he "grab[s] them by the pussy" (Garcia, 2016). Trump's comments about women, allegations of sexual abuse against him by multiple women, and his victory over Clinton, the first female presidential nominee in US history, generated anger and galvanized protests. On January 21, 2017, Trump's first full day as president, millions of people took part in the Women's March on Washington and in other cities worldwide to support gender equality and civil rights. Many wore pink "pussy" hats with cat ears referencing Trump's comment. Several months before #MeToo going viral, high-profile men in media were ousted from their positions following accusations of sexual misconduct. *Fox News* founder and CEO Roger Ailes resigned and Bill O'Reilly, host of the *O'Reilly Factor* on *Fox News*, was fired after allegations against them were made public (Steel & Schmidt, 2017).

The public demonstrations protesting the mistreatment of women and high-profile men being held accountable for sexually exploitive behavior informed schemas with fresh information regarding a shift in responses to sexual assault; victims who come forward will be taken seriously and perpetrators will be held accountable. This shift was legitimized when #MeToo went viral.

After #MeToo went viral a wave of sexual misconduct allegations against celebrities and politicians surfaced at a rapid-fire pace. Matt Lauer, host of the Today Show on NBC was fired, and CBS CEO Leslie Moonves resigned after being publicly accused of sexually inappropriate behavior (Anderson & Toor, 2018). Actor Kevin Spacey was accused of initiating sexual contact with a minor and fired from the Netflix show he was starring in at the time, House of Cards. Alabama's Republican candidate for Senate Roy Moore lost an election after allegations of sexual assault against him surfaced and the hashtag #NoMoore spread quickly across social media. Democratic Senator for Minnesota, Al Franken was pressured to resign after allegations of sexually inappropriate behavior and posts and images to that effect went viral on social media. Comedian Louis C.K., Prairie Home Companion creator Garrison Keillor, longtime television host Charlie Rose (Carmon I. & Brittain, 2017), and numerous other politicians, business leaders, and celebrities lost their jobs or reputations after allegations of sexual misconduct.[7]

The activity before #MeToo went viral made the #MeToo frame more accessible in people's minds. When evoked, Superframes like #MeToo are easily activated and retrieved from memory (Minsky, 1974). Once #MeToo went viral, people were more easily able to reference these past activities as a way to evaluate the legitimacy of #MeToo. Case after case of people coming forward and prominent men being held to account for sexually exploitive behavior memorialized #MeToo as a turning point where sexual assault would no longer be tolerated and perpetrators would be held accountable and victims were empowered to come forward to talk about and seek justice for the sexual abuse they have suffered.

[7]On October 18, 2017, gymnast McKayla Maroney tweeted she had been sexually assaulted by Larry Nassar, the doctor for the US female Olympic gymnastics team.

#FakeNews?

The internet has made news more accessible and given rise to many competitive voices, it's also become harder to figure out the integrity of the news source. In what Pew Researchers called a "striking finding from 2018," most news posts on Twitter were posted by fake accounts. They estimated that two-thirds (66%) of tweeted links to popular news and media websites were posted by Twitter "bots" or automated accounts with a relatively small number of highly active bots generating many of the posts (Wojcik et al., 2018).[8] A "Bot" can play a valuable part in the social media ecosystem; they can answer questions in real time and generate automated updates about news stories or events. "Bots" have also been used in exploitive ways to alter perceptions of political discourse on social media, spread misinformation, and manipulate online rating and review systems (Wojcik et al., 2018). Twitter has set rules outlining proper and improper uses of automation. Proper usage includes broadcasting helpful information, generating interesting or creative content, and automatically replying to users via direct message. Twitter prohibits any circumventing of the platform's software protocols, spamming, and violating user privacy.

Twitter "bots" can be extremely influential in promoting certain understandings underpinning the #MeToo movement (Garkey, 2017). *Newsweek* detailed a sophisticated social media campaign, a "botnet" to generate opposition against Senator Al Franken which later lead to his resignation. Amidst the wave of sexual misconduct allegations against powerful men at the end of 2017, model and LA radio host, Leanne Tweeden accused Franken of groping her on a USO trip in 2005. After the allegations surfaced Twitter was immediately inundated with the hashtags such as "#frankenfondles," a photo of Franken miming grabbing Tweeden's breasts, and a "meme" or image with the phrase "Franken is a groper." The hashtags and images originated thousands of "bot" accounts. The fake Twitter accounts also shared a link to a news article criticizing Franken. The website for the news article was based in Japan and had been created the day before the allegations against Franken became public. Prominent right-wing activists with millions of Twitter followers joined in to denounce Franken. One tweeted, "Thinking of offering money to people who go on tv and say Al Frank is a predator" (Burleigh, 2018). The Alliance for Securing Democracy, an organization that tracks Russian social media accounts and discourse, found that "Al Franken" was a top trending topic in the days following the allegations. The agency also detected counter-bots that were planted to defend Franken to keep the conversation going (Garkey, 2017). The notion of "Al Franken is a groper" dominated in the US and effectively silenced the testimonies of eight former female staffers defending Franken and other supporters. A similar manipulation is believed to have affected the 2016 US presidential election.

[8] Pew researchers used a "Botometer" algorithm to identify bot accounts.

Social Media as a Justice-Seeking Tool

Social media has the potential to be an effective or risky justice-seeking tool. The #MeToo movement has opened up vast resources online that help victims of sexual assault seek justice, network with allies and other survivors, and recover emotionally from their trauma. However, individuals who share their experiences publicly may lose control of their story or face legal consequences.

Disclosing Sexual Assault

#MeToo has galvanized the notion that the response to disclosing sexual abuse is that of unconditional support, admiration for being brave, and insistence that it was not their fault. Research finds that disclosing abuse results in a positive impact psychologically (Andalibi, Haimson, De Choudhury, & Forte, 2016; McClain & Amar, 2013). #MeToo founder Tarana Burke indicated that the #MeToo movement allows people to create community with shared experiences which can satisfy emotional and social gains linked to self-esteem and identity such as recognition, attention and validation. Burke described, "You have a built-in group of people who automatically gets you, who automatically believes you, who automatically wants to hear you. That's the wildfire of it" (Rowley, 2018). Disclosing can be liberating for a survivor, promote a sense of taking control, and perhaps preventing bad things from happening to someone else.

Cyber Vigilantism

People who turn to social media for justice may also put themselves at risk. The #MeToo era has seen dozens of high-profile people lose their jobs and reputations. Social media can be a platform for sexual assault victims to seek justice when victims feel the legal system has come up short or is inadequate to meet their needs. When an accusation fails to destroy the accused as seen in the Hollywood version of #MeToo, victims may feel their only recourse may be to turn to vigilante justice via social media, a practice called *cyber vigilantism* (e.g., Smallridge, Wagner, & Crowl, 2016).

Publicly accusing someone of sexual assault or harassment can backfire. Once allegations are public, a person risks losing control of the story and increases vulnerability to public scrutiny. Whitney Phillips (2015), author of *This is Why We Can't Have Nice Things*, a book on internet trolls, is wary of the unintended consequences of social media vigilantism. Phillips explains, "Something that you do or say or post now can be taken and recombined and re-harnessed for negative ends and without your knowledge or consent. It sets people up to be re-violated, and if the original harm is a violation, that's really scary" (p. 27).

Public disclosure can lead to defamation lawsuits as a way for the accused to restore their reputation. Even if the accused loses in civil court, the accuser would have to spend money to defend themselves. The details of the alleged attack would be aired publicly, and the victims would have to relive the trauma (Wong & La Ganga, 2016). An October 2018 lawsuit highlighted the potential consequences of speaking out about sexual misconduct. Stephen Elliott, a writer and founder of the literary site the Rumpus, sued "Shitty Media Men" list creator Moira Donegan for $1.5 million in damages, alleging that the accusations next to his name in the now-offline list were unsubstantiated, false, and defamatory (Sherman, 2018).[9]

Unintended Consequences of the #MeToo Movement

All movements, no matter how virtuous in intent, may result in unintended consequences. While the #MeToo movement has encouraged awareness of and sensitivity to sexually exploitive behavior, studies suggest it has also intensified anxieties around being wrongfully held liable for sexual misconduct.

As the public sharing of "injustices" garners far more attention and emotional outpouring than most other events on social media, some suggest that #MeToo incentivizes disclosures of sexual victimization. Critics argue that #MeToo, by situating victimhood as a privileged and coveted status, may encourage exaggerated or false claims of sexual assault and harassment.

One year into the #MeToo movement, an October 2018 poll of 2201 adults in the US found that 57% were equally worried about men facing false accusations of sexual assault as they were about women being subjected to sexual harassment and assault (Piacenza, 2018). During the same month an analysis of Reddit forums found that of the posts containing the word "rape," 60% of them mentioned false accusations. Two-thirds expressed concerns about men being falsely accused while the remaining third contained accounts of men who had reportedly been falsely accused of rape (Reddit, 2018).

False disclosures may happen for a host of reasons such as to belong, for a sense of purpose,

[9]The suit is still pending at the time of writing.

to make friends or promote trusting bonds with others (see O'Callaghan, Lorenz, Ullman, & Kirkner, 2018). De Zutter, Horselenberg, and Van Koppen (2017) found that false complainants were primarily motivated by emotional gain with 20% of complainants reporting they did not know why they filed a false allegation.[10] Studies have found that false allegations of sexual assault can function to produce an alibi, to exact or gain sympathy and attention, often when under stress (Kanin, 1994). Other pathways to false sexual assault and harassment claims include lying, false interpretations, false memories, intoxication, substance abuse, biased or flawed investigations, personality disorders, or other form of mental dysfunction (Engel & O'Donohue, 2012; O'Donohue & Bowers, 2006).

All false allegations aren't necessarily false but rather may reflect the complexities inherent to human interactions and variations from one individual to another. Consent rules that dictate whether a sexual violation has occurred may be part of the problem. The National Council for Higher Education and Risk Management (NCHERM) one of the country's largest higher-education consulting practices specializing in Title IX, argues that consent as a construct is imperfect in both theory and practice, "Our consent rules need to be malleable to account for the vagaries of the human experience, and we need to be flexible enough to allow for the fact that human communication and interaction are imperfect" (Black et al., 2017). NCHERM points out, "Having less-than-ideal sex is unfortunate, but probably universal at some point for all people who are sexually active" (Black et al., 2017). The anxieties in relation to accusations of sexual misconduct may have the unintended effect of men actively avoiding women and harming women in the long run. A study presented at a meeting for the American Heart Association found that bystanders are less likely to perform CPR on women for fear of being accused of sexual assault (Norton, 2018).

Studies focused on workplace interactions between men and women reflect a similar anxiety. A Pew Research survey revealed that 51% of US adults felt that the recent focus on sexual harassment made it harder for men to know how to interact with women in the workplace (Graf, 2018). Kim Elsesser (2015), author of "Sex and the Office," predicts that if men start to back away from women in the workplace, the result would be a "sex partition" that would adversely impact female workers' career advancement. A 2018 article in *Bloomberg* titled "Wall Street Rule for the #MeToo Era: Avoid Women at All Costs" found men are taking extra precautions to keep their distance from women. Interviews with more than 30 senior executives revealed men are avoiding one-on-one meetings and dinners with female colleagues, sitting next to them on flights, and are booking hotel rooms on different floors. One respondent noted that just hiring a woman these days is "an unknown risk" that she might take something the wrong way (Tan & Porzecanski, 2018). Texas Sheriff Jim Kaelin dubbed "Sheriff Hugs" made a similar statement in a viral Facebook post in the month after #MeToo went viral when allegations were publicized nearly every day. The Sheriff announced that #MeToo made him discontinue receiving and giving hugs from anyone outside of his family and close friends. He explained, "[Y]ou just don't know when this hug might come back and bite you. The workplace, for one, can become hostile if an employee "feels" threatened by your hugs" (Zeisler, 2017). A common hashtag, #MGTOW meaning "Men Go The Other Way," refers to men avoiding interactions with women out of fear of being accused of sexually inappropriate behavior.

Andi Zeisler (2017) author and cofounder of a feminist blog site argues that focusing on the discomfort of a man rather than his behavior toward women discredits those who speak up about harassment. She emphasizes that acting as though women "frivolously point fingers" trivializes the reality that women who come forward with accu-

[10] Complainants file a false allegation out of material gain, emotional gain, or a disturbed mental state. The list can be subdivided into eight different categories: material gain, alibi, revenge, sympathy, attention, a disturbed mental state, relabeling, or regret.

sations often risk losing their job or ostracization by their colleagues.

Applying Framing to the #MeToo Movement: The Injustices, the Victims and Who's to Blame

Framing in the context of social movements involves identifying an injustice, the victims of the injustice, and where to direct blame (Benford, 1997). The #MeToo frame assigns meaning to articulations and interpretations intended to mobilize potential adherents, garner support, and demobilize antagonists (Snow & Benford, 1988). This section identifies the injustices, victims, protagonists, and antagonists of the #MeToo movement. Counter injustice claims, injustices that the #MeToo is said to have caused, are also discussed.

Injustice Claims of the #MeToo Movement

Before collective action is likely to occur, a critical mass of people must socially construct a sense of injustice (Hunt & Benford, 1992; Gamson, Fireman, & Rytina, 1982). *Diagnostic framing* refers to the identification of an injustice, identifying the victims of a given injustice and amplifying their victimization (Benford & Hunt, 1992). The widespread participation in #MeToo over social media drew attention to injustices related to the universality and normalization of sexual assault and harassment including the history of women being silenced, dismissed, and not supported after coming forward, and the underreporting of sexual assault to police.

#BelieveWomen and #BelieveVictims are mantras of the #MeToo movement to address injustices. Thus, they constitute *prognostic framing;* the articulation of proposed solutions to the problem that takes place among activists, opponents, targets of influence, media, and bystanders (Benford & Hunt, 1992). Like #MeToo, #BelieveWomen and #BelieveVictims are also Superframes, highly resonant frames for evaluating issues and judging others (Benford & Hunt, 1992; Minsky, 1974).

#BelieveVictims is about being supportive of those who make claims of sexual assault and acknowledging that they are entitled to support, advocacy, and help. The "Believe the Victim" movement originated in the 1970s in the context of psychological treatment to recognize the harm suffered by sexual assault victims and the need for therapists to believe clients claiming sexual assault was necessary and appropriate for therapeutic purposes (Bourke, 2012). Taken literally, the #BelieveWomen and #BelieveVictims hashtags promote the assumption that all sexual assault accusations are automatically true or rarely false. The #MeToo directive to "believe the victim" is supported by the "false accusations are rare" frame and relies on the widely cited statistic from National Sexual Violence Resource Center (2012) that 2–10% of sexual assault reports are false. However, this research has been scrutinized for using unreliable data and unscientific methodologies.[11] There is no clear consensus on the prevalence of "false" or "true" rape accusations. Rape accusations cannot always be classified as either "false" or "true," in reality far more cases fall outside this binary and are never pursued for various reasons (see O'Donohue, Chap. 32, this volume). According to researchers studying false allegations, "To classify a case as a false allegation, a thorough investigation must yield evidence that a crime did not occur" (Lisak, Gardinier, Nicksa, & Cote, 2010). Using the same logic, classifying an allegation as "true" also requires a thorough investigation that yields evidence that a crime *did* occur (Schow, 2018). This would not be a fair assessment either.

Framing literature shows that judgments are not based just on the facts, but on frames. According to George Lakoff (2004) "To be

[11]Turvey, Savino, and Mares (2017) quotes a study by researcher Edward Greer, past president of the Association American Law Schools. Greer traced the one and only source for the "2%" statistic to Susan Brownmiller's (1975) book, "Against Our Will: Men, Women and Rape." Brownmiller cited findings by female police officers in a New York City rape squad. Their methods are unknown and the finding was never verified.

accepted the facts must fit the frame. If the facts don't fit the frame, the facts bounce off" (Lakoff, 2004, p. 17). While the #BelieveWomen and #BelieveVictims frames promote respectful treatment of persons who report sexual assault crimes, they may also encourage the presumption that persons accused of sexual assault are automatically guilty. Framing scholars caution against applying socially constructed frames to specific situations as this ignores the variations in individual experiences and risks causing further injustices (Benford, 1997). The presumption of innocence is part of the "due process" frame and is often misconstrued as being anti-victim. For proponents for of the #BelieveVictims frame, any facts that suggest the accused is innocent, "bounce off." Supporting victims and respecting constitutional protections should exist in the same space but given the strength of the #BelieveWomen / #BelieveVictims frames this is often not the case.

Victims of the #MeToo Movement

Frames reflect existing biases, prejudice, and ideology in society (Edelman, 1993). Women and girls are overwhelmingly victims of sexual abuse and are prominently displayed as victims in the #MeToo movement. Boys and men, while they are also victims of sexual assault, they are also more often the perpetrators of sexual abuse and depicted as such. Women who are poor, are from certain ethnic minorities, and who have intellectual disabilities are disproportionately likely to be victims of rape (USDOJ, 2017). Those who are more likely to be victims of sexual exploitation are also more likely to be marginalized or discounted altogether as victims in the #MeToo movement.

Sex workers, who are at significant risk for sexual victimization, claim their voices had been left out of the #MeToo movement (Cooney, 2018). "Sex workers" refers to people who choose to participate in a range of sex-based work, including prostitutes, escorts, strippers, pornography actors, dominatrixes, erotic massage therapists, and nude webcam models, among other jobs (Cooney, 2018).[12] Confusion among #MeToo activists regarding how to frame support for sex workers was evident during the Women's March in January 2017. Janet Mock, sex worker, author and transgender activist helped draft the guiding principles for the March. She wrote a line stating "…we must stand in solidarity with sex workers' rights." "Sex workers" was later deleted and the line was edited to say that sex exploitation "in all forms is a violation of human rights." It was eventually changed back to Mock's original wording (Vagianos, 2017). The day after the Women's March a group of sex trade survivors and advocates issued an open letter criticizing the March's "pro-sex trade" position as "thoroughly anti-feminist" and condemned March leaders for "ignoring and erasing" the voices of sex trade survivors and for "perpetuat[ing] the status quo of women as commodified goods" (Burris, 2017).

Sex workers criticized Ashley Judd, one of the actresses at the forefront of #MeToo for her activism to abolish all sex work for being "inherently harmful" to women. In angry posts on Twitter, they blasted Judd's "simple-minded" assumptions that all sex workers are women and all their clients are men and that sex workers cannot give consent because the presence of money is proof of coercion (Zimmerman, 2018). They argued that the sex work structure and sex worker experiences are complex and that Judd "lacks the cognitive ability to fully grasp [its] complexity" (Zimmerman, 2018). The backlash from sex workers reflects that #MeToo activists treated sex workers as though their voices represented a unified whole, a tendency that framing scholars caution against as it ignores the uniqueness of individual experiences (Benford, 1997).

#MeToo founder Tarana Burke started the #MeToo movement for black women and girls but feels their voices and their suffering has been ignored (Burke, 2017). She writes, "In 2006, I launched the #MeToo movement because I wanted to find ways to bring healing into the lives of black women and girls. But a year after the

[12] Consensual sex work is not to be confused with sex trafficking when people are forced into sex work by violence, threats or other forms of coercion.

movement they have not felt seen" (Burke, 2018a; Burke, 2018b). Burke told the *Huffington Post*, "It's about the 60% of black girls like me who will be experiencing sexual violence before they turn 18 (Vagianos, 2018).

Writing in the *Yale Law Journal,* Angela Onwuachi-Willig (2018) chastised the #MeToo movement for ignoring the contributions and experiences of women of color, particularly black women, and for failing to recognize the unique forms of harassment and the heightened vulnerability to harassment that women of color frequently face in the workplace. The public perception that Alyssa Milano started #MeToo rather than its actual founder, Tarana Burke, a black woman, highlights a common concern about the ways that black women's contributions can be ignored or dismissed, only to have the same ideas lauded when they are presented by white women (White, 2017).

Journalist Emily Yoffe describes in a September 2017 article in *The Atlantic* how race is almost completely unacknowledged by the government with regard to campus sexual assault. She explains, black males don't fit the archetypal image of the campus rapist—a rich, white fraternity athlete (Yoffe, 2017b). Though black men make up only about 6% of college undergraduates, they are vastly overrepresented in sexual assault cases on college campuses (Yoffe, 2017b). Supporting evidence for this is anecdotal since the Office for Civil Rights (OCR), which regulates how colleges respond to sexual assault, doesn't document the race of the accused and accuser in sexual assault complaints. Harvard Law School professor, Jeannie Suk Gersen (2017) wrote in the *New Yorker* that in general, the campus personnel she'd spoken with who routinely work on sexual-misconduct cases said that most of the complaints they see are against minorities. Michael Jones (2018) writing for the *CollegeFix* profiled 11 cases where black students suffered under false allegations or poorly administered campus tribunals. Many were suspended or expelled, and many had their promising sports careers derailed.

Janet Halley, a professor at Harvard Law School, is one of the few people who have publicly addressed the role of race in campus sexual assault. Halley (2015) argues in the *Harvard Law Review* that interracial assault allegations are a category that bears particular scrutiny given that "American racial history is laced with vendetta-like scandals in which black men are accused of sexually assaulting white women" (p. 106). The social disadvantage black men continue to carry in our culture may make it easier to blame black men and may make it harder for black men to defend themselves against sexual assault allegations (Halley, 2015). Unconscious racial biases might influence some women to view a regretted encounter with a man of a different race as an assault (Yoffe, 2017b). Racial biases, coupled with the lack of resources common among minority students on campus, might systematically disadvantage men of color in adjudication (Yoffe, 2017b). Gersen (2017) noted in her *New Yorker* article, "[If] we have learned from the public reckoning with the racial impact of over-criminalization, mass incarceration, and law enforcement bias, we should heed our legacy of bias against black men in rape accusations."

Policies reacting to the notion that a "rape culture" on campuses that reduce protections for the accused may exacerbate injustices for black students accused of sexual assault. In 2011 the Obama administration issued its "Dear Colleague Letter" (DCL) calling to put an end to "rape culture" on college and university campuses using Title IX, the federal law that prevents discrimination in education (USDOJ, 2011). Definitions of what constitutes sexual misconduct were broadened, and procedures to investigate and adjudicate misconduct were often stacked against the accused; overwhelmingly young men. The DCL guidance warned that every college that receives federal funding (most of them) would risk having that money pulled for noncompliance. In a 2017 *California Law Review* article "The Sex Bureaucracy" about the regulation of sexual assault on college and university campuses, Harvard Law professors Gersen and Suk (2016) argue that, "[C]onduct classified as illegal by the sex bureaucracy has grown substantially and indeed, it plausibly covers almost all sex students are having today" (p. 930).

To support the "rape culture" frame, the DCL guidance cited a study that 1 in 5 females will be raped while at college. The "1 in 5" statistic came from a 2007 study funded by the National Institute of Justice called the Campus Sexual Assault Study (CSA) (Krebs, Lindquist, Warner, Fisher, & Martin, 2007). Lead author of the CSA study, Christopher Krebs cautioned against the reliability of the data stating, "We don't think one in five is a nationally representative statistic" since they had only sampled two schools in their study. Krebs added, "[T]here will never be a definitive estimate of the prevalence of sexual assault" (Yoffe, 2014).[13] Another widely cited and more alarming statistic supporting the "rape culture" frame was a 2000 study commissioned by the U.S. Department of Justice claiming that 1 in 4 college women will be raped while at college.[14] The authors of the study included a disclaimer that their projections were "suggestive" stating, "To assess accurately the victimization risk for women throughout a college career, longitudinal research following a cohort of female students across time is needed" (Fisher, Cullen, & Turner, 2000).

Victim politics in the #MeToo movement reflect elite bias, the tendency for framings to focus on movement elites while neglecting others (Benford, 1997). The most prominent voices on social media and in academia behind #MeToo—white, well-off, able-bodied graduates—are less likely than average to experience sexual violence. Sex workers and black women, though at increased risk for sexual exploitation, tend to be left out as victims. Frames are not based just on the facts, but on frames. The "rape culture" frame, while not necessarily supported by the facts, may subject black male college students accused of sexual misconduct to unfair campus policies a racialized bias.

[13] Krebs noted that the response rate was 42% and there was no way to know if there was response bias, if victims of sexual assault were more likely to participate in the study or not (Krebs & Lindquist, 2014).

[14] An activist organization, One in Four, takes its name from the finding.

Who's to Blame?

Since social movements seek to remedy some problem or issue, directed action is contingent on identification of the source of causality or blame (Benford, 1997). Social movement actors engage in *adversarial framing* (Gamson, 1995) in the construction of antagonists and protagonists. As a Superframe, #MeToo provides "the interpretive medium" in which actors will assign blame for a particular problem (Benford & Hunt, 1992). Framing enables people to "locate, perceive, identify and label" (Goffman, 1974, p. 21). The #MeToo frame draws on already existing cultural anxieties and diagnostic claims to "fortify the identity of their targets by delivering a strong negative identity" (Gamson, 1992, p. 135; Snow & Benford, 1988). A sexual misconduct accusation in the context of #BelieveVictims presumes guilt and the individual is placed in a stigmatized category that can "engulf the total field" or define the individual (Heider, 1958, p. 54). Most people have a certain "picture in their head" of a "sexual predator" (Lippmann, 1946). The "sexual predator" resonates with themes of threat, danger, and low morals, which hypermobilizes blame.

#MeToo founder Tarana Burke says that in the year since the #MeToo movement began, she observed an unwavering obsession with the perpetrators—a cyclical circus of accusations, culpability, and indiscretions (Rowley, 2018). She blames the media for latching onto every salacious detail in #MeToo stories and a culture that fixates on high drama (Rowley, 2018).

Burke (2018b) pointed out on Twitter that #MeToo has been fixated on individuals rather than on the systems of oppression that allow sexual violence, patriarchy, racism and sexism to persist. Burke insists the movement needs to "shift from talking about individuals … and begin to talk about power."

Media scholar, Shanto Iyengar (1996) indicates that news viewers prefer "episodic framing" focused on individuals over "thematic framing" about social contexts. "Episodic framing" is #MeToo news stories are often told using "episodic framing" and point viewers to a specific individual to blame (e.g., Harvey Weinstein) for a certain problem (i.e., sexually exploitive treatment of women). #MeToo stories using "thematic framing" offer a broader theme (i.e., patriarchal systems of power) as the cause of a particular problem (i.e., sexually exploitive treatment of women). "Episodic frames" are more dramatic and cognitively resonant while "thematic frames" tend to be more dull they are often more accurate (Iyengar, 1996). Iyengar found that "episodic frames" promote "individual responsibility" explaining, "It is easier to see cause and treatment in the person depicted than in the context" (Feinburg, 2009).[15]

The #MeToo, #BelieveWomen, #BelieveVictims frames also extend blame to others. In campus Title IX proceedings, witnesses who *defend* the accused pay a social and professional price. Harvard PhD student Tanaya Devi was ostracized by her peers and faculty in her own department for defending Harvard Economics Professor Roland Fryer, who was being investigated in December 2018 for verbal harassment (Taylor, 2019). Devi, who is a dark-skinned native of India and who was present for many of the allegedly harassing comments insisted she saw no harassment and spoke very highly of Fryer, who is black. Racial identity accelerates moral culpability toward antagonists. Race-based stereotypes are culturally embedded and inherent in attitudes about culpability (Jones, 2009). Fryer's lawyer, Harvard Law School Dean Ronald S. Sullivan, also black, stated Fryer "was portrayed as an over-sexualized black man who no one could tell no" (Taylor, 2019).

Reports about the allegations against Fryer highlighted research he had published where he found no evidence of racial bias in police shootings (see Fryer Jr, 2018). According to Fryer, "To make me seem less human they highlighted the part of my research that was the most controversial and failed to mention that the same paper also found racial bias in the form of huge racial differences on lower-level uses of force" (Taylor, 2019). Alex Bell, a PhD student who supports Fryer said, "It's not just white people who think Roland is too black; black people also think Roland is too white, especially after his police shootings paper."

Fryer was found guilty of sexual harassment despite the Harvard investigator concluding that the complainant was probably not telling the truth and multiple eyewitnesses contradicting her claims. Stuart Taylor, coauthor of *Campus of Campus Rape Frenzy*, Harvard Law School graduate, and writer for the *New York Times* criticized the finding against Fryer. He also criticized the *New York Times* coverage of the story for casting Fryer as a criminal and discounting Tanaya Devi's outspoken support of Fryer. Taylor (2019) writes:

> This conclusion seems driven less by evidence than by sympathy for the complainant and a need to win applause from people steeped in "believe-the-woman"—and disbelieve-the-man—ideology by finding Fryer guilty of something. For an ever-expanding, and surely costly, investigation to do less would not have played well in, say, the *New York Times*.

Harvard Dean Ronald Sullivan, while already unpopular for representing Fryer, faced further scrutiny after he joined Harvey Weinstein's legal team as the film producer faces criminal charges of sexual abuse in New York. Students protested calling for Sullivan, to step down as dean citing that representing Weinstein signaled he was unsupportive of survivors of sexual assault and his role as dean made them feel unsafe (Harris, 2019). Sullivan defended his decision to represent Weinstein, saying even "unpopular defendants" have the right to legal representation. In March 2019 52 Harvard faculty members signed an open letter contextualizing Sullivan's decision to represent Weinstein (Avi-Yonah, 2019). The letter states, "[L]egal advocacy in service of constitutional principles is not only fully consistent with Sullivan's roles of law professor and dean ... but one of the many possible models that resident deans can provide in teaching, mentoring, and advising students."

#MeToo critics are deemed antagonists. Journalist Nancy Rommelmann (2019) wrote in the *LA Times* that she was branded hostile to

[15]Iyengar's comments are from an interview with the FrameWorks institute about his work on framing in the media.

sexual assault survivors for discussing frustrations about the #MeToo movement, among other topics on her YouTube series. She described that feminist activists stalked her, took pictures of her and posted them to social media sites. Her husband was driven out of business. Activists called her husband's vendors urging them to stop working for a company that supports "rape culture." Rommelmann pointed out an irony that "so-called feminists," defending a cause to empower women drove a man out of business because his wife voices opinions of her own.

Rommelmann (2019) expressed that she doesn't hate the people who waged the attack, but rather "see[s] them as afraid of ideas of others" and "unwilling to confront the world beyond their small chosen groups." She extended offers to have conversations about the issues they felt were dangerous enough to go to war over but never received a response. Benford (1997) warns against treating frames as though they are a single reality. The #MeToo movement risks becoming oversimplified when nuances and complexities of varied perspectives are neglected.

The attack on Rommelmann represents a broader issue with outrage. The impacts of #MeToo activism rooted in fear and hate traps women in victimhood, demonizes men, and dismisses dissenting women as "man-pleasing collaborators" (Young, 2019).

#MeToo founder Tarana Burke said in a Ted Talk, "Suddenly a movement that was started to support all survivors of sexual violence is being talked about like it's a vindictive plot against men" (Vagianos, 2018). #HimToo has emerged on social media through hashtags and memes as #MeToo's first major inversion; male pushback against #MeToo. #HimToo has been dubbed a "hashtag-slinging countermovement," the #AllLivesMatter of sexual assault (Ellis, 2018). #HimToo serves as a reminder that males can be victims of sexual assault who face similar stigmas and suffer privately. As one user on Twitter wrote, "Sexual harassment and assault are not limited to cis gender women #metoo #hertoo #himtoo #themtoo" (Ellis, 2018). Tarana Burke tweeted, "I've said repeatedly that the #metooMVMT is for all of us, including these brave young men who are now coming forward" (Burke, 2018b).

#HimToo frames the #MeToo movement as "a widespread feminist witch hunt falsely accusing men of sexual misconduct" (Ellis, 2018). Many women, including mothers of boys, are using the hashtag #ProtectOurBoys to denounce what they consider false claims. *Families Advocating for Campus Equality* was founded in 2013 by "three mothers of sons who had been falsely accused of sexual misconduct at their respective colleges," says the group's website, which describes the group as an unbiased, gender-neutral resource for families going through the sexual misconduct disciplinary process on campus. *Save Our Sons* advocates for men's rights by publicizing stories and legal cases about college men and schoolboys who have been acquitted of sexual misconduct charges or to have suffered unjustly at the hands of accusers (Save Our Sons, 2019).[16]

Counter Injustice Claims

Disputes often erupt between and within social movement organizations. "Framing contests," or square offs between movements and their detractors with detractors making counter injustice claims (Ryan, 1991).

Sexual Misconduct, One Term Fits All?

"Sexual misconduct" is the most commonly used term to define unacceptable sexual behavior. Use of such a broad term can be problematic when it is used to describe nearly every behavior deemed sexually inappropriate and is regarded with the same level of seriousness and the same consequences as sexual assault (Davis, 2018a, 2018b). Masha Gessen (2017) writing for the *New Yorker* said, "the distinctions between rape and coercion are meaningful, in the way it is meaningful to distinguish between, say, murder and battery."

[16]More information about Save Our Sons can be found at https://helpsaveoursons.com/

Actor Matt Damon faced social media backlash when he suggested that a "spectrum" of sexual misconduct needs to be taken into account when evaluating the men who have faced allegations (Gans, 2017). Though Damon himself had never been accused of sexual misconduct, his comments were highly publicized, and he was immediately attacked.[17] Damon was accused of "mansplaining," where a man explains something in a way that is oversimplified and condescending to women. The backlash against Damon represented antagonism toward men and revealed a #MeToo double standard. When #MeToo founder Tarana Burke (Davis, 2018a, 2018b) made a similar argument in an article she penned for *Variety* magazine social media paid little attention. Burke wrote, "Sexual violence happens on a spectrum, so accountability has to happen on a spectrum. And that means various ways of being accountable are necessary." The backlash against Damon illustrates the strength of the #MeToo frame and resistance to complexities. A possible explanation for the resistance to distinguish between different sexual behaviors under the #MeToo frame traces back to frames encouraging a single reality and simplifying the issue of sexual assault. And thus, reducing the ability to address the problem of sexual violence in a critical way. Psychologist Deborah L. Davis (2018a, 2018b) writing in *Psychology Today* points out, "[T]reating all transgressions as equally criminal is foolish and destructive. [I]f we can't do the hard work of differentiating between degrees of transgression, the #MeToo movement can't do the hard work of changing social norms."

[17]The first to call Damon out was ex-girlfriend Minnie Driver, his and co-star in their 1997 film Good Will Hunting. After more than a year of dating, Driver learned that the two were no longer a couple from when Matt Damon in an appearance on "The Oprah Winfrey Show" told Oprah that he was single. A construct coined by Greg Matoesian (1995), "the patriarchal logic of sexual rationality" in his analysis of the William Kennedy Smith trial describes a strategy employed by Kennedy's lawyer with the premise that women who are rejected allege rape for revenge.

#MeToo Backlash

Allegations against comedian Aniz Ansari were a catalyst for the first notable backlash against the #MeToo movement for its promotion of gendered frames that remove female agency and paint women as helpless victims. The allegations against Ansari were by an anonymous woman, "Grace," and published in the online publication *Babe* in January 2018. Grace described going to Ansari's home after a date. They kissed and had oral sex until she put on the brakes. They got dressed, watched TV and he started kissing her again. She told him "You guys are all the same" and cried on way home. Ansari texted Grace the next day, saying it was fun meeting her. She responded that he had ignored her nonverbal cues and made her cry. "I'm so sad to hear this," he wrote back. "Clearly, I misread things in the moment and I'm truly sorry." After talking to friends, Grace concluded that Ansari had sexually assaulted her. She told the *Babe* reporter, "I was debating if this was an awkward sexual experience or sexual assault. And that's why I confronted so many of my friends and listened to what they had to say" (Way, 2018).

After the allegations against Ansari went viral, the internet was awash with claims and counterclaims about the rights and wrongs of what had taken place. Some believed his behavior exemplified the aggressive, entitled, chauvinistic attitude that too many men show towards women (Roberts, 2018). Others felt Ansari was the victim of a witch hunt, persecuted by an internet mob with no respect for due process and didn't deserve to be publicly humiliated and professionally assassinated (Weiss, 2018).

Counter Injustice Claim: #MeToo Hurts Women and Victims

Some fear that the #MeToo frame has been trivialized by partisan and reactionary discourse and that this will harm women, particularly victims of sexual abuse, and be detrimental to feminist gains. The #MeToo mantra to "Believe all women" has been criticized for being condescending to women and fetishizing them. “Women are no longer human and flawed. They are Truth personified. They are above reproach… it’s condescending to think that women and their claims can’t stand up to interrogation and can’t handle skepticism” (Weiss, 2017).

Social movements are comprised of interacting, coacting, and reacting human beings (Benford, 1993; Buechler, 1993; Hunt & Benford, 2004). As such, Benford (1997) criticizes the tendency to treat socially constructed frames as though they are *real* and exist independent of the actors involved. He states, “Social movements do not frame issues; their activists or other participants do the framing” (Benford, 1997, p. 418). This reification, he argues, neglects human agency where “human action and interaction are stripped from the text” (p. 418).

Following the allegations against Ansari, high-profile women in the media blamed #MeToo and #BelieveWomen for imposing victimhood on young women. Bari Weiss (2018) in her *New York Times* article, “Aniz Ansari is Guilty. Of Not Being a Mind Reader” writes, “I’m apparently the victim of sexual assault. And if you’re a sexually active woman in the 21st century, chances are that you are, too.”

Female commentators warned the allegations against Ansari infantilized women as incapable of enforcing personal boundaries. Christine Hoff Sommers, author of “The War Against Boys” and “Who Stole Feminism?,” argues that *equity feminism* has been eclipsed by what she calls *fainting couch feminism* or *victim feminism* which views women as fragile, easily traumatized and as an oppressed and silenced class (Saul, 2017). Weiss (2018) argues #MeToo is reflective of Grace’s narrative where Ansari is depicted as the only one having agency while Grace is merely acted upon. She writes, “[W]hat ought to be a movement for women’s empowerment [was turned] into an emblem for female helplessness.” Cable news host Ashleigh Banfield criticized Grace’s inability to distinguish between a “bad date” and “sexual assault” (Baragona, 2018). Meghan Holstein (2018) in her piece for *Medium* argued that conflating negative feelings with lack of consent may lead women to mischaracterize awkward sexual encounters as sexual assault. She writes, “When she processes her emotions, later on, she will experience regret. That doesn’t make that interaction rape.” Holstein (2018) suggests that awkward sexual experiences can be avoided by “clearly communicat[ing] what they want (or didn’t want), *when* they wanted it (or didn’t want it).”

Grace’s comment about talking to her friends to determine if she had been sexually assaulted offers insight into her ability to make decisions on her own about what happens in her life. Research finds that each time we recall an event, it is being reassembled, and sometimes changed by the very process of recall. A 2015 study by the education insurance group United Educators analyzing 305 student claims of sexual assault at 104 colleges found that 40% delayed reporting an assault and “in most cases [the student] labeled the incident a sexual assault only after talking with friends or attending prevention training” (Keehan, Caputo, Pettegrew, & Bennett, 2015). The study, which was conducted before #MeToo went viral, suggests that decision-making among many young people regarding sexual victimization is subject to outside influence. The increase in discourse and prevention training following #MeToo may further “prime” decisions about victimhood.

The #MeToo movement has caused sexual assault advocacy, training, and education efforts to proliferate. Programs often apply trauma-informed approaches that send the message to young people that they are biologically programmed to become helpless during unwanted sexual encounters and to suffer mental impairment afterward (Yoffe, 2017a). Alcohol can further impact memory. Given that he majority of sexual assaults on college campuses (78%) involve alcohol, young people may inadvertently be encouraged to view consensual late-night, alcohol-fueled encounters that might produce disjointed memories and some regret as something more sinister (Keehan et al., 2015).

Disputes among women about the Ansari allegations and positions regarding #MeToo were quickly characterized in the media as generational. Older feminists (anyone over 40) were considered sinisterly complicit, laughably outdated, or just too scared of overstepping. Younger women are either righteously passionate, naively idealistic, or out for blood. Feminist icon and author of the Handmaid's Tale, 78-year-old Margaret Atwood was criticized by young feminists for speaking out against #MeToo. Atwood (2018) responded by writing a piece called, "Am I a Bad Feminist?" in the UK's *Globe and Mail* where she gave her perspective of the dangers and consequences of treating women as though they have limited agency. Atwood (2018) writes:

> My fundamental position is that women are human beings. Nor do I believe that women are children, incapable of agency or of making moral decisions. If they were, we're back to the 19th century, and women should not own property, have credit cards, have access to higher education, control their own reproduction or vote. There are powerful groups in North America pushing this agenda, but they are not usually considered feminists... they are just feeding into the very old narrative that holds women to be incapable of fairness or of considered judgment, and they are giving the opponents of women yet another reason to deny them positions of decision-making in the world.

Overall, the allegations against Ansari were said to damage the #MeToo movement and served to discredit women and trivialize victimhood. Bari Weiss (2018) of *The New York Times* called the Ansari allegations "the worst thing that has happened to the #MeToo movement since it began."

Surveys suggest that the storm of sexual assault allegations, confessions, and firings in the wake of #MeToo has actually made Americans more skeptical about sexual misconduct. A poll in the *Economist* surveying 1500 Americans in November 2017 and September 2018 revealed a small but clear shift against victims of sexual assault and misconduct ("Measuring the #MeToo backlash," 2018). In a column for the *Atlantic*, contributing editor Caitlin Flanagan (2018) called the allegations against Ansari "proof that women are angry, temporarily powerful—and very, very dangerous".

Counter Injustice Claim: #BelieveWomen Undermines Due Process

A prominent counter injustice frame alleges that the #MeToo directive to "believe all women" with claims of sexual abuse undermines the presumption of innocence for the accused. The #BelieveEvidence hashtag is used to reject that women should always be believed and signals a perspective in favor of due process for the accused. As most victims of sexual violence are women and most of those accused of sexual violence are men, the two hashtags pit women and men against each other.

Commentators argue that asserting that women are always telling the truth and that accused men are always guilty is irresponsible, uncritical, and destructive. Writing for *New York Magazine* Andrew Sullivan (2018) likened the #MeToo movement to McCarthyism stating, "[Activists] believe they are fighting an insidious, ubiquitous evil—the patriarchy—just as the extreme anti-Communists in the 1950s believed that commies were everywhere and so foul they didn't deserve a presumption of innocence, or simple human decency." In an interview for *The Guardian*, Margaret Atwood likens the #MeToo politics of ignoring due process to the Salem Witch Trials. Atwood points out that "'innocent until proven guilty' is the key to a civilized society" and worries that "guilt by accusation" has at times been used justify new forms of oppression" (Kassam, 2018). In an editorial for *The Harvard Crimson*, Elizabeth Bartholet writes that while she "applaud[s] the removal of many alleged perpetrators who have clearly abused their positions of power" and "celebrate[s] those who have stepped forward to call out sexual misconduct" what she finds "deeply troubling" is the argument that "if some innocent men must be sacrificed to the cause of larger justice, so be it" (Bartholet, 2018).

#MeToo and #DueProcess are effectively competing frames. In a rational world, proponents of #MeToo don't want innocent men to be punished for a rape they didn't commit just as those who advocate for #DueProcess don't want those who commit rape to escape accountability and hurt others. Therein lies the power of frames. The strength of the #MeToo frame has caused many to be reticent about speaking out against due process in the for the accused for fear of being accused themselves of siding with rapists. Within the #MeToo frame, advocating for due process is viewed as a category of "rape myth acceptance." #DueProcess has become a proxy for favoring the accused, being an apologist of inappropriate behavior, and as generally being unsupportive of women and victims of sexual assault.

The Obama-era guidance to end "rape culture" on college and university campuses called for more vigorous investigation of campus sexual-assault claims using Title IX, the federal law that prevents discrimination in education (USDOJ, 2011). The letter didn't specify procedural safeguards or rules for the examination of evidence. As a result, colleges and universities developed and implemented their own procedures, which vary widely from campus to campus. The Obama-era guidance, while well intentioned, subjected victims and the accused to an unreliable process. A 2019 survey of college and university presidents by *Inside Higher Ed* and Gallup found that 42% of public university leaders and 60% of those at private colleges agree or strongly agree that "the Obama administration's approach did not place enough emphasis on due process for those accused of sexual assault or harassment (Piper, 2019). A 2018 report by the Foundation for Individual Rights in Education (FIRE) revealed that nearly three quarters (73.6%) of America's top 53 universities do not guarantee presumption of innocence in campus proceedings regarding sexual misconduct (FIRE, 2018).

Some schools have implemented procedures that may be considered arbitrary and capricious, ultimately opening the gate for lawsuits from either an alleged victim who may feel that he or she was not adequately heard or from an accused individual who feels unjustly punished. According to a 2015 study by United Educators (a large national insurance provider for colleges and universities), about one-third of all Title IX-related lawsuits against institutions are brought by those accused of sexual misconduct (Keehan et al., 2015).

As of 2018 nearly 400 accused students have taken their schools to court citing violations of due process and gender bias against males (of which is a violation of Title IX) and courts are increasingly finding in their favor. The National Center for Higher Education Risk Management (NCHERM) a law firm that provides Title IX consulting to hundreds of colleges and universities urged that higher-education institutions are "losing case after case in federal court on what should be very basic due process protections" (NCHERM, 2017). KC Johnson and Stuart Taylor (Johnson & Taylor Jr, 2017) in their book *Campus Frenzy* discuss how since Obama's 2011 Title IX guidance universities have lost more than 100 federal and state court decisions in lawsuits brought by students accused of sexual assault, and that 53 more lawsuits (at the federal level alone) were settled before a court could render any decision. Seventy-two percent of accused students who sued the institution also sued the victim for defamation or slander (Keehan et al., 2015). Given the strength of the #BelieveVictim frame, this suggests that litigation may also be a means to repair the reputation of the accused. The lawsuits revealed that the accused students, mostly males, faced investigations characterized by anti-male bias and pro-accuser bias among academic officials. In a 2016 decision involving a student from Brandeis University, U.S. District Judge F. Dennis Saylor criticized victim-centric investigative practices. He wrote, "Whether someone is a 'victim' is a conclusion to be reached at the end of a fair process, not an assumption to be made at the beginning" (*Doe v Brandeis*, 2016, p. 12).

Lawsuits cited other unfair procedures such as secret training of adjudicators to believe accusers even in the face of discrediting evidence; concealment of exculpatory evidence; bans of meaningful cross-examination; designation of a single investigator; and in some cases the accused were not allowed to know what they were being accused of, who was accusing them, evidence against them, or given the opportunity to defend themselves. Many schools also limit the ability of the accused to present evidence and call witnesses in their defense. Schools impose campus bans prohibiting the accused from being on campus or gag orders directing the accused to not speak with anyone affiliated with the school including students, staff, and faculty. Title IX investigators use the lowest standard of proof, the preponderance of evidence (50% plus a feather) to determine the likelihood of a sexual misconduct violation, including sexual assault, a violent criminal offense. The Foundation for Individual Rights in Education (FIRE) which advocates for civil liberties on campus noted, "Given the marked lack of core due process protections in the vast majority of campus judicial systems, the adjudication of such serious, life-altering accusations requires more than our lowest standard of proof." The American Association of University Professors and the American College of Trial Lawyers have made similar points (Johnson & Taylor, 2018a).

The debate over due process protections for those accused of sexual misconduct on college campuses exhibited the strength of the #MeToo frame while simultaneously exposing its flaws. The "rape culture" frame promotes an artificially inflated sense of justice denied which creates incentives for a separate justice system for sexual-abuse cases that minimizes due process for the accused (e.g., Title IX sexual assault tribunals on college campuses). The overwhelmingly liberal campus climate in the US reflects a dedication to the "rape culture" and "believe the victim" frames and opposition to due process protections for those accused of sexual misconduct.

Liberal politicians operate on frames over facts regarding legislation to address the "rape culture" on college campuses. Kirsten Gillibrand, a Democratic senator from New York who cosponsored CASA (the Campus Accountability and Safety Act) in 2015, took the "rape culture" frame to a new level of danger.[18] Gillibrand announced, "We should never accept the fact that women are at a greater risk of sexual assault as soon as they step onto a college campus. But today they are." Government statistics say the opposite. The US Bureau of Justice's National Crime Victimization Survey (NCVS) shows that women in college are *less* likely to be sexually assaulted than women not attending college. From 1995 to 2011 NCVS found that of females aged 18–24 who reported being victims of threatened, attempted, or completed rape/sexual assault, 0.6% were in college and 0.8% were not in college (Sinozich & Langton, 2014).

Senator Gillibrand had invited "Mattress Girl" Emma Sulkowicz to the State of the Union where she introduced the CASA legislation. Emma Sulkowicz, a Columbia University student, became a symbol of "rape culture" and the failure to address sexual assault on college campuses. Sulkowicz began carrying a 50-pound mattress around campus after her Title IX rape accusation was determined to be invalid. Sulkowicz was the subject of multiple profiles in *The New York Times*. After messages between Sulkowicz and her "rapist" surfaced, it became apparent that Sulkowicz had likely falsified her rape claim because her "rapist" was not interested in a romantic relationship with her (Bauer-Wolf, 2017).

In September 2017, Betsy Devos, the US Secretary of Education appointed by Trump rescinded the Obama administration's Title IX guidelines for adjudicating sexual misconduct on college campuses (USDOJ, 2017). In November 2018, Devos released new guidelines designed to restore fairness to campus Title IX sexual assault and harassment investigations, guided by legal precedents from lawsuits brought by accused students (USDOE, 2018). These guidelines include the right for accused students to be presumed innocent; a proposal granting accusers and the accused the right to cross-examine witnesses through a lawyer or an advocate; and the right of the accused to examine all the evidence uncovered in the campus investigation, and all the materials used to train campus adjudicators. Her proposals were met with strong opposition by #MeToo activists, with the most

[18]The guidance would, among other things, require all colleges provide a confidential adviser to guide victims through the entire process of bringing an accusation while no guidance or assistance is mandated for the accused.

vocal being liberal college students and university leaders.

Devos proposed implementing cross-examination which the Supreme Court described as the "greatest legal engine ever invented for the discovery of truth" (*California v Green*, 1970, p. 11). In *Doe v Baum* (2018) a lawsuit brought by a University of Michigan student found guilty of sexual assault and expelled, the judge determined that in "he-said, she-said" cases the university must allow cross-examination to satisfy due process. University students and leaders argued that cross examination would deter sexual assault victims from reporting sexual assault and would retraumatize the accuser.

Devos opposed the single investigator model where one person serves as prosecutor, detective, judge, and executioner. A federal court ruling against Brandeis University, cited the "obvious" dangers "of combining in a single individual the power to investigate, prosecute, and convict" (*Doe v Brandeis University*, p. 70). University leaders praised the single investigator model and criticized Devos for micromanaging campus handling of sexual assault (Johnson, 2019).

Devos's new guidelines proposed that trauma-informed training for title IX investigators be public given that training programs use unsupported science on trauma that rationalizes inconsistencies in the accuser's account, gaps or lack of memory, and that "freezing" is a common response to sexual advances regardless of whether violence or threats of violence were present (Yoffe, 2017a). Harvard law professor Janet Halley has ridiculed the trauma-informed training used at her university. Halley told Emily Yoffe in an interview for *The Atlantic* that the trauma-informed Title IX training materials at Harvard were "100% aimed to convince them to believe complainants, precisely when they seem unreliable and incoherent" (Yoffe, 2017a).

The American Civil Liberties Union (ACLU) ironically voiced opposition to *civil liberty* initiatives outlined by Devos' new Title IX guidelines stating they promote an "unfair process" The ACLU stated in a tweet (ACLU, 2018):

> It promotes an unfair process, inappropriately favoring the accused and letting schools ignore their responsibility under Title IX to respond promptly and fairly to complaints of sexual violence.

Senator Claire McCaskill, a Democrat from Missouri and a cosponsor of the CASA bill, said to the *Washington Post* stated, "I don't think we are anywhere near a tipping point where the people accused of this are somehow being treated unfairly" (Anderson, 2014). Democratic senator Dianne Feinstein tweeted that allowing cross-examination and equal access to evidence would "silence" and "drown out the voices of victims" (Johnson & Taylor, 2018b). Rejecting Devos's Title IX guidelines appears to be less about balancing fair procedures in campus investigations and more about rejecting the Trump administration.

Framing and Partisan Politics in the #MeToo Era

Competing interpretations of #MeToo discourse has become highly polarized among political lines. Framing activity and the extent of its resonance are affected by the cultural and political environment (McAdam, 1999). An October 2017 Pew Research poll of US adults found that 69% of Democrats felt that the country hasn't gone far enough in granting women equal rights with men while only 26% of Republicans agreed with the sentiment (Horowitz, Parker, & Stepler, 2017). Framing processes and political opportunity are linked interactively, the extent to which they constrain or facilitate collective action depends on how they are framed by movement actors and others (Koopmans & Duyvendak, 1995). A December 2017 Pew Research poll revealed that Democratic women were more likely to identify as a victim compared to Republican women, suggesting a relationship between political identity and identifying as a victim. While half of Democratic women said that they experienced at least one form of gender discrimination at work while only a third of Republican women felt the same way (Parker & Funk, 2017).

In August 2018, Trump's nominee for the US Supreme Court, Brett Kavanaugh was accused of sexual misconduct. Kavanaugh's accuser, Christine Blasey Ford testified before the US Senate. The hearings politicized #MeToo with conservatives calling for due process while liberals insisted "#BelieveWomen," and reflected the tone and line of questioning from senators posed to Kavanaugh and Ford. Emily Yoffe (2018) writing in *The Atlantic* summed up the politicization of sexual assault, "Sexual violence is a serious national problem. But in the wake of the Kavanaugh hearing, it has joined the list of explosively partisan issues." After the Kavanaugh hearings #DueProcess and #BelieveWomen hashtags were memorialized as a way to signal political allegiances.

The politically charged due process vs #BelieveWomen debate during Kavanaugh's confirmation hearing was compared to campus Title IX tribunals. John Davidson (2018) writing for the *Federalist* stated that Democrats are trying to turn the Kavanaugh Supreme Court confirmation hearing into "a Kafkaesque version of a Title IX tribunal" where "the accused is presumed guilty, may not know the identity of the accuser, and is not permitted to mount a defense." During the Kavanaugh hearings Trump fueled the "due process" frame calling it a "Scary Time" for young men generating the #scarytime hashtag on Twitter. In his tweet Trump declared (Trump, 2018):

> It's a very scary time for young men in America when you can be guilty of something that you may or may not be guilty of. Peoples (sic) lives are being shattered and destroyed by a mere allegation [...] There is no recovery for someone falsely accused—life and career are gone. Is there no such thing any longer as Due Process?

This arguably marked the moment when "due process" became a firmly partisan frame, not equated with fairness and justice but signaled being pro-Trump and thus hostile to sexual assault survivors. The "due process" frame is now liable for nearly any other grievance about Trump.

Republican Senate majority leader Mitch McConnell weighed in on the importance of due process during Kavanaugh's confirmation process stating, "[T]otally uncorroborated allegations [must not be] enough to destroy an American's life" (Johnson & Taylor, 2018b). Republican Senator Susan Collins said, "In evaluating any given claim of misconduct, we will be ill served in the long run if we abandon the presumption of innocence and fairness, tempting though it may be. It is when passions are most inflamed that fairness is most in jeopardy" (Johnson & Taylor, 2018b).

Senator Mazie Hirono, a Democrat from Hawaii warned that Kavanaugh's confirmation will "send a message to every victim of sexual violence that their pain doesn't matter, that they do not deserve justice, and that for them, fair treatment is out of reach" (*CNN*, 2018). Richard Blumenthal, a Democrat Senator from Connecticut asserted that Kavanaugh's confirmation was threatening women's rights (Nilsen & Zhou, 2018).

Is #MeToo a Moral Panic?

#MeToo appears to be characteristic of a moral panic, where a social condition or group of persons is defined as a grave threat to societal values and interests (Cohen, 1972). Stages of a moral panic include defining a threat which is depicted in a simple and recognizable symbol by the media (i.e., #MeToo), a response by policy makers (i.e., Title IX guidance) and the moral panic itself resulting in social changes (Cohen, 1972).

A moral panic involves a heightened level of concern about an issue and its impact on the rest of society (i.e., gender inequality, "campus rape culture"), and reflects simple, punitive solutions to complex problems (i.e., #BelieveWomen, "guilt by accusation," rejecting due process). Fear tends to produce emotional, reactionary responses rather than a rational assessment of a problem. This leads to increased hostility directed toward a person or group and/or their problematic behavior and a consensus in society about who this "evildoer" is (i.e., those accused of sexual misconduct and their supporters; anyone who criticizes #MeToo) (Cohen, 1972).

For individuals who regularly view #MeToo stories and posts and have tailored the news to their belief system, that information can engender the belief that a greater portion of the population is engaged in this disturbing behavior than actually is, or that the harm incurred is greater than what has occurred. Existing research has portrayed college campuses as such bastions of "rape culture" and discriminatory toward women when at the same time, female enrollment in colleges has surpassed that of males. While theory and reality suggest that moral panic exaggerates the threat, fierce support of the campus "rape culture" frame in spite of facts, and the intense opposition to due process in campus rape proceedings reflect tangible consequences of the #MeToo moral panic.

Conclusion

Social media has become an important part of our personal, public, professional, and political lives. The #MeToo movement is clearly having an important impact that will help to shape how we publicly discuss sexual assault for years to come. Going forward there are some "counter frames" or challenges to the versions of reality promoted by #MeToo that activists, participants, and supporters might consider in order to better address the injustice claims of the #MeToo movement and to minimize unintended consequences and related injustices that the #MeToo movement promotes (Benford, 1987).

First, just because #MeToo is popular doesn't mean that #MeToo can solve every problem overnight. Social media allowed #MeToo to gain in popularity very quickly. #MeToo founder Tarana Burke expressed, "Part of the challenge of Me Too getting so popular is that people think that the popularity is a solution" (Smola, 2018). Burke cautions however that #MeToo has been spread too thin. She observes that people are "taking the infrastructure that already exists—#MeToo, the movement and the hashtag—and appending additional ideas to it." Burke is describing "frame extension," a frame alignment process from social movements literature that involves "extending the boundaries" of a frame (Snow, Rochford Jr, Worden, & Benford, 1986, p. 469). Extending the frame too far risks straying from its original purpose which can result in loss of support for the cause. Burke believes that extending the boundaries of #MeToo asks too much of the movement by "weighing it down with the inevitable freight of hope and expectation" (Garber, 2018, p. 1).

Second, humans and their interactions are complex and far more nuanced than the #MeToo movement accounts for. #MeToo is a socially constructed frame, made by humans, experienced by humans. Humans must not be stripped from the context. We must resist applying socially constructed frames to individual-level explanations as this neglects the complexities of humans and the issues being addressed by the #MeToo movement. We should keep in mind that our brain simplifies information often without our knowledge. We are all subject to unconscious biases. In a 2019 interview Supreme Court Justice Ruth Bader Ginsberg pointed to acknowledgment of "unconscious biases" as her message to the next generation of feminists (Rosen, 2019). This includes the racial and social biases that exist in culture that marginalizes those who are victimized the most. Failure to acknowledge the ways in which unconscious bias influences judgements and evaluations others hinders addressing #MeToo injustices in an effective way.

Furthermore, Burke argues that failing to center marginalized voices in our movements relegates these voices to "no more than a footnote" and that "it will require those whose voices are most often heard to find ways to amplify those voices that often go unheard" (Burke, 2017). We know that those voices who are most heard in the #MeToo movement are white, educated women. An analysis of partisan prejudice by Predictwise, a polling and analytics firm, found in a ranking of counties in the U.S. that the most politically *intolerant* Americans tend to be white, highly educated and more partisan themselves (Ripley, Tenjarla, & He, 2019). Burke urges, "We have to shift the narrative that it's a gender war, that it's anti-male, that it's men against women, that it's only for a certain type of person—that it's for white, cisgender, heterosexual, famous women. That has to shift… that's a part of our work, too" (Rowley, 2018, p. 1).

Third, things need to be fair. For the #MeToo movement to influence change for the better, it must seek justice, not perpetuate injustice. Supporting victims of violence and due process for those accused of violent crimes are fundamental values in our society. According to Ginsburg (Rosen, 2019, p. 1):

> Supporting survivors of sexual assault and establishing systems of equitable justice are not mutually exclusive. Due process is not an obstruction to justice, it is a foundation of the American rule of law and was meant to be a barrier to hasty judgment and conviction by public opinion". (Rosen, 2019, p. 1)

The CEO of TIME'S UP Lisa Borders resigned in February 2019 following sexual misconduct allegations against her son (French, 2019). Borders resigned because TIME'S UP, an organization that addresses sexual assault and harassment in the workplace, viewed support for survivors and support for the accused as a zero-sum game (TIME'S UP, 2019).[19] This reflected a missed opportunity to contextualize support for survivors of sexual assault and due process for accused in the same space as Ginsburg suggests.

The #MeToo movement aims to address unfair and biased practices that invalidate women who spoke out about sexual abuse. Real equality for men and women means procedures that do not presume either side is innocent or guilty. The solution is to eliminate unfair and biased processes, not simply shift them to those accused of sexual assault. Ginsburg offers that young people play a significant role in upholding fairness in the #MeToo era. Ginsburg states (Rosen, 2019):

> The person who is accused has a right to defend herself or himself, and we certainly should not lose sight of that… Young people should appreciate the values on which our nation is based and how precious they are, and if they don't become part of the crowd that seeks to uphold them … Learned Hand said—if the spirit of liberty dies in the hearts of the people, there is no court capable of restoring it. (p. 1)

[19]To learn more about TIME'S UP refer to this link: https://www.timesupnow.com/about_times_up

Court decisions have become so problematic for universities that many campuses are being forced to change policies to restore due process regardless of whether the Trump administration implements its new Title IX regulations or not. In February 2019, court rulings deemed existing procedures for investigating Title IX cases in California so unfair that colleges and universities across the state were forced to halt ongoing Title IX proceedings and reevaluate ways to implement more balanced policies (Watanabe & Hussain, 2019).

Finally, change requires male participation. #MeToo activities, definitions, and processes that criminalize or demonize men can lead to the unintended consequence of turning men and women into opposing camps. According to Burke, "[T]he [#MeToo] movement is actually working when the public understands that there is no expected narrative, standard perpetrator and victim, or archetypical story of abuse". (Rowley, 2018. p. 1)

References

Allport, G. W. (1954). *The nature of prejudice*. New York, NY: Perseus Publishing.

ACLU. (2018, November 16). [Twitter entry]. https://twitter.com/ACLU/status/1063456843706585089

Andalibi, N., Haimson, O. L., De Choudhury, M., & Forte, A. (2016, May). Understanding social media disclosures of sexual abuse through the lenses of support seeking and anonymity. In *Proceedings of the 2016 CHI conference on human factors in computing systems* (pp. 3906–3918). New York: ACM.

Anderson, M., & Toor, S. (2018, October 11). *How social media users have discussed sexual harassment since #MeToo went viral*. Retrieved from http://www.pewresearch.org/fact-tank/2018/10/11/how-social-media-users-have-discussed-sexual-harassment-since-metoo-went-viral/

Anderson, N. (2014, August 24). *The Washington Post*. Men punished in sexual misconduct cases on college campuses are fighting back. Retrieved from https://www.washingtonpost.com/local/education/men-punished-in-sexual-misconduct-cases-on-colleges-campuses-are-fighting-back/2014/08/20/96bb3c6a-1d72-11e4-ae54-0cfe1f974f8a_story.html

Ardovini-Brooker, J., & Caringella-MacDonald, S. (2002). Media attributions of blame and sympathy in ten rape cases. *The Justice Professional, 15*, 3–18. https://doi.org/10.1080/08884310212826

Atwood, M. (2018). Am I a bad feminist? *The Globe and Mail.* Retrieved May 15, 2018, from: https://www.theglobeandmail.com/opinion/am-i-a-bad-feminist/article37591823/?utm_source=facebook.com&utm_medium=Referrer%3A+Social+Network+%2F+Media&utm_campaign=Shared+Web+Article+Links

Avi-Yonah, S. S. (2019, February 4). Winthrop dean Sullivan defends Fryer, criticizes Harvard investigation. *The Harvard Crimson.* Retrieved from https://www.thecrimson.com/article/2019/2/4/sullivan-defends-freyer/

Baragona, J. (2018, January 15). HLN host Ashleigh Banfield destroys Aniz Ansari accuser: "You have chipped away at a movement". *Mediaite.* Retrieved from https://www.mediaite.com/tv/ashleigh-banfield-blasts-aziz-ansaris-accuser-you-have-chiseled-away-at-the-metoo-movement/

Bartlett, F. C. (1932). *Remembering: A study in experimental and social psychology*. Cambridge, UK: Cambridge University Press.

Bartholet, E. (2018, January 16). #MeToo excesses. *The Harvard Crimson.* Retrieved from https://www.thecrimson.com/article/2018/1/16/bartholet-metoo-excesses/

Bauer-Wolf, J. (2017, July 24). Mattress protest and its aftermath. *Inside Higher Ed.* Retrieved from https://www.insidehighered.com/news/2017/07/24/media-circus-surrounding-mattress-girl-case-changed-conversation-sexual-assault

Benford, R. D. (1997). An insider's critique of the social movement framing perspective. *Sociological Inquiry, 67*(4), 409–430.

Benford, R. D., & Hunt, S. A. (1992). Dramaturgy and social movements: The social construction and communication of power. *Sociological Inquiry, 62*(1), 36–55.

Benford, R. D. (1993). "You could be the hundredth monkey": Collective action frames and vocabularies of motive within the nuclear disarmament movement. *Sociological Quarterly, 34*(2), 195–216.

Benford, R. D., & Snow, D. A. (2000). Framing processes and social movements: An overview and assessment. *Annual Review of Sociology, 26*(1), 611–639.

Black, N., Henry, M., Lewis, W. S., Morris, L., Oppenheim, A., Schuster, S. K., Sokolow, B. A., Swinton, D. C. (2017). *Due process and the sex police*. The National Council for Higher Education and Risk Management (NCHERM). Retrieved from https://cdn.tngconsulting.com/website-media/ncherm.org/unoffloaded/2017/04/TNG-Whitepaper-Final-Electronic-Version.pdf

Bourke, J. (2012, May 1). Sexual violence, bodily pain, and trauma: A history theory. *Culture and Society, 29*(3), 25.

Brownmiller, S. (1975). *Against our will: men, women and rape*. New York: Simon & Schuster.

Buechler, S. M. (1993). Beyond resource mobilization? Emerging trends in social movement theory. *The Sociological Quarterly, 34*(2), 217–235.

Burke, T. (2017, November 9). #MeToo was started for Black and Brown women and girls. They're still being ignored. *Washington Post*. Retrieved from https://www.washingtonpost.com/news/post-nation/wp/2017/11/09/the-waitress-who-works-in-the-diner-needs-to-know-that-the-issue-of-sexual-harassment-is-about-her-too

Burke, T. (2018a). #MeToo Founder Tarana Burke on the Rigorous Work That Still Lies Ahead. *Variety.* Retrieved from https://variety.com/2018/biz/features/tarana-burke-metoo-one-year-later-1202954797/

Burke, T. (2018b, August 20). [*Twitter entry*]. Retrieved from https://twitter.com/TaranaBurke/status/1031498206260150272

Burleigh, N. (2018, February 20). The social media Psy-op that took down Al Franken. *Newsweek.* https://www.msn.com/en-us/news/politics/the-social-mediapsy-op-that-took-down-al-franken/ar-BBJjJpC

Burns, R., & Crawford, C. (1999). School shootings, the media, and public fear: Ingredients for a moral panic. *Crime, Law and Social Change, 32*(2), 147–168.

Burris,A.(2017,January22).Openletterfromsextradesurvivors. Medium. Retrieved from https://medium.com/@autumnburris/open-letter-from-sex-trade-survivors-b18b3781d101

California v Green, 387 S.Ct 399 U.S. 149. (Sup. Ct. 1970).

Caputi, T. L., Nobles, A. L., & Ayers, J. W. (2018, December). Internet searches for sexual harassment and assault, reporting, and training since the #MeToo movement. *JAMA Internal Medicine.* https://doi.org/10.1001/jamainternmed.2018.5094.

Carmon, I., & Brittain, A. (2017, November 20). Eight women say Charlie rose sexually harassed them — With nudity, groping and lewd calls. *The Washington Post.* https://www.washingtonpost.com/investigations/eight-women-say-charlie-rose-sexually-harassed-them%E2%80%94with-nudity-groping-and-lewdcalls/2017/11/20/9b168de8-caec-11e7-8321-481fd63f174d_story.html?utm_term=.2e1d50623554

CNN (2018, September 27). *Wolf Blitzer coverage of Brett Kavanaugh Confirmation Hearing for Supreme Court*. Retrieved from http://www.cnn.com/TRANSCRIPTS/1809/27/wolf.02.html

Cohen, S. (1972). *Folk devils and moral panics: The creation of the mods and rockers*. London: Paladin.

Cooney, S. (2018, February 13). 'They Don't Want to Include Women Like Me.' Sex workers say they're being left out of the #MeToo movement. *Time.* Retrieved from http://time.com/5104951/sex-workers-me-too-movement/

Davidson, J. D. (2018, September 19). Don't turn the Kavanaugh confirmation into a title IX Kangaroo Court. *The Federalist.* Retrieved from https://thefederalist.com/2018/09/19/dont-let-kavanaugh-confirmation-turn-title-ix-kangaroo-court/

Davis, D. L. (2018a, January 19). Has the #MeToo movement gone overboard with Aziz Ansari? *Psychology*

Today. Retrieved March 13, 2018, from https://www.psychologytoday.com/us/blog/laugh-cry-live/201801/has-the-metoo-movement-gone-overboard-aziz-ansari

Davis, J. (2018b, October 5). How many rape accusations are false? *Medium*. Retrieved from https://medium.com/@jimpreston_36730/how-many-rape-accusations-are-false-f52e4c675f2a

De Zutter, A. W. E. A., Horselenberg, R., & Van Koppen, P. J. (2017). Filing false vice reports: Distinguishing true from false allegations of rape. *The European Journal of Psychology Applied to Legal Context, 9*(1), 1–14.

Doe v. (2016). Brandies University, 1:15-cv-11557-FDS (D. Mass). https://kcjohnson.files.wordpress.com/2013/08/brandeis-decision.pdf

Doe v. (2018) Baum et al., 17-2213 (6th Cir.). http://www.opn.ca6.uscourts.gov/opinions.pdf/18a0200p-06.pdf

Donath, J., & Boyd, D. (2004). Public displays of connection. *BT Technology Journal, 22*(4), 71–82.

Edelman, M. (1964). *The symbolic uses of power*. Urbana-Champagne, IL: University of Illinois Press.

Edelman, M. J. (1993). Contestable categories and public opinion. *Political Communication, 10*(3), 231–242.

Ellis, E. G. (2018, September 27). How #HimToo became the anti #MeToo of the Kavanaugh hearings. *Wired*. Retrieved from https://www.wired.com/story/brett-kavanaugh-hearings-himtoo-metoo-christine-blasey-ford/

Elsesser, K. (2015). *Sex and the office: Women, men, and the sex partition that's dividing the workplace*. Lanham: Rowman & Littlefield.

Engel, J., & O'Donohue, W. (2012). Pathways to false allegations of sexual assault. *Journal of Forensic Psychology Practice, 12*(2), 97–123.

Entman, R. M. (1993, Autumn). Framing: toward clarification of a fractured paradigm. *Journal of Communication, 43*(4), 51–58.

Farrow, R. (2017, October 10). From aggressive overtures to sexual assault: Harvey Weinstein's accusers tell their stories. *The New Yorker*. Retrieved from https://www.newyorker.com/news/news-desk/from-aggressive-overtures-to-sexual-assault-harvey-weinsteins-accusers-tell-their-stories

Feinburg, J. (2009, March). *How framing influences citizen understanding of public issues an interview with Shanto Iyengar, a leading scholar on frame effects*. Washington, DC: Frameworks Institute.

Fisher, B. S., Cullen, F. T., & Turner, M. G. (2000). *The sexual victimization of college women. Series*. Washington, DC: National Institute of Justice, US Department of Justice.

Fiske, S., & Taylor, S. (1991). *Social cognition* (2nd ed.). New York, NY: McGrawHill.

Flanagan, C. (2018, January 14). The humiliation of Aziz Ansari. *The Atlantic*. Retrieved May 15, 2018, from https://www.theatlantic.com/entertainment/archive/2018/01/the-humiliation-of-aziz-ansari/550541/.

Foundation for the Individual Rights in Education (FIRE). (2018, December 18). *Spotlight on due process*. Retrieved from https://www.thefire.org/spotlight/due-process-reports/due-process-report-2018/

French, D. (2019, February 25). The great due-process revival. *National Review*. Retrieved from https://www.nationalreview.com/corner/due-process-protections-metoo-movement/amp/?__twitter_impression=true

Fryer Jr, R. G. (2018). Reconciling results on racial differences in police shootings. In AEA *papers and proceedings* (Vol. 108, pp. 228–33).

Gamson, W. A., Fireman, B., & Rytina, S. (1982). *Encounters with unjust authority*. Homewood, IL: Dorsey.

Gamson, W. A., & Modigliani, A. (1987). The changing culture of affirmative action. In R. D. Braungart (Ed.), *Research in political sociology* (Vol. 3, pp. 137–177). Greenwich, CT: JAI.

Gamson, W. A., & Modigliani, A. (1989). Media discourse and public opinion on nuclear power: A constructionist approach. *American Journal of Sociology, 95*(1), 37.

Gamson, W. A. (1992). *Talking politics*. New York: Cambridge University Press.

Gamson, W. A. (1995). Constructing social protest. In *Social movements and culture* (Vol. 4, pp. 85–106).

Gans, F. (2017, December 15). Matt Damon faces backlash after saying there's a 'spectrum' when it comes to allegations of sexual misconduct. *Boston Globe*. Retrieved from https://www.bostonglobe.com/arts/2017/12/15/matt-damon-says-there-spectrum-behavior-when-comes-allegations-sexual-misconduct/Fcq4pKMDKQzVfnxmnr3LLJ/story.html?comments=all&sort=OLDEST_CREATE_DT&page=3

Garber, M. (2018, July 4). Is #MeToo Too Big? *The Atlantic*. Retrieved August 20, 2018, from https://www.theatlantic.com/entertainment/archive/2018/07/is-metoo-too-big/564275/

Garcia, A. (2016, October 7). Trump gets caught saying "Grab Her by the Pussy". *YouTube* [Video]. Retrieved from https://www.youtube.com/watch?v=o21fXqguD7U

Garkey, O. (2017, November 16). Heads up: Russians boosting Franken story per Hamilton 68. Daily Kos. https://www.dailykos.com/stories/2017/11/16/1716247/-Heads-up-Russians-boosting-Franken-story-per-Hamilton-68

Gersen, J., & Suk, J. (2016). The sex bureaucracy. *California Law Review, 104*(4), 881–948. Retrieved from https://scholarship.law.berkeley.edu/cgi/viewcontent.cgi?article=4327&context=californialawreview.

Gersen, J. S. (2017, September 8). Betsy DeVos, Title IX, and the "both sides" approach to sexual assault. *The New Yorker*. Retrieved July 6, 2018, from https://www.newyorker.com/news/news-desk/betsy-devos-title-ix-and-the-both-sides-approach-to-sexual-assault

Gessen, M. (2017, November 14). When does a watershed become a sex panic? *The New Yorker*. Retrieved March 13, 2018, from https://

www.newyorker.com/news/our-columnists/when-does-a-watershed-become-a-sex-panic

Goffman, E. (1974). *Frame analysis: An essay on the organization of experience*. Cambridge, MA: Harvard University Press.

Graber, D. A. (1988). *Processing the news: How people tame the information tide*. Boston, MA: Addison-Wesley Longman Ltd.

Graf, N. (2018, April 4). Sexual harassment at work in the era of #MeToo. Pew Research Center. Retrieved from http://www.pewsocialtrends.org/2018/04/04/sexual-harassment-at-work-in-the-era-of-metoo/

Halley, J. (2015). Trading the megaphone for the Gavel in Title IX enforcement. *Harvard Law Review Forum, 128*, 103.

Harris, S. (2019, February 26). Harvard attacks a defense attorney for doing his job: Ronald Sullivan could be penalized for daring to represent Harvey Weinstein. *New York Daily News*. Retrieved from https://www.nydailynews.com/opinion/ny-oped-harvard-attacks-a-defense-attorney-for-doing-his-job-20190226-story.html?outputType=amp&__twitter_impression=true

Heider, F. (1958). *The psychology of interpersonal relations*. Hillsdale, NJ: Lawrence Erlbaum Associates.

Hodge, A. (2018, February 5). Every feminist hashtag you need to know, from #metoo to #timesup. [Blog]. *YourDreamblog*. Retrieved from https://yourdream.liveyourdream.org/2018/02/feminist-hashtags-metoo-timesup/

Holstein, M. (2018, July 13). Why women make false rape accusations and why they think their accusations are true. *Medium*. Retrieved from https://medium.com/@meholstein/why-women-make-false-rape-accusations-938ffdf9a181

Horowitz, J. M., Parker, K., & Stepler, R. (2017, October 18). Wide Partisan gaps in U.S. over how far the country has come on gender equality. *Pew Research Center*. Retrieved August 20, 2018, from http://www.pewsocialtrends.org/2017/10/18/wide-partisan-gaps-in-u-s-over-how-far-the-country-has-come-on-gender-equality/

Hunt, S. A., & Benford, R. D. (1992). Social movements and the social construction of reality: An emergent paradigm. In *American Sociological Association section on collective behavior and social movements workshop on culture and social movements*. San Diego, California, June (Vol. 18).

Hunt, S. A., & Benford, R. D. (2004). Collective identity, solidarity, and commitment. In *The Blackwell companion to social movements* (pp. 433–457).

Iyengar, S. (1996). Framing responsibility for political issues. *The Annals of the American Academy of Political and Social Science*, 59–70.

Johnson, K. C. (2019, February 27). Title IX has a cross-examination crisis. *Minding the Campus*. Retrieved from https://www.mindingthecampus.org/2019/02/27/title-ix-has-a-cross-examination-crisis/

Johnson, K. C., & Taylor, S., Jr. (2017). *The Campus Rape Frenzy: The attack on due process at America's universities*. New York: Encounter Books.

Johnson, K. C., & Taylor Jr S. (2018a, December 12). It's time for republicans to show they truly care about due process. *The Weekly Standard*. Retrieved from https://www.weeklystandard.com/k-c-johnson/why-arent-republicans-more-vocal-in-supporting-title-ix-reform

Johnson, K. C., & Taylor Jr S. (2018b, November, 30). The ACLU's J'Accuse. *The Weekly Standard*. Retrieved from https://www.weeklystandard.com/k-c-johnson/with-its-response-to-devos-title-ix-changes-the-aclu-comes-out-openly-against-due-process

Jones, A. (2009). *Women who kill*. New York, NY: Feminist Press.

Jones, M. (2018, November 7). *Believe the survivor? Here's 11 times young black men were railroaded by campus sexual assault claims*. Retrieved from https://www.thecollegefix.com/believe-the-survivor-heres-11-times-young-black-men-were-railroaded-by-campus-sexual-assault-claims/

JustBeInc. (2013a). Tarana Burke, Founder and Director. Retrieved from http://justbeinc.wixsite.com/justbeinc/board

JustBeInc. (2013b). The Inception. Retrieved from https://justbeinc.wixsite.com/justbeinc/the-me-too-movement-cmml

Kanin, E. J. (1994). False rape allegations. *Archives of Sexual Behavior, 23*(1), 81–92.

Kantor, J. & Twohey, M. (2017, October 5). Harvey Weinstein paid off sexual harassment accusers for decades. *The New York Times*. Retrieved from https://www.nytimes.com/2017/10/05/us/harvey-weinstein-harassment-allegations.html

Kassam, A. (2018, January 15). Margaret Atwood faces feminist backlash on social media over #MeToo. *The Guardian*. Retrieved from https://amp.theguardian.com/books/2018/jan/15/margaret-atwood-feminist-backlash-metoo?__twitter_impression=true

Keehan, A., Caputo, E., Pettegrew, H., Bennett, M. (2015, October). *Confronting campus sexual assault: An examination of higher education claims. United educators*. Retrieved from http://www.ncdsv.org/ERS_Confronting-Campus-Sexual-Assault_2015.pdf

Kinder, D. R., & Sanders, L. M. (1990). Mimicking political debate with survey questions: The case of white opinion on affirmative action for blacks. *Social Cognition, 8*(1), 73–103.

Koopmans, R., & Duyvendak, J. W. (1995). The political construction of the nuclear energy issue and its impact on the mobilization of anti-nuclear movements in Western Europe. *Social Problems, 42*(2), 235–251.

Krebs, C. & Lindquist, C. (2014). Setting the Record Straight on '1 in 5'. *Time*. Retrieved from http://time.com/3633903/campus-rape-1-in-5-sexual-assault-setting-record-straight/

Krebs, C. P., Lindquist, C. H., Warner, T. D., Fisher, B. S., & Martin, S. L. (2007). *The campus sexual assault (CSA) study: Final report*. Washington, DC: National Institute of Justice, US Department of Justice.

Lakoff, G. (2004). *Don't think of an elephant: Know your values and frame the debate*. White River Junction, VT: Chelsea Green Publishing.

Lippmann, W. (1946). *Public opinion*. New York, NY: Transaction Publishers.

Lisak, D., Gardinier, L., Nicksa, S. C., & Cote, A. M. (2010). False allegations of sexual assault: An analysis of ten years of reported cases. *Violence Against Women, 16*, 1318–1334. https://doi.org/10.1177/1077801210387747

Matsa, K. E. & Shearer, E. (2018, September 10). News Use Across Social Media Platforms 2018. *Pew Research Center*. Retrieved from http://www.journalism.org/2018/09/10/news-use-across-social-media-platforms-2018/

McAdam, D. (1999). *Political process and the development of Black insurgency, 1930–1970*. Chicago: University of Chicago Press.

McClain, N., & Amar, A. F. (2013). Female survivors of child sexual abuse: Finding voice through research participation. *Issues in Mental Health Nursing, 34*(7), 482–487.

"Measuring the #MeToo backlash" (2018, October 20). *The Economist*. Retrieved from https://www.economist.com/united-states/2018/10/20/measuring-the-metoo-backlash

Minsky, M. (1974). Artificial Intelligence, Memo No. 306. *Artificial Intelligence*.

Nicolaou, E. (2018, October 4). A #MeToo timeline to show how far we've come — & how far we need to go. Refinery29. https://www.refinery29.com/enus/2018/10/212801/me-too-movement-history-timeline-year-weinstein

National Center for Higher Education Risk Management. (2017). *The 2017 NCHERM Group Whitepaper: Due process and sex police*. Retrieved from https://www.ncherm.org/wp-content/uploads/2017/04/TNG-Whitepaper-Final-Electronic-Version.pdf

Nelson, T. E., Clawson, R. A., & Oxley, Z. M. (1997). Media framing of a civil liberties conflict and its effect on tolerance. *American Political Science Review, 91*(03), 567–583.

Nilsen, E. & Zhou, L. (2018, October 7). 12 senators on what kind of message Brett Kavanaugh's confirmation sends to America's women. *Vox*. Retrieved from https://www.google.com/amp/s/www.vox.com/platform/amp/policy-and-politics/2018/10/7/17946218/brett-kavanaugh-senate-confirmation-senators

Norton, A. (2018, November 5). Bystanders less likely to give CPR to women. *UPI*. Retrieved from https://www.upi.com/Health_News/2018/11/05/Bystanders-less-likely-to-give-CPR-to-women/3721541447788/?mp=3

O'Callaghan, E., Lorenz, K., Ullman, S. E., & Kirkner, A. (2018). A dyadic study of impacts of sexual assault disclosure on survivors' informal support relationships. *Journal of Interpersonal Violence*, 886260518795506.

O'Donohue, W., & Bowers, A. H. (2006). Pathways to false allegations of sexual harassment. *Journal of Investigative Psychology and Offender Profiling, 3*(1), 47–74.

Onwuachi-Willig, A. (2018, June 2018). What about #UsToo?: The invisibility of race in the #MeToo Movement. *The Yale Law Journal*, **128**. Retrieved from https://www.yalelawjournal.org/forum/what-about-ustoo

Parker, K., & Funk, C. (2017, December 14). Gender discrimination comes in many forms for today's working women. *Pew Research Center*. Retrieved May 11, 2018, from http://www.pewresearch.org/fact-tank/2017/12/14/gender-discrimination-comes-in-many-forms-for-todays-working-women/

Phillips, W. (2015). *This is why we can't have nice things: Mapping the relationship between online trolling and mainstream culture*. Cambridge: MIT Press.

Piacenza, J. (2018, October 11). A year into #MeToo, public worried about false allegations. *Morning Consult*. Retrieved from https://morningconsult.com/2018/10/11/a-year-into-metoo-public-worried-about-false-allegations/

Piper, G. (2019, March 19). Survey: University presidents support due process but are too scared to speak up. *The College Fix*. Retrieved from https://helpsaveoursons.com/survey-university-presidents-support-due-process-but-are-too-scared-to-speak-up/

Plous, S. (1993). *The psychology of judgment and decision making*. New York: McGraw-Hill Book Company.

Reddit. (2018, October 20). Reddit is obsessed with false accusations of rape. Meanwhile, 2/3 rapes goes unreported. *Redditt*. Retrieved from https://imgur.com/KWpDWwi

Ripley, A., Tenjarla, R., & He, A. Y. (2019, March 4). The Geography of Partisan prejudice. *The Atlantic*. Retrieved from https://www.theatlantic.com/amp/article/583072/?__twitter_impression=true

Roberts, R. (2018, October 21). A mother of a son's middle path in the #MeToo era. *Chicago Tribune*. Retrieved from http://www.chicagotribune.com/lifestyles/parenting/ct-life-metoo-era-mother-son-20181020-story.html

Rommelmann, N. (2019, February 22). Outrage culture is out of control. *LA Times*. Retrieved from https://www.latimes.com/opinion/op-ed/la-oe-rommelmann-me-too-portland-20190222-story.html?outputType=amp&__twitter_impression=true

Rosen, J. (2019, February 15). Ruth Bader Ginsburg opens up about #MeToo, voting rights, and millennials. *The Atlantic*. Retrieved from https://www.theatlantic.com/politics/archive/2018/02/ruth-bader-ginsburg-opens-up-about-metoo-voting-rights-and-millenials/553409/

Rowley, L. (2018, October 23). The architect of #MeToo says the movement has lost its way. *The Cut*. Retrieved from https://www.thecut.com/2018/10/tarana-burke-me-too-founder-movement-has-lost-its-way.html

Ryan, C. (1991). *Prime time activism: Media strategies for grassroots organizing*. Boston, MA: South End Press.

Saul, S. (2017, November 3). *'Victim feminism' and sexual assault on campus. New York Times*. Retrieved March 13, 2018, from https://www.nytimes.com/2017/11/03/education/edlife/christina-hoff-sommers-sexual-assault-feminism.html

Save Our Sons. (2019). [website]. Retrieved from https://helpsaveoursons.com/

Scheufele, D. A. (1999). Framing as a theory of media effects. *Journal of Communication, 49*(1), 103–122.

Schow, A. (2018, August 31). Lies, damned lies, and campus sexual assault statistics. *The Daily Wire*. Retrieved from https://www.dailywire.com/news/35309/lies-damned-lies-and-campus-sexual-assault-ashe-schow

Shah, A. K., & Oppenheimer, D. M. (2008). Heuristics made easy: An effort-reduction framework. *Psychological Bulletin, 134*(2), 207.

Sherman, C. (2018, October 17). The "Shitty Media Men" list lawsuit is freaking out women in media. *Vice News*. Retrieved from https://news.vice.com/en_us/article/evw7mj/the-shitty-media-men-list-lawsuit-is-freaking-out-women-in-media

Sinozich, S., & Langton, L. (2014, December). *Rape and sexual assault victimization among college-age females, 1995–2013*. United States Department of Justice, Bureau of Justice Statistics.

Smallridge, J., Wagner, P., & Crowl, J. N. (2016). Understanding cyber-vigilantism: A conceptual framework. *Journal of Theoretical & Philosophical Criminology, 8*(1).

Smola, J. (2018, April 23). Founder of 'Me Too' movement fears narrative being hijacked from helping survivors heal. *The Columbus Dispatch*. Retrieved from https://www.dispatch.com/news/20180423/founder-of-me-too-movement-fears-narrative-being-hijacked-from-helping-survivors-heal

Snow, D. A., & Benford, R. D. (1988). Ideology, frame resonance, and participant mobilization. *International Social Movement Research, 1*(1), 197–217.

Snow, D. A., & Benford, R. D. (1992). Master frames and cycles of protest. *Frontiers in Social Movement Theory, 133*, 155.

Snow, D. A., Rochford, E. B., Jr., Worden, S. K., & Benford, R. (1986). Frame alignment processes, micromobilization, and movement participation. *American Sociological Review, 5*(1), 464–481.

Statista. (2018a). *Social media usage in the United States*. Retrieved from https://www.statista.com/topics/3196/social-media-usage-in-the-united-states/

Statista. (2018b). *Number of social media users worldwide from 2010 to 2021 (in billions)*. Retrieved from https://www.statista.com/statistics/278414/number-of-worldwide-social-network-users/

Steel, E., & Schmidt, M. (2017). *The New York Times*. Sebastopal: O'Reilly.

Tajfel, H. (1974). Social identity and intergroup behaviour. *Social Science Information, 13*, 65–93.

Tan, G., & Porzecanski, K. (2018, December 3). Wall street rule for the #MeToo era: Avoid women at all cost. *Bloomberg*. Retrieved from https://www.bloomberg.com/news/articles/2018-12-03/a-wall-street-rule-for-the-metoo-era-avoid-women-at-all-cost

Taylor, S. (2019, January 27). Harvard, the NY Times and the #MeToo Takedown of a Black Academic Star. *RealClearInvestigations*. Retrieved from https://www.realclearinvestigations.com/articles/2019/01/27/harvard_the_new_york_times_and_the_metoo_takedown_of_a_black_academic_star.html

TIME'S UP. (2019). [webpage] Retrieved from https://www.timesupnow.com/about_times_up

Trump. (2018, October 2). [Twitter entry]. Retrieved from https://twitter.com/realDonaldTrump/status/962348831789797381?ref_src=twsrc%5Etfw%7Ctwcamp%5Etweetembed%7Ctwterm%5E962348831789797381&ref_url=https%3A%2F%2Fwww.cnn.com%2F2018%2F02%2F10%2Fpolitics%2Ftrump-tweets-on-porter%2Findex.html

Turvey, B., Savino, J. O., & Mares, A. C. (2017). *False allegations: Investigative and forensic issues in fraudulent reports of crime*. London: Elsevier, Inc.

United States Department of Education, Office for Civil Rights. (2011, April 4). *Dear colleague letter on sexual violence*. Retrieved from https://www2.ed.gov/about/offices/list/ocr/letters/colleague-201104.pdf

United States Department of Education, Office for Civil Rights. (2017, September 22). *Interim Guidelines for Title IX of Education Amendments of 1972*. Retrieved from https://www2.ed.gov/about/offices/list/ocr/letters/colleague-title-ix-201709.pdf

United States Department of Education, Office for Civil Rights. (2018, November). *Notice of Proposed Rulemaking; Title IX of the Education Amendments of 1972*. Retrieved from https://www2.ed.gov/about/offices/list/ocr/docs/title-ix-nprm.pdf

Vagianos, A. (2017, January 18). Janet mock: Sex workers' rights must be part of the women's march. *Huffington Post*.

Vagianos, A. (2018, November 30). Tarana Burke: 'We have moved so far away from the origins' of Me Too. *Huffington Post*. Retrieved from https://www.huffingtonpost.com/entry/tarana-burke-me-too-backlash_us_5c014658e4b0d04f48b373b3

Watanabe, T. & Hussain, S. (2019, February 14). Ruling affirming the rights of students accused of sexual misconduct roiles California colleges. *LA Times*. Retrieved from https://www.latimes.com/local/education/la-me-california-universities-title-ix-20190215-story.html

Way, K. (2018, January 14). I went on a date with Aziz Ansari. It turned into the worst night of my life. *Babe*. Retrieved from https://babe.net/2018/01/13/aziz-ansari-28355

Weiss, B. (2017, November 28). The limits of 'believing all women. *The New York Times*. Retrieved May 13, 2018, from https://www.nytimes.com/2017/11/28/opinion/metoo-sexual-harassment-believe-women.html

Weiss, B. (2018, January 15). Aziz Ansari is guilty. Of not being a mind reader. *The New York Times*. Retrieved January 15, 2018, from https://www.nytimes.com/2018/01/15/opinion/aziz-ansari-babe-sexual-harassment.html

White, G. B. (2017, November 22). The glaring blind spot of the 'Me Too' movement issues overview. *The Atlantic*. Retrieved from https://www.theatlantic.com/entertainment/archive/2017/11/the-glaring-blind-spot-of-the-me-too-movement/546458/

Winter, N. J. (2005). Framing gender: Political rhetoric, gender schemas, and public opinion on US health care reform. *Politics & Gender, 1*(03), 453–480.

Wojcik, S., Messing, S., Smith, A., Rainie, L., & Hitlin, P. (2018, April 9). Bots in the Twittersphere. Pew Research. http://www.pewinternet.org/2018/04/09/bots-inthe-twittersphere/

Wong, J. C., & La Ganga, M. L. (2016, September 13. 'My own form of justice': rape survivors and the risk of social media 'vigilantism'. *The Guardian.* Retrieved from https://www.google.com/amp/s/amp.theguardian.com/society/2016/sep/13/social-media-rape-survivors-justice-legal-system

Yoffe, E. (2014, December 7). The college rape overcorrection. *Slate.* Retrieved from http://www.slate.com/articles/double_x/doublex/2014/12/college_rape_campus_sexual_assault_is_a_serious_problem_but_the_efforts.html

Yoffe, E. (2017a, September 8). The bad science behind campus response to sexual assault. *The Atlantic.* Retrieved from https://www.theatlantic.com/education/archive/2017/09/the-bad-science-behind-campus-response-to-sexual-assault/539211/

Yoffe, E. (2017b, September 11). The question of race in campus sexual-assault cases. *The Atlantic.* Retrieved from https://www.theatlantic.com/education/archive/2017/09/the-question-of-race-in-campus-sexual-assault-cases/539361/

Yoffe, E. (2018, October 13). Does anyone still take both sexual assault and due process seriously? *The Atlantic.*

Young, C. (2019, February 22). The future of women is female. And she's furious. *Reason.com.* Retrieved from https://helpsaveoursons.com/category/hunting-ground-debunked/

Zeisler, A. (2017, December 7). #Metoo isn't about hugging or male discomfort with women. *Newsweek.* Retrieved from https://www.newsweek.com/metoo-isnt-about-hugging-or-male-discomfort-touching-women-741236

Zimmerman, A. (2018, November 27). Ashley Judd's anti-prostitution crusade angers sex workers: 'you are harming people'. *The Daily Beast.* Retrieved from https://www.thedailybeast.com/sex-workers-blast-ashley-judds-anti-prostitution-crusade-you-are-harming-people

7 Pornography and Sexual Violence

John D. Foubert, Will Blanchard, Michael Houston,
and Richard R. Williams Jr.

Pornography and Sexual Violence

Approximately 20 years ago if people desired to look at pornography, they would have limited options. One could purchase a magazine, video, or some other hard copy medium from a retailer (often brick and morter), find a hard copy form of pornography around the house, or borrow a copy from a friend or family member. For decades, magazines, videos, and other media were utilized for porn consumption. All of this changed a couple of decades ago with the mass production and ubiquitous availability of desktop, laptop, and handheld personal computers. Pornography was then available direct to the viewers without having to interact with another person (Braithwaite, Coulson, Keddington, & Fincham, 2015). Although pornography is not new, this mass exposure to pornography, particularly high-speed internet pornography, ushered in by technological advances over the past 20 years is a game changer. It is no longer necessary to go to a store to purchase and view pornography. Using the internet is now the primary means for viewing pornography (Wery & Billieux, 2016). In addition, the international nature of pornography websites makes shutting down sites illegal in the US difficult in cases where they are hosted overseas.

J. D. Foubert (✉)
Union University, Jackson, TN, USA

W. Blanchard · M. Houston · R. R. Williams Jr.
Oklahoma State University, Stillwater, OK, USA

This explosion of the availability of pornography to the general public has led to many studies finding significant social ills directly related to pornographic use. Viewing pornography is not harmless as some would lead to believe, in fact, the violence and exploitation in pornography leads to numerous negative effects (Foubert, 2017). The next sections will explore these negative effects of pornography on society.

Pornography and Violence

Prior to high-speed internet pornography, there was a broader range of images available, many which were not overtly violent. Magazines like Playboy featured more playful images, while Hustler and Penthouse tested the bounds of obscenity (Dines, 2010). Over time, most pornography has included violence in some form, with 88% of images containing violent acts (Bridges, Wosnitzer, Scharrer, Sun, & Liberman, 2010) and its harmful effects are not surprising. The violence depicted in pornography leads to numerous negative effects on viewers. Pornography is largely degrading and depicts acts of sexual violence toward women (Sun, Bridges, Johnson, & Ezzell, 2016). Pornographic images and scenes in videos routinely depict the objectification of women and its logical result, violence. For consumers of pornography, these images can create abnormal

W. T. O'Donohue and P. A. Schewe (eds.), *Handbook of Sexual Assault and Sexual Assault Prevention*,
https://doi.org/10.1007/978-3-030-23645-8_7

sexual expectations and unwanted sexual advances that can lead to violent behavior (Sun, Ezzell, & Kendall, 2017).

When reviewing the best-selling pornographic videos, Bridges et al. (2010) found that 88% of the scenes depicted sex acts with physical aggression including slapping, choking, and bondage. Furthermore, 70% of these aggressive acts were perpetrated by men, and 87% of the physically violent acts were against women. These depictions create a sense of expected reality in viewers which can lead to violent, nonconsensual sexual encounters (Bridges et al., 2010).

Sun et al. (2016) use Cognitive Script Theory to help explain why viewers of pornography are more likely to perpetrate acts of violence in sexual encounters. The authors of Cognitive Script Theory propose that the more an individual consumes similar scripts, codes are created in the brain pertaining to the behaviors depicted, and sometimes experienced. The more codes that are created associated with particular behaviors, the more likely it is that the individual exhibits that behavior in real-life experiences. Pertaining to pornography, habitual viewers of pornography have sexually explicit codes or scripts created in cognition that are called upon when sexual encounters are presented. These scripts are rooted in violence, objectification, and skewed gender norms (Sun et al., 2016).

Relatedly, exposure to pornography leads to more rigid views of gender roles. In the large majority of pornography, restrictive gender stereotypes are perpetuated leading to the notion of violent, domineering men and women who are subservient to every violent act a man can come up with to demean her (Brown & L'Engle, 2009; Häggström-Nordin, Sandberg, Hanson, & Tyde'n, 2006; Malamuth & Impett, 2001). This notion is a contributor to higher incidents of sexual violence in those who view pornography regularly (Brown & L'Engle, 2009). Furthermore, research shows relationships between consistent viewers of pornography and perpetration of higher levels of sexual harassment in the workplace (Brown & L'Engle, 2009; Häggström-Nordin et al., 2006; Malamuth & Impett, 2001). The violence associated with sex in pornography is impacting viewers and is related to real-life sexual violence and harassment (Foubert, 2017). For the general public this is a problem, but another segment of the population is greatly impacted as well. Emerging adults or adolescents are also impacted by pornography.

Pornography and Adolescents

The age that a person first views pornography continues to be younger as compared to previous generations. Ninety-seven percent of males and 62% of females have viewed pornography by the age of 17 (Sabina, Wolak, & Finkelhor, 2008). Studies are finding when adolescents view pornography, numerous negative effects are presented. Viewing pornography at a young age causes adolescents to begin to believe that what they are watching depicts real life, and young men and women begin to expect similar sexual encounters (Peter & Valkenburg, 2008, 2010). This is problematic because this leads many adolescents to view relationships more instrumentally and less relationally (Valkenburg, 2010).

Research is also showing that adolescents who view pornography are more likely to begin sexual activity at earlier ages, when they may not be developmentally ready for such activity. This early onset of sexual activity is due to the adolescents' more permissive attitudes or views toward casual sex that are directly linked to their pornography use (Van, Jochen, & Vandenbosch, 2017). Additionally, because of the violence and proclivity of drug and alcohol use in pornography, adolescents who view pornography show higher rates of risky behaviors including the use of drugs and alcohol and risky sex practices including unprotected sex and sex with multiple partners (Braun-Courville & Rojas, 2009; Brown & L'Engle, 2009; Peter & Valkenburg, 2006). Although one can't claim that these relationships are causal given the near impossibility of an experimental study in this area, the strong relationships between pornography and adolescent behavior are striking.

Other Negative Relationships

Along with the perpetuation of sexual violence and harassment, and the negative effects pornography has on adolescents, users of pornography experience other negative thoughts and physiological experiences. Wery and Billieux (2016) found that people who watch pornography experience decreased levels of sexual satisfaction and experience erectile dysfunction at higher rates as compared to those who do not watch pornography regularly. Sun et al. (2016) contend that regular consumers of pornography report lower levels of satisfaction with sexual performance. This lack of sexual satisfaction leads to questions about virility, and lower levels of self-esteem and creates body image issues.

Additionally, researchers are finding that habitual users of pornography experience lower levels of general motivation and problems with working memory. Laier, Schulte, and Brand (2012) found that pornographic users reported losing sleep and missing important appointments after viewing pornography. The study found that viewers of pornography who experienced sexual arousal reported problems with memory. The researchers contend that sexual arousal from pornography use directly interfered with working memory.

Pornography is typically a violent form of media with a variety of negative effects. These effects are witnessed by viewers from adolescence through adulthood. This chapter examines the violent content of pornography and target audiences, how men's perpetration of sexual violence is directly related to pornography and increases in men who exhibit higher risk factors for sexual violence, how the effects of pornography are both direct and indirect and have strong associations with sexually violent behaviors, pornography and the effects on women, how pornography and sexual violence impact the development of the adolescent brain, and child pornography and the exploitation of children and the relation to child abuse and sexual violence.

Pornography as Violence

Pornography is produced and consumed across multiple genres and subgenres, cultures, and demographics (Fritz & Paul, 2017). Moreover, pornography is often catered to different audiences (men, women, gay men, lesbians) and governed by a complex mix of intents (mostly capitalist and political). Industry data suggest that worldwide the profits of the porn industry are at 100 billion dollars (Ropelato, 2010). Regardless of source, purpose, or label, pornography is consistently linked to violence through themes of objectification, degradation, exploitation, power inequality, verbal abuse, and outright physical aggression (Bridges et al., 2010; Gorman, Monk-Turner, & Fish, 2010; Whisnant, 2016).

On-Camera "Consent" Normalizes Violence

Authors disagree on how to define violence in pornography. One significant point of contention is whether consent absolves a behavior from being classified as "violent." Bridges et al. (2010) found that the three most common physically aggressive behaviors in pornography—spanking, gagging, and open-hand slapping—were greeted, on camera, with pleasure or neutrality 95.9% of the time by women and 84% of the time by men. This indifference to aggressive behaviors in porn is cited in other studies (Klaassen & Peter, 2015; Whisnant, 2016) and effectively renders "violence" as invisible in these contexts. Moreover, acts of verbal abuse, psychological abuse, and emotional abuse have gone under-acknowledged in many studies of porn and its violent tendencies (Bridges et al., 2010). As a case in point on how these research practices influence violent findings in porn, Bridges et al. (2010), in analyzing 304 scenes of top-selling mainstream pornography, found that 88.2% of scenes contained physical aggression including slapping, hitting, gagging, and bondage, and 48.7% of scenes contained verbal aggression including calling a woman a bitch or a slut who likes a particular demeaning activity.

When controlling for "consent," however, all instances of aggression dropped to just 12.2%. Yet violent behavior with alleged consent is still violent behavior.

Whisnant (2016) illuminates the "consent" issue by arguing that men and women in the porn industry are paid actors in a profit-driven industry and, therefore, are often coerced into responding positively or neutrally to acts that they might not otherwise enjoy or even welcome. Whisnant cites the work of self-proclaimed feminist pornographer, Tristan Taormino. Taormino, who touts her work as "guilt-free" and empowering pornography, self-describes her work as profit-driven. Moreover, Whisnant notes that Taormino's work often celebrates themes of pain, dominance, and power as allegedly authentic desires of her actors. Taormino's philosophy is difficult to justify in a capitalist industry; however, if her actors were not willing to engage in these experiences, they would quickly be out of work. In fact, many porn agencies will only represent actors who have purged their "no list," meaning they will engage in any act on set, regardless of their comfort level or preferences (Whisnant, 2016). Saying "no" in porn narratives is also trivialized. Vannier, Currie, and O'Sullivan (2014) found that in a sample of 100 top free online videos, in every instance in which a character resisted a sexual act, violent or otherwise, that character ultimately relented to the forced experience. Many authors argue that patterns like this in pornography normalize a sexual script of violence and "token resistance."

Violence Across Cultures

Some authors argue that porn is not inherently violent, but rather that violence in porn flows out of larger contexts of culture, audience, and purpose. Arakawa, Flanders, and Hatfield (2012), for example, studied pornography across egalitarian and non-egalitarian societies. They studied popular softcore still images from the United States, Japan, and Norway. Their hypothesis was that in countries scoring high on the United Nations' gender empowerment measure (GEM) women would be less disempowered and more empowered in mainstream pornography. However, despite their hypothesis, they found that in all three countries women were often bound, placed in submissive poses, or dehumanized through emphasis on their genitalia to the marginalization of their faces. Norway did showcase a greater variety in body types, meaning the female form was less extremely idealized, but the researchers noted that, regardless of a country's GEM score, most images failed to show a healthy respect for women.

One cultural sub-genre, the Asian women category, has showcased fewer instances of outright physical aggression and nonnormative behavior than other categories (Zhou & Paul, 2016). Studies have shown that this category averages .33 aggressive acts per scene as opposed to .83 aggressive acts per scene in other genres. Researchers suggest that this reduction in outright physical violence is due to the docile and obedient "Lotus Blossom" narrative archetype. Unfortunately, this archetype fundamentally showcases power imbalance, as well. Aggressive acts in this category are perpetrated 68.3% of the time by men and target women 88% of the time. Zhou and Paul (2016) postulate that careful domination is a prevailing theme in this context. Whereas some strands of pornography treat women—particularly women of color—like animals, Asian pornography treats women like human dolls.

Gender Inequality

Gender inequality is common in pornography, and some have argued that this inequality feeds violence on screen (Arakawa et al., 2012). For example, Klaassen and Peter (2015) studied 400 videos from top sites (Pornhub, RedTube, YouPorn, and xHamster) and found that women were far more likely than men to be used as instruments of sexual gratification. Men were depicted as achieving orgasm in 75.5% of scenes, while women were only depicted as achieving orgasm in 16.8%. Men received oral sex in 80.5% of scenes, while women received oral sex in 47.5%. Women were featured in sexualized close-ups in 60.8% of scenes, while men were featured in 18.8%. Moreover, while scripts put men and women in equally powerful roles (teacher, boss, etc.), men were more likely to assume control and appear dominant during sexual activity (38.5% male dominance; 13.2% female dominance) and women were more likely to behave submissive (42.5% female submission; 10.2% male submission). In acts of outright physical violence, 37.2% of scenes portrayed violence, such as hitting or slapping, toward women, while only 2.8% showed violence toward men.

Klaassen and Peter's (2015) findings track with other recent studies in internet pornography. Gorman et al. (2010) studied a sample of free, highly accessible videos using the most popular search terms on the web. They found similar disparities in how men and women were portrayed, particularly with regard to men being more likely to receive oral sex. However, they also found that in these videos 13% depicted explicit force, 55% had themes of domination or exploitation, 47% showed submission and always by a female, 55% showed women naked more often than men, 49% depicted women as eager to do anything asked, 45% showed men "marking territory" by ejaculating on a woman's face, and, in all cases, women responded neutrally or favorably to violent or coercive acts. Vannier et al. (2014) echoed these results in studying two popular subgenres, teen and MILF videos, with one interesting exception: men were portrayed nude more often than women (74% to 47%). Their research clarifies, though, that this distinction is largely due to women wearing costumes to denote their age and status as moms, schoolgirls, secretaries, and other roles. Moreover, they report that men are more often in control of the pace and direction of sexual activity and that male actors are consistently the same age and build regardless of the female's age or role. This phenomenon is painfully explicit in the "casting couch" subgenre, in which young women are manipulated into sex with fake casting agents under the illusion that they are trying out for paying roles.

"Feminist," Queer, and Porn "For Women"

If violence enjoys a symbiotic relationship with gender inequality, then it could be hypothesized that less male-centric pornography should also be less violent. However, while studies have shown that feminist, queer, and For Women pornography do showcase higher instances of reciprocity in power and sexual pleasure (Shim, Kwon, & Cheng, 2015), violence persists. Coding instances of agency, authenticity, objectification, and aggression, Fritz and Paul (2017) compared these women-centric genres against mainstream pornography and found that a gender gap appeared across all categories. Women were less overtly objectified in feminist pornography than in other kinds of pornography but equally objectified in For Women porn. In fact, "gaping," or an emphasis on the spread open genitals, was most common in the For Women genre. Women were depicted as having less agency than men in all genres except the queer feminist category, and even in this category, 54% of scenes with aggressive behavior had violence directed toward women. Physical aggression, particularly toward women, occurred with relative frequency across all women-centric genres. Shim et al. (2015) offer one of the only rebuttals to this finding. Comparing 200 images across men's and women's pornography sites, their research team found that sexually unequal themes were much higher on men's sites (25%) than women's sites (4%). Interestingly, though, their team also found that instances of objectification were more frequent on women's sites than men's. They posit that this finding could reveal how the concept of the female body as a sexual object is becoming normalized across gender cultures.

One of the most indicting studies on this phenomenon—women (not) abdicating violence toward women—again comes from Whisnant's (2016) review of feminist Tristan Taormino. In reviewing a small cross-section of Taormino's work, Whisnant reveals common tropes of racially explicit and demeaning language, domination, "gang bang" anal sex, ejaculation on women, strangulation, gagging, spanking, and slapping. Taormino argues that these tropes are exciting to many women and that her work is empowering women to combat puritanical attitudes toward sex. However, as Whisnant illustrates, Taormino's work also communicates that power hierarchies are a given, that violent actions that injure and kill women daily can and should be treated as gameplay, and that resisting painful and previously nonnormative activities, such as anal sex, makes one a prude. In fact, Taormino appears to adopt an alarming "anything goes" mentality in her approach to sex. She describes an instance in which a woman was bound, hit with tomatoes, and urinated on by a group prior to sex. Taormino classifies this episode as appropriate and nonviolent because it was consensual. This faulty logic is extended further when she even suggests that her initial alarm at this humiliating scene showcased her own narrow-mindedness and baggage more than anything inherently damaging in the activity.

This closing example offers a vivid illustration of how the notion of "violence" can be twisted. If the parties involved *appear* neutral toward an act or if an act is normative for even the smallest subset of the population, Taormino suggests that act is nonviolent. This stance precludes the idea that some activities, no matter how normalized, are intrinsically damaging. Pornography—across cultures, genres, and audiences—dehumanizes, objectifies, exploits, degrades, and abuses. Pornography is inescapably violent and, worse still, it perpetuates a cultural narrative that says sexual violence is okay.

Pornography and Men's Perpetration of Sexual Violence: The Importance of Individual Differences

Men are much more likely than women to consume pornography, with most studies showing men consuming at a rate at least twice that of women (Carroll, Busby, Willoughby, & Brown, 2017; Lo & Wei, 2005) Men's consumption of pornography impacts their views of women in measurable ways—including, but not limited to, objectification and acceptance of sexual mistreatment of women (Malamuth, Hald, & Koss, 2012; Mikorski & Szymanski, 2017; Wright & Bae, 2015). However, does pornography's impact on men extend beyond attitudes to acts of sexual violence? In this section, we assert that pornography is a significant predictor of men's sexual violence toward women, particularly when men possess preexisting risk factors for sexual violence.

Pornography as Predictor of Sexual Violence

Societal pressure exerted against committing and/or reporting acts of sexual violence makes examining a direct link between pornography and sexual violence challenging. Furthermore, little work has been done to scrutinize how perpetrators' consumption of pornography informs or incites their actions. Yet, a growing multiplicity of studies have demonstrated clear connections between pornography and perpetration from a variety of approaches. Frequent viewing of pornography is associated with escalating dissatisfaction with sexual relationships and increasing attitudes of sexual aggression (Simons, Simons, Lei, & Sutton, 2012; Vega & Malamuth, 2007). The confluence of these two results alone—sexual dissatisfaction and sexual aggression—points to the potential for acts of sexual violence. However, more explicit links are available. According to Rudman and Mescher (2012), men who view objectifying images of women are not just more likely to accept acts of sexual violence against women; they are more likely to endorse these acts. Finally, Alexy, Burgess, and Prentky (2009) found that some men viewing pornography are more likely to step beyond sexually aggressive attitudes and to engage in coerced and forced sexual acts; this is shown by higher rates of pornography use among sex offenders than a nonoffending population.

Although the evidence points to pornography as a predictor of sexual violence—even when controlling for other variables (Malamuth & Huppin, 2005), it is important to note inconsistencies in the data, including a strong degree of heterogeneity among studies (Malamuth et al., 2012). Clearly and reasonably, not every male that views pornography will commit a real act of sexual violence. How, then, can the inherent evidence of both correlation and discrepancies be accurately described? The most reasonable explanation is that pornography does, in fact, function as a predictor for sexual violence but that three important types of risk factors are likely to mediate and/or to moderate the connection: (1) other direct and indirect behavioral choices such as use of especially violent pornography, (2) sociocultural/environmental factors such as peer support for sexual violence and (3) individual/personality differences such as hypermasculinity and an emphasis on impersonal sex (Hald & Malamuth, 2015). In other words, pornography is a significant predictor of sexual violence when additional factors are also true of a consumer of pornography.

Behavioral Factors

Behavioral decisions accompanying pornography—both those directly related to the pornography itself, as well as those seemingly unrelated to pornography—can impact pornography's connection to sexual violence. First and most clearly among these behavioral factors is the frequency with which pornography is consumed. Higher than average consumption of pornography adds a statistically significant amount to pornography's prediction of sexual aggression, while infrequent pornography consumption demonstrates a less significant relationship (Vega & Malamuth, 2007). Another important influencer is the type of pornography being viewed. Pornography depicting violent or other extreme actions is more likely to produce an increased level of sexual aggression in the viewer than pornography without violent content (Malamuth et al., 2012; Vega & Malamuth, 2007). However, those exposed to softer forms of pornography still manifested significantly greater rape myth acceptance than those unexposed and greater rape propensity in hypothetical scenarios (Romero-Sanchez, Toro-Garcia, Horvath, & Megias, 2017). Alcohol consumption, as a seemingly unrelated behavioral choice, still influences sexual behaviors when combined with intake of pornography. Acts of sexual coercion and dominance are statistically more common in men who recurrently consume both pornography and alcohol before or during sexual encounters (Wright, Sun, Steffen, and Tokunaga, 2015). Finally, even usage of Facebook, when combined with other behaviors such as association with abusive male peers, has been associated as with pornography as a predictor of unwanted sexual overtures (Mikorski & Szymanski, 2017).

Sociocultural/Environmental Factors

Factors surrounding the men who view pornography still bear connection to pornography's potential impact. For example, increasing access to pornography, as a broader cultural dynamic, intensifies both the frequency and severity of pornography available to would-be consumers. In fact, Wright (2011) reports that pornographic media makes sexual and violent content ubiquitously accessible to both youth and adults. More particular to individual users, though, are a series of more intimate, even familial, environmental factors. Because there is often a discrepancy in partners' use of pornography (with male partners consuming significantly more pornography than females), the partner with greater use of pornography is associated with increased levels of sexual aggression (Carroll et al., 2017; Willoughby, Carroll, Busby, and Brown, 2016). Men who received frequent corporeal punishment in their homes of origin, in combination with subsequent or concurrent use of pornography, were more likely to engage in sexual victimization of women (Simons et al., 2012). Adolescents who experience a generally troubled home life are more prone to view pornography frequently, and frequent use of pornography is, in turn, a predictor of sexual aggression (Peter & Valkenburg, 2016; Vega & Malamuth, 2007).

Individual Differences

Each individual is unique; therefore, it is only reasonable to suggest each male's processing of pornographic material is, in some ways, unique (Malamuth & Huppin, 2005; Wright & Bae, 2015). Underlying this premise are data that contend for the importance of individual differences when applying connections between pornography and sexual violence. In a study on "agreeableness" as an inherent personality factor, Hald and Malamuth (2015) found that experimental exposure to pornography only increased acceptance of sexual violence when men were also low in agreeableness. Conversely, lower levels of agreeableness combined with greater past usage of pornography provided significant prediction of attitudes supporting violence against women. In addition to inherent personality traits, a man's preexisting sexual preference for certain types of pornography appears to be a powerful factor in predicting aggression outcomes. In both adolescents and adults, men who reported or manifested sexual arousal from violent or extreme pornography were more commonly associated with expressions of sexual aggression (Hald & Malamuth, 2015; Malamuth & Huppin, 2005). Furthermore, what seems to be true of personal differences in agreeableness and natural sexual arousal is also true of preexisting tendencies of aggression. When a man is already predisposed to aggression in other realms, violent pornography is particularly influential in producing increased sexual aggression (Baer, Kohut, & Fisher, 2015; Kingston, Malamuth, Fedoroff, & Marshall, 2009).

When various behavioral choices, environmental factors, and personal differences are overlapped to produce a clear understanding of the relationship between pornography and sexual violence, it becomes obvious that the relationship must be defined by an accounting for individual differences. However, the unifying presence of pornography at the nexus of these factors seems to communicate a clear message: the surrounding environmental and personality variables react with the presence of frequent and/or violent pornography to direct the disparate factors toward the perpetration of sexual violence.

Relationship of Porn to Predictors of Sexual Violence

In 2010 there were roughly four million pornography sites on the internet. By 2015 it was estimated that 10,000 porn sites were added to the internet every week (DeKeseredy & Olsson, 2011). Additionally DeKeseredy and Olsson (2011) present that the internet has virtually eliminated former media of pornography consumption. Today, it is difficult to even examine the online growth of pornography because profits are not monitored as strictly as other businesses, and the online mediums are more numerous than ever (DeKeseredy, 2015).

The proliferation of pornography over the internet not only changed the amount of pornography available, studies show that the levels of violence and racism also have increased (DeKeseredy, 2015). Scholars along with workers in the porn industry report that over the past decade the levels of violent porn, gore porn, child porn, and racist acts depicted in porn have increased exponentially (DeKeseredy, 2015). Furthermore, scholars warn that the increase in violent and racist pornography may just be the beginning, and these increases are likely to continue with the continued growth of the porn industry (Bridges & Anton, 2013).

Studies are beginning to reveal this increased violence is affecting consumers in negative ways. Some examples of these are negative gender stereotypes including entitlement, objectification, and viewing men as dominant and women as subservient in sexual encounters. Unnatural sexual expectations are also a byproduct of pornography consumption. Viewers of porn create mental images and expectation of what sex should be and attempt to play those out in real-life (Dines, 2010). Many times behavior mirrors the violence of the pornography leading to sexually violent acts (Foubert, 2017). Also, higher levels of pornography consumption creates a desensitization relating to sexual violence which leads to less willingness to stop sexually violent or explicit acts (Foubert, Brosi, & Bannon, 2011). This section will address each of these and provide evidence to the harmful ways they are impacting society.

Negative Gender Stereotypes and Entitlement

Regular consumers of pornography report flawed views of gender roles and stereotypes (Hald, Malamuth, & Lange, 2013). Men who watch pornography at higher rates present lower levels of egalitarian thoughts toward women (Hald et al., 2013). Men who watch pornography also typically view the man as domineering and the woman as subservient in sexual encounters (Hald et al., 2013). Additionally, higher consumers of pornography report higher instances of sexism leading to aggressive sexual encounters (Hald et al., 2013).

Studies have shown that males consuming heavy amounts of pornography exhibit higher levels of sexual entitlement. Bouffard (2010) describes sexual entitlement as attitudes fostering male dominance and hostility toward women in sexual encounters. Sexually entitled men use more pornography, buy into rape myths, and are more sexually aggressive. Sexually entitled men objectify women and largely expect submission in sexual encounters (Bouffard, 2010).

Along with negative gender stereotypes, entitlement issues, and objectification, watching pornography also leads to confusion between fantasies and real life for heavy pornographic consumers. The disconnect between what is viewed virtually between what relationships look like in real life leads some heavy porn users to higher levels of sexual violence against women and even children (DeKeseredy, 2016). The following section discusses the disconnect between fantasy expectations and reality.

Fictional Expectation vs. Reality Leads to Sexual Violence

Consumption of sexually explicit materials directly affects sexual behaviors (Hald, Kuyper, Adam, & Wit, 2013). Watching pornography often leads to acts of sexual violence or risky sexual behaviors such as multiple partners and unprotected sex (Van et al., 2017). As was explained previously, the violence in pornography continues to increase, oftentimes leading pornography consumers down a violent sexual path. DeKeseredy (2015) found that pornography consumption was a key risk factor for women who experienced sexual violence and pornography played a role in the violence men exhibited toward women in sexual acts.

Pornography use is a predictor of unwanted sexual advances (Mikorski & Szymanski, 2017). These unwanted sexual advances oftentimes stem from a desire to recreate what was seen on a video or other pornographic medium (Mikorski & Szymanski, 2017). Researchers reported that men pressured sexual partners into imitating what was viewed on pornographic videos. When this took place, the sexual encounters were routinely violent or at least outside of a consensual sexual relationship (DeKeseredy, 2015). The victims of these sexually violent encounters were in casual sexual relationships, dating relationships, marriage relationships and even recently divorced (DeKeseredy & Olsson, 2011).

Furthermore, researchers are finding that higher levels of consumption of pornography create a sort of callousness to sexual violence and nonconsensual sexual practices. This callousness often times leads individuals into not recognizing sexually violent behavior and an unwillingness to intervene when experiencing or witnessing nonconsensual or violent sexual behaviors (Foubert & Bridges, 2017). The following section reviews this desensitized state.

Flipping the Script: An Unwillingness to Recognize and Stop Sexual Violence

Researchers are finding that higher levels of porn consumption over time desensitize individuals to a point where the likelihood of men intervening in sexually violent situations is diminished. This diminished sense of bystander intervention was similar between men and women (Foubert & Bridges, 2017). In addition to being less likely to intervene in nonconsensual situations, men who watch higher amounts of porn are more likely to believe rape myths and have increased levels of behavioral intent to rape and are more likely to believe rape myths (Foubert et al., 2011).

Studies show that regular viewing of pornography changes the sexual script for individuals. A sexual script is a belief system developed from social norms and experiences that help dictate what roles people play in sexual encounters (Gagnon & Simon, 2005). Higher consumption of pornography alters the sexual script oftentimes in detrimental ways. Braithwaite et al. (2015) contend that pornography changes the sexual script leading to riskier sex practices, higher levels of nonconsensual sex acts and lower levels of sexual intimacy.

A major limitation to pornography research is that scholars are hesitant or not able to keep pace with the rapid growth of pornography on the internet. Academic scholars and university leaders have long deemed pornography research as not fitting in the academic setting (Ullen, 2014). However, this hesitancy is beginning to be met with more studies analyzing the effects pornography has on consumers. This is much needed research and as this section highlights, failure to address the issues pornography creates, may have severe and in some cases, life altering consequences.

Pornography and Women

Despite the existence of self-described "feminist" pornographers (Whisnant, 2016), scholarship has yet to bear out that pornography can be more empowering than disempowering to women (Arakawa et al., 2012). In fact, a number of feminist scholars actually argue that pornography is implicitly discriminatory and violent toward women (Romito & Beltramini, 2011). The previously cited study conducted by Bridges et al. (2010) of mainstream pornography in 2005 is informative here. Analyzing 304 scenes, the researchers found that 88.2% of scenes were violent. Within those scenes, 94.4% of aggressive acts were directed toward women, 70.3% of those acts were perpetrated by men, and 95.9% of the time women expressed pleasure or neutrality toward this aggression. Violence toward men was minimal and when it occurred, men were four-times more likely than their female counterparts to show displeasure on screen.

Unfortunately, the common scripts of both mainstream and niche pornography not only portray physical aggression toward women, but they also perpetuate notions of objectification and degradation (Gorman et al., 2010). The larger societal impact of these scripts, as they normalize violent sexual and relational behavior, is still under study, but cases from around the world are beginning to reveal the damaging effects of pornography for women.

Abuse in Intimate Relationships

One of the most significant risks to women in a "pornified" relationship is abuse from a partner (DeKeseredy, 2014). In a qualitative study of 55 women from rural Ohio, DeKeseredy and Hall-Sanchez (2017) uncovered a cohort of women trapped by small-town cultures, economics, and social pressures in dangerous, porn-informed relationships. Many of these women were pressured to watch—or, at the very least, allow their partners to watch—what is colloquially known as "gonzo," a form of ultra-aggressive pornography. While the study could not verify a causal relationship between this porn use and abuse, all of the women studied shared stories of nonnormative sexual behavior and 80% were victims of at least two types of nonsexual abuse, as well. They reported being stalked, blackmailed, psychologically degraded and manipulated, and having their possessions taken, damaged, or destroyed.

DeKeseredy and Hall-Sanchez (2017) uncovered five themes in their interviews, which they linked with abusive tendencies. Primarily men were (1) learning about sex and sexual "norms" through pornography, (2) seeking to imitate pornography and to compare their partners in terms of body type and sexual proclivity to characters in pornography, (3) introducing other sexual partners in their relationships, (4) filming sexual acts without consent, and (5) adopting the broader culture of pornography in everyday life. These trends, coupled with a strong male peer support system that favored pornography use and sexual subjugation and objectification of women, fed a perilous environment for women in these rural communities.

Emotional and Psychological Damage

Pornography use puts women at risk of psychological and emotional trauma, as well. Wright and Tokunaga (2017) studied a cohort of women who perceived their partners to be pornography users and found that the presence of pornography in a relationship, whether implicit or explicit, impacts a woman's feelings of self. Prior to their study, Wright and Tokunaga unpacked common arguments for and against pornography use in intimate relationships. They expected that women might be satisfied by their partners' pornography use based on three factors: (1) pornography could provide "educational" value, leading to more fulfilling sex; (2) pornography could provide a sexual catharsis for men, reducing their inclination toward physical infidelity; and (3) pornography could empower women in their sexual expression.

Existing literature and anecdotal evidence suggested to the researchers, however, that there could be more reasons for women to be dissatisfied than satisfied. Pornography use could be suggestive of virtual infidelity, it could display a lack of relational commitment, damage the sense of a partner's character, create dissonance between private and public life, cause a partner to feel "like leftovers," force a partner to vie for sexual attention, create high-pressure contexts to imitate painful sexual acts, damage body image, and erode self-esteem. Consistent with their hypotheses, through an extensive meta-analysis of quantitative and qualitative literature, Wright and Tokunaga (2017) found a strong correlation between pornography use and dissatisfaction. Women who perceived their partners to be pornography users were less relationally satisfied, less sexually satisfied, and less satisfied with their bodies. Impact on self-satisfaction was not found to be statistically significant, but it is important to note that no correlation surfaced on any front between pornography use and satisfaction for women. In all cases, just the perception of pornography use led to emotional and psychological damage for women.

A Vicious Cycle of Harm

Studies show that as women are exposed to and victimized by pornography, they are increasingly likely to enter into a cycle of high-risk sexual behavior, nonnormative sexual attitudes, and abuse (Davis, Norris, George, Martell, & Heiman, 2006; Kernsmith & Kernsmither, 2009). Romito and Beltramini (2011), in a study of Italian youth, found that young girls were three times more likely than boys to be pressured into watching pornography by their romantic partners. Once exposed, Kernsmith and Kernsmither (2009) found that pornography use among women is a significant predictor of all forms of sexual aggression except for physical violence and intimidation. Female pornography users were more likely to leverage extortion, bargaining, sweet talk, deceit, obligation, and emotional manipulation for sex. Researchers theorize that in these instances women could be imitating what they see in pornography, which does not often depict women as physically aggressive but does typically depict them as sexually willing and often insatiable.

Unfortunately, the damage of porn consumption goes further than sexual aggressiveness for women. Davis et al. (2006) found that women who consume aggressive pornography, particularly when this behavior is positively reinforced and consumed alongside alcohol, develop calloused attitudes toward female-directed violence and victimization. In their study, a group of sober and intoxicated women were exposed to an eroticized rape depiction in which the victim's response was left ambiguous. This depiction was intentionally counter to what is often shown in rape myth supportive pornography, in which female victims ultimately "enjoy" being raped. Instead, study participants were asked to assert their own value judgment on the episode. What the researchers discovered was disturbing in considering cycles of abuse fostered by pornography. Intoxicated women were more likely to describe the rape episode as socially acceptable and were more likely to envision themselves as "enjoying" being the victim. Intoxicated women reported more arousal at the depiction and were less likely than their sober counterparts to label the event as "rape."

Making these outcomes of sexual aggressiveness and acceptance of violent "norms" worse is the fact that these patterns seem to be self-perpetuating. Romito and Beltramini (2011) found that young girls who experienced family psychological violence were 5.8 times more likely to watch pornography. Girls who experienced sexual violence were 4.24 times more likely to watch pornography. A third of these girls reported watching pornography that depicted strong violence toward women and the majority of these girls reported that, in part, they were watching pornography to "learn about sex." Interestingly, girls with a history of psychological violence were almost twice as likely to watch violent pornography than their peers. Romito and Beltramini (2011) offer two theories as to why this might be. It could be that some women have heightened interest or preoccupation with sex following abuse. This could be particularly salient among young women who were coerced into watching pornography as a "learning" exercise by their abusers. Second, women could be watching violent pornography as a coping strategy. Seeing violent sexual behavior frequently and broadly across pornography could normalize their abusive experiences, numbing the emotional and psychological pain of those episodes.

A movement exists that claims that some pornography can be sexually exciting and liberating for women (Whisnant, 2016), and it is true that not all pornography is as extreme or explicit in its violence as "gonzo" (DeKeseredy & Hall-Sanchez, 2017). However, as Bridges et al. (2010) have illustrated, even mainstream, soft core pornography is overwhelmingly gender-biased and steeped in narratives that normalize aggression toward women. These on-screen narratives can lead to a host of off-screen abuses. From physical and psychological damage in intimate relationships, to predicaments of life satisfaction and identity, to dangerous cycles of sexual aggression and the acceptance of violent sexual myths, women in pornified contexts live in the crosshairs of what many authors have called a public crisis (Romito & Beltramini, 2011).

Adolescents, Pornography, and Sexual Violence

Pornography has shown a substantial impact on the minds and behaviors of adolescents. Due to the developing nature of the adolescent brain, we hold that adolescents are particularly susceptible to the negative effects of pornography consumption. These negative effects are manifested in both sexual and societal attitudes and behaviors. It is especially concerning that adolescent use of pornography is a significant predictor of sexual violence (Ybarra & Thompson, 2018).

Adolescent Access to Pornography

Suggesting that the advent of recent technology has increased young people's access to sexual content is a significant understatement. Pornography, once requiring physical transmission through production and purchase, can now be accessed limitlessly and freely through a few keystrokes in a Google search bar (Walker, Makin, & Morczek, 2016). Even society's recent ties to desktop computers have been replaced by mobile phones. Most teenagers can access pornography at will—anytime, anywhere (Owens, Behun, Manning, & Reid, 2012; Stanley et al., 2018). Of course, adolescents do not have to seek sexually charged content; they often encounter it involuntarily through participation in other forms of entertainment. Paul Wright (2011) assembled data from multiple studies to demonstrate that mass media's sexual content so invades young people's lives that its effects cannot be easily avoided. Malamuth and Huppin (2005) concur that television is a significant source of adolescents' exposure to sex-saturated material. Although not all sexual content can be strictly labeled as pornographic, social media, YouTube, and other supposedly filtered environments still enable adolescents to be exposed to far more sexual content than even centerfold magazines of the past could have offered. Furthermore, the pornography industry is a multibillion dollar enterprise that is actively utilizing a variety of new means (such as interactive gaming systems and personal digital assistants) to make pornography accessible to a new, emerging generation of consumers—even if this generation is still underage (Alexy et al., 2009).

Adolescent Usage of Pornography

The wide and increasing availability of pornography ensures that adolescent rates of consuming it will also be high and increasing. According to one study, as many as 91% of adolescents acknowledge having purposefully read, watched, or listened to some form of sexual media; in another study, as many as 70% of teenagers report unintentional exposure to pornography (Malamuth & Huppin, 2005). It is almost certain these percentages are supported strongly by adolescent males, who are known to consume pornography in numbers disproportionate to females (Landripet, 2016). In fact, adolescent consumers of pornography are more likely to be male, older (within the stages of puberty), sensation seekers, and have disturbed family relationships (Peter & Valkenburg, 2016). However, when all types of pornography and forms of contact are combined, half or more of all adolescents can be categorized as having viewed pornography.

Pornography's Impact on Adolescents

What impact does adolescents' exposure to pornography have upon them? Do the unique qualities of adolescence produce a unique impact? Adolescence, as a stage of development, involves transitional changes in body, mind, emotions, social interactions, sexuality, and more. That these changes are occurring while exposure to pornography is taking place suggests something different might be happening in the adolescent than what would be happening in those whose maturation is relatively stable (Owens et al., 2012). When considering pornography's impact on a variety of developing attitudes and behaviors, adolescents' susceptibility becomes apparent.

Sexual Attitudes

Even though most adults who are exposed to pornography experience some changes in attitudes regarding matters of sexuality, pornography's impact upon adolescents' sexual attitudes appears to be even stronger. In adolescents, pornography use is directly associated with permissive sexual attitudes and stronger gender-stereotypical beliefs (Peter & Valkenburg, 2016). Adolescent males who regularly view pornography are more likely to hold negative gender attitudes (Stanley et al., 2018). Youth who consume pornography develop unrealistic ideals about sexuality, including sexual preoccupation, with females experiencing feelings of inferiority and males fearing inability to perform sexually (Owens et al., 2012). Frequent viewing of pornography is associated with adolescents' plans to have more sexual partners in the future (Alexy et al., 2009).

Sexual Behaviors

Mass media's sexual content almost certainly impacts adolescents' sexual behavior (Wright, 2011). Exposure to pornographic content, therefore, would be expected to demonstrate significant impact, which it does. Greater frequency in viewing pornography is associated with higher incidences of "hooking up" with a higher number of "hookup partners"; it is also associated with having had more sexual partners and more single occasion sexual partners (Alexy et al., 2009).

Boys who view pornography are more likely to be involved in sexting—sending sexually explicit messages and images (Stanley et al., 2018). Adolescent consumption of violent pornography is linked to increased aggression in sexual relationships (Owens et al., 2012; Landripet, 2016).

Sexual Violence

Adolescents' use of pornography is directly connected to sexual behaviors extending beyond mutual consent. Boys' regular viewing of pornography is associated with increased sexual coercion and abuse (Stanley et al., 2018). In young people, ages 10–21, continuing exposure to violent pornography is a strong predictor of five types of sexual violence: sexual harassment, sexual assault, coercive sex, attempted rape, and rape (Ybarra & Thompson, 2018). Alexy et al. (2009) found that sexually reactive adolescents using pornography are more likely to engage in coerced sexual acts, forced sexual acts, sex with animals, and exposing themselves to strangers.

Societal Attitudes and Behaviors

In addition to pornography's connection to negative outcomes in matters of developing sexuality, pornography has also been linked to negative societal impacts, as well. Owens et al. (2012) found that young people who view pornographic material report that doing so decreases their self-confidence; they manifest higher incidences of depressive symptoms; they also are more inclined to delinquent behaviors. Among children and adolescents who are considered sexually reactive, exposure to pornography makes them more inclined to lying, stealing, truancy, manipulation, and arson (Alexy et al., 2009). Ultimately, adolescents using pornography report diminished life satisfaction (Willoughby, Young-Petersen, & Leonhardt, 2018).

These overwhelming signs of adolescent maladjustment associated with exposure to pornography point to just how damaging pornography can be to the developing mind. Adolescents' strong and increasing consumption of pornography continues to be a matter of public importance and should remain a matter of public concern.

Children

In this section, we discuss the intersections between children (those under 18), pornography and violence. Obviously, because of their age, children cannot consent to being in pornography. Thus, we classify child pornography as an act of sexual violence. Indeed, the content of child pornography is often overtly violent (McKibbin, Humphreys, & Hamilton, 2017).

Children Viewing Pornography

Many individuals age 10–17 view pornography, including about half in this age range, with more of this population using as they get older. The pornography they see includes behaviors that most parents would not want their kids acting out, for example, unprotected sex, nonrelational and recreational sex exchanges, group sex, and sex with strangers. Other depictions include women as sexual objects subordinate to men as well as male to female aggression. Moreover, nearly 90% of scenes in pornographic movies include aggressive behavior such as choking, gagging, or spanking—almost always toward a woman (Wright, 2014).

What is the impact of watching this pornography? Children exposed to it are less likely to use contraceptives, have more nonrelational and recreational sexual attitudes and behaviors, and have a higher likelihood of engaging in group sex. Exposure to porn also correlates with the perception that women are sex objects and with perpetration of sexually aggressive behavior (Brown & L'Engle, 2009; Wright, 2014).

Children in Pornography

During the last decade, interest in pornography featuring teens (above and below the age of consent) has significantly increased (Walker et al.,

2016). Internationally, there is a 70% increase in pictures of girls under 10 and a 25% increase in those over 10 appearing in online pornography (Smith, Thompson, & Davidson, 2014). If one accepts the definition of child sexual abuse proffered by the World Health Organization, defining it essentially as involving children in sexual activity they cannot fully understand, consent to, for which they are not developmentally prepared, or otherwise violates the laws or taboos of society, then the making of child pornography constitutes child sexual abuse (World Health Organization, 2006). About half of the child sexual abuse that is perpetrated today is carried out by children or other people under the age of 21 (McKibbin et al., 2017). When people under 21 who have committed child sexual abuse have been studied, researchers find that this population has difficulty controlling their pornography use and often cite such use as a factor leading to their abuse of other children (McKibbin et al., 2017).

A common producer of child pornography is young people themselves. Among those people under 21 who upload nude or nearly nude sexual images to the internet, one in six images depicts a child 15 or under. Nearly all images are created using webcams and nearly all images feature girls. A majority of the behavior commonly depicted in images made by girls 15 years old and younger included pictures of naked genitalia; nearly half included nonpenetrative sexual activity. Nearly all such images are located on websites that primarily host sexual pictures of young girls. It is noteworthy that most of the images of girls under 15 were taken with a webcam rather than a phone. This suggests that taking the photos may have been coerced by a third party who is either present with them or chatting online (Internet Watch Foundation, Microsoft, 2015).

Adults Who View Child Pornography

When discussing child pornography offenders, there is such diversity in their personality characteristics that an exact profile is difficult to pinpoint. Though some assume that offenders begin with viewing online child porn and escalate to contact offending, researchers have found that some offenders are contact offenders first and then later start downloading child pornography. Thus, a single offender type is difficult to put forth (Henshaw, Ogloff, and Clough, 2017). However, commonalities in several studies do point to limited characteristics where offender types can be roughly distinguished.

Aside from other children, child pornography viewers are almost all men, Caucasian, in their late 30s to mid-40s, employed, and well educated (Henshaw et al. 2017; McKibbin et al., 2017; Wolak, Finkelhor, & Mitchell, 2011). When people in the general, non-incarcerated population, have been questioned about their child pornography usage, they have been found to be more antisocial and sexually deviant than the general population. Some characteristics that are associated with a higher likelihood of viewing child pornography include ever having sex with a male, holding the perception of children as seductive, having friends who have watched child pornography, frequent pornography use, greater than average aggressive tendencies, ever viewing violent pornography, and engaging in sexually coercive behavior (Seto et al., 2014).

Toward an Offender Typology

Three groups of people who exploit children are identifiable by their behavior. They include (a) people who view child pornography, (b) people who both look at child pornography and carry out hands on offenses, and (c) those do not look at child pornography but do commit hands-on offenses. Given the high volume of notifications police departments get of people looking at child pornography, police desire a method to identify men at high risk of a contact offense so that they can prioritize saving children from hands-on offenses. Among men arrested for possession of child pornography, variables that predicted their committing a contact offense include prior police contacts, charges, or convictions concerning non-contact sexual offending, the confiscation of more than two computers during a house search, having victims under 5 years old, and having intrusive or violent content in the material confiscated (Smid, Schepers, Kamphuis, van Linden, & Bartling, 2015). Researchers determined that past victimization of a child is the strongest predictor of future victimization of a child. In addition, people who have sexual contact with children have more cognitive distortions and more emotional identification with children (Babchishin, Hanson, & VanZuylen, 2014).

Although it appears heterogeneity exists among child porn only offenders, there do appear to be key differences between child porn offenders and contact sexual offenders. A distinguishing characteristic between child pornography offenders and hands-on offenders is that child pornography offenders tend to be otherwise high functioning members of society who are prosocial individuals and who can exercise self-control (Clevenger, Navarro, and Jasinski, 2016; Henshaw et al., 2017). Contact sex offenders, when compared to child porn only offenders, have lower socioeconomic status, are older, have less education, have lower occupational standing and are more likely to be mentally ill. A higher portion of child porn only offenders are single than their married contact offender counterparts. Child porn only offenders also have a lower interest in romantic relationships and may also be less skilled than contact offenders in initiating and maintaining intimate relationships (Henshaw et al., 2017).

Interestingly, child pornography only offenders score higher on victim empathy than contact offenders, suggesting that empathy may play a protective role in preventing hands-on offenses. Offenders who use both child pornography and who have contact offenses score higher than any group on pedophilia (Babchishin et al., 2014). Online child pornography offenders are more likely to have deviant sexual interests, yet, the online only offender had lower victim access, and lower antisociality (Babchishin et al., 2014).

Conclusion

In conclusion, it is clear that the connection between sexual violence and pornography is strong. While not a one-to-one causal connection, the use of pornography, especially frequent use of violent pornography, is a major risk factor for committing sexual violence. As this chapter comes to a close, it seems fitting to report on a few studies that show signs that the impact of pornography can be inhibited. For example, some level of education about pornography, even briefing or debriefing a study, can lessen some of the harms (Allen, D'Alessio, Emmers, & Gebhardt, 1996; Isaacs & Fisher, 2008; Vandenbosch & Van Oosten, 2018). Furthermore, it seems that intrinsic religiosity—a type of religious commitment where one reads religious texts and frequently attends religious services—also mitigates some of the impact of pornography (Foubert & Rizzo, 2013). Studying these personality and environmental variables are ripe areas for future studies.

References

Alexy, E. M., Burgess, A. W., & Prentky, R. A. (2009). Pornography use as a risk marker for an aggressive pattern of behavior among sexually reactive children and adolescents. *Journal of the American Psychiatric Nurses Association, 14*, 442.

Allen, M., D'Alessio, D., Emmers, T. M., & Gebhardt, L. (1996). The role of educational briefings in mitigating effects of experimental exposure to violent sexually explicit material: A meta-analysis. *The Journal of Sex Research, 33*(2), 135–141.

Arakawa, D. R., Flanders, C., & Hatfield, E. (2012). Are variations in gender equality evident in pornography? A cross-cultural study. *International Journal of Intercultural Relations, 36*(2), 279–285.

Babchishin, K. M., Hanson, R. K., & VanZuylen, H. (2014). Online child pornography offenders are different: A meta-analysis of the characteristics of online and offline sex offenders against children. *Archives of Sexual Behavior, 44*(1), 45–66.

Baer, J. L., Kohut, T., & Fisher, W. A. (2015). Is pornography use associated with anti-woman sexual aggression? Re-examining the Confluence Model with third variable considerations. *The Canadian Journal of Human Sexuality, 24*(2), 160–173.

Bouffard, L. A. (2010). Exploring the utility of entitlement in understanding sexual aggression. *Journal of Criminal Justice, 38*(5), 870–879.

Braithwaite, S., Coulson, G., Keddington, K., & Fincham, F. (2015). The influence of pornography on sexual scripts and hooking up among emerging adults in college. *Archives of Sexual Behavior, 44*(1), 111–123.

Braun-Courville, D. K., & Rojas, M. (2009). Exposure to explicit web sites and adolescent sexual attitudes and behaviors. *Journal of Adolescent Health, 45*, 156–162.

Bridges, A. J., & Anton, C. (2013). Pornography and violence against women. In *Violence against girls and women: international perspectives* (pp. 183–206).

Bridges, A. J., Wosnitzer, R., Scharrer, E., Sun, C., & Liberman, R. (2010). Aggression and sexual behavior in best-selling pornography videos: A content analysis update. *Violence Against Women, 16*(10), 1065–1085.

Brown, J. D., & L'Engle, K. L. (2009). X-rated: Sexual attitudes and behaviors associated with U.S. early adolescents' exposure to sexually explicit media. *Communication Research, 36*(1), 129–151.

Carroll, J., Busby, D., Willoughby, B., & Brown, C. (2017). The porn gap: Differences in men's and women's pornography patterns in couple relationships. *Journal of Couple and Relationship Therapy, 16*(2), 146–163.

Clevenger, S. L., Navarro, J. N., & Jasinski, J. L. (2016). A matter of low self-control? Exploring differences between child pornography possessors and child pornography producers/distributers using self-control theory. *Sexual Abuse, 28*, 555–571.

Davis, K. C., Norris, J., George, W. H., Martell, J., & Heiman, J. R. (2006). Rape-myth congruent beliefs in women resulting from exposure to violent pornography: Effects of alcohol and sexual arousal. *Journal of Interpersonal Violence, 21*(9), 1208–1223.

DeKeseredy, W. S. (2014). *Thinking critically about adult pornography and woman abuse: New progressive directions in research, theory, and policy.* Paper presented at the National Deviancy Conference, Teeside University.

DeKeseredy, W. S. (2015). Critical criminological understandings of adult pornography and woman abuse new progressive directions in research and theory. *International Journal for Crime, Justice and Social Democracy, 4*(4).

DeKeseredy, W. S. (2016). Pornography and violence against women. In C. A. Cuevas & C. M. Dennison (Eds.), *The Wiley handbook on the psychology of violence* (1st ed.). Hoboken, NJ: John Wiley & Sons, Ltd.

DeKeseredy, W. S., & Hall-Sanchez, A. (2017). Adult pornography and violence against women in the heartland: Results from a rural Southeast Ohio study. *Violence Against Women, 23*(7), 830–849.

DeKeseredy, W. S., & Olsson, P. (2011). Adult pornography, male peer support, and violence against women: The contribution of the "dark side" of the internet. In M. V. Martin, M. A. Garcia-Ruiz, & A. Edwards (Eds.), *Technology for facilitating humanity and combating social deviations: Interdisciplinary perspectives*. Hershey, PA: Information Science Reference.

Dines, G. (2010). *Pornland: How porn has hijacked our sexuality*. Boston, MA: Beacon Press.

Foubert, J. D. (2017). *How pornography harms: What teens, Young adults, parents and pastors need to know*. Boston: LifeRich Publishers.

Foubert, J. D., & Bridges, A. J. (2017). What is the attraction? Pornography use motives in relation to bystander intervention. *Journal of Interpersonal Violence, 32*(20), 3071–3089.

Foubert, J. D., Brosi, M. W., & Bannon, R. S. (2011). Pornography viewing among fraternity men: Effects on bystander intervention, rape myth acceptance and behavioral intent to commit sexual assault. *Sexual Addiction & Compulsivity, 18*(4), 212–231.

Foubert, J. D., & Rizzo, A. J. (2013). Integrating religiosity and pornography use into the prediction of bystander efficacy and willingness to prevent sexual assault. *Journal of Psychology and Theology, 41*(3), 242–251.

Fritz, N., & Paul, B. (2017). From orgasms to spanking: A content analysis of the agentic and objectifying sexual scripts in feminist, for women, and mainstream pornography. *Sex Roles, 77*(9–10), 639–652.

Gagnon, J. H., & Simon, W. (2005). *Sexual conduct: The social sources of human sexuality*. Chicago: Aldine.

Gorman, S., Monk-Turner, E., & Fish, J. N. (2010). Free adult internet web sites: How prevalent are degrading acts? *Gender Issues, 27*(3–4), 131–145.

Häggström-Nordin, E., Sandberg, J., Hanson, U., & Tyde'n, T. (2006). "It's everywhere": Young Swedish people's thoughts and reflections about pornography. *Scandinavian Journal of Caring Sciences, 20*, 386–393.

Hald, G., & Malamuth, M. (2015). Experimental effects of exposure to pornography: The moderating effect of personality and mediating effect of sexual arousal. *Archives of Sexual Behavior, 44*(1), 99–109.

Hald, G. M., Kuyper, L., Adam, P. C. G., & Wit, J. B. F. (2013). Does viewing explain doing? Assessing the association between sexually explicit materials use and sexual behaviors in a large sample of Dutch adolescents and young adults. *Journal of Sexual Medicine, 10*(12), 2986–2995.

Hald, G. M., Malamuth, N. N., & Lange, T. (2013). Pornography and sexist attitudes among heterosexuals. *Journal of Communication, 63*(4), 638–660.

Henshaw, M., Ogloff, J. R. P., & Clough, J. A. (2017). Looking beyond the screen: A critical review of the literature on the online child pornography offender. *Sexual Abuse, 29*(5), 416–445.

Internet Watch Foundation & Microsoft. (2015). *Emerging Patterns and Trends Report #1 Youth-Produced Sexual Content*.

Isaacs, C., & Fisher, W. (2008). A computer based educational intervention to address potential negative effects of Internet pornography. *Journal of Communication Studies, 59*(1), 1–18.

Kernsmith, P. D., & Kernsmither, R. M. (2009). Female pornography use and sexual coercion perpetration. *Deviant Behavior, 30*, 589–610.

Kingston, D., Malamuth, N., Fedoroff, P., & Marshall, W. (2009). The importance of individual differences in pornography use: Theoretical perspectives and implications for treating sexual offenders. *Journal of Sex Research, 46*(2–3), 216–232.

Klaassen, M. J., & Peter, J. (2015). Gender (in) equality in Internet pornography: A content analysis of popular pornographic Internet videos. *The Journal of Sex Research, 52*(7), 721–735.

Laier, C., Schulte, F., & Brand, M. (2012). Pornographic picture processing interferes with working memory performance. *The Journal of Sex Research, 50*(7), 642–652.

Landripet, I. (2016). Perceived pornography realism as a mediator of the association between pornography use and problematic sexual behavior among male adolescents. In *13th Congress of the European Federation of Sexology*.

Lo, V., & Wei, R. (2005). Exposure to internet pornography and Taiwanese Adolescents' sexual attitudes and behavior. *Journal of Broadcasting & Electronic Media, 49*(2), 221–237.

Malamuth, N., Hald, M., & Koss, G. (2012). Pornography, individual differences in risk and men's acceptance of violence against women in a representative sample. *Sex Roles, 66*(7), 427–439.

Malamuth, N., & Huppin, M. (2005). Pornography and teenagers: The importance of individual differences. *Adolescent Medicine Clinics, 16*(2), 315.

Malamuth, N. M., & Impett, E. A. (2001). Research on sex and the media: What do we know about effects on children and adolescents? In D. G. Singer & J. L. Singer (Eds.), *Handbook of children and the media* (pp. 269–287). Thousand Oak, CA: Sage.

McKibbin, G., Humphreys, C., & Hamilton, B. (2017). "Talking about child sexual abuse would have helped me": Young people who sexually abused reflect on preventing harmful sexual behavior. *Child Abuse & Neglect, 70*, 210–221.

Mikorski, R. M., & Szymanski, D. (2017). Masculine norms, peer group, pornography, Facebook, and men's sexual objectification of women. *Psychology of Men and Masculinity, 18*(4), 257–267.

Owens, E., Behun, R., Manning, J., & Reid, R. (2012). The impact of internet pornography on adolescents: A review of the research. *Sexual Addiction & Compulsivity, 19*(1–2), 99–122.

Peter, J., & Valkenburg, P. (2016). Adolescents and pornography: A review of 20 years of research. *The Journal of Sex Research, 53*(4–5), 509–531.

Peter, J., & Valkenburg, P. M. (2006). Adolescents' exposure to sexually explicit material on the internet. *Communication Research, 33*, 178–204.

Peter, J., & Valkenburg, P. M. (2008). Adolescents' exposure to sexually explicit internet material and sexual preoccupancy: A three-wave panel study. *Media Psychology, 11*, 207–234.

Peter, J., & Valkenburg, P. M. (2010). Adolescents' use of sexually explicit internet material and sexual uncertainty: The role of involvement and gender. *Communication Monographs, 77*, 357–375.

Romero-Sánchez, M., Toro-García, V., Horvath, M., & Megías, J. (2017). More than a magazine: Exploring the links between lads' mags, rape myth acceptance, and rape proclivity. *Journal of Interpersonal Violence, 32*(4), 515–534.

Romito, P., & Beltramini, L. (2011). Watching pornography: Gender differences, violence and victimization. An exploratory study in Italy. *Violence Against Women, 17*(10), 1313–1326.

Ropelato, J. (2010). *Internet pornography statistics*. Retrieved from TopTenReviews.com

Rudman, L., & Mescher, K. (2012). Of animals and objects. *Personality and Social Psychology Bulletin, 38*(6), 734–746.

Sabina, C., Wolak, J., & Finkelhor, D. (2008). The nature and dynamics of internet pornography exposure for youth. *Cyber Psychology and Behavior, 11*, 691–693.

Seto, M. C., Hermann, C. A., Kjellgren, C., Priebe, G., Sveden, C., & Langstro, N. (2014). Viewing child pornography: Prevalence and correlates in a representative community sample of young Swedish men. *Archives of Sexual Behavior, 44*(1), 67–79.

Shim, J. W., Kwon, M., & Cheng, H. I. (2015). Analysis of representation of sexuality on women's and men's pornographic websites. *Social Behavior and Personality: An International Journal, 43*(1), 53–62.

Simons, L., Simons, R., Lei, M.-K., & Sutton, T. (2012). Exposure to harsh parenting and pornography as explanations for males' sexual coercion and females' sexual victimization. *Violence and Victims, 27*(3), 378–395.

Smid, W., Schepers, K., Kamphuis, J. H., van Linden, S., & Bartling, S. (2015). Prioritizing child pornography notifications: Predicting direct victimization. *Sexual Abuse, 27*(4), 398–413.

Smith, P. K., Thompson, F., & Davidson, J. (2014). Cyber safety for adolescent girls: Bullying, harassment, sexting, pornography, and solicitation. *Current Opinion in Obstetrics & Gynecology, 26*(5), 360–365.

Stanley, N., Barter, C., Wood, M., Aghtaie, N., Larkins, C., Lanau, A., & Overlien, C. (2018). Pornography, sexual coercion and abuse and sexting in young people's intimate relationships: A European study. *Journal of Interpersonal Violence, 33*(19), 2919–2944.

Sun, C., Bridges, A., Johnson, J., & Ezzell, M. (2016). Pornography and the male sexual script: An analysis of consumption and sexual relations. *Archives of Sexual Behavior, 45*(4), 995–995.

Sun, C., Ezzell, M., & Kendall, O. (2017). Naked aggression: The meaning and practice of ejaculating on a Woman's face. *Violence Against Women; Thousand Oaks, 23*(14), 1710–1729.

Ullen, M. (2014). Pornography and its critical reception: Toward a theory of masturbation. *Jump Cut: A Review of Contemporary Media, 51*.

Valkenburg, P. M. (2010). Processes underlying the effects of adolescents' use of sexually explicit internet material: The role of perceived realism. *Communication Research, 37*, 375–399.

Van Oosten, J., Jochen, P., & Vandenbosch, L. (2017). Adolescents' Sexual Media Use and willingness to engage in casual sex: differential relations and underlying processes. *Human Communication Research, 43*(1), 127–147.

Vandenbosch, L., & Van Oosten, M. (2018). Explaining the relationship between sexually explicit internet material and casual sex: A two-step mediation model of perceived utility and instrumental attitudes. *Archives of Sexual Behavior, 34*(2), 150–159.

Vannier, S. A., Currie, A. B., & O'Sullivan, L. F. (2014). Schoolgirls and soccer moms: A content analysis of free "teen" and "MILF" online pornography. *The Journal of Sex Research, 51*(3), 253–264.

Vega, V., & Malamuth, N. (2007). Predicting sexual aggression: The role of pornography in the context of general and specific risk factors. *Aggressive Behavior, 33*(2), 104–117.

Walker, A., Makin, D., & Morczek, A. (2016). Finding Lolita: A comparative analysis of interest in youth-oriented pornography. *Sexuality & Culture, 20*(3), 657–683.

Wery, A., & Billieux, J. (2016). Online sexual activities: An exploratory study of problematic and non-problematic usage patterns in a sample of men. *Computers in Human Behavior, 56*(March), 257.

Whisnant, R. (2016). "But what about feminist porn?" Examining the work of Tristan Taormino. *Sexualization, Media, & Society, 2*(2), 1–12.

Willoughby, B., Carroll, J., Busby, J., & Brown, S. (2016). Differences in pornography use among couples: Associations with satisfaction, stability, and relationship processes. *Archives of Sexual Behavior, 45*(1), 145–158.

Willoughby, B., Young-Petersen, B., & Leonhardt, N. (2018). Exploring trajectories of pornography use through adolescence and emerging adulthood. *The Journal of Sex Research, 55*(3), 297–309.

Wolak, J., Finkelhor, D., & Mitchell, K. (2011). Child pornography possessors: Trends in offender and case characteristics. *Sexual Abuse, 23*(1), 22–42.

World Health Organization. (2006). *Preventing child maltreatment: A guide to taking action and generating evidence*. Geneva: World Health Organization and International Society for Prevention of Child Abuse and Neglect.

Wright, P. (2011). Mass media effects on youth sexual behavior assessing the claim for causality. *Annals of the International Communication Association, 35*(1), 343–385.

Wright, P., & Bae, J. (2015). A national prospective study of pornography consumption and gendered attitudes toward women. *Sexuality & Culture, 19*(3), 444–463.

Wright, P., Sun, C., Steffen, N., & Tokunaga, R. (2015). Pornography, alcohol, and male sexual dominance. *Communication Monographs, 82*(2), 252–270.

Wright, P. J. (2014). Pornography and the sexual socialization of children: Current knowledge and a theoretical future. *Journal of Children and Media, 8*(3), 305–312.

Wright, P. J., & Tokunaga, R. S. (2017). Women's perceptions of their male partners' pornography consumption and relational, sexual, self, and body satisfaction: Toward a theoretical model. *Annals of the International Communication Association, 42*(1), 55–73.

Ybarra, M., & Thompson, R. (2018). Predicting the emergence of sexual violence in adolescence. *Prevention Science, 19*(4), 403–415.

Zhou, Y., & Paul, B. (2016). Lotus blossom or dragon lady: A content analysis of "Asian women" online pornography. *Sexuality & Culture, 20*(4), 1083–1100.

Pornography and Sexual Assault

8

Ana J. Bridges

Pornography and Sexual Assault

Sexual assault is defined as any sexual act that is nonconsensual, including sexual acts that occur with people who are unable to consent by virtue of age (e.g., a minor) or cognitive status (e.g., a person who is intoxicated or unconscious; a person who by virtue of a cognitive deficit is unable to consent) (U.S. Department of Justice, 2016). In its most extreme form, sexual assault includes forcible penetration or rape. However, nonconsensual sexual assaults do not necessarily involve physical contact between victim and perpetrator; for instance, exposing oneself to an unsuspecting person ("flashing") or showing someone pornographic material when this is unwanted also meets the definition of sexual assault (Breiding, Basile, Smith, Black, & Mahendra, 2015). Approximately one in four women and one in nine men in the US have experienced some sort of unwanted sexual contact, although underreporting of assaults remains problematic (Breiding et al., 2015). Specifically, an estimated 32% of US women have experienced unwanted sexual attention, 28% experienced unwanted sexual contact, and 19% experienced forced or substance-use facilitated rape that included genital penetration (Smith et al., 2017). In men, the rates are 13% for unwanted sexual attention, 11% for unwanted sexual contact, and 1.5% for penetrative rape (Smith et al., 2017). Most sexual assaults are perpetrated by men and in approximately 80% of cases the perpetrator is known to the victim (Smith et al., 2017).

Understanding the causes of sexual assault requires a broad and multifaceted approach; singular explanations are insufficient (Ward, Fisher, & Beech, 2016). Causes can include: biological/genetic predispositions; adverse childhood experiences such as experiences of abuse and neglect; psychological traits such as a lack of empathy, attitudes supportive of violence, difficulties with emotion regulation, or interpersonal conflict; sociocultural factors such as gender role socialization, violence and conflict, and economic strain; and contextual factors such as provocation or alcohol or drug intoxication (Ward et al., 2016). To focus on any one factor runs the risk of ignoring the myriad other causes of sexual assault, and to potentially miss how these different factors interact. Nevertheless, this chapter concerns itself with how the viewing of pornography in particular relates to sexual assault through mechanisms such as shaping sociocultural norms about gender, shifting attitudes about sexual violence and objectification of women, and modeling aggressive sexual behavior. I begin by providing a definition of pornography and detail the scope of the industry, especially as it

A. J. Bridges (✉)
Department of Psychological Science, University of Arkansas, Fayetteville, AR, USA
e-mail: abridges@uark.edu

W. T. O'Donohue and P. A. Schewe (eds.), *Handbook of Sexual Assault and Sexual Assault Prevention*,
https://doi.org/10.1007/978-3-030-23645-8_8

has moved increasingly to web-based dissemination. Next, theories that articulate why pornography might relate to sexual violence against women are presented. Evidence about the role pornography may play in sexual assault is reviewed according to three primary methods of scientific investigation: laboratory studies, surveys, and crime statistics. I end with some suggestions for additional research to address key gaps in the literature.

What is Pornography?

Pornography is often defined as sexually explicit material that is designed to arouse the viewer/user (Ferguson & Hartley, 2009; Hald, Malamuth, & Yuen, 2010). Since the late 1800s, the US has regulated the distribution of materials considered "obscene" (*Act for the Suppression of Trade in, and Circulation of, Obscene Literature and Articles of Immoral Use; 17 Stat. 598, 1873).* This act was first challenged when, in 1957, the US Supreme Court heard arguments for two cases, both challenging whether the obscenity act was a violation of the right to free speech, guaranteed under the US constitution's First Amendment (*Roth* vs. *US; Alberts* vs. *California*). Although the Supreme Court ruled obscene materials were not protected under the First Amendment, its decisions redefined obscene materials as those that violated contemporary community standards and whose primary aim or theme was to arouse excessive sexual interests. Defining pornography therefore became a matter of its normative content *and* its primary purpose, but both of these components have remained difficult to quantify in a reliable manner (Gould, 2010).

While the content of pornography is highly variable, mainstream pornography that is marketed towards heterosexual male viewers tends to follow a rather predictable pattern (Tarrant, 2016). The focus of the medium (initially print materials such as books and magazines, then video home system or VHS, and increasingly now digital videos available on the internet) is on the male gaze and male sexual pleasure. For instance, many films are shot using "point of view" (or POV), a pornography film style that attempts to place the viewer into the scene as though he or she were a camera person or main character; most POV pornography is shot from the male actor's perspective (Bakonyi, 2012). The videos often open directly onto a scene with two (or more) people naked or nearly naked and quickly progress to include oral sex, anal sex, vaginal sex, and end with male ejaculation. Female pleasure is not the primary focus, although verbally female performers spend much of the video time expressing pleasure at every touch and position. Consent is rarely depicted explicitly—although this is often also true in nonpornographic films (Jozkowski, Rhoads, Canan, & Hunt, 2016)— and discussions of safe sex or expressions of affection are infrequent (Bridges et al., 2010; Willis, Canan, Jozkowski, & Bridges, 2018). Women tend to meet traditional standards of beauty and much of mainstream pornography may include elements of subtle or overt racism and sexism, such as depicting Black actors as lower status and greater instance of aggressive behavior in cross-race scenes compared to same-race scenes (Bridges et al., 2010; Cowan, & Campbell, 1994; Klaassen & Peter, 2015). Despite these undertones of racism, over time Black Americans are more likely to view pornography than Whites and their rate of use is increasing faster than any other racial demographic group (Perry & Schleifer, 2017).

Much of popular pornography depicts acts of aggression or degradation. For instance, a content analysis of 50 popular pornographic films from 2004 to 2005 found nearly 50% of scenes contained verbal aggression (mostly insults), 75% of scenes contained spanking, 54% of scenes depicted gagging, 37% showed hair pulling, and 27% showed choking (Bridges et al., 2010). Atkinson and Rodgers (2016) noted "insertion of objects, gagging and vomiting resulting from forceful oral sex, simulated rape, strangulation, anal sex and spitting have become merely choices from drop-down menus on many popular porn websites" (p. 1298). Furthermore, social networks may promote a sense of shared interest and normalization, which can result in a reduced perception of harm (Atkinson & Rodgers, 2016).

Despite the appearance of variety, the majority of internet pornography is being offered by a single corporation, MindGeek (Johnson, 2010; Tarrant, 2016). MindGeek owns and manages over 150 pornography websites, including popular sites such as PornHub, RedTube, and YouPorn, as well as many pornography film production and distribution companies.

Pornography is big business, although precise revenue data are difficult to obtain. Some estimate the industry to generate between $5–12 billion per year (for a review, see Tarrant, 2016). Internet piracy and the ease of availability of low- or no-cost pornography on the internet have resulted in significant declines in profits. Estimates are that in 2013, 78% of a mixed-gender sample of internet-using adults in the US had accessed a pornographic website (Tarrant, 2016). Users are more likely to be men, younger, and more highly educated (Buzzell, 2005). In a study of approximately 200 heterosexual couples, Bridges and Morokoff (2011) found 71% of men and 56% of women had viewed pornography at some point in the past year; the frequency of use among men and women was significantly different, with men on average accessing pornography once per week and women on average accessing pornography once per month. In another study of over 600 heterosexual couples, Poulsen, Busby, and Galovan (2013) found 36% of women and 73% of men reported any pornography use, with men's frequency of use greater than women's.

Three of the top 10 most trafficked websites are pornography sites (https://www.similarweb.com). During the first half of 2018, xvideos.com ranked sixth highest in the US for web traffic (behind Google, Facebook, YouTube, Amazon, and Yahoo), with an estimated 3.07 billion visits. PornHub, another popular website, reported that in 2017, over 81 million people per day visited their website (the majority of these visitors were located in the US; https://www.pornhub.com/insights/2017-year-in-review). A great deal of the content on PornHub is provided by users themselves who upload homemade videos to the website. In 2017, PornHub reported their users and content partners provided over four million pornographic videos to the website, approximately 20% of which they considered "amateur" videos (those produced by individuals unassociated with a commercial organization). The top five search terms on PornHub by US users in 2017 were lesbian, MILF (moms I'd like to f***), step sister, ebony, and step mom. The growth of the mobile phone industry is reflected in statistics detailing how pornography is accessed: in 2008, 99% of PornHub users accessed pornography through their desktop computers and only 1% through mobile devices. One decade later, 75% of PornHub users accessed the website through mobile devices (https://www.pornhub.com/insights/10-years).

Historical Perspectives on Pornography's Effects

As technology enhanced its availability, an increased number of scholars and policy makers began asking what might be the effects of pornography use. The first Presidential Commission on Obscenity and Pornography (commonly referred to as the *Lockhart Commission*) was formed in 1967 to evaluate existing laws related to and recommend definitions of obscenity and pornography. Because little scientific work had been done in this area, they also commission two national surveys and some laboratory studies (Bates & Donnerstein, 1990). In its final report in 1970, the Lockhart Commission concluded benefits of existing laws regulating the sale and distribution of pornography lacked community consensus and were largely unsuccessful. They further suggested it was not the role of Congress to determine what adults should and should not read or view or to legislate morality, and recommended a lifting of restrictions. After the Lockhart Commission released its reports, many scholars noted a dearth of scientific research to inform questions of the effects of pornography access on the public (Gould, 2010). Academics therefore began exploring these questions in earnest.

Perhaps in part because of dissatisfaction with the recommendations made by the Lockhart

Commission, in 1985 President Reagan created a second Commission on Pornography (referred to as the *Meese Commission*) (Bates & Donnerstein, 1990). The Meese Commission was tasked with determining the nature, extent, and impact of pornography on society. The Meese Commission concluded there was a *causal* association between violent or degrading pornography and aggressive behaviors and attitudes. In contrast, the Commission was unable to reach consensus regarding whether nonviolent, nondegrading pornography was harmful. The Meese Commission, in particular, has been criticized for its biased methodology and selective inclusion of research (Bates & Donnerstein, 1990).

It is clear pornography has been part of human history for as long as humans have had the capacity to document sexuality (Tarrant, 2016), although recently the distribution has increased with technology to unprecedented levels. Since the early 1970s, there has been concern among scholars, lawmakers, and others about what role, if any, pornography may play in society's ills including violence against women. Most well-known are efforts to categorize pornography as "obscenity" (U.S. Attorney General's Commission on Pornography, 1986). Still in existence today, these obscenity laws make the possession, sale, and distribution via US postal service of some pornographic materials that might meet the legal definition of obscenity illegal, although they are rarely enforced and the context of enforcement has become increasingly narrow (Rowbottom, 2018). Taking a different tactic, Andrea Dworkin and Catherine MacKinnon drafted legislation in the 1980s for the city of Minneapolis that would classify pornography as a form of sex discrimination and a violation of women's civil rights. Although vetoed by the mayor, the city council reintroduced the ordinance, finding that "pornography is central in creating and maintaining the civil inequality of the sexes" and provides a "systematic practice of exploitation and subordination based on sex which differentially harms women" (Baldwin, 1984, p. 630). Other cities also passed the ordinance, but passages were vetoed by city mayors or overturned by US courts. More recently, states such as Florida, Utah, and Kansas have declared pornography constitutes a public health risk, and others, such as Rhode Island, are considering the same, in part because of arguments suggesting viewing pornography can have negative impacts on the user and others.

Critiques of these efforts (obscenity laws, civil rights ordinances, or declarations of public health crises) have suggested these efforts are evidence of "moral panic" that is not rooted in the scientific literature (Klein, 2015). In fact, there has been and continues to be a group of scholars, clinicians, policy makers, and activists who highlight the benefits of pornography. For instance, Watson and Smith (2012) suggested pornography can decrease sexual anxiety, encourage sexual exploration, and increase personal well-being. Hald and Malamuth (2008) found people who used pornography reported being better sexual partners and more open-minded about sex. One study reported young adults saw pornography as empowering, especially feminist and sex-positive pornography that emphasized diversity, modeled sexual consent, and appeared more genuinely enjoyable to performers (Weinberg, Williams, Kleiner, & Irizarry, 2010). Lim, Carrotte, and Hellard (2015) note most of the studies highlighting the benefits of pornography use self-report and focus on perceived benefits and satisfaction; little laboratory work has been done.

Theories Relating Pornography Use to Sexual Assault

Why might people believe pornography use is linked to sexual assault? The question is part of a larger academic effort to understand possible links between consumption of media and behavior (Ferguson & Hartley, 2009). On the one hand, some have argued pornography *reduces* sexual violence because it offers users, primarily men, an outlet to "vent" their sexual urges (Kendall, 2007; Posner, 1994), or have discussed pornography access is associated with greater freedoms (such as free speech) and gender equality, making it a marker of a more open, liberal society that is associated with reduced violence against women (Baron, 1990). On the other hand, some have argued pornography is associated with greater aggression, include sexual assault. These theories range from relatively straightforward (e.g., social modeling) to more complex (e.g., socioecological models). These diverse perspectives are reviewed below.

Theories positing a negative association between pornography and sexual assault. Outlet theories that pornography use provides a substitute for sexual assault rest on an assumption of rational decision-making (Posner, 1994). According to these theories, the biological drive to procreate can be met in multiple ways. Ideally, this drive is met by engaging in consenting sexual relations with a willing partner. However, when this option is not available, people will seek other means of meeting this biological need. In deciding which alternative means a person might pursue, he or she weighs the relative costs and benefits of each option. If the costs of some approaches are low (e.g., viewing pornography and masturbating, which is not illegal and can be typically accessed for free) compared to other approaches (e.g., sexually assaulting someone who is not consenting, which is illegal and has the potential to result in significant financial, personal, and environmental costs), then the person will rationally select the lowest cost option. It stands to reason, then, that decriminalizing pornography and increasing its ease of access would reduce rates of sexual assault (D'Amato, 2006).

A second group of theories argues for a negative relation between pornography access and sexual assault. These theories focus on the relative freedoms people within a society have. Societies with greater freedoms, including free access to sexually explicit material, also tend to be more liberal regarding gender roles and sexual behavior, show greater gender equality, and lower rates of sexual assault (Baron, 1990). Proponents of these theories also focus on how representations of sexuality, especially diverse sexualities of marginalized populations such as people who identify as queer or transgender, have typically been criminalized and maintain power imbalances disfavoring repressed groups (Stardust, 2014). Accordingly, greater access to pornography is seen as both a marker of and perhaps even a causal contributor to greater freedoms and equality. Some pornographers have argued for the value of feminist pornography, in particular, as a way to upend traditional gender roles and increase gender equality (Liberman, 2015).

Theories positing a positive association between pornography and sexual assault. The major theories that have suggested pornography is positively associated with sexual aggression, including sexual assault, rely on social learning theory (Bandura, 1978) and its derivations, feminist theories, and individual differences/risk theories. Social learning theory (Bandura, 1978) states people can and do learn how to behave by watching models. According to this theory, pornography users learn sexual and aggressive behaviors from the materials they watch and, particularly when those behaviors are rewarded, are then more likely to do the same things in their own lives when faced with a similar situation. Bandura (1978) emphasized the difference between learning that could happen as a result of modeling through media (*acquisition*) and the subsequent demonstration of that learning through action (*application*). Learning is broadly construed and may involve learning new sexual behaviors or positions, facilitating already learned manners of behaving sexually, or decreasing inhibitions of previous learning about socially acceptable and unacceptable forms of behavior (Check & Malamuth, 1986).

More updated versions of social learning theory include sexual scripts theory (Simon & Gagnon, 1986) and the 3 AM model (Wright, 2011). Both theories argue pornography is used as one source for learning about sexual behavior—it provides a "script," much like a script an actor in a play might use, for how to behave during a sexual encounter. When faced with a situation that might entail sexual behavior, the user relies on the pornographic script to guide their actions. However, acquiring scripts for sexual behavior does not necessarily mean they will be acted upon—the person has to be in a situation they see as one that matches the script and then apply it to their behavior. As an analogy, people may have some idea about how a soldier might behave in a wartime situation, but lacking an environment that mimics that situation, they would never act in that manner (Check & Malamuth, 1986). Given how often popular pornography includes acts of mild aggression (Bridges et al., 2010, as reviewed above) and lacks modeling of consent or even context to determine implicit consent (Willis et al., 2018), greater consumption of pornography is theorized to result in greater sexual aggression. Indeed, studies of sex offenders find they have greater physiological responses to depictions of explicit sexual assaults than do non-offenders (Abel, Barlow, Blanchard, & Guild, 1977; Seto & Kuban, 1996). However, most pornography does not depict overt acts of sexual violence or rape (Bridges et al., 2010); it is illegal in many countries and most men do not become sexually aroused when rape is depicted as clearly abhorrent to the victim (Malamuth & Check, 1980), so simple modeling is unlikely to explain associations between pornography use and sexual assault.

Theories that have emphasized the role of cultural factors elevating the status of men over women are broadly considered feminist theories. Feminist theorists have argued that materials that objectify and degrade women, including many genres of pornography (Cowan & Campbell, 1994), contribute to a general cultural climate where aggression towards women is seen as the norm (see Baron & Straus, 1987). These theorists argue that such a climate, then, is one in which all forms of violence against women are more tolerated. Feminist theories focus more on how media consumption may shift attitudes supporting notions of women as sex objects, available for male pleasure, and reinforce cultural stereotypes about rape (such as the idea that "no" means "yes" and other rape myths; Lonsway & Fitzgerald, 1994; see also Wright & Tokunaga, 2016). Furthermore, some argue portrayals of women as sex objects may lead viewers to feel violence against women is not as egregious and need not require the same measure of punishment as other crimes (e.g., Mullin & Linz, 1995). Compared to social modeling theories, feminist theories are broader and do not suggest there are necessarily direct links between pornography and sexual violence. Instead, pornography both reflects and creates a cultural climate in which violence against women is tolerated.

Malamuth et al. (1996) developed the confluence model to explain how individual differences relate to risk of sexual violence perpetration. The confluence model states that *for people already predisposed to act violently* (e.g., people high in hostile masculinity and with an impersonal sexual orientation), *pornography can elevate the risk of aggression.* Hostile masculinity is defined as having a domineering and distrustful view of women, while impersonal sexual orientation is defined as the ability to engage in sexual relations without intimacy or a sense of closeness (Baer, Kohut, & Fisher, 2015). The theory suggests that pornography can activate beliefs or stereotypes the person already possesses, thereby potentiating sexual violence. Importantly, the theory (and some research evidence, reviewed below) suggests pornography use does not have these potentiating effects in the absence of preexisting risk factors.

Reviewing the Research Evidence

What, then, is the evidence for an association between pornography and sexual assault? The rest of this chapter concerns itself with reviewing the evidence, providing additional data from 2016 statistics, and suggesting priorities for addressing remaining questions. The studies are divided into three general types: laboratory, correlational, and sociological. Each type has certain strengths and weaknesses (Table 8.1); in combination, they can inform the question of whether, and how, pornography might relate to sexual assault.

Evidence from Laboratory Studies

Laboratory studies represent the most rigorous scientific approaches to measuring how one variable may *cause* something- in fact, it is the only method that can prove causation. A typical

Table 8.1 Types of research studies

Study type	Example	Strengths	Weaknesses
Laboratory	Bring a group of participants into the lab, one at a time Randomly assign participants to either view pornography or view neutral media Measure participants on some outcome, such as willingness to convict a perpetrator of rape	Ability to isolate the effects of an independent variable and measure its impact on a dependent variable Only study design able to discern cause/effect relationships	Low external validity (since you cannot measure actual sexual assault perpetration, researchers must use proxy variables that may not translate well to the real world) Limited sample characteristics (mostly college-aged males)
Correlational-cross-sectional	Give a group of people questionnaires that assess pornography use and sexual assault perpetration attitudes and behaviors	Large samples can be representative of populations Allows more direct measure of the variables of interest	Self-report biases Lack of manipulation of the independent variable means you cannot draw cause–effect conclusions Third variable problem (are associations due to some third variable?) Since all data are collected at the same time point, no ability to discern if pornography use precedes, follows, or coincides with sexual assault attitudes and behaviors
Correlational-longitudinal	Give a group of people questionnaires that assess pornography use and sexual assault perpetration attitudes and behaviors At a later point in time, re-administer questionnaires	Large samples can be representative of populations Allows more direct measure of the variables of interest Allows for temporal ordering of variables (e.g., does pornography use come before or after attitudes and behaviors supportive of sexual assault?)	Self-report biases Lack of manipulation of the independent variable means you cannot draw cause–effect conclusions Third variable problem
Sociological-secondary analyses	Obtain large-scale data from existing sources at regional, state, national, or international levels (e.g., pornography distribution rates and crime statistics) Correlate the variables of interest Can compare across regions (e.g., in different countries) or across time (e.g., before and after passage of laws permitting sales of pornography)	Large data sets allow for strong tests of hypotheses No need to collect original data, so less expensive Allow for comparisons across cultures or subcultures and time	Data may not correspond precisely to variables of interest (e.g., may be difficult to obtain estimates of pornography use, or crime that is underreported) Lack of manipulation of the independent variable means you cannot draw cause–effect conclusions Third variable problem

laboratory study examining whether pornography *causes* aggression will include (1) random assignment of participants to experimental or control conditions, (2) manipulation of the independent variable (typically pornography exposure), (3) measurement of the dependent variable (typically some measure of aggression), and (4) the use of statistical significance testing (and, ideally measures of effect size) to examine group differences. Studies examining how pornographic material affects sexual aggression are necessarily limited in how aggression can be measured. It is not ethical, possible, or desirable to have participants actually harm another person, sexually or otherwise, so proxy variables must be used that are thought to index sexual aggression. For instance, some studies have operationalized sexual aggression by changes in self-reported attitudes (such as acceptance of rape myths; Donnerstein & Berkowitz, 1981), self-reported likelihood of willingness to rape if assured they would not be caught (Check, 1985), willingness to convict an accused sexual perpetrator in the context of a mock trial (Zillman & Bryant, 1982), adding hot sauce to someone's food (Fischer & Greitemeyer, 2006), or showing a person a dirty joke or picture they believe the person will find offensive (Nagayama Hall & Hirschman, 1994). In a review of laboratory paradigms to examine sexual aggression, Davis et al. (2014) summarize evidence of the reliability (i.e., consistency) and validity (i.e., theoretical associations and predictive power) of these analogues. Most lack information about reliability; however, the majority show evidence of theoretical associations with related concepts (and, importantly, lack of associations with theoretically unrelated concepts) and predictive power. With technological advances, some studies are now indexing sexually aggressive behavior using virtual reality (Abbey & Wegner, 2015) or instant messaging (Angelone, Mitchell, & Carola, 2009) with the hope this will expand the behavioral responses participants may exhibit in a lab and will provide greater external validity to real-world behavior. However, because these methods are just beginning to emerge, they have not yet been evaluated for their reliability or validity.

The earliest empirical study I could find examining pornography and aggression was conducted by Meyer in 1972. Forty-eight male college students participated in this experiment. Each participant arrived at the lab individually to participate in a study on grading using electrical shocks. The participant was given 5 min to write an essay on the importance of obtaining a college education, then told they would be graded on their essay by another participant (in reality, the other participant was a study confederate). The participant was then given a "bad" grade by the confederate in the form of eight electric shocks (where a maximum was 10, and higher number of shocks meant a worse grade). This was done to provoke the participant into experiencing anger. After the shocks, it was the confederate's "turn" to write an essay which the participant would then grade. During the five-minute wait period in which the confederate was presumably writing their essay, most participants were shown a film that was ostensibly part of another study and would make "good use" of their five-minute wait time. The three types of film clips used in the study were (a) violent but not sexual (i.e., a knife fight), (b) sexually explicit (a scene described as hard-core pornographic from a "stag" film), or (c) exciting but not violent or sexual (a cowboy riding a half-broken horse). One-fourth of participants saw no film and served as the control condition. After viewing the film, participants were asked to grade the confederate's essay (in the form of assigning electric shocks). Meyer found participants in the violent film group gave the greatest number of shocks (average of 7.50 out of a possible 10). Participants in the sexually arousing (pornographic) film gave the second highest number of shocks (average of 6.00), while participants in the control (average of 4.67) and nonviolent, nonsexual film (average of 4.83) conditions gave the least number of shocks. The author concludes that sexual arousal from pornographic media can result in increased retaliatory aggressive behavior in subjects who had been previously provoked.

A more recent study by Hald and Malamuth (2015) of 201 Danish adults (100 men, 101 women) invited participants to attend a laboratory session where participants were randomly assigned to view either pornography or a neutral film and complete self-report measures of agreeableness and attitudes supporting violence against women (comprised of acceptance of interpersonal violence and acceptance of rape myths). The pornographic film included explicit depictions of oral sex, vaginal sex, anal sex, double penetration, and facial ejaculation. One scene was between one man and one woman, while another scene was between two men and one woman. None of the films depicted explicit violence or degradation and both depicted actors signaling sexual pleasure. In the control condition, the participants viewed film scenes about nature. Participants were divided into groups based on their trait-level agreeableness. Analyses revealed no differences between the experimental and control groups on measures of attitudes supporting violence against women; however, for men classified as low in agreeableness, participants in the pornography film condition rated their attitudes supporting violence against women as significantly higher ($M = 43.66$, SD = 10.49) than low agreeableness men in the control condition ($M = 33.45$, SD = 8.89), a large effect.

A meta-analysis of 16 experimental studies found a significant effect of exposure to pornography in the lab and subsequent rape myth acceptance scores, $r = 0.15$ (Allen et al., 1995), which corresponds with a small effect size. These effects were present whether experiments compared control participants who viewed neutral films or no films to: (a) participants who viewed violent pornography ($r = 0.11$, 5 studies), or (b) participants who viewed nonviolent pornography ($r = 0.13$, 7 studies). Because the differences between these two effect sizes does not reflect a direct comparison of violent and nonviolent pornography, Allen et al. (1995) also calculated an average effect size for studies comparing participants who viewed violent to nonviolent pornography, finding that viewing violent pornography increased rape myth acceptance more than viewing nonviolent pornography ($r = 0.16$, 8 studies). In all cases, however, effect sizes for the association between pornography viewing and rape myth acceptance were small. In short, rigorous laboratory studies that are true experiments find small but significant effects of pornography use on aggression-supportive attitudes and behaviors.

Evidence from Correlational Studies

Cross sectional. Studies exploring pornography use with sexual assault perpetration (or proxy variables that are related to sexual assault perpetration, like attitudes supporting sexual violence, rape myth acceptance, and willingness to intervene in a potentially assaultive situation as a witness) represent the bulk of research on this topic. It is helpful to note research suggests differing methods of assessing sexual aggression tend to be highly correlated with one another (average $r = 0.28$, range 0.03–0.62; Bouffard & Goodson, 2017). Cross-sectional studies involve surveying a group of people at one time period, asking about both pornography use and sexual assault variables, and then examining whether pornography use and sexual assault variables are correlated. Because the data are collected all at once, the ability to discern temporal ordering is impossible (meaning perhaps pornography use precedes later sexual violence, or perhaps people who engage in sexual assault later seek out pornography, or some third factor relates to both pornography use and sexual violence). Data are also typically collected using self-report, meaning participant responses are subject to biases such as socially desirable responding (answering questions in a way that would meet with societal approval) or recall biases (e.g., not being able to recall some events, or over-reporting other events if they were particularly salient). Nevertheless, these studies help inform the question of whether pornography use may relate to sexual assault potential.

Numerous studies have assessed whether pornography use is associated with attitudes supporting violence against women (Hald et al., 2010). These attitudes are typically captured with questionnaires that assess things like (a) condoning violence in interpersonal relationships (such as beliefs that sometimes men are justified in hitting their wives); (b) adversarial relationships between men and women (such as believing women take advantage of men); and (c) rape myths (such as the idea that women who dress provocatively are "asking" for rape, or that women initially refuse sex in order not to appear "easy," even if they are sexually interested). A meta-analysis of nine studies ($N = 2309$ men) exploring the average correlation between pornography use and violence-supportive attitudes found a significant positive association, $r = 0.18$, $p < 0.001$ (Hald et al., 2010), a small effect. The findings were strongest when correlating violent pornography use to violence-supportive attitudes ($r = 0.24$, $p < 0.001$) but remained significant even when exploring nonviolent pornography and sexual assault attitudes ($r = 0.13$, $p < 0.001$).

Some studies have examined how self-reported pornography use relates to self-reported likelihood of engaging in sexual assault or willingness to rape or sexually coerce someone if guaranteed not to get caught. Published research in this area generally finds a small but positive association between the two variables. For instance, Foubert, Brosi, and Bannon (2011) found small positive correlations between use of sadomasochist ($r = 0.17$) or rape pornography ($r = 0.19$) and self-reported behavioral intentions to sexually assault someone in a sample of 489 college men, all members of fraternities. In studies examining whether pornography use is associated with intervening in the context of witnessing a possible sexual assault, researchers again tend to find higher violent/degrading pornography use is associated with lower bystander behavioral intentions in men, but not women (Foubert & Bridges, 2017). Notably, use of nonviolent sexually explicit pornography did not show the same association.

The most direct answer to the question of whether pornography use is associated with sexual assault can be gleaned by asking study participants about both pornography use and history of sexual assault perpetration. For instance, Stanley et al. (2016) conducted a survey of 4564 European adolescents. Participants completed the paper and pencil surveys in their schools. The surveys assessed, among other things, pornography use (did the participant regularly watch online pornography) and history of sexual coercion perpetration (had the participant ever pressured a partner into kissing, touching, or something else; had they ever pressured or physically forced someone into have sexual intercourse). The researchers found teens who regularly used pornography were twice as likely to report engaging in sexual coercion than teens who did not regularly use pornography, even after controlling for other variables (such as age, academic achievement, and other sexual behaviors).

Although the bulk of studies examine male perpetrators, studies with women also find pornography use relates to sexual coercion perpetration (Kernsmith & Kernsmith, 2009). A meta-analysis of 17 studies cross-sectional studies of both men and women found a small-to-moderate significant association between pornography use and self-reported history of sexual aggression (both physical and verbal), $r = 0.28$, $p < 0.001$ (Wright, Tokunaga, & Kraus, 2016). Higher use of pornography was associated with higher self-reported sexual aggression and this association did not vary as a function of gender (men vs. women), age group (adolescents vs. adults), publication outlets (published vs. unpublished studies), or country (US vs. other countries).

Longitudinal. Longitudinal data exploring pornography use and sexual assault related variables are helpful to inform a temporal ordering of variables. While the literature reviewed above suggested associations between pornography use and variables related to sexual assault, these studies are unable to discern the extent to which one may precede the other in time. Critical to this inquiry is whether there is some self-selection bias- that is, whether people who already hold violence-supportive attitudes against women are more likely to seek media that comport to their preexisting beliefs or if exposure to media relates to subsequent changes in attitudes. Although longitudinal studies cannot confirm causality (does pornography *cause* sexual assault?), it can inform one of the preconditions of causality—ordering of variables in time. Something cannot *cause* something else if it happens *after* the thing it supposedly causes. Given how difficult it is to design good laboratory simulations of sexual aggression, longitudinal studies are important to answering the question of how pornography may influence sexual assault potential.

Peter and Valkenburg (2009) conducted a year-long, three-wave longitudinal study of 962 Dutch adolescents and young adults (aged 13–20 years). Participants completed survey measures online at three time points that included questions about their use of pornography, their liking of pornography, and their views of women as sex objects (e.g., "Unconsciously, girls always want to be persuaded to have sex" and "There is nothing wrong with boys being primarily interested in a woman's body"). Analyses revealed pornography use at time 1 was a significant predictor of viewing women as sex objects 1 year later for both boys and girls (standardized path coefficient = 0.15, $p < 0.01$), while viewing women as sex objects at time 1 was a significant predictor of greater pornography use 1 year later (standardized path coefficient = 0.09, $p < 0.01$), but for boys only. Furthermore, the link between time 1 pornography use and time 3 views of women as sex objects was partially mediated by increased liking for pornography. These results suggest while there is some truth that people select media that comports with their preexisting beliefs, media like pornography may also shape attitudes and beliefs.

Similar findings occur when examining adults. Using national representative samples of adults in the US, Wright and Funk (2014) conducted a longitudinal analysis using the General Social Survey, finding pornography use at time 1 is associated with lower support for policies such as affirmative action and equal rights for women at time 2 (standardized regression coefficient = 0.13, $p < 0.05$), and these associations are stronger than when using policy opposition at time 1 to predict pornography use at time 2 (odds ratio = 0.81, $p > 0.05$). In a meta-analysis of five studies examining the association between pornography use at time 1 and sexually aggressive behavior at time 2, Wright et al. (2016) find a correlation of $r = 0.27$, $p < 0.001$ (moderate effect size). In summary, longitudinal data in general support cross-sectional associations between pornography use and sexual aggression, and suggest the temporal ordering of these associations is such that pornography use precedes later aggression-supportive attitudes, beliefs, and behaviors. These effects were generally small to moderate in size and many held for both men and women.

Evidence from Sociological Secondary Data Studies

One final method researchers have utilized to investigate whether there is an association between pornography use and sexual assault is to examine existing population-based data sources that report on some pornography-related distribution or access variable (e.g., circulation rates of pornographic magazines, pornographic movie rentals, Google searches for terms like "porn," access to high-speed internet, or changes in laws limiting access to pornography) and population-level crime statistics (rates of rape, sexual assault, or sex crimes). The strength of such studies is they provide a macro-level analysis of what happens to *communities* when pornography is more accessible. Limitations include the inability to tie *individual* use of pornography with sexual assault, the frequent need for proxy variables to assess pornography access since these sorts of records are not kept publicly, and the need to limit analyses to reported sexual assaults, a crime which is grossly underreported (Kilpatrick, Resnick, Ruggiero, Conoscenti, & McCauley, 2007). Nevertheless, their findings are informative.

On the whole, and in contrast to much of the experimental and correlational research, findings from population-based studies are more mixed and more likely to find no associations, or even a significant *negative* association, between pornography access and reported sexual assaults (for a review, see Ferguson & Hartley, 2009). For instance, Kutchinsky (1991) examined rates of rape and aggravated assault in four countries over a 20-year period, from 1964 to 1984. Three of the countries (Denmark, Sweden, West Germany) had legalized pornography while one (United States) had not, although pornography remained accessible in the US at that time. The author found rape rates remained stable and low in the three countries where pornography was legal, while rates over the 20-year span were rising dramatically in the US. When examining rates of rape versus rates of nonsexual assaults, Kutchinsky found the rates of both types of crimes increased similarly over time, which he argues suggests the increases in rape are due to general increases in aggressive crime. In the other countries, while rates of aggravated assault were generally moderately increasing over the 20-year time period, rates of reported rape were not increasing or were increasing at a slower pace. The author argued this provides evidence that access to legal pornography does not increase incidents of rape. One important limitation of this study is that it did not measure actual access to pornography- the author assumed legalization equated to increased access and consumption, but also noted pornography was easily accessible in the US during that same time period. The author also suggests increased willingness to report crimes, including rape, may account for some of the changes. Furthermore, at the same time that pornography was decriminalized, many sexual behaviors were also decriminalized (such as same-sex prostitution and voyeurism; Check & Malamuth, 1986). Therefore, the decline in sex offenses may have been due to fewer behaviors meeting the definition of an offense. In fact, rape rates may have actually increased following legalization of pornography in Denmark (Check & Malamuth, 1986).

In six states in the US, Kimmel and Linders (1996) found correlations between circulation rates of nine pornographic magazines and rates of reported rape varied tremendously, from a large negative association (in Ohio, $r = -0.82$) to a moderate positive association (in Florida, $r = 0.30$). Rape rates in general were slowly rising in most states over the 11-year period of the study (1979–1989), but circulation rates of pornographic magazines were declining rapidly over that same time period, likely due to the advent of the home video player. That is, the index of pornography consumption was limited to magazine circulation rates at a time when people began moving away from magazines and towards video tapes as the preferred medium of pornography consumption. In Japan, a non-Western industrialized country with a rich history of producing violent pornography and *manga* (cartoon pornography), increased access to pornography over 20+ year period (from 1970s to 1990s) coincided with a decrease in reported rapes, murder, and violent crimes, but a slight increase in sexual assaults (Diamond & Uchiyama, 1999). The authors conclude not only is pornography access not associated with an increase in sex crimes, but may actually *reduce* sex crimes by giving people a more appropriate outlet to meet sexual needs. (This argument, of course, presupposes sexual assaults are driven by sexual urges and not by a desire to dominate, aggress against, debase, or punish someone; Cowan & Quinton, 1997.) Similar lack of associations between rape and access to pornography have been reported in the Czech Republic (Diamond, Jozifkova, & Weiss, 2011) and in four US states that ceased to enforce obscenity statutes (Winick & Evans, 1996). Notable is that nearly all of these studies examined trends in sexual assault over time but did not provide quantitative measures of pornography consumption from which to then calculate correlations.

Others however have found the opposite relationship. For instance, Baron and Straus (1984) examined rape rates (as reported in the FBI Uniform Crime Reports) and magazine circulation rates for eight pornographic magazines (such as *Playboy* and *Hustler,* all soft-core, since none showed erect penises or penetrative sex) in US states, finding a strong positive correlation between magazine sales and rapes ($r = 0.63$, $p < 0.001$ for 1979 data, and $r = 0.58$ for 1980 data) that remained significant even after controlling for other variables that may relate to rape, such as poverty, race, male gender, and young adult age. Rape rates were strongly associated with other aspects of what Baron and Straus called a “macho culture” that included gender and economic inequality, a culture which may account for both increases in pornography consumption and crimes against women such as sexual assault. Scott and Schwalm (1988) found similar associations when examining rates of reported rape and circulation of 10 popular pornographic magazines in 1982, $r = 0.54$, $p < 0.05$. The association between pornography magazine circulation rates and reported sexual assaults remained significant even after controlling for numerous variables such as poverty, alcohol use, rurality, race, and gender inequality. Gentry

(1991), using standard metropolitan statistical areas as the unit of analysis (instead of states, which are largely heterogeneous in make-up), also found a positive correlation between rates of reported rapes and circulation of three popular pornographic magazines (from 1979 to 1981), $r = 0.25$, $p < 0.01$, but after controlling for variables such as the percentage of the population in that area that was between 18 and 34 years of age, the association between the two variables was no longer significant.

More recently, researchers have used internet access (and broadband access specifically) to index pornography use in communities. Since much of pornography is now accessed through the internet and involves downloading or streaming relatively large video files that require greater internet bandwidth and speed, these studies suggest technology advances that make such streaming less cumbersome are likely to relate to increased pornography use. Bhuller, Havnes, Leuven and Mogstad (2013) analyzed broadband access in Norway over a 10-year period and rates of diverse crime statistics, including rape and child sexual abuse. Unlike many other studies, Bhuller and colleagues included reports, criminal charges, and convictions to index criminal activity. They also collected potential control variables (see below). The authors found increased access to broadband internet was associated with increased sex crimes ($p < 0.05$). Specifically, the authors found that as internet user rates increased by 1 percentage point, the overall rate of sex crimes increased by 1.15 per 100,000 inhabitants. These results remained significant even after controlling for potential covariates including demographic characteristics (percent of population that is female, age, percent of population that is immigrant, population density, education, income, poverty, and unemployment; $p < 0.01$), police density, and rates of other crimes. In follow-up analyses, the authors determine facilitation of reporting was not responsible for the increased reporting of sex crimes (specifically, they found no changes in the ratio of reports of rape to charges of rape across the 10-year period of this study). However, in Germany these results failed to replicate (Nolte, 2017).

In the literature I reviewed, there was no pattern I could discern regarding whether a study was likely to show a positive (vs. no or negative) association between pornography access and reported sexual assaults. In studies that looked at historical data of rape rates (e.g., Diamond et al., 2011 reporting from 1970s to 2000s; Diamond & Uchiyama, 1999 reporting from 1970s to 1990s; Kutchinsky, 1991 reporting from 1960s to 1980s), there is evidence that over time reported rapes are declining. This historically overlaps with technological advances and lifting of legal bans that are presumed to make pornography more accessible, but they also coincide with other important factors that might relate to crime overall, such as improved economic conditions and the rise of women's civil rights efforts in the 1970s and 1980s that increased awareness of sexual assault. There have also been changes in how crimes are categorized and prosecuted. While some of these studies suggested other types of crimes were increasing or occurring at similar rates during the time period in which reported sexual assaults were decreasing (e.g., Diamond et al., 2011 in Croatia; Kutchinsky, 1991 in Denmark, Sweden, and West Germany), others find drops in violent crimes of all types (e.g., Diamond & Uchiyama, 1999 in Japan; Kutchinsky, 1991 in the US). Studies that have indexed pornography access more directly (e.g., Baron & Straus, 1984; Scott & Schwalm, 1988) typically find significant positive correlations, although they may shift after controlling for more proximal variables associated with sexual assault perpetration (e.g., Gentry, 1991).

Secondary Analyses: Predicting State-Level Rates of Reported Forcible Rate from Google Searches for Porn

The contradictory findings between correlation and laboratory-based studies, that generally support small but significant associations between higher pornography use and sexual assault related outcomes, and large-scale sociological and crime statistics studies, that often fail to find evidence between greater pornography distribution rates and sexual assault related crimes, suggest some method-related factors are at play. Fundamentally these different sources of data provide answers to different questions; that is, studies with individuals see whether *within a person* we find higher pornography use is associated with greater sexual assault-related variables, while sociological studies see whether *geographic areas* with higher access to or distribution of pornographic materials also experience higher levels of sex-related crimes. Nevertheless, that a literature review would result in essentially opposite conclusions if we divide studies up by their methodological approaches leads to interpretive challenges. What are we to make of this?

Individual studies certainly, and different approaches to research studies generally, have limitations, which is why it is important to investigate matters utilizing multiple methods. To date, the majority of studies utilizing pornography distribution and crime statistics suffer from two major limitations. Setting aside the issue of the accuracy of crime statistics (which are highly problematic, especially given how often sexual assault is unreported; Kilpatrick et al., 2007), the operationalizations of pornography access have generally been lacking and the associations have failed to control for other variables that may relate to *both* pornography access and crime. In terms of operationalizations of pornography access, studies have either evaluated crime rates pre- and post-legalization of pornography (e.g., Kutchinsky, 1991) or have used number of paid subscriptions to pornographic media, such as magazines, to index pornography access (e.g., Baron & Straus, 1984). Given most pornography is accessed for free and, especially in the last decade, through the internet, these indices are problematic. Some more recent studies examined access to high-speed internet as a proxy for pornography access (Bhuller et al., 2013; Kendall, 2007); however, these studies failed to assess the extent to which internet access was related to actual searches for pornography.

To investigate further the question of how pornography access relates to crime in a given region, and to overcome prior methodological limitations of sociological studies, I examined how internet searches for "pornography" related to reported sexual assault rates in all 50 states and the District of Columbia. I obtained relative search values (RSVs) for 2016 from Google Trends. Google Trends permits users to query how often a given search term occurred in a given time period. The user can specify regions (e.g., states), time periods (e.g., years, months, weeks), and search terms. Google Trends provides normalized scores that range from 0 to 100, which 100 representing the highest interest in that search term over the specified period of time. A score of 50 would mean that that region had half as many search terms as the highest region with a score of 100. Although absolute search queries are not provided, these data do give an index of relative frequency of searches by region and time. This served as the primary independent variable.

I also extracted data from the U.S. Census Bureau (2016) for all 50 states and the District of Columbia for potential covariates in the analysis. Data included: percent of population living in poverty, percent of population age 25+ who had obtained a college education, and percent of population that identified as non-Hispanic White. The primary dependent variable was the number of reported forcible rapes per 100,000 in 2016, extracted from the U.S. Department of Justice (2016).

Descriptive statistics and correlations among study variables are presented in Table 8.2. There was a significant positive bivariate correlation between the states' number of Google Trend searches for "porn" in 2016 and the number of forcible rapes in that state, $r = 0.26$, $p = 0.033$, moderate effect size. Searches for "porn" were also significantly correlated with poverty and educational attainment; states with higher poverty rates and with fewer residents holding a Bachelor's degree or higher had significantly greater Google Trend searches for "porn." The percent of racial/ethnic minorities in a state was unassociated with Google Trend searches for "porn."

A standard multiple regression analysis revealed that after controlling for the three demographic variables (poverty, % non-Hispanic

Table 8.2 Descriptive statistics and correlations among study variables

Variable	1	2	3	4	5
1. Google Trend RSV for "porn"	1.00	–	–	–	–
2. % population living at or below federal poverty level	0.65***	1.00	–	–	–
3. % population age 25+ with Bachelor's degree or higher	−0.83***	−0.46***	1.00	–	–
4. % population non-Hispanic White	0.05	−0.24*	−0.23	1.00	–
5. Number of forcible rapes reported, per 100,000	0.26*	0.22	−0.05	−0.16	1.00
Mean	74.53	12.45	30.04	68.67	43.73
Standard deviation	11.41	3.11	6.12	16.18	13.85

Note. *$p < 0.05$, **$p < 0.01$, ***$p < 0.001$. All variables are from 2016. $N = 51$ (all 50 states and the District of Columbia)

Table 8.3 Standard multiple regression predicting number forcible rapes from pornography Google searches, controlling for demographic variables

Variable	*B* (SE)	*β*	*t*	*p*
1. Google Trend RSV for "porn"	0.86 (0.35)	0.71	2.47	0.017
2. % population living at or below federal poverty level	−0.12 (0.84)	−0.03	−0.14	0.891
3. % population age 25+ with Bachelor's degree or higher	1.17 (0.59)	0.52	2.00	0.052
4. % population non-Hispanic White	−0.07 (0.13)	−0.08	−0.53	0.601

White, and college educated), Google Trend searches for pornography were significantly associated with rates of forcible rape in each state, $\beta = 0.71$, $p = 0.017$. In fact, only searches for "porn" related to sexual assault rates; poverty, educational attainment, and race/ethnicity did not. Results are presented in Table 8.3.

Summary and Future Directions

Research on media effects have been of special interest to scholars for decades, with the question of whether and how pornography use might relate to sexual assault being of particular interest. Across time and methods, the general finding is that pornography, especially violent pornography, appears to be associated with small but significant increases in sexual assault-related variables, such as rape myth acceptance, negative attitudes towards women, self-reported willingness to rape, and past history of assaultive behavior. These effects appear to be more pronounced in some people, especially people who have traits that already place them at risk for increased assault potential (e.g., hostile masculinity, trait-level aggression). At the level of geographic analysis, however, associations are inconsistent.

Key Gaps in the Literature

Despite nearly 50 years of research into the question of how pornography use is associated with sexual assault, key gaps remain. First, the most rigorous scientific approach to answering this question relies on laboratory experiments that include manipulation of the independent variable and observations of the dependent variable. Given studies cannot ethically or feasible examine actual sexual assault perpetration, researchers have had to get creative at developing alternative behaviors that are proxies for assault (e.g., putting hot sauce in someone's food). The degree to which these proxy measures of aggression are valid for indexing actual sexual assault perpetration potential remains questionable. In addition, laboratory studies, although able to manipulate exposure to pornography, do not mimic the ways in which pornography is actually used by people (that is, typically people use pornography to aid masturbation). The potency of pairing pornography with orgasm, which happens frequently outside of the lab but never (or almost never) in the lab means the effects under investigation in these research studies are limited to really answering whether pornography viewing *without masturbation and orgasm* increases aggression.

Second, most studies, especially correlational studies, have participants self-report both pornography use and sexual assault perpetration histories. Self-report data are problematic because of difficulties with accurate recall of past behavior and social desirability responding (Brener, Billy, & Grady, 2003), differing definitions of what "counts" as pornography (Willoughby & Busby, 2016), and a reluctance to report illegal behavior. It is likely technological advances that increase a sense of anonymity, such as computer-assisted surveys, more behaviorally specific questions, and clear time frames can reduce these biases (Fenton, Johnson, McManus, & Erens, 2001; Turner et al., 1998).

Third, particularly for sociological studies, the inability to find accurate estimates of pornography consumption (and users, and types of materials being distributed) in a geographic area creates challenges. Unlike other types of statistics that are regularly kept by governments and municipalities, private industries rarely share distribution statistics. Furthermore, since the vast majority of pornography is now accessed online, anonymously, and for free, estimates of consumption that rely on circulation rates of magazines, store video rentals, or even website subscriptions will largely underestimate use. Fortunately, new metrics such as Google Trends can provide some approximations of pornography access, but the data are not in raw numbers such as the total number of actual Google searches for the word "pornography," nor do they include searches conducted through other search engines or times when people may have accessed a site directly by typing in the URL. Similarly, crime statistics data are limited by crimes that are reported to law enforcement. Many crimes, particularly sexual assaults, are grossly underreported (Kilpatrick et al., 2007). In addition, definitions of crimes change over time, making longitudinal trend research difficult.

Fourth, evaluations of pornography effects on sexual assault tend to evaluate few variables at a single time, such as examining pornography use and objectification of women. However, as Malamuth et al. (1996) articulated in their model, how pornography influences sexual behavior is theoretically quite complex. On the occasions when people have examined three or more variables together, especially over time, interesting caveats to the pornography → sexual assault link emerge (e.g., Hald & Malamuth, 2015; Peter & Valkenburg, 2010). A greater emphasis on exploring more complex relations is important for future research. Relatedly, few studies explore how pornography use *adds* to the prediction of sexual assault potential above and beyond other variables (for an exception, see Vega & Malamuth, 2007). It will be important to continue examining the relative value of assessing pornography use in the prediction of sexual assault potential in relation to other variables.

Last, but not least, the research on pornography and sexual assault has largely been carried out with relatively young, US, primarily White men. This is true of research on sexual aggression in general, which largely ignores the role of culture and ethnic group differences (Nagayama Hall, Teten, DeGarmo, Sue, & Stephens, 2005). However, cultural factors certainly shape variables related to masculinity/femininity, sexual behavior, attitudes towards women, and consequences of violating social norms. In addition, sociocultural differences in exposure to violence and aggression, economic opportunities, familial risk factors, and discrimination experiences can translate into different risks of delinquency in general, and sexual aggression in particular. For instance, Nagayama Hall et al. (2005) found hostile masculinity, a critical component of the confluence model (Malamuth et al., 1996), predicted sexual aggression in Hawaiian Asian Americans, but not in European Americans or mainland Asian Americans). Greater attention to cultural factors and attempts to replicate findings in diverse cultural groups will be critical moving forward.

Conclusion

So, what can we conclude about the link between pornography and sexual assault? Does pornography cause sexual assault? Not directly, no. Other proximal factors such as hostile masculinity and substance use are the most direct and clear causes of sexual assault (Casey et al., 2017; Haikalis, Leone, Parrott, & DiLillo, 2018; Ward et al., 2016). However, the question is whether pornography may contribute in general to a climate that tolerates or even promotes sexual assault. The answer here is more like *yes, with caveats* (for a thorough legal analysis see Adams, 2000). Experimental studies (that allow for tight control of variables, manipulations, and determinations of how pornography *causes* an effect), correlational studies (that allow for self-report of what is typically private behavior, assessment of attitudes and beliefs, and analyses over time), and sociological studies (that allow for community-level effects instead of just focusing on individual-level effects) show increases in rape-supportive attitudes and sexual assault with increased access to pornography, especially violent and degrading pornography (Oddone-Paolucci, Genuis, and Violato, 2000). However, these findings appear to be stronger for some people than for others, such as for people who already possess personal traits that make them at risk for assault and aggression (specifically, people who are high in hostile masculinity; Malamuth, Sockloskie, Koss, & Tanaka 1991), is stronger in people who perceive pornography as being more real (Peter & Valkenburg, 2010), and for people who do not identify or empathize with the effort of performers (Parvez, 2006). Further, effects such as these can be mitigated when participants are debriefed and informed about the possible negative consequences of viewing pornography (Malamuth & Check, 1984). Sexual assault rates are therefore better explained by variables other than pornography use, although pornography use does provide a unique contribution to prediction of sexual assault perpetration (Vega & Malamuth, 2007).

Taken together, research suggests a ban on pornography is not warranted, but rather efforts to increase media literacy, including educating the populace to be more critical consumers of pornography, to limit attempts to enhance realism perceptions, and to peel back the "fun" veneer of pornography production, distribution, and consumption are important. Pornography literacy classes can be infused in sexual education courses; in fact, some have already been doing so with preliminary outcomes being quite positive (Rothman et al., 2018). Continuing to address the gender inequities that promote violence against women and efforts to promote reporting of sexual assault, punishment of perpetrators, and protection of victims remain priorities.

References

Abbey, A., & Wegner, R. (2015). Using experimental paradigms to examine alcohol's role in men's sexual aggression: Opportunities and challenges in proxy development. *Violence Against Women, 21*, 975–996. https://doi.org/10.1177/1077801215589378

Abel, G. G., Barlow, D. H., Blanchard, E. B., & Guild, D. (1977). The components of rapists' sexual arousal. *Archives of General Psychiatry, 34*, 895–903. https://doi.org/10.1001/archpsyc.1977.01770200033002

Adams, D. (2000). Can pornography cause rape. *Journal of Social Philosophy, 31*, 1–43. https://doi.org/10.1111/0047-2786.00029

Allen, M., Emmers, T., Gebhardt, L., & Giery, M. (1995). Exposure to pornography and acceptance of rape myths. *Journal of Communication, 45*, 5–26. https://doi.org/10.1111/j.1460-2466.1995.tb00711.x

Angelone, D. J., Mitchell, D., & Carola, K. (2009). Tolerance of sexual harassment: A laboratory paradigm. *Archives of Sexual Behavior, 38*, 949–958. https://doi.org/10.1007/s10508-008-9421-2

Atkinson, R., & Rodgers, T. (2016). Pleasure zones and murder boxes: Online pornography and violent video games as cultural zones of exception. *British Journal of Criminology, 56*, 1291–1307. https://doi.org/10.1093/bjc/azv113

Baer, J. L., Kohut, T., & Fisher, W. A. (2015). Is pornography use associated with anti-woman sexual aggression? Re-examining the Confluence Model with third variable considerations. *Canadian Journal of Human Sexuality, 24*, 160–173. https://doi.org/10.3138/cjhs.242-A6

Bakonyi, B. (2012). *Gender ideologies on adult video-sharing websites* (unpublished master's thesis). Erasmus University Rotterdam, Netherlands. Retrieved from https://thesis.eur.nl/pub/12318/Bakony.pdf

Baldwin, M. (1984). The sexuality of inequality: The Minneapolis pornography ordinance. *Law & Inequality: A Journal of Theory and Practice, 2*, 629–653.

Bandura, A. (1978). Social learning theory of aggression. *Journal of Communication, 28*, 12–29. https://doi.org/10.1111/j.1460-2466.1978.tb01621.x

Baron, L. (1990). Pornography and gender equality: An empirical analysis. *Journal of Sex Research, 27*, 363–380.

Baron, L., & Straus, M. A. (1984). Sexual stratification, pornography, and rape in the United States. In N. Malamuth & E. Donnerstein (Eds.), *Pornography and sexual aggression* (pp. 185–209). Orlando, FL: Academic Press.

Baron, L., & Straus, M. A. (1987). Four theories of rape: A macrosociological analysis. *Social Problems, 34*, 467–489. https://doi.org/10.1525/sp.1987.34.5.03a00060

Bates, B. J., & Donnerstein, E. I. (1990). Public opinion and the two pornography commissions: Comparing the incomparable. *Southwestern Mass Communication Journal, 6*, 1–14.

Bhuller, M., Havnes, T., Leuven, E., & Mogstad, M. (2013). Broadband internet: An information superhighway to sex crime? *Review of Economic Studies, 80*, 1237–1266. https://doi.org/10.1093/restud/rdt013

Bouffard, L., & Goodson, A. (2017). Sexual coercion, sexual aggression, or sexual assault: How measurement impacts our understanding of sexual violence. *Journal of Aggression, Conflict and Peace Research, 9*, 269–278. https://doi.org/10.1108/jacpr-05-2017-0292

Breiding, M. J., Basile, K. C., Smith, S. G., Black, M. C., & Mahendra, R. R. (2015). *Intimate partner violence surveillance: Uniform definitions and recommended data elements (Version 2.0)*. Atlanta, GA: Centers for Disease Control and Prevention.

Brener, N. D., Billy, J. O., & Grady, W. R. (2003). Assessment of factors affecting the validity of self-reported health-risk behavior among adolescents: Evidence from the scientific literature. *Journal of Adolescent Health, 33*, 436–457. https://doi.org/10.1016/S1054-139X(03)00052-1

Bridges, A. J., Wosnitzer, R., Scharrer, E., Sun, C., & Liberman, R. (2010). Aggression and sexual behavior in best-selling pornography videos: A content analysis update. *Violence Against Women, 16*, 1065–1085. https://doi.org/10.1177/1077801210382866

Bridges, A. J., & Morokoff, P. J. (2011). Sexual media use and relational satisfaction in heterosexual couples. *Personal Relationsips, 18*, 562–585. https://doi.org/10.1111/j.1475-6811.2010.01328.x

Buzzell, T. (2005). Demographic characteristics of persons using pornography in three technological contexts. *Sexuality & Culture, 9*, 28–48. https://doi.org/10.1007/BF02908761

Casey, E. A., Masters, N. T., Beadnell, B., Hoppe, M. J., Morrison, D. M., & Wells, E. A. (2017). Predicting sexual assault perpetration among heterosexually active young men. *Violence Against Women, 23*, 3–27. https://doi.org/10.1177/1077801216634467

Check, J. (1985). *The effects of violent and nonviolent pornography*. Ottawa, Canada: Department of Justice (Department of Supply and Services Contract No. 05SV 19200-3-0899).

Check, J. V. P., & Malamuth, N. M. (1986). Pornography and sexual aggression: A social learning theory analysis. *Annals of the International Communication Association, 9*, 181–213. https://doi.org/10.1080/23808985.1986.11678607

Cowan, G., & Campbell, R. R. (1994). Racism and sexism in interracial pornography: A content analysis. *Psychology of Women Quarterly, 18*, 323–338. https://doi.org/10.1111/j.1471-6402.1994.tb00459.x

Cowan, G., & Quinton, W. J. (1997). Cognitive style and attitudinal correlates of the Perceived Causes of Rape scale. *Psychology of Women Quarterly0, 21*, 227–245. https://doi.org/10.1111/j.1471-6402.1997.tb00110.x

D'Amato, A. (2006). *Porn up, rape down*. Northwestern Public Law Research Paper No. 913013 (June 23).

Davis, K. C., George, W. H., Nagayama Hall, G. C., Parrott, D. J., Tharp, A. T., & Stappenbeck, C. A. (2014). Studying sexual aggression: A review of the evolution and validity of laboratory paradigms. *Psychology of Violence, 4*, 462–476. https://doi.org/10.1037/a0037662

Diamond, M., Jozifkova, E., & Weiss, P. (2011). Pornography and sex crimes in the Czech Republic. *Archives of Sexual Behavior, 40*, 1037–1043. https://doi.org/10.1007/s10508-010-9696-y

Diamond, M., & Uchiyama, A. (1999). Pornography, rape, and sex crimes in Japan. *International Journal of Law and Psychiatry, 22*, 1–22. https://doi.org/10.1016/s0160-2527(98)00035-1

Donnerstein, E., & Berkowitz, L. (1981). Victim reactions in aggressive erotic films as a factor in violence against women. *Journal of Personality and Social Psychology, 41*, 710–724. https://doi.org/10.1037/0022-3514.41.4.710

Fenton, K., Johnson, A., McManus, S., & Erens, B. (2001). Measuring sexual behavior: Methodological challenges in survey research. *Sexually Transmitted Infections, 77*, 84–92. https://doi.org/10.1136/sti.77.2.84

Ferguson, C. J., & Hartley, R. D. (2009). The pleasure is momentary… the expense damnable? The influence of pornography on rap and sexual assault. *Aggression and Violent Behavior, 14*, 323–329. https://doi.org/10.1016/j.avb.2009.04.008

Fisher, P., & Greitemeyer, T. (2006). Music and aggression: The impact of sexual-aggressive song lyrics on aggression-related thoughts, emotions, and behavior toward the same and the opposite sex. *Personality and Social Psychology Bulletin, 32*, 1165–1176. https://doi.org/10.1177/0146167206288670

Foubert, J. D., & Bridges, A. J. (2017). Predicting bystander efficacy and willingness to intervene in college men and women: The role of exposure to varying levels of violence in pornography. *Violence Against Women, 23*, 692–706. https://doi.org/10.1177/1077801216648793

Foubert, J. D., Brosi, M. W., & Bannon, R. S. (2011). Pornography viewing among fraternity men: Effects on bystander intervention, rape myth acceptance and behavioral intent to commit sexual assault. *Sexual*

Addiction & Compulsivity, 18, 212–231. https://doi.org/10.1080/10720162.2011.625552

Gentry, C. S. (1991). Pornography and rape: An empirical analysis. *Deviant Behavior, 12*, 277–288. https://doi.org/10.1080/01639625.1991.9967879

Gould, G. B. (2010). *Obscenity and pornography: A historical look at the American Library Association, the Commission on Obscenity and Pornography, and the Supreme Court* (Unpublished master's thesis). University of Northern Iowa, Cedar Falls, IA.

Haikalis, M., Leone, R. M., Parrott, D. J., & DiLillo, D. (2018). Sexual assault survivor reports of missed bystander opportunities: The role of alcohol, sexual objectification, and relational factors. *Violence Against Women, 24*, 1232–1254. https://doi.org/10.1177/1077801218781941

Hald, G. M., & Malamuth, N. M. (2008). Self-perceived effects of pornography consumption. *Archives of Sexual Behavior, 37*, 614–625.

Hald, G. M., & Malamuth, N. M. (2015). Experimental effects of exposure to pornography: The moderating effect of personality and mediating effect of sexual arousal. *Archives of Sexual Behavior, 44*, 99–109. https://doi.org/10.1007/s10508-014-0291-5

Hald, G. M., Malamuth, N. M., & Yuen, C. (2010). Pornography and attitudes supporting violence against women: Revisiting the relationship in nonexperimental studies. *Aggressive Behavior, 36*, 14–20. https://doi.org/10.1002/ab.20328

Johnson, J. A. (2010). To catch a curious clicker: A social network analysis of the online pornography industry. In K. Boyle (Ed.), *Everyday pornography* (pp. 147–163). New York: Routledge.

Jozkowski, K. N., Rhoads, K. E., Canan, S. C., & Hunt, M. (2016, November). Consent and refusal cues depicted by characters engaging in sexual behavior in popular mainstream films. Presented as part of a symposium, *Understanding the Action in "Lights, Camera, Action": Examining Sexual Behaviors and Sexual Consent Portrayals in Mainstream Films*. Annual Meeting of the Society for the Scientific Study of Sexuality, Phoenix, AZ.

Kendall, T. D. (2007). *Pornography, rape, and the internet*. Mimeo. Retrieved from www.yapaka.be/sites/yapaka.be/files/actualite/pornography-rape-and-the-internet.pdf

Kernsmith, P. D., & Kernsmith, R. M. (2009). Female pornography use and sexual coercion perpetration. *Deviant Behavior, 30*, 589–610. https://doi.org/10.1080/01639620802589798

Kilpatrick, D. G., Resnick, H. S., Ruggiero, K. J., Conoscenti, L. M., & McCauley, J. (2007). *Drug-facilitated, incapacitated, and forcible rape: A national study*. Charleston, SC: National Crime Victims Research & Treatment Center.

Kimmel, M. S., & Linders, A. (1996). Does censorship make a difference? An aggregate empirical analysis of pornography and rape. *Journal of Psychology and Human Sexuality, 8*, 1–20. https://doi.org/10.1300/J056v08n03_01

Klaassen, M. J. E., & Peter, J. (2015). Gender (in)equality in internet pornography: A content analysis of popular pornographic internet videos. *Journal of Sex Research, 52*, 721–735. https://doi.org/10.1080/00224499.2014.976781

Klein, M. (2015). Pornography, the narrative of public health. In A. Bolin & P. Whelehan (Eds.), *The international encyclopedia of human sexuality* (pp. 965–968). London: Wiley-Blackwell.

Kutchinsky, B. (1991). Pornography and rape: Theory and practice? Evidence from crime data in four countries where pornography is easily available. *International Journal of Law and Psychiatry, 14*, 47–64. https://doi.org/10.1016/0160-2527(91)90024-H

Liberman, R. (2015). 'It's a really great tool': Feminist pornography and the promotion of sexual subjectivity. *Porn Studies, 2*, 174–191. https://doi.org/10.1080/23268743.2015.1051913

Lim, M. S. C., Carrotte, E. R., & Hellard, M. E. (2015). The impact of pornography on gender-based violence, sexual health and well-being: What do we know? *Journal of Epidemiological Community Health, 70*, 3–5.

Lonsway, K. A., & Fitzgerald, L. F. (1994). Rape myths: In review. *Psychology of Women Quarterly, 18*, 133–164. https://doi.org/10.1111/j.1471-6402.1994.tb00448.x

Malamuth, N. M., & Check, J. V. P. (1980). Penile tumescence and perceptual responses to rape as a function of victim's perceived reactions. *Journal of Applied Social Psychology, 10*, 528–547.

Malamuth, N. M., & Check, J. V. P. (1984). Debriefing effectiveness following exposure to pornographic rape depictions. *Journal of Sex Research, 20*, 1–13. https://doi.org/10.1080/00224498409551203

Malamuth, N. M., Heavey, C. L., & Linz, D. (1996). The confluence model of sexual aggression: Combining hostile masculinity and impersonal sex. *Journal of Offender Rehabilitation, 23*, 13–37. https://doi.org/10.1300/J076v23n03_03

Malamuth, N. M., Sockloskie, R. J., Koss, M. P., & Tanaka, J. S. (1991). Characteristics of aggressors against women: Testing a model using a national sample of college students. *Journal of Consulting and Clinical Psychology, 59*, 670–681. https://doi.org/10.1037/0022-006x.59.5.670

Meyer, T. P. (1972). The effects of sexually arousing and violent films on aggressive behavior. *Journal of Sex Research, 8*, 324–333. https://doi.org/10.1080/00224497209550766

Mullin, C. R., & Linz, D. (1995). Desensitization and resensitization to violence against women: Effects of exposure to sexually violent films on judgments of domestic violence victims. *Journal of Personality and Social Psychology, 69*, 449–459. https://doi.org/10.1037/0022-3514.69.3.449

Nagayama Hall, G. C., & Hirschman, R. (1994). The relationship between men's sexual aggression inside and outside the laboratory. *Journal of Consulting and Clinical Psychology, 62*, 375–380. https://doi.org/10.1037/0022-006x.62.2.375

Nagayama Hall, G. C., Teten, A. L., DeGarmo, D. S., Sue, S., & Stephens, K. A. (2005). Ethnicity, culture, and sexual aggression: Risk and protective factors. *Journal of Consulting and Clinical Psychology, 73*, 830–840. https://doi.org/10.1037/0022-006X.73.5.830

Nolte, A. (2017). *The internet effects on sex crime and murder: Evidence from the broadband internet expansion in German*. Centre for European Economic Research, Discussion paper no. 17-050. Retrieved from https://papers.ssrn.com/sol3/papers.cfm?abstract_id=3072289.

Oddone-Paolucci, E., Genuis, M., & Violato, C. (2000). A meta-analysis of the published research on the effects of pornography. In C. Violator, E. Oddone-Paolucci, & M. Genuis (Eds.), The changing family and child development (pp. 48-59). Aldershot, England: Ashgate Publishing Ltd.

Parvez, Z. F. (2006). The labor of pleasure: How perceptions of emotional labor impact women's enjoyment of pornography. *Gender & Society, 20*, 605–631. https://doi.org/10.1177/0891243206291109

Perry, S. L., & Schleifer, C. (2017). Race and trends in pornography viewership, 1973–2016: Examining the moderating roles of gender and religion. *Journal of Sex Research, 56*, 62. https://doi.org/10.1080/00224499.2017.1404959

Peter, J., & Valkenburg, P. M. (2009). Adolescents' exposure to sexually explicit internet material and notions of women as sex objects: Assessing causality and underlying processes. *Journal of Communication, 59*, 407–433. https://doi.org/10.1111/j.1460-2466.2009.01422.x

Peter, J., & Valkenburg, P. M. (2010). Processes underlying the effects of adolescents' use of sexually explicit internet material: The role of perceived realism. *Communication Research, 37*, 375–399. https://doi.org/10.1177/0093650210362464

Posner, R. A. (1994). *Sex and reason*. Cambridge, MA: Harvard University Press.

Poulsen, F. O., Busby, D. M., & Galovan, A. M. (2013). Pornography use: Who uses it and how it is associated with couple outcomes. *Journal of Sex Research, 50*, 72–83. https://doi.org/10.1080/00224499.2011.648027

Rothman, E. F., Adhia, A., Christensen, T. T., Paruk, J., Alder, J., & Daley, N. (2018). A pornography literacy class for youth: Results of a feasibility and efficacy pilot study. *American Journal of Sexuality Education, 13*, 1–17. https://doi.org/10.1080/15546128.2018.1437100

Rowbottom, J. (2018). The transformation of obscenity law. *Information & Communications Technology Law, 27*, 4–29. https://doi.org/10.1080/13600834.2017.1393929

Scott, J. E., & Schwalm, L. A. (1988). Rape rates and the circulation rates of adult magazines. *Journal of Sex Research, 24*, 241–250. https://doi.org/10.1080/00224498809551419

Seto, M. C., & Kuban, M. (1996). Criterion-related validity of a phallometric test for paraphilic rape and sadism. *Behaviour Research and Therapy, 34*, 175–183. https://doi.org/10.1016/0005-7967(95)00056-9

Simon, W., & Gagnon, J. H. (1986). Sexual scripts: Permanence and change. *Archives of Sexual Behavior, 15*, 97–120. https://doi.org/10.1007/BF01542219

Smith, S. G., Chen, J., Basile, K. C., Gilbert, L. K., Merrick, M. T., Patel, N. …., et al. (2017). *The National Intimate Partner and sexual violence survey: 2010–2012 state report*. Atlanta, GA: Centers for Disease Control and Prevention.

Stanley, N., Barter, C., Wood, M., Aghtaie, N., Larkins, C., Lanau, A., & Överlien, C. (2016). Pornography, sexual coercion and abuse and sexting in young people's intimate relationships: A European study. *Journal of Interpersonal Violence*,. online ahead of print, *33*, 2919. https://doi.org/10.1177/0886260516633204

Stardust, Z. (2014). Fisting is not permitted': Criminal intimacies, queer sexualities and feminist porn in the Australian legal context. *Porn Studies, 1*, 242–259. https://doi.org/10.1080/23268743.2014.928643

Tarrant, S. (2016). *The pornography industry: What everyone needs to know*. New York: Oxford University Press.

Turner, C. F., Ku, L., Rogers, S. M., Lindberg, L. D., Pleck, J. H., & Sonenstein, F. L. (1998). Adolescent sexual behavior, drug use, and violence: Increased reporting with computer survey technology. *Science, 280*, 867–873. https://doi.org/10.1126/science.280.5365.867

U.S. Attorney General's Commission on Pornography. (1986). *Attorney General's commission on pornography: Final report*. Retrieved from https://catalog.hathitrust.org/Record/000824987.

U.S. Census Bureau. (2016). *Fact Finder.* Retrieved from https://factfinder.census.gov

U.S. Department of Justice. (2016). *Rape and sexual assault*. Retrieved from https://www.bjs.gov/index.cfm?ty=tp&tid=317

Vega, V., & Malamuth, N. M. (2007). Predicting sexual aggression: The role of pornography in the context of general and specific risk factors. *Aggressive Behavior, 33*, 104–117. https://doi.org/10.1002/ab.20172

Ward, T., Fisher, S., & Beech, A. (2016). An integrated theory of sexual offending. In A. Phenix & H. Hoberman (Eds.), *Sexual offending*. New York: Springer.

Watson, M. A., & Smith, R. D. (2012). Positive porn: Educational, medical, and clinical uses. *American Journal of Sex Education, 7*, 122–145.

Weinberg, M. S., Williams, C. J., Kleiner, S., & Irizarry, Y. (2010). Pornography, normalization, and empowerment. *Archives of Sexual Behavior, 39*, 1389–1401. https://doi.org/10.1007/s10508-009-9592-5

Willis, M., Canan, S. N., Jozkowski, K. N., & Bridges, A. J. (2018). *How is sexual consent modeled in popular pornography?* Paper presented at the annual meeting of the International Academy of Sex Research, Madrid, Spain.

Willoughby, B. J., & Busby, D. M. (2016). In the eye of the beholder: Exploring variations in the perceptions of pornography. *Journal of Sex Research, 53*, 678–688. https://doi.org/10.1080/00224499.2015.1013601

Winick, C., & Evans, J. T. (1996). The relationship between nonenforcement of state pornography laws and rates of sex crime arrests. *Archives of Sexual Behavior, 25*, 439–453. https://doi.org/10.1007/BF02347541

Wright, P. J. (2011). Mass media effects on youth sexual behavior: Assessing the claim for causality. *Annals of the International Communication Association, 35*, 343–385. https://doi.org/10.1080/23808985.2011.11678121

Wright, P. J., & Funk, M. (2014). Pornography consumption and opposition to affirmative action for women: A prospective study. *Psychology of Women Quarterly, 38*, 208–221. https://doi.org/10.1177/0361684313498853

Wright, P. J., & Tokunaga, R. S. (2016). Men's objectifying media consumption, objectification of women, and attitudes supportive of violence against women. *Archives of Sexual Behavior, 45*, 955–964. https://doi.org/10.1007/s10508-015-0644-8

Wright, P. J., Tokunaga, R. S., & Kraus, A. (2016). A meta-analysis of pornography consumption and actual acts of sexual aggression in general population studies. *Journal of Communication, 66*, 183–205. https://doi.org/10.1111/jcom.12201

Zillman, D., & Bryant, J. (1982). Pornography and sexual callousness, and the trivialization of rape. *Journal of Communication, 32*, 10–21. https://doi.org/10.1111/j.1460-2466.1982.tb02514.x

9 Rape Mythology and Victim Blaming as a Social Construct

Kathryn M. Ryan

Rape Myths and the Social Construction of Rape

Rape myths are stereotypes about rape that undermine victims', rapists', and society's ability to correctly identify events as rape. These myths presuppose that some events are *real* rapes and that others are not real rapes (e.g., they reflect unfortunate miscommunication, victim manipulation, or sexual prerogatives). Common rape myths include: men cannot be raped, there must be physical resistance for it to be rape, and rape victims are responsible for their rape. Rape myths serve to protect rapists and perpetuate sexual aggression (e.g., Edwards, Turchik, Dardis, Reynolds, & Gidycz, 2011; Gerger, Kley, Bohner, & Siebler, 2007). They are deeply embedded in culture (e.g., Brownmiller, 1975/1981; Lonsway & Fitzgerald, 1994) and can be found in religious doctrine and cultural prescriptions that can apply to both female and male rape victims (e.g., Lonsway & Fitzgerald, 1994; Struckman-Johnson & Struckman-Johnson, 1992; Turchik & Edwards, 2012). Rape myths vary in the popularity with which they are held, but can be impactful even when held by a small minority. Rape myths often suggest that victims are responsible for their rapes (e.g., they engaged in risky and seductive behavior or their appearance caused the event). Rape myths also suggest that "unfortunate" circumstances contribute to purported rape (e.g., the supposed inability to control sexual urges or the presence of alcohol). At their core, rape myths involving female victims are influenced by gender, traditional beliefs, and hostile attitudes toward women (Lonsway & Fitzgerald, 1994, 1995). Rape myths involving male victims are a product of gender stereotypes and sexual norms (Turchik & Edwards, 2012).

Background, History, and the Development of Measures of Rape Myths

Social science theory and research on rape myths are a product of a cultural revolution in Western societies that began in the 1960s. This brought the second wave of the Women's Movement and a concomitant interest in Women's Studies (Evans, 1995). It also brought an interest in the personal and political nature of violence against women (Brown, 2017). It is in this context that social science research on rape flourished. This research noted the widespread presence of rape, the attempted moral justifications for rape, and rape myths.

In 1975, Brownmiller published, *Against Our Will: Men, Women and Rape* (Brownmiller,

K. M. Ryan (✉)
Department of Psychology, Lycoming College, Williamsport, PA, USA
e-mail: ryan@lycoming.edu

W. T. O'Donohue and P. A. Schewe (eds.), *Handbook of Sexual Assault and Sexual Assault Prevention*,
https://doi.org/10.1007/978-3-030-23645-8_9

1975/1981). Brownmiller's book documented the widespread presence of rape and its patriarchal origins, resting on the view of women as property. She noted the use of rape as a weapon of hegemony in wars, pogroms, and subjugation (e.g., slavery). She also described the cultural and political ramifications of rape, "Rape is to women as lynching was to blacks: the ultimate physical threat by which all men keep all women in a state of psychological intimidation" (p. 281). Brownmiller exposed many rape myths (e.g., women lie about rape, women are responsible for rape, and women who do not actively physically resist are not victims of rape). She noted what she called the four *deadly male myths of* (female) *rape* which were: all women want to be raped; no woman can be raped against her will; she was asking for it; and if you're going to be raped, you might as well relax and enjoy it. A central theme of the book was that rape myths promote and foster rape.

At approximately the same time, Koss and her colleagues (e.g., Koss, Dinero, Seibel, & Cox, 1988; Koss & Oros, 1982; Warshaw, 1988/1994) conducted a large-scale study of US college students. This research suggested that there were many victims of rape (as legally defined) who did not label their personal experience as rape (they were *unacknowledged rape victims).* Nevertheless, unacknowledged rape victims often showed the same symptoms as women who were acknowledged rape victims (e.g., sexual dysfunction issues, psychological distress, and problematic alcohol use) (e.g., Frazier & Seales, 1997; Koss et al., 1988; McMullin & White, 2006; Schwartz & Leggett, 1999). This leads to the questions: "Could someone be raped (or rape) and not know it?" and "Why would they not know it?" One answer is found in the widespread misunderstanding concerning the nature of many rapes (e.g., Kanin, 1984; Warshaw, 1988/1994) and the adherence to a real-rape script that assumes that rapes are physically violent events that occur between strangers (e.g., Ryan, 1988). Many rapes involve acquaintances (not strangers); perpetrators use size, strength, and weight to disarm and neutralize the victim (not weapons or extreme physical aggression); there is often prior consensual sexual foreplay; and alcohol and other drugs are often involved. It is likely that rape myths create ideas about the nature of sex that prevent individuals from understanding the reality of rape for many (e.g., Edwards et al., 2011; Ryan, 2011).

Goodchilds and her colleagues added research on adolescents' views concerning the legitimate use of force during sex on dates (e.g., Goodchilds, Zellman, Johnson, & Giarrusso, 1988). Goodchilds et al. asked a mixed-race group of adolescents who were between 14 and 18 years old about the circumstances that legitimized the use of force for sex. Most participants (72%) said that force was never acceptable. Nevertheless, in response to other questions, many said they believed that some circumstances could legitimize the use of force. These circumstances included: he's so turned on he cannot stop, she's had sexual intercourse with other guys, she is stoned or drunk, and she led him on. All of these would be rape myths. Only 34% of the participants said never to all of nine circumstances listed. Goodchilds et al. also found that many boys believed that some situations (e.g., a girl going to a guy's house or to the beach with him) and behaviors (e.g., ticking, professing love, or talking about sex) signaled a girl's interest in sex, a view that might not be shared by their dating partners. Finally, participants were more likely to label nonconsensual sex as rape when the couple wasn't dating.

It is in this larger cultural and scholarly context that research on rape myths emerged. Two of the earliest researchers on rape myth acceptance were Burt (1980) and Feild (Barnett & Felid, 1977; Feild, 1978). Burt and Feild both looked at rape myth acceptance in adult citizens, but Feild also looked at police, victim advocates, and a small number of men who were convicted of rape and currently incarcerated in a mental institution. Both measures explored female rape myth acceptance (i.e., they assumed that perpetrators were male and the victims were female) and were initially validated on college students. Burt's items were drawn from feminist theory and social psychology research and the measure was called the *Rape Myth Acceptance* scale. Burt included two additional scales, *Adversarial Sexual Beliefs* (e.g., "In a dating relationship a woman is largely out to take advantage of a man" p. 222) and *Acceptance of Interpersonal Violence (*e.g., "Sometimes the only way a man can get a cold woman turned on is to used force" p. 222), which were highly correlated with rape myth acceptance. Follow-up research suggested there were potentially three major factors of the *Rape Myth Acceptance Scale* (e.g., Briere, Malamuth, & Check, 1985; Jones, Russell, & Bryant, 1998). They were: Doubts concerning claims of rape, Rape victim blame, and Beliefs that women lie about rape (an additional factor in the Briere et al. study was Rape only happens to certain kinds of women).

Feild's items were drawn from a review of popular and scholarly publications and the measure was called *Attitudes toward Rape*. There were two measures—an initial 25-item measure (Barnett & Felid, 1977) and a final 32-item measure (Feild, 1978). These measures are virtually identical. Feild sought to include items about the act, the victims, and the rapist. Feild also included a test which attempted to measure knowledge about the circumstances of rape; however, there was no correlation between rape knowledge and rape myth acceptance in Feild's study. Barnett and Feild found significant gender differences on 18 items from the 25-item *Attitudes toward Rape* scale, with most of these items indicating that males were more likely than females to believe rape myths. This gender difference has been supported in later research. Gender differences often emerge indicating that females are less likely than males to believe rape myths (e.g., Anderson, Cooper, & Okamura, 1997; Hockett, Smith, Klausing, & Saucier, 2016; Lonsway & Fitzgerald, 1994). Meta-analyses show effect sizes are often in the small-medium range (e.g., Anderson et al. found an average correlation $r = .33$ for gender differences in rape myth acceptance and Hockett et al. found an average $d = .23$ in perceptions of rape victims).

Feild (1978) found eight sub-factors for the 32-item *Attitudes toward Rape* scale. The largest factor was labeled "Women's Responsibility in Rape Prevention" and included items such as "A woman should be responsible for preventing her own rape" (R) and "A raped woman is a responsible victim, not an innocent one" (R) (all items are from Table 1, pp. 161–164). The other factors were: the relationship between rape and sex (e.g., "The reason most rapists commit rape is for sex" (R) and "Rape is the expression of an uncontrollable desire for sex" (R)), punishment for rapists (e.g., "A convicted rapist should be castrated" (R) and "A man who has committed rape should be given at least 30 years in prison" (R)), women's culpability in rape (e.g., "In forcible rape, the victim never causes the crime" and "Women provoke rape by their appearance or behavior" (R)), the perceived normality of rape (e.g., "Rapists are 'normal' men" (R) and "All rapists are mentally sick"), power motivations for rape (e.g., "Women are trained by society to be rape victims" (R) and "All rape is an exercise of male power over women" (R)), perceptions of women after rape (e.g., "A woman should not feel guilty following a rape" (R) and "A raped woman is a less desirable woman"), and women's resistance during rape (e.g., "During a rape, a woman should do everything she can do to resist" (R) and "If a woman is going to be raped, she might as well relax and enjoy it"). Feild found several important group differences in rape myth acceptance. Most notably, victim advocates frequently showed lower rape myth acceptance than the other groups and police officers showed similar attitudes toward rape as rapists on four of the eight factors. Finally, gender differences emerged on seven of the eight factors with females showing more negative attitudes towards rape.

Payne, Lonsway, and Fitzgerald (1999) reviewed the literature and found 24 measures of rape myth acceptance, but Lonsway and Fitzgerald (1995) suggested that Burt's measure was the most widely used. Payne et al. noted that most measures concentrated on beliefs about rape victims and had problems with question wording. They developed the *Illinois Rape Myth Acceptance* scale in response. Their participants were mostly college students, but Payne et al. also distributed the *Illinois Rape Myth Acceptance Scale* to a small number of victim advocates and police cadets. The *Illinois Rape Myth Acceptance Scale* had seven factors: she asked for it, it wasn't really rape, he didn't mean it, she wanted it, she lied, rape is a trivial event, and rape is a deviant event.

The *Illinois Rape Myth Acceptance* scale was later updated to provide a subtler measure of rape myths (McMahon & Farmer, 2011). Based on focus group feedback, McMahon and Farmer updated the wording of items and kept four of the original seven factors: she asked for it, it wasn't really rape, he didn't mean it, and she lied. They also added items that reflected the role of alcohol in unintentionality (i.e., "If a guy is drunk, he might rape someone unintentionally;" "If both people are drunk, it can't be rape;" and "It shouldn't be considered rape if a guy is drunk and didn't realize what he was doing" p. 75). This became a fifth factor. Females were more rejecting of rape myths than males. Only one item showed general agreement: "If a girl acts like a slut, eventually she is going to get into trouble" (54.2% agreed). The other items that were agreed on by at least 33% of the participants were: "If a girl is raped while she is drunk, she is at least somewhat responsible for letting things get out of control" (37%), "When girls go to parties wearing slutty clothes, they are asking for trouble" (34.9%), "If a girl initiates kissing or hooking up, she should not be surprised if a guy assumes she wants to have sex" (36.2%), "When guys rape, it is usually because of their strong desire for sex" (36.2%), "Guys don't usually intend to force sex on a girl" (34.4%), and "If a girl doesn't say "no" she can't claim rape" (33.2%).

Gerger et al. (2007) suggested that most measures of rape myths were outdated and produced highly skewed distributions (i.e., most participants strongly disagreed). In response, they developed the *Acceptance of Modern Myths about Sexual Aggression* scale. It was a 30-item measure and is available in English and German. The *Acceptance of Modern Myths about Sexual Aggression* scale produced higher levels of item acceptance and less skewed distributions than the *Illinois Rape Myth Acceptance Scale*. Sample items include: "It is a biologically necessity for men to release sexual pressure from time to time," "Although the victims of armed robbery have to fear for their lives, they receive far less psychological support than do rape victims," and "If a woman invites a man to her home for a cup of coffee after a night out this means that she wants to have sex" (pp. 439–440). The *Acceptance of Modern Myths about Sexual Aggression* Scale added items that reflected a denial of the scope of sexual assault and a lack of support for relevant policies, along with more traditional rape myth acceptance items assessing antagonism towards its victims, beliefs that male coercion is normal, and beliefs that blame the victim or circumstances (Eyssel & Bohner, 2008).

Finally, Struckman-Johnson and Struckman-Johnson (1992) argued that there are also male rape myths (e.g., adult men cannot be raped) and they developed a measure of *Male Rape Myth Acceptance*. The items were created by face value to reflect the beliefs that males cannot be raped (two items), male rape victims are somewhat to be blamed (two items), and rape is not traumatic for male rape victims (two items). There were six items written with a male perpetrator and six items with a female perpetrator. All items were rated by college students on 6-point Likert scales with higher numbers indicating greater agreement. The items were preceded by a definition of rape. Results showed that most participants disagreed with male rape myths, especially when there were male perpetrators. In addition, female participants showed lower male rape myth acceptance than male participants. The lowest levels of acceptance were found for the traumatic items (i.e., "Most men who are raped by a man (woman) are upset by the incident" (R) and "Most men who are raped by a man (woman) do not need counseling after the incident" (p. 90)); however, some participants agreed that a male rape victim would not be upset when raped by a female (35% of males and 22% of females). For the myth that men cannot be raped, 22% of males and 18% of females agreed (30% of the males and 18% of the females agreed that a strong man could not be raped by a woman). Nevertheless, some of these results might be due to the fact that participants saw a definition of rape before they responded to the measure.

In conclusion, measures of rape myths have evolved along with the larger culture. Most measures suggest some form of victim culpability, desire for perpetrator exoneration, and beliefs that certain types of rape do not occur. They also suggest that rape is a product of sexual urges and people should be skeptical of claims of rape, especially when there is a delay in reporting. We can expect measures to continue to evolve as rape myths change. Many older rape myths (e.g., the trivialization of rape and blatant victim blaming) are now socially unacceptable and have been replaced with the beliefs that some victims contribute to their victimization and that rape can be an unintentional consequence of sexual interactions (McMahon & Farmer, 2011). Alcohol and miscommunication are often invoked (Deming, Covan, Swan, & Billings, 2013; McMahon & Farmer, 2011), along with sexually provocative behaviors and a lack of physical resistance (McMahon & Farmer, 2011; Peterson & Muehlenhard, 2004). Thus, there is a shift from automatically exonerating purported assailants and blaming rape victims to expressing concerns that some behaviors can impair judgment and make individuals vulnerable to victimization/perpetration. Even the earliest research on rape myth acceptance found that some items were endorsed infrequently. For example, the Feild (1978) data showed low levels of agreement with "If a woman is going to be raped, she might as well relax and enjoy it" (p. 162) and "'Nice' women do not get raped" (p. 163). Three subscales from the *Illinois Rape Myth Acceptance Scale* also showed low levels of agreement (i.e., It wasn't really rape, Rape is a trivial event, and Rape is a deviant event; Payne et al., 1999). More recent examples of infrequently endorsed beliefs are "Any woman who is careless enough to walk through 'dark alleys' at night is partly to be blamed if she is raped" (p. 439, Gerger et al., 2007) and "If the accused 'rapist' doesn't have a weapon, you really can't call it rape" (p. 77, McMahon & Farmer, 2011).

It is possible that, much like modern racism and benevolent sexism (e.g., Glick & Fiske, 1996; McConahay, 1983), modern Western rape myths are framed in terms of seemingly more benign issues such as unfairness to the accused (and a possible rush to judgment), beliefs that rape victims get more funding and attention than they deserve, and concern that society has gone too far in challenging old norms. In addition, contemporary rape myths suggest that rape can result from alcohol abuse, slutty behaviors, and sexual urges (McMahon & Farmer, 2011), but they still blame the victims and exonerate the perpetrators. Contemporary rape myths also place limits on the acceptable behaviors for women (and some men). Thus, they support the old adage that potential victims are responsible for rape prevention.

There is also a need for more culturally sensitive measures of rape myth acceptance. For example, Huang (2016) developed a Chinese version of rape myth acceptance based on Burt's *Rape Myth Acceptance* scale and the *Illinois Rape Myth Acceptance Scale*. Huang and Lin (2017) argue that rape myths in Taiwan are influenced by traditional Chinese values such as an orientation toward family and the need for chastity. Oh and Neville (2004) also found that the importance of chastity influenced responses on the Korean Rape Myth Acceptance Scale. They suggest that some beliefs (e.g., victim culpability) are cross-cultural, whereas others are culturally specific (e.g., the tragic loss of virginity). Family and culture can also influence rape myth acceptance in Hispanic males (Lawson, Munoz-Rojas, Gutman, & Siman, 2012).

Finally, the question should be asked: Do rape myths largely operate at a conscious level, as is supported by current measures and most research, or might they reflect unconscious processes? Cognitive psychology suggests that there may be different levels of processing (e.g., Evans & Stanovich, 2013). Judgments are frequently made at a default level that is rapid and intuitive. Some judgments may be later followed by conscious reflection. Both conscious and unconscious thoughts can be biased and rape myths might operate at both levels. If rape myths operate at an unconscious level, then they might influence individuals even in the absence of awareness. There are a variety of attitudes (e.g., ageism, racism, sexism) where implicit biases have been found (Nosek, Banaji, &

Greenwald, 2010). Implicit Association Measures examine the unconscious connections that people make between constructs by rapidly presenting pairs of words and examining reaction times in responses. Implicit measures of rape myths may be needed (Edwards et al., 2011). For example, Edwards et al. note the possibility of an implicit power–dominance association that could be related to rape myth acceptance. There could also be research exploring individuals' unconscious associations with a real-rape stereotype and rape myths (e.g., real rapes are physically violent events, rapists are strangers, and strong resistance is essential in real rapes; alcohol use, sexual urges, miscommunication, and later regret are indications that it was possibly not a real rape).

Temkin and Krahé (2008) believe that rape myths (and the real-rape stereotype) act as heuristics that induce schematic processing at every stage of legal decision-making (e.g., police, juries, judges). Bohner and colleagues (e.g., Bohner, Eyssel, Pina, Siebler, & Viki, 2009; Süssenbach, Eyssel, & Bohner, 2013) argue that rape myths act as cognitive schemas (i.e., mental frameworks for organizing experience and memory) and that rape myth-inconsistent cues (e.g., the presence of alcohol) can impact judgments of culpability, especially for those who strongly hold rape myths. Rape myths may be chronically accessible in sexually coercive males (Bohner, Jarvis, Eyssel, & Siebler, 2005) and tied to dominance motives for sex (Chiroro, Bohner, Viki, & Jarvis, 2004). Finally, White, Donat, and Humphrey (1995) found that affectively based attitudes toward rape (i.e., value judgments, descriptions of character, or injunctions such as "Women who get raped while hitchhiking get what they deserve" p. 34) showed a stronger association with sexual coercion than did cognitively based attitudes (i.e., statements that could be verified as factual (or not) such as "In forcible rape the victim never causes the crime" p. 34). This suggests a stronger link between emotionally based rape myths and behavior than with cognitively based rape myths and behavior. And, Huang (2016) found that sexual aggression in Taiwanese males was associated with two rape victim myths (i.e., women secretly wish to be raped and victims exhibit improper demeanors) but not rape perpetrator myths (i.e., perpetrators are sexually impulsive and rapists are the minority who are deviants). Thus, the underlying relationship between rape myths and related behaviors might be quite complex.

Rape Myths Prevent Victims from Understanding That They Were Raped

Weis and Borges (1973) argued that rape is the perfect crime to get away with because cultural beliefs and norms delegitimize purported victims. They noted that sex-role socialization produces masculine men and feminine women who interact in private in a dating game that could easily result in nonconsensual sex. Society taught the woman that she was "both defenseless and responsible for the prevention of her victimization" (p. 94). Because of rape myths (e.g., rapists are strangers, rapists are lower class), it can take a long time for a woman to know the true intentions of her assailant as he shifts from seduction to rape. She might respond to the intimidation with incredulity, embarrassment, and/or paralyzing fear. Because the woman knows her assailant and does not want to be stigmatized as a victim, she could hesitate to define her experience with forced sex as rape. Thus, societal beliefs create the *justifiable rape* and the *legitimate* (i.e., culpable) victim. Moreover, typical social responses to rape (e.g., the police) further delegitimize the victim's experience and make it unlikely that she will disclose or report the event. Thus, she becomes the *safe* victim who tells no one.

Research shows that the majority of rapes are not reported, especially acquaintance rapes (e.g., Fisher, Daigle, Cullen, & Turner, 2003; Littleton, Rhatigan, & Axsom, 2007; Temkin, 1987/2002). Wilson and Miller (2016) conducted a meta-analysis of 28 articles and found that 60% of women did not acknowledge the rape. This could be because the woman was concerned with the repercussions of reporting. It is also possible that she had not labeled the event as a rape (Peterson & Muehlenhard, 2004, 2007). Rape myths create rape scripts that suggest that rape is an extremely physically violent event that occurs between strangers (Ryan, 2011). The assailant is clearly in the wrong and the victim is completely blameless. Because stereotyped rape scripts do not match a victim's personal experience with force and coercion, she won't acknowledge that her experience of sex without consent was rape (Littleton et al., 2007). In support of this, Kahn, Mathie, and Torgler (1994) found that women who held stereotyped rape scripts were less likely to label their personal experience with forced sex as rape. Women were also less likely to acknowledge their experience as rape if the assailant was their boyfriend, if they did not engage in intercourse, and if they were impaired by alcohol or drugs (Kahn, Jackson, Kully, Badger, & Halvorsen, 2003). Women who acknowledged rape were more likely to report they felt dirty, confused, sad, and detached from reality after the experience. They also reported more forceful aggression, threat/intimidation, and greater assailant blame. Bondurant (2001) found that participants were more likely to acknowledge an event as rape if it was aggressive and they were less likely to acknowledge an event as rape if they endorsed more items from a real-rape script (e.g., physical attacks, weapon use, and severe physical harm to victims). Finally, rape victims were more likely to report a rape to police if it matched some features of a real-rape script (i.e., the presence of a weapon, physical force, injuries, and multiple assaults) but not others (e.g., there was prior drinking or a prior relationship) (Du Mont, Miller, & Myhr, 2003).

Peterson and Muehlenhard (2004) found that two common rape myths influenced the acknowledgement of rape (i.e., it's not rape if women don't fight back and women who sexually tease men deserve the consequences of their behavior). Peterson and Muehlenhard also found that inconsistencies between the sex acts and the definition of rape as penile-vaginal penetration inhibited rape acknowledgment. In addition, their data suggested that rape acknowledgement might not be a dichotomous decision. They suggest that rape myths provide a series of *hurdles* that must be overcome in order to label an event as rape. Definitions of sex in which issues of consent and willingness must be negotiated can make self-definitions of rape ambiguous for potential victims (Peterson & Muehlenhard, 2007). This is especially true when alcohol is involved. Furthermore, defining an event as rape has implications for understanding of the self, the relationship, and the other person. For example, labeling an incident as rape might imply that people should report it, increase their feelings of vulnerability and trauma, and/or require that they label the other person as a rapist and themselves as rape victims.

Peterson and Muehlenhard (2011) developed a theory of self-labeling of nonconsensual sex in terms of whether the event closely matched the victim's rape script (or a different sex script) and the consequences she anticipated in applying the rape victim label. Their research showed that participants who were unacknowledged rape victims rejected the rape victim label, often matching their experience to several stereotyped rape script elements that were lacking. These include characteristics of the assailant (e.g., he was their boyfriend, he was a nice guy), their own behavior (e.g., she was intoxicated or engaging in sexual foreplay), low levels of force and resistance, and/or their motivation to avoid the *rape victim* label.

In conclusion, rape myth acceptance can interfere with the ability to label a personal experience as rape. This can have detrimental ramifications for mental and physical health (Ullman, 2010). Rape myth acceptance can also place women at risk for future victimization (Littleton, Grills, Layh, & Rudolph, 2017). Rape myths are a part of a general cognitive schema that influences emotions and behavior (Bohner et al., 2009). Rape myths serve different functions in males and females. Rape myths decrease the perceived threat of rape for females. And, because females are more likely to identify with rape victims, rape myths can support defensive victim-blaming attributions (Grubb & Turner, 2012). When rape victims blame themselves for their experiences, it can delay rape acknowledgment and the healing process (Ullman, 2010).

Rape Myths Prevent Assailants from Understanding That They Raped

Rape myths are an important determinant of assailants' self-labelling. Ryan (2004) suggested that rape myths are a central element in the belief systems of rapists. She cited evidence for rape myths in convicted rapists and acquaintance rapists who were not convicted offenders. Weis and Borges (1973) noted that men are socialized to initiate sexual activity as an act of power and dominance. "The man learns the same basic mythology of rape as the woman. He is aware of the notion that rape can only be committed by a stranger" (p. 87). This myth helps men to rationalize and justify sexual aggression at the same time that it prevents victims from reporting their experience.

Kanin (1984) found that the majority of self-disclosed date rapists said that they ignored the victim's attempts at resistance because of prior sexual foreplay (and their belief that the victim was aroused), they implicated alcohol as a "causal factor," and they used "physical overpowering" rather than threats or weapons to coerce sex (p. 101). "Put simply, a substantial number of these rapes occurred because the 'right man' (sexually aggressive and determined) did the 'right thing' (presented a level of force not usually encountered in dating) to the 'right girl' (easily frightened or inebriated)" (p. 102).

Kanin (1967) also found that men who engaged in more extreme sexual pressure were likely to believe that sexual aggression was sometimes justified (e.g., the woman was a teaser, gold-digger, or loose). Real or imagined promiscuity elicited male demands for sex (Kanin, 1969). Sexually aggressive men held a sexual double standard and exploited a partner's willingness to engage in sexual foreplay as provocation and an excuse for rape.

Anderson et al. (1997) found that a predisposition towards perpetrating rape was a strong predictor of rape myth acceptance in males. They included 32 reports in a meta-analysis. They predicted that rape myths (and other rape-supportive attitudes) would correlate with measures of sexual coercion. Cognitive predisposition measures (e.g., a desire to rape and coercive fantasies) correlated .59 with rape myths. A self-reported likelihood to rape correlated .38 with rape myth acceptance and sexual force/coercion showed a lower but still highly significant correlation with rape myths ($r = .19$).

Schewe, Adam, and Ryan (2009) studied the relationship between rape myth acceptance and a personal temptation to sexually aggress in college males. Responses on the *Rape Myth Acceptance* scale were not related to an acknowledgement of the temptation to use force; however, men who were sexually coercive or aggressive showed a greater belief in the manipulativeness of women compared with the other tempted participants. In addition, several sexual aggressors blamed the victim for their behavior (e.g., she was a tease, she had a weak no). And, several nonsexually aggressive participants endorsed rape myths when trying to explain how other men could be tempted to sexually aggress.

In sum, rape myths can serve to rationalize aggressive tendencies in males, creating *techniques of neutralization* that include denial of victimization, injury, or responsibility (Bohner et al., 2009). Rape myths can reflect a self-serving bias in males that serves to dismiss the possibility of rape (Grubb & Turner, 2012). This could be because males are more likely to identify with perpetrators than with victims. Rape myths are associated with the proclivity to rape (e.g., Bohner et al., 2005; Chiroro et al., 2004). Sexually coercive males are more likely to hold rape myths (e.g., Bohner et al., 2005; Carr & VanDeusen, 2004; DeGue & DiLillo, 2004; Truman, Tokar, & Fischer, 1996). They are also more likely to repeat sexual aggression if they minimize the severity of rape and blame the victim (Abbey & McAuslan, 2004). Sexually aggressive males are also more likely than others to believe that most men share their rape-supportive attitudes (Kroner, Boer, & Mills, 2004). And, feedback that other men believe rape myths increased rape proclivity in males, especially those who themselves believe rape myths (Bohner, Siebler, & Schmelcher, 2006).

Rape Myths Prevent Society from Understanding the Nature of Rape and Can Create a Lucifer Effect

Rape myths also operate at a systemic level. Historical, cultural, and religious forces support rape myths (Edwards et al., 2011; Franiuk & Shain, 2011). These forces impact society at many levels, including peer groups and legal institutions. This can lead to a *Lucifer Effect* in which the social power structure directs individuals' behavior and leads to rape (Zimbardo, 2007/2008). Rape myths play a central role in constructing legitimate and illegitimate sexual aggression. They can operate in peer-group support of rape (e.g., fraternities, sports teams, and members of the military) and influence societal responses to rape (e.g., legal, religious, and cultural).

Peer Groups

College Fraternities and Sports Teams. Peer groups influence sexual aggression in males (e.g., Mikorski & Szymanski, 2017). Two groups that have been associated with sexual aggression in college are fraternities and sports teams (e.g., Benedict, 1998; Kingree & Thompson, 2013; Schwartz & DeKeseredy, 1997; Young, Desmarais, Baldwin, & Chandler, 2017). Both groups show greater rape myth acceptance (e.g., Benedict, 1998; Boeringer, 1999; McMahon, 2010, 2015; Seabrook, Ward, & Giaccardi, 2018) and are influenced by a cultural context that encourages entitlement and demeans women (Martin, 2016). Rape myth acceptance has been linked to sexual coercion in high school and college athletes (e.g., Forbes, Adams-Curtis, Pakalka, & White, 2006; Young et al., 2017) and fraternity members (e.g., Kingree & Thompson, 2013; Seabrook, McMahon, & O'Connor, 2018).

Schwartz and DeKeseredy (1997) presented a model that suggests that male peer support for rape and heavy alcohol use are part of a culture that promotes the abuse of women in college. Nevertheless, it is unclear whether sexually aggressive men seek specific groups or whether the groups change the men. It is likely that both forces occur. Research shows higher levels of rape myth acceptance in males who intended to pledge a fraternity or play in college sports (McMahon, 2010). In addition, longitudinal data showed that males who joined a fraternity held more rape myths than a comparison group of males (Seabrook, McMahon, & O'Connor, 2018). Research also showed that perceived peer approval and heavy alcohol use influenced the likelihood of later sexual aggression in fraternity members (Kingree & Thompson, 2013). Rape myth acceptance was associated with perceived peer pressure to have sex, perceived approval of forced sex, heavy drinking, and sexual aggression. Perceived peer-pressure and rape myth acceptance were also associated with sexual deception in fraternity members (Seabrook, McMahon, & O'Connor, 2018). And, rape myth acceptance was correlated with the sexual objectification of women.

It appears that pornography might play a role in promoting coercive sex in fraternities. Bleecker and Murnen (2005) found that fraternity members were more likely to display degrading sexual images of women than were nonmembers and there was a correlation between the use of degrading images and rape myth acceptance. Foubert, Brosi, and Bannon (2011) found that 83% of fraternity members viewed pornography (27% viewed sadomasochistic pornography). Both were associated with rape myth acceptance, especially sadomasochistic pornography. Finally, fraternity members and athletes might be more likely than other men to believe that group sex is appropriate (Benedict, 1998; Sanday, 1990). This can have dangerous consequences for women.

Gang rapes are especially heinous. Fraternities and athletic teams are relatively common sources of gang rape in college (e.g., Benedict, 1998; O'Sullivan, 1993; Warshaw, 1988/1994). Sanday (1990) studied a fraternity gang rape at the University of Pennsylvania ("pulling a train" p. 1). She suggested that the rape was a male bonding ritual in which a drugged, drunk, and comatose woman was later held as responsible for her victimization. Loyalty, brotherhood, and the dehumanization and objectification of women are causal factors in fraternity gang rape (e.g., Martin & Hummer, 1995; Sanday, 1990). Athletic teams can also promote a rape culture (Warshaw, 1988/1994). Benedict suggests that athletes often assume consent in potential sexual partners because of the adulation they receive and the presence of groupies. "It is the suddenness and abundance of special treatment that instills in the student-athlete a sense of elitism" (p. 50). Benedict cites peer pressure and entitlement as factors in the gang-rape of a woman by the members of a professional football team. The team's lawyers portrayed the victim as responsible for the incident.

The military. Rape is also associated with the military. Brownmiller (1975/1981) dedicates an entire book chapter to rape in war (including both world wars, Bangladesh, and Vietnam) and another on riots, pogroms, and revolutions. She said that, "men who rape in war are ordinary Joes" (p. 25) and "a simple rule of thumb in war is that the winning side is the side that does the raping" (p. 27). Rape is the ultimate humiliation of an objectified enemy and the victim is a symbol. Rape is one of the rewards of winning. Rape can be part of the arsenal of war.

Turchik and Edwards (2012) noted that most reported sexual assaults in members of the military were from other members of the military. Research shows that sexual harassment and sexual assaults are more common in the military than in civilian society (e.g., Allard, Nunnink, Gregory, Klest, & Platt, 2011). In a literature review of research on military sexual trauma, Allard et al. reported prevalence rates between 22 and 45%. Prevalence rates were lower for male than for female victims. Nevertheless, military sexual trauma was associated with psychological, medical, and physical complaints in both males and females. Street and colleagues (i.e., Street, Mahan, Hendricks, Gardner, & Stafford, 2003; Street, Stafford, Mahan, & Hendricks, 2008) studied a random sample of military reservists. They found that 3.5% of the males and 23.3% of the females reported sexual assault and 1.2% of the males and 11.1% of the females reported an attempted or completed rape while they were in the military (Street et al., 2003). The estimated prevalence of any military sexual trauma (including sexual harassment) was 27.2% for males and 60% for females. There was a higher prevalence rate for military sexual trauma for females in the Marines than for those in other groups (75%).

Skinner et al. (2000) studied a random sample of female veterans in a VA hospital and found that 23% said that someone had "used force or the threat of force to have sexual relations with you against your will while you were in the military (p. 295)." Fifty-five percent suggested that they were "subjected to uninvited or unwanted sexual attention" (p. 295). O'Brien, Keith, and Shoemaker (2015) suggest that rape myths are part of a military culture that derogates women (e.g., joking, insult talk, homophobic language).

Turchik and Edwards (2012) suggested that the military perpetuates the myth that men cannot be raped. Voller et al. (2015) examined the role of male rape myth acceptance in Gulf War veterans who were victims of sexual abuse. Male rape myth acceptance was correlated with the devaluation of emotions and lower self-efficacy. Voller et al. suggested that the rejection of male rape myths was associated with increased self-efficacy in all of the veterans (not just those who were sexually victimized).

O'Brien et al. (2015) interviewed male veterans who were in treatment programs who had a history of military sexual assault. They suggested that the most important male rape myth stated that men cannot be raped (or *real men* cannot be raped). This myth promotes shame and steals the victim's manhood. O'Brien et al. also cited several other male rape myths: Male rape is not serious, Male rape is homosexual, and Females cannot rape males. These rape myths lead victims to question their own culpability and delay treatment.

Carroll and Clark (2006; Carroll, Rosenstein, Foubert, Clark, & Korenman, 2016) studied military cadets and compared them with civilian college students. They found that male cadets shared many rape scripts with civilian college males, but they also had a few distinctive scripts. Most importantly, the cadets focused more on the female victim's culpable behaviors (e.g., seductive dress, event mislabeling). A later study using the short form of the *Illinois Rape Myth Acceptance Scale* suggested that civilian fraternity/sorority students and students in military/naval academies showed similar rape myths (e.g., females lie about rape and females' behaviors make them culpable). As in other research, females had lower rape myth acceptance than males. Interestingly, students in the military academy showed lower rape myth acceptance than those in the naval academy and civilian fraternity and sorority members.

In conclusion, there is evidence to suggest that some peer groups act to support rape myths. They include male-dominated groups such as fraternities, sports teams, and the military. These groups can act to support a rape-prone individual and encourage rape in those who are not rape-prone. When rape myths are held by powerful people and systems are corrupt, they can create a Lucifer Effect. The Lucifer Effect refers to an individual's transformation of character from ordinary to evil in the face of potent situational pressures (Zimbardo, 2007/2008). The Lucifer Effect can cause average people to become rapists. "Reasonable people act irrationally, independent people act in mindless conformity, and peaceful people act as warriors" (p. 11). One example is rape in war. One consequence of corrupt political and military authorities is that they encourage the average GI Joe to rape. Another example could be found in some fraternities and athletic teams. Group bonding rituals and the presence of rape myths (e.g., women enjoy a *train*) can produce sexual aggression that is exalted—even exaggerated. The individuals who rape are left with the memory of their own despicable behavior and must deal with the psychological, moral, and emotional consequences on their own. How can an average Joe deal with the fact that they raped—that they were a rapist—that they are a rapist? Cognitive dissonance theory predicts that they must believe those rape myths that justified their behavior. To do otherwise is to risk their identity as a moral person. Thus, rape myths might cause sexual aggression, but they also might be a product of sexual aggression.

Justice System

Rape myths operate throughout the criminal justice system creating a *justice gap* in which victims of sexual assault are denied justice (Temkin & Krahé, 2008). Stereotypes (e.g., rapists are strangers and there must be considerable physical resistance for it to be a rape) operate at every stage of the legal process: victims' decisions to report, the police response, lawyers' decisions to prosecute, how defense attorneys defend the case, jury decision making, and judges' behavior. In each stage, rape myths decrease the likelihood that purported perpetrators will be reported, prosecuted, or convicted. Furthermore, beliefs about other people's rape myths can also negatively influence individuals' responses (e.g., the police anticipate jury decision making in rejecting some cases). Rape myths operate at the core of victim-blaming attributions that can occur in police officers, juries (and the general public), lawyers, and judges. Rape myths operate at both an individual and an institutional level to create the justice gap.

Justice system—the police. Police hold several rape myths (e.g., Feild, 1978; Krahé, 1991; Parratt & Pina, 2017). Most attrition in rape cases occurs at the police investigation phase (Hamilton (2004) as cited in Brown & Horvath, 2009 (p. 328); Temkin & Krahé, 2008). Brown and Horvath describe a vicious cycle in which rape myths trigger a *real-rape* stereotype, which in turn influences attrition that then feeds into and fosters further acceptance of rape myths. Police see rape as serious and they understand the negative consequences of rape, but they also perceive the *typical* rape and the *credible* rape to be the stereotyped real rape (Krahé, 1991). Police were more dubious about rape when victims were drunk, when there was little resistance or attempted escape, when the victim and assailant were previously acquainted, and when the rape took place in someone's home.

Parratt and Pina (2017) did a systematic review of research on rape myths in police officers. Characteristics of the crime, the police officers (e.g., gender, age, and personal experience), beliefs and attitudes (e.g., rape myths), and professional training all influenced decisions about rape. Research showed that "officers had a preconceived idea of what the ideal victim would be; leading them to question the victims' credibility and increase victim blame if victims did not fit officers' pre-conceptions" (p. 80). For example, the presence of a prior relationship led to greater victim blame. Research showed that there were many factors that interacted to yield complicated outcomes; however, female police officers often had lower rape myth acceptance than male officers.

Temkin and Krahé (2008) describe a process called *downstreaming* in which police officers decided whether to proceed with a particular case (or treat it with suspicion) based on their assumptions concerning juries' real-rape stereotypes. Moreover, when rape victims anticipated dealing with suspicious police officers, they were less likely to report the event. Thus, beliefs about other people's rape myths can influence police and victim behavior even when they do not share the rape myth.

O'Keeffe, Brown, and Lyons (2009) studied police decision making on rape cases in Ireland (the police are called the Garda). They described a skeptical mindset in which the Garda assumed there were a relatively high proportion of false claims and a need for collaborative evidence. O'Keeffe et al. described a heuristic process in which the Garda looked for cues of deception in purported victims, including inappropriate affect, inconsistent information, information that did not match a story line that was consistent with a stereotyped real rape, and other characteristics about the purported victim (e.g., promiscuity and social class). O'Keeffe et al. suggested that there is a strong confirmation bias and need for evidence that matched the real-rape stereotype. Thus, rape myths can influence the Garda's interviewing process as well as their final recommendations.

Finally, Cook and Lane (2017) demonstrated that male rape myth acceptance in jail correctional officers was associated with victim blame of incarcerated sexual assault victims. Jail correction officers from Florida were distributed surveys and 376 participated in the study. Rape myths were assessed by 4 items from the *Male Rape Myth Acceptance Scale* and victim blame was assessed by a 7-item measure (e.g., "Some inmates deserve to be sexually assaulted in jail because of the way they act" p. 355). Attitudes toward homosexuality were also assessed. Two of the 4 male rape myths were significantly associated with victim blame (i.e., "It is impossible for a man to rape a man" and "Most men who are raped by a man do not need counselling after the incident" p. 359). Regression analyses were complex but showed that victim blaming was associated with male rape myth acceptance and homophobia.

Justice system—lawyers, juries, and judges. Research also demonstrates the common use in rape myths in criminal trials. Research on the role of rape myths in criminal trials often uses vignettes and mock juries (e.g., Temkin & Krahé, 2008). It is more difficult to find research on real-life decisions; however, some researchers have used court observations (e.g., Smith & Skinner, 2017; Temkin, Gray, & Barrett, 2018) and others have interviewed participants (e.g., judges and barristers were interviewed by Temkin & Krahé).

Ellison and Munro (2009) used a mock jury paradigm involving 27 jury deliberations to study typical jurists' responses to an acquaintance rape. Mini-trials were enacted based on scripts created by experts. The trials took approximately 75 min and juries deliberated for another 90 min. Nine scenarios were presented. Ellison and Munro varied the victim's resistance, delay in reporting, and the amount of victim distress expressed during the trial. Several themes emerged that are consistent with the juries' use of rape myths. For example, many jurors blamed the purported victim for sending mixed signals prior to the rape, inviting the man into her home, and talking to him for an extensive period of time. The jurors suggested that men have a difficult time controlling their sexual behavior, but force (and bruising) was not acceptable and might be an indication of rape. Jurors spent a lot of time discussing the role of alcohol in sexual behavior, even though the individuals only had one drink. They also suggested that an abrupt departure of the purported assailant might be consistent with rape.

Rape myths can also influence the jury's decision-making process. Ellison and Munro

(2010) studied the dynamics of decision making using the mock jury trials noted in the previously reviewed study. Results showed a pronounced trend toward acquittal during the deliberation process. Jurors often influenced other jurors by noting inconsistencies with the real-rape stereotype (e.g., a lack of resistance) and they underscored the need for 100% certainty for a guilty verdict (a misreading of the mandate to find *beyond a reasonable doubt*).

These findings were replicated in a 2013 study of mock jury responses to a purported rape by an ex-partner, even though jurors were instructed by the judge that a prior relationship did not imply a lack of guilt (Ellison & Munro, 2013). "The jurors in this study invoked a number of acceptable 'scripts', forged in the context of contemporary socio-(hetero)sexual relationships, against which the conduct of the parties, and the allegations of sexual assault, were measured. These scripts often positioned women as having primary responsibility for acting as sexual gatekeepers, communicating their willingness or refusal clearly and unequivocally, whilst bearing in mind the presumed predisposition of 'red-blooded' men to 'push their luck' as sexual initiators" (pp. 309–310). Jury deliberations influenced the final adjudged innocence of the defendant.

Gray (2006) studied the influence of judicial instructions on decisions concerning perpetrator guilt. University students took the *Rape Myth Acceptance* scale and were given a vignette describing a date rape. The guidance instructions were varied (pro-rape myths, anti-rape myths, and neutral). Males showed greater rape myth acceptance than females. In addition, responses on the *Rape Myth Acceptance* scale were significantly correlated with judgments of perpetrator innocence (r = .46). Finally, participants who were given guidance instructions involving rape myths were more likely to believe that the accused assailant was innocent than were participants who were given instructions refuting rape myths. This was especially true for males who initially supported rape myths.

Ellison and Munro (2009) studied the influence of guidance instructions on jury decision-making using a mock-jury paradigm. They included expert testimony or expansive instructions that dealt with and refuted some common rape myths (e.g., individual differences in reactions to rape, levels of resistance, delays in reporting, and emotional responses). A content analysis of the jury discussions and later self-report measures showed that jurors were impacted by both expert testimony and expansive instructions to show lower rape myth acceptance in judgments of guilt, except for the case where there was a lack of resistance and absence of injury. Thus, some rape myths persisted in the face of expert guidance to the contrary.

Krahé, Temkin, Bieneck, and Berger (2008) studied rape myths in future lawyers (study 1 had undergraduate law students and study 2 had post-graduate lawyer trainees). Both studies used 6 rape vignettes that varied perpetrator-victim relationships and coercive strategies (physical force versus alcohol-induced incapacitation). Results showed that prospective lawyers held several rape myths and rape myth acceptance was associated with victim blame (especially when the purported victim and assailant had a prior relationship or when alcohol was involved).

Temkin et al. (2018) engaged in rape trial observations in England and developed themes involving rape myths. They found that the defense often invoked rape myths and the real-rape stereotype to highlight inconsistencies and discredit the victim. Prosecutors and judges rarely countered the rape myths (and some judges even affirmed rape myths).

Smith and Skinner (2017) did a discourse analysis of court observations in the UK. They found a pattern in which the arguments that lawyers used assumed that people responded rationally even in exigent circumstances (e.g., the decision to rape or the proper response must be completely logical). The most common rape myths referred to victims' inappropriate demeanor, delays in reporting, failure to cut contact with the accused, and (lack of) physical resistance.

Zydervelt, Zajac, Kaladelfos, and Westera (2017) coded transcripts from rape trials in New Zealand and New South Wales to test for changing trends in defense lawyers' cross-examination of rape complainants. They noted that cross examinations are by nature adversarial and found that the lawyers often used rape myths to challenge purported victims' credibility/plausibility (e.g., relationships with the accused perpetrator before or after the event, delayed reporting, a lack of resistance, and prior sexual history). Defense attorneys also questioned the victim's reliability and consistency (e.g., intoxication or inconsistencies in her account).

Finally, Temkin and Krahé (2008, Chap. 6) interviewed 17 judges and seven barristers, all of whom worked on rape trials. Temkin and Krahé noted that rape myths influenced some behaviors. For example, some judges told jurors to seek independent corroboration of the victim's testimony. Others believed that the victim's sexual history was relevant. Thus, some judges and prosecutors were also influenced by rape myths.

In conclusion, research shows the presence of rape myths throughout the justice system (e.g., Horvath & Brown, 2009; Temkin & Krahé, 2008). There is a consistent pattern in which rape myths increase victim blame and decrease the likelihood of prosecution and convictions, creating a justice gap. Rape myths occur at the individual level but they are also a part of institutions. When rape myths are present in the training of professionals or in the instructions to a jury, they can impact victim reporting, police recommendations, and/or jury decisions. When jury members invoke rape myths to convince other jury members to vote for an acquittal, they can lead to the exoneration of the guilty. Unfortunately, the use of rape myths might be inherent in a criminal justice system that assumes an adversarial process. Police are skeptical of potential rape victims and defense attorneys base victim cross-examination on rape myths, causing secondary victimization. Thus, rape myths operate at the core of the current justice system and have ramifications throughout.

Religion and Culture

Rape myths also operate at a cultural level. Religion and culture impact social beliefs that justify and sustain sexual aggression (e.g., Edwards et al., 2011; Franiuk & Shain, 2011). Definitions of rape are culturally specific and they determine the meaning of behavior (Martin, 2003). Support for rape myths are embedded in laws, language, and social policies (Edwards et al., 2011; Turchik & Edwards, 2012). Culture may be even more important than gender in understanding attitudes toward sexual aggression (Nayak, Byrne, Martin, & Abraham, 2003). Rape myth acceptance is associated with restrictive beliefs about women (Costin & Schwarz, 1987). And, rape myth acceptance might be related to other prejudicial beliefs, including homophobia, ageism, classism, and religious intolerance (Aosved & Long, 2006). Finally, male rape myths are common and this results in the invisibility and marginalization of male rape victims in war (Grey & Shepherd, 2013).

Edwards et al. (2011) described the impact of Western cultural and Judeo-Christian beliefs on four female rape myths. The myths are: husbands cannot rape their wives, women enjoy rape, women asked to be raped, and women lie about being raped. Edwards et al. cited long-standing tradition and three institutions (i.e., legal, religious, and media) that support rape myths. In addition, Franiuk and Shain (2011) added evidence of religious and cultural support for rape myths (e.g., husbands cannot rape their wives and women ask to be raped) in Hinduism and Islam and their related cultures. Religious texts, cultural traditions that promote family honor, and the lower status of women justify punishment for rape victims, especially when religion and cultural traditions are conflated (and supported by law).

Sheldon and Parent (2002) suggest that "most clergy blame the victim and adhere to rape myths" (p. 233). They found that Christian religious fundamentalism correlated with responses to an acquaintance rape vignette. A content analysis showed that the clergy sometimes blamed the victim of a date rape for showing inadequate resistance and the victim of an acquaintance rape for showing poor judgment. A small number of clergy mentioned the wife's duty to submit and be sexually competent when responding to a wife rape vignette.

Klement and Sagarin (2017) studied Christian dating-advice books directed toward women. A thematic analysis showed strong beliefs that women must remain pure and negative consequences for violating social norms. The books suggested that women were responsible for sexual aggression (e.g., flirting, provocative dress), that women should accept that some sexual aggression is normal, and that nonsubmissive women should be derogated.

Ward (1988) was one of the first rape myth researchers to focus on culture. She validated an *Attitudes toward Rape Victims* scale on a variety of groups (e.g., university students, police, lawyers, and social workers) in Singapore and university students in the US. The *Attitudes toward Rape Victims* measure concentrated on victim credibility, denigration, trivialization, deservingness, and blame. Males had more unfavorable views of rape victims than did females on 23 of 25 items. Interestingly, Singaporean students showed more negative attitudes toward rape victims than US students. In addition, there were also differences within the Singaporean sample: police were the least favorable, lawyers and doctors were in the middle, and social workers and psychologists were the most favorable in their attitudes toward rape victims.

Many researchers have shown cultural effects on rape myths. For example, Scottish university students showed lower rape myth acceptance than US college students (Muir, Lonsway, & Payne, 1996) and Asian American college males showed greater misogyny, less perpetrator blame, and more victim blame than Caucasian American students (Koo, Stephens, Lindgren, & George, 2012). In addition, Japanese males showed greater rape myth acceptance than US males, perhaps because Japan is a male-dominant culture (Stillman, Yamawaki, Ridge, White, & Copley, 2009). And, rape myth acceptance appeared to be higher in a Turkish participant sample than in comparison groups from the west and Israel (Costin & Kaptanoğlu, 1993). Thus, it is clear that some cultures are more supportive of rape myths than others. Nevertheless, cultural differences are not always found. For example, ethnic identity did not predict rape myth acceptance in Asian Indians in the US (Tummala-Narra, Houston-Kolnik, Sathasivam-Rueckert, & Greeson, 2017) and Scandinavians (a relatively liberal group) did not show lower rape myth acceptance than individuals from North America (Bendixen, Henriksen, & Nøstdahl, 2014).

Other researchers have explored the underlying reasons for cultural differences in rape myth acceptance. For example, Hill and Marshall (2018) found that Indians showed greater rape myth acceptance than Britons at least partially because of more negative attitudes toward women. Canto, Perles, and Martín (2017) found that belief in an honor culture correlated with victim blame in Spanish college students who were judging an acquaintance rape and marital rape vignette (but not a stranger rape vignette). In addition, Rebeiz and Harb (2010) studied Lebanese students and found that conservative and traditional beliefs were associated with rape myth acceptance on the *Attitudes toward Rape Victims* scale. Interestingly, the same data did not show differences in rape myth acceptance between Christian and Muslim students.

Research has also showed that similarity in ethnic identity can influence reactions to perpetrators of rape. Bongiorno, McKimmie, and Masser (2016) found that white Australians took ethnic similarity into account when judging acquaintance rape vignettes that did not adhere to the real-rape stereotype. Perpetrators were described as English or American (culturally similar) or Indian or Pakistani (culturally dissimilar). The vignettes were identical except for perpetrator information and two details that were inconsistent with a real-rape script (i.e., a lower level of physical resistance and a lack of cooperation with the police). It appears that perpetrator and victim blame mediated the effects of cultural similarity and script elements on judgments of perpetrator guilt and punishment. Thus, ethnic similarity might influence responses to some rapes (and rapists).

In conclusion, religion and culture play an important role in rape myth acceptance. Culture and religion help to shape society's views of normal and abnormal behavior. Rape myths are used to caution individuals about the appropriateness of behavior and they can entitle some individuals to rape. This can have lasting negative effects on rape victims. Unfortunately, the presence of rape myths at a deep cultural level also makes it very likely that secondary victimization will occur and rape will remain a hidden crime.

Best Practice

Education and Prevention

Rape myths are often discussed in college education and prevention efforts; however, they might still exist in some college training. For example, an examination of college websites showed that most of the messages were aimed at females and many suggested that rape prevention was up to them (e.g., there is no safe place, you can't trust anyone, and you must communicate sexual limits) (Bedera & Nordmeyer, 2015). These rape myths clearly reflected the old adage that women are vulnerable, but they also are responsible for rape prevention. Rape prevention efforts have showed some success in educating participants about rape myths (e.g., Kress et al., 2006; O'Donohue, Yeater, & Fanetti, 2003). And, Rape myths should continue to be a primary target of rape prevention work (Schewe, 2002). However, rape myth acceptance scores can rebound over time, sometimes to their original levels (e.g., Davis & Liddell, 2002; Heppner, Humphrey, Hillenbrand-Gunn, & DeBord, 1995) and sometimes to levels that are somewhat lower than the original levels (Foubert & Marriott, 1997). Even when there are significant long-term program effects, programs may be better at reducing rape myth acceptance than at reducing actual sexual aggression (e.g., Foubert, 2000; Gidycz et al., 2001). Moreover, the benefits of rape prevention might be lower in males who are at higher risk for sexual aggression (e.g., Stephens & George, 2009) and rape prevention programs might not reduce rape myths in high-risk males to the levels that are found in low-risk males (Schewe & O'Donohue, 1993a). Finally, there are problems with some of the outcome measures used in prevention work, as many rape myth acceptance scales are outdated and have issues with validity (Baldwin-White, Thompson, & Gray, 2016; Heppner et al., 1995; Schewe & O'Donohue, 1993b). There is also the question of the *clinical significance* (as opposed to statistical significance) of changes in rape myth acceptance found in prevention work (Schewe & O'Donohue, 1993b) and an absence of criteria for acceptable levels of rape myth acceptance. In addition, there is a need for culturally sensitive measures.

Still, some argue that it is good to use rape myth education in bystander intervention programs (e.g., McMahon, 2010), although it is a mistake to list potentially outdated rape myths as this can backfire (Krahé, 2016). It appears that longer programs work better than shorter programs (e.g.,Anderson & Whiston, 2005 ; Flores & Hartlaub, 1998). Some suggest that same-sex audiences work better than mixed-sex audiences (e.g., Brecklin & Forde, 2001; Schewe, 2002). Theory-testing research performs better than atheoretical programs (Schewe, 2002; Schewe & O'Donohue, 1993b). And, motivated audiences show better retention than unmotivated audiences (Foubert & Marriott, 1997; Foubert & Newberry, 2006). Finally, responding to rape myth acceptance scales may in itself attune participants to their stereotypes and decrease later rape myth acceptance (e.g., Foubert & Marriott, 1997; Rau et al., 2010).

The outdated nature of many rape myth measures and the presence of newer rape scripts (e.g., Clark & Carroll, 2008; Littleton, Tabernik, Canales, & Backstrom, 2009) argues that myths and scripts have changed and will continue to change over time. Thus, it is important for rape education and prevention efforts to recognize the evolving nature of our understanding of rape and the nuances of sexual negotiation (Frith, 2009).

- Any rape prevention efforts must include contemporary rape myths in outcome measures (e.g., alcohol-induced "mistakes" are not real rapes, victims' promiscuous behavior leads to rape, and rape is due to sexual urges). Old-fashioned rape myths (e.g., rape victims should relax and enjoy it, rapists are deviants, and all women want to be raped) should be avoided. Rape myths must be perceived to be personally relevant, although the real-rape stereotype can and should be acknowledged.

- Any rape prevention efforts must include myths about male rape victims.
- Culturally relevant rape myth measures should be developed.
- Rape prevention programs must address potentially unconscious determinants in understanding sexual behavior (including heuristics and schema) and ask participants to acknowledge their own sexual assumptions, especially those concerning normal and abnormal sexual behaviors. Educators might consider using examples of implicit associations and/or priming to illustrate the possibility of unconscious associations (e.g., Devine, 1989; Nosek et al., 2010).
- Rape prevention programs must go beyond the overly simplistic "no means no" messages to acknowledge the complexities and nuances of negotiating sexual behavior.
- Rape prevention programs should include warnings about the Lucifer Effect, especially for those in male-dominated peer groups.

Medicine, Religion, and Psychotherapy

There is some evidence that therapists and counselors hold fewer rape myths than other professional groups (e.g., Ward, 1988). Nevertheless, there is a danger of secondary victimization, as therapists assist victims and perpetrators in working through their own and society's rape myths. Rape myths can be used as a tool to educate and to advocate for rape survivors (Ullman, 2010). Rape myths can also protect individuals from believing that they are victims or perpetrators (Bohner et al., 2009). Thus, the discussion of rape myths and scripts must be done very carefully and efforts must be made at avoiding the imposition of personal rape myths on rape victims. Rape myths can delay acknowledgment and treatment for rape survivors (Ullman, 2010) and they can leave individuals vulnerable to future victimization or perpetration (Littleton et al., 2017).

- Rape myth theory and research should be part of the education and training of professionals, especially those who will likely deal with the aftermath of rape (e.g., college counselors, emergency room personnel, and victim advocates). Training should include a feminist therapeutic orientation because it enhances a victim-oriented perspective and understanding concerning the social and political context of rape (e.g., Brown, 2017; Hutchinson & McDaniel, 1986), including the presence of rape myths.
- There needs to be more research on rape myths and rape-myth prevention in counselors, therapists, and medical personnel.
- Counselors, therapists, and medical personnel need to be aware of their own rape myths (and real-rape stereotypes) in an effort to avoid secondary victimization This will require continuous vigilance. They should be especially attuned to unconscious (implicit) associations that suggest that the rape victim was culpable in rape.
- Clergy must challenge the use of religious scripture to condemn and punish rape victims and they must become aware of their own real-rape stereotypes.

Justice Systems

Researchers have focused on the need to reform the justice system in order to reduce attrition, eliminate the justice gap, and decrease secondary victimization (Temkin & Krahé, 2008). Because police act as gatekeepers and have a pivotal role in determining which cases are prosecuted, one could argue that they are the most important element in the criminal justice system response to rape. Police should be educated about rape myths, but training alone will not eliminate bias (Parratt & Pina, 2017). Parratt and Pina note that several factors influence attitudes toward rape in the police (e.g., level of education, gender, and experience with rape victims). These factors can interact to influence perceptions of rape victims (e.g., female police officers benefit more than male police officers from sexual assault training, they are more likely to know rape victims, and they are more likely to use rape victim advocates). Most police officers reported an absence of clear guidelines for rape investigations. Guidelines should be provided. In addition, police should be encouraged to examine the impact of their personal beliefs every time they interview a purported victim of rape. They should also be encouraged to include victim advocates when taking rape complaints. It is crucial that police and correctional officers be made aware of the roles that male rape myths and homophobia have in their treatment of men who are raped outside of prison or while incarcerated. Officers must be made aware of the danger of secondary victimization and the justice gap.

Researchers have also noted problems with jury decisions (e.g., Krahé & Temkin, 2009; Temkin & Krahé, 2008). Krahé and Temkin suggest several possible solutions. For example, jurors could be pre-screened to eliminate those with strong rape myth acceptance and/or juries could be required to provide an account for their decisions (thus reducing heuristic processing). It is also possible to replace juries with educated judges, especially female judges. In addition, it appears that expert testimony and judicial instructions can reduce rape myth acceptance and may inhibit a group dynamic that favors acquittal. Finally, educating juries (and the larger public) about rape myths is essential to reducing the impact of rape myths in trials.

In addition, rape myth education is essential in the training of judges and lawyers (Temkin et al., 2018). This is especially important for anyone serving in sexual assault trials. Professionals must be warned against using rape myths in either prosecution or defense, as this opens the door for juries to entertain their own rape myths. Most importantly, jurists must move from a system that assumes rational thought (Smith & Skinner, 2017). Judges are an essential element in rape trials and should be encouraged to use jury instructions and allow expert testimony to reduce the justice gap for rape.

- It is essential that education about rape myths and realities occurs throughout the justice system, including the police, lawyers, judges, and juries. Special efforts must be made to educate police and custodial officers about their prejudices concerning rape victims that results in high attrition rates. Nevertheless, since past research showed mixed results for sexual assault training programs on police officers (Parratt & Pina, 2017), more research is needed. Research on rape prevention in college students might be useful in implementing programs for police officers. For example, research shows that motivated participants retain more information (e.g., Foubert & Marriott, 1997; Foubert & Newberry, 2006), longer programs work better (Anderson & Whiston, 2005; Flores & Hartlaub, 1998), and *The men's program,* which features a male sexual assault victim who is a police officer, is quite successful at increasing understanding and empathy for rape victims in college males (e.g., Foubert & Perry, 2007).
- In addition, officers must be made aware of the roles of male rape myths and homophobia in the poor treatment of male rape victims both in- and outside of prison.
- Special efforts also must be made to ensure that the adversarial process inherent in the justice system and group dynamics favoring acquittal in jury decision making are not allowed to rely on rape myths and the real-rape stereotype.

Overall Conclusion

Rape myths play a pivotal role in the social construction of rape. Continued research is essential to address the changing nature of rape myths. Rape myths can be held at a cultural level, at an institutional level, and at the individual level. Rape myths legitimize sexual aggression and in so doing foster sexual aggression. Rape myths help to create the *legitimate* victim who is blamed for the event and lead to secondary victimization when victims disclose or report the rape. Recognizing rape mythology helps people to understand the true nature of many rapes and is essential in the fight against rape.

References

Abbey, A., & McAuslan, P. (2004). A longitudinal examination of male college students' perpetration of sexual assault. *Journal of Consulting and Clinical Psychology, 72*, 747–756. https://doi.org/10.1037/0022-006X.72.5.747

Allard, C. B., Nunnink, S., Gregory, A. M., Klest, B., & Platt, M. (2011). Military sexual trauma research: A proposed agenda. *Journal of Trauma & Dissociation, 12*, 324–345.

Anderson, K. B., Cooper, H., & Okamura, L. (1997). Individual differences and attitudes toward rape: A meta-analytic review. *Personality and Social Psychology Bulletin, 23*, 295–315. https://doi.org/10.1177/0146167297233008

Anderson, L. A., & Whiston, S. C. (2005). Sexual assault education programs: A meta-analytic examination of their effectiveness. *Psychology of Women Quarterly, 29*, 374–388. https://doi.org/10.1111/j.1471-6402.2005.00237.x

Aosved, A. C., & Long, P. J. (2006). Co-occurrence of rape myth acceptance, sexism, racism, homophobia, ageism, classism, and religious intolerance. *Sex Roles, 55*, 481–492. https://doi.org/10.1007/s11199-006-9101-4

Baldwin-White, A., Thompson, M. S., & Gray, A. (2016). Pre- and postintervention factor analysis of the Illinois Rape Myth Acceptance Scale. *Journal of Aggression, Maltreatment & Trauma, 25*, 636–651. https://doi.org/10.1080/10926771.2015.1107173

Barnett, N. J., & Felid, H. S. (1977). Sex differences in university students' attitudes toward rape. *Journal of College Student Personnel, 18*, 93–96.

Bedera, N., & Nordmeyer, K. (2015). 'Never go out alone': An analysis of college rape prevention tips. *Sexuality and Culture: An Interdisciplinary Quarterly, 19*(3), 533–542. https://doi.org/10.1007/s12119-015-9274-5

Bendixen, M., Henriksen, M., & Nøstdahl, R. K. (2014). Attitudes toward rape and attribution of responsibility to rape victims in a Norwegian community sample. *Nordic Psychology, 66*(3), 168–186. https://doi.org/10.1080/19012276.2014.931813

Benedict, J. R. (1998). *Athletes and acquaintance rape*. Thousand Oaks, CA: Sage.

Bleecker, E. T., & Murnen, S. K. (2005). Fraternity membership, the display of degrading sexual images of women, and rape myth acceptance. *Sex Roles, 53*, 487–493. https://doi.org/10.1007/s11199-005-7136-6

Boeringer, S. B. (1999). Associations of rape-supportive attitudes with fraternal and athletic participation. *Violence Against Women, 5*, 81–90. https://doi.org/10.1177/10778019922181167

Bohner, G., Eyssel, F., Pina, A., Siebler, F., & Viki, G. T. (2009). Rape myth acceptance: Cognitive, affective and behavioural effects of beliefs that blame the victim and exonerate the perpetrator. In M. Horvath, J. Brown, M. Horvath, & J. Brown (Eds.), *Rape: Challenging contemporary thinking* (pp. 17–45). Devon, UK: Willan Publishing.

Bohner, G., Jarvis, C. I., Eyssel, F., & Siebler, F. (2005). The causal impact of rape myth acceptance on men's rape proclivity: Comparing sexually coercive and noncoercive men. *European Journal of Social Psychology, 35*, 819–828. https://doi.org/10.1002/ejsp.284

Bohner, G., Siebler, F., & Schmelcher, J. (2006). Social norms and the likelihood of raping: Perceived rape myth acceptance of others affects men's rape proclivity. *Personality and Social Psychology Bulletin, 32*, 286–297. https://doi.org/10.1177/0146167205280912

Bondurant, B. (2001). University women's acknowledgment of rape. *Violence Against Women, 7*, 294–314. https://doi.org/10.1177/1077801012218245l

Bongiorno, R., McKimmie, B. M., & Masser, B. M. (2016). The selective use of rape-victim stereotypes to protect culturally similar perpetrators. *Psychology of Women Quarterly, 40*, 398–413. https://doi.org/10.1177/0361684316631932

Brecklin, L. R., & Forde, D. R. (2001). A meta-analysis of rape education programs. *Violence and Victims, 16*, 303–321.

Briere, J., Malamuth, N., & Check, J. V. (1985). Sexuality and rape-supportive beliefs. *International Journal of Women's Studies, 8*, 398–403.

Brown, J. M., & Horvath, M. H. (2009). Do you believe her and is it real rape? In M. Horvath, J. Brown, M. Horvath, & J. Brown (Eds.), *Rape: Challenging contemporary thinking* (pp. 325–342). Devon, UK: Willan Publishing.

Brown, L. S. (2017). Contributions of feminist and critical psychologies to trauma psychology. In S. N. Gold & S. N. Gold (Eds.), *APA handbook of trauma psychology: Foundations in knowledge* (pp. 501–526). Washington, DC: American Psychological Association. https://doi.org/10.1037/0000019-025

Brownmiller, S. (1975/1981). *Against our will: Men, women, and rape*. New York: Bantam.

Burt, M. R. (1980). Cultural myths and supports for rape. *Journal of Personality and Social Psychology, 38*, 217–230. https://doi.org/10.1037/0022-3514.38.2.217

Canto, J. M., Perles, F., & Martín, J. S. (2017). Culture of honour and the blaming of women in cases of rape/La cultura del honor y la inculpación de la mujer en casos de violación. *Revista de Psicología Social, 32*, 80–107. https://doi.org/10.1080/02134748.2016.1250488

Carr, J. L., & VanDeusen, K. M. (2004). Risk factors for male sexual aggression on college campuses.

Journal of Family Violence, 19, 279–289. https://doi.org/10.1023/B:JOFV.0000042078.55308.4d

Carroll, M. H., & Clark, M. D. (2006). Men's acquaintance rape scripts: A comparison between a regional university and a military academy. *Sex Roles, 55*, 469–480. https://doi.org/10.1007/s11199-006-9102-3

Carroll, M. H., Rosenstein, J. E., Foubert, J. D., Clark, M. D., & Korenman, L. M. (2016, April 11). Rape myth acceptance: A comparison of military service academy and civilian fraternity and sorority students. *Military Psychology, 28*, 306. https://doi.org/10.1037/mil0000113

Chiroro, P., Bohner, G., Viki, G. T., & Jarvis, C. I. (2004). Rape myth acceptance and rape proclivity: Expected dominance versus expected arousal as mediators in acquaintance-rape situations. *Journal of Interpersonal Violence, 19*, 427–441. https://doi.org/10.1177/0886260503262081

Clark, M. D., & Carroll, M. H. (2008). Acquaintance rape scripts of women and men: Similarities and differences. *Sex Roles, 58*, 616–625. https://doi.org/10.1007/s11199-007-9373-3

Cook, C. L., & Lane, J. (2017). Blaming the victim: Perceptions about incarcerated sexual assault victim culpability among a sample of jail correctional officers. *Victims & Offenders, 12*(3), 347–380. https://doi.org/10.1080/15564886.2015.1065531

Costin, F., & Kaptanoğlu, C. (1993). Beliefs about rape and women's social roles: A Turkish replication. *European Journal of Social Psychology, 23*, 327–330. https://doi.org/10.1002/ejsp.2420230308

Costin, F., & Schwarz, N. (1987). Beliefs about rape and women's social roles: A four-nation study. *Journal of Interpersonal Violence, 2*, 46–56. https://doi.org/10.1177/088626087002001003

Davis, T. L., & Liddell, D. L. (2002). Getting inside the house: The effectiveness of a rape prevention program for college fraternity men. *Journal of College Student Development, 43*(1), 35–50.

DeGue, S., & DiLillo, D. (2004). Understanding perpetrators of nonphysical sexual coercion: Characteristics of those who cross the line. *Violence and Victims, 19*, 673–688. https://doi.org/10.1891/vivi.19.6.673.66345

Deming, M. E., Covan, E. K., Swan, S. C., & Billings, D. L. (2013). Exploring rape myths, gendered norms, group processing, and the social context of rape among college women: A qualitative analysis. *Violence Against Women, 19*, 465–485. https://doi.org/10.1177/1077801213487044

Devine, P. G. (1989). Stereotypes and prejudice: Their automatic and controlled components. *Journal of Personality and Social Psychology, 56*, 5–18. https://doi.org/10.1037/0022-3514.56.1.5

Du Mont, J. D., Miller, K., & Myhr, T. L. (2003). The role of 'real rape' and 'real victim' stereotypes in the police reporting practices of sexually assaulted women. *Violence Against Women, 9*, 466–486. https://doi.org/10.1177/1077801202250960

Edwards, K. M., Turchik, J. A., Dardis, C. M., Reynolds, N., & Gidycz, C. A. (2011). Rape myths: History, individual and institutional-level presence, and implications for change. *Sex Roles, 65*, 761–773. https://doi.org/10.1007/s11199-011-9943-2

Ellison, L., & Munro, V. E. (2009). Of 'normal sex' and 'real rape': Exploring the use of socio-sexual scripts in (mock) jury deliberation. *Social & Legal Studies, 18*(3), 291–312.

Ellison, L., & Munro, V. E. (2010). Getting to (not) guilty: Examining jurors' deliberative processes in, and beyond, the context of a mock rape trial. *Legal Studies, 30*(1), 74–97.

Ellison, L., & Munro, V. E. (2013). Better the devil you know? 'Real rape' stereotypes and the relevance of a previous relationship in (mock) juror deliberations. *The International Journal of Evidence & Proof, 17*(4), 299–322.

Evans, J. (1995). *Feminist theory today: An introduction to second-wave feminism*. Thousand Oaks, CA: Sage.

Evans, J. S. B. T., & Stanovich, K. E. (2013). Dual-process theories of higher cognition: Advancing the debate. *Perspectives on Psychological Science, 8*, 223–241.

Eyssel, F., & Bohner, G. (2008). Modern rape myths: The Acceptance of Modern Myths about Sexual Aggression (AMMSA) Scale. In M. A. Morrison, T. G. Morrison, M. A. Morrison, & T. G. Morrison (Eds.), *The psychology of modern prejudice* (pp. 261–276). Hauppauge, NY: Nova Science Publishers.

Feild, H. S. (1978). Attitudes toward rape: A comparative analysis of police, rapists, crisis counselors, and citizens. *Journal of Personality and Social Psychology, 36*, 156–179. https://doi.org/10.1037/0022-3514.36.2.156

Fisher, B. S., Daigle, L. E., Cullen, F. T., & Turner, M. G. (2003). Reporting sexual victimization to the police and others: Results from a national-level study of college women. *Criminal Justice and Behavior, 30*(1), 6–38. https://doi.org/10.1177/0093854802239161

Flores, S. A., & Hartlaub, M. G. (1998). Reducing rape-myth acceptance in male college students: A meta-analysis of intervention studies. *Journal of College Student Development, 39*, 438–448.

Forbes, G. B., Adams-Curtis, L. E., Pakalka, A. H., & White, K. B. (2006). Dating aggression, sexual coercion, and aggression-supporting attitudes among college men as a function of participation in aggressive high school sports. *Violence Against Women, 12*, 441–455. https://doi.org/10.1177/1077801206288126

Foubert, J. D. (2000). The longitudinal effects of a rape-prevention program on fraternity men's attitudes, behavioral intent, and behavior. *Journal of American College Health, 48*(4), 158–163. https://doi.org/10.1080/07448480009595691

Foubert, J. D., Brosi, M. W., & Bannon, R. S. (2011). Pornography viewing among fraternity men: Effects on bystander intervention, rape myth acceptance and behavioral intent to commit sexual assault. *Sexual Addiction & Compulsivity, 18*, 212–231. https://doi.org/10.1080/10720162.2011.625552

Foubert, J. D., & Marriott, K. A. (1997). Effects of a sexual assault peer education program on men's belief in rape myths. *Sex Roles, 36*, 259–268. https://doi.org/10.1007/BF02766271

Foubert, J. D., & Newberry, J. T. (2006). Effects of two versions of an empathy-based rape prevention program on fraternity Men's survivor empathy, attitudes, and behavioral intent to commit rape or sexual assault. *Journal of College Student Development, 47*(2), 133–148. https://doi.org/10.1353/csd.2006.0016

Foubert, J. D., & Perry, B. C. (2007). Creating lasting attitude and behavior change in fraternity members and male student athletes: The qualitative impact of an empathy-based rape prevention program. *Violence Against Women, 13*, 70–86. https://doi.org/10.1177/1077801206295125

Franiuk, R., & Shain, E. A. (2011). Beyond Christianity: The status of women and rape myths. *Sex Roles, 65*, 783–791. https://doi.org/10.1007/s11199-011-9974-8

Frazier, P. A., & Seales, L. M. (1997). Acquaintance rape is real rape. In M. D. Schwartz & M. D. Schwartz (Eds.), *Researching sexual violence against women: Methodological and personal perspectives* (pp. 54–64). Thousand Oaks, CA: Sage Publications, Inc.. https://doi.org/10.4135/9781483327907.n4

Frith, H. (2009). Sexual scripts, sexual refusals and rape. In M. Horvath, J. Brown, M. Horvath, & J. Brown (Eds.), *Rape: Challenging contemporary thinking* (pp. 99–122). Devon, UK: Willan Publishing.

Gerger, H., Kley, H., Bohner, G., & Siebler, F. (2007). The Acceptance of Modern Myths about Sexual Aggression Scale: Development and validation in German and English. *Aggressive Behavior, 33*, 422–440. https://doi.org/10.1002/ab.20195

Gidycz, C. A., Layman, M. J., Rich, C. L., Crothers, M., Gylys, J., Matorin, A., & Jacobs, C. D. (2001). An evaluation of an acquaintance rape prevention program: Impact on attitudes, sexual aggression, and sexual victimization. *Journal of Interpersonal Violence, 16*, 1120–1138. https://doi.org/10.1177/088626001016011002

Glick, P., & Fiske, S. T. (1996). The ambivalent sexism inventory: Differentiating hostile and benevolent sexism. *Journal of Personality and Social Psychology, 70*, 491–512. https://doi.org/10.1037/0022-3514.70.3.491

Goodchilds, J. D., Zellman, G. L., Johnson, P. B., & Giarrusso, R. (1988). *Adolescents and their perceptions of sexual interactions. Rape and sexual assault* (Vol. 2, pp. 245–270).

Gray, J. M. (2006). Rape myth beliefs and prejudiced instructions: Effects on decisions of guilt in a case of date rape. *Legal and Criminological Psychology, 11*(1), 75–80. https://doi.org/10.1348/135532505X68250

Grey, R., & Shepherd, L. J. (2013). "Stop rape now?" Masculinity, responsibility, and conflict-related sexual violence. *Men and Masculinities, 16*, 115–135.

Grubb, A., & Turner, E. (2012). Attribution of blame in rape cases: A review of the impact of rape myth acceptance, gender role conformity and substance use on victim blaming. *Aggression and Violent Behavior, 17*, 443–452. https://doi.org/10.1016/j.avb.2012.06.002

Heppner, M. J., Humphrey, C. F., Hillenbrand-Gunn, T. L., & DeBord, K. A. (1995). The differential effects of rape prevention programming on attitudes, behavior, and knowledge. *Journal of Counseling Psychology, 42*, 508–518. https://doi.org/10.1037/0022-0167.42.4.508

Hill, S., & Marshall, T. C. (2018). Beliefs about sexual assault in India and Britain are explained by attitudes toward women and hostile sexism. *Sex Roles, 79*, 421. https://doi.org/10.1007/s11199-017-0880-6

Hockett, J. M., Smith, S. J., Klausing, C. D., & Saucier, D. A. (2016). Rape myth consistency and gender differences in perceiving rape victims: A meta-analysis. *Violence Against Women, 22*, 139–167. https://doi.org/10.1177/1077801215607359

Horvath, M., & Brown, J. (2009). *Rape: Challenging contemporary thinking*. Devon, UK: Willan Publishing.

Huang, J. (2016). Rape myths and rape by juveniles. *Journal of Forensic Psychiatry & Psychology, 27*(4), 489–503. https://doi.org/10.1080/14789949.2016.1158848

Huang, J., & Lin, Y. (2017). Development of Chinese rape myths concept and scale [Abstract]. *Chinese Journal of Psychology, 59*(2), 63–87. Abstract received from PsycINFO Accession Number: 2017-41359-001.

Hutchinson, C. H., & McDaniel, S. A. (1986). The social reconstruction of sexual assault by women victims: A comparison of therapeutic experiences. *Canadian Journal of Community Mental Health, 5*(2), 17–36. https://doi.org/10.7870/cjcmh-1986-0013

Jones, M. E., Russell, R. L., & Bryant, F. B. (1998). The structure of rape attitudes for men and woman: A three-factor model. *Journal of Research in Personality, 32*, 331–350. https://doi.org/10.1006/jrpe.1998.2217

Kahn, A. S., Jackson, J., Kully, C., Badger, K., & Halvorsen, J. (2003). Calling it rape: Differences in experiences of women who do or do not label their sexual assault as rape. *Psychology of Women Quarterly, 27*, 233–242. https://doi.org/10.1111/1471-6402.00103

Kahn, A. S., Mathie, V. A., & Torgler, C. (1994). Rape scripts and rape acknowledgment. *Psychology of Women Quarterly, 18*, 53–66.

Kanin, E. J. (1967). Reference groups and sex conduct norm violations. *Sociological Quarterly, 8*, 495–504. https://doi.org/10.1111/j.1533-8525.1967.tb01085.x

Kanin, E. J. (1969). Selected dyadic aspects of male sex aggression. *Journal of Sex Research, 5*(1), 12–28.

Kanin, E. J. (1984). Date rape: Unofficial criminals and victims. *Victimology, 9*, 95–108.

Kingree, J. B., & Thompson, M. P. (2013). Fraternity membership and sexual aggression: An examination of mediators of the association. *Journal of American College Health, 61*, 213–221. https://doi.org/10.1080/07448481.2013.781026

Klement, K. R., & Sagarin, B. J. (2017). Nobody wants to date a whore: Rape-supportive messages in women-directed Christian dating books. *Sexuality and Culture: An Interdisciplinary Quarterly, 21*(1), 205–223. https://doi.org/10.1007/s12119-016-9390-x

Koo, K. H., Stephens, K. A., Lindgren, K. P., & George, W. H. (2012). Misogyny, acculturation, and ethnic identity: Relation to rape-supportive attitudes in Asian American college men. *Archives of Sexual Behavior, 41*, 1005–1014. https://doi.org/10.1007/s10508-011-9729-1

Koss, M. P., Dinero, T. E., Seibel, C. A., & Cox, S. L. (1988). Stranger and acquaintance rape: Are there differences in the victim's experience? *Psychology of Women Quarterly, 12*, 1–24. https://doi.org/10.1111/j.1471-6402.1988.tb00924.x

Koss, M. P., & Oros, C. J. (1982). Sexual experiences survey: A research instrument investigating sexual aggression and victimization. *Journal of Consulting and Clinical Psychology, 50*, 455–457. https://doi.org/10.1037/0022-006X.50.3.455

Krahé, B. (1991). Police officers' definitions of rape: A prototype study. *Journal of Community & Applied Social Psychology, 1*(3), 223–244. https://doi.org/10.1002/casp.2450010305

Krahé, B. (2016). Societal responses to sexual violence against women: Rape myths and the 'real rape' stereotype. In H. Kury, S. Redo, & E. Shea (Eds.), *Women and children as victims and offenders: Background, prevention, reintegration: Suggestions for succeeding generations* (pp. 671–700). Cham, Switzerland: Springer International Publishing.

Krahé, B., & Temkin, J. (2009). Addressing the attitude problem in rape trials: Some proposals and methodological considerations. In M. Horvath, J. Brown, M. Horvath, & J. Brown (Eds.), *Rape: Challenging contemporary thinking* (pp. 301–321). Devon, UK: Willan Publishing.

Krahé, B., Temkin, J., Bieneck, S., & Berger, A. (2008). Prospective lawyers' rape stereotypes and schematic decision making about rape cases. *Psychology, Crime & Law, 14*(5), 461–479. https://doi.org/10.1080/10683160801932380

Kress, V. E., Shepherd, J. B., Anderson, R. I., Petuch, A. J., Nolan, J. M., & Thiemeke, D. (2006). Evaluation of the impact of a coeducational sexual assault prevention program on college students' rape myth attitudes. *Journal of College Counseling, 9*(2), 148–157. https://doi.org/10.1002/j.2161-1882.2006.tb00101.x

Kroner, D. G., Boer, D. P., & Mills, J. F. (2004). Explaining rape-supportive attitudes among rapists. *American Journal of Forensic Psychology, 22*, 65–76.

Lawson, S. L., Munoz-Rojas, D., Gutman, L. S., & Siman, M. N. (2012). Changing attitudes and perceptions of Hispanic men ages 18 to 25 about rape and rape prevention. *Issues in Mental Health Nursing, 33*, 864–870. https://doi.org/10.3109/01612840.2012.728279

Littleton, H., Grills, A., Layh, M., & Rudolph, K. (2017). Unacknowledged rape and re-victimization risk: Examination of potential mediators. *Psychology of Women Quarterly, 41*, 437–450. https://doi.org/10.1177/0361684317720187

Littleton, H., Tabernik, H., Canales, E. J., & Backstrom, T. (2009). Risky situation or harmless fun? A qualitative examination of college women's bad hook-up and rape scripts. *Sex Roles, 60*, 793–804. https://doi.org/10.1007/s11199-009-9586-8

Littleton, H. L., Rhatigan, D. L., & Axsom, D. (2007). Unacknowledged rape: How much do we know about the hidden rape victim? *Journal of Aggression, Maltreatment & Trauma, 14*, 57–74. https://doi.org/10.1300/J146v14n04_04

Lonsway, K. A., & Fitzgerald, L. F. (1994). Rape myths: In review. *Psychology of Women Quarterly, 18*, 133–164. https://doi.org/10.1111/j.1471-6402.1994.tb00448.x

Lonsway, K. A., & Fitzgerald, L. F. (1995). Attitudinal antecedents of rape myth acceptance: A theoretical and empirical reexamination. *Journal of Personality and Social Psychology, 68*, 704–711. https://doi.org/10.1037/0022-3514.68.4.704

Martin, E. (2003). What is 'rape?'—Toward a historical, ethnographic approach. In C. B. Travis & C. B. Travis (Eds.), *Evolution, gender, and rape* (pp. 363–381). Cambridge, MA: MIT Press.

Martin, P. Y. (2016). The rape prone culture of academic contexts: Fraternities and athletics. *Gender & Society, 30*, 30–43. https://doi.org/10.1177/0891243215612708

Martin, P. Y., & Hummer, R. A. (1995). Fraternities and rape on campus. In P. Searles & R. J. Bergen (Eds.), *Rape and society: Readings on the problem of sexual assault* (pp. 139–151). Boulder: Westview.

McConahay, J. B. (1983). Modern racism and modern discrimination: The effects of race, racial attitudes, and context on simulated hiring decisions. *Personality and Social Psychology Bulletin, 9*, 551–558. https://doi.org/10.1177/0146167283094004

McMahon, S. (2010). Rape myth beliefs and bystander attitudes among incoming college students. *Journal of American College Health, 59*, 3–11. https://doi.org/10.1080/07448481.2010.483715

McMahon, S. (2015). Participation in high school sports and bystander intentions, efficacy to intervene, and rape myth beliefs. *Journal of Interpersonal Violence, 30*, 2980–2998. https://doi.org/10.1177/0886260514555009

McMahon, S., & Farmer, G. L. (2011). An updated measure for assessing subtle rape myths. *Social Work Research, 35*(2), 71–81.

McMullin, D., & White, J. W. (2006). Long-term effects of labeling a rape experience. *Psychology of Women Quarterly, 30*(1), 96–105. https://doi.org/10.1111/j.1471-6402.2006.00266.x

Mikorski, R., & Szymanski, D. M. (2017). Masculine norms, peer group, pornography, Facebook, and men's sexual objectification of women. *Psychology of Men & Masculinity, 18*(4), 257–267. https://doi.org/10.1037/men0000058

Muir, G., Lonsway, K. A., & Payne, D. L. (1996). Rape myth acceptance among Scottish and American students. *The Journal of Social Psychology, 136*, 261–262. https://doi.org/10.1080/00224545.1996.9714002

Nayak, M. B., Byrne, C. A., Martin, M. K., & Abraham, A. G. (2003). Attitudes toward violence against women: A cross-nation study. *Sex Roles, 49*, 333–342. https://doi.org/10.1023/A:1025108103617

Nosek, B., Banaji, M. R., & Greenwald, A. G. (2010). Project implicit. *Project Implicit.*

O'Brien, C., Keith, J., & Shoemaker, L. (2015). Don't tell: Military culture and male rape. *Psychological Services, 12*, 357–365. https://doi.org/10.1037/ser0000049

O'Donohue, W., Yeater, E. A., & Fanetti, M. (2003). Rape prevention with college males: The roles of rape myth acceptance, victim empathy, and outcome expectancies. *Journal of Interpersonal Violence, 18*, 513–531. https://doi.org/10.1177/0886260503251070

Oh, E., & Neville, H. (2004). Development and validation of the Korean Rape Myth Acceptance Scale. *The Counseling Psychologist, 32*, 301–331. https://doi.org/10.1177/0011000003261351

O'Keeffe, S., Brown, J. M., & Lyons, E. (2009). Seeking proof or truth: Naturalistic decision-making by police officers when considering rape allegations. In M. Horvath, J. Brown, M. Horvath, & J. Brown (Eds.), *Rape: Challenging contemporary thinking* (pp. 229–254). Devon, UK: Willan Publishing.

O'Sullivan, C. (1993). Fraternities and the rape culture. In Buchwald, E., Fletcher, P. R., & Roth, M. (Eds.). *Transforming a rape culture* (pp. 23–20). Minneapolis, MN: Milkweed Editions.

Parratt, K. A., & Pina, A. (2017). From 'real rape' to real justice: A systematic review of police officers' rape myth beliefs. *Aggression and Violent Behavior, 34*, 68–83. https://doi.org/10.1016/j.avb.2017.03.005

Payne, D. L., Lonsway, K. A., & Fitzgerald, L. F. (1999). Rape myth acceptance: Exploration of its structure and its measurement using the Illinois Rape Myth Acceptance Scale. *Journal of Research in Personality, 33*, 27–68. https://doi.org/10.1006/jrpe.1998.2238

Peterson, Z. D., & Muehlenhard, C. L. (2004). Was it rape? The function of women's rape myth acceptance and definitions of sex in labeling their own experiences. *Sex Roles, 51*, 129–144. https://doi.org/10.1023/B:SERS.0000037758.95376.00

Peterson, Z. D., & Muehlenhard, C. L. (2007). Conceptualizing the 'wantedness' of women's consensual and nonconsensual sexual experiences: Implications for how women label their experiences with rape. *Journal of Sex Research, 44*(1), 72–88.

Peterson, Z. D., & Muehlenhard, C. L. (2011). A match-and-motivation model of how women label their nonconsensual sexual experiences. *Psychology of Women Quarterly, 35*, 558–570. https://doi.org/10.1177/0361684311410210

Rau, T. J., Merrill, L. L., McWhorter, S. K., Stander, V. A., Thomsen, C. J., Dyslin, C. W., … Milner, J. S. (2010). Evaluation of a sexual assault education/prevention program for male U.S. Navy personnel. *Military Medicine, 175*, 429–434. https://doi.org/10.7205/MILMED-D-09-00218

Rebeiz, M. J., & Harb, C. (2010). Perceptions of rape and attitudes toward women in a sample of Lebanese students. *Journal of Interpersonal Violence, 25*, 735–752. https://doi.org/10.1177/0886260509334410

Ryan, K. M. (1988). Rape and seduction scripts. *Psychology of Women Quarterly, 12*, 237–245. https://doi.org/10.1111/j.1471-6402.1988.tb00939.x

Ryan, K. M. (2004). Further evidence for a cognitive component of rape. *Aggression and Violent Behavior, 9*, 579–604. https://doi.org/10.1016/j.avb.2003.05.001

Ryan, K. M. (2011). The relationship between rape myths and sexual scripts: The social construction of rape. *Sex Roles, 65*, 774–782. https://doi.org/10.1007/s11199-011-0033-2

Sanday, P. R. (1990). *Fraternity gang rape: Sex, brotherhood, and privilege on campus.* New York, NY: New York University Press.

Schewe, P. (2002). Guidelines for developing rape prevention and risk reduction interventions. *Preventing Violence in Relationships.* https://doi.org/10.1037/10455-005

Schewe, P., & O'Donohue, W. (1993b). Rape prevention: Methodological problems and new directions. *Clinical Psychology Review, 13*, 667–682. https://doi.org/10.1016/0272-7358(93)90032-H

Schewe, P. A., Adam, N. M., & Ryan, K. M. (2009). A qualitative analysis of the temptation to use force in sexual relationships. *Violence and Victims, 24*, 219–231. https://doi.org/10.1891/0886-6708.24.2.219

Schewe, P. A., & O'Donohue, W. (1993a). Sexual abuse prevention with high-risk males: The roles of victim empathy and rape myths. *Violence and Victims, 8*, 339–351.

Schwartz, M. D., & DeKeseredy, W. S. (1997). *Sexual assault on the college campus: The role of male peer support.* Thousand Oaks, CA: Sage Publications, Inc..

Schwartz, M. D., & Leggett, M. S. (1999). Bad dates or emotional trauma? The aftermath of campus sexual assault. *Violence Against Women, 5*(3), 251–271. https://doi.org/10.1177/1077801992218121

Seabrook, R. C., McMahon, S., & O'Connor, J. (2018). A longitudinal study of interest and membership in a fraternity, rape myth acceptance, and proclivity to perpetrate sexual assault. *Journal of American College Health, 66*, 510. https://doi.org/10.1080/07448481.2018.1440584. (online.

Seabrook, R. C., Ward, L. M., & Giaccardi, S. (2018). Why is fraternity membership associated with sexual assault? Exploring the roles of conformity to masculine norms, pressure to uphold masculinity, and objectification of women. *Psychology of Men & Masculinity, 19*, 3–13. https://doi.org/10.1037/men0000076

Sheldon, J. P., & Parent, S. L. (2002). Clergy's attitudes and attributions of blame toward female rape victims. *Violence Against Women, 8*, 233–256. https://doi.org/10.1177/10778010222183026

Skinner, K. M., Kressin, N., Frayne, S., Tripp, T. J., Hankin, C. S., Miller, D. R., & Sullivan, L. M. (2000). The prevalence of military sexual assault among female Veterans' Administration outpatients. *Journal of Interpersonal Violence, 15*, 291–310. https://doi.org/10.1177/088626000015003005

Smith, O., & Skinner, T. (2017). How rape myths are used and challenged in rape and sexual assault trials. *Social & Legal Studies, 26*, 441–466.

Stephens, K. A., & George, W. H. (2009). Rape prevention with college men: Evaluating risk status. *Journal of Interpersonal Violence, 24*, 996–1013. https://doi.org/10.1177/0886260508319366

Stillman, T. F., Yamawaki, N., Ridge, R. D., White, P. H., & Copley, K. J. (2009). Comparing predictors of sexual harassment proclivity between Japanese and U.S. men. *Psychology of Men & Masculinity, 10*, 30–43. https://doi.org/10.1037/a0013918

Street, A., Mahan, C., Hendricks, A., Gardner, J., & Stafford, J. (2003). Military sexual trauma among the reserve components of the armed forces. US D. o. V. Affairs (Ed.).

Street, A. E., Stafford, J., Mahan, C. M., & Hendricks, A. (2008). Sexual harassment and assault experienced by reservists during military service: Prevalence and health correlates. *Journal of Rehabilitation Research and Development, 45*, 409.

Struckman-Johnson, C., & Struckman-Johnson, D. (1992). Acceptance of male rape myths among college men and women. *Sex Roles, 27*, 85–100. https://doi.org/10.1007/BF00290011

Süssenbach, P., Eyssel, F., & Bohner, G. (2013). Metacognitive aspects of rape myths: Subjective strength of rape myth acceptance moderates its effects on information processing and behavioral intentions. *Journal of Interpersonal Violence, 28*, 2250–2272. https://doi.org/10.1177/0886260512475317

Temkin, J. (1987/2002). *Rape and the legal process*. 2nd ed. Oxford: Oxford University Press.

Temkin, J., Gray, J. M., & Barrett, J. (2018). Different functions of rape myth use in court: Findings from a trial observation study. *Feminist Criminology, 13*(2), 205–226.

Temkin, J., & Krahé, B. (2008). *Sexual assault and the justice gap: A question of attitude*. Portland, OR: Hart Publishing.

Truman, D. M., Tokar, D. M., & Fischer, A. R. (1996). Dimensions of masculinity: Relations to date rape supportive attitudes and sexual aggression in dating situations. *Journal of Counseling & Development, 74*, 555–562. https://doi.org/10.1002/j.1556-6676.1996.tb02292.x

Tummala-Narra, P., Houston-Kolnik, J., Sathasivam-Rueckert, N., & Greeson, M. (2017). An examination of attitudes toward gender and sexual violence among Asian Indians in the United States. *Asian American Journal of Psychology, 8*, 156–166. https://doi.org/10.1037/aap0000078

Turchik, J. A., & Edwards, K. M. (2012). Myths about male rape: A literature review. *Psychology of Men & Masculinity, 13*, 211–226. https://doi.org/10.1037/a0023207

Ullman, S. E. (2010). *Talking about sexual assault: Society's response to survivors*. Washington, DC, US: American Psychological Association. https://doi.org/10.1037/12083-000

Voller, E., Polusny, M. A., Noorbaloochi, S., Street, A., Grill, J., & Murdoch, M. (2015). Self-efficacy, male rape myth acceptance, and devaluation of emotions in sexual trauma sequelae: Findings from a sample of male veterans. *Psychological Services, 12*, 420–427. https://doi.org/10.1037/ser0000046

Ward, C. (1988). The attitudes toward rape victims scale: Construction, validation, and cross-cultural applicability. *Psychology of Women Quarterly, 12*, 127–146. https://doi.org/10.1111/j.1471-6402.1988.tb00932.x

Warshaw, R. (1988/1994). *I never called it rape* (2nd ed.). New York: HarperPerennial.

Weis, K., & Borges, S. S. (1973). Victimology and rape: The case of the legitimate victim. *Issues in Criminology, 8*(2), 71–115.

White, J. W., Donat, P. N., & Humphrey, J. A. (1995). An examination of the attitudes underlying sexual coercion among acquaintances. *Journal of Psychology and Human Sexuality, 8*, 27–47. https://doi.org/10.1300/J056v08n01_03

Wilson, L. C., & Miller, K. E. (2016). Meta-analysis of the prevalence of unacknowledged rape. *Trauma, Violence, and Abuse, 17*, 149–159. https://doi.org/10.1177/1524838015576391

Young, B., Desmarais, S. L., Baldwin, J. A., & Chandler, R. (2017). Sexual coercion practices among undergraduate male recreational athletes, intercollegiate athletes, and non-athletes. *Violence Against Women, 23*, 795–812. https://doi.org/10.1177/1077801216651339

Zimbardo, P. (2007/2008). *The Lucifer effect: Understanding how good people turn evil.* New York, NY: Random House.

Zydervelt, S., Zajac, R., Kaladelfos, A., & Westera, N. (2017). Lawyers' strategies for cross-examining rape complainants: Have we moved beyond the 1950s? *British Journal of Criminology, 57*, 551–569.

Part III

Risk Factors of Sexual Victimization and Perpetration

10 Who Is at High Risk for Victimhood?

Ebru Yucel, Nicole Cantor, Meredith Joppa, and D. J. Angelone

Introduction

This chapter provides an overview of sexual violence (SV) victimology by attempting to answer the question of *who is at high risk for victimhood?*. We have tried to provide a clear definition of this construct as it relates to sexual violence but also acknowledge that other researchers have used a variety of terms to represent the behaviors under study. Indeed, one issue for the field is the problem of terminology (e.g., sexual assault, rape, sexual coercion), which can potentially lead to inferred differences in the behaviors in question. Nonetheless, as we attempt to describe in this chapter, sexual violence victimization is an unfortunately common experience for many individuals. Given the negative sequelae associated with experiences of sexual violence victimization, we hope that future iterations of this chapter provide a more optimistic outlook. However, the existence of many group- and individual-level risk factors for sexual violence victimization should serve as an ongoing call for change. In addition to risk factors associated with increased prevalence rates, we also discuss some potential gaps in the literature and consider the need to examine the intersectionality of person and situational factors to reveal a more comprehensive picture of risk for sexual violence. Finally, it is important to note that while the focus of this chapter is on sexual violence victimization, we do not suggest that an individual is ever responsible for their victimhood. We fully acknowledge that any person who perpetrates these behaviors on another person is completely responsible for their actions and any consequences experienced by the victim.

We begin with an overview of SV victimization prevalence in the US, summarize the consequences of SV victimization, and consider the impact of revictimization. We then identify three major domains of risk for SV victimization covering multiple factors that may contribute to victimology: (1) demographic and individual risk factors, (2) behavioral risk factors, and (3) environmental risk factors. Naturally, considering these categories separately can potentially lead to an incomplete conceptualization of victimization. As such, we recognize that different SV victimization risk factors can interact and are not always additive; thus, the role of intersectionality in victimization research is discussed at the end of the chapter.

Ways to Consider Victimology

Victimization refers to any situation where an individual is treated unfairly or unjustly. For the purposes of this chapter, we focus on sexual

E. Yucel · N. Cantor · M. Joppa · D. J. Angelone (✉)
Rowan University, Glassboro, NJ, USA
e-mail: angeloned@rowan.edu

W. T. O'Donohue and P. A. Schewe (eds.), *Handbook of Sexual Assault and Sexual Assault Prevention*,
https://doi.org/10.1007/978-3-030-23645-8_10

victimization, which refers to situations in which someone attempts, threatens, or completes forced sexual advances without first receiving consent (Carlson & Duckworth, 2019). These sexual advances can span a wide continuum, including less severe behaviors such as telling sexually inappropriate jokes, to more severe behaviors, such as sexual assault and rape. A term that captures this continuum, sexual violence, has been defined by the Centers for Disease Control as any form of sexual contact or behavior that occurs without the consent of the recipient (CDC, 2012). SV victimization among adults can occur in a variety of interpersonal contexts, including intimate partners, friends, family members, colleagues, or strangers. It is worth noting that most research on SV victimization in adults has focused on sexual assault; however, for purposes of this chapter, we review findings related to the broader spectrum of SV victimization when applicable.

Prevalence of Sexual Violence Victimization in the United States

SV victimization occurs at different rates in different populations. Consistent findings regarding the universal frequency of SV victimization are therefore limited. The national prevalence rates described below reflect primarily SV victimization experiences among adult victims. Traditionally, the United States Bureau of Justice Statistics (BJS) releases national data annually through the National Crime Victimization Survey (NCVS) on criminal victimization. These reports concern not only adults but also individuals who age 12 or older from a nationally representative sample of US households. While these data present one estimate of the frequency of SV victimization, it is not uncommon for victims of SV to either delay reporting or decide not to report these crimes. In response, the BJS has begun examining incidents of SV victimization that are reported and not reported to police.

According to the 2016 Criminal Victimization Survey, 323,450 individuals over the age of 12 in the US experienced SV victimization in 2016 alone (Morgan & Kena, 2017). A mere 22.9% of those incidents were reported to the police, leaving 77.1% of SV victimization instances unreported. These incidence rates cannot be compared to previous year's data as the NCVS survey sample went through a routine redesign in 2016. However, it is possible to compare data from previous years. For example, 284,350 individuals over the age of 12 experienced SV victimization in 2015, as compared to 207,760 individuals in 2014, suggesting an increase in reported SV victimization.

Another representative national survey, the 2011 National Intimate Partner and Sexual Violence Survey (NISVS), almost one in five adult women (19.3%) and one in 59 men (1.7%) reported a lifetime history of rape (Breiding et al., 2014). These numbers represent an increase from the 2010 NISVS data, where the prevalence rates for lifetime rape were 18.3% for women and 1.4% for men (Black et al., 2011a, 2011b). The 2011 NISVS also reported that 1.6% of women had been raped in the past year, but the prevalence of rape in the past 12 months for men was too small to report (Breiding et al., 2014). In contrast to the NCVS data, the NISVS estimate suggests that 1.9 million women were raped in the year preceding the survey (Breiding et al., 2014). Other forms of SV examined by the NISVS include being made to penetrate a partner, sexual coercion, unwanted sexual contact, and noncontact unwanted sexual experiences. These other forms of SV were reported in 2011 by 43.9% of women in their lifetimes (5.5% in the past year), and 23.4% of men in their lifetimes (5.1% in the past year) (Breiding et al., 2014). We will further discuss gender differences in SV, as well as other demographic and individual risk factors, in the following sections.

Consequences of Sexual Violence Victimization

There are multiple mental and physical health consequences to SV victimization that are both immediate and long-term; thus, SV victimization can be considered both a public health and a public safety problem. Well over half of rape victims experience some severe medical or mental health consequence of SV victimization (Krebs, Lindquist, Warner, Fisher, & Martin, 2007). Within a male and female undergraduate sample, anywhere from 25% to 45% of rape victims suffer from nongenital physical trauma, while 19% to 22% suffer from genital trauma (Krebs et al., 2007). Up to 32% of women and 16% of men experience physical injury such as bruises, welts, and even broken bones as a result of a rape (Tjaden & Thoennes, 2006). Medical consequences of nonconsensual sex also include high cholesterol, stroke, and heart disease (Smith & Breiding, 2011). In fact, female victims of nonconsensual sex are more likely to report heart attack and heart disease in their lifetime as compared to nonvictims (Smith & Breiding, 2011). In addition, anywhere between 1% and 5% of female victims become pregnant following rape (Krebs et al., 2007), with close to 32,000 pregnancies resulting from rape each year (Holmes, Resnick, Kilpatrick, & Best, 1996). A more recent study reported that 26% of women who had been raped reported at least one pregnancy as the result of the rape (McFarlane & Malecha, 2005), but very limited data are available regarding pregnancies and their outcomes following SV, particularly pregnancies associated with rape by intimate partners (McFarlane, 2007). Finally, up to 40% of rape victims contract a sexually transmitted disease following the assault (Krebs et al., 2007).

In reference to mental health consequences, there is an increased lifetime risk of anxiety, depression, eating disorders, posttraumatic stress disorder, sleep disorders, substance abuse, psychosis, dissociation, somatization, personality disorders, and suicide attempts for individuals who experience SV victimization (Browne & Finkelhor, 1986; Chen et al., 2010; Maniglio, 2009). In addition, rape victims are 13 times more likely to commit suicide than people who have not experienced rape (Krebs et al., 2007). Trauma symptoms commonly experienced after SV victimization include self-destructiveness, isolation, low self-esteem, physical health problems, and suicidality (Browne & Finkelhor, 1986). Sexual risk behaviors exhibited by individuals who experience SV victimization at an early age include condomless sex, having multiple sexual partners, early involvement in sexual activity, prostitution, and sexual maladjustment (Browne & Finkelhor, 1986; Chen et al., 2010; Maniglio, 2009).

Understanding the consequences of SV victimization is critical for the field of victimology, as it sheds light on the scope of this far-reaching problem. Having identified the extant of effects of SV victimization, researchers have been guided towards identifying prevention interventions in an effort to preclude future SV victimization. That said, there are continuous efforts to identify where this prevention is needed, and what the mechanisms of change may be. To this end, we will identify certain factors that may increase one's risk of experiencing SV victimization. However, it is important to note that the scope of our knowledge regarding these factors is still developing.

Demographic and Individual Risk Factors

Demographic risk factors for SV victimization refer to innate characteristics that tend to remain stable over time. For the purposes of this chapter, we conceptualize demographic risk factors using the ADDRESSING framework (Hays, 2008), which includes age, developmental and acquired disabilities, religion, ethnicity, socioeconomic status, sexual orientation, indigenous heritage, national origin, and gender (Hays, 2008). This widely used framework moves beyond a unidimensional view of diversity toward a multidimensional conceptualization of identity with intersecting cultural components (Hays, 2008). In addition, this section identifies individual risk factors, which include attitudes, beliefs, or characteristics that may increase an individual's risk of SV victimization.

Age. In terms of the adult population, 20% of women have experienced adult sexual assault, similar to the 1 in 5 statistic most commonly reported for female college students who have experienced SV victimization (Muehlenhard, Peterson, Humphreys, & Jozkowski, 2017). SV victimization which occurs under the age of 18 is typically called childhood sexual abuse (CSA), and has been defined as any sexual activity with a child where consent cannot be given (Saul & Audage, 2007). More than half (50–54%) of female rape victims are under the age of 18 (Humphrey & White, 2000; Peipert & Domagalski, 1994; Silverman, Raj, Mucci, & Hathaway, 2001; Tjaden & Thoennes, 2000b). Other researchers report that up to 27% of women and 16% of men have experienced CSA before the age of 18 (Finkelhor, Shattuck, Turner, & Hamby, 2014). Specifically, victimization occurred before the age of eight in 22% of women who report CSA and 22% of men, although perpetrators of CSA differ by gender, with 40% of men reporting perpetration by a stranger and 29% of women reporting perpetration by a family member (Finkelhor et al., 2014). Most research on SV victimization has focused on young people, and we know little about SV victimization in middle and older adulthood.

Gender. Incidence rates of SV victimization vary by gender. In general, women in the US are more likely to be victims of rape than men, with estimates from the CDC in 2012 noting 302,091 female victims of rape compared to 92,748 male victims of rape (CDC, 2012). These differences replicate previous findings regarding gender differences from the National Violence Against Women survey, which noted an estimated 876,064 rapes perpetrated against women during 12 months between 1995 and 1996 as compared to 111,298 rapes perpetrated against men during the same period (Tjaden & Thoennes, 2006). With regard to prevalence rates, 18.3% of women and 1.4% of men experience rape at some point in their lifetime (Black et al., 2011a). Among female rape victims, the majority of perpetrators were intimate partners (51.1%) followed by family members (12.5%), acquaintances (40.8%) and strangers (13.8%) (Black et al., 2011b). Additionally, men have been shown to perpetrate the majority of SV victimization (Smith et al., 2017). Of the women who reported experiencing rape in their lifetime, 97.3% of perpetrators were men (Smith et al., 2017). Among male rape victims, the majority of perpetrators were acquaintances (52.4%), followed by strangers (15.1%) (Black et al., 2011b). Men have been shown to perpetrate the majority of rapes against other men, representing 86.5% of perpetrators. Within the US, 5.3% of men and 5.6% of women experience SV victimization other than rape, such as unwanted sexual contact in the previous 12 months (Black et al., 2011b). Of the women who experience unwanted sexual contact in their lifetime, 94.9% of perpetrators were men (Smith et al., 2017). Of the men who reported experiencing sexual contact in their lifetime, 14.5% of perpetrators were men and 81.6% were women (Smith et al., 2017). Additionally 13% of women and 6% of men experienced sexual coercion: unwanted sexual contact that occurs due to feeling pressured, tricked, threatened, or forced in a non-physical way, during their lifetime (Black et al., 2011b). Of the women who reported experiencing sexual coercion in their lifetime, 96.3% of perpetrators were men (Smith et al., 2017). Of the men who reported experiencing unwanted sexual coercion in their lifetime, 36.7% of perpetrators were men and 53.0% were female (Smith et al., 2017).

The literature suggests that individuals whose gender identity and/or expression differs from their sex assigned at birth are at high risk for SV victimization. The frequency of transgender individuals' experiences with SV victimization varies between studies, perhaps reflective of differences in research methods or a calling for a greater focus on transgender individuals' experiences with SV victimization to establish consistent findings. One study suggests that up to 50% of transgender individuals experience SV victimization (Stotzer, 2009). Compared to cisgender adults, predicted probabilities for SV victimization are higher among transgender people: heterosexual cisgender men have a predicted probability of experienced SV victimization of 2.9%, cisgender women's predicted probability is 7.7%, and transgender individuals' predicted probability is 12.2% (Coulter et al., 2017). The highest predicted probability of sexual assault (57.7%) is among black transgender individuals (Coulter et al., 2017). Transgender individuals who have engaged in sex work, experienced homelessness, or are disabled maintain high levels of lifetime SV victimization risk (James et al., 2016). Finally, upwards of 12% of youth who identified as gender nonconforming or transgender in kindergarten experience SV victimization prior to 12th grade (Grant et al., 2011).

Sexual Orientation. The LGB+ population includes a wide range of sexual orientations including, but not limited to, lesbian, gay, and bisexual. Overall, the LGB+ population has been identified as a high-risk population for SV victimization (Ford & Soto-Marquez, 2016). More specifically, men and women who identify as gay, lesbian, bisexual, or questioning are about twice as likely to experience some form of SV than their heterosexual counterparts (Coulter et al., 2017). Additionally, bisexual female college students are at highest risk of SV victimization in comparison to straight, gay, lesbian, and bisexual male peers (Ford & Soto-Marquez, 2016). Reasons underlying increased risk for victimization in the LGB+ community are not well understood, although risk for violence among this population is much higher in comparison to heterosexual individuals (CDC, 2012). One explanation is "corrective rape," a hate crime with the goal of "changing" the victim's orientation to heterosexual, while forcing them to conform to gender stereotypes (Bartle, 2000; Martin, Kelly, Turquet, & Ross, 2009). It is important to note that although research tends to focus on the victimization of heterosexual women, women and men in the LGB+ community often face higher risk in comparison, with almost half of all bisexual women experiencing some form of SV within their lifetimes (CDC, 2012). Bisexual or questioning men are at three times more risk of SV victimization than heterosexual men (Coulter et al., 2017), and men who identify as gay are about 3.5 times more likely to experience sexual assault in comparison to heterosexual cisgender men (Coulter et al., 2017).

Race, Ethnicity, and Indigenous Heritage. Non-white women are most likely to be victims of rape: American Indian and Alaska Native women are at highest risk, followed by mixed race, African-American, white, and Asian/Pacific Islander women (Tjaden & Thoennes, 2000a). American Indian, Alaska Native, and Hispanic women are more likely to report experiencing rape than their Non-Hispanic, Caucasian, African-American, and mixed-raced counterparts (CDC, 2012). At current, there is a lack of data with regard to intra- vs. interracial perpetrators and victims. However, estimates of SV victimization among specific racial and ethnic groups does vary by age. Among high school students, 13.5% of mixed-race students, 12.5% of American Indian/Alaska Natives, 10.5% of Native Hawaiian/Pacific Islander students, 8.6% of black students, 8.2% of Hispanic students, and 7.4% of white students are victims of sexual assault by being forced to have sexual intercourse at some time in their lives (CDC, 2012). Among adult women, 35.5% of mixed-race women, 26.9% of American Indian/Alaska Natives, 22% of Non-Hispanic blacks, 18.8% of Non-Hispanic whites, and 14.6% of Hispanics, experienced an attempted or a completed rape at some time in their lives (CDC, 2012).

There are also unique patterns of risk for SV victimization among American Indians and Alaska Natives (Yuan, Koss, Polacca, & Goldman, 2006). Male victims report that the most common perpetrator is a male relative (45%), followed by a stranger (43%), contrary to the high rates of acquaintance rape seen in nonindigenous cultures (Yuan et al., 2006). However, existing studies have not indicated whether the perpetrators in these interactions are of the same or different culture as the victim. For female victims, 14% report being raped during adulthood, a rate much higher than that of male participants (2%). For female victims of sexual assault, most perpetrators were a male relative (55%), followed by a romantic partner (46%). The strongest predictor for sexual assault in women was being separated or divorced. Other significant risk factors included being the victim of emotional abuse during childhood, cohabitating, sexual abuse during childhood, physical neglect during childhood, and a lifetime diagnosis of alcohol dependence. Women who highly identified with their tribe were at increased risk of being raped; however, women with more experiences living within or near tribal lands were less likely to be raped (Yuan et al., 2006).

Religion. Little research exists on religion as a risk factor for SV victimization; however, most research has focused on Abrahamic religions (faiths which identify Abraham as a biblical patriarch), most commonly Judaism, Christianity, and Islam. The general themes of female celibacy, wifely duties, the ideal woman outlined in Abrahamic religions may contribute to male violence against women (Narasimhan-Madhavan, 2006; Niaz, 2003). While prevalence estimates of SV victimization in the US do not identify differences by religious affiliation, international research suggests that religion may be an important factor. For example, in Bangladesh, a predominantly Muslim country, approximately 55% of women in rural areas and 40% of women in urban areas believe that a woman cannot refuse her husband sex just because she does not want to have sex (Krug, Dahlberg, Mercy, Zwi, & Lozano, 2002). Not inconsequentially, 50% of rural Bangladeshi women and 37% of urban Bangladeshi women reported experiencing sexual violence from an intimate partner in their lifetime (Krug et al., 2002). For a review of the international sexual violence literature, see the World Health Organization's *World Report on Violence and Health* (Krug et al., 2002).

Socioeconomic Status. There is a strong link between poverty and SV (Bassuk, Melnick, & Browne, 1998; Greco & Dawgert, 2007). Individuals with a household income of less than $25,000 per year are at least twice as likely to experience sexual assault in comparison to other income brackets (Morgan & Kena, 2016). For example, among a sample of African American women living in poverty, 41% of women who were living in shelters and 21% of women living in low-income housing reported being sexually assaulted at some point in their lifetime (Wenzel, Tucker, Hambarsoomian, & Elliott, 2006). It is important to note that, as a result of societal barriers, African American citizens are disproportionately affected by poverty in comparison to white European citizens, making it difficult to tease apart the relative risks of racial and/or ethnic minority status from socioeconomic status. It appears that the relationship between SV victimization and socioeconomic status is cyclical in nature: victimization increases the likelihood of unemployment and decreased income (Byrne, Resnick, Kilpatrick, Best, & Saunders, 1999), perhaps because of the mental and physical health consequences of experiencing SV victimization. In addition, people who are less able to meet their basic needs may be targeted for victimization due to their vulnerability (Greco & Dawgert, 2007).

Developmental & Acquired Disabilities. Developmental and acquired disabilities include learning disabilities, physical illnesses, and mental illnesses that impair functioning (Hays, 2008). According to a meta-analysis conducted in 2012, the pooled prevalence rate of SV victimization for adults with mental illness ranges from 1.3% to 12.2% (Plummer & Findley, 2012). However, studies that evaluate SV victimization among individuals with disabilities typically ask general questions about limitations in daily activities and the need for assistive equipment (Loiselle & Fuqua, 2007; Mason, Riger, & Foley, 2004). Thus, existing research on SV victimization among individuals with disabilities has generally only covered people who experience problems in functioning, whether it is physical, mental, or developmental. There are higher rates of victimization among women with a disability in comparison to men with or without a disability, and women without a disability (Powers et al., 2002). For example, there is a fourfold risk of sexual assault victimization for women with severe disability impairments (i.e., injuries, chronic diseases, or mental health conditions that extremely limit normal activities) as opposed to women without disabilities (Casteel, Martin, Smith, Gurka, & Kupper, 2008). Factors such as marital status, age, and race also appear to increase risk of sexual assault among women with disabilities (Martin et al., 2006). Given the overall devaluation of individuals with disabilities, dehumanization has led to disproportionately low rates of reporting, which may be due to a lack of sensitivity from law enforcement and health workers (Hassouneh-Phillips & McNeff, 2005; Swedlund & Nosek, 2000). Despite these risks, this area of research continues to remain understudied (Plummer & Findley, 2012).

History of victimization. Perhaps one of the most important and notable sequelae of SV victimization is increased risk for future victimization. Individuals who are revictimized may experience more severe consequences. Experiencing CSA increases one's likelihood to experience adult victimization; women who experience rape under the age of 18 are twice as likely to report experiencing rape as an adult (Tjaden & Thoennes, 2000a). Depending on the type of CSA, women are between 3 and 11 times more likely to be victims of sexual assault as an adult (Black et al., 2011a, 2011b; Maniglio, 2009). In addition, there is growing evidence to suggest that experiencing SV victimization in adolescence can also increase the likelihood of a subsequent assault in adulthood (Angelone, Marcantonio, & Melillo, 2017; Humphrey & White, 2000). In fact, female college students who reported SV victimization were four times more likely to experience SV victimization in high school than those without a college SV victimization experience (Himelein, Vogel, & Wachowiak, 1994; Katz, May, Sörensen, & DelTosta, 2010; Miller, Markman, & Handley, 2007).

Overall, the greatest number of trauma symptoms are reported by sexually abused children who are later sexually assaulted as adults (Gold, Milan, Mayall, & Johnson, 1994). Further, experiencing SV victimization in adolescence and again in adulthood is associated with greater levels of alcohol and drug consumption, frequency of use, and level of consequences than women who never experienced SV victimization (Angelone et al., 2017). Women who are revictimized report more trauma symptoms, greater engagement in sexual risk behaviors, and significant mental health issues as compared individuals who experienced an isolated incident of SV victimization (Gold et al., 1994).

Attitudes and Beliefs. Rape myths, commonly known as rape supportive attitudes, are defined as prejudicial, stereotyped, or false beliefs about rape and rapists that are persistently held and deny or justify sexual violence against women (Burt, 1980; Lonsway & Fitzgerald, 1995). Rape myths stem from the ideals of a patriarchal society where women are encouraged to adhere to traditional gender norms; failure to abide by traditional gender norms results in guilty and blame for sexual behavior (Angelone, Cantor, Marcantonio, & Joppa, in press). Those who endorse rape myths believe that victims deserve experiencing sexual assault because their behaviors allowed for the assault to happen. Women who endorse rape myths, relative to women who do not, are less inclined to blame the perpetrator of SV victimization and more inclined to blame the victim (Loiselle & Fuqua, 2007; Mason et al., 2004). These women also believe that they are less susceptible to sexual assault and rape (Bohner & Lampridis, 2004). However, women who endorse rape myths are less likely to rely on victimization risk information when appraising a situation, therefore leaving them susceptible victimization (Yeater, Treat, Viken, & McFall, 2010). Similarly, men who endorse rape myths are less sensitive to women's affective cues (Farris, Viken, Treat, & McFall, 2006). Rape supportive attitudes also interfere with both women's and men's use of helpful information such as victimization risk that drives effective decision making within potential sexual encounters (Yeater et al., 2010). Finally, women who have been victimized and endorse rape myths experience worse outcomes during the recovery process as compared to women who reject such attitudes (Burt & Katz, 1988).

Sexist attitudes also impact SV victimization. Individuals who harbor sexist beliefs or attitudes maintain that men and women must subscribe to certain gender roles (Glick & Fiske, 2002; Hamilton & Armstrong, 2009; Kitzinger & Frith, 1999). These roles describe women as subservient, innocent, pure, fragile, and submissive, and men as aggressive, dominant, and in control (Canan, Jozkowski, & Crawford, 2016; Jozkowski, Marcantonio, & Hunt, 2017; Yamawaki, 2007). As such, it is up to men to initiate sexual encounters with women, who are the sexual gatekeepers (Hamilton & Armstrong, 2009; Jozkowski et al., 2017; Jozkowski & Peterson, 2013). Such attitudes can result in a series of provocative beliefs, such as the idea that women want to be forced into sex because initiating sexual activity goes against a women's role as innocent and submissive (Canan et al., 2016; Joskowski et al., 2017).

Cognitive and Behavioral Risk Factors

Behavioral risk factors comprise individual actions that increase risk for SV victimization. The predominant behavioral risk factor that we focus on is substance use, particularly alcohol use. While we provide evidence to suggest that certain actions may increase a person's risk for SV victimization, it is important to reiterate a specific point from our introduction: we do not suggest that an individual is ever responsible for their victimhood. We fully acknowledge that any person who perpetrates SV on another person is completely responsible for their actions and any consequences experienced by the victim. We also refer the reader to Chaps. 16 and 17 in this volume.

Cognitive Processing. As described above, any victimization experience increases risk for being revictimized (Messman-Moore & Long, 2003). One explanation is that victimized women are not perceiving risk as actively as women who have not been victimized (Yeater et al., 2010). Given that severe victimization history predicts a higher threshold for risk perception, cognitive risk factors appear related to victimization. Women who have been previously victimized and are not adequately or accurately perceiving risk are less likely to leave a dangerous situation. Women who have been victimized require greater evidence that a situation is risky, and rely less on victimization risk information when appraising a situation (Yeater et al., 2010). Further, women who have been victimized experience deficits in information processing (Yeater et al., 2010). Others have hypothesized that fear of losing a relationship may obscure women's risk recognition (Norris, Nurius, & Dimeff, 1996; Nurius & Norris, 1996; Turchik, Probst, Chau, Nigoff, & Gidycz, 2007).

Risk Perception and Alcohol Use. An individual's perception of risk can be divided into threat appraisal and behavioral response. Identifying when you feel uncomfortable and leaving a situation is threat appraisal, while the point at which you leave the situation is behavioral response (Davis et al., 2009; Meadows, Jaycox, Orsillo, & Foa, 1997; Messman-Moore & Brown, 2006; Norris et al., 2006). Alcohol is involved in at least half of all sexual assaults (Abbey, 2011; Abbey, Zawacki, Buck, Clinton, & McAuslan, 2004). Because alcohol decreases cognitive capacity, it may limit the ability to recognize abstract risk cues, thus increasing the threshold for threat appraisal and making a behavioral response (Davis Cue, Hendershot, George, Norris, & Heiman, 2007). Some researchers suggest that alcohol may be consumed by SV victimization perpetrators as a means for excusing hookup behavior and not having to justify that behavior (Paul, McManus, & Hayes, 2000). In addition, women who experience sexual assault are at risk for utilizing substances as a coping tool, which augments the risk of revictimization (Angelone et al., 2017; Krebs et al., 2007). In addition, substances other than alcohol may also be related to SV victimization and may follow early victimization experiences (Gidycz, Hanson, & Layman, 1995). For example, marijuana use in the past 30 days is associated with both SV victimization and rape (Champion et al., 2004; Messman-Moore, Coates, Gaffey, & Johnson, 2008). Regardless of the type of substance involved, there is a complex relationship with SV victimization that warrants further study.

Environmental Risk Factors

Environmental risk factors, such as college or occupational settings, include situations or circumstances that increase susceptibility to SV victimization. These settings may promote SV victimization through a variety of factors, such as increased access to alcohol, unequal power dynamics, or rape supportive culture. The environmental factors discussed in this chapter include college, athletic involvement, Greek life, study abroad, relationship status, hookup culture, prison and community confinement settings, and occupational settings.

Higher Education. Given the frequency of SV victimization within a nationally representative sample, some specific populations may face increased risk for experiencing SV victimization (Coulter et al., 2017). College and university students are one such group, with roughly 4.1% of undergraduate women and 0.8% of undergraduate males reporting being raped in the 2014–2015 academic year (Morgan & Kena, 2016). Consistent with the frequently reported 1 in 5 statistic (Muehlenhard et al., 2017), 20.5% of undergraduate females and 7% of undergraduate males report experiencing sexual assault in college (Krebs, Lindquist, Warner, Fisher, & Martin, 2009). Overall, college is a high-risk environment with college women maintaining three times the risk for sexual assault than noncollege women (Koss, Gidycz, & Wisniewski, 1987). One way to predict SV victimization in a college population is by examining high-risk behavior: students who participate in high-risk behaviors such as condomless sex or using alcohol before sex, are more likely to experience SV victimization (Stephens, 2016). Some groups of college students may be at greater risk for SV victimization because of their social or leisure activities including athletics, participation in Greek life, and studying abroad.

Intercollegiate Athletes. Athletes differ in their susceptibility to sexual perpetration and victimization in comparison with their nonathlete counterparts. Athletes may differ in their susceptibility to SV involvement based on their sport: males who play contact sports are more likely to engage in aggressive behaviors towards their partner (Burns, 2009), but we do not yet know how type of sport might be related to SV victimization for either men or women. Although uncommon, athletes are also more likely to experience SV victimization when engaging in sexual relationships with their coaches (Johansson, 2013). Previous studies suggest that male college athletes sometimes exhibit high rates of sexual risk behaviors that may lead to SV victimization, such as condomless sex and having multiple sexual partners, along with dating aggression, sexual activity, abusive behaviors, sexually aggressive behaviors, and sexual violence (Chandler, Johnson, & Carroll, 1999; Forbes, 2006; Grossbard, Lee, Neighbors, Hendershot, & Larimer, 2007; Locke & Mahalik, 2005). For example, college athletes have reported a greater likelihood than nonathletes to sexually victimize someone through fondling the opposite sex against their will, and having forced sex with someone of the opposite sex (Chandler et al., 1999). Male college athletes sometimes exhibit high rates of sexual risk behaviors that may increase their risk for SV victimization or perpetration, such as condomless sex and having multiple sexual partners, along with dating aggression, sexual activity, abusive behaviors, sexually aggressive behaviors, and sexual violence (Chandler et al., 1999; Forbes, 2006; Grossbard et al., 2007; Locke & Mahalik, 2005). Currently, the majority of research on NCAA intercollegiate athletes examines men as perpetrators and women as victims, although there continues to be a deficit in the literature that clearly identifies prevalence rates of SV.

Greek Life. Sorority members are more likely to have experienced attempted or completed rape than nonsorority members (Minow & Einolf, 2009). Alcohol consumption plays a role in the relationship between SV victimization and Greek life involvement, with sorority members consuming far more alcohol then nonmembers (Curtis, 2011; Minow & Einolf, 2009). Alcohol consumption, particularly the frequency of blacking out due to alcohol, is not only positively associated with Greek life (fraternities and sororities) involvement but also incapacitated SV victimization (Voloshyna et al., 2018). One explanation for the increase in SV victimization experienced by sorority women may be their exposure to fraternity houses, which provides easy access to alcohol (Copenhaver & Grauerholz, 1991). This easy access to alcohol induces increased risk for experiencing SV victimization, which may be due to an inability to provide or perceive consent and decreased inhibitions and risk recognition.

Study Abroad. Most 4-year colleges and universities offer students the opportunity to earn credits towards their degrees at institutions in other countries. Students who travel abroad typically increase their alcohol consumption and risky sexual behaviors while they are abroad (Pedersen, Larimer, & Lee, 2010). More specifically, students who reported high immersion in their environment and an inconsistent history of condom use may be more likely to engage in risky sexual behaviors, even if they do not intend to (Marcantonio, Angelone, & Sledjeski, 2016). It has been hypothesized that the concept of a "backspace" may be the driving factor in the behavior of students who study abroad (Milhausen, Reece, & Perera, 2006). Backspace refers to the removal of typical norms and restraints, such as the fear of judgment from peers (Maticka-Tyndale, Herold, & Oppermann, 2003). The addition of alcohol and like-minded co-travelers may also catalyze the effects of being away from "normal" life (Sönmez et al., 2006). Previous studies have identified estimates of the prevalence of sexual assault victimization between 18% and 38% (Flack et al., 2014; Marcantonio, Angelone, & Joppa, 2018).

Relationship Status. Although relationship status has not been extensively studied as a risk factor for sexual assault, there are some components of relationships that may lead to more or less risk for SV. For instance, SV is more likely to occur in romantic relationships where sex occurs on a regular basis, rather than relationships where intercourse is nonexistent or uncommon (Kaestle & Halpern, 2005). Intimate partner sexual violence (IPSV) refers to unwanted sexual contact that occurs within the context of an intimate relationship, and is fairly common, with national rates estimated at about 32.9% among women and 9.9% among men (Black et al., 2011a, 2011b). Typically, 9% to 13% of women from community and national samples report experiencing sexual assault by an intimate partner (McFarlane & Malecha, 2005). Among young adults, these rates increase to approximately 47% (Renner & Whitney, 2012). Some studies suggest that jealousy has been linked to IPV, and may be the instigator of perpetration (Goetz & Shackelford, 2006). According to the CDC, intimate partners perpetrate the majority of female rape (51.1%) in the US (Black et al., 2011a, 2011b). Nearly 41% of female rape victims report perpetration by acquaintances, 12.5% by family members, and 13.8% by strangers (Black et al., 2011a, 2011b). These rates differ for males and females, with 52.4% of male rape victims reporting being victimized by an acquaintance, followed by 15.1% report being victimized by strangers. Among men who were forced to perpetrate a sexual partner, 44.8% were forced to perpetrate a dating partner while 44.7% were forced to perpetrate an acquaintance (Black et al., 2011a, 2011b). Women who are in physically abusive relationships also report high rates of SV victimization. Among physically abused women, 68% experienced sexual assault, defined in this case as forced vaginal, oral, or anal sex, by their intimate partner (McFarlane & Malecha, 2005). Other studies suggest that anywhere from 40% to 50% of physically abused women have also been sexually assaulted (McFarlane & Malecha, 2005).

Hookup Culture. Casual sex is becoming more ingrained in American society, potentially leading to both positive and negative outcomes (Garcia, Reiber, Massey, & Merriwether, 2012). While casual sex may instigate positive affect in both men and women (Owen & Fincham, 2011), it can also lead to scenarios where the sexual encounter may not be consensual. Approximately 8% of college students had experienced a hookup in which they did not or were not able to give consent (Lewis, Granato, Blayney, Lostutter, & Kilmer, 2012). There are also cases where individuals may consent to sexual activity, despite not wanting to have sex (Peterson & Muehlenhard, 2007). For instance, most college students report engaging in unwanted sex during a hookup (77.8%), versus an ongoing relationship (13.9%) or a date (8.3%) with someone known (Flack et al., 2007). Further, 70% of students reported experiencing unwanted sex in the context of a hookup (Garcia et al., 2012). It has been hypothesized that nonconsensual sex is more likely to occur in contexts involving alcohol and substance use. There can also be cases where individuals may consent to sexual activity, despite not wanting to have sex (Peterson & Muehlenhard, 2007).

Prison and Community Confinement Settings. The culture of the prison system in the US is inherently different from the culture outside of prison walls. In addition, it is important to mention that rates of SV within prison settings may be underreported. For instance, the majority of prison wardens reported sexual assault rates between 0% and 1% within their prisons (Moster & Jeglic, 2009). However, sexual assault rates within prisons typically fall between 19% and

25% (Bell et al., 1999). One problematic attitude is the idea that prison rape is acceptable, as it is the price that criminals are paying for their wrongdoing (Struckman-Johnson, Struckman-Johnson, Rucker, Bumby, & Donaldson, 1996). As is expected, there are differences between male and female inmates, with male inmates typically experience more violence in their victimization (Morash, Jeong, Bohmert, & Bush, 2012). Male inmates who do not identify as heterosexual, in addition to those who have previously experienced victimization, have higher probability of being victimized while incarcerated (Morash et al., 2012). Similarly, female inmates are also at increased risk of SV victimization. In fact, female inmates are twice as likely to have experienced sexual violence in comparison to nonprisoner females (Sable, Fieberg, Martin, & Kupper, 1999). In a study conducted with three Midwestern prisons, between 19% and 90% of female inmates had experienced sexual coercion from a male guard (Norris et al., 1996; Nurius & Norris, 1996; Turchik et al., 2007; VanNatta, 2010).

Occupational settings. An individual's career may have an impact on their level of risk for SV victimization as well. The work that one does may force them to be in an environment that leaves them accessible to perpetrators, or there might be a power dynamic that forces the individual involuntary into sexual interactions. Overall, there are several occupations that have been identified as increasing risk for SV victimization. For example, sex workers have been identified as a group that is particularly susceptible to experiencing sexual assault (Mont & McGregor, 2004). Sex workers include anyone who engages in sexual activity in exchange for goods or money. Some may argue that this increased risk may be related to more frequent engagement in sex; however, this increased risk may also be a result of the stigma and dehumanization of sex workers (Mont & McGregor, 2004). A lack of empathy and increased victim-blaming is associated with sexual assault involving a sex worker as the victim (McCabe & Hardman, 2005). Relative to other victims of sexual assault, sex workers tend to be younger, come from a lower socioeconomic status, and are more likely to engage in cocaine and heroin use than non-sex worker victims (Mont & McGregor, 2004). In addition, sex workers are less likely to report their sexual assault to authorities than non-sex workers because of the fear that they will not be taken seriously, or that they will be prosecuted for prostitution if they come forward (Jordan, 2004).

Another occupation that may involve higher risk for victimization is military service. Female veterans experience higher rates of SV than women in the general population (Katz, Huffman, & Cojucar, 2017). In fact, SV estimates among female veterans range from 2.8% to 47% (Ormerod & Steel, 2018). Estimates vary partly due to the fact the rates of reporting tend to be extremely low among women in the military (Holland, Rabelo, & Cortina, 2016). Women in the military have also reported that the military service is very difficult to leave, especially after developing a passion for the career. Thus, victims become consistently accessible to their perpetrators and often experience sexual assault more than once from the same person (Ormerod & Steel, 2018). Another problematic aspect of victimization in the military is that, although men also report high levels of victimization, they are less likely to report their sexual assault than female military personnel (Gurung et al., 2018).

Recently, the film industry has come under fire for becoming a breeding ground for SV. A recent survey conducted by USA Today recruited 843 women who work in the entertainment industry. Approximately 94% of women who took part in the survey reported experiencing some type of sexual harassment or assault (Puente & Kelly, 2017). More than one fifth of respondents (21%) reported being forced to engage in sexual contact at least once during their career. Under the category of "incidents that happened at least once," 87% of women surveyed reported experiencing unwelcome sexual comments, jokes or gestures, while 69% of respondents reported that they were touched in a sexual way. Only one in four women surveyed said they reported their experiences to someone, and only 29% of women who reported their experience saw improvement in their workplace as a result of their reporting (Puente & Kelly, 2017).

There are several other careers that may have a potential for risk of SV victimization, although they remain understudied. For example, according to one study, approximately 8% of those who work in the hospitality industry report some form of sexual assault from a supervisor or a customer (Ineson, Yap, & Whiting, 2013). However, there is room for more investigation into national prevalence rates and the mechanisms behind the assaults.

Future Directions

While the extant literature has much to tell us about risk factors for SV victimization, there is still much work to be done in this area. First, our knowledge of risks for SV victimization related to specific facets of human diversity, such as those in the ADDRESSING framework (Hays, 2008), is still developing. In terms of demographic risk factors, we know little about specific SV victimization risk factors among Black/African American, Hispanic, and Pacific Islander populations in the US. In addition to a need for a greater understanding on SV victimization prevalence and risk internationally (see Chap. 11, this volume), little research exists on SV victimization among recent immigrants and refugees in the US.

Regarding gender, while there is some research on transgender women's risk for SV victimization (Coulter et al., 2017), we know less about SV victimization among transgender men or individuals whose gender identity falls outside the male/female dichotomy. There is a clear need for SV victimization research to use more inclusive definitions of gender, such as gender nonconforming, nonbinary, and genderqueer, and to explore SV victimization more broadly along the continuum of gender expression, not just identity. A less categorical approach is also needed in terms of sexual orientation and SV victimization risk: in addition to a need for more research on risk for SV victimization among lesbian women, a more inclusive approach should conceptualize sexual orientation along a continuum, including people who identify as asexual, to build a more comprehensive portrait of SV victimization among members of the LGBTQ community.

Second, an important direction for future research is to move beyond identifying specific risk factors in isolation, and toward an intersectional approach to risk for victimization experiences. The framework of intersectionality goes beyond individual risk factors and addresses how intersecting systems of oppression and inequality create conditions of privilege and vulnerability. Intersectionality has its roots in twentieth century Black feminist thought (Collective, 1986; Collins, 1989; Crenshaw, 1989) and has been applied to research in many fields, including psychology (Moradi, 2017) and the study of violence against women of color (Crenshaw, 1991). Applying an intersectional lens to contemporary SV victimization research is a critical avenue for furthering the field. We need to examine how the confluence of sociopolitical systems of oppression like sexism, racism, wealth inequality, heterosexism, and transphobia affect risks for SV victimization among individuals with minority status. For example, it appears that being Black and transgender lead to the highest rate of victimization. According to recent research, those who identify as transgender are about four times more likely to be victimized in comparison to the general population (Coulter et al., 2017). This number more than doubles to 8.3 times for transgender individuals who also identify as African-American. One reason for this serious increase in SV victimization risk is that the oppression and dehumanization faced by both transgender and African-American people increases their risk of victimization via experiences of both social (i.e., bullying) and institutional (i.e., state and federal laws) oppression.

Much of our knowledge of cognitive, behavioral, and environmental risk factors for SV victimization comes from research with college students. While research on settings, cognitions, and behaviors associated with increased SV victimization risk has been critical in advancing our knowledge of targets for prevention interventions, many samples have limited diversity. It is unclear how generalizable the findings may be to individuals of different age, socioeconomic status, and occupations, among other variables. Integrating what we know about cognitive (e.g., risk perception) and behavioral (e.g., substance use) SV victimization risk factors to identify which thoughts and actions might be most protective for certain individuals in specific settings will be an important next step in developing targeted and tailored prevention programming.

Finally, recent cultural shifts in the US present important avenues for future research. The #MeToo movement has recently changed the way the public thinks about SV victimization, gender, and power, particularly in the workplace. Furthermore, research on relationship qualities and characteristics associated with SV victimization is still in its infancy. Although we know that individuals in relationships, and particularly abusive relationships, are at increased risk for SV victimization, the impact of the online dating, mobile technology like hook-up apps and sites that allow potential partners to hypothetically obtain "consent" in advance of sexual encounters are changing the landscape of sex and dating in the twenty-first century and will undoubtedly present a world of novel risk factors we have yet to investigate.

References

Abbey, A. (2011). Alcohol's role in sexual violence perpetration: Theoretical explanations, existing evidence and future directions: Alcohol and sexual violence perpetration. *Drug and Alcohol Review, 30*(5), 481–489. https://doi.org/10.1111/j.1465-3362.2011.00296.x

Abbey, A., Zawacki, T., Buck, P. O., Clinton, A. M., & McAuslan, P. (2004). Sexual assault and alcohol consumption: What do we know about their relationship and what types of research are still needed? *Aggression and Violent Behavior, 9*(3), 271–303. https://doi.org/10.1016/S1359-1789(03)00011-9

Angelone, D. J., Cantor, N., Marcantonio, T., & Joppa, M. C. (in press). An examination of the mediating role of sexism on the gender and rape myth acceptance relationship. *Violence Against Women*.

Angelone, D. J., Marcantonio, T., & Melillo, J. (2017). An evaluation of adolescent and young adult (re)victimization experiences: Problematic substance use and negative consequences. *Violence Against Women, 24*, 586. https://doi.org/10.1177/1077801217710001

Bartle, E. E. (2000). Lesbians and hate crimes. *Journal of Poverty, 4*(4), 23–43. https://doi.org/10.1300/J134v04n04_02

Bassuk, E. L., Melnick, S., & Browne, A. (1998). Responding to the needs of low-income and homeless women who are survivors of family violence. *Journal American Medical Womens Association, 53*, 57–64.

Bell, C., Coven, M., Cronan, J. P., Garza, C. A., Guggemos, J., & Storto, L. (1999). Rape and sexual misconduct in the prison system: Analyzing America's most "open" secret. *Yale Law and Policy Review, 18*(1), 195–223.

Black, M. C., Basile, K. C., Breiding, M. J., Smith, S. G., Walters, M. L., Merrick, M. T., & Stevens, M. R. (2011a). *National intimate partner and sexual violence survey*. Atlanta, GA: Centers for Disease Control and Prevention. Retrieved from http://vawnet.org/Assoc_Files_VAWnet/NRCWebinar_NISVSBriefingHandout.pdf

Black, M. C., Basile, K. C., Breiding, M. J., Smith, S. G., Walters, M. L., Merrick, M. T., ... Stevens, M. R. (2011b, November). *The National Intimate Partner and Sexual Violence Survey: 2010 summary report*. National Center for Injury Prevention and Control Centers for Disease Control and Prevention. Retrieved from http://www.cdc.gov/violenceprevention/pdf/nisvs_report2010-a.pdf

Bohner, G., & Lampridis, E. (2004). Expecting to meet a rape victim affects women's self-esteem: The moderating role of rape myth acceptance. *Group Processes & Intergroup Relations, 7*, 77–88. https://doi.org/10.1177/1368430204039974

Breiding, M. J., Smith, S. G., Basile, K. C., Walters, M. L., Chen, J., & Merrick, M. T. (2014). Prevalence and characteristics of sexual violence, stalking, and intimate partner violence victimization—National intimate partner and sexual violence survey, United States, 2011. *Morbidity and Mortality Weekly Report. Surveillance Summaries (Washington, DC: 2002), 63*(8), 1–18.

Browne, A., & Finkelhor, D. (1986). Impact of child sexual abuse: A review of the research. *Psychological Bulletin, 99*(1), 66–77. https://doi.org/10.1037/0033-2909.99.1.66

Burns, D. (2009). *Experience and expression of anger and aggression in dating relationships for male college athletes in contact and non-contact sports*. Retrieved from https://shareok.org/handle/11244/7330

Burt, M. R. (1980). Cultural myths and supports for rape. *Journal of Personality and Social Psychology, 38*(2), 217. https://doi.org/10.1037/0022-3514.38

Burt, M. R., & Katz, B. L. (1988). Coping strategies and recovery from rape. *Annals of the New York Academy of Sciences, 528*(1), 345–358. https://doi.org/10.1111/j.1749-6632.1988.tb50876.x

Byrne, C. A., Resnick, H. S., Kilpatrick, D. G., Best, C. L., & Saunders, B. E. (1999). The socioeconomic impact of interpersonal violence on women. *Journal of Consulting and Clinical Psychology, 67*(3), 362–366. https://doi.org/10.1037/0022-006X.67.3.362

Canan, S. N., Jozkowski, K. N., & Crawford, B. L. (2016). Rape myth acceptance and token resistance in greek and non-greek college students from two university samples in the United States. *Journal of Interpersonal Violence, 33*, 1–29. https://doi.org/10.1177/0886260516636064

Carlson, G. C., & Duckworth, M. P. (2019). Sexual victimization and benefit expectations of risky behavior among female college students. *Journal of Interpersonal Violence, 34*(8), 1543–1562. https://doi.org/10.1177/0886260516651626

Casteel, C., Martin, S. L., Smith, J. B., Gurka, K. K., & Kupper, L. L. (2008). National study of physical and sexual assault among women with disabilities. *Injury Prevention, 14*(2), 87–90. https://doi.org/10.1136/ip.2007.016451

CDC. (2012). *Sexual violence*. Retrieved from https://www.cdc.gov/violenceprevention/pdf/sv-datasheet-a.pdf

Champion, H. L. O., Foley, K. L., DuRant, R. H., Hensberry, R., Altman, D., & Wolfson, M. (2004). Adolescent sexual victimization, use of alcohol and other substances, and other health risk behaviors. *The Journal of Adolescent Health, 35*(4), 321–328. https://doi.org/10.1016/j.jadohealth.2003.09.023

Chandler, S. B., Johnson, D. J., & Carroll, P. S. (1999). Abusive behaviors of college athletes. *College Student Journal, 33*(4), 638–645.

Chen, L. P., Murad, M. H., Paras, M. L., Colbenson, K. M., Sattler, A. L., & Goranson, E. N. (2010). Sexual abuse and lifetime diagnosis of psychiatric disorders: Systematic review and meta-analysis. *Mayo Clinic Proceedings, 85*(7), 618–629. https://doi.org/10.4065/mcp.2009.0583

Collective, C. R. (1986). *The Combahee River Collective statement: Black Feminist organizing in the seventies and eighties*. Albany, NY: Kitchen Table: Women of Color Press.

Collins, P. H. (1989). The social construction of Black feminist thought. *Signs, 14*(4), 745–773.

Copenhaver, S., & Grauerholz, E. (1991). Sexual victimization among sorority women: Exploring the link between sexual violence and institutional practices. *Sex Roles, 24*(1–2), 31–41. https://doi.org/10.1007/BF00288701

Coulter, R. W. S., Mair, C., Miller, E., Blosnich, J. R., Matthews, D. D., & McCauley, H. L. (2017). Prevalence of past-year sexual assault victimization among undergraduate students: Exploring differences by and intersections of gender identity, sexual identity, and race/ethnicity. *Prevention Science, 18*(6), 726–736. https://doi.org/10.1007/s11121-017-0762-8

Crenshaw, K. (1989). Demarginalizing the intersection of race and sex: A Black feminist critique of antidiscrimination doctrine, feminist theory and antiracist politics. *University of Chicago Legal Forum, 1989*, 139.

Crenshaw, K. (1991). Mapping the margins: Intersectionality, identity politics, and violence against women of color. *Stanford Law Review, 43*(6), 1241–1299. https://doi.org/10.2307/1229039

Curtis, J. K. (2011). *Sexual assault on a college campus: The influences of alcohol consumption, alcohol expectancies, risky behaviors, and sorority membership*. Theses and Dissertations. Available from ProQuest. Retrieved from https://docs.lib.purdue.edu/dissertations/AAI3479460

Davis Cue, K., Hendershot, C. S., George, W. H., Norris, J., & Heiman, J. R. (2007). Alcohol's effects on sexual decision making: An integration of alcohol myopia and individual differences. *Journal of Studies on Alcohol and Drugs, 68*, 843–851. https://doi.org/10.15288/jsad.2007.68.843

Davis, K. C., George, W. H., Norris, J., Schacht, R. L., Stoner, S. A., Hendershot, C. S., & Kajumulo, K. F. (2009). Effects of alcohol and blood alcohol concentration limb on sexual risk-taking intentions. *Journal of Studies on Alcohol and Drugs, 70*(4), 499. https://doi.org/10.15288/jsad.2009.70.499

Farris, C., Viken, R. J., Treat, T. A., & McFall, R. M. (2006). Heterosocial perceptual organization: Application of the choice model to sexual coercion. *Psychological Science, 17*(10), 869–875. https://doi.org/10.1111/j.1467-9280.2006.01796.x

Finkelhor, D., Shattuck, A., Turner, H. A., & Hamby, S. L. (2014). The lifetime prevalence of child sexual abuse and sexual assault assessed in late adolescence. *Journal of Adolescent Health, 55*(3), 329–333. https://doi.org/10.1016/j.jadohealth.2013.12.026

Flack, W. F., Daubman, K. A., Caron, M. L., Asadorian, J. A., D'Aureli, N. R., Gigliotti, S. N., … Stine, E. R. (2007). Risk factors and consequences of unwanted sex among university students: Hooking up, alcohol, and stress response. *Journal of Interpersonal Violence, 22*(2), 139–157. https://doi.org/10.1177/0886260506295354

Flack, W. F., Kimble, M. O., Campbell, B. E., Hopper, A. B., Petercă, O., & Heller, E. J. (2014). Sexual assault victimization among female undergraduates during study abroad: A single campus survey study. *Journal of Interpersonal Violence, 30*, 3453. https://doi.org/10.1177/0886260514563833

Forbes, G. B. (2006). Dating aggression, sexual coercion, and aggression-supporting attitudes among college men as a function of participation in aggressive high school sports. *Violence Against Women, 12*(5), 441–455. https://doi.org/10.1177/1077801206288126

Ford, J., & Soto-Marquez, J. G. (2016). Sexual assault victimization among straight, gay/lesbian, and bisexual college students. *Violence and Gender, 3*(2), 107–115. https://doi.org/10.1089/vio.2015.0030

Garcia, J. R., Reiber, C., Massey, S. G., & Merriwether, A. M. (2012). Sexual hookup culture: A review. *Review of General Psychology, 16*(2), 161–176. https://doi.org/10.1037/a0027911

Gidycz, C. A., Hanson, K., & Layman, M. J. (1995). A prospective analysis of the relationships among sexual assault experiences an extension of previous findings. *Psychology of Women Quarterly, 19*(1), 5–29. https://doi.org/10.1111/j.1471-6402.1995.tb00276.x

Glick, P., & Fiske, S. T. (2002). Ambivalent responses. *APA PsycNET, 57*(6–7), 444b. https://doi.org/10.1037/0003-066X.57.6-7.444b

Goetz, A. T., & Shackelford, T. K. (2006). Sexual coercion and forced in-pair copulation as sperm competition tactics in humans. *Human Nature, 17*(3), 265–282. https://doi.org/10.1007/s12110-006-1009-8

Gold, S. R., Milan, L. D., Mayall, A., & Johnson, A. E. (1994). A cross-validation study of the trauma symptom checklist: The role of mediating variables. *Journal of Interpersonal Violence, 9*(1), 12–26. https://doi.org/10.1177/088626094009001002

Grant, J. M., Mottet, L., Tanis, J., Harrison, J., Herman, J. L., & Keisling, M. (2011). *Injustice at every turn: A report of the National Transgender Discrimination Survey*. Washington. Retrieved from http://www.thetaskforce.org/reports_and_research/ntds

Greco, D., & Dawgert, S. (2007). *Poverty and sexual violence: Building prevention and intervention responses*. Enola, PA. Retrieved from http://www.pcar.org/sites/default/files/pages-pdf/poverty_and_sexual_violence.pdf

Grossbard, J. R., Lee, C. M., Neighbors, C., Hendershot, C. S., & Larimer, M. E. (2007). Alcohol and risky sex in athletes and nonathletes: What roles do sex motives play? *J Stud Alcohol Drugs, 68*(4), 566–574. Retrieved from http://www.jsad.com/doi/pdf/10.15288/jsad.2007.68.566

Gurung, S., Ventuneac, A., Rendina, H. J., Savarese, E., Grov, C., & Parsons, J. T. (2018). Prevalence of military sexual trauma and sexual orientation discrimination among lesbian, gay, bisexual, and transgender military personnel: A descriptive study. *Sexuality Research and Social Policy, 15*(1), 74–82. https://doi.org/10.1007/s13178-017-0311-z

Hamilton, L., & Armstrong, E. (2009). Gendered sexuality in young adulthood: Double binds and flawed options. *Gender and Society, 23*(5), 589–616. https://doi.org/10.1177/0891243209345829

Hassouneh-Phillips, D., & McNeff, E. (2005). "I thought I was less worthy": Low sexual and body esteem and increased vulnerability to intimate partner abuse in women with physical disabilities. *Sexuality and Disability, 23*(4), 227. https://doi.org/10.1007/s11195-005-8930-3

Hays, P. A. (2008). *Addressing cultural complexities in practice: Assessment, diagnosis, and therapy* (2nd ed.). Washington, DC: American Psychological Association. https://doi.org/10.1037/11650-000

Himelein, M. J., Vogel, R. E., & Wachowiak, D. G. (1994). Nonconsensual sexual experiences in precollege women: Prevalence and risk factors. *Journal of Counseling & Development, 72*(4), 411–415. https://doi.org/10.1002/j.1556-6676.1994.tb00959.x

Holland, K. J., Rabelo, V. C., & Cortina, L. M. (2016). Collateral damage: Military sexual trauma and help-seeking barriers. *Psychology of Violence, 6*(2), 253–261. https://doi.org/10.1037/a0039467

Holmes, M. M., Resnick, H. S., Kilpatrick, D. G., & Best, C. L. (1996). Rape-related pregnancy: Estimates and descriptive characteristics from a national sample of women. *American Journal of Obstetrics and Gynecology, 175*(2), 320–325. https://doi.org/10.1016/S0002-9378(96)70141-2

Humphrey, J. A., & White, J. W. (2000). Women's vulnerability to sexual assault from adolescence to young adulthood. *Journal of Adolescent Health, 27*(6), 419–424. https://doi.org/10.1016/S1054-139X(00)00168-3

Ineson, E. M., Yap, M. H. T., & Whiting, G. (2013). Sexual discrimination and harassment in the hospitality industry. *International Journal of Hospitality Management, 35*, 1–9. https://doi.org/10.1016/j.ijhm.2013.04.012

James, S. E., Herman, J. L., Rankin, S., Keisling, M., Mottet, L., & Anafi, M. (2016). *The report of the 2015 U.S. Transgender Survey*. Washington, DC: National Center for Transgender Equality. Retrieved from https://www.transequality.org/sites/default/files/docs/USTS-Full-Report-final.pdf

Johansson, S. (2013). Coach–athlete sexual relationships: If no means no does yes mean yes? *Sport, Education and Society, 18*(5), 678–693. https://doi.org/10.1080/13573322.2013.777662

Jordan, J. (2004). Beyond belief?: Police, rape and Women's credibility. *Criminal Justice, 4*(1), 29–59. https://doi.org/10.1177/1466802504042222

Joskowski, K., Marcantonio, T. L., & Hunt, M. E. (2017). College students' sexual consent communication and perceptions of sexual double standards: A qualitative investigation. *Perspectives on Sexual and Reproductive Health, 49*(4), 237–244. https://doi.org/10.1363/psrh.12041

Jozkowski, K. N., & Peterson, Z. D. (2013). College students and sexual consent: Unique insights. *Journal of Sex Research, 50*(6), 517–523. https://doi.org/10.1080/00224499.2012.700739

Kaestle, C. E., & Halpern, C. T. (2005). Sexual intercourse precedes partner violence in adolescent romantic relationships. *Journal of Adolescent Health, 36*(5), 386–392. https://doi.org/10.1016/j.jadohealth.2004.02.030

Katz, J., May, P., Sörensen, S., & DelTosta, J. (2010). Sexual revictimization during women's first year of college: Self-blame and sexual refusal assertiveness as possible mechanisms. *Journal of Interpersonal Violence, 25*(11), 2113–2126. https://doi.org/10.1177/0886260509354515

Katz, L. S., Huffman, C., & Cojucar, G. (2017). In her own words: Semi-structured interviews of women veterans who experienced military sexual assault. *Journal of Contemporary Psychotherapy, 47*(3), 181–189. https://doi.org/10.1007/s10879-016-9349-0

Kitzinger, C., & Frith, H. (1999). Just say no? The use of conversation analysis in developing a feminist perspective on sexual refusal. *Discourse & Society, 10*(3), 293–316. https://doi.org/10.1177/0957926599010003002

Koss, M. P., Gidycz, C. A., & Wisniewski, N. (1987). The scope of rape: Incidence and prevalence of sexual aggression and victimization in a national sample of higher education students. *Journal of Consulting and Clinical Psychology, 55*(2), 162–170. https://doi.org/10.1037/0022-006X.55.2.162

Krebs, C. P., Lindquist, C. H., Warner, T. D., Fisher, B. S., & Martin, S. L. (2007). *Campus sexual assault (CSA)*

study, final report. Retrieved from https://www.ncjrs.gov/pdffiles1/nij/grants/221153.pdf

Krebs, C. P., Lindquist, C. H., Warner, T. D., Fisher, B. S., & Martin, S. L. (2009). College women's experiences with physically forced, alcohol- or other drug-enabled, and drug-facilitated sexual assault before and since entering college. *Journal of American College Health, 57*(6), 639–647. https://doi.org/10.3200/JACH.57.6.639-649

Krug, E. G., Dahlberg, L., Mercy, J., Zwi, A., & Lozano, R. (Eds.). (2002). *World report on violence and health*. Geneva: World Health Organisation.

Lewis, M. A., Granato, H., Blayney, J. A., Lostutter, T. W., & Kilmer, J. R. (2012). Predictors of hooking up sexual behaviors and emotional reactions among U.S. college students. *Archives of Sexual Behavior, 41*(5), 1219–1229. https://doi.org/10.1007/s10508-011-9817-2

Locke, B. D., & Mahalik, J. R. (2005). Examining masculinity norms, problem drinking, and athletic involvement as predictors of sexual aggression in college men. *Journal of Counseling Psychology, 52*(3), 279–283. https://doi.org/10.1037/0022-0167.52.3.279

Loiselle, M., & Fuqua, W. R. (2007). Alcohol's effects on women's risk detection in a date-rape vignette. *Journal of American College Health, 55*(5), 261–266. https://doi.org/10.3200/JACH.55.5.261-266

Lonsway, K. A., & Fitzgerald, L. F. (1995). Attitudinal antecedents of rape myth acceptance: A theoretical and empirical reexamination. *Journal of Personality and Social Psychology, 68*(4), 704. https://doi.org/10.1037/0022-3514.68.4.704

Maniglio, R. (2009). The impact of child sexual abuse on health: A systematic review of reviews. *Clinical Psychology Review, 29*(7), 647–657. https://doi.org/10.1016/j.cpr.2009.08.003

Marcantonio, T., Angelone, D. J., & Joppa, M. (2018). Understanding contributing factors to verbal coercion while studying abroad. *Journal of American College Health, 66*(6), 440–444. https://doi.org/10.1080/07448481.2018.1431912

Marcantonio, T., Angelone, D. J., & Sledjeski, E. (2016). Using a pattern-centered approach to assess sexual risk-taking in study abroad students. *Journal of American College Health, 64*(3), 165–173. https://doi.org/10.1080/07448481.2015.1085058

Martin, A., Kelly, A., Turquet, L., & Ross, S. (2009). *Hate crimes: The rise of corrective rape in South Africa*. Retrieved February 7, 2018, from https://www.actionaid.org.uk/sites/default/files/publications/hate_crimes_the_rise_of_corrective_rape_in_south_africa_september_2009.pdf

Martin, S. L., Ray, N., Sotres-Alvarez, D., Kupper, L. L., Moracco, K. E., Dickens, P. A., … Gizlice, Z. (2006). Physical and sexual assault of women with disabilities. *Violence Against Women, 12*(9), 823–837. https://doi.org/10.1177/1077801206292672

Mason, G. E., Riger, S., & Foley, L. A. (2004). The impact of past sexual experiences on attributions of responsibility for rape. *Journal of Interpersonal Violence, 19*(10), 1157–1171. https://doi.org/10.1177/0886260504269094

Maticka-Tyndale, E., Herold, E. S., & Oppermann, M. (2003). Casual sex among Australian schoolies. *Journal of Sex Research, 40*(2), 158–169. https://doi.org/10.1080/00224490309552177

McCabe, M. P., & Hardman, L. (2005). Attitudes and perceptions of workers to sexual harassment. *The Journal of Social Psychology, 145*(6), 719–740. https://doi.org/10.3200/SOCP.145.6.719-740

McFarlane, J. (2007). Pregnancy following partner rape: What we know and what we need to know. *Trauma, Violence, & Abuse, 8*(2), 127–134. https://doi.org/10.1177/1524838007301222

McFarlane, J., & Malecha, A. (2005). Sexual assault among intimates: Frequency, consequences and treatments. *Obstetrics and Gynecology., 105*, 99. https://doi.org/10.1097/01.AOG.0000146641.98665.b6

Meadows, E. A., Jaycox, L. H., Orsillo, S., & Foa, E. B. (1997, November). *The impact of assault on risk recognition in ambiguous situations*. Presented at the 31st annual meeting of the Association for the Advancement of Behavior Therapy, Miami Beach, FL.

Messman-Moore, T. L., & Brown, A. L. (2006). Risk perception, rape, and sexual revictimization: A prospective study of college women. *Psychology of Women Quarterly, 30*(2), 159–172. https://doi.org/10.1111/j.1471-6402.2006.00279.x

Messman-Moore, T. L., Coates, A. A., Gaffey, K. J., & Johnson, C. F. (2008). Sexuality, substance use, and susceptibility to victimization. *Journal of Interpersonal Violence, 23*, 1730. https://doi.org/10.1177/0886260508314336

Messman-Moore, T. L., & Long, P. J. (2003). The role of childhood sexual abuse sequelae in the sexual revictimization of women: An empirical review and theoretical reformulation. *Clinical Psychology Review, 23*(4), 537–571. https://doi.org/10.1016/S0272-7358(02)00203-9

Milhausen, R. R., Reece, M., & Perera, B. (2006). A theory-based approach to understanding sexual behavior at Mardi Gras. *Journal of Sex Research, 43*(2), 97–106. https://doi.org/10.1080/00224490609552304

Miller, A. K., Markman, K. D., & Handley, I. M. (2007). Self-blame among sexual assault victims prospectively predicts revictimization: A perceived sociolegal context model of risk. *Basic and Applied Social Psychology, 29*(2), 129–136. https://doi.org/10.1080/01973530701331585

Minow, J. C., & Einolf, C. J. (2009). Sorority participation and sexual assault risk. *Violence Against Women, 15*(7), 835. https://doi.org/10.1177/1077801209334472

Mont, J. D., & McGregor, M. J. (2004). Sexual assault in the lives of urban sex workers: A descriptive and comparative analysis. *Women & Health, 39*(3), 79–96. https://doi.org/10.1300/J013v39n03_06

Moradi, B. (2017). (Re)focusing intersectionality: From social identities back to systems of oppression and privilege. In K. A. DeBord, A. R. Fischer, K. J. Bieschke, R. M. Perez, K. A. DeBord, A. R. Fischer, et al.

(Eds.), *Handbook of sexual orientation and gender diversity in counseling and psychotherapy* (pp. 105–127). Washington, DC: American Psychological Association. https://doi.org/10.1037/15959-005

Morash, M., Jeong, S., Bohmert, M. N., & Bush, D. R. (2012). Men's vulnerability to prisoner-on-prisoner sexual violence: A state correctional system case study. *The Prison Journal, 92*(2), 290–311. https://doi.org/10.1177/0032885512439185

Morgan, R. E., & Kena, G. (2016). *Criminal victimization 2016*. Washington, DC: U.S. Department of Justice.

Morgan RE, & Kena, G. (2017). *Criminal victimization, 2016* (Bureau of Justice Statistics No. 251150). Washington, DC: U.S. Department of Justice.

Moster, A. N., & Jeglic, E. L. (2009). Prison warden attitudes toward prison rape and sexual assault: Findings since the Prison Rape Elimination Act (PREA). *The Prison Journal, 89*(1), 65–78. https://doi.org/10.1177/0032885508329981

Muehlenhard, C. L., Peterson, Z. D., Humphreys, T. P., & Jozkowski, K. N. (2017). Evaluating the one-in-five statistic: Women's risk of sexual assault while in college. *Journal of Sex Research, 54*(4–5), 549–576. https://doi.org/10.1080/00224499.2017.1295014

Narasimhan-Madhavan, D. (2006). Gender, sexuality and violence: Permissible violence against women during the partition of India and Pakistan. *Hawwa, 4*(2), 396–416. https://doi.org/10.1163/156920806779152237

Niaz, U. (2003). Violence against women in South Asian countries. *Archives of Women's Mental Health, 6*(3), 173–184. https://doi.org/10.1007/s00737-003-0171-9

Norris, J., George, W. H., Stoner, S. A., Masters, N. T., Zawacki, T., & Davis, K. C. (2006). Women's responses to sexual aggression: The effects of childhood trauma, alcohol, and prior relationship. *Experimental and Clinical Psychopharmacology, 14*(3), 402–411. https://doi.org/10.1037/1064-1297.14.3.402

Norris, J., Nurius, P. S., & Dimeff, L. A. (1996). Through her eyes: Factors affecting women's perception of and resistance to acquaintance sexual aggression threat. *Psychology of Women Quarterly, 20*(1), 123–145. https://doi.org/10.1111/j.1471-6402.1996.tb00668.x

Nurius, P. S., & Norris, J. (1996). A cognitive ecological model of women's response to male sexual coercion in dating. *Journal of Psychology and Human Sexuality, 8*(1–2), 117–139. https://doi.org/10.1300/J056v08n01_09

Ormerod, A. J., & Steel, J. (2018). Sexual assault in the military. In C. B. Travis, J. W. White, A. Rutherford, W. S. Williams, S. L. Cook, K. F. Wyche, et al. (Eds.), *APA handbook of the psychology of women: Perspectives on women's private and public lives* (pp. 195–213). Washington, DC: American Psychological Association. https://doi.org/10.1037/0000060-011

Owen, J., & Fincham, F. D. (2011). Young adults' emotional reactions after hooking up encounters. *Archives of Sexual Behavior, 40*(2), 321–330. https://doi.org/10.1007/s10508-010-9652-x

Paul, E. L., McManus, B., & Hayes, A. (2000). "Hookups": Characteristics and correlates of college students' spontaneous and anonymous sexual experiences. *The Journal of Sex Research; New York, 37*(1), 76–88. https://doi.org/10.1080/00224490009552023

Pedersen, E. R., Larimer, M. E., & Lee, C. M. (2010). When in Rome: Factors associated with changes in drinking behavior among American college students studying abroad. *Psychology of Addictive Behaviors, 24*(3), 535–540. https://doi.org/10.1037/a0019863

Peipert, J. F., & Domagalski, L. R. (1994). Epidemiology of adolescent sexual assault. *Obstetrics and Gynecology, 84*(5), 867–871. https://doi.org/10.1177/0886260511421674

Peterson, Z. D., & Muehlenhard, C. L. (2007). Conceptualizing the "wantedness" of women's consensual and nonconsensual sexual experiences: Implications for how women label their experiences with rape. *Journal of Sex Research, 44*(1), 72–88. https://doi.org/10.1080/00224490709336794

Plummer, S.-B., & Findley, P. A. (2012). Women with disabilities' experience with physical and sexual abuse: Review of the literature and implications for the field. *Trauma, Violence, and Abuse, 13*(1), 15–29. https://doi.org/10.1177/1524838011426014

Powers, L. E., Curry, M. A., Oschwald, M., Maley, S., Saxton, M., & Eckels, K. (2002). Barriers and strategies in addressing abuse: A survey of disabled women's experiences. (PAS Abuse Survey). *The Journal of Rehabilitation, 68*(1), 4. https://doi.org/10.1177/1524838011426014

Puente, M., & Kelly, C. (2017). *How common is sexual misconduct in Hollywood?* Retrieved April 24, 2018, from https://www.usatoday.com/story/life/people/2018/02/20/how-common-sexual-misconduct-hollywood/1083964001/

Renner, L. M., & Whitney, S. D. (2012). Risk factors for unidirectional and bidirectional intimate partner violence among young adults. *Child Abuse & Neglect, 36*(1), 40–52. https://doi.org/10.1016/j.chiabu.2011.07.007

Sable, M. R., Fieberg, J. R., Martin, S. L., & Kupper, L. L. (1999). Violence victimization experiences of pregnant prisoners. *American Journal of Orthopsychiatry, 69*(3), 392–397. https://doi.org/10.1037/h0080413

Saul, J., & Audage, N. C. (2007). *Preventing child sexual abuse within youth-serving organizations: Getting started on policies and procedures [Data set]*. American Psychological Association. https://doi.org/10.1037/e587062010-001

Silverman, J. G., Raj, A., Mucci, L. A., & Hathaway, J. E. (2001). Dating violence against adolescent girls and associated substance use, unhealthy weight control, sexual risk behavior, pregnancy, and suicidality. *JAMA, 286*(5), 572–579. https://doi.org/10.1001/jama.286.5.572

Smith, S. G., Basile, K. C., Gilbert, L. K., Merrick, M. T., Patel, N., Walling, M., & Jain, A. (2017). *The National Intimate Partner and Sexual Violence Survey (NISVS):*

2010–2012 state report. Atlanta, GA: National Center for Injury Prevention and Control, Centers for Disease Control and Prevention.

Smith, S. G., & Breiding, M. J. (2011). Chronic disease and health behaviours linked to experiences of non-consensual sex among women and men. *Public Health, 125*(9), 653–659. https://doi.org/10.1016/j.puhe.2011.06.006

Sönmez, S., Apostolopoulos, Y., Yu, C. H., Yang, S., Mattila, A., & Yu, L. C. (2006). Binge drinking and casual sex on spring break. *Annals of Tourism Research, 33*(4), 895–917. https://doi.org/10.1016/j.annals.2006.06.005

Stephens, S. G. (2016). *Relationship of sexual violence and high-risk behaviors among male and female U.S. college students*. Retrieved from http://fsu.digital.flvc.org/islandora/object/fsu%3A366123/

Stotzer, R. L. (2009). Violence against transgender people: A review of United States data. *Aggression and Violent Behavior, 14*(3), 170–179. https://doi.org/10.1016/j.avb.2009.01.006

Struckman-Johnson, C., Struckman-Johnson, D., Rucker, L., Bumby, K., & Donaldson, S. (1996). Sexual coercion reported by men and women in prison. *Journal of Sex Research, 33*(1), 67–76. https://doi.org/10.1080/00224499609551816

Swedlund, N. P., & Nosek, M. (2000). An exploratory study on the work of independent living centers to address abuse of women with disabilities. *Journal of Rehabilitation, 66*, 57–64.

Tjaden, P., & Thoennes, N. (2000a). *Full report of the prevalence, incidence, and consequences of violence against women*. U.S. Department of Justice. Retrieved from https://www.ncjrs.gov/pdffiles1/nij/183781.pdf

Tjaden, P., & Thoennes, N. (2000b). Prevalence and consequences of male-to-female and female-to-male intimate partner violence as measured by the National Violence Against Women Survey. *Violence Against Women, 6*(2), 142–161. https://doi.org/10.1177/10778010022181769

Tjaden, P., & Thoennes, N. (2006). *Extent, nature, and consequences of rape victimization: Findings from the National Violence Against Women Survey*. National Institue of Justice. Retrieved from https://www.ncjrs.gov/pdffiles1/nij/210346.pdf

Turchik, J. A., Probst, D. R., Chau, M., Nigoff, A., & Gidycz, C. A. (2007). Factors predicting the type of tactics used to resist sexual assault: A prospective study of college women. *Journal of Consulting and Clinical Psychology, 75*(4), 605–614. https://doi.org/10.1037/0022-006X.75.4.605

VanNatta, M. (2010). Conceptualizing and stopping state sexual violence against incarcerated women. *Social Justice, 37*(1), 27–52.

Voloshyna, D. M., Bonar, E. E., Cunningham, R. M., Ilgen, M. A., Blow, F. C., & Walton, M. A. (2018). Blackouts among male and female youth seeking emergency department care. *American Journal of Drug & Alcohol Abuse, 44*(1), 129–139. https://doi.org/10.1080/00952990.2016.1265975

Wenzel, S. L., Tucker, J. S., Hambarsoomian, K., & Elliott, M. N. (2006). Toward a more comprehensive understanding of violence against impoverished women. *Journal of Interpersonal Violence, 21*(6), 820–839. https://doi.org/10.1177/0886260506288662

Yamawaki, N. (2007). Rape perception and the function of ambivalent sexism and gender-role traditionality. *Journal of Interpersonal Violence, 22*(4), 406–423. https://doi.org/10.1177/0886260506297210

Yeater, E. A., Treat, T. A., Viken, R. J., & McFall, R. M. (2010). Cognitive processes underlying women's risk judgments: Associations with sexual victimization history and rape myth acceptance. *Journal of Consulting and Clinical Psychology, 78*(3), 375–386. https://doi.org/10.1037/a0019297

Yuan, N. P., Koss, M. P., Polacca, M., & Goldman, D. (2006). Risk factors for physical assault and rape among six native American tribes. *Journal of Interpersonal Violence, 21*(12), 1566–1590. https://doi.org/10.1177/0886260506294239

Alcohol and Sexual Assault

11

Emily R. Mouilso and Lauren F. Wilson

Definitions and Prevalence

About half of all sexual assaults involve alcohol consumption either by the victim, the perpetrator, or both (see Abbey, Zawacki, Buck, Clinton, & McAuslan, 2004; Lorenz & Ullman, 2016 for reviews). In fact, college women who monitored their alcohol use and experiences of victimization were 19 times more likely to be sexually assaulted on days when they drank heavily than on sober days (Parks, Hsieh, Bradizza, & Romosz, 2008). Similarly, for college men the odds of perpetrating sexual assault increase as alcohol consumption increases (Shorey, Stuart, McNulty, & Moore, 2014).

The term *rape* is typically defined as unwanted oral, anal, or vaginal penetration obtained by physical force (Bureau of Justice Statistics, 2016). Although state laws vary, at the federal level and in most states instances in which the victim is unable to give consent because of alcohol intoxication are included in the definition of rape. *Sexual assault* is a broader term that encompasses a wide range of unwanted sexual experiences, including attempted or completed rape, penetration obtained via verbal coercion or misuse of authority, and unwanted grabbing or fondling (Bureau of Justice Statistics, 2016). Estimates of the prevalence of rape and sexual assault are based on a variety of sources, including police reports, general population surveys, and surveys of male and female college students. Conservative estimates suggest that at least 25% of American women have been sexually assaulted and at least 20% of American men have perpetrated sexual assault. Furthermore, at least 10% of American women report having been raped and at least 5% of American men report having committed rape (Abbey & McAuslan, 2004; Kilpatrick, Resnick, Ruggierio, Conoscenti, & McCauley, 2007; Tjaden & Thoennes, 2000).

The vast majority of American adults have consumed alcohol at least once and approximately half report drinking in the past month (Center for Behavioral Health Statistics and Quality, 2016). *Binge drinking* is typically defined as drinking five or more alcoholic drinks for men or four of more alcoholic drinks for women on one occasion (NIAAA, 2004; SAMHSA, 2017). Approximately 13% of American adults report engaging in binge drinking in the past year (Grant et al., 2017). When compared to other patterns of alcohol consumption, binge drinking is associated with particularly negative outcomes, including social, legal, medical, and occupational consequences (Kraus, Baumeister, Pabst, & Orth, 2009; Vicary & Karshin, 2002).

E. R. Mouilso (✉) · L. F. Wilson
University of Georgia, Athens, GA, USA

W. T. O'Donohue and P. A. Schewe (eds.), *Handbook of Sexual Assault and Sexual Assault Prevention*,
https://doi.org/10.1007/978-3-030-23645-8_11

The Connection Between Sexual Assault and Alcohol Use

Alcohol use is involved in about half of all violent crimes (Collins & Messerschmidt, 1993), including sexual assault. However, the fact that alcohol consumption and sexual assault frequently co-occur does not mean that alcohol use causes sexual assault. Drinking cannot cause a person to be sexually assaulted because experiencing experiences differs across a number of significant dimensions, including the setting in which the assault occurs, the perpetrator's tactic(s), and victim–perpetrator relationship. It is likely that if alcohol impacts vulnerability to one kind of victimization it may not confer the same risk (or any risk) to another kind of victimization. For example, acquaintances are more likely to use alcohol as a sexual assault tactic than are intimate partners because intimate partners can rely on the greater physical access to the victim afforded by the relationship and verbal coercion (Cleveland, Koss, & Lyons, 1999). Thus it is highly unlikely that there is one way in which alcohol use confers risk for sexual assault or that alcohol use confers risk in all circumstances.

Physiological and Pharmacological Effects

Perhaps the most straightforward explanation for the link between alcohol use and sexual assault is that a perpetrator may exploit someone who is unconscious as a result of heavy drinking or may not understand what is happening or is too incapacitated to physically object or resist. Victimizations of this type are generally referred to as *alcohol-facilitated* or *incapacitated* sexual assaults and are common, especially for college women (McCauley, Ruggiero, Resnick, Conoscenti, & Kilpatrick, 2009; Testa, Livingston, VanZile-Tamsen, & Frone, 2003).

Even less-significant levels of alcohol intoxication may increase a potential victim's vulnerability to sexual assault because alcohol conveys physical, so-called pharmacological, effects that may alter perception, slow reaction time, and impair decision-making (Monks, Tomaka, Palacios, & Thompson, 2010a, 2010b). These changes may make it more difficult for a victim to identify and effectively navigate risky situations, communicate clearly, and resist physically. Pharmacological effects may also increase the risk of perpetration by altering a potential perpetrator's cognitions and decreasing impulsive control (Abbey & Ortiz, 2008; Abbey, 2011a, 2011b). These effects may interact with a perpetrator's individual traits and risk factors; for instance, higher trait impulsivity differentiated heavy drinking sexual assault perpetrators from other sexual assault perpetrators in a sample of college men (Zawacki, Abbey, Buck, McAuslan, & Clinton-Sherrod, 2003).

According to the *alcohol myopia* model, intoxication makes attending to multiple cues more difficult and focuses the individual on the most salient cues in a given situation (Steele & Southwick, 1985). Thus inhibiting cues (e.g., fear of assault, fear of punishment or rejection) become less salient and compelling cues (e.g., interest in sex, pleasure, or a relationship) dominate one's attention. For example, an intoxicated perpetrator may misinterpret friendly cues as a desire for sexual activity or an intoxicated victim may discount risk cues and not engage in self-protective behaviors.

Consistent with this model, in laboratory studies, women who have ingested a moderate amount of alcohol are less accurate in perceiving risky situations and express lower intentions to resist sexual advances (Stoner et al., 2007; Testa, Livingston, & Collins, 2000). These changes may be particularly true for women with a history of sexual assault (George et al., 2015). Laboratory studies and alcohol administration studies, specifically, also provide support for the alcohol myopia theory for perpetration. For instance, men administered alcohol generally reported greater misperceptions around women's interest in sex and their sexual arousal compared to men not administered alcohol, and alcohol-receiving men also reported a stronger entitlement to sex (see Abbey & Wegner, 2015 for a review). Although Abbey and Wegner (2015) did not review dosage effects related to misperceptions of women's interest in sex, men's feelings of entitlement to sex was found for both low (i.e., blood alcohol content of 0.05) and high (i.e., blood alcohol content of 0.10; Davis et al., 2012). Findings via survey have corroborated these laboratory studies; for instance, a study by Parkhill, Abbey, and Jacques-Tiura (2009) found that perpetrators who reported heavy drinking also described longer periods of misperceiving their victim's behavior as signaling sexual desire than non-heavy drinkers.

Alcohol Use Expectations, Motivations, Settings, and Misperceptions

Beyond its physical effects, alcohol consumption has powerful influence on our social perceptions, experiences, and environments. In particular, Americans tend to have gendered beliefs and expectations about alcohol use that support men's sexual aggression towards women, for instance, associating alcohol consumption with perpetration of aggressive behavior (Reinarman & Levine, 1997) and, for men, sexually aggressive behavior specifically (Cowley, 2014). As a result, intoxicated men may believe that they are less able to control their behavior and more likely to aggress. These beliefs may help to explain the consistent finding that men who have been drinking are more likely than sober men to perpetrate sexual assault, especially if they believe they have been rejected, deceived, or wronged (see Abbey, 2002 for review).

There are also widely held beliefs around alcohol consumption and sexual assault victims. College men perceive women who drink in bars to be more promiscuous and believe that women use alcohol consumption to signal sexual interest (Abbey, 2002; Cowley, 2014). Together with the before-mentioned effects of alcohol myopia, these social beliefs create a particularly dangerous interaction. Intoxicated women may be vulnerable to sexual assault because men are more likely to misperceive ambiguous or friendly cues as sexual interest, make sexual advances, and ignore any attempts at resistance. In analyzing college student interviews about their experiences with unwanted sexual contact, Cowley (2014) found that most respondents attributed the sexual assault to an interaction between alcohol use and unhealthy gendered beliefs (e.g., norms and scripts, rape myths). For example, both male and female participants described alcohol as disinhibiting existing gendered traits, such as aggression in men, and regarded alcohol use as a means of signaling sexual availability for women who would not otherwise be interested in casual sex. This was further supported in a subsample of men who reported various levels of justification of their assaultive behaviors, as their attitudes around rape and their observation of the victim's alcohol intake were both significantly associated with post-assault justification (Wegner, Abbey, Pierce, Pegram, & Woerner, 2015).

Social situations, locations, and experiences are also shaped by individuals' alcohol beliefs. For instance, if it is true that social expectations tell men that women who drink are more promiscuous, men may purposefully seek out situations where alcohol is served, such as bars or parties, intending to have sex (Purcell & Graham, 2005; Zawacki et al., 2003). Additionally, beliefs surrounding alcohol may permit sexually aggressive behavior in these spaces, for instance groping may be seen by perpetrators and bystanders as more permissible in bars than in other social situations (Becker & Tinkler, 2015).

Exposure to risky drinking settings, such as bars or fraternity parties, may be a stronger predictor of sexual victimization than alcohol consumption itself (Parks & Miller, 1997; Schwartz & Pitts, 1995). Because drinking can only confer risk for assault in the presence of a potential perpetrator, the setting in which alcohol is consumed is an important factor in the link between alcohol use and sexual assault. Consistent with this idea, Schwartz and Pitts (1995) proposed a feminist version of *routine activities theory* (Cohen & Felson, 1979), which suggests that frequent drinking confers risk for sexual assault by exposing individuals to situations that include a high number of potential perpetrators and few suitable guardians (e.g., parents, teachers). Research supports the idea that sexual assaults often occur after drinking in bars or parties (Mohler-Kuo, Dowdall, Koss, & Wechsler, 2004;

Testa et al., 2003) and particularly fraternity parties (Chevalier & Einolf, 2009) relative to other drinking settings. These hypotheses are further supported by findings related to perpetration, such as Testa and Cleveland's (2017) longitudinal studies finding that frequency of party attendance predicted sexual assault perpetration.

Long-Term Associations and Reciprocity

It is important to not assume that the relationship between alcohol and sexual assault is unidirectional. Since alcohol has arousal- and anxiety-reducing properties, it may be used by a victim as a means of self-medication following a traumatic event (Stewart & Conrod, 2003). Experiencing a sexual assault (or other traumatic event) may lead to initiation or increase in alcohol consumption, which may increase the risk of future sexual assault (Lorenz & Ullman, 2016). Although it is not clear that victimization increases alcohol use generally, consumption does seem to increase for some victims (see Lorenz & Ullman, 2016; Testa & Livingston, 2009 for reviews). Women with a history of victimization are more likely than other women to use alcohol to cope with distress (Ullman, Filipas, Townsend, & Starzynski, 2005). Exposure to personalized trauma cues has been found to prompt craving for alcohol in alcohol-dependent individuals (Coffey et al., 2002). In a sample of men with a history of sexual assault victimization, drinking to cope partially mediated the link between victimization and problematic drinking behavior (Fossos, Kaysen, Neighbors, Lindgren, & Hove, 2011). Fossos et al. (2011) found both direct and indirect relationships between victimization history and consequences of drinking for men but only indirect relationships for women. Thus, some elements of the self-medication model have been supported.

Empirically testing the possible bidirectional relationship will require prospective studies measuring how sexual assault and drinking influence each other over time. To date several such studies have been described but results are inconsistent. For example, in a large sample of young women Bryan et al. (2015) found that history of childhood sexual abuse and/or adult sexual assault predicted alcohol use, alcohol use predicted later victimization, and victimization in turn predicted increased alcohol use. Additionally, there is evidence that previous victimization may influence behaviors, such as decreasing protective behaviors, when intoxicated and/or when faced with risky interpersonal situations (George et al., 2015; Gilmore, Stappenbeck, Lewis, Granato, & Kaysen, 2015). Among studies that did not support a bidirectional relationship, some concluded that sexual assault was not predictive of increased alcohol use (Gidycz et al., 2007) while others concluded that post-assault drinking did not predict revictimization (Parks, Hsieh, Taggart, & Bradizza, 2014). Additionally some studies have found that alcohol use did not predict revictimization but alcohol problems (Testa & Livingston, 2000) or binge drinking (Mouilso, Fischer, & Calhoun, 2012) did. Given these conflicting results, it seems a bidirectional relationship may exist only for some individuals and/or only under some circumstances; however, additional data are necessary.

How Are Alcohol-Involved Sexual Assaults Different?

Sexual assaults that involved alcohol use by the victim, perpetrator, or both often differ in important ways from assaults that do not involve alcohol use. Contrary to the "stranger danger" stereotype, the vast majority of sexual assaults are perpetrated by someone known to the victim, such as a romantic partner, friend, or acquaintance (Abbey & McAuslan, 2004; Tjaden & Thoennes, 2000). As noted above, assaults that involve alcohol are more likely to be perpetrated by acquaintances (e.g., classmate, friend-of-a-friend, first date) rather than romantic partners (Kilpatrick et al., 2007; Testa & Livingston, 2009). In sexual assaults when the victim is drinking, offenders are virtually always drinking, but around half of assaults involve drinking by the perpetrator alone (Ullman & Brecklin, 2000). Drinking by either the victim or perpetrator is associated with more severe assaults (e.g., more physical injuries, multiple perpetrators) relative to assaults that do not involve drinking. Perpetrator-only drinking is associated with the most severe physical injury and greatest perceived threat of death for the victim (Ullman & Najdowski, 2009). Indeed, perpetrators who are heavy drinkers are more likely to use more aggressive perpetration tactics and to engage in behaviors designed to isolate and control their potential victims (Abbey et al., 2004; Parkhill et al., 2009). However, higher levels of perpetrator intoxication reduce the likelihood of completed rape (Testa, VanZile-Tamsen, & Livingston, 2004), perhaps because victims more effectively resist perpetrators who are physically and mentally compromised by alcohol. Regarding victims, binge drinking seems to increase risk for sexual assault relative to other patterns of alcohol consumption (McCauley, Calhoun, & Gidycz, 2010; Mouilso, Fischer, & Calhoun, 2012).

Victims of alcohol-involved sexual assaults seem to experience more post-assault distress and self-blame, especially if they were drinking (Littleton, Grills-Taquechel, & Axsom, 2009; Ullman & Najdowski, 2009). However, if the assault involved alcohol, victims are less likely to label their experience as rape or acknowledge that a crime has been committed (Bondurant, 2001; Littleton et al., 2009). Instead, they may consider the experience to be a miscommunication or a bad date or be unsure how to label the experience at all. Perhaps this difference is due to the generally accepted myth that rape always involves a stranger and use of physical force, which is rarely the case in alcohol-involved sexual assaults. Labeling is important because it is linked to seeking and receiving support (e.g., from friends, family, medical professionals, mental health professionals, police). Despite the possible positive outcomes of disclosure (e.g., access to social and practical support), there are often negative outcomes as well (e.g., disbelief, blame). Victims of alcohol-involved sexual assault seem to be more likely than other victims to experience negative outcomes when they disclose (Ullman & Najdowski, 2009) although this pattern may not exist for college women (Littleton et al., 2009) or in cases of perpetrator-only drinking (Ullman & Najdowski, 2009).

Continued Misunderstandings, Key Gaps, and Future Directions

Study Design and Measurement

Many different types of studies have been used to understand the link between alcohol use and sexual assault. Cross-sectional studies ask participants if they drink and if they have experienced or perpetrated a sexual assault. Event-based studies ask participants to report whether drinking occurred at the time of a sexual assault. Prospective studies measure drinking and sexual assault overtime to determine if earlier behavior or experiences predict later behavior or experiences. Laboratory studies generally test the impact of drinking on participants' beliefs, behaviors, or behavioral intentions in a laboratory setting. Each type of study provides a different type of information and has its own strengths and weaknesses. The majority of studies in this area are cross-sectional, which is helpful in establishing that a link exists but does not provided much useful information about the nature or directionality of the link between alcohol and sexual assault.

To establish true causality, laboratory studies, such as alcohol administration studies, are required because only these studies can employ random assignment to control for possible alternative explanations (Abbey, 2017). However, laboratory studies may lose real world applicability by overlooking important variables due to sampling limitations and the necessity of relying on proxies for sexual assault (see Abbey & Wegner, 2015, for a review). Additionally, gaps remain in the types of completed or published laboratory studies. For instance, laboratory studies to date have tended to focus on casual sexual relationships (meaning intimate and stranger relationships are less well understood) and have tended to rely on physical pressure rather than the more commonly used verbal pressure or alcohol tactics for sexual assault perpetration (Abbey & Wegner, 2015). Further understanding of the role alcohol plays in sexual assault may be achieved through laboratory paradigms that address these gaps along with expanding their methods to better account for a variety of potential victim reactions, validating new and innovative methods, and expanding upon the individual difference variables that are measured (Abbey & Wegner, 2015).

This review has highlighted the importance of additional prospective studies measuring how sexual assault and drinking influence each other over time. In order to provide the richest data, such studies should include a multitude of individual and situational variables that may moderate, intensify, or explain the alcohol and sexual assault connection. Diary studies and timeline followback methodologies provide a promising perspective means of establishing temporal relationship between sexual assault and alcohol use. Both timeline follow back and diary studies provide data that can be sequenced in order to identify antecedents and their consequences; this type of approach enables better understanding of which alcohol consumption effects are proximal to and which are distally predictive of sexual assault, as well as increase understanding of other factors that may amplify the connection between alcohol and sexual assault. Diary studies also provide a means of collecting in vivo data, which can help elucidate factors that predict sexual assault without the bias of retrospective report. Diary methods have been used to both understand the relationship between alcohol use and perpetration (e.g., Shorey et al., 2014) and alcohol use and victimization, along with its associated deleterious sequelae (e.g., Neal & Fromme, 2007; Parks & Fals-Stewart, 2004; Parks, Hsieh, et al., 2008). Lastly, the nuanced aspects of human belief, social norms, attitudes, and thought are difficult to fully capture in standardized surveys and retrospective reports. Therefore, nuance and key elements may be found through qualitative methods, such as analyzing interviews (e.g., Becker & Tinkler, 2015; Cowley, 2014; Koo, Nguyen, Andrasik, & George, 2015).

Regardless of the type of study, part of the confusion around the relationship between alcohol use and sexual assault lies in measurement limitations. Different operationalizations of the variables of interest lead to conflicting results. This may be in part because different measures are confounded with other important factors (e.g., impulsivity). For instance, alcohol use may be conceptualized in a variety of ways, with so-labeled distal, proximal, and event-level effects (see Abbey, Wegner, Woerner, Pegram, & Pierce, 2014 for a review). Even within each of these categories, there are a variety of metrics used for both distal (e.g., alcohol problems, dependency symptoms) and proximal (e.g., heavy episodic drinking, binge drinking) measures. Different metrics may influence understanding of causal relationships or prevalence rates, such as the example of mixed findings between sexual assault victimization and later drinking. Therefore, researchers should carefully consider what labels they use and what conclusions are drawn based on their methods. Additionally, reliance on distal and proximal measures is insufficient for drawing causal conclusions not only because of potential confounds but also because it is unclear if alcohol was used (and in what quantities) during the sexual assault, as would be captured with event-level measurement. Measurement precision for sexual assault outcomes is equally essential and just as varied within the existing literature. Many different types of and labels for sexual assault exist (e.g., sexual coercion, sexual aggression, sexual assault, rape, forced penetration, sodomy), and the findings related to prevalence rates, risk factors, and related environmental variables depend on the definitions used (see Bouffard, Bouffard, Goodson, & Goodson, 2017 for a review). Therefore, it is clear that, without measurement precision and clarity, findings are muddled.

Of course, alcohol is not the only substance associated with sexual assault. Hindmarch and Brinkmann (1999) conducted urinalysis of 1033 samples supplied by victims of rape where drugs were allegedly involved and 37% of samples tested positive for alcohol, 19% tested positive for cannabinoids, 5% tested positive for other substances [e.g., gamma-hydroxybutyrate (GHB), cocaine, morphine, flunitrazepam (Rohypnol)].

Similar to the research on alcohol, sexual assault victims are more likely to report use of illicit substances cross-sectionally (McCauley, Ruggiero, Resnick, & Kilpatrick, 2010; Zinzow et al., 2012) and at the time of the assault (Resnick et al., 2012) and experiencing a sexual assault may be associated with initiation of or increased substance use (Sturza & Campbell, 2005). Illicit drug use also shares a relationship with sexual assault perpetration, though findings are mixed or weak compared to alcohol effects (Testa, 2004). Amongst adolescents, perpetrators are much more likely to report illicit drug use than non-perpetrators (Borowsky, Hogan, & Ireland, 1997). In a sample of young adults, illicit drug use, both directly before the encounter and distally, has been linked to increased severity of sexual aggression, even after controlling for proximal alcohol use (Swartout & White, 2010). However, epidemiological studies have found that illicit drugs appear to be commonly used alongside alcohol and uncommonly used in comparison to alcohol alone (Hurley, Parker, & Wells, 2006).

Given that alcohol and marijuana seem to be the substances most frequently involved in drug-facilitated or incapacitated rape (Hindmarch & Brinkmann, 1999; Kilpatrick et al., 2007), recent changes in laws related to marijuana that impact its availability may impact the occurrence of sexual assault, and this could be a topic for future research. Additionally, despite media attention given to illicit drugs, such as so called date-rape drugs like GHB and Rohypnol, alcohol is much more frequently related to sexual assault (Abbey & Jacques-Tiura, 2011). Given the influential role of alcohol, it is important that future research investigating the relationship between substance use and sexual assault also assess alcohol use. Generally, a best practice for future research is to engage with multiple types of methodologies with heavy focus on experimental, longitudinal, diary, and qualitative studies. Combining tactics helps identify nuance, isolate driving variables, and clarify areas of confusion. Additionally, future research must be clear and precise regarding how variables are operationalized, and event-level measurements will provide more causal understanding than proximal or distal variations on the same theme.

Study Sample Selection

Of course, even with appropriate methods, research findings are limited by the study sample. Frequently, studies in this area lack diversity in participants. For instance, although most sexual assaults involve a male perpetrator and a female victim, individuals of all genders can be victims and perpetrators (see Turchik, Hebenstreit, & Judson, 2016 for review). Nearly 5% of American men report rape victimization (Centers for Disease Control and Prevention, 2011), and sexual assault victimization is even more common (Bureau of Justice Statistics, 2016; Navarro & Clevenger, 2017). Approximately half of male victims report the sexual assault was perpetrated by a female intimate partner (Centers for Disease Control and Prevention, 2011), and a substantial minority of women report perpetrating sexual assault (Russell, Doan, & King, 2017; Struckman-Johnson, Struckman-Johnson, & Anderson, 2003). Although data are limited, alcohol use seems to increase risk of victimization for men (Navarro & Clevenger, 2017), and women report exploitation of intoxication as a common perpetration tactic (Russell et al., 2017). However, theories and research focus almost exclusively on male perpetrators and female victims (Turchik et al., 2016). Similarly, the majority of perpetration studies have focused on college men. The limited data that do exist suggest variable rates of reported sexual assault perpetration in other groups (e.g., 22–27% in community samples, 15% in US Navy recruits, and 3–8% in youth under 18; Abbey et al., 2004).

Some evidence exists that factors such as race, ethnicity, or background play important roles in alcohol-involved sexual assault rates, reporting, and consequences. Koo et al. (2015) found that Asian-identifying college students reported a low likelihood to report alcohol-involved rape. Another study found that Asian-identifying college women with a history of incapacitated rape had fewer drinking problems than White-identifying college women with a similar history (Nguyen, Kaysen, Dillworth, Brajcich, & Larimer, 2010). Monks et al. (2010a, 2010b) found that, in a sample of predominantly Hispanic students, alcohol use and expectancies predicted sexual victimization reports, but, notably, sensation seeking also independently predicted sexual victimization. Importantly, these studies suggest that better understanding racial, ethnic, and cultural factors, particularly when there may be culturally specific alcohol expectancies. The possible impact of sexual orientation has also been understudied. In a national sample of lesbian and bisexual-identifying women, experiencing sexual assault victimization predicted higher levels of alcohol use and more alcohol-related problems (Rhew, Stappenbeck, Bedard-Gilligan, Hughes, & Kaysen, 2017). Clearly, demographic factors and identity play a role in how alcohol and sexual assault interrelate; thus, fully capturing the complex interplay between alcohol and sexual assault requires research with diverse samples.

Prevention Implications

Researchers who study risk factors for sexual assault, including factors related to alcohol, are often accused of blaming the victim (Abbey, 2011a, 2011b). Victim blaming is a pernicious reality in our society that contributes to many negative outcomes, including increased distress and self-blame for victims and decreased reporting of sexual assault. Rather than conferring blame on victims, identification of risk factors provides information that can empower victims and, perhaps, contribute to empirically supported risk reduction and prevention efforts.

Despite being thoroughly debunked, the myth that most sexual assaults are perpetrated by a deranged stranger who ambushes his victim in a dark alley and overwhelms her with physical force persists. More than 30 years of research has consistently concluded that most sexual assaults are committed by someone known to the victim and physical force is often absent. As a result of this common misunderstanding, the role of alcohol consumption is often undervalued as a perpetration tactic and risk factor. One consequence is that many sexual assault risk reduction programs do not include information about the role of alcohol use or teach alcohol-related self-protection behaviors (Testa & Livingston, 2009). Instead, many programs include components like self-defense training that are better suited to resisting physical attacks.

Because binge drinking may confer additional risk for sexual assault beyond frequency and volume of alcohol consumed, this pattern seems to be a particularly important intervention target. In the substance use literature, many strategies have been shown to reduce binge drinking in college students (Larimer & Cronce, 2002, 2007) and these strategies can be incorporated into sexual assault risk reduction programs. For example, Gilmore, Lewis, and George (2015) conducted a randomized control trial of a web-based sexual assault risk reduction program with binge drinking college women. Among participants at highest risk of revictimization, receiving personalized feedback and recommendations related to sexual assault risk and drinking behavior reduced revictimization (both alcohol involved and non-alcohol involved) and the frequency of binge drinking reported at follow up. Bystander strategies that address the role of alcohol beliefs, expectancies, and scripts in sexual assault are another promising approach to sexual assault prevention. Existing strategies that are supported by evidence include a range of methodologies, such as online training (e.g., RealConsent; Salazar, Vivolo-Kantor, Hardin, & Berkowitz, 2014), performance-based programs (e.g., Sex Signals; Rothman & Silverman, 2007), and workshops (The Men's Program; Foubert & Marriott, 1996).

The growing concern about alcohol use, particularly on college campuses, has spurred the development and implementation of many drinking reduction programs. There is some evidence that interventions focusing on reducing alcohol use also reduce sexual assault (Clinton-Sherrod, Morgan-Lopez, Brown, McMillen, & Cowells, 2011). However, 26% of the high school students report having been drunk at least once (Johnston, O'Malley, Miech, Bachman, & Schulenberg, 2017), and there seems to be a high degree of stability between an individual's high school and college pattern of alcohol use (Reifman & Watson, 2003; Wechsler, Davenport, Dowdall, Moeykens,

& Castillo, 1994). Thus intervention efforts that occur before college seem likely to have the most impact on alcohol use and, by extension, sexual assault. Given that a history of sexual victimization (either child sexual abuse or adult victimization) is a consistent and strong risk factor for revictimization (see Arata, 2002; Classen, Palesh, & Aggarwal, 2005 for reviews), early intervention may be the most effective method of breaking this cycle. Despite this evidence, a review of adolescent intimate partner and sexual violence prevention programs found none that addressed alcohol use (Lundgren & Amin, 2015).

Prevention strategies targeting broader community and societal-level factors yield promising results. To date, alcohol and sexual assault policies are variable. A review of state legislation from Richards and Kafonek (2016) found that many institutes of higher education lack sexual misconduct policies, including affirmative consent standards (i.e., explicitly stating that consent must be given for each specific sexual engagement rather than implied). Additionally, legal statues continue to vary dramatically across states in terms of whether consent and incapacity are defined and whether/how the gender of victims and perpetrators is addressed (DeMatteo, Galloway, Arnold, & Patel, 2015). Previous work has suggested that policy change recommendations may include limiting the availability of alcohol at certain times or in certain places (e.g., college campuses), increasing prices or taxes of alcohol, reducing the density of alcohol outlets in certain locations, intervening to reduce alcohol use by problem users, reducing overservice or refusing service to aggressive individuals, changing alcohol marketing, and implementing community interventions to manage individuals in alcohol-use situations (Lippy & DeGue, 2016; World Health Organization, 2009). Further evaluation of policies is required to understand their effectiveness with contextual nuances, local practices, and alcohol scripts (Lippy & DeGue, 2016).

Together, these prevention strategies provide intervention points at multiple levels (e.g., individually, relationally, community-wide, societally). Because of its complexity, preventing alcohol-related sexual assault will likely require a multifaceted approach that utilizes many strategies at these various levels. This is in alignment with findings from the literature; for instance, a review of interventions for reducing and preventing violence against women found that interventions with the most promise to achieve widespread prevention also provided comprehensive programming at multiple levels of the social ecology (e.g., at individual, relational, community, and societal levels) and continuously engaged with diverse stakeholders (Arango, Morton, Gennari, Kiplesund, & Ellsberg, 2014). Therefore, preventions with the highest impact will likely be multifaceted, addressing the behaviors, attitudes, and policies that all contribute to alcohol-related sexual assault perpetration.

Clinical Implications

Sexual assault can result in negative outcomes for victims, including increased negative affect, self-blame, and posttraumatic stress disorder symptoms (Littleton et al., 2009; Ullman & Najdowski, 2009). Several interventions have been found to effectively reduce these symptoms and improvements are generally maintained (Kline, Cooper, Rytwinksi, & Feeny, 2017). Given the differences between alcohol-involved and other types of sexual assaults, one might expect treatment outcomes to differ based on assault type. Treatment outcomes have not been found to differ based on related dimensions (e.g., child vs. adult victimization, sexual vs. physical victimization, Kline et al., 2017), but the role of alcohol involvement as a predictor of treatment outcome has not been widely studied. Regardless, it seems likely that treatment tailoring may be important for victims of alcohol-involved assaults. For example, exposure-based treatments in which victims recount the trauma in detail may be ill suited to victims of incapacitated rape who have limited memory of the event. Higher rates of self-blame among victims of alcohol-involved assaults may require specific challenging of societal myths that view women as sexually available and, thus, appropriate targets if drinking or drunk. Finally, the disconnect between what is considered a "typical" or "legitimate" rape and the experience of an alcohol-involved assault likely contributes to the tendency of victims to discount or explain away this type of victimization and to victims experience of more negative reactions when they do disclose. Challenging the underlying myths, attitudes, and expectations at a societal level would likely help reduce the frequency of these assaults and improve outcomes for victims.

For perpetrators who have some engagement with the legal system, proven or at least promising treatments exist for reducing recidivism (Kim, Benekos, & Merlo, 2016). While surgical castration and hormonal medication have significantly larger effects, psychological treatments consistently produce small reductions in recidivism (Kim et al., 2016). Cognitive behavioral therapy and relapse prevention (CBT-RP; Moster, Wnuk, & Jeglic, 2008) is the most commonly used psychological treatment for sexual offenders (Losel & Schmucker, 2005). CBT-RP includes various techniques to correct thoughts, feelings, and behaviors that promote sexual assault and develop more prosocial patterns, including challenging cognitive distortions and teaching empathy and social skills. The goal of RP is to teach offenders to recognize high-risk situations and to use coping skills to reduce the likelihood of reoffending. Results of the current review suggest the importance of challenging alcohol-related offense-supportive cognitive distortions (e.g., I can't control myself when I drink, Women use alcohol to signal sexual interest). The physical effects of alcohol (e.g., impaired decision-making, alcohol myopia) should be considered as they relate to an offender's likelihood of effectively implementing a RP plan. Finally, regardless of whether the offender is drinking, exposure to risky drinking setting should be considered a high-risk behavior and should be addressed in treatment.

Conclusion

Sexual assault is an endemic problem in our society, and alcohol use is consistently connected to sexual assault perpetration and victimization. However, the link between alcohol use and sexual assault is complex with a host of associated factors likely contributing to the relationship (e.g., gendered scripts around alcohol use, being in places where alcohol is served). The complexity of this relationship is in part confused by the varied and inconsistent means of measuring, labeling, and describing both alcohol use and sexual assault. Additionally, when the linkage between alcohol use and sexual assault is only studied in limited samples, it is more difficult to draw meaningful conclusion. To better understand this multifactorial association, future research will benefit from diverse samples, experimental paradigms to parse apart pharmacological effects of alcohol from social scripts surrounding its use, and prospective, longitudinal designs to understand the interplay between alcohol and sexual assault over time in context of other influential variables.

From what we do understand about alcohol's role in sexual assault, population-level prevention will require careful programming that addresses multiple levels of the social ecology. A combination of bystander interventions, norms change, and local and statewide policies will likely be required. Intervening early in adolescence to address alcohol use and its relationship to sex and gender-related beliefs will likely be important. When sexual assaults do occur, addressing the role of alcohol with victims and perpetrators may be helpful for reducing negative outcomes for victims and continued unhealthy expectations from perpetrators. As researchers, preventionists, and clinicians, we must cease to undervalue the role that alcohol plays in sexual assault and become more accustomed to discussing gendered social scripts and alcohol use patterns that are closely tied to alcohol use.

References

Abbey, A. (2002). Alcohol-related sexual assault: A common problem among college students. *Journal of Studies on Alcohol, 14*, 118–128.

Abbey, A. (2011a). Alcohol and dating risk factors for sexual assault: Double standards are still alive and well entrenched. *Psychology of Women Quarterly, 35*(2), 362–368. https://doi.org/10.1177/0361684311404150

Abbey, A. (2011b). Alcohol's role in sexual violence perpetration: Theoretical explanations, existing evidence, and future directions. *Drug and Alcohol Review, 30*, 481–489. https://doi.org/10.1111/j.1465-3362.2011.00296.x

Abbey, A. (2017). Moving beyond simple answers to complex questions: How does context affect alcohol's role in sexual assault perpetration? A commentary on Testa and Cleveland (2017). *Journal of Studies on Alcohol and Drugs, 78*(1), 14–15. https://doi.org/10.15288/jsad.2017.78.14

Abbey, A., & Jacques-Tiura, A. J. (2011). Sexual assault perpetrators' tactics: Associations with their personal characteristics and aspects of the incident. *Journal of Interpersonal Violence, 26*(14), 2866–2889. https://doi.org/10.1177/0886260510390955

Abbey, A., & McAuslan, P. (2004). A longitudinal examination of male college students' perpetration of sexual assault. *Journal of Consulting and Clinical Psychology, 72*, 747–756. https://doi.org/10.1037/0022-006x.72.5.747

Abbey, A., & Ortiz, L. G. (2008). *Alcohol and sexual violence perpetration*. Harrisburg, PA: VAWnet, a project of the National Resource Center on Domestic Violence/Pennsylvania Coalition Against Domestic Violence.

Abbey, A., & Wegner, R. (2015). Using experimental paradigms to examine alcohol's role in men's sexual aggression: Opportunities and challenges in proxy development. *Violence Against Women, 21*(8), 975–996. https://doi.org/10.1177/1077801215589378

Abbey, A., Wegner, R., Woerner, J., Pegram, S. E., & Pierce, J. (2014). Review of survey and experimental research that examines the relationship between alcohol consumption and men's sexual aggression perpetration. *Trauma, Violence & Abuse, 15(4)*, 265–282. https://doi.org/10.1177/1524838014521031

Abbey, A., Zawacki, T., Buck, P. O., Clinton, A. M., & McAuslan, P. (2004). Sexual assault and alcohol consumption: What do we know about their relationship and what types of research are still needed? *Aggression and Violent Behavior, 9*, 271–303. https://doi.org/10.1016/s1359-1789(03)00011-9

Arango, D. J., Morton, M., Gennari, F., Kiplesund, S., & Ellsberg, M. (2014). *Interventions to prevent or reduce violence against women and girls: A systematic review of reviews*. Washington, DC: World Bank. https://openknowledge.worldbank.org/handle/10986/21035

Arata, C. M. (2002). Child sexual abuse and sexual revictimization. *Clinical Psychology: Science and Practice, 9*, 135–164. https://doi.org/10.1093/clipsy.9.2.135

Becker, S., & Tinkler, J. (2015). "Me getting plastered and her provoking my eyes" young people's attribution of blame for sexual aggression in public drinking spaces. *Feminist Criminology, 10*(3), 235–258. https://doi.org/10.1177/1557085114541142

Bondurant, B. (2001). University women's acknowledgement of rape: Individual, situational, and social factors. *Violence Against Women, 7*, 294–314. https://doi.org/10.1177/1077801201007003004

Borowsky, I. W., Hogan, M., & Ireland, M. (1997). Adolescent sexual aggression: Risk and protective factors. *Pediatrics, 100*(6), e7–e7.

Bouffard, L., Bouffard, L., Goodson, A., & Goodson, A. (2017). Sexual coercion, sexual aggression, or sexual assault: How measurement impacts our understanding of sexual violence. *Journal of Aggression, Conflict and Peace Research, 9*(4), 269–278. https://doi.org/10.1108/jacpr-05-2017-0292

Bryan, A. E., Norris, J., Abdallah, D. A., Stappenbeck, C. A., Morrison, D. M., Davis, K. C., … Zawacki, T. (2015). Longitudinal change in women's sexual victimization experiences as a function of alcohol consumption in sexual victimization history: A latent transition analysis. *Psychology of Violence, 6(2)*, 271–279. https://doi.org/10.1037/a0039411

Bureau of Justice Statistics. (2016). *Criminal Victimization. (NCJ 251150)*. Washington, DC: Department of Justice.

Center for Behavioral Health Statistics and Quality. (2016). 2015 National Survey on Drug Use and Health: Detailed Tables. Substance Abuse and Mental Health Services Administration.

Centers for Disease Control and Prevention. (2011). *National intimate partner and sexual violence survey: 2010 Summary report*. Atlanta, GA: Centers for Disease Control and Prevention.

Chevalier, M. J., & Einolf, C. J. (2009). Sorority participation and sexual assault risk. *Violence Against Women, 15*, 835–851. https://doi.org/10.1177/1077801209334472

Classen, C. C., Palesh, O. G., & Aggarwal, R. (2005). Sexual revictimization: A review of the empirical literature. *Trauma, Violence & Abuse, 6*, 103–129. https://doi.org/10.1177/1524838005275087

Cleveland, H. H., Koss, M. P., & Lyons, J. (1999). Rape tactics from the survivors' perspective. *Journal of Interpersonal Violence, 14*, 532–547. https://doi.org/10.1177/088626099014005005

Clinton-Sherrod, M., Morgan-Lopez, A., Brown, J. M., McMillen, B. A., & Cowells, A. (2011). Incapacitated sexual violence involving alcohol among college women: The impact of a brief drinking intervention. *Violence Against Women, 17*, 135–154. https://doi.org/10.1177/1077801210394272

Coffey, S. F., Saladin, M. E., Drobes, D. J., Brady, T., Dansky, B. S., & Kilpatrick, D. G. (2002). Trauma and substance cue reactivity in individuals with comorbid posttraumatic stress disorder and cocaine or alcohol dependence. *Drug and Alcohol Dependence, 65*, 115–127. https://doi.org/10.1016/s0376-8716(01)00157-0

Cohen, L. E., & Felson, M. (1979). Social change and crime rate trends: A routine activity approach. *American Sociological Review, 44*, 488–608.

Collins, J. J., & Messerschmidt, P. M. (1993). Epidemiology of alcohol-related violence. *Alcohol Health & Research World, 17*, 93–100. https://doi.org/10.1002/9781118411094.ch16

Cowley, A. (2014). "Let's get drunk and have sex": The complex relationship of alcohol, gender, and sexual victimization. *Journal of Interpersonal Violence, 29*, 1258–1278. https://doi.org/10.1177/0886260513506289

Davis, K. C., Schraufnagel, T. J., Jacques-Tiura, A. J., Norris, J., George, W. H., & Kiekel, P. A. (2012). Childhood sexual abuse and acute alcohol effects on men's sexual aggression intentions. *Psychology of Violence, 2*, 179–193. https://doi.org/10.1037/a0027185

DeMatteo, D., Galloway, M., Arnold, S., & Patel, U. (2015). Sexual assault on college campuses: A 50-state survey of criminal sexual assault statutes and their relevance to campus sexual assault. *Psychology, Public Policy, and Law, 21*(3), 227–238. https://doi.org/10.1037/law0000055

Fossos, N., Kaysen, D., Neighbors, C., Lindgren, K. P., & Hove, M. C. (2011). Coping motives as a mediator of the relationship between sexual coercion and problem drinking in college students. *Addictive Behaviors, 36*(10), 1001–1007. https://doi.org/10.1016/j.addbeh.2011.06.001

Foubert, J. D., & Marriott, K. A. (1996). Overcoming men's defensiveness toward sexual assault programs: Learning to help survivors. *Journal of College Student Development, 37*, 470–472. https://doi.org/10.1353/csd.2006.0016

George, W. H., Davis, K. C., Masters, N. T., Jacques-Tiura, A. J., Heiman, J. R., Norris, J., … Andraisk, M. P. (2015). Sexual victimization, alcohol intoxication, sexual-emotional responding, and sexual risk in heavy episodic drinking women. *Archives of Sexual Behavior, 43*, 645–658. https://doi.org/10.1007/s10508-013-0143-8

Gidycz, C. A., Loh, C., Lobo, T., Rich, C., Lynn, S. J., & Pashdag, J. (2007). Reciprocal relationships among alcohol use, risk perception, and sexual assault: A prospective analysis. *Journal of American College Health, 56*, 5–14. https://doi.org/10.3200/JACH.56.1.5-14

Gilmore, A. K., Lewis, M. L., & George, W. H. (2015). A randomized controlled trial targeting alcohol use and sexual assault risk among college women at high risk for victimization. *Behaviour Research and Therapy, 7(4)*, 38–49. https://doi.org/10.1016/j.brat.2015.08.007

Gilmore, A. K., Stappenbeck, C. A., Lewis, M. A., Granato, H. F., & Kaysen, D. (2015). Sexual assault history and its association with the use of drinking protective behavioral strategies among college women. *Journal of Studies on Alcohol and Drugs, 76*, 459–464. https://doi.org/10.15288/jsad.2015.76.459

Grant, B. F., Chou, S. P., Saha, T. D., Pickering, R. P., Kerridge, B. T., Ruan, W. J., … Hasin, D. S. (2017). Prevalence of 12-month alcohol use, high-risk drinking, and *DSM-IV* alcohol use disorder in the United States, 2001–2002 to 2012–2013: Results from the national epidemiologic survey on alcohol and related conditions. *JAMA Psychiatry, 74(9)*, 911–923. https://doi.org/10.1001/jamapsychiatry.2017.2161

Hindmarch, I., & Brinkmann, R. D. (1999). Trends in the use of alcohol and other drugs in cases of sexual assault. *Human Psychopharmacology, 14*, 225–231. https://doi.org/10.1002/(SICI)1099-1077(199906)14:4<225::AID-HUP92>3.0.CO;2-3

Hurley, M., Parker, H., & Wells, D. L. (2006). The epidemiology of drug facilitated sexual assault. *Journal of Clinical Forensic Medicine, 13*(4), 181–185. https://doi.org/10.1016/j.jcfm.2006.02.005

Johnston, L. D., O'Malley, P. M., Miech, R. A., Bachman, J. G., & Schulenberg, J. E. (2017). *Monitoring the Future national survey results on drug use, 1975–2016: Overview, key findings on adolescent drug use*. Ann Arbor, MI: Institute for Social Research, The University of Michigan.

Kilpatrick, D. G., Resnick, H. S., Ruggierio, K. J., Conoscenti, L. M., & McCauley, J. (2007). *Drug-facilitated, incapacitated, and forcible rape: A national study (NCJ 219181)*. Charleston, SC: Medical University of South Carolina, National Crime Victims Research & Treatment Center.

Kim, B., Benekos, P. J., & Merlo, A. (2016). Sex offender recidivism revisited: Review of recent meta-analyses on the effects of sex offender treatment. *Trauma, Violence & Abuse, 17(1)*, 105–117. https://doi.org/10.1177/1524838014566719

Kline, A. C., Cooper, A. A., Rytwinksi, N. K., & Feeny, N. C. (2017). Long-term efficacy of psychotherapy for posttraumatic stress disorder: A meta-analysis of randomized controlled trials. *Clinical Psychology Review, 59*, 30–40. https://doi.org/10.1016/j.cpr.2017.10.009

Koo, K. H., Nguyen, H. V., Andrasik, M. P., & George, W. H. (2015). The cultural context of nondisclosure of alcohol-involved acquaintance rape among Asian American college women: A qualitative study. *The Journal of Sex Research, 52*(1), 55–68. https://doi.org/10.1080/00224499.2013.826168

Kraus, L., Baumeister, S. E., Pabst, A., & Orth, B. (2009). Association of average daily alcohol consumption, binge drinking and alcohol-related social problems: Results from the German Epidemiological Surveys of Substance Abuse. *Alcohol and Alcoholism, 44(3)*, 314–320. https://doi.org/10.1093/alcalc/agn110

Larimer, M. E., & Cronce, J. M. (2002). Identification, prevention, and treatment: A review of individual focused strategies to reduce problematic alcohol consumption by college students. *Journal of Studies on Alcohol*, (Suppl 14), 148–163. https://doi.org/10.15288/jsas.2002.s14.148

Larimer, M. E., & Cronce, J. M. (2007). Identification, prevention, and treatment revisited: Individual focused college drinking prevention strategies 1999–2006. *Addictive Behaviors, 32*, 2439–2468. https://doi.org/10.1016/j.addbeh.2007.05.006

Lippy, C., & DeGue, S. (2016). Exploring alcohol policy approaches to prevent sexual violence perpetration. *Trauma, Violence & Abuse, 17*(1), 26–42. https://doi.org/10.1177/1524838014557291

Littleton, H., Grills-Taquechel, A., & Axsom, D. (2009). Impaired and incapacitated rape victims: Assault characteristics and post-assault experiences. *Violence and Victims, 24*, 439–457. https://doi.org/10.1891/0886-6708.24.4.439

Lorenz, M. A. & Ullman, S. E. (2016). Alcohol and sexual assault victimization: Research findings and future directions. *Aggression and Violent Behavior, 31*, 82–94. https://doi.org/10.1016/j.avb.2016.08.001

Losel, F., & Schmucker, M. (2005). The effectiveness of treatment for sexual offenders: A comprehensive meta-analysis. *Journal of Experimental Criminology, 1*, 117–146. https://doi.org/10.1007/s11292-004-6466-7

Lundgren, R., & Amin, A. (2015). Addressing intimate partner violence and sexual violence among adolescents: Emerging evidence of effectiveness. *Journal of Adolescent Health, 56*(1), S42–S50. https://doi.org/10.1016/j.jadohealth.2014.08.012

McCauley, J. L., Calhoun, K. S., & Gidycz, C. A. (2010). Binge drinking and rape: A prospective examination of college women with a history of previous sexual assault. *Journal of Interpersonal Violence, 25*, 1655–1668. https://doi.org/10.1177/0886260509354580

McCauley, J. L., Ruggiero, K. J., Resnick, H. S., Conoscenti, L. M., & Kilpatrick, D. G. (2009). Substance abuse among college women as a function of rape experiences: Results from a national study of college women. *Addictive Behaviors, 34*, 458–462.

McCauley, J. L., Ruggiero, K. J., Resnick, H. S., & Kilpatrick, D. G. (2010). Incapacitated, forcible, and drug/alcohol-facilitated rape in relation to binge drinking, marijuana use, and illicit drug use: A national survey. *Journal of Traumatic Stress, 23*, 132–140. https://doi.org/10.1002/jts.20489

Mohler-Kuo, M., Dowdall, G. W., Koss, M. P., & Wechsler, H. (2004). Correlates of rape while intoxicated in a national sample of college women. *Journal of Studies on Alcohol, 65*, 37–45. https://doi.org/10.15288/jsa.2004.65.37

Monks, S. M., Tomaka, J., Palacios, R., & Thompson, S. E. (2010a). Sexual assault in female and male college students: Examining the roles of alcohol use, alcohol expectancies, and sexual sensation seeking. *Substance Use & Misuse, 45*, 2258–2280. https://doi.org/10.3109/10826081003694854

Monks, S. M., Tomaka, J., Palacios, R., & Thompson, S. E. (2010b). Sexual victimization in female and male college students: Examining the roles of alcohol use, alcohol expectancies, and sexual sensation seeking. *Substance Use & Misuse, 45*(13), 2258–2280. https://doi.org/10.3109/10826081003694854

Moster, A., Wnuk, D. W., & Jeglic, E. L. (2008). Cognitive behavioral therapy interventions with sex offenders. *Journal of Correctional Health Care, 14*(2), 109–121. https://doi.org/10.1177/1078345807313874

Mouilso, E. R., Fischer, S., & Calhoun, K. S. (2012). A prospective study of sexual assault and alcohol use among first-year college women. *Violence and Victims, 27*(1), 78–94. https://doi.org/10.1891/0886-6708.27.1.78

National Institute on Alcohol Abuse and Alcoholism. (2004). Helping patients who drink too much: A clinician's guide. Rockville, MD: National Institutes of Health.

Navarro, J. N., & Clevenger, S. (2017). Calling attention to the importance of assisting male survivors of sexual victimization. *Journal of School Violence, 16*(2), 222–235. https://doi.org/10.1080/15388220.2017.1284478

Neal, D. J., & Fromme, K. (2007). Event-level covariation of alcohol intoxication and behavioral risks during the first year of college. *Journal of Consulting and Clinical Psychology, 75*, 294–306. https://doi.org/10.1037/0022-006x.75.2.294

Nguyen, H. V., Kaysen, D., Dillworth, T. M., Brajcich, M., & Larimer, M. E. (2010). Incapacitated rape and alcohol use in White and Asian American college women. *Violence Against Women, 16*(8), 919–933. https://doi.org/10.1177/1077801210377470

Parkhill, M. R., Abbey, A., & Jacques-Tiura, A. J. (2009). How do sexual assault characteristics vary as a function of perpetrators' level of intoxication? *Addictive Behaviors, 34*, 331–333. https://doi.org/10.1016/j.addbeh.2008.11.003

Parks, K. A., & Fals-Stewart, W. (2004). The temporal relationship between college women's alcohol consumption and victimization experiences. *Alcoholism: Clinical and Experimental Research, 28*, 625–629. https://doi.org/10.1097/01.alc.0000122105.56109.70

Parks, K. A., Hsieh, Y.-P., Bradizza, C. M., & Romosz, A. M. (2008). Factors influencing the temporal relationship between alcohol consumption and experiences with aggression among college women. *Psychology of Addictive Behaviors, 22*, 210–218. https://doi.org/10.1037/0893-164x.22.2.210

Parks, K. A., & Miller, B. A. (1997). Bar victimization of women. *Psychology of Women Quarterly, 21*, 509–525. https://doi.org/10.1111/j.1471-6402.1997.tb00128.x

Parks, K. A., Hsieh, Y.-P., Taggart, C., & Bradizza, C. M. (2014). A longitudinal analysis of drinking and victimization in college women: Is there a reciprocal relationship? *Psychology of Addictive Behaviors, 28*(4), 943–951. https://doi.org/10.1037/a0036283

Purcell, J., & Graham, K. (2005). A typology of Toronto nightclubs at the turn of the millennium. *Contemporary Drug Problems, 32*(1), 131–167. https://doi.org/10.1177/009145090503200109

Reifman, A., & Watson, W. K. (2003). Binge drinking during the first semester of college: Continuation and desistance from high school patterns. *Journal of American College Health, 52*(2), 73–81. https://doi.org/10.1080/07448480309595727

Reinarman, C., & Levine, H. G. (1997). *Crack in America: Demon Drugs and Social Justice*. Berkeley, CA: University of California Press.

Resnick, H. S., Walsh, K., McCauley, J. L., Schumacher, J. A., Kilpatrick, D. G., & Acierno, R. E. (2012). Assault related substance use as a predictor of substance use over time within a sample of recent victims of sexual assault. *Addictive Behaviors, 37*, 914–921. https://doi.org/10.1016/j.addbeh.2012.03.017

Rhew, I. C., Stappenbeck, C. A., Bedard-Gilligan, M., Hughes, T., & Kaysen, D. (2017). Effects of sexual assault on alcohol use and consequences among young adult sexual minority women. *Journal of Consulting and Clinical Psychology, 85*(5), 424–433. https://doi.org/10.1037/ccp0000202

Richards, T. N., & Kafonek, K. (2016). Reviewing state legislative agendas regarding sexual assault in higher education: Proliferation of best practices and points of caution. *Feminist Criminology, 11*(1), 91–129. https://doi.org/10.1177/1557085115621163

Rothman, E., & Silverman, S. (2007). The effect of a college sexual assault prevention program on first-year students' victimization rates. *Journal of American College Health, 55*(5), 283–290. https://doi.org/10.3200/JACH.55.5.283-290

Russell, T. D., Doan, C. M., & King, A. R. (2017). Sexually violent women: The PID-5, everyday sadism, and adversarial sexual attitudes predict female sexual aggression and coercion against male victims. *Personality and Individual Differences, 111*, 242–249. https://doi.org/10.1016/j.paid.2017.02.019

Salazar, L. F., Vivolo-Kantor, A., Hardin, J., & Berkowitz, A. (2014). A web-based sexual violence bystander intervention for male college students: Randomized controlled trial. *Journal of Medical Internet Research, 16*(9). https://doi.org/10.2196/jmir.3426

Schwartz, M. D., & Pitts, V. L. (1995). Exploring a feminist routine activities approach to explaining sexual assault. *Justice Quarterly, 12*, 9–31. https://doi.org/10.1080/07418829500092551

Shorey, R. C., Stuart, G. L., McNulty, J. K., & Moore, T. M. (2014). Acute alcohol use temporally increases the odds of male perpetrated dating violence: A 90-day diary analysis. *Addictive Behaviors, 39*(1), 365–368. https://doi.org/10.1016/j.addbeh.2013.10.025

Steele, C. M., & Southwick, L. (1985). Alcohol and social behavior, I: The psychology of drunken excess. *Journal of Personality and Social Psychology, 48*, 18–34. https://doi.org/10.1037/0022-3514.48.1.18

Stewart, S. H., & Conrod, P. J. (2003). Psychosocial models of functional associations between posttraumatic stress disorder and substance use disorder. In P. C. Ouimette & P. J. Brown (Eds.), *Trauma and substance abuse: Causes, consequences, and treatment of comorbid disorders* (pp. 29–55). Washington, DC: American Psychological Association.

Stoner, S. A., Norris, J., George, W. H., Davis, K. C., Masters, N. T., & Hessler, D. M. (2007). Effects of alcohol intoxication and victimization history on women's sexual assault resistance intentions: The role of secondary cognitive appraisals. *Psychology of Women Quarterly, 31*, 344–356. https://doi.org/10.1111/j.1471-6402.2007.00384.x

Substance Abuse and Mental Health Services Administration. (2017). Key substance use and mental health indicators in the United States: Results from the 2016 National Survey on Drug Use and Health (HHS Publication No. SMA 17-5044, NSDUH Series H-52). Rockville, MD: Center for Behavioral Health Statistics and Quality, Substance Abuse and Mental Health Services Administration. Retrieved from https://www.samhsa.gov/data/

Struckman-Johnson, C., Struckman-Johnson, D., & Anderson, P. (2003). Tactics of sexual coercion: When men and women won't take no for an answer. *The Journal of Sex Research, 40*(*1*), 76–86. https://doi.org/10.1080/00224490309552168

Sturza, M. L., & Campbell, R. (2005). An exploratory study of rape survivors' prescription drug use as a means of coping with sexual assault. *Psychology of Women Quarterly, 29*, 353–363. https://doi.org/10.1111/j.1471-6402.2005.00235.x

Swartout, K. M., & White, J. W. (2010). The relationship between drug use and sexual aggression in men across time. *Journal of Interpersonal Violence, 25*(9), 1716–1735. https://doi.org/10.1177/0886260509354586

Testa, M. (2004). The role of substance use in male-to-female physical and sexual violence: A brief review and recommendations for future research. *Journal of Interpersonal Violence, 19*(12), 1494–1505. https://doi.org/10.1177/0886260504269701

Testa, M., & Cleveland, M. J. (2017). Does alcohol contribute to college men's sexual assault perpetration? Between-and within-person effects over five semesters. *Journal of Studies on Alcohol and Drugs, 78*(1), 5–13. https://doi.org/10.15288/jsad.2017.78.5

Testa, M., & Livingston, J. A. (2000). Alcohol and sexual aggression: Reciprocal relationships over time in a sample of high risk women. *Journal of Interpersonal Violence, 15*, 413–427. https://doi.org/10.1177/088626000015004005

Testa, M., Livingston, J. A., & Collins, R. L. (2000). The role of women's alcohol consumption in evaluating vulnerability to sexual aggression. *Experimental and Clinical Psychopharmacology, 8*, 185–191. https://doi.org/10.1037/t38000-000

Testa, M., Livingston, J. A., VanZile-Tamsen, C., & Frone, M. R. (2003). The role of women's substance use in vulnerability to forcible and incapacitated rape. *Journal of Studies on Alcohol, 64*, 756–764. https://doi.org/10.15288/jsa.2003.64.756

Testa, M. & Livingston, J. A. (2009). Alcohol consumption and women's vulnerability to sexual victimization: Can reducing women's drinking prevent rape? *Substance Use & Misuse, 44*, 1349–1376. https://doi.org/10.1080/10826080902961468

Testa, M., VanZile-Tamsen, C., & Livingston, J. A. (2004). The role of victim and perpetrator intoxication on sexual assault outcomes. *Journal of Studies on Alcohol, 65*, 320–329. https://doi.org/10.15288/jsa.2004.65.320

Tjaden, P., & Thoennes, N. (2000). Full report of the prevalence, incidence, and consequences of violence against women: Findings from the National Violence against Women Survey (NCJ 183781). National Institute of Justice and the Centers for Disease Control and Prevention.

Turchik, J. A., Hebenstreit, C. L., & Judson, S. S. (2016). An examination of the gender inclusiveness of current theories of Sexual violence in adulthood: Recognizing male victims, female perpetrators, and same-sex violence. *Trauma, Violence & Abuse, 17*(2), 133–148. https://doi.org/10.1177/1524838014566721

Ullman, S. E., & Brecklin, L. R. (2000). Alcohol and adult sexual assault in a national sample of women. *Journal of Substance Abuse, 11,* 405–420. https://doi.org/10.1016/S0899-3289(00)00036-5.

Ullman, S. E., Filipas, H. H., Townsend, S. M., & Starzynski, L. (2005). Trauma exposure, PTSD, and problem drinking among sexual assault survivors. *Journal of Studies on Alcohol, 66*, 610–619.

Ullman, S. E., & Najdowski, C. J. (2009). Revictimization as a moderator of psychosocial risk factors for problem drinking in female sexual assault survivors. *Journal of Studies on Alcohol and Drugs, 70*(1), 41–49. https://doi.org/10.15288/jsad.2009.70.41

Vicary, J. M., & Karshin, C. M. (2002). College alcohol abuse: A review of the problems, issues, and prevention approaches. *The Journal of Primary Prevention, 22*(3), 299–331. https://doi.org/10.1023/A:1013621821924

Wechsler, H., Davenport, A., Dowdall, G., Moeykens, B., & Castillo, S. (1994). Health and behavioral consequences of binge drinking in college: A national survey of students at 140 campuses. *Journal of the American Medical Association, 272*(21), 1672–1677. https://doi.org/10.1001/jama.1994.03520210056032

Wegner, R., Abbey, A., Pierce, J., Pegram, S. E., & Woerner, J. (2015). Sexual assault perpetrators' justifications for their actions: Relationships to rape supportive attitudes, incident characteristics, and future perpetration. *Violence Against Women, 21*(8), 1018–1037. https://doi.org/10.1177/1077801215589380

World Health Organization. (2009). Preventing violence by reducing the availability and harmful use of alcohol. Retrieved from http://apps.who.int/iris/bitstream/10665/44173/1/9789241598408_eng.pdf

Zawacki, T., Abbey, A., Buck, P. O., McAuslan, P., & Clinton-Sherrod, A. M. (2003). Perpetrators of alcohol-involved sexual assaults: How do they differ from other sexual assault perpetrators and nonperpetrators? *Aggressive Behavior, 29*, 366–380. https://doi.org/10.1002/ab.10076

Zinzow, H. M., Resnick, H. S., McCauley, J. L., Amstadter, A. B., Ruggiero, K. J., & Kilpatrick, D. G. (2012). Prevalence and risk of psychiatric disorders as a function of variant rape histories: Results from a national survey of women. *Social Psychiatry and Psychiatric Epidemiology, 4*, 893–902. https://doi.org/10.1007/s00127-011-0397-1

Risk Perception and Sexual Assault

12

Terri L. Messman-Moore and Selime R. Salim

You were alone, isolated, and weak. The three of them had been watching girls all night, waiting for someone to separate from the group. It happened to be you, but it could've been anyone. Opportunity is what matters, nothing else...
I'm telling you...Watch the nature channel. Predators go for the easy prey.

—Mindy McGinnis, The Female of the Species (2016, p. 157)

Introduction

According to the National Intimate Partner and Sexual Violence Survey, approximately 1 in 5 women will experience rape during their lifetimes, compared to 1 in 71 men (Black et al., 2011). In a large, multi-institutional investigation of the prevalence of rape and sexual assault among 14,989 female college students, over one-third of college women experienced completed or attempted sexual assault in their lifetime, and 10.3% were sexually assaulted during one academic year (Krebs, Lindquist, Berzofsky, Shook-Sa, & Peterson, 2016). Sexual assault carries significant negative consequences for women's mental health, and is associated with increased risk for development of posttraumatic stress disorder (PTSD), depression and suicidality, anxiety, disordered eating, and substance use disorders (for review and meta-analysis, see Dworkin, Menon, Bystrynski, & Allen, 2017).

The vast majority of sexual violence perpetrators are men. Men commit 98% of rapes against women, and 93.3% of rapes against men (Berkowitz, 2002; Black et al., 2011). Thus, sexual aggression prevention efforts should focus on men. A recent meta-analytic review concluded that male-targeted sexual assault prevention programs do have positive impacts on attitudes and intentions to engage in future sexual aggression, although there is no evidence that such programs actually reduce the incidence of sexual assault perpetrated by men (Wright, Zounlome, & Whiston, 2018). Given this, a broad and multi-pronged approach must encompass not only sexual aggression prevention programs for men (Wright et al., 2018) but also bystander intervention programming (Moynihan et al., 2015) and risk-reduction programs designed for women (Banyard, 2013).

Teaching girls and women to recognize and respond to risk is an important component of any comprehensive effort for sexual assault prevention. One of the primary means a woman has at her disposal to reduce her risk for sexual assault is to learn to identify, and respond effectively to, risky situations that may increase her vulnerability to assault. Indeed, the earlier a woman is able to detect risk the more options available for her to escape a risky situation or, if necessary, to mount an effective defense (Norris, Zawacki,

T. L. Messman-Moore (✉) · S. R. Salim
Department of Psychology, Miami University, Oxford, OH, USA
e-mail: messmat@miamioh.edu

W. T. O'Donohue et al. (eds.), *Handbook of Sexual Assault and Sexual Assault Prevention*, https://doi.org/10.1007/978-3-030-23645-8_12

Davis, & George, 2018). Research on sexual assault risk factors among women, and the translation of such findings into risk-reduction programs, is a cornerstone of a trauma-informed empowerment programming (DePrince & Gagnon, 2018). Such programs empower women by providing information about sexual assault risk that can inform choices regarding control and safety in interpersonal situations. It is particularly important that interventions include information about contextual and individual factors that increase risk for sexual assault, including risk perception.

Risk perception involves perceived vulnerability for sexual assault among women (i.e., for self and others), as well as contextual and situational factors that involve identifying risk in specific settings and with particular actors. Thus, it is critical to focus on risk perception in relation to sexual assault among women, with one caveat. Such information does not imply, under any circumstances, that women are responsible for sexual assault perpetrated against them. We must hold perpetrators accountable for their actions. Blaming victims for failure to take action to avoid sexual assault is damaging and must be avoided at all costs (see Bhuptani & Messman-Moore, this volume). However, in the absence of effective male-focused prevention programs, research as well as programming aiming to empower women to reduce their risk for sexual assault is warranted.

Because primary prevention efforts with men so far have not proven effective in reducing rates of sexual violence (Gidycz, Orchowski, & Edwards, 2011; Yeater & O'Donohue, 1999), it is imperative that we empower women with the knowledge and skills they can use to identify and respond to sexual victimization risk. Risk-reduction programming efforts with women are effective (Hollander, 2014; Senn et al., 2015). Furthermore, a core component of these programs is to place the responsibility and blame for sexual violence with the perpetrator and not the victims (Hollander, 2016). Contrary to concerns raised by opponents of prevention efforts focused on women, women who experience rape after participation in prevention programs actually evidence reductions in their self-blame and increases in perpetrator blame (Gidycz et al., 2015; Gidycz, Rich, Orchowski, King, & Miller, 2006). Therefore, carefully designed programs that empower women and reinforce that the responsibility and blame for sexual violence lies with perpetrators can be effective in preventing sexual assault, as well as minimize victims' perceptions of self-blame.

Chapter Overview

This chapter presents research on sexual assault and risk perception among women. We first describe different paradigms for research on risk perception. We then focus on studies examining perceived risk for sexual assault and optimistic bias as it pertains to women's understanding of general risk for sexual assault and personal vulnerability. Next, we examine situational risk perception, including research on risk recognition as well as behavioral response to risk. We discuss research on the link between women's alcohol consumption and impaired risk perception, with a particular focus on lab-based analog experiments regarding the role of alcohol intoxication on women's risk recognition and response. Studies of global alcohol consumption and risk perception are also included. Throughout our review of research on risk perception, we discuss the role of previous victimization history and the impact of revictimization on risk perception and related factors. We end the chapter discussing how traumatic distress may influence women's risk recognition and responses, including the unique role of specific forms of psychopathology such as PTSD. We conclude with a critique of the research and suggestions for future investigations.

Definitions and Conceptualization of Risk Perception

Research on risk perception and sexual assault is a broad literature comprised of studies investigating distinct but related concepts. In a review of the literature, Gidycz, McNamara, and Edwards (2006) identified two different areas of risk perception research. The first domain pertains to research examining a more general estimate of perceived vulnerability, whereas the second domain pertains to research on perception of situational risk. Investigations of general estimates of perceived vulnerability assess women's awareness and knowledge of risk factors for sexual assault in general for all women (population-based) and for the self (individual-based). Such investigations examine general risk factors applicable to all women and women's perceived personal risk estimate rating in which individuals estimate the likelihood they will experience sexual victimization in the future (Gidycz et al., 2007). Estimating the likelihood of sexual victimization in general, or indicators of vulnerability for oneself or others, is one manner in which risk perception is assessed directly, explicitly asking participants to identify risk. A second distinct literature examines situational risk perception, with studies focused on women's recognition of risk cues as well as purported behavioral responses to such risk using implicit (as opposed to explicit) methodologies. Implicit methods reduce levels of demand characteristics regarding expected responses or the purpose of the research. Given differences in conceptualization of risk perception and methodology result in a heterogeneous literature, we discuss these two literatures separately.

Perceived Risk for Sexual Assault

Overall, women have high levels of awareness of sexual assault risk and possess knowledge of self-protective behaviors. In addition, women are generally accurate in distinguishing risk for different types of sexual assault (Orchowski, Creech, Reddy, Capezza, & Ratcliff, 2012; Untied, Orchowski, & Lazar, 2013). Women identify greater risk for coercion related to alcohol (or drug) impairment or intoxication compared to other forms of coercion (e.g., physical force, misuse of authority). In one study, 71% of college women thought it was likely they would encounter a man who would deliberately provide alcohol or drugs to increase their level of intoxication in an attempt to engage in sexual intercourse (Orchowski et al., 2012). However, despite consistent research indicating women understand that sexual assault occurs and risk factors for it, women also display complex responses to risky situations. These potentially counterintuitive responses may result from optimistic bias, or factors that impair women's ability to generate effective responses.

Optimistic Bias

In spite of widespread recognition of sexual assault risk, women tend to perceive themselves at relatively lower risk for sexual assault compared to other women (Chapin & Pierce, 2012; Cue, George, & Norris, 1996; Hickman & Muehlenhard, 1997; Norris, Nurius, & Graham, 1999; but not Brown, Messman-Moore, Miller, & Stasser, 2005). The optimistic bias—a discrepancy between perceived risk for others vs. the self—has been demonstrated in relation to numerous negative experiences beyond sexual assault, including intimate partner violence, crime victimization, and cancer (Vitek, Lopez, Ross, Yeater, & Rinehart, 2018). Such beliefs may stem from perceived abilities to handle sexually aggressive encounters. In one study, women reported lower perceived personal vulnerability to future sexual assault because of beliefs that they are uniquely equipped (compared to other women) to respond to such risk (Parks, Miller, Collins, & Zetes-Zanatta, 1998). This discrepancy between acknowledged general vulnerability and perceived personal vulnerability for sexual assault is illustrative of the phenomenon of optimistic bias. In a particularly rigorous study of sexual assault optimistic bias, Yeater, Viken, Hoyt, and Dolan (2009) examined women's perceived vulnerability to sexual assault by experimentally manipulating the participants' perspective in the vignette. Two groups of female college students were randomly assigned to take on the perspective of the self (or others) by imagining herself (or an anonymous woman) in a particular scenario. Results showed evidence of optimistic bias—participants who responded to vignettes written in second person (imagine yourself scenario) estimated lower risk for themselves compared to participants who responded to the same vignette written in the third person (imagine an anonymous woman scenario). Although this difference was statistically significant, women did acknowledge risk for unwanted sexual experiences in the first person vignettes as well as the anonymous woman scenario. Interestingly, differences in risk ratings for the self vs. an anonymous woman emerged for the high-impact vignette scenarios, where the risk for adverse consequences was greatest. These findings suggest that the optimistic bias may come into play in situations that contain *more* risk for adverse outcomes in which women may perceive their own skills to thwart negative experiences from occurring as greater compared to other women. These results provide evidence for the optimistic bias phenomenon, and suggest that the perspective from which women experience a potentially risky scenario affects their assessments of sexual assault risk in experimental or laboratory settings.

Women's optimistic bias for sexual assault risk may be especially problematic if such beliefs inhibit self-protective responses in risky situations. Untied and Dulaney (2015) utilized a video intervention for college women and manipulated perceived similarity to a portrayed sexual assault survivor (the narrator of the video) to test whether perceived similarity affected shifts in optimistic bias. The video intervention significantly reduced optimistic bias, but only for individuals in the high similarity condition (when the sexual assault survivor was of similar age). Furthermore, findings also highlighted that race dissimilarity (between the respondent and portrayed rape victim) may *increase* optimistic bias, as there was a reduction in White participants' optimistic bias from pre- to posttest but an increase for Black participants. Thus, tailored intervention content may only reduce optimistic bias *if* respondents perceive similarity.

History of Sexual Victimization

Perceptions of vulnerability or risk for future sexual assault appears related to women's previous experiences with interpersonal victimization. In general, women who reported never experiencing sexual assault report lower levels of perceived risk for sexual victimization compared to those who have (Orchowski et al., 2012; Untied et al., 2013). This may be because, having already experienced sexual assault, women perceive themselves to be highly similar to a typical victim (Brown et al., 2005). Indeed, a history of sexual assault is associated with women's perceptions of increased vulnerability to future sexual assault (Brown et al., 2005; Norris et al., 1999; Norris, Nurius, & Dimeff, 1996; Orchowski et al., 2012; Untied et al., 2013). Previously victimized women also report lower levels of self-efficacy regarding their ability to respond effectively or assertively to future sexual assault or coercion (Untied et al., 2013). Moreover, previous experience with specific forms of sexual assault are associated with a significantly increased sense of vulnerability *for those same types of sexual assault*, including different unwanted acts (e.g., unwanted sexual contact vs. intercourse), and acts that would occur in particular contexts (e.g., coercion in the context of high levels of intoxication vs. forcible coercion) (Orchowski et al., 2012). However, not all studies have shown that previously victimized women differ from nonvictimized women in terms of perceived risk (Brown et al., 2005; Yeater et al., 2009).

Summary

Research shows that women, while knowledgeable about sexual assault risk, tend to believe their own risk is lower than that of other women. This display of optimistic bias may be amenable to intervention if the victim is more relatable (Helweg-Larsen & Shepperd, 2001; Untied & Dulaney, 2015), although more research is needed in this area. Moreover, women who experienced sexual assault report a heightened sense of vulnerability for future assault, particularly for the same type of assault that occurred earlier, and decreased self-efficacy for effective responses compared to nonvictimized women. However, findings are mixed, and not all research shows this effect among previously victimized women.

Studies that examine perceived personal risk and general vulnerability to sexual assault are important contributions to the risk perception literature. Methodologies that involve explicit instruction to identify risk factors may elicit demand characteristics among participants, influencing the likelihood that research participants will detect risk cues. For example, when researchers give instructions to identify risk cues or label the degree of risk in a situation, then the participant is aware that the researcher is assessing risk perception, or at least is aware that the stimuli presented likely contain risk cues. In order to avoid possible demand characteristics, other methods involve an indirect or implicit approach to infer women's risk perception without directly requesting participants to report on it.

Situational Risk Perception

The assessment of situational risk perception includes two components: risk recognition and risk response (i.e., behavioral response to risk recognition cues) (Messman-Moore & Brown, 2006). Risk recognition can involve the respondent's ability to identify *personal* risk in a risky situation, often indirectly measured by proxy variables such as "feeling uncomfortable" in a potentially risky hypothetical scenario (Breitenbecher, 1999; Messman-Moore & Brown, 2006). Risk recognition can also be assessed from an *observer* perspective. In this case, participants view or listen to stimuli depicting two individuals interacting in a social or intimate situation, and are asked to provide judgments about risk and sexual aggression. Some researchers focus only on risk recognition. However, risk perception also involves a *behavioral response*, or the actions the respondent takes once potential risk is recognized. The ability to recognize risk is important, but the behavioral response of leaving is crucial to reducing victimization risk.

Methodological Considerations

Research on risk perception reflects diverse methodology that typically involve hypothetical vignettes, including those in a written format (Messman-Moore & Brown, 2006; Walsh, DiLillo, & Messman-Moore, 2012; Yeater & Viken, 2010), an audio format (Marx & Gross, 1995; Soler-Baillo, Marx, & Sloan, 2005), or a video format (Breitenbecher, 1999; Parks, Levonyan-Radloff, Dearing, Hequembourg, & Testa, 2016). In addition to differences in presentation format, assessment of risk perception also varies based upon the research participant's perspective (as the participant in the scenario or an observer). Varied approaches involve immersion via instructions to "pretend that you are participating in each activity as it is described" to assess personal risk (Messman-Moore & Brown, 2006, p. 171). Another perspective involves asking participants to listen to interactions between actors and indicate if sexual aggression had occurred (the observer perspective), typically utilizing the Marx vignette (Marx & Gross, 1995). This audio-recording portrays a heterosexual couple interacting, which escalates to sexual assault when the male actor apparently forces sexual behavior despite the female actor's verbal refusal. Within this paradigm, Marx, Calhoun, Wilson, and Meyerson (2001) instructed women to press a button to indicate, "if and when they thought the man has gone too far" (p. 27). This approach assesses situational risk perception via response latency, as longer duration indicates more impaired risk perception to the audio-based scenario.

Empirical Studies of Situational Risk Perception

The majority of studies indicate impaired risk perception is associated with sexual victimization, a pattern robust to the numerous methodological differences across studies. Indeed, poor risk perception is both a correlate and predictor of sexual victimization in multiple studies (Breitenbecher, 2008; Messman-Moore & Brown, 2006; Soler-Baillo et al., 2005; Testa, Livingston, & Collins, 2000; Walsh et al., 2012), although findings are sometimes mixed (see Breitenbecher, 1999). Using a restrictive definition of risk perception as entailing only risk recognition may explain why some studies show no association between sexual victimization and risk perception. Methods that disentangle risk recognition and risk response are useful for this reason. For example, in two different studies of college women using the Risk Perception Survey (a written vignette in which the participant immerses herself), there were no differences between victimized and nonvictimized women with regard to risk recognition. However, sexually victimized women were more likely to exhibit impaired behavioral risk response, that is, delayed responses to a risky scenario with a stranger and another with an acquaintance, staying significantly later in the scenario than women who did not experience sexual victimization (Messman-Moore & Brown, 2006; Walsh et al., 2012). Another study revealed a similar pattern utilizing different vignette methodology with community women (VanZile-Tamsen, Testa, & Livingston, 2005). In that investigation, a history of CSA or adult sexual assault was not related to risk recognition in any of three scenarios (which only varied by perpetrator type—a male friend, a date, or a boyfriend). However, sexually victimized women had lower levels of sexual assertiveness, and were less likely to use active forms of resistance in the hypothetical vignette (i.e., impaired behavioral risk response). A third study of college women that used videotaped vignettes (one with an acquaintance, one with a romantic partner) did not find evidence of a link between sexual victimization (CSA or adult sexual assault) and risk recognition (Breitenbecher, 1999). However, behavioral risk response was not assessed.

Utilizing the audiotaped Marx vignette within the observer paradigm, Soler-Baillo et al. (2005) found that sexually victimized women exhibited significantly longer response latencies relative to nonvictimized women. Thus, conclusions regarding risk perception in cross-sectional studies are complex. Most studies show no relation between sexual victimization and risk recognition, although with some methodologies sexual assault is associated with longer response latencies (indicative of poor risk recognition). More consistently, studies indicate that regardless of risk recognition, impaired behavioral risk response is consistently associated with sexual victimization. Unfortunately, temporal inferences regarding vulnerability or risk for assault are limited given cross-sectional designs, making it difficult to determine if impaired risk perception is a risk factor or outcome of sexual assault.

Two prospective studies, which can demonstrate temporal relations, suggest impaired risk perception increases vulnerability to sexual assault. One prospective study found that impaired risk perception—delayed risk recognition and behavioral response (i.e., indicating that they would stay longer in the vignette scenario)—predicted sexual victimization and rape over an 8-month follow-up (Messman-Moore & Brown, 2006). In addition, Marx et al. (2001) found that delayed response latency (to the Marx vignette) predicted risk for rape during a 2-month follow-up period among college women with a previous history of sexual assault. Prospective studies that examine both risk recognition and behavioral risk response frequently indicate that behavioral response does predict (or was associated with) sexual victimization, even when risk recognition did not. Thus, sexual victimization is a likely outcome as well as a consistent predictor of impaired risk perception in the form of less effective behavioral responses to risk, but is inconsistently associated with situational risk recognition.

Alcohol Consumption and Risk Perception

Alcohol use is often inextricably entwined with sexual assault. Women's risk for sexual assault is associated with the physiological effects of alcohol and the context in which alcohol is consumed, which may include risky social situations with motivated perpetrators (Lorenz & Ullman, 2016). Alcohol-related physiological changes including disruption of higher-order cognitive processes, decreased reaction time, and impaired decision-making (Monks, Tomaka, Palacios, & Thompson, 2010) may significantly increase women's vulnerability for sexual assault through negative impacts on women's risk perception, including interpretation of cues, communication, resistance, and perceptions and responses to threat (Lorenz & Ullman, 2016). In a literature review of risk perception and alcohol intoxication that did not examine sexual assault, Melkonian and Ham (2018) concluded that intoxication does interfere with risk perception in terms of attention to risk cues, appraisal or interpretation of such cues, and generation of behavioral responses. Importantly, alcohol intoxication not only interferes with risk recognition but also may dampen fear associated with perceived risk, which could motivate self-protective action. Such effects may explain how alcohol intoxication influences women's risk perception and responses in risky situations.

There is a growing literature examining the interaction between alcohol use, risk perception, and sexual assault. Women's alcohol use may increase their vulnerability to sexual assault via its impact on reduced risk recognition and impaired responses to potential danger (Davis, Stoner, Norris, George, & Masters, 2009; Parks et al., 2016; Testa, Livingston, VanZile-Tamsen, & Frone, 2003). Moreover, negative effects of alcohol use on risk perception are more pronounced among women who are heavy drinkers or who have a history of sexual assault (e.g., George et al., 2014). Several studies focus on establishing links between alcohol use and risk perception, whereas others examine the association among all variables. Experimental studies involving administration of alcohol in laboratories have helped to establish an understanding of how alcohol intoxication may affect women's ability to perceive risk. In correlational studies, researchers examine associations between risk perception and general alcohol use patterns (or propensity to engage in heavy drinking). Both types of studies contribute valuable and different information to the literature on risk perception and sexual assault.

Alcohol Administration Experiments

Analog designs permit direct observation of the physiological effects of alcohol consumption on women's risk recognition and behavioral responses to sexual assault risk. These studies are valuable because the controlled setting and standardized administration of alcohol permits precise measurement of alcohol-related impairment, and experimental designs permit causal interpretation of risk perception effects when noted. Furthermore, administering doses of alcohol and a placebo beverage in the laboratory allows researchers to control for actual and perceived levels of intoxication. In one such analog study (Testa et al., 2000), alcohol consumption was not related to risk recognition. However, alcohol use did predict riskier behavioral responses. Women who consumed alcohol perceived more benefits and fewer negative consequences of entering a hypothetical risky situation and reported a higher likelihood of participating in potentially risky behaviors such as inviting the man in and engaging in sexual activity with him (e.g., kissing) compared to women who had not consumed alcohol. Moreover, women who consumed alcohol also report lower levels of resistance during a hypothetical sexual assault.

Kelly Cue Davis et al. (2009) conducted two experimental, laboratory-based studies to examine the potential impact of women's alcohol consumption on sexual assault risk perception. Davis et al. then examined women's responses to hypothetical vignettes, which varied level of intimacy with the male depicted in the scenario. Risk perception was assessed in terms of risk appraisals for ambiguous risk cues (e.g., male–female size differential, presence of a male in an isolated setting) and clear risk cues (e.g., sexually aggressive remarks or verbal demands for intercourse, physical restraint). Women intoxicated at low or high levels (BAC = 0.04 or BAC = 0.08) were less aware of the ambiguous risk cues than women who had not had any alcohol; however, both sober and intoxicated women were equally aware of clear risk cues. Intoxicated women's levels of discomfort (i.e., risk recognition) did not increase as risk in the situation became more apparent, in contrast to sober women who reported significantly increased levels of discomfort as clear risk cues (i.e., sexual aggression) in the situation increased. Detection of clear or ambiguous risk cues was unrelated to relationship intimacy depicted in the vignette; however, participants in the established relationship condition reported less discomfort in the presence of clear and ambiguous risk cues. Women who consumed alcohol reported significantly lower risk recognition and impaired behavioral risk response (i.e., anticipated increased compliance with unwanted sexual activity) (Davis et al., 2009; Norris et al., 2006). Findings suggest that alcohol intoxication impairs women's ability to detect specific types of risk cues, and also may numb or dampen women's discomfort and fear in response to such cues.

In another series of laboratory-based experiments, Kathleen Parks et al. (2016) examined women's responses to videos depicting risk cues for sexual assault, and in one study examined risk perception among 60 intoxicated women (BAC = 0.08). Compared to sober participants, intoxicated women were less likely to recognize sexual assault risk cues in the higher risk videos. However, there were no differences between intoxicated and sober women in their intentions to leave the situation. Loiselle and Fuqua (2007) utilized the Marx vignette, and found that women who consumed alcohol had significantly longer response latencies (indicating when the man should stop) than women in the placebo group (who were deceived to believe they had received alcohol when they had not).

Overall, findings from analog studies indicate that alcohol intoxication impairs risk perception in hypothetical scenarios. Moreover, alcohol use decreases the likelihood that women will leave, respond assertively, or engage in resistance. Generalization of these findings is limited given the laboratory setting and the drawback that these studies include older research participants compared to other sexual violence research, given legal mandates regarding administration of alcohol in a laboratory setting. In contrast, risk for college sexual victimization decreases significantly after the first year (Humphrey & White, 2000; Krebs, Lindquist, Warner, Fisher, & Martin, 2009), thus other types of studies are critical to understanding links among alcohol consumption, risk perception, and sexual victimization.

Self-Reported Alcohol Consumption

Researchers have examined risk perception in relation to women's report on their typical consumption patterns for alcohol or other substances (e.g., marijuana, other drugs), as well as self-reported substance-related difficulties, problems, or negative outcomes. Studies regarding general patterns of women's alcohol use (as opposed to in vivo, laboratory administration) in relation to risk perception show consistent, yet complex, relations among variables. Alcohol use is associated with women's perceived vulnerability or risk estimate ratings. Mitchell, MacLeod, and Cassisi (2017) found that women's high levels of problematic alcohol use were associated with *decreased* perceptions of *personal* risk in specific scenarios (e.g., the man's sexual entitlement; the man paying for the date) but *increased* perceptions of *global* risk factors (e.g., social, economic, and environmental conditions that increase risk for sexual assault). In contrast, Gidycz et al. (2007) found women who typically engaged in heavy drinking perceived themselves at greater risk for future sexual assault.

Within the situational risk perception framework, Eshelman, Messman-Moore, and Sheffer (2015) reported that both substance use and substance-related problems were associated with impaired risk perception in college women. In that study, impaired risk perception (risk recognition and behavioral responses) was associated with greater substance use, including higher levels of heavy episodic drinking and marijuana use, higher alcohol tolerance, and more alcohol blackouts. Greater heavy episodic drinking (but not marijuana use) mediated the link between substance-related sexual assault and impaired risk recognition. In contrast, increased alcohol tolerance, higher number of alcohol-related blackouts, and greater heavy episodic drinking and marijuana use mediated the link between substance-related sexual assault and delayed behavioral responses in the risk vignette. In other words, several substance use variables, including heavy consumption levels and negative effects such as blackouts and tolerance may explain why alcohol-related sexual assault is associated with impaired risk recognition and with riskier behavioral responses.

In a study examining both perceived vulnerability and situational risk perception among college women who are regular drinkers, sexual victimization appears to be associated with decreased behavioral response to a risky scenario, partly because victimization is associated with two alcohol-related variables: drinking to cope with anxiety and average weekly alcohol consumption (Neilson et al., 2018). Interestingly, different patterns emerged depending upon conceptualizations of risk perception. In terms of risk estimate ratings, perceived risk for incapacitated sexual assault was *not* directly associated with weekly drinking nor with drinking to cope (in contrast to the findings of Mitchell et al., 2017). However, weekly drinking directly predicted *behavioral response* to the risk vignette (drinking to cope indirectly predicted behavioral response via weekly drinking), consistent with research by Eshelman et al. (2015). These findings suggest that female drinkers with a history of sexual assault are likely to use alcohol to cope with anxiety, and that global levels of alcohol consumption are proximal predictors of decreased behavioral responses in risk scenarios.

Numerous studies examine alcohol use and intoxication in relation to risk perception and sexual victimization. Associations between women's alcohol use and sexual victimization (Fisher, Cullen, & Turner, 2000; Mohler-Kuo, Dowdall, Koss, & Wechsler, 2004), and the impairing effects of alcohol consumption on recognizing sexual aggression risk cues (Abbey, Zawacki, Buck, Clinton, & McAuslan, 2004) have been widely documented. However, more research is needed on how other substances and multiple drug use may influence risk perception and sexual victimization. With the increased legalization of marijuana in the United States, its availability and use are likely to increase and it may be particularly important to assess how marijuana use affects risk perception for sexual victimization.

Summary

Research indicates sexual assault, women's alcohol consumption, and situational risk perception are frequently associated. Laboratory studies indicate that alcohol intoxication consistently impairs behavioral responses to risk, and in some cases, interferes with detection of risk cues. Impairment in risk perception is generally greater among women with histories of sexual victimization and among heavier drinkers. Women's self-reported patterns of alcohol consumption are also associated with impaired risk recognition and risk response, although findings regarding women's typical alcohol use and their perceived personal risk for sexual victimization is mixed. Findings suggest that women who experience sexual assault may drink to cope with anxiety or other distress, and that this type of drinking may be a specific risk factor for sexual assault via impaired risk perception. Additional studies are needed to determine whether women's alcohol use and intoxication affects risk perception in all scenarios, and whether specific forms of sexual assault, such as alcohol-related or incapacitated assaults, are more likely to be linked to both risk perception deficits and hazardous substance use.

The Importance of Context in Risk Perception

Sexual victimization occurs in a sociocultural context amid situational factors that inevitably influence women's risk perception, including risk recognition, risk appraisals, and decisions regarding their subsequent behaviors. The Cognitive Ecological Model framework proposed by Nurius and Norris (1996) emphasizes the importance of contextual factors in women's risk recognition and response, focusing on two types of cognitive appraisals: primary and secondary. In this model, risk recognition is a component of primary appraisals, which refer to an initial assessment of a situation as either neutral, posing benefit, or posing threat, and lead to women's detection of risk for victimization. Once a woman identifies that she may be in a dangerous situation, she engages in secondary appraisals to further determine the nature of the threat, as well as assess her ability to respond to the threat and the response options available to her. These secondary appraisals also involve assessment of the potential consequences of each response, thus influencing her decision-making process and ultimate behavioral response. This theory suggests that women are processing two related but distinct issues, the detection of risk, and then a relative risk-benefit analysis of responding to risk with particular strategies. Research disentangling risk recognition from risk response falls within this framework.

The social context, including relationship to a potential perpetrator, may affect risk recognition. Although women acknowledge acquaintance rape is more common than stranger rape, they generally fear stranger rape more (Hickman & Muehlenhard, 1997). Davis et al. (2009) found that women had greater awareness of risk in vignettes with an acquaintance or casual date than with a man in an established dating relationship, and that women's drinking amplified this difference. A history of sexual assault or childhood sexual abuse influences women's cognitive appraisals in ways that may lead to less effective responses to risk of sexual victimization. For example, women with victimization histories appear to have higher thresholds for classifying a situation as risky, and thus need more clear risk cues in the environment for their primary cognitive appraisals of risk (Yeater, Treat, Viken, & McFall, 2010). More severely victimized women may prioritize the potential costs to popularity when considering responses to risk (Yeater et al., 2010; Yeater, Treat, Viken, & Lenberg, 2018). Thus, social aspects of situations (i.e. fear of losing social acceptance of peers/men) may impede women's assessment of risk or affect behavioral responses to risk cues.

Contextual factors also influence women's decisions regarding how to respond after risk is detected. Women's social and intimacy goals affect their risk appraisals in the relational context, and some appraisals may hinder women's ability to form effective responses to sexual victimization risk. According to VanZile-Tamsen et al. (2005), women's reported likelihood of direct verbal and physical resistance responses to a vignette decreased as the level of prior intimacy with a potential perpetrator increased. Secondary cognitive appraisals that may inhibit self-protective behavioral responses in risky situations include fear of rejection (by the man or by one's peers), a desire for social acceptance or popularity, self-consciousness, and fear of physical injury (Norris et al., 1996; Nurius, Norris, Young, Graham, & Gaylord, 2000; Stoner et al., 2007).

Sexual Assault Characteristics and Risk Perception

History of sexual victimization appears to influence risk perception, particularly secondary cognitive appraisals and behavioral responses. For example, women who experienced childhood sexual abuse believe they have less control in sexual situations, which is associated with alcohol consumption to alleviate sexual anxiety (Walsh et al., 2013). Women with sexual victimization histories also differ in the perceived social benefits (e.g., affection) or negative social consequences if they reject men's sexual advances that may lead them to be less assertive in their responses to risk (Porter, Koch, Saules, & Sexton, 2015). Furthermore, appraisals related to embarrassment, fear of rejection, and the impairing effects of alcohol may be more likely to interfere with assertive responding in victims compared to nonvictims (Nurius, Norris, Dimeff, & Graham, 1996; Stoner et al., 2007).

Severity of sexual assault and type of sexual coercion appears to influence the association between sexual assault and risk perception. Risk recognition is more likely to be associated with more severe forms of sexual assault. Earlier studies with broad definitions of victimization including noncontact experiences (such as exhibitionism) or low-level severity acts (e.g., kissing) (Breitenbecher, 1999; Cue et al., 1996), are less likely to show an association between sexual victimization and risk perception, whereas studies comparing types of victimization show significant associations for rape but not verbally coerced intercourse (Marx et al., 2001). Related, some researchers claim that risk perception is more relevant to particular forms of sexual assault, namely alcohol- or substance-related sexual assault. Eshelman et al. (2015) reported that only substance-related sexual assault, and not forcible assault, was associated with risk perception (decreased risk recognition and decreased behavioral responses) assessed with a written vignette. Thus, the link between risk perception and sexual assault appears to vary in relation to characteristics of sexual assault, factors that may explain mixed findings in the current literature.

Revictimization and Risk Perception

Researchers generally conceptualize the relationship between sexual assault and risk perception in two ways: (1) risk perception deficits as a risk factor for subsequent assault, or (2) risk perception as an outcome of previous victimization. Both explanations are plausible, especially given most studies are cross-sectional, which prohibits inferences regarding proximal relations among variables. An additional consideration is that repeated sexual assault or sexual revictimization may show unique, significant relations with impaired risk perception as well as explain earlier disparate findings across multiple studies. When studies examine revictimization, researchers find more nuanced and complex relationships. Wilson, Calhoun, and Bernat (1999) found that women who experienced revictimization (i.e., repeated sexual assault) show more impaired risk recognition compared to women who experience a single sexual assault or to nonvictims. However, Yeater and O'Donohue (2002) found that single-incident victims took significantly longer than nonvictims and revictimized women (multiple-incident victims) to be trained to recognize risk. In the only prospective research in this area, impaired risk perception predicted sexual revictimization, and was more impaired among these women. Messman-Moore and Brown (2006) reported that *revictimized* women demonstrated *worse* risk recognition, but sexually victimized women reported *better* risk recognition than nonvictims. Women with childhood victimization only identified threat cues significantly earlier in the vignette than did revictimized women or women without a history of sexual victimization. They theorize that women sexually abused during childhood (but who were *not* revictimized) may actually be more sensitive or alert to potential danger cues, and that this sensitization may serve to buffer risk for future revictimization.

Most research on risk perception focuses on college samples, but a recent cross-sectional study examined the impact of revictimization on risk recognition among female psychiatric inpatients in Germany (Bockers, Roepke, Michael, Renneberg, & Knaevelsrud, 2014). Risk recognition was significantly more impaired among women experiencing revictimization (two or more incidents of interpersonal violence [sexual or physical maltreatment] across two distinct developmental periods [i.e., childhood, adolescence, or adulthood]) compared to women experiencing victimization (sexual or physical maltreatment) during childhood or adolescence only. Moreover, risk recognition was a significant predictor of revictimization in a multivariate model. These findings extend research on risk perception and victimization to include different types of interpersonal violence, and importantly study risk perception among women beyond a college sample, in this case female psychiatric inpatients.

Traumatic Distress and Risk Perception

Several consequences of sexual assault and childhood sexual abuse may be relevant to risk perception (DePrince & Gagnon, 2018). Neurocognitive correlates of victimization such as executive functioning deficits (e.g., difficulties sustaining or directing attention, conflict-monitoring; Stein, Kennedy, & Twamley, 2002) will likely negatively affect recognition of risk, as well as interfere with the ability to engage effective and assertive behavioral risk responses (DePrince & Gagnon, 2018). Diminished executive control and attention may explain links between risk perception and emotional consequences of sexual victimization, including depression, dissociation, anxiety, and PTSD. Emotion dysregulation, particularly lack of emotion regulation strategies and impulsive behavior when distressed, is one mechanism underlying the association between lifetime sexual victimization and impaired risk perception, and appears to increase vulnerability for revictimization (Walsh et al., 2012). Moreover, global emotion dysregulation is associated with impaired risk perception as well, but was not associated with revictimization or frequency of sexual assault (Carlson & Duckworth, 2016).

Psychological distress associated with sexual victimization such as symptoms of PTSD impact women's ability to detect risk (e.g., Wilson et al., 1999; Yeater, Hoyt, Leiting, & Lopez, 2016). According to Gidycz, Rich, et al. (2006), specific aspects of PTSD such as dissociative and numbing symptoms of PTSD decrease overall levels of awareness, which may translate into impaired risk recognition, whereas intrusive thoughts about prior trauma may impair attention to outside cues that signal potential risk toward individuals. Wilson et al. (1999) found that women with elevated hyperarousal symptoms reported better risk recognition, thus some facets of PTSD may increase sensitivity to threat cues. However, clinical levels of distress associated with PTSD hyperarousal may result in less confidence in risk recognition abilities, leading to a decreased likelihood of self-protective responses when risk is detected (Messman-Moore & Resick, 2002).

Distress may also affect how women respond to risk. In one study of 334 college women, symptoms of PTSD were negatively associated with women's generation of self-protective responses to a hypothetical scenario, as well as their perceived efficacy to engage in self-protection (Yeater et al., 2016). Importantly, however, this finding held only for non-Hispanic white women, and was not significant for Hispanic women. Moreover, Messman-Moore and Brown (2006) failed to find cross-sectional or prospective associations between psychological distress and risk perception, perhaps because they assessed general traumatic stress rather than PTSD symptoms specifically.

At least one study suggests that different forms of psychological distress may show unique associations with risk recognition, finding differences between PTSD and depression, for example. Volkert, Randjbar, Moritz, and Jelinek (2013) examined risk recognition among German victims of trauma (defined as exposure to any type of potentially traumatic experience meeting both DSM-IV Criterion A1 and A2) across a variety of scenarios using the Marx audiotape vignette (Marx & Gross, 1995). Results indicated that higher levels of PTSD symptoms were associated with more impaired risk recognition, whereas higher levels of depressive symptoms were associated with less impaired risk recognition (an apparent buffering effect). Because trauma experience and risk scenarios reflected heterogeneous trauma types in the Volkert study, we may not be able to apply these results unequivocally to our understanding of risk perception and sexual assault. However, such findings should prompt additional research in this area.

Conclusions

Impaired risk perception is frequently associated with sexual assault. Although more research is needed, there is preliminary evidence risk perception is a risk factor for future sexual victimization. Associations between sexual assault and risk perception are consistent across studies for impaired risk response, whereas results regarding risk recognition are often mixed. Unfortunately, few studies utilizing prospective designs are available, thus we know less about causal and proximal relations, or how risk perception and sexual assault may influence one another. Factors such as the severity of sexual assault and the presence of sexual revictimization appear to influence risk perception, with more severe and extensive sexual violence associated with more impairment in detecting and responding to risk cues. Psychological distress related to victimization—particularly PTSD symptoms—is associated with impaired risk perception, and may explain why women with more extensive sexual assault histories typically demonstrate more impaired risk perception.

Future studies should utilize prospective designs to examine mediators and moderators of the link between sexual assault and risk perception. Additional studies focused on the role of alcohol use and intoxication in relation to both risk perception and sexual assault will help to clarify relevant mechanisms. We must design new studies to clarify whether specific types of sexual assault show stronger associations to risk perception via alcohol intoxication or substance use problems. The research to date using vignette methods has focused exclusively on heterosexual interactions within a female-victim male-perpetrator paradigm with predominantly White samples, limiting generalization of findings to more ethnically and racially diverse samples and for trans-women, lesbians, and bisexual women. Research indicates that racial/ethnic, gender, and sexual minority populations experience increased rates of sexual victimization (Coulter et al., 2017; Rennison & Rand, 2003; Rothman, Exner, & Baughman, 2011; Stotzer, 2009; Walters, Chen, & Breiding, 2013). Further, gender and sexual minority populations experience higher rates of depression, PTSD, and substance use (Balsam, Beauchaine, Mickey, & Rothblum, 2005; Cochran, Mays, Alegria, Ortega, & Takeuchi, 2007; Roberts, Austin, Corliss, Vandermorris, & Koenen, 2010) that may impact risk perception. Finally, some differences in risk perception and sexual victimization are associated with ethnic and racial identity (Rinehart, Yeater, Musci, Letourneau, & Lenberg, 2014; Untied & Dulaney, 2015; Yeater et al., 2016). Therefore, it is important to continue examining and clarifying how the experiences of minority populations may be related to risk perception. It is also of interest to expand research regarding the link between psychological distress and risk perception among victims, in order to identify relative buffering vs. impairment effects of distress on risk perception (e.g., for distinct clusters of PTSD symptoms), and whether different types of distress affect risk perception in unique ways (e.g., PTSD vs. depression). Random clinical trials investigating efficacy of treatment for PTSD among sexual assault survivors should also assess risk perception to determine whether effective PTSD treatment will ameliorate deficits in risk perception, decreasing risk for subsequent revictimization.

Lest we forget, we must leave this topic with a reminder: victims are not responsible for their sexual assault. Even if a woman has impaired risk perception, or fails to take what from an omnipotent view is the most effective self-protective response, we must not blame her for sexual assault. Women who experience blaming responses upon rape disclosure experience heightened levels of shame, which lead to PTSD and depression (Bhuptani, Kaufman, Messman-Moore, Gratz, & DiLillo, 2019; DeCou, Cole, Lynch, Wong, & Matthews, 2017). As a society, it is imperative that we shift the focus of responsibility for sexual assault back to the perpetrator and attend to the needs of victims by providing education, support, and encouragement for recovery.

References

Abbey, A., Zawacki, T., Buck, P. O., Clinton, M. A., & McAuslan, P. (2004). Sexual assault and alcohol consumption: What do we know about their relationship and what types of research are still needed. *Aggression and Violent Behavior, 9*, 271–303.

Balsam, K. F., Beauchaine, T. P., Mickey, R. M., & Rothblum, E. D. (2005). Mental health of lesbian, gay, bisexual, and heterosexual siblings: Effects of gender, sexual orientation, and family. *Journal of Abnormal Psychology, 114*, 471–476.

Banyard, V. L. (2013). Go big or go home: Reaching for a more integrated view of violence prevention. *Psychology of Violence, 3*, 115–120. https://doi.org/10.1037/a0032289

Berkowitz, A. (2002). Fostering men's responsibility for preventing sexual assault. In American Psychological Association (Ed.), *Preventing violence in relationships: Interventions across the life span* (pp. 163–196). Washington, DC: APA Publishing.

Bhuptani, P. H., Kaufman, J. S., Messman-Moore., T. L., Gratz, K. L. & DiLillo, D. (2019). Rape disclosure and depression among community women: The mediating roles of shame and experiential avoidance. *Violence Against Women, 25*, 1226–1242. https://doi.org/10.1177/1077801218811683

Black, M. C., Basile, K. C., Breiding, M. J., Smith, S. G., Walters, M. L., Merrick, M. T., … Stevens, M. R. (2011). The national intimate partner and sexual violence survey: 2010 summary report. The Centers of Disease Control and Prevention, National Center for Injury Prevention and Control. Retrieved January 22, 2019 from http://www.cdc.gov/ViolencePrevention/pdf/NISVS_Report2010-a.pdf

Bockers, E., Roepke, S., Michael, L., Renneberg, B., & Knaevelsrud, C. (2014). Risk recognition, attachment anxiety, self-efficacy, and state dissociation predict revictimization. *PLoS One, 9*(9), e108206.

Breitenbecher, K. H. (1999). The association between the perception of threat in a dating situation and sexual victimization. *Violence and Victims, 14*, 135–146. Retrieved from http://psycnet.apa.org/record/1999-03303-001

Breitenbecher, K. H. (2008). The convergent validities of two measures of dating behaviors related to risk for sexual victimization. *Journal of Interpersonal Violence, 23*, 1095–1107. https://doi.org/10.1177/088626050731397

Brown, A. L., Messman-Moore, T. L., Miller, A. G., & Stasser, G. (2005). Sexual victimization in relation to perceptions of risk: Mediation, generalization, and temporal stability. *Personality and Social Psychology Bulletin, 31*, 963–976.

Carlson, G. C., & Duckworth, M. P. (2016). Sexual victimization and benefit expectations of risky behavior among female college students. *Journal of Interpersonal Violence, 34*, 1543. https://doi.org/10.1177/0886260516651626

Chapin, J. R., & Pierce, M. (2012). Optimistic bias, sexual assault, and fear. *The Journal of General Psychology, 139*, 19–28. https://doi.org/10.1080/00221309.2011.635724

Cochran, S. D., Mays, V. M., Alegria, M., Ortega, A. N., & Takeuchi, D. (2007). Mental health and substance use disorders among Latina/o and Asian American lesbian, gay, and bisexual adults. *Journal of Consulting and Clinical Psychology, 75*, 785–794.

Coulter, R. W. S., Mair, C., Miller, E., Blosnich, J. R., Matthews, D. D., & McCauley, H. L. (2017). Prevalence of past-year sexual assault victimization among undergraduate students: Exploring differences by and intersections of gender identity, sexual identity, and race/ethnicity. *Prevention Science, 18*, 726–736. https://doi.org/10.1007/s11121-017-0762-8

Cue, K. L., George, W. H., & Norris, J. (1996). Women's appraisals of sexual-assault risk in dating situations. *Psychology of Women Quarterly, 20*, 487–504. https://doi.org/10.1111/j.1471-6402.1996.tb00318.x

Davis, K., Stoner, S., Norris, J., George, W., & Masters, T. (2009). Women's awareness of and discomfort with sexual assault cues: Effects of alcohol consumption and relationship type. *Violence Against Women, 15*, 1106–1125. https://doi.org/10.1177/1077801209340759

DeCou, C. R., Cole, T. T., Lynch, S. M., Wong, M. M., & Matthews, K. C. (2017). Assault-related shame mediates the association between negative social reactions to disclosure of sexual assault and psychological distress. *Psychological Trauma: Theory, Research,. Practice, and Policy, 9*, 166–172. https://doi.org/10.1037/tr000018

DePrince, A. P., & Gagnon, K. L. (2018). Understanding the consequences of sexual assault: What does it mean for prevention to be trauma informed? In L. Orchowski & C. Gidycz (Eds.), *Sexual assault risk reduction and resistance* (pp. 15–30). Amsterdam: Elsevier. https://doi.org/10.1016/B978-0-12-805389-8.00002-5

Dworkin, E. R., Menon, S. V., Bystrynski, J., & Allen, N. E. (2017). Sexual assault victimization and psychopathology: A review and meta-analysis. *Clinical Psychology Review, 56*, 65–81.

Eshelman, L. R., Messman-Moore, T. L., & Sheffer, N. (2015). The importance of substance-related sexual victimization impact on substance use and risk perception in female college students. *Journal of Interpersonal Violence, 30*, 2616–2635. https://doi.org/10.1177/0886260514553630

Fisher, B. S., Cullen, F. T., & Turner, M. G. (2000). *The sexual victimization of college women.* Washington, DC: U.S. Department of Justice, National Institute of Justice and Bureau of Justice Statistics.

George, W. H., Davis, K. C., Masters, N. T., Jacques-Tiaura, A. J., Heiman, J. R., Norris, J., … Andrasik, M. P. (2014). Sexual victimization, alcohol intoxication, sexual-emotional responding, and sexual risk in heavy episodic drinking women. *Archives of Sexual Behavior, 43*, 645–658. https://doi.org/10.1007/s10508-013-0143-8

Gidycz, C. A., Loh, C., Lobo, T., Rich, C., Lynn, S. J., & Pashdag, J. (2007). Reciprocal relationships among alcohol use, risk perception, and sexual victimization: A prospective analysis. *Journal of American College Health, 56*, 5–14. https://doi.org/10.3200/JACH.56.1.5-14

Gidycz, C. A., McNamara, J. R., & Edwards, K. M. (2006). Women's risk perception and sexual victimization: A review of the literature. *Aggression and Violent Behavior, 11*, 441–456. https://doi.org/10.1016/j.avb.2006.01.004

Gidycz, C. A., Orchowski, L. M., & Edwards, K. M. (2011). Primary prevention of sexual violence. In M. Koss & J. White (Eds.), *Violence against women and children: Navigating solutions* (Vol. 2, pp. 159–179). Washington, DC: American Psychological Association.

Gidycz, C. A., Orchowski, L. M., Probst, D. R., Edwards, K. M., Murphy, M., & Tansill, E. (2015). Concurrent administration of sexual assault prevention and risk reduction programming outcomes for women. *Violence Against Women, 21*, 780–800. https://doi.org/10.1177/1077801215576579

Gidycz, C. A., Rich, C. L., Orchowski, L. M., King, C., & Miller, A. K. (2006). The evaluation of a sexual assault self-defense and risk-reduction program for college women: A prospective study. *Psychology of Women Quarterly, 30*, 173–186. https://doi.org/10.1111/j.1471-6402.2006.00280.x

Helweg-Larsen, M., & Shepperd, J. A. (2001). Do moderators of the optimistic bias affect personal or target risk estimates? A review of the literature. *Personality and Social Psychology Review, 5*, 74–95. https://doi.org/10.1207/S15327957PSPR0501_5

Hickman, S. E., & Muehlenhard, C. L. (1997). College women's fears and precautionary behaviors relating to acquaintance rape and stranger rape. *Psychology of Women Quarterly, 21*, 527–547.

Hollander, J. A. (2014). Does self-defense training prevent sexual violence against women? *Violence Against Women, 20*, 252–269. https://doi.org/10.1177/1077801214526046

Hollander, J. A. (2016). The importance of self-defense training for sexual violence prevention. *Feminism & Psychology, 26*, 207–226. https://doi.org/10.1177/0959353516637393

Humphrey, J. A., & White, J. W. (2000). Women's vulnerability to sexual assault from adolescence to young adulthood. *Journal of Adolescent Health, 27*, 419–424. https://doi.org/10.1016/S1054-139X(00)00168-3

Krebs, C., Lindquist, C., Berzofsky, M., Shook-Sa, B., & Peterson, K. (2016). Campus climate survey validation study final technical report. Bureau of Justice Statistics Research and Development Series. Retrieved January 22, 2019 from https://www.bjs.gov/content/pub/pdf/ccsvsftr.pdf

Krebs, C. P., Lindquist, C. H., Warner, T. D., Fisher, B. S., & Martin, S. L. (2009). College women's experiences with physically forced, alcohol- or other drug-enabled, and drug- facilitated sexual assault before and since entering college. *Journal of American College Health, 57*, 639–647. https://doi.org/10.3200/jach.57.6.639-649

Loiselle, M., & Fuqua, W. R. (2007). Alcohol's effects on women's risk detection in a date- rape vignette. *Journal of American College Health, 55*, 261–266. https://doi.org/10.3200/JACH.55.5.261-266

Lorenz, K., & Ullman, S. E. (2016). Alcohol and sexual assault victimization: Research findings and future directions. *Aggression and Violent Behavior, 31*, 82–94. https://doi.org/10.1016/j.avb.2016.08.001

Marx, B. P., Calhoun, K. S., Wilson, A. E., & Meyerson, L. A. (2001). Sexual revictimization prevention: An outcome evaluation. *Journal of Consulting and Clinical Psychology, 69*, 25–32. https://doi.org/10.1037/0022-006X.69.1.25

Marx, B. P., & Gross, A. M. (1995). Date rape: An analysis of two contextual variables. *Behavior Modification, 19*, 451–463. https://doi.org/10.1177/01454455950194003

McGinnis, M. (2016). *The female of the species*. New York: Harper Collins.

Melkonian, A. J., & Ham, L. S. (2018). The effects of alcohol intoxication on young adult women's identification of risk for sexual assault: A systematic review. *Psychology of Addictive Behaviors, 32*, 163–172. https://doi.org/10.1037/adb0000349

Messman-Moore, T. L., & Brown, A. L. (2006). Risk perception, rape, and sexual revictimization: A prospective study of college women. *Psychology of Women Quarterly, 30*, 159–172. https://doi.org/10.1111/j.1471-6402.2006.00279.x

Messman-Moore, T. L., & Resick, P. A. (2002). Brief treatment of complicated PTSD and peritraumatic responses in a client with repeated sexual victimization. *Cognitive and Behavioral Practice, 9*(2), 89–99.

Mitchell, J. C., MacLeod, B. P., & Cassisi, J. E. (2017). Modeling sexual assault risk perception among heterosexual college females: The impact of previous victimization, alcohol use, and coping style. *Violence Against Women, 23*, 143–162. https://doi.org/10.1177/1077801216638767

Mohler-Kuo, M., Dowdall, G. W., Koss, M. P., & Wechsler, H. (2004). Correlates of rape while intoxicated in a national sample of college women. *Journal of Studies on Alcohol, 65*, 37–45.

Monks, S. M., Tomaka, J., Palacios, R., & Thompson, S. E. (2010). Sexual assault in female and male college students: Examining the roles of alcohol use, alcohol expectancies, and sexual sensation seeking. *Substance Use & Misuse, 45*, 2258–2280. https://doi.org/10.3109/10826081003694854

Moynihan, M. M., Banyard, V. L., Cares, A. C., Potter, S. J., Williams, L. M., & Stapleton, J. G. (2015). Encouraging responses in sexual and relationship violence prevention: What program effects remain one year later. *Journal of Interpersonal Violence, 30*, 110–132. https://doi.org/10.1177/0886260514532719

Neilson, E. C., Bird, E. R., Metzger, I. W., George, W. H., Norris, J., & Gilmore, A. K. (2018). Understanding sexual assault risk perception in college: Associations among sexual assault history, drinking to cope, and alcohol use. *Addictive Behaviors, 78*, 178–186. https://doi.org/10.1016/j.addbeh.2017.11.022

Norris, J., George, W. H., Stoner, S. A., Masters, N. T., Zawacki, T., & Davis, K. C. (2006). Women's responses to sexual aggression: The effects of childhood trauma, alcohol, and prior relationship. *Experimental and Clinical Psychopharmacology, 14*, 402–411. https://doi.org/10.1037/1064-1297.14.3.402

Norris, J., Nurius, P. S., & Dimeff, L. A. (1996). Through her eyes: Factors affecting women's perception of and resistance to acquaintance sexual aggression threat. *Psychology of Women Quarterly, 20*, 123–145.

Norris, J., Nurius, P. S., & Graham, T. L. (1999). When a date changes from fun to dangerous: Factors affecting women's ability to distinguish. *Violence Against Women, 5*, 230–250. https://doi.org/10.1177/10778019922181202

Norris, J., Zawacki, T., Davis, K. C., & George, W. H. (2018). The role of psychological barriers in women's resistance to sexual assault by acquaintances. In L. Orchowski & C. Gidycz (Eds.), *Sexual Assault Risk Reduction and Resistance* (pp. 87–110). Elsevier. https://doi.org/10.1016/B978-0-12-805389-8.00002-5

Nurius, P. S., & Norris, J. (1996). A cognitive ecological model of women's response to male sexual coercion in dating. *Journal of Psychology and Human Sexuality, 8*, 117–139. https://doi.org/10.1300/JO56v08n01-09

Nurius, P. S., Norris, J., Dimeff, L. A., & Graham, T. L. (1996). Expectations regarding acquaintance sexual aggression among sorority and fraternity members. *Sex Roles, 35*, 427–444.

Nurius, P. S., Norris, J., Young, D. S., Graham, T. L., & Gaylord, J. (2000). Interpreting and defensively responding to threat: Examining appraisals and coping with acquaintance sexual aggression. *Violence and Victims, 15*, 187–208.

Orchowski, L. M., Creech, S. K., Reddy, M. K., Capezza, N. M., & Ratcliff, T. (2012). College women's perceived risk to experience sexual victimization: A prospective analysis. *Violence and Victims, 27*, 194–214. https://doi.org/10.1891/0886-6708.27.2.194

Parks, K. A., Levonyan-Radloff, K., Dearing, R. L., Hequembourg, A., & Testa, M. (2016). Development and validation of a video measure for assessing women's risk perception for alcohol-related sexual assault. *Psychology of Violence, 6*, 573–585. https://doi.org/10.1037/a0039846

Parks, K. A., Miller, B. A., Collins, R. L., & Zetes-Zanatta, L. (1998). Women's descriptions of drinking in bars: Reasons and risks. *Sex Roles, 38*, 701–717.

Porter, K. E., Koch, E. I., Saules, K., & Sexton, M. B. (2015). The impact of sexual assault history on perceived consequences of risky dating scenarios. *Acta Psychopathologica, 1*(4), 1–9.

Rennison, C. M., & Rand, M. R. (2003). *Bureau of justice statistics national crime victimization survey: Criminal victimization, 2002* (NCJ 199994). Retrieved from Bureau of Justice Statistics website http://www.bjs.gov/content/pub/pdf/cv02.pdf

Rinehart, J. K., Yeater, E. A., Musci, R. J., Letourneau, E. J., & Lenberg, K. L. (2014). The role of ethnicity, sexual attitudes, and sexual behavior in sexual revictimization during the transition to emerging adulthood. *Child Maltreatment, 19*, 178–187. https://doi.org/10.1177/1077559514551946

Roberts, A. L., Austin, S. B., Corliss, H. L., Vandermorris, A. K., & Koenen, K. C. (2010). Pervasive trauma exposure among US sexual orientation minority adults and risk of posttraumatic stress disorder. *American Journal of Public Health, 100*, 2433–2441. https://doi.org/10.2105/AJPH.2009.168971

Rothman, E. F., Exner, D., & Baughman, A. L. (2011). The prevalence of sexual assault against people who identify as gay, lesbian, or bisexual in the United States: A systematic review. *Trauma, Violence & Abuse, 12*, 55–66. https://doi.org/10.1177/1524838010390707

Senn, C. Y., Eliasziw, M., Barata, P. C., Thurston, W. E., Newby-Clark, I. R., Radtke, H. L., & Hobden, K. L. (2015). Efficacy of a sexual assault resistance program for university women. *New England Journal of Medicine, 372*, 2326–2335. https://doi.org/10.1056/NEJMsa1411131

Soler-Baillo, J. M., Marx, B. P., & Sloan, D. M. (2005). The psychophysiological correlates of risk recognition among victims and non-victims of sexual assault. *Behaviour Research and Therapy, 43*, 169–181. https://doi.org/10.1016/j.brat.2004.01.004

Stein, M. B., Kennedy, C. M., & Twamley, E. W. (2002). Neuropsychological function in female victims of intimate partner violence with and without posttraumatic stress disorder. *Biological Psychiatry, 52*, 1079–1088. https://doi.org/10.1016/j.psychres.2004.01.008

Stoner, S. A., Norris, J., George, W. H., Davis, K. C., Masters, N. T., & Hessler, D. M. (2007). Effects of alcohol intoxication and victimization history on women's sexual assault resistance strategies: The role of secondary cognitive appraisals. *Psychology of Women Quarterly, 31*, 344–356.

Stotzer, R. L. (2009). Violence against transgender people: A review of United States data. *Aggression and Violent Behavior, 14*, 170–179. https://doi.org/10.1016/j.avb.2009.01.006

Testa, M., Livingston, J. A., & Collins, R. L. (2000). The role of women's alcohol consumption in evaluation of vulnerability to sexual aggression. *Experimental and Clinical Psychopharmacology, 8*, 185. https://doi.org/10.1037/1064-1297.8.2.185

Testa, M., Livingston, J. A., VanZile-Tamsen, C., & Frone, M. R. (2003). The role of women's substance use in vulnerability to forcible and incapacitated rape. *Journal of Studies on Alcohol, 64*, 756–764. https://doi.org/10.15288/jsa.2003.64.756

Untied, A. S., & Dulaney, C. L. (2015). College students' perceived risk of sexual victimization and the role of optimistic bias. *Journal of Interpersonal Violence, 30*, 1417–1431. https://doi.org/10.1177/0886260514540326

Untied, A. S., Orchowski, L. M., & Lazar, V. L. (2013). College men's and women's respective perceptions of risk to perpetrate or experience sexual assault: The role of alcohol use and expectancies. *Violence Against Women, 19*, 903–923. https://doi.org/10.1177/1077801213498216

VanZile-Tamsen, C., Testa, M., & Livingston, J. A. (2005). The impact of sexual assault history and relationship context on appraisal of and responses to acquaintance sexual assault risk. *Journal of Interpersonal Violence, 20*, 813–832. https://doi.org/10.1177/0886260505276071

Vitek, K. N., Lopez, G., Ross, R., Yeater, E. A., & Rinehart, J. K. (2018). Women's appraisals of victimization risk: Current status, methodological challenges, and future directions. In L. Orchowski & C. Gidycz (Eds.), *Sexual assault risk reduction and resistance* (pp. 67–86). Amsterdam: Elsevier. https://doi.org/10.1016/B978-0-12-805389-8.0004-9

Volkert, J., Randjbar, S., Moritz, S., & Jelinek, L. (2013). Risk recognition and sensation seeking in revictimization and posttraumatic stress disorder. *Behavior Modification, 37*, 39–61. https://doi.org/10.1177/0145445512449647

Walsh, K., Messman-Moore, T. L., Zerubavel, N., Chandley, R. B., DeNardi, K. A., & Walker, D. P. (2013). Perceived sexual control, sex-related alcohol expectancies and behavior predict substance-related sexual revictimization. *Child Abuse & Neglect, 37*, 353–359.

Walsh, K. L., DiLillo, D., & Messman-Moore, T. L. (2012). Lifetime sexual victimization and poor risk perception: Does emotion dysregulation account for the links? *Journal of Interpersonal Violence, 27*, 3054–3071. https://doi.org/10.1177/0886260512441081

Walters, M. L., Chen, J., & Breiding, M. J. (2013). *The National Intimate Partner and Sexual Violence Survey (NISVS): 2010 findings on victimization by sexual orientation*. Atlanta, GA: National Center for Injury Prevention and Control, Centers for Disease Control and Prevention.

Wilson, A. E., Calhoun, K. S., & Bernat, J. A. (1999). Risk recognition and trauma-related symptoms among sexually revictimized women. *Journal of Consulting and Clinical Psychology, 67*, 705–710. https://doi.org/10.1037/0022-006X.67.5.705

Wright, L. A., Zounlome, N. O. O., & Whiston, S. C. (2018). The effectiveness of male-targeted sexual assault prevention programs: A meta-analysis. *Trauma, Violence, & Abuse*, 1524838018801330. https://doi.org/10.1177/1524838018801330

Yeater, E. A., Hoyt, T., Leiting, K. A., & Lopez, G. (2016). Association between sexual victimization history, posttraumatic stress symptoms, and women's decision making in risky social situations: The moderating role effect of ethnicity. *Journal of Psychopathological Behavior, 38*, 666–680. https://doi.org/10.1007/s10862-016-9557-7

Yeater, E. A., & O'Donohue, W. T. (1999). Sexual assault prevention programs: Current issues, future directions, and the potential efficacy of interventions with women. *Clinical Psychology Review, 19*, 739–771.

Yeater, E. A., & O'Donohue, W. T. (2002). Sexual revictimization: The relationship among knowledge, risk perception, and ability to respond to high-risk situations. *Journal of Interpersonal Violence, 17*, 1135–1144.

Yeater, E. A., Treat, T. A., Viken, R. J., & Lenberg, K. L. (2018). Sexual attitudes moderate the effects of alcohol intoxication on women's risk judgments. *Journal of Interpersonal Violence, 33*(2), 228–249. https://doi.org/10.1177/0886260515604414

Yeater, E. A., Treat, T. A., Viken, R. J., & McFall, R. M. (2010). Cognitive processes underlying women's risk judgments: Associations with sexual victimization history and rape myth acceptance. *Journal of Consulting and Clinical Psychology, 78*, 375–386.

Yeater, E. A., Viken, R. J., Hoyt, T., & Dolan, J. L. (2009). Self-other perspective and sexual attitudes affect estimates of sexual risk. *Sex Roles, 61*, 110–119. https://doi.org/10.1007/s11199-009-9618-4

Yeater, E. A., & Viken, R. J. (2010). Factors affecting women's response choices to dating and social situations. *Journal of Interpersonal Violence, 25*(8), 1411–1428.

13 Empathy and Sexual Offending: Theory, Research and Practice

William L. Marshall and Liam E. Marshall

Empathy has been a focus of theory, research, and practice since the beginning of the modern period of work with sex offenders (Laws & Marshall, 2003; Marshall & Laws, 2003). In particular deficits in empathy have been invoked to explain how sex offenders can persist in their abusive acts in the face of their victims' evident suffering. We will refer to this idea as the "empathy deficit hypothesis," although it has rarely been viewed as such; it has mostly been accepted as fact. Treatment providers have assumed that sensitizing sex offenders to victim suffering will begin a process that will lead to the development of empathy which will, as a result, inhibit future offending. The logic of this has typically been seen to be compelling by treatment providers. The more general psychological literature views empathic responses as an initial step in an unfolding process that leads to a compassionate response such as offering reassurance to people who are clearly distressed. In the case of sex offenders, this process is expected to result in either the termination of ongoing abuse or, more hopefully, a desistance in the propensity to sexually offend.

Within the sex offender field, difficulties in empathy have been conceptualized by theorists, researchers, and treatment providers, as restricted only towards the victims of sexual abuse. These deficits have been viewed as either applying to all sexual abuse victims or as being limited only to the offenders' own victims. This restricted focus seems rather odd since a deficit in generalized (i.e., trait) empathy would be evident toward all people, not just the general category of victims of sexual abuse. Since problems in forging and maintaining intimate relationships with adults have been shown to predict sexual reoffending, building the skills involved in these relationships has been seen as a critical target of sex offender treatment (Hanson & Morton-Bourgon, 2005). Since both Saarni (1990) and Brehm (1992) have shown that empathy is a critical feature of the skills involved in intimate relationships, empathy enhancement might be included in this segment of sex offender treatment. Unfortunately, we could not locate any article on intimacy skills training for sex offenders that included an empathy enhancement component. Perhaps it is assumed that the prior efforts to instill empathy at the beginning of treatment will automatically generalize to this component of treatment.

In order to examine the empathy deficit hypothesis, we need to identify the components of empathy and its related concepts. Empathy has

W. L. Marshall
Rockwood Psychological Services,
Kingston, ON, Canada

L. E. Marshall (✉)
Rockwood Psychotherapy & Consulting and
Waypoint Centre for Mental Health Care,
Penetanguishene, ON, Canada
e-mail: liammarshall@waypointcentre.ca

W. T. O'Donohue and P. A. Schewe (eds.), *Handbook of Sexual Assault and Sexual Assault Prevention*,
https://doi.org/10.1007/978-3-030-23645-8_13

been a focus of research in general psychology for many years so an examination of that literature may help to place our consideration of the empathy deficit hypothesis in a broader context. After identifying how empathy has been conceptualized in the broader literature, we will then examine how theorists in the sex offender field have considered its role, what the research has revealed about this presumed lack of empathy, and how therapists have gone about enhancing empathy in their attempts to reduce reoffending.

The Features of Empathy and Related Concepts

In the broader psychological literature, empathy is viewed as initiating a sequence of responses that may, or may not, result in action intended to avert or reduce the suffering of another person. When empathic feelings are experienced, they may trigger sympathetic feelings which may, in turn, initiate a compassionate response aimed at ameliorating the observed person's suffering. There have been numerous attempts to define each of these steps but there is sufficient commonality to justify a brief summary.

Zhou, Valiente, and Eisenberg (2003) define empathy as "a state of emotional arousal that stems from the apprehension or comprehension of another's affective state" (p. 269). This view of empathy acknowledges that the observer must recognize the other person's distress (i.e., a cognitive component) and experience feelings in response to that recognition (i.e.., an emotional component). Sympathy, according to Zhou et al. is triggered by the experience of empathy and involves an "other-oriented, emotional response… (that may include)… the desire to alleviate the other's negative emotion" (p. 269. section in parentheses added). Compassion, according to Cassell (2009), is an action that is directed outward and transcends any "preoccupation with the centrality of the self" (p. 397). In this view compassion, initially provoked by an empathic response, involves actions aimed at reducing another person's discomfort. Thus, a set of interconnected responses intervenes between the initial recognition of distress in another person and actions that are intended to ameliorate that distress. In the general literature it is typically assumed that the observer is not the instigator of the distress. This, of course, is not the case when we are considering sex offenders but nevertheless it seems reasonable to assume that the processes involved are the same.

Despite the general implication that an empathic recognition of grief will lead to sympathetic feelings and perhaps to compassionate action, there are situations where distress in another person, far from generating empathy, produces feelings of satisfaction. When a villain in a movie or novel gets his due desserts, the reader or viewer is not expected to feel sympathy; quite the contrary she is expected to feel satisfaction. Furthermore, when an observer has an angry or hostile relationship with a clearly distressed person, it is unlikely that empathy, sympathy, and a compassionate response will ensue (Batson, Fultz, & Schoenrade, 1987). This point is, of course, relevant in the case of some sex offenders such as rapists and sexual sadists who in the course of their offenses, appear to intend to cause distress. Thus, sensitizing these particular offenders to distress in their victims would seem to be counterproductive. Nevertheless this is the way in which most programs have addressed the assumed deficits in empathy and theorists and researchers have, for the most part, accepted the assumptions of treatment providers.

Empathy in Sex Offenders

Theory

While treatment programs had been attempting to enhance empathy among sex offenders for some years, it was not until the mid-1990s that a theory was outlined in an attempt to encourage more specific research aimed at elucidating the nature of this presumed deficit. Marshall, Hudson, Jones, and Fernandez (1995) proposed a model that viewed the recognition of distress in another person as the first stage in an unfolding process that finally results in an attempt to alleviate the observed person's suffering. This model included the steps outlined in the previous section: empathic responding leading to feelings of sympathy which in turn produce compassionate action. Marshall et al. suggested that sex offenders might have deficits at any, or all, of these stages. They suggested that research efforts should be directed at determining the capacity of sex offenders to experience each of the three unfolding processes rather than being limited to an evaluation of empathy alone. Both research and treatment, they suggested, should shift from what was seen as a narrow focus on empathy to a broader conceptualization of the issues. Furthermore, if treatment was to be effective, Marshall et al. declared, this range of skills (empathy, sympathy and compassion) would have to be implemented by the offender during the stage at which he was contemplating an offense. Once an offense was initiated, they said, the possible inhibitory processes of empathic feelings and compassionate responding would be unlikely to occur. Practitioners, for the most part, ignored these suggestions.

Not surprisingly, Marshall and colleagues' theory did not go unchallenged. Both Barnett and Mann (2017) and Polaschek (2003) pointed out that the concept of empathy does not include a sympathetic and compassionate response. While this is an appropriate criticism, these critics did not take up the implications that empathic responses alone will not necessarily inhibit abusive behavior. In elaborating their alternative view, Barnett and Mann (2017) suggested that the notion of empathy involves four responses: (1) the ability to take the perspective of another person; (2) a respectful view of other people; (3) the capacity for an emotional response that is manageable; and (4) the application of these skills to a specific situation. Barnett and Mann identified a series of blocks that could forestall an empathic response to a victim of sexual abuse, including particularly the failure of an offender to apply his capacity in the offense circumstances. This same concern was identified earlier by Polaschek (2003) in her chapter on theories of empathy.

Polaschek (2003) in fact questioned whether empathy is even possible during an offense. She pointed out that empathy may be present in sex offenders when they are not contemplating an offense or after an offense is completed, but she thought it unlikely that empathy could occur during the narrowing of the offender's focus that occurs when he is enacting the abuse. Among her many cogent points, Polaschek suggested that the simplest explanation is that sex offenders simply suspend any capacity they might have for empathy in order to offend. She claimed there is a problem with the plausibility of empathy acting as an inhibitor once an offense is initiated. Sex offenders, Polaschek said, either disregard signs of distress in their victim or these signs serve to enhance their arousal.

Many sex offenders, Polaschek notes, rarely acknowledge during assessment, or in the early stages of treatment, that their offense caused harm. Some may even acknowledge observing distress in their victim but feel no sympathy because, as we noted earlier, this distress serves to further excite them. Given that rapists typically express anger toward their victim (Groth, Burgess, & Holmstrom, 1977), and seek to humiliate them (Darke, 1990), we would expect evidence of distress to enhance rather than impede the assaults of these offenders. Similar issues would apply to sexual sadists who clearly seek to inflict pain and suffering during their offense (Nitschke & Marshall, 2018). Thus, Polaschek does not simply criticize the views expressed by Marshall et al., she calls into question the relevance of empathy as either an explanatory concept or as a legitimate target of treatment. Two plausible alternative explanations are consistent with Polaschek's simple idea.

Noting that sex offenders must initiate a series of steps prior to offending in order to access a victim, Ward, Hudson, and Marshall (1995) invoked Baumeister's (1991) notion of "cognitive deconstruction." Cognitive deconstruction describes a process whereby people avoid self-awareness when they intend to engage in a forbidden behavior. Baumeister suggested there are hierarchical levels of meaning which we attach to our actions. When people engage in acceptable behaviors, Baumeister says, they operate at a high level of meaning involving full awareness of what they are doing and the implications of their behavior for their view of themselves. However, when they intend to engage in behaviors that are otherwise unacceptable to them, and that have potential negative consequences for them, they deliberately operate at a more concrete level of awareness. In such circumstance the focus is narrowed to just the steps required to satisfy their immediate desires. In this state, the needs and well-being of others are disregarded, as are the potential judgments of other people, and the possible consequences to themselves. Ward et al. claimed that when sex offenders decide to offend, they deliberately enter a cognitively deconstructed state which effectively suspends all concerns about the effects on their victim. In this state they ignore the possibility of subsequent prosecution and conviction and their likely fall from grace among family and friends. This cognitively deconstructed state continues into their abusive act making them unresponsive to their victim's distress. Unfortunately this appealing proposal has not received the research attention it deserves nor has it, along with Polaschek's suggestion, had any impact on treatment.

Accepting that sex offenders do not display empathy for their victims during assessment or treatment (Bumby, 2000; Bumby, Marshall, & Langton, 1999) suggested that this is simply another aspect of their well-established "cognitive distortions" (Murphy & Page, 2014). Bumby does not suggest that these distortions arise during the abusive act. He is more concerned to explain why it is that sex offenders resist, at the points of assessment and treatment, the idea that their victim suffered during the abuse. O'Shaughnessy (2009) has similarly proposed that sex offenders "are very effective at rationalizing their conduct to believe that their behavior is not harmful to their victims" (p. 150). In fact, Bumby (2000) views all cognitive distortions as strategies by which sex offenders attempt to protect their sense of self-worth and to avoid feelings of shame. Sex offenders, he says, are acutely aware of the harm they have caused and that their cognitively distorted way of presenting themselves during prosecution and trial, and at assessment and treatment, is simply a way to avoid any further erosion of their sense of self-esteem. Support for Bumby's idea comes from studies showing a significant relationship between empathy deficits and cognitive distortions among sex offenders (Marshall, Champange, Brown, & Miller, 1997; Marshall, Hamilton, & Fernandez, 2001), as well as by evidence that sex offenders experience strong feelings of shame concerning their offenses (Sparks, Bailey, Marshall, & Marshall, 2003).

As we have seen, the accounts of Marshall et al. (1995) and Barnett and Mann (2017) do not question the empathy deficit hypothesis. Ward et al. (1995), Polaschek (2003), and Bumby (2000) on the other hand, consider the apparent lack of empathy among sex offenders to be better understood in terms of other processes. For Ward et al., this apparent deficit is viewed as essentially irrelevant since the offenders, by narrowing their focus, are not in a position to recognize distress in their victims. Polaschek's explanation is the most parsimonious. She dismisses the empathy deficit hypothesis by maintaining that sex offenders simply deliberately withhold any capacity for empathy they may have in order to offend. Bumby's idea is that apparent empathy deficits are simply one aspect of the tendency of sex offenders to present in various distorted ways in order to avoid further increases in shame. Both Bumby's and Polaschek's views imply that research attempts to identify empathy deficits in sex offenders are misplaced and that treatment aimed at enhancing empathy among sex offenders is unnecessary. Indeed, in Bumby's view such treatment, in so far as it depends on successful attempts to sensitize offenders to the harm they have caused, will further increase the offenders' feelings of shame, which is almost certain to be counter-productive. In view of these various views on the nature of empathy in sex offending, we need to consider what the research tells us about the occurrence and nature of empathy deficits among sex offenders.

Research

As we have seen, ideas about how it is that sex offenders are able to abuse others despite the evident suffering of their victims has been that these offenders are bereft of empathy. Several early authorities (Araji & Finkelhor, 1985; Hildebran & Pithers, 1989; Salter, 1988) advanced this empathy deficit hypothesis, although they stated it as an obvious fact rather than a theory. Because of their status in the field, the empathy deficit hypothesis came to be widely accepted. However, there were some discrepancies in the application of this idea to research and practice. These disagreements centered on whether the presumed deficit was in the offenders' capacity to feel empathy toward all victims of sexual abuse or only toward their own victims. These differences in the scope of the hypothesis came to be described as deficits in either general (or trait) empathy or a victim-specific deficit in empathy.

The idea of more general empathy deficits appeared to be supported by the results of a meta-analysis conducted by Miller and Eisenberg (1988). They found that deficits in trait empathy were associated with displays of aggression. Vachon, Lyman, and Johnson (2014) later replicated these findings. In both cases, however, this relationship was quite small. While Jolliffe and Farrington (2007) also found a lack of empathy to be related to violent offending, this relationship was not evident in their assessment of sexual offending. Consistent with this latter observation, Smallbone, Wheaton, and Hourigan (2003) found that while empathy deficits were predictive of criminal versatility among sex offenders, these deficits were unrelated to the offenders' sexual crimes.

Research examining the notion of a general empathy deficit among sex offenders, while not extensive, failed to clarify the issue. For example, three reports assessing sex offenders (Chaplin, Rice, & Harris, 1995; Marshall & Maric, 1996; Rice, Chaplin, Harris, & Coutts, 1994) identified deficiencies in trait empathy while two other studies (Langevin, Wright, & Handy, 1988; Marshall, Jones, Hudson, & McDonald, 1993) found no such apparent deficits. While the results of a recent meta-analysis by Morrow (2018) offer some perspective on the issue, it is hard to know what to make of his findings. Morrow found that 67.87% of the studies failed to show any differences in trait empathy between sex offenders and matched samples from the general population. While 25% of the studies entering Morrow's analysis found sex offenders to have lower levels of general empathy, 7.14% of the reports revealed higher empathy among sex offenders compared to the comparison subjects. It may be that these observed discrepancies are due to problems with the measures used to identify empathy.

For example, Serran's (2002) review of the psychometric status of the measures of general empathy used in these various studies, revealed serious flaws in each of the assessment procedures. Two of the most commonly employed measures, the *Hogan Empathy Scale* (Hogan, 1969) and Mehrabian and Epstein's (1972) questionnaire, were both shown to be multifactorial and thus appeared to be measuring a variety of features that may or may not be related to empathy. In addition both these measures failed to meet acceptable standards for validity and reliability. Serran found that the other measure of trait empathy employed in a small number of studies of sex offenders fared rather better in terms of its psychometric status. She reported that Davis' (1983) *Interpersonal Reactivity Index* appeared to meet reasonable psychometric standards. This measure has subscales that are meant to be viewed as assessments of four aspects of empathy: perspective taking, fantasy, personal distress, and empathic concern. In one often-cited study of sex offenders using this scale (Pithers, 1994), scores on these four concepts were collapsed to produce an overall estimate of empathy. This may be a questionable strategy since each of these features appears to be measuring different, and perhaps independent, aspects of empathy.

Given the confusing results and the problems with measurement in the assessment of trait empathy, as well as a growing disenchantment with the idea that sex offenders lack such generalized empathic skills, some researchers began to consider the possibility that the presumed deficits may be victim-specific. Beckett and Fisher (1994) were the first to voice to this idea. As a result of their idea, Beckett and Fisher developed a measure aimed at evaluating "victim-specific" empathy deficits in sex offenders. This assessment procedure was later employed by Beech, Fisher, and Beckett (1998) and was shown to be sensitive to changes in victim empathy arising from treatment.

Following this original idea, Fernandez and her colleagues (Fernandez, Marshall, Lightbody, & O'Sullivan, 1999) developed a unique measure that assessed three potential categories of empathy deficits: (1) toward all people, (2) toward all victims of sexual abuse, and (3) toward only their own victim. Studies employing this measure (Fernandez & Marshall, 2003; Marshall et al., 1997, 2001; Marshall & Moulden, 2001) showed that sex offenders did not lack empathy toward people in general but were somewhat deficient in empathy toward all victims of sexual abuse. However, their most marked deficits were shown to be toward their own victims.

Taken together with Beech and colleagues' findings, the results using Fernandez's measure appear to indicate that it is a lack of empathy toward their own victims that characterizes sex offenders. However, these results could also be perhaps more parsimoniously construed in terms of Bumby's (2000) suggestion that apparent victim-specific deficits among sex offenders simply reflect a strategy adopted to avoid shame and to reduce any further erosions of self-worth. Nevertheless, these findings on victim-specific deficits served to encourage treatment providers to target the enhancement of victim empathy among sex offenders.

Treatment

In the treatment of all types of offenders, Andrews and Bonta (2010) point to a broad range of evidence indicating that for such treatment to be effective, it must adhere to what they call *The Principles of Effective Offender Treatment*. These principles were originally derived from a pair of meta-analyses of a large number of reports of treatment outcomes (Andrews et al., 1990; Andrews, Bonta, & Hoge, 1990). Some years later, Hanson, Bourgon, Helmus, and Hodgson (2009) demonstrated that these principles also applied to the treatment of sex offenders.

These ideas involve three subordinate principles described as Risk, Needs, and Responsivity. However, it is only the Needs Principle that concerns us here. This principle states that in order for treatment to be effective it must address those features of sex offenders that are both potentially modifiable and that have been shown to predict reoffending. These problematic aspects of offenders are known as "criminogenic factors." Andrews and Bonta (2010) additionally note that targeting non-criminogenic features, takes away time that might otherwise be spent on the more appropriate issues, and might, therefore, reduce the effectiveness of treatment. It follows from these ideas that in order to justify addressing empathy deficits in sex offender treatment, these deficits must be shown to be criminogenic. Unfortunately, the evidence does not support the idea that empathy is a criminogenic factor.

Hanson and Morton-Bourgon (2005), for example, reported the results of a comprehensive meta-analysis of various features of sex offenders that had, up to that point, been targets of treatment. Hanson and Morton-Bourgon found that empathy deficits did not predict reoffending. Mann and Barnett (2012) took issue with this conclusion. They correctly pointed out that the assessments of empathy in the five reports entering the meta-analysis were based on therapist ratings conducted after treatment was completed. As Mann and Barnett pointed out, such ratings are notoriously unreliable so cannot, therefore, serve as a basis for inferences about the criminogenic status of empathy. Mann and Barnett might also have noted that the ratings were completed after treatment was complete which, if treatment was effective, would necessarily have markedly reduced the range of potential scores. As a consequence this would have rendered these ratings unsuitable to serve as a basis for any predictions. While these considerations are important, the results leave the criminogenic status of empathy deficits unclear. However, it is important to be clear that there is, to this date, no evidence indicating that empathy deficits are, in fact, criminogenic.

Mann and Barnett (2012) provided the most comprehensive analysis up to that time, of the treatment implications of the empathy deficit hypothesis. In their attempt to be fair to the persistent efforts by treatment providers to address empathy, Mann and Barnett pointed to the results of three reports of sex offender treatment (Garrett, Oliver, Wilcox, & Middleton, 2003; Levenson & Prescott, 2009; Wakeling, Webster, & Mann, 2005). In each of these studies sex offenders were asked to identify the feature of treatment they considered to be the most important. In each case the offenders declared the empathy component to be the most helpful and enlightening. In particular, these clients said that addressing empathy for their victim helped them take responsibility for their crimes.

In considering the relevance of these remarks by offenders, we note again that empathy deficits have not, as yet, been shown to be criminogenic nor has the offenders' failure to accept responsibility for their crimes. Perhaps of equal importance, there was no indication that these positive evaluations by clients had any impact on their subsequent risk to reoffend. In fact Maruna (2001) has shown that offenders who readily take responsibility for their crimes have higher post-release recidivism rates than do offenders who deny having committed an offense. Thus the fact that sex offenders find the empathy component to be helpful is irrelevant to the consideration of what needs to be addressed in the treatment of these clients.

Approaches to the Enhancement of Victim Empathy

Given the evidence presented in the previous section, it may seem redundant to provide details of how therapists have gone about enhancing sex offenders' empathy for their victims. However, for the sake of completeness, and given that almost all current programs continue to address this issue (see survey by McGrath, Cumming, Burchard, Zeoli, & Ellerby, 2010), we will provide an account of the strategies that have been employed.

Salter (1988) outlined several procedures she considered essential and the majority of programs have followed her suggestions. Sex offenders, she said, should be required to engage in discussions with survivors of sexual abuse or their advocates, with the aim of making it clear to the offenders that victims of sexual abuse typically display extensive signs of distress. Salter also recommended that offenders be required to read literature detailing these negative consequences and then write hypothetical letters of apology to their victims. Salter believed these procedures would not only enhance the empathy of sex offenders for their victims, it would also lead the offenders to accept responsibility for their crimes both of which she declared were essential before treatment could be fully engaged. Some variations on Salter's proposals were almost immediately thereafter incorporated into the majority of treatment programs for sex offenders (Knopp, Freeman-Longo, & Stevenson, 1992) and have been retained as a component in current programs (McGrath et al., 2010).

Many programs added to Salter's proposed methods, a requirement that sex offenders write hypothetical letters from their victims indicating what these victims might say regarding the suffering they experienced during and after the crime. In response to these letters, offenders have typically been required to write another note that not only acknowledges the harm they have done, but that also offers an apology to their victims. Furthermore, it has been common to require the clients to engage in role-plays where they take the part of the offender and then reverse role-play their victim. These additional components are apparently meant to further sensitize the offenders to the harm they have done. While Pithers (1994) showed that this combination of procedures resulted in enhancements of victim empathy, he later discovered to his dismay these role-plays are fraught with problems and can readily lead to civil law suits filed by the offenders against their therapists and program managers (Pithers, 1997). Furthermore, Webster, Bowers,

Mann, and Marshall (2005) showed that role-plays added little to any of the observed changes in empathy.

Aside from these issues, we (Marshall & Marshall, 2017) have expressed concerns regarding the typical current strategies aimed at enhancing empathy along with the concurrent requirement that these clients acknowledge the veracity of the official version of their crimes. Aside from the issue of the dubious criminogenic status of these two factors, we also questioned the wisdom of the location of these strategies. Typically it is considered necessary to address these two factors at the onset of treatment, because it is assumed that treatment cannot proceed prior to the offenders taking full responsibility for their crimes. There is, however, no empirical basis for this assumption and it seems entirely reasonable that these clients could overcome well-established criminogenic factors in the absence of acknowledging their guilt. For example, the skills involved in effective intimate relationships are not dependent upon an acknowledgement of guilt, nor are the capacities necessary to overcome sexual preoccupation, or to develop more effective ways to cope so that impulsiveness can be diminished. We also pointed to concerns about the de-motivational effects of aggressively challenging clients at the very beginning of treatment. There is clear evidence from both the sex offender literature (Prescott, 2014) and the more general treatment literature (Miller & Rollnick, 2002), that the early establishment of motivation is critical to subsequent engagement and completion of treatment.

None of these concerns is meant to imply that sex offender treatment is so effective as to not require further development. The potential for further development, however, must rely on evidence not on the common sense intuitions of therapists. While there is evidence as we have seen indicating that sex offenders' empathy for their victims can be enhanced (Beech et al., 1998; Marshall, O'Sullivan, & Fernandez, 1996), Landenberger and Lipsey (2005) demonstrated that the inclusion of a victim empathy component in the treatment of non-sex offenders was associated with poorer, not better, outcomes.

If treatment providers are to persist in their attempts to enhance empathy and have their clients accept responsibility for their crimes, then it is incumbent upon these clinicians to demonstrate that these factors are, indeed, criminogenic. Otherwise treatment providers will be in danger of committing what Gendreau, Smith, and Therault (2009) derisively call "correctional quackery" by which they meant treatment based on common sense rather than on evidence. Mann and Barnett (2012) echoed this sentiment when they concluded, after their thorough review, that although empathy has been, and continues to be, considered an important treatment target with sex offenders "such enthusiasm is not founded on empirical evidence" (p. 297).

Conclusions

In this chapter, we initially identified what we have called the "empathy deficit hypothesis." This hypothesis, although not stated as such in the literature, proposes that sex offenders suffer from an inadequate capacity for empathy and that this incapacity is what allows them to abuse their victims despite the evident suffering of these unfortunate people. In order to set a framework for considering the implications of this hypothesis, we described the ways in which empathy has been viewed in the general psychological literature. In this literature, empathy is seen as a necessary first step in an unfolding process that leads to sympathy for the distressed person and to compassionate action to ameliorate that person's suffering. We noted that in the sex offender literature, these two subsequent issues of sympathy and compassion have received no direct attention, it being apparently assumed that once an empathic response occurs, ameliorative action will automatically follow.

From the mostly unqualified acceptance of the empathy deficit hypothesis, theories of the nature and relevance of empathic difficulties among sex offenders have been elaborated. Only two theorists, Bumby and Polaschek, called into question the idea that sex offenders actually suffer from a lack of the capacity to feel empathy. Ward et al. (1995) dismissed any consideration of empathy by suggesting that when a sex offender decides to abuse someone, he deliberately enters a state where he sets aside all other concerns and focuses only on those actions needed to offend.

Research efforts have proceeded on the acceptance of the empathy deficit hypothesis, again without actually articulating it as such. Studies examining the idea that sex offenders lack empathy toward all people (i.e., a trait deficit) have produced equivocal results, whereas those addressing the idea that sex offenders have more limited victim-specific deficits, have generated more consistent findings.

Treatment efforts meant to address these presumed problems have mostly followed strategies derived from Salter's (1988) original proposals despite the fact that these deficits have yet to be shown to be criminogenic (i.e., predict reoffending). Furthermore, there is no evidence demonstrating that effectively enhancing empathy has any impact on reducing subsequent re-offense rates. On the face of currently available evidence, then, we do not believe that continued efforts directed at theorizing, researching, and treating assumed deficits in empathy among sex offenders is justified.

References

Andrews, D. A., & Bonta, J. (2010). *The psychology of criminal conduct* (5th ed.). New Providence, , NJ: Lexis Nexis.

Andrews, D. A., Bonta, J., & Hoge, R. D. (1990). Classification for effective rehabilitation: Rediscovering psychology. *Criminal Justice and Behavior, 17*, 19–52.

Andrews, D. A., Zinger, I., Hoge, R. D., Bonta, J., Gendreau, P., & Cullen, F. T. (1990). Does correctional treatment work? A clinically relevant and psychologically informed meta-analysis. *Criminology, 28*, 369–404.

Araji, S., & Finkelhor, D. (1985). Explanations of pedophilia: Review of empirical research. *Bulletin of the American Academy of Psychiatry & the Law, 13*, 17–37.

Barnett, G. D., & Mann, R. E. (2017). Theories of empathy deficits in sex offenders. In A. R. Beech & T. Ward (Eds.), *The Wiley handbook on the theories, assessment, and treatment of sexual offending* (Vol. 1, pp. 223–244). Chichester: John Wiley & Sons.

Batson, C. D., Fultz, J., & Schoenrade, P. A. (1987). Distress and empathy: Two qualitatively distinct emotions with different motivational consequences. *Journal of Personality, 55*, 19–39.

Baumeister, R. F. (1991). *Escaping the self.* New York, NY: Basic Books.

Beckett, R.C., & Fisher, D. (1994, September). *Assessing victim empathy: A new measure.* Paper presented at the 13th Annual Conference of the Association for the Treatment of Sexual Abusers. San Francisco, CA.

Beech, A. R., Fisher, D., & Beckett, R. C. (1998). *Step 3: An evaluation of the prison sex offender treatment program.* London: Home Office.

Brehm, S. S. (1992). *Intimate relationships* (2nd ed.). New York, NY: McGraw-Hill.

Bumby, K. M. (2000). Empathy inhibition, intimacy deficits, and attachment difficulties in sex offenders. In D. R. Laws, S. M. Hudson, & T. Ward (Eds.), *Remaking relapse prevention with sex offenders: A sourcebook* (pp. 143–166). Thousand Oaks, CA: Sage Publications.

Bumby, K. M., Marshall, W. L., & Langton, C. M. (1999). A theoretical model of the influence of shame and guilt on sexual offending. In B. K. Schwartz (Ed.), *The sex offender. Vol.3. Theoretical advances, treating special populations, and legal developments* (pp. 5.1–5.12). Kingston, NJ: Civic Research Institute.

Cassell, E. J. (2009). Compassion. In S. J. Lopez & C. R. Snyder (Eds.), *Oxford handbook of positive psychology* (pp. 393–403). New York, NY: Oxford University Press.

Chaplin, T. C., Rice, M. E., & Harris, G. T. (1995). Salient victim suffering and the sexual responses of child molesters. *Journal of Consulting and Clinical Psychology, 3*, 249–255.

Darke, J. L. (1990). Sexual aggression: Achieving power through humiliation. In W. L. Marshall, D. R. Laws, & H. E. Barbaree (Eds.), *Handbook of sexual assault: Issues, theories and treatment of the offender* (pp. 55–72). New York, NY: Plenum Press.

Davis, M. H. (1983). Measuring individual differences in empathy: Evidence for a multidimensional approach. *Journal of Personality and Social Psychology, 9*, 223–229.

Fernandez, Y. M., & Marshall, W. L. (2003). Victim empathy, social self-esteem and psychopathy in rapists. *Sexual Abuse: A Journal of Research and Treatment, 15*, 11–26.

Fernandez, Y. M., Marshall, W. L., Lightbody, S., & O'Sullivan, C. (1999). The child molester empathy measure: Description and an examination of its reliability and validity. *Sexual Abuse: A Journal of Research and Treatment, 11*, 17–31.

Garrett, T., Oliver, C., Wilcox, D. T., & Middleton, D. (2003). Who cares? The views of sexual offenders about the group treatment they receive. *Sexual Abuse: A Journal of Research and Treatment, 15*, 323–338.

Gendreau, P., Smith, P., & Therault, Y. L. (2009). Chaos theory and correctional treatment: Common sense, correctional quackery and the law of fart catchers. *Journal of Contemporary Criminal Justice, 25*, 384–396.

Groth, A. N., Burgess, A. W., & Holmstrom, L. L. (1977). Rape: Power, anger, and sexuality. *American Journal of Psychiatry, 134*, 1239–1243.

Hanson, R. K., Bourgon, G., Helmus, L., & Hodgson, S. (2009). The principles of effective correctional treatment also apply to sexual offenders: A meta-analysis. *Criminal Justice and Behavior, 36*, 865–891.

Hanson, R. K., & Morton-Bourgon, K. E. (2005). The characteristics of persistent sexual offenders: A meta-analysis of recidivism studies. *Journal of Consulting and Clinical Psychology, 73*, 1154–1163.

Hildebran, D., & Pithers, W. D. (1989). Enhancing offender empathy for sexual abuse victims. In D. R. Laws (Ed.), *Relapse prevention with sex offenders* (pp. 236–243). New York, NY: Guilford Press.

Hogan, R. (1969). Development of an empathy scale. *Journal of Consulting and Clinical Psychology, 33*, 307–316.

Jolliffe, D., & Farrington, D. P. (2007). Empathy and offending: A systematic review and meta-analysis. *Aggression and Violent Behavior, 9*, 441–476.

Knopp, F. H., Freeman-Longo, R. E., & Stevenson, W. (1992). *Nationwide survey of juvenile and adult sex-offender treatment programs*. Orwell, VT: Safer Society Press.

Landenberger, N. A., & Lipsey, M. W. (2005). The positive effects of cognitive-behavioral programs for offenders: A met-analysis of factors associated with effective treatment. *Journal of Experimental Criminology, 1*, 451–476.

Langevin, R., Wright, M. A., & Handy, L. (1988). Empathy, assertiveness, aggressiveness, and defensiveness among sex offenders. *Annals of Sex Research, 1*, 533–547.

Laws, D. R., & Marshall, W. L. (2003). A brief history of behavioral and cognitive behavioral approaches to sex offenders: Part 1. Early developments. *Sexual Abuse: A Journal of Treatment and Research, 15*, 75–92.

Levenson, J. S., & Prescott, D. (2009). Treatment experiences of civilly committed sex offenders: A consumer satisfaction survey. *Sexual Abuse: A Journal of Treatment and Research, 21*, 6–20.

Mann, M. E., & Barnett, G. D. (2012). Victim empathy intervention with sexual offenders: Rehabilitation, punishment, or correctional quackery? *Sexual Abuse: A Journal of Treatment and Research, 25*, 282–301.

Marshall, L. E., & Marshall, W. L. (2017). Motivating sex offenders to enter and effectively engage in treatment. In D. Wilcox, R. Gray, R. Donathy, & B. Brim (Eds.), *Working with sex offenders: A guide for practitioners* (pp. 98–112). Oxford: Routledge.

Marshall, W. L., Champange, F., Brown, C., & Miller, S. (1997). Empathy, intimacy, loneliness, and self-esteem in nonfamilial child molesters. *Journal of Child Sexual Abuse, 6*, 87–97.

Marshall, W. L., Hamilton, K., & Fernandez, Y. M. (2001). Empathy deficits and cognitive distortions in child molesters. *Sexual Abuse: A Journal of Treatment and Research, 13*, 123–131.

Marshall, W. L., Hudson, S. M., Jones, R., & Fernandez, Y. M. (1995). Empathy in sex offenders. *Clinical Psychology Review, 15*, 99–113.

Marshall, W. L., Jones, R., Hudson, S. M., & McDonald, E. (1993). Generalized empathy in child molesters. *Journal of Child Sexual Abuse, 2*, 61–68.

Marshall, W. L., & Laws, D. R. (2003). A brief history of behavioral and cognitive behavioral approaches to sexual offender treatment: Part 2. The modern era. *Sexual Abuse: A Journal of Treatment and Research, 15*, 93–120.

Marshall, W. L., & Maric, A. (1996). Cognitve and emotional components of generalized empathy deficits in child molesters. *Journal of Child Sexual Abuse, 5*, 101–110.

Marshall, W. L., & Moulden, H. (2001). Hostility toward women and victim empathy in rapists. *Sexual Abuse: A Journal of Treatment and Research, 13*, 249–255.

Marshall, W. L., O'Sullivan, C., & Fernandez, Y. M. (1996). The enhancement of victim empathy among incarcerated child molesters. *Legal and Criminological Psychology, 1*, 95–102.

Maruna, S. (2001). *Making good: How ex-convicts reform and rebuild their lives*. Washington, DC: American Psychological Association.

McGrath, R. J., Cumming, G. F., Burchard, B. L., Zeoli, S., & Ellerby, L. (2010). *Current practices and trends in sexual offender management. The Safer Society 2009 North American Survey*. Brandon, VT: Safer Society Press.

Mehrabian, A., & Epstein, N. (1972). A measure of emotional empathy. *Journal of Personality, 40*, 525–543.

Miller, P. A., & Eisenberg, N. (1988). The relation of empathy to aggressive and externalizing/antisocial behavior. *Psychological Bulletin, 103*, 324–344.

Miller, W. R., & Rollnick, S. (Eds.). (2002). *Motivational interviewing: Preparing people for change* (6th ed.). New York, NY: Guilford Press.

Morrow, E. (2018). Cognitive, affective, and general empathy in sexual offenders: A meta-analysis. Doctoral thesis, Chicago School of Professional Psychology.

Murphy, W. D., & Page, I. J. (2014). The role of cognitive factors in sexual offending. In M. S. Carich & S. E. Mussack (Eds.), *The Safer Society handbook of sexual abuser assessment and treatment* (pp. 151–175). Brandon, VT: Safer Society Press.

Nitschke, J., & Marshall, W. L. (2018). An evaluation of assessments for sexual sadism. In J. Proulx, E. Beauregard, A. J. Carter, A. Mokros, R. Darjee, & J. James (Eds.), *Routledge international handbook of sexual homicide studies* (pp. 303–316). New York, NY: Routledge.

O'Shaughnessy, R. J. (2009). The role of personality disorder in sexual offending. In F. M. Saleh, A. J. Grudzinskas, J. M. Bradford, & D. J. Brodsky (Eds.), *Sex offenders: Identification, risk assessment, treatment, and legal issues* (pp. 144–155). New York, NY: Oxford University Press.

Pithers, W. D. (1994). Process evaluation of a group therapy component designed to enhance sex offenders empathy for sexual abuse survivors. *Behaviour Research and Therapy, 32*, 565–570.

Pithers, W. D. (1997). Maintaining treatment integrity with sexual abusers. *Criminal Justice and Behavior, 24*, 34–51.

Polaschek, D. L. (2003). Empathy and victim empathy. In T. Ward, D. R. Laws, & S. M. Hudson (Eds.), *Sexual deviance: Issues and controversies* (pp. 172–189). Thousand Oaks, CA: Sage Publications.

Prescott, D. S. (2014). Motivating clients to change. In M. S. Carich & S. E. Musack (Eds.), *The Safer Society Handbook of sexual abuser assessment and treatment* (pp. 103–124). Brandon, VT: Safer Society Press.

Rice, M. E., Chaplin, T. C., Harris, G. T., & Coutts, J. (1994). Empathy for the victim and sexual arousal among rapists and nonrapists. *Journal of Interpersonal Violence, 9*, 435–449.

Saarni, C. (1990). Emotional competence: How emotions and relationships become integrated. In R. A. Thompson (Ed.), *Socioemotional development* (pp. 115–182). Lincoln, NB: University of Nebraska Press.

Salter, A. C. (1988). *Treating child sex offenders and victims: Assessment and treatment of child sex offenders: A practical guide*. Beverley Hills, CA: Sage Publications.

Serran, G. A. (2002). The measurement of empathy. In Y. M. Fernandez (Ed.), *In their shoes: Examining the issue of empathy and its place in the treatment of offenders* (pp. 16–35). Oklahoma City, OK: Wood'N'Barnes.

Smallbone, S. W., Wheaton, J., & Hourigan, D. (2003). Trait empathy and criminal versatility in sexual offenders. *Sexual Abuse: A Journal of Research and Treatment, 15*, 49–60.

Sparks, J., Bailey, W., Marshall, W.L., & Marshall, L.E. (2003, October). *Shame and guilt in sex offenders*. Paper presented at the 22nd. Annual Research and Treatment Conference of the Association for the Treatment of Sexual Abusers. St.Louis.

Vachon, D. D., Lyman, D. R., & Johnson, J. A. (2014). The (non) relation between empathy and aggression: Surprising results from a meta-analysis. *Psychological Bulletin, 140*, 16.

Wakeling, H. C., Webster, S. D., & Mann, R. E. (2005). Sexual offenders' treatment experience: A qualitative and quantitative investigation. *Journal of Sexual Aggression, 11*, 171–186.

Ward, T., Hudson, S. M., & Marshall, W. L. (1995). Cognitive distortions and affective deficits in sex offenders: A cognitive deconstructionist interpretation. *Sexual Abuse: A Journal of Treatment and Research, 7*, 67–83.

Webster, S. D., Bowers, L. E., Mann, R. E., & Marshall, W. L. (2005). Developing empathy in sexual offenders: The value of offense re-enactments. *Sexual Abuse: A Journal of Research and Treatment, 17*, 63–77.

Zhou, Q., Valiente, C., & Eisenberg, N. (2003). Empathy and its measurement). In S. J. lopez & C. R. Snyder (Eds.), *Positive psychological assessment: A handbook of models and measures* (pp. 269–284). Washington, DC: American Psychological Association.

Overview of Adult Sexual Offender Typologies

14

Michelle L. Wojcik and Bonnie S. Fisher

The often violent and profane nature of sex crimes can instill fear into individuals and blanket communities with distrust (Levenson, Brannon, Fortney, & Baker, 2007) which can either erode or mobilize collective efficacy. Though rates of sexual violence have been declining since the early 1990s (Planty, Langton, Krebs, Berzofsky, & Smiley-McDonald, 2013), public perception studies have demonstrated that sexual violence and sexual offenders remain a salient area of concern for the general public (Button, Tewksbury, Mustaine, & Payne, 2013; Levenson et al., 2007; Proctor, Badzinski, & Johnson, 2002). Despite research questioning the effectiveness of harsh punishments reducing recidivism (e.g., Agan, 2011), sanctions for convicted sex offenders have become harsher over the years and remain favored by the general public (Button et al., 2013). Legislators and the general public often view sexual offenders as one homogenous population all with a high risk of recidivism (Levenson et al., 2007). However, research suggests that sexual offenders constitute a heterogeneous population that varies in offending behavior, motivations, and risk for recidivism (e.g., Hanson, Harris, Helmus, & Thornton, 2014; Wortley & Smallbone, 2013). A considerable amount of clinical speculation and empirically based typological research has been conducted to explain and measure the characteristics and motivations of those who perpetrate acts of sexual violence (e.g., Groth, 1979; Knight & Prentky, 1990; Tener, Wolak, & Finkelhor, 2015; Vandiver & Kercher, 2004).

Sexual offender typologies have developed using a variety of methods such as: (1) clinical descriptions, (2) demographic clusters (univariate or multivariate), (3) psychometric profiles, and (4) theory-derived classifications (Bickley & Beech, 2001). Traditionally, researchers have classified sexual offenders into typologies based upon characteristics and motivation of the offender and their age preference for victims. Most separate sexual offenders by those who offend against children and those whose victims are age appropriate or adults. Many other typologies also specify between male and female offenders and adults and juveniles. Likewise, many classification systems distinguish between subtypes of offenders (e.g., Holmes & Holmes, 1996). Recently developed typologies have differentiated between offenders who commit contact offenses versus those who only offend online (e.g., Krone, 2004; Sullivan & Beech, 2004; Tener et al., 2015). Emerging research also has brought attention to offenders who sexually assault both child and adult victims (Rice & Knight, 2018). Despite the diverse assortment of typologies available, there is no universally accepted typological system for sexual offenders.

M. L. Wojcik (✉) · B. S. Fisher
School of Criminal Justice, University of Cincinnati, Cincinnati, OH, USA
e-mail: wojcikml@mail.uc.edu

W. T. O'Donohue and P. A. Schewe (eds.), *Handbook of Sexual Assault and Sexual Assault Prevention*,
https://doi.org/10.1007/978-3-030-23645-8_14

Additionally, the empirical research on existing typologies is limited and has produced inconsistent results concerning reliability, validity, and intervention development (see Bickley & Beech, 2001).

The current body of research suggests that some sex offenders do not fit precisely into one typology, but share characteristics with multiple typologies, or none at all (e.g., Beech, Elliott, Birgden, & Findlater, 2008; Bickley & Beech, 2001; Rice & Knight, 2018; Robertillo & Terry, 2007). For example, several typologies describe types of cyber sexual offenders by their use of child pornography, their motivation for offending, and whether they offend solely online (e.g., Krone, 2004; Lanning, 2010; Tener et al., 2015). Lanning's (2001, 2010) description of the diverse offender who has deviant sexual interests but no specific interest in minors may also qualify as Tener et al.'s (2015) sex-focused type who search the internet for casual or transactional sexual encounters.

Understanding the characteristics and offense patterns common to sexual offenders and classifying them correctly through adequate typological systems can aid researchers and practitioners in developing more effective treatment, supervision, management, and prevention policy. This chapter provides a review of the typologies for adult rapists, child abusers, female offenders, and cyber sexual offenders, discusses the limitations of traditional typologies, and offers suggestions for future research.

Adult Male Rapists

Like all sexual offenders, adult male rapists make up a diverse homogenous group. Though rapists have unique personal and criminal histories, they often share some common characteristics. When attempting to understand rapists' behavior and motivation, one should consider issues of power, anger, level of physical force used, and sexual interests of the offender (Groth, 1979). Research has produced many adult rapist typologies in which offenders are classified by the primary motivation of their offense, which is broadly described as sexual or nonsexual in nature (Knight & Prentky, 1990; Robertillo & Terry, 2007).

Groth, Burgess, and Holmstrom (1977; Groth, 1979) were among the first to develop a typology based on the amount of aggression used, the motivation of the offender, and the manifestation of other antisocial behaviors (e.g., poor social skills, other criminality, distorted perception of his masculinity). Future research further expanded upon or developed similar classification schemes (e.g., Berger, 2000; Knight, 1999; Knight & Prentky, 1990). Many of the existing typologies of male rapists have similar themes or overlapping categories (e.g., the sadistic type discussed by Groth, 1979; Knight & Prentky, 1990; Prentky, Cohen, & Seghorn, 1985; Rada, 1978). For the purposes of this chapter, traditional adult male rapist typologies were summarized into five classifications by motivation and behavioral and offense characteristics, as presented in Table 14.1: (1) compensatory, (2) sadistic, (3) anger, (4) power/control, and (5) opportunistic/antisocial.

The compensatory rapist, also referred to as the power reassurance or gentleman rapist, doubts their desirability and has feelings of inadequacy and poor social skills. Such individuals may have a "courtship disorder" resulting in the inability to form healthy relationships with same age partners (Freund, 1990). They commit rape in an effort to achieve social competence, improve self-esteem, and make their feelings of inadequacy dissipate (Rada, 1978). The compensatory rapist may perceive that the victim has displayed sexual interest in him or that through the use of force, the victim will grow to like him (Craissati, 2005). Compensatory rapists use the level of force necessary to assault the victim, only display anger in response to resistance, and may run away if the victim screams or fights back. They show concern for the well-being of their victim and do not want to harm them. As such, they show less aggression in both sexual and nonsexual situations compared to other classifications of rapists (Budrionis & Jongsma, 2003; Cohen, Seghorn, & Calmas, 1969; Groth et al., 1977; Prentky et al., 1985; Robertillo & Terry, 2007).

Table 14.1 Summary of adult male rapist typologies

Classification	Motivation	Behavioral and offense characteristics
Compensatory	Sexual	• Rape to relieve feelings of inadequacy • Uses minimal physical aggression
Sadistic	Sexual	• Sexually aroused by the victim's fear and pain • High rates of psychopathy
Anger/retaliation	Nonsexual	• Motivated by power, anger, aggression, and hatred • High levels of physical and sexual aggression to "get even" with women
Power/control	Nonsexual	• Wants power and dominance over victim • Use aggression to restore inner fears about their own masculinity
Opportunistic/antisocial	Nonsexual	• Impulsively rapes during the commission of another nonsexual crime • Poor impulse control

Sources: Groth (1979); Cohen et al. (1969); Knight and Prentky (1990); Robertillo & Terry (2007)

Like the compensatory rapist, the sadistic rapist is motivated by sexual fantasies. However, the sadistic rapist's fantasies are sexually aggressive as they are aroused by the pain the fear they cause their victims (Groth, 1979; Groth et al., 1977; Knight, 1999; Rada, 1978; Robertillo & Terry, 2007). They spend time and effort planning their attacks, their victims are almost always strangers, and they show no remorse for their actions. The sadistic rapist may torture their victims, and their attacks can lead to sexual murder. Research has shown that sadistic rapists have higher rates of psychopathy and weapon use compared to nonsadistic rapists (Barbaree, Seto, Serin, Amos, & Preston, 1994).

A third type of offender is the anger retaliation rapist, also referred to as vindictive rapists. These offenders have long histories of antisocial aggressive behavior and are motivated by power, anger, aggression, revenge, and hatred rather than sexual desire (Craissati, 2005). They use high levels of physical and sexual aggression and try to "get even" for the real or imagined injustices they have experienced by using rape as a weapon to punish women (Groth et al., 1977; Knight, 1999). Attacks by such individuals are often impersonal and involve degrading and humiliating behavior motivated by the need for power and aggression. As such, they often cause their victims high levels of physical injury (Knight, 1999). They may plan an attack against a specific person or "blitz" attack an individual who sparks their rage.

Like the anger retaliation rapist, power/control or power assertive rapists are typically motivated by nonsexual needs. Rather, they are motivated by a desire to achieve power and dominance through gaining control over their victim. They use aggressive but nonlethal behavior to restore their inner fears about their sexuality and masculinity (Groth, 1979; Prentky et al., 1985; Robertillo & Terry, 2007). These offenders often use alcohol and/or drugs before they attack and are geographically mobile (Craissati, 2005). Their rapes are impulsive and opportunistic; as such, their attacks are often unplanned and usually do not involve a weapon. They often rape their victims on the day they meet them, meet them at a public place (e.g., bar) and are likely to leave their victims emotionally traumatized (Robertillo & Terry, 2007).

The final traditional adult male rapist classification, the opportunistic/antisocial offender, is motivated by nonsexual needs and impulsively rapes during the commission of another crime (Knight, 1999). These individuals have poor impulse control and often engage in impulsive and adventure-seeking lifestyles. Their offenses are unplanned predatory acts and are primarily motivated by situational and contextual factors (e.g., encountering a victim during a burglary). Opportunistic/antisocial rapists exhibit little anger except in response to victim resistance. They generally have a more antisocial disposition than other types of rapists and engage in general crime more so than sex-related crime. For these individuals, rape is one of many antisocial and predatory behaviors they engage in (Knight, 1999; Prentky et al., 1985; Robertillo & Terry, 2007).

There has been little published research and evaluation on the psychometric properties of these early typologies of adult male rapists (e.g., Knight, 1999). Some early typologies used a psychodynamic approach to classify rapists by their motivations to offend (e.g., Groth et al., 1977), while others were constructed using empirical data from clinical samples (Knight & Prentky, 1990). In an early evaluation of the Massachusetts Treatment Center Rapist Typology, Version 3 (MTC:R3), Knight (1999) found evidence of concurrent validity, cross-temporal stability, and predictive potency for several types of offenders. Though, Knight (1999) notes that the typology was in need of some "fine-tuning," and similar studies have failed to classify rapists according to the nine subtypes described in the MTC:R3 without refinement (Barbaree et al., 1994). More recent research has shown support for the MTC:R3 in producing distinct types, but a small sample size ($n = 10$) limits the generalizability of these results (Reid, Wilson, & Boer, 2010).

Serious methodical concerns such as low sample size, social desirability in self-reports, sampling bias due to an over reliance on convicted offenders, low reoffense rates, and inconsistent measures of recidivism (i.e., committing a general offense versus committing a new sexual offense) threaten the validity and reliability of traditional adult male rapist typologies (Bickley & Beech, 2001; Gannon & Ward, 2008; Jennings & Fox, 2016). In practice, these early typologies, have little value in clinical assessment and treatment as they exclude irrational cognitions (i.e., offense-supportive beliefs) displayed by many men who commit rape (Hudson & Ward, 1997). Gannon and Ward (2008, p. 349) suggest that for the scientific knowledge of rapists to be improved researchers must develop valid and clinically meaningful etiological models to guide forensic practice.

Adult Child Abusers

Individuals who sexually abuse children vary in sex, sexual orientation, race, and economic status. Child abusers are often characterized as exhibiting poor social skills, having feelings of vulnerability, worthlessness, inadequacy, humiliation, and loneliness (e.g., Beech, 1998; Terry & Tallon, 2004). They often experience passive or frustrating adult relationships and view themselves as unattractive (Groth, 1979; Robertillo & Terry, 2007). Child abusers are most often classified into typologies based upon the magnitude of their preference for sexual relationships exclusively with children (e.g., Groth & Gary, 1982; Knight & Prentky, 1990). Further, adult male child abusers are commonly classified as either preferential or situational. Preferential abusers, also referred to as fixated abusers, have a persistent, continual, and compulsive attraction to children and often have victim age and gender preferences. Whereas situational, or regressed, offenders are primarily attracted to adults and tend to be triggered by external stressors (Groth & Birnbaum, 1978; Groth & Gary, 1982; Terry & Tallon, 2004).

Preferential offenders, those that are exclusively attracted to children, typically report that their attraction to children began in adolescence. They identify with children socially (Simon, Sales, Kasniak, & Kahn, 1992) and do not develop past the point where they find children attractive and desirable (Finkelhor, 1984). Many preferential offenders are diagnosed with pedophilia, which is the presence of recurrent, intense sexually arousing fantasies, sexual urges, or behaviors involving sexual activity involving pre-pubescent children (American Psychiatric Association, 2013). These individuals are often unable to reach psychosexual maturity to the extent that during adulthood, they have no age-appropriate sexual relationships (Finkelhor, 1984). The preferential offender's acts tend to be premeditated and do not result from enduring stressful life events (Robertillo & Terry, 2007). The majority of preferential offenders abuse extrafamilial male children (Priest & Smith, 1992).

Simon et al. (1992) attempted to empirically validate the preferential-situational (fixated-regressed) typology using a sample of 136 cases of convicted child abusers. They operationalized a detailed list of criteria for defining preferential versus situational offenders using Groth and Birnbaum's (1978) suggested dichotomy. For example, preferential offenders were measured using criteria such as having no indication of at least one sexual relationship with an adult, having never been married or in a cohabitating relationship, and having past convictions or allegations of child sexual abuse. If Groth and Birnbaum's (1978) dichotomous typology were valid, the criteria defining offenders would produce a bimodal distribution, with offenders falling into one category or the other. Rather, the authors found the opposite of what Groth and Birnbaum's (1978) typology predicted, a unimodal and continuous distribution. Such findings caused Simon et al. (1992) to question the clinical utility of the typology and caution its use in making legal or therapeutic decisions.

In part, due to research demonstrating that the preferential-situational typology is unfit to describe all types of child sexual abusers, scholars further distinguish between types of offenders. As shown in Table 14.2, preferential/fixated offenders are often further classified into three distinct types: (1) manipulative, (2) introverted, and (3) sadistic based on their primary attraction and behavioral characteristics. Manipulative child molesters often seek relationships with vulnerable children and will recruit and groom children for an extended period to lower resistance (Conte, 1991). These offenders typically do not use weapons or aggression (Kaseweter, Woodworth, Logan, & Freimuth, 2016). Rather, they give children much affection, love, gifts, and enticements to maintain a sexual "relationship" (Terry & Tallon, 2004). Likewise, the introverted child molester has poor psychosexual development and desires affection from children but lacks the social skills necessary to effectively groom and manipulate access to victims (Knight & Prentky, 1990). Finally, the sadistic child molester is sexually aroused by inflicting pain on children and uses force to gain access to victims. These offenders are aggressive, often use weapons, and target stranger victims (Groth & Gary, 1982; Kaseweter et al., 2016; Terry & Tallon, 2004).

In contrast to preferential offenders, situational offenders are not solely attracted to children but prefer social and sexual interaction with adults. Instead, their secondary attraction to children emerges in adulthood and is often brought on by external stressors such as unemployment, marital problems, substance abuse,

Table 14.2 Summary of adult male child abuser typologies

Classification	Primary attraction	Behavioral and offense characteristics
Preferential	Children	
Manipulative		• Groom vulnerable children for a long period of time to lower resistance • Give children affection and gifts to maintain sexual relationship
Introverted		• Poor psychosexual development, desire affection from children • Lacks social skills to groom or manipulate access to victim
Sadistic		• Sexually aroused by inflicting pain on children • Aggressive and uses force to gain access to victims
Situational	Adults	
Inadequate		• Low self-esteem and poor social skills • Children become a substitute for adult sexual relationships
Indiscriminate		• Abuse children both physically and sexually • Antisocial in nature and use children for their own interests
Experimental		• Driven by desire to experiment with sexual behavior • Victimizes children out of boredom

Sources: Groth and Gary (1982); Holmes and Holmes (1996); Knight and Prentky (1990)

loneliness, stress, isolation, or anxiety (Robertillo & Terry, 2007). These stressors reduce the offender's confidence in themselves and their sexual involvement with children is temporary (Simon et al., 1992). Situational offenders typically victimize children whom they can easily access, such as their own children or those in which they have frequent unsupervised contact. This type is not necessarily motivated by sexual desire and primarily consists of incest offenders or offenders who sexually assault female adolescents (Priest & Smith, 1992; Robertillo & Terry, 2007; Terry & Tallon, 2004). Situational child molesters are often described according to three types: (1) inadequate, (2) indiscriminate, and (3) experimental (Holmes & Holmes, 1996).

Inadequate abusers have a primary sexual attraction to age-appropriate adults, but low self-esteem and poor social skills restrict them from forming age-appropriate sexual relationships. For these offenders, children are their only sexual outlet and become a substitute for an adult relationship. Indiscriminate offenders are more antisocial in nature and abuse children both physically and sexually. They do not prefer children over adults and tend to use children (or anyone accessible) for their own interests. Finally, the experimental child molester is driven by their desire to experiment with almost any type of sexual behavior and tends to sexually victimization children out of boredom (Groth & Gary, 1982; Holmes & Holmes, 1996; Terry & Tallon, 2004).

Knight and Prentky (1990) and Knight, Carter, and Prentky (1989) built upon this preferential-situational typology and developed multidimensional typologies of offenders on two axes. This system, known as the Massachusetts Treatment Center: Child Molester Typology, version 3 (MTC:CM3), assigns each offender a separate Axis I and Axis II typology. As described in Table 14.3, Axis I assesses the extent that an offender fixates on children and the offender's level of social competence. Axis II considers the level of contact an offender has with children and is analyzed based on the meaning (i.e., interpersonal or sexual) of that contact. This axis also evaluates the amount and type of physical injury involved in the contact (Robertillo & Terry, 2007; Terry & Tallon, 2004).

Looman, Gauthier, and Boer (2001) attempted to replicate the MTC:CM3 typology using 109 child abusers in Canada. Their results showed that all abuse types, other than the sadistic types, were able to be reliably classified into all subgroups. The authors note (p. 764) that this exception may be the result of a small number of offenders (n = 33) who fell into the sadistic subgroups, rather than flaws in the typology. Their findings further indicated that it was possible to apply the MTC:CM3 typology to sexual offenders outside of Knight and Prentky's (1990) Massachusetts sample. Looman et al. (2001) suggest that the MTC:CM3 may be used by clinicians to identify offenders with a high risk of sexual recidivism to then enroll them into intensive treatment programs. While this typology has been empirically evaluated, some researchers have questioned its clinical utility concerning recidivism or treatment; additional research on predictive validity and treatment relevance is needed (e.g., Camilleri & Quinsey, 2008; Gannon & Ward, 2008).

Table 14.3 MTC:CM3 Classification of child abusers

Axis	Description of axis measurement
Axis I	• Assess the extent to which the offender is fixated with children (on a continuum) • Measure the level of social competence of the offender
Axis II	• Assesses the amount of contact the offender has with children (e.g., abuses own children) • Meaning of the contact (sexual and interpersonal) • Amount and the type of physical injury involved in the contact (i.e., threats and use of force)

Source: Knight and Prentky (1990); Terry and Tallon (2004)

Female Sex Offenders

In 2015, women made up just 1.2% of all sexual offenders under the jurisdiction of state correctional authorities (Carson & Anderson, 2016). Despite low prevalence, as with male offenders, there is significant heterogeneity among the population of female sexual offenders. Female offenders vary in their motivation, patterns of offending, characteristics, and experiences (Nathan & Ward, 2002; Sandler & Freeman, 2009). Despite the vast amount of research on male sex offenders, most of the existing typologies are not applicable to female sexual offenders, hence why several female-specific typologies have been developed (e.g., Mathews, Matthews, & Speltz, 1989; Vandiver & Kercher, 2004). Compared to male sexual offenders, females are more likely to initiate their behavior at an early age (Bourke, Doherty, McBride, Morgan, & McGee, 2014), admit their behavior (Matthews, 1993), commit their offense with a male co-offender and sexually assault male victims (Nathan & Ward, 2002; Vandiver, 2006). Female sexual offenders are also more likely to be motivated by coercion, threats, and fear of abuse, and to gain the attention and affection of an intimate partner (Matthews, Mathews, & Speltz, 1991). Some research has also suggested that female offenders are less likely to have offended during adolescence or use force during the commission of the offense (Matthews et al., 1991).

Matthews and colleagues (Mathews et al., 1989, 1991) developed one of the most well-known female sexual offender typologies. Using interviews with a clinical sample of 16 women, the researchers identified three types of female sex offenders, as summarized in Table 14.4: (1) teacher/lover, (2) male coerced/male accompanied, and (3) predisposed/self-initiated. Teacher/lover offenders abuse adolescents through their position of power (e.g., high school teacher, mentorship role). They often exhibit dependency needs, abuse substances, experienced a traumatic upbringing, and attempt to meet intimacy and/or sexual needs through offending. These offenders have a difficult time seeing themselves as criminals, but rather see themselves as an equal in a consenting romantic and sexual relationship with an adolescent.

The male coerced/male accompanied offenders are often subordinate and passive women who are coerced by a male they fear. They may be victims of domestic violence and accompany their male partner in abuse that he had been previously committing alone. As such, they tend to victimize their own children (Matthews et al., 1991). These offenders often have low self-esteem, low intelligence, exhibit feelings of powerlessness, fear being alone, and experienced sexual abuse during childhood (Mathews et al., 1989; Syed & Williams, 1996).

Table 14.4 Summary of female sexual offender typologies

Classification	Behavioral and offense characteristics
Teacher/lover	• Abuse adolescents through their position of power • Attempt to meet intimacy and/or sexual needs by offending
Male coerced/male accompanied	• Subordinate woman coerced or accompanied by a male accomplice • Low self-esteem, low intelligence, and feelings of powerlessness • Some witness the abuse without intervening, others take an active role in perpetrating abuse
Predisposed/self-initiated	• Were physically and/or sexually abused as children • May exhibit symptoms of PTSD, depression, addictive behavior, and be suicidal • May be motivated by sadistic fantasies
Source: Matthews et al. (1991)	
Homosexual criminal	• Motivated by financial gain • Engage in the exploitation or forced prostitution of other females • Have high number of arrests for no sexual crimes
Aggressive homosexual	• Victimize adult females, often as a form of intimate partner violence • Motivated by anger, retaliation, and jealousy
Source: Vandiver and Kercher (2004)	

More recent research has differentiated between women who take an active role in abuse by engaging in direct sexual contact with the victim and those who participate passively by watching the abuse, procuring victims for others, and exposing children to sexual interaction or pornography (Grayston & De Luca, 1999). Research also has shown that some women who take an active role in abuse while accompanied by a male, may not necessarily be coerced but motivated by jealousy and anger (Nathan & Ward, 2002).

Similar to the male accompanied offender, predisposed offenders also referred to as self-initiated offenders, victimize their own children or prepubescent children in their care, but do not offend with a male accomplice. Many of predisposed offenders were physically and/or sexually abused as children, have severe psychological disorders, exhibit addictive behavior, and find it difficult to establish healthy sexual relationships as adults (Mathews et al., 1989, 1991). They are more likely than other types of female offenders to display symptoms of posttraumatic stress disorder (PTSD), depression, and be chronically suicidal (Johansson-Love & Fremouw, 2005; Matthews et al., 1991). These offenders may be motivated by sadistic fantasies produced by anger and are more likely to cause harm to their victims (Matthews, 1993; Matthews et al., 1991).

Early female sex offender typologies primarily focused on the sexual abuse of prepubescent children and relied on clinical samples. Recent research developed new typologies to describe female offenders who sexually assault adult or postpubescent females. Using a large sample of 471 convicted female sex offenders, Vandiver and Kercher (2004) established six classifications: (1) heterosexual nurturer, (2) noncriminal homosexual, (3) female sexual predator, (4) young child exploiter, (5) homosexual criminal, and (6) aggressive homosexual. Several of their classifications echoed Matthews and colleagues work (Mathews et al., 1989, 1991) but they added types describing female offenders who offend against adult or postpubescent females, as presented in Table 14.4. The homosexual criminal type is older and more motivated by economic gain than by sexual desire. These offenders engage in the exploitation or forced prostitution of other females who are over 30 years old, display antisocial personality traits and have a higher number of arrests for nonsexual crimes. Whereas aggressive homosexual offenders tend to victimize adult females, often as a form of intimate partner violence; these offenders are older, and are motivated by anger, retaliation, and jealousy (Simons, 2014; Vandiver & Kercher, 2004).

Sandler and Freeman (2009) attempted to test the findings of Vandiver and Kercher (2004) using a sample of 390 female sexual offenders who shared similar demographic characteristics with the original sample. Their study was one of the first empirical tests of a typology for female sexual offenders as past typologies typically relied on small samples sizes (e.g., Matthews et al., 1991). As with the original typology, Sandler and Freeman also found six distinct types of female sexual offender, but the types themselves differed substantially from those found by Vandiver and Kercher. While Vandiver and Kercher (2004) identified six types with a definite preference for one victim gender over the other, only one type in Sandler and Freeman's (2009) analyses showed a strong gender preference. However, their results reinforced the importance of victim and offender age in classifying female offenders.

Female-specific typologies provide a foundation for prevention research and treatment interventions by offering insight into the pathways to offending, motivation, and behavior of female offenders. These typologies assist researchers in understanding the extent that female offenders are similar to, or different from, male sexual offenders. When comparing female to male sexual offender typologies, several similarities emerge (e.g., sexual motivation). However, there are also some notable differences between male and female offenders, such as the prevalence of a co-offender/accomplice during the abuse event (Mathews et al., 1989; Nathan & Ward, 2002; Vandiver, 2006).

Cyber Sexual Offenders

The anonymity, accessibility, and affordability of the internet have led many offenders to use the web as a vehicle for the commission of sexual abuse (Cooper, 1998). As described by Robertiello and Terry (2007, p. 9) the internet serves as a tool for committing child sexual abuse in at least three ways: (1) taking pornographic images of children and distributing them through the internet, (2) sending and consuming pornographic images of children, and (3) luring or soliciting children online. Beech and colleagues (2008) add that the internet also serves as a tool for maintaining and developing online pedophilic networks. The internet allows for easy access to large amounts of sexually abusive media and allows those who are sexually interested in children to organize, maintain, and increase their collection of abusive content (Quayle & Taylor, 2007). The internet not only provides an opportunity for offenders to access abusive content, but it also facilitates a subculture of child sex offenders. Through the use of technology, child sex offenders have been able to form large virtual communities where the abuse of children is acceptable and normal (Taylor, Holland, & Quayle, 2001). These communities reinforce the belief that sexual attraction to children is an expression of "love" rather than abuse, and that children enjoy sexual acts with adults (Quayle & Taylor, 2002).

Sexual offenders often use the internet to "seduce" or otherwise facilitate contact with potential victims (Wolak, Finkelhor, Mitchell, & Ybarra, 2008). To gain compliance, some child sex offenders groom potential victims by showing them pictures of other children having sex. These images are used to show the child what the offender wants the victim to do and to encourage hesitant children to participate in the acts (Alsan, 2011). Several typologies have been created to describe cyber offenders. An important commonality across internet-related typologies is the distinction between offenders who access and download abusive content of children but do not engage in contact offenses and offenders who sexually abuse children offline. Many of these typologies also describe the behavioral move from internet offenses to contact sexual offenses against children, often termed "crossover offending" (Beech et al., 2008).

Lanning (2001, 2010) was among the first to develop a typology which defines three categories, with subtypes within each category, of offenders who use the internet for sexually abusive purposes. Table 14.5 presents a summary of Lanning's (2001, 2010) typology. The situational offender subtypes include those who are not

Table 14.5 Typology of information-technology sexual offenders

Classification	Behavioral and offense characteristics
Situational offenders	
"Normal" adolescent/adult	• An adolescent searching for pornography or impulsive/curious adult with newly found access to sexual opportunities • May include adolescents engaging in "sexting"
Morally indiscriminate	• History of varied criminal offenses • Parents/guardians who make their children available for sex online
Profiteers	• Criminal trying to make easy money through trafficking child pornography • Includes those who blackmail victims after subjecting them to embarrassing sexual contact
Preferential offenders	
Pedophile (Hebephile)	• Definite sexual preference for children or minors
Diverse	• Has a wide variety of paraphilic or deviant sexual interests • Willing to try anything sexual • No strong preferences towards children
Latent	• Criminally act out on their sexual preferences after their inhibitions weaken and arousal patterns fueled through online communication
Miscellaneous "offenders"	
Media reporters	• Mistakenly believe they can go online to traffic child pornography or arrange meetings with suspected abusers as part of an authorized news expose
Pranksters	• Disseminate false or incriminate information to embarrass targets
Older "boyfriends"	• In their late teens or early twenties • Attempt to sexually interact with adolescents
Overzealous citizens	• Members of society who take on their own investigations of online child sexual abuse

Source: Lanning (2001, 2010)

typically motivated by sexual desire. Their sexual activity can be related to bullying or extortion activity. For example, the morally indiscriminate subtype often has a history of criminal offenses and is motivated by power and anger. In contrast, the "normal" adolescent/adult type is typically searching online for pornography and discovers a wide range of sexually explicit materials and sexual opportunities. Most notably, this type also includes adolescents who use the internet to share sexually explicit images of adolescent children, which may include images they created themselves (i.e., through sexting). While against the law, situational offenders' behavior is as not long-term, persistent, and predictable as the preferential type (Lanning, 2010).

Preferential cyber offenders tend to be serial offenders who victimize children through the operation of child sex rings and/or the collection, creation, or distribution of child pornography (Lanning, 2010). These offenders tend to have above average intelligence and come from a middle-class or high socioeconomic background. Within the preferential offender types, Lanning distinguishes between the pedophile/hebephile type and the diverse type of offender. The pedophile type has a primary sexual interest in children. Whereas, the diverse type is primarily interested in a variety of deviant sexual behaviors that sometimes involve children. This type may victimize children to minimize confronting challenges or embarrassment regarding their deviant sexual interests (Lanning, 2010).

Unlike most other typologies (e.g., Krone, 2004), Lanning (2010) described a miscellaneous "offenders" type. These offenders break the law by accessing sexually abusive content of children on the internet but often do so with nonmalicious or vigilante motives. This category includes media reporters who genuinely believe they can traffic child pornography online and arrange meetings with suspected child molesters as part of an all-access news exposé. Prankers who distribute false or incriminating information to embarrass targets of their "dirty tricks" are also included in this category. Lanning (2001, 2010) offered an extensive typology which considers the many reasons an individual decides to use the internet to facilitate sexual offenses. However, as Beech and colleagues (2008) noted, some of Lanning's types are not discrete categories and some overlap. For example, older "boyfriend" offenders may attempt to satisfy their deviant sexual interests by soliciting adolescents online. Lanning claims that while some offenders may exhibit characteristics from multiple types, there will be a dominant theme to an offender's behavior and background characteristics, allowing the offender to be classified under one category. However, as Alsan (2011) points out, Lanning does not provide criteria to determine which type an offender ought to be classified if he exhibits a combination of characteristics.

Krone (2004) developed a comprehensive behavioral-based typology that placed types on a continuum of increasing seriousness of offending. Krone described seriousness using three online behavioral factors: (1) the level of networking by the offender, (2) the level of security they employ to avoid detection, and (3) the nature of abuse, from indirect to contact victimization. Krone (2004) defined nine types of internet sex offenders described in Table 14.5. This typology emphasized several important distinctions between different types of online offending behaviors. For example, the nonsecure collector actively seeks child pornography through peer-to-peer networks. Whereas, the secure collector actively seeks material but only through secure networks (e.g., encryption, protective group entry requirements). Unlike the nonsecure and secure collector types who actively search for abuse content, the browser type unintentionally comes across child pornography (e.g., through spam) but purposefully saves/downloads the material. Krone (2004) discussed the offender's progression from the use abusive online content to crossing-over and committing direct contact offenses. His typology has been recognized as useful in guiding the work of police officers (Wortley & Smallbone, 2006) as it makes the important distinction between offenders who use the internet as part of a broader pattern of contact offending and those who are exclusively accessing abusive content. However, like other cyber sexual offender typologies, Krone's typology

(2004) has been criticized for including categories that are not mutually exclusive (Alsan, 2011).

Upon reviewing previous typologies (e.g., Krone, 2004; Lanning, 2001; Sullivan & Beech, 2004) and noting several overlapping categories, Beech and colleagues (2008) summarized cyber sexual offenders into four distinct types. The first type includes individuals who access abusive images sporadically, impulsively and/or out of curiosity. The second type consists of individuals who access/trade abusive images of children to fuel their sexual interest in children. The third type represents individuals who use the internet as part of a pattern of offline contact offending, including those who use the internet to locate and/or groom contact victims and those who use the internet to disseminate images they have produced. The final type includes individuals who access abusive images for seemingly nonsexual reasons (e.g., for financial profit).

Tener and colleagues (2015) argued for a more complex description of cyber offenders. The scholars resisted the stereotypical view that cyber offenders are expert predators who use technology to identify victims, contact them using fabricated identities, and seduce them to offline meetings for the purpose of sexual exploitation. Though some fit into this stereotype, they argued that it only represents a small portion of offenders. To better understand the complex dynamics between cyber offenders and their victims, the authors developed a typology of cyber sexual offenders based on their patterns of online communication, offline and online identities, their relationship to the victim, and their level of sex crime expertise.

Tener and colleagues (2015) interviewed law enforcement investigators about specific cases involving internet-related child sexual exploitation crimes. Using a grounded theory and constant comparisons approach they analyzed 75 case narratives collected from the interviews. Four types of cyber sexual offender were identified: (1) the experts, (2) the cynical, (3) the affection-focuses, and (4) the sex focused. Expert offenders always have more than one victim and usually meet victims online, with some of their relationships existing solely online. These offenders use both true and fabricated identities when soliciting victims and may present victims with money or gifts to get their cooperation. Experts demonstrate a high level of sex crime expertise, have large collections of child pornography, and target victims who are most vulnerable to exploitation because they are overweight, have acne or experience other problems.

The cynical offenders have similar characteristics to the expert type but have lower expertise and are less extreme. These offenders often have one or few victims who they usually have met face-to-face. Other relationships are based online or started online and advanced to in-person meetings. A sexual relationship may develop immediately or progress gradually, and many of their relationships are reciprocal at first. These offenders may possess child pornography but not on as large a scale as the experts (Tener et al., 2015). The third type, the affection-focused, are characterized by having genuine feelings of love, care, and affections for victims. It is rare for this type to possess child pornography. Most often, their relationships begin online and develop into a close romantic relationship, with both the victim and offender interested in meeting face-to-face. Sometimes these offenders were unaware that they were involved with a minor (e.g., a minor lied about their age) and upon learning about their actual age, felt that they were too emotionally involved to end communication with the victim (Tener et al., 2015). In other cases, the affection-focused offender was an older teen who was unaware that their reciprocal relationship with a younger teen was illegal. Unlike other types, these offenders do not coerce or manipulate their victims.

The sex-focused type described offenders who were looking on the internet for immediate sexual encounters. These offenders have a low level of sex crime expertise and generally present their real identities. The relationships of sex-focused offenders can be viewed as exchanges or deals, and they are not interested in forming romantic or emotional relationships. They do not necessarily seek out underage adolescents but are willing to engage in sexual interactions with a minor if approached by one.

For example, sex-focused offenders may initially communicate (sometimes unknowingly) with minors on a sexually oriented networking site then meet face-to-face for a planned sexual encounter.

Several typologies highlight the countless ways the internet can be used to manipulate and gain access to victims and connect and exchange abusive content with networks of sexual offenders (e.g., Krone, 2004; Lanning, 2010). While some offenders seek illegal content and interactions online, others are unaware that they are sexually involved and/or have a romantic relationship with an underage person (Tener et al., 2015). More recent typologies (e.g., Tener et al., 2015) demonstrate that some offenders are not motivated by deviant sexual thoughts and beliefs. Rather, to both the offender and the victim, some of these relationships may have appeared genuine and reciprocal. Given the heterogeneous nature of the population, no cyber sexual offender typology has universal validity; they are not comprehensive and overlap in many ways (Alsan, 2011). However, typologies can aid in enhancing the understanding of dynamics between cyber sexual offenders and their victims so that researchers and policymakers can attempt to develop effective prevention programs and treatment for both the offender and their victim.

Sexual Predators or Criminal Opportunists?

Sexual offender typologies have been met with skepticism within the criminological literature because of the implicit assumption that sex offenders are different from conventional, nonsexual offenders (e.g., Smallbone & Wortley, 2004a, 2004b). This perspective assumes that sexual offenders commit sexual offenses persistently and almost exclusively throughout their criminal careers (Harris, Mazerolle, & Knight, 2009). Alternatively, criminologists have argued that offenders who commit sexual offenses are just as likely to engage in many different crimes (e.g., substance use, physical assault) during their criminal career as those who commit nonsexual crimes (e.g., Gottfredson & Hirschi, 1990; Wortley & Smallbone, 2013). According to this criminological perspective, most sexual offenses represent one of many manifestations of an offender's antisocial nature (Harris et al., 2009).

Research supporting this general offending perspective has shown that most sexual offenders engage in both sexual and nonsexual offenses (Lussier, 2005; Smallbone & Wortley, 2004a, 2004b; Wortley & Smallbone, 2013). Harris and colleagues (2009; Harris, Knight, Dennison, and Smallbone, 2011) studied the criminal histories of sexual offenders and consistently found versatility in offenses across types of sexual offenders. Both rapists and child abusers engaged in multiple types of crime over their criminal careers. Similarly, in a series of studies, Smallbone and Wortley (2000, 2001, 2004a, 2004b) examined the criminal careers of convicted child abusers and consistently found that of the offenders with a previous conviction, the vast majority were convicted of a nonsexual offense.

While many sexual abusers also engage in general offending, research has identified a small but notable group of persistent sexual offenders. Wortley and Smallbone (2013) described a small category of persistent specialists who generally do not have nonsexual convictions but are more likely to have multiple sexual convictions. These serial sexual offenders started offending at a later age than other sexual offenders and often report having a nonheterosexual orientation. Persistent sexual offenders often abuse nonfamilial male victims, report a higher number of victims, and are likely to have frequent and extended contact with victims. Harris and colleagues (2009, 2011) also identified a small subgroup of child molesters and mixed age offenders as crime specialists. They suggest that group may warrant a sexually specific classification and specialized treatment as they appear to be substantially different from the rest of offenders.

Collectively, these studies' findings suggest that while there is a small group of sexually specialized offenders, most sexual offenders are not persistent specialists. Rather, sexual abuse is a limited or occasional activity in the offender's general involvement in crime (Wortley & Smallbone, 2013). Instead of an underlying motivation to sexually offend these general offenders may struggle to exhibit self-control and fail to restrain their behavior in the face of particular opportunities and temptations.

Limitations to Traditional Typologies

Typologies can act as a useful investigative, assessment, and treatment tool and offer considerable insight on the motivations and behavioral and offense characteristics of male and female sexual offenders. However, the heterogeneity of the sexual offender population has made it difficult to develop a comprehensive model of sexual offending. The methodological limitations of typology development such as issues of sampling methods (e.g., clinical samples, drawing a sample by victim sex, convicted offenders), low base rates of sexual reoffense, and social desirability in self-reports (e.g., omitting offenses involving same-sex victims) have limited the validity and reliability of many existing typologies and inspired criticism (Bickley & Beech, 2001). Many existing typologies are not mutually exclusive, and offenders share characteristics of multiple classifications. Similarly, sex offenders do not always specialize in one type of offending (e.g., adult rape or child abuse) but engage in multiple types of sexual and nonsexual offenses (i.e., crossover offending; Heil, Simons, & Burton, 2010; Smallbone & Wortley, 2004a, 2004b; Wortley & Smallbone, 2013).

The occurrence of crossover offending challenges the validity of traditional sex offender typologies, many of which are based on one victim type (e.g., children; Simons, 2014). Research has shown that sexual offenders often admit to victimizing considerably more persons than recorded in official arrest and court records. Male sexual offenders engage in high rates of crossover offending with their victims varying in age (i.e., children and adults), relationship to the offender (i.e., family member) and gender (e.g., Heil, Ahlmeyer, & Simons, 2003). Female offenders also report patterns of both age and relationship crossover offending (Heil et al., 2010).

Examining the occurrence of crossover offending has become even more crucial with the development of cyber sexual offender typologies. Some internet offenders solely offend online (i.e., viewing or collecting child pornography) and do not attempt contact sexual abuse (Beech et al., 2008). Making this distinction between offenders is important for classification systems because strictly cyber offenders may not pose a direct threat to children. A meta-analysis examining the prevalence of contact child sexual abuse among cyber offenders found that 12 percent of cyber offenders engaged in known contact abuse as indicated by official records (i.e., arrests, charges, and/or convictions). However, this rate increased to approximately 50 percent when using self-report data, suggesting that there may be a distinct group on online-only offenders (Seto, Hanson, & Babchishin, 2011).

Emerging sexual offender typology research has begun to recognize the importance of understanding the motivation and behavior of crossover offenders in an effort to enhance prevention and treatment efforts. Using a sample of 567 sexual offenders committed for treatment, Rice and Knight (2018) compared the characteristics of adults with mixed aged sexual offense victims (MASOVs) with that of adults who exclusively offend against children (CSOVs) or adults (ASOVs). Overall, their results show that MASOVs were not significantly different from CSOVs or ASOVS in their trauma history (e.g., childhood neglect and physical abuse, family stability, and sexual assault victimization). However, they did experience more cumulative abuse than both groups. MASOVs also displayed lower self-esteem and higher levels of psychopathy compared to CSOVs. Rice and Knight's (2018) findings demonstrate the need to develop treatment plans specific to mixed aged sexual offenders because they display different characteristics than offenders who exclusively offender against adults or children.

Future Directions

Findings from studies on crossover and mixed age offending suggest the traditional typologies based on age preference for victims may not be a useful tool for allocating resources, evaluating risk, or constructing individualized treatment interventions (Simons, 2014). Research has shown that specialized sexual offenders do exist, but they make up the minority of sexual offenders (Harris et al., 2009; Wortley & Smallbone, 2013). Many of the current policies aimed at preventing and managing sexual offenders were implemented under the assumption that sexual offending is a distinct and specialized type of offending. This led to the implementation of universal and selective crime control policies that target convicted sexual offenders such as community registration and notification, and resident restrictions (Harris et al., 2009). To most effectively treat and prevent sexual offending, it is important to classify and treat offenders based on characteristics that have been shown to increase the risk of recidivism. Rather than applying strict sexual-offense-specific policy and treatment to all sexual offenders, it may be most beneficial to target general-offense related factors such as antisocial beliefs and attitudes, poor self-control, and weak problem-solving, and anger-management skills (Wortley & Smallbone, 2013). Sexual-offense-specific treatment should be uniquely designed for specialized sex offenders.

To address the issues of heterogeneity and crossover offending, Robertiello and Terry (p. 10, 2007) suggest that perhaps the best way to view typologies of sexual offenders is as a continuum rather than mutually exclusive, exhaustive categories. Typologies should be seen as a tool for enhancing the understanding of the motivations and tactics of sexual offenders. They have the potential to aid researchers and practitioners in developing treatment and supervision strategies tailored to the offender. As sexual offender typology advances, researchers and practitioners should be cautious when regarding sexual offenders as having different risks and needs from non-sexual offenders. Future research should also address crossover and mixed age offending when developing classification systems and treatment and prevention interventions.

References

Agan, A. Y. (2011). Sex offender registries: Fear without function? *Journal of Law and Economics, 54*, 207–239.

Alsan, D. (2011). Critically evaluating typologies of internet sex offenders: A psychological perspective. *Journal of Forensic Psychology Practice, 11*, 406–431.

American Psychiatric Association. (2013). *Diagnostic and statistical manual of mental disorders* (5th ed.). Washington, DC: American Psychiatric Association.

Barbaree, H. E., Seto, M. C., Serin, R. C., Amos, N. L., & Preston, D. L. (1994). Comparison between sexual and nonsexual rapist subtypes. *Criminal Justice and Behavior, 21*, 95–114.

Beech, A. R. (1998). A psychometric typology of child abusers. *International Journal of Offender Therapy and Comparative Criminology, 42*, 391–339.

Beech, A. R., Elliott, I. A., Birgden, A., & Findlater, D. (2008). The internet and child sexual offending: A criminological review. *Aggression and Violent Behavior, 13*, 216–228.

Berger, R. D. (2000). Successfully investigating acquaintance sex assault. National Center for Women and Policing: OJP.

Bickley, J., & Beech, A. R. (2001). Classifying child abusers: Its relevance to theory and clinical practice. *International Journal of Offender Therapy and Comparative Criminology, 45*, 51–69.

Bourke, A., Doherty, S., McBride, O., Morgan, K., & McGee, H. (2014). Female perpetrators of child sexual abuse: Characteristics of the offender and victim. *Psychology, Crime & Law, 20*, 769–780.

Budrionis, R., & Jongsma, A. E. (2003). *The sexual abuse victim and sexual offender treatment planner*. West Sussex: John Wiley & Sons.

Button, D. M., Tewksbury, R., Mustaine, E. E., & Payne, B. K. (2013). Factors contributing to perceptions about policies regarding the electronic monitoring of sex offenders: The role of demographic characteristics, victimization experiences, and social disorganization. *International Journal of Offender Therapy and Comparative Criminology, 57*, 25–54.

Camilleri, J. A., & Quinsey, V. L. (2008). Pedophilia: Assessment and treatment. In D. R. Laws & W. O'Donohue (Eds.), *Sexual deviance: Theory, assessment, and treatment* (Vol. 2, pp. 183–212). New York: Guilford Press.

Carson, E. A. & Anderson, E. (2016). Prisoners in 2015. U.S. Department of Justice: Bureau of Justice Statistics. Retrieved from http://www.bjs.gov/index.cfm?ty=pbdetail&iid=5869

Cohen, M. L., Seghorn, T., & Calmas, W. (1969). Sociometric study of sex offenders. *Journal of Abnormal Psychology, 74*, 249–255.

Conte, J. R. (1991). The nature of sexual offences against children. In C. R. Hollin & K. Howells (Eds.), *Clinical Approaches to Sex Offenders and Their Victims*. West Sussex, England: John Wiley & Sons.

Cooper, A. (1998). Sexuality and the internet: Surfing into the new millennium. *Cyber Psychology and Behavior, 1*, 187–193.

Craissati, J. (2005). Sexual violence against women: A psychological approach to the assessment and management of rapists in the community. *Probation Journal: The Journal of Community and Criminal Justice, 52*, 401–422.

Finkelhor, D. (1984). *Child sexual abuse*. New York: Free Press.

Freund, K. (1990). Courtship disorder. In W. L. Marshall, D. R. Laws, & H. E. Barbaree (Eds.), *Handbook of sexual assault: Issues, theories and treatment of the offender*. New York: Plenum Press.

Gannon, T.A., & Ward, T. (2008). Rape: Psychopathology and theory. In D.R. Laws & W. O'Donohue (Eds.), Sexual Deviance: Theory, Assessment, and Treatment, vol. 2 (pp. 336–355). New York: Guilford Press.

Gottfredson, M. R., & Hirschi, T. (1990). *A general theory of crime*. Stanford, CA: Stanford University Press.

Grayston, A. D., & De Luca, R. V. (1999). Female perpetrators of child sexual abuse: A review of the clinical and empirical literature. *Aggression and Violent Behaviour, 4*, 93–106.

Groth, A. N. (1979). *Men who rape: The psychology of the offender*. New York: Plenum Press.

Groth, A. N., & Birnbaum, H. J. (1978). Adult sexual orientation and attraction to underage persons. *Archives of Sexual Behavior, 7*, 175–181.

Groth, A. N., Burgess, A. W., & Holmstrom, L. L. (1977). Rape: Power, anger, and sexuality. *American Journal of Psychiatry, 134*, 1239–1243.

Groth, A. N., Hobson,W. F., & Gary, T. S. (1982). The child molester: Clinical observations. In J. Conte & D.A. Shore (Eds.), Social work and child sexual abuse. New York: Haworth, 1, 129.

Hanson, R. K., Harris, A. J., Helmus, L., & Thornton, D. (2014). High-risk sex offenders may not be high risk forever. *Journal of Interpersonal Violence, 29*, 2792–2813.

Harris, D. A., Knight, R. A., Dennison, S., & Smallbone, S. (2011). Post release specialization and versatility in sexual offenders referred for civil commitment. *Sexual Abuse: A Journal of Research and Treatment, 23*, 243–259.

Harris, D. A., Mazerolle, P., & Knight, R. A. (2009). Understanding male sexual offending: A comparison of general and specialist theories. *Criminal Justice and Behavior, 36*, 1051–1069.

Heil, P., Ahlmeyer, S., & Simons, D. (2003). Crossover sexual offenses. *Sexual Abuse: A Journal of Research and Treatment, 15*, 221–236.

Heil, P., Simons, D. A., & Burton, D. (2010). Using the polygraph with female sexual offenders. In T. A. Gannon & F. Cortoni (Eds.), *Female sexual offending: Theory, assessment, & treatment*. Hoboken, NJ: John Wiley & Sons.

Holmes, R. M., & Holmes, S. T. (1996). *Profiling violent crimes: An investigative tool*. Thousand Oaks, CA: Sage Publications.

Hudson, S. M., & Ward, T. (1997). Rape: Psychopathology and theory. In D. R. Laws & W. O'Donohue (Eds.), *Sexual deviance: Theory, assessment, and treatment* (Vol. 1, pp. 322–355). New York: Guilford Press.

Jennings, W. G., & Fox, B. H. (2016). Rape and other sexual offending behaviors. In B. M. Huebner & T. S. Bynum (Eds.), *Handbook of measurement issues in criminology and criminal justice* (pp. 69–91). West Sussex: John Wiley & Sons, Inc.

Johansson-Love, J., & Fremouw, W. (2005). A critique of the female sexual perpetrator research. *Aggression and Violent Behavior, 11*, 12–26.

Kaseweter, K., Woodworth, M., Logan, M., & Freimuth, T. (2016). High-risk sexual offenders: Towards a new typology. *Journal of Criminal Justice, 47*, 123–132.

Knight, R. A. (1999). Validation of a typology for rapists. *Journal of Interpersonal Violence, 14*, 297–323.

Knight, R. A., Carter, D. L., & Prentky, R. A. (1989). A system for the classification of child molesters: Reliability and application. *Journal of Interpersonal Violence, 4*, 3–23.

Knight, R. A., & Prentky, R. A. (1990). Classifying sexual offenders. In W. L. Marshall, D. R. Laws, & H. E. Barbaree (Eds.), *Handbook of sexual assault* (pp. 23–52). New York, NY: Springer.

Krone, T. (2004). A typology of online child pornography offending. *Trends and Issues in Crime and Criminal Justice, 279*, 1–6.

Lanning, K. V. (2001). Child molesters: A behavioral analysis, 4th ed. Retrieved from https://www.mjfacts.com/resources/NC70.pdf

Lanning, K. V. (2010). Child molesters: A behavioral analysis, 5th ed. Retrieved from http://www.missingkids.com/content/dam/ncmec/en_us/desktop/publications/nc70.pdf

Levenson, J. S., Brannon, Y. N., Fortney, T., & Baker, J. (2007). Public perceptions about sex offenders and community protection policies. *Analyses of Social Issues and Public Policy, 7*, 137–161.

Looman, J., Gauthier, C., & Boer, D. (2001). Replication of the Massachusetts treatment center child molester typology in a Canadian sample. *Journal of Interpersonal Violence, 16*, 753–767.

Lussier, P. (2005). The criminal activity of sexual offenders in adulthood: Revisiting the specialization debate. *Sexual Abuse: A Journal of Research and Treatment, 17*, 269–292.

Mathews, R., Matthews, J., & Speltz, K. (1989). Female sexual offenders: An exploratory study. Orwell, VT: The Safer Society Press.

Matthews, J. K. (1993). Working with female sexual abusers. In M. Elliott (Ed.), *Female sexual abuse of children*. New York: Guilford Press.

Matthews, J. K., Mathews, R., & Speltz, K. (1991). Female sexual offenders: A typology. In M. Q. Patton (Ed.), *Family sexual abuse: Frontline research and evaluation*. Newbury Park: Sage Publications.

Nathan, P., & Ward, T. (2002). Female sex offenders: Clinical and demographic features. *Journal of Sexual Aggression, 8*, 5–21.

Planty, M., Langton, L., Krebs, C., Berzofsky, M., & Smiley-McDonald, H. (2013). Female victims of sexual violence, 1994–2010. Retrieved from https://www.bjs.gov/content/pub/pdf/fvsv9410.pdf

Prentky, R. A., Cohen, M. L., & Seghorn, T. K. (1985). Development of a rational taxonomy for the classification of sexual offenders: Rapists. *Bulletin of the American Academy of Psychiatry and the Law, 13*, 39–70.

Priest, R., & Smith, A. (1992). Counseling adult sexual offenders: Unique challenges and treatment paradigms. *Journal of Counseling & Development, 71*, 27–32.

Proctor, J. L., Badzinski, D. M., & Johnson, M. (2002). The impact of media on knowledge and perceptions of Megan's law. *Criminal Justice Policy Review, 13*, 356–379.

Quayle, E., & Taylor, M. (2002). Paedophiles pornography and the internet: Assessment issues. *British Journal of Social Work, 3*, 863–875.

Quayle, E., & Taylor, M. (2007). *Internet and child pornography*. London: Psychology Press Ltd.

Rada, R. T. (1978). *Clinical aspects of the rapist*. New York: Grune & Stratton.

Reid, S. L., Wilson, N. J., & Boer, D. P. (2010). Application of the Massachusetts treatment center revised rapist typology to New Zealand high-risk rapists: A pilot study. *Sexual Abuse in Australia and New Zealand, 2*, 77–84.

Rice, J., & Knight, R. A. (2018). Differentiating adults with mixed age victims from those who exclusively sexually assault children or adults. *Sexual Abuse, 0*, 1–21.

Robertillo, G., & Terry, K. (2007). Can we profile sex offenders? A review of sex offender typologies. *Aggression and Violent Behavior, 12*, 508–519.

Sandler, J. C., & Freeman, N. J. (2009). Female sex offender recidivism: A large-scale empirical analysis. *Sexual Abuse: A Journal of Research and Treatment, 21*, 455–473.

Seto, M. C., Hanson, K. R., & Babchishin, K. M. (2011). Contact sexual offending by men with online sexual offenses. *Sexual Abuse: A Journal of Research and Treatment, 23*, 124–145.

Simon, L. M. J., Sales, B., Kasniak, A., & Kahn, M. (1992). Characteristics of child molesters: Implications for the fixated-regressed dichotomy. *Journal of Interpersonal Violence, 7*, 211–225.

Simons, D. A. (2014). Sex offender typologies. *Office of Justice Programs: Sex Offender Management Assessment and Planning Initiative* (Chapter 3). Retrieved from https://www.smart.gov/SOMAPI/printerFriendlyPDF/adult-sec3.pdf

Smallbone, S. W., & Wortley, R. K. (2000). *Child sexual abuse in Queensland: Offender characteristics and modus operandi*. Brisbane: Queensland Crime Commission.

Smallbone, S. W., & Wortley, R. K. (2001). *Child sexual abuse: Offender characteristics and modus operandi (Australian Institute of Criminology Trends and Issues in Crime and Criminal Justice, No. 193)*. Canberra: Australian Institute of Criminology.

Smallbone, S. W., & Wortley, R. K. (2004a). Criminal versatility and paraphilic interests among adult males convicted of sexual offenses against children. *International Journal of Offender Therapy and Comparative Criminology, 48*, 175–188.

Smallbone, S. W., & Wortley, R. K. (2004b). Onset, persistence and versatility of offending among adult males convicted of sexual offenses against children. *Sexual Abuse: A Journal of Research and Treatment, 16*, 285–298.

Sullivan, J., & Beech, A. R. (2004). Assessing Internet sex offenders. In M. C. Calder (Ed.), *Child sexual abuse and the Internet: Tackling the new frontier* (pp. 69–83). Lyme Regis: Russell House.

Syed, F., & Williams, S. (1996). Case studies of female sex offenders in the Correctional Service of Canada. Ottawa: Correctional Service Canada.

Taylor, M., Holland, G., & Quayle, E. (2001). Typology of paedophile picture collections. *The Police Journal, 74*, 97–107.

Tener, D., Wolak, J., & Finkelhor, D. (2015). A typology of offenders who use online communications to commit sex crimes against minors. *Journal of Aggression, Maltreatment & Trauma, 24*, 319–337.

Terry, K., & Tallon, J. (2004). *Child sexual abuse: A review of the literature. The nature and scope of the problem of sexual abuse of minors by priests and deacons* (pp. 1950–2002). Washington, DC: United States Conference of Catholic Bishops.

Vandiver, D. M. (2006). Female sex offenders: A comparison of solo offenders and co-offenders. *Violence and Victims, 21*, 339–354.

Vandiver, D. M., & Kercher, G. (2004). Offender and victim characteristics of registered female sexual offenders in Texas: A proposed typology of female sexual offenders. *Sexual Abuse: A Journal of Research and Treatment, 16*, 121–137.

Wolak, J., Finkelhor, D., Mitchell, K. J., & Ybarra, M. L. (2008). Online "predators" and their victims. *American Psychologist, 63*, 111–128.

Wortley, R., & Smallbone, S. (2013). A criminal careers typology of child sexual abusers. *Sexual Abuse: A Journal of Research and Treatment, 26*, 569–585.

Wortley, R. K., & Smallbone, S. (2006). Applying situational principles to sexual offenses against children. In R. K. Wortley & S. Smallbone (Eds.), *Situational prevention of child sexual abuse* (pp. 7–36). Monsey, NY: Criminal Justice Press.

The Role of Hypermasculinity as a Risk Factor in Sexual Assault Perpetration

15

Catalina Vechiu

Sexual assault victimization continues to pose a significant public health concern in the United States. National prevalence rates estimate that 19.3% of women and 1.7% of men have been sexually assaulted at some point in their lifetime (Breiding et al., 2014). The high prevalence of sexual assault victimization on college campuses and the extensive psychological consequences associated with sexual assault have garnered increased attention from researchers, policymakers, and the media. Part of the increased media attention in recent years is due to international movements against sexual assault such as #MeToo and the mishandling of well-known cases involving college football teams or fraternities that serve to increase public awareness of the widespread prevalence and far-reaching consequences of sexual violence. The identification of risk factors for sexual violence is fundamental for the development of prevention and intervention efforts. Yet, investigations of preventative methods for sexual assault perpetration have largely focused on victim characteristics and contextual factors. These investigations have yet to lead to a consensus on the optimal approach for sexual assault prevention. Prevention programs borne out of this literature have not undergone rigorous empirical evaluation and are largely ineffective (see Newlands & O'Donohue, 2016 for a review). It may be more prudent to examine perpetrator characteristics that increase the likelihood of sexual violence perpetration. Although such data exist, most focus on perpetrator personality traits, alcohol consumption, and beliefs and attitudes about sexuality. A significantly smaller number of studies have examined the role of hypermasculinity in sexual assault perpetration. Hypermasculinity refers to the exaggeration of male stereotypical behavior such that hypermasculine men engage in callous sexual behavior towards women, endorse beliefs that violence is manly, and experience danger as exciting (Mosher & Sirkin, 1984). Hypermasculinity has been found to be associated with endorsement of rape myths and sexual assault perpetration (Locke & Mahalik, 2005; Zinzow & Thompson, 2015). This chapter provides an overview of the theoretical framework of hypermasculinity, identifies the sociocultural correlates of hypermasculinity that are associated with the perpetration of sexual assault, and reviews limitations in the literature as well as promising prevention programs and intervention strategies.

C. Vechiu (✉)
University of Nevada, Reno, Reno, NV, USA

W. T. O'Donohue and P. A. Schewe (eds.), *Handbook of Sexual Assault and Sexual Assault Prevention*,
https://doi.org/10.1007/978-3-030-23645-8_15

Theoretical Conceptualization of Hypermasculinity

Hierarchy of Masculinities

The prevention of gendered violence requires an understanding of the impact of differential socialization on the development of masculinities and gendered power relations. The study of masculinities was brought to the forefront of scholarly discourse by Connell's (1987) seminal paper on hegemonic masculinity. The concept of *hegemony* is derived from Gramsci's (1971) analysis of class relations and refers to a position of dominance in social life that is culturally dynamic. Connell (1987) proposed that there are multiple masculinities that are fluid, dynamic, and vary across cultures and individuals and serve to legitimize gender inequality. One form of masculinity is perpetuated over another at any given time by those who benefit from it and those who are oppressed by it (Jewkes et al., 2015). To further understand men's dominant position in society and the subordination of women, Connell (2005) posited that it is necessary to examine the dynamic gender relations between the embodiments of multiple masculinities. According to Connell (2005), the hierarchy of masculinities includes:

- *Hegemonic masculinity*: can be defined as the "configuration of gender practice which embodies the currently accepted answer to the problem of the legitimacy of patriarchy, which guarantees (or is taken to guarantee) the dominant position of men and the subordination of women" (Connell, 2005, p. 77). Hegemonic masculinity is a culturally idealized manifestation of manhood that refers to economically privileged men who exhibit socially dominant and accepted characteristics of traditional masculinity. This may not be the most prevalent form of masculinity, but it is often the most culturally valued. Hegemonic masculinity is a display of successful claim to authority that upholds the patriarchy. Bearers of hegemonic masculinity are those who hold institutional power or great wealth, are often White, heterosexual, and wealthy.
- *Subordinate masculinity*: can be defined in opposition to hegemonic masculinity, such that it is the exhibition of values and characteristics that are expelled from hegemonic masculinity. Bearers of subordinate masculinity are those who are physically weak, engage in overt expression of emotions, are not heterosexual, or are effeminate. Connell (2005) states that gay men are the exemplary form of subordinate masculinity due to the cultural stigmatization of homosexuality. Gay men are subjugated to political and cultural exclusion, legal and street violence, economic discrimination, and personal boycott (Connell, 2005). Subordinate masculinity is assimilated to femininity.
- *Complicit masculinity*: can be defined "in ways that realize the patriarchal dividend, without the tensions or risks of being the frontline troops of patriarchy" (Connell, 2005, p. 79). Bearers of complicit masculinity are those who do not embody the characteristics of hegemonic masculinity but often benefit from and admire it. Connell (2005) specifically refers to the advantage men in general gain from the overall subordination of women.
- *Marginalized masculinity*: can be defined as a form of masculinity that idealizes characteristics normative of hegemonic masculinity but is applied to men who are marginalized in society, such as men from minority groups or disabled men. Bearers of marginalized masculinity are those who value characteristics such as physical strength and aggression and wealth but are not identified as hegemonic due to their ethnicity or social status. Connell (2005) posits that African-American athletes are exemplars of marginalized masculinity, such that their individual wealth and fame does not yield social authority to all black men.

Some scholars have expanded Connell's (1987) hierarchy of masculinities to include *toxic masculinity*, which refers to "the constellation of socially regressive male traits that serve to foster domination, the devaluation of women, homophobia, and wanton violence" (Kupers, 2005, p. 714). Toxic masculinity delineates the characteristics of hegemonic masculinity that are the most socially destructive, such as extreme competition and greed, the need to dominate and control others, particularly women, gay or effeminate men, readiness to resort to violence, and need for respect (Kupers, 2005). According to Kupers (2005), although desiring respect is not inherently toxic, the repeated frustration of a man's need to be respected can lead to toxicity. Toxic masculinity has been subject to considerable theoretical analyses, primarily focusing on (1) the factors that lead to the development of toxic masculinity within prison contexts and (2) deconstruction of various television shows that highlight the development and impact of toxic masculinity. Empirical studies examining its utility and association with sexual assault perpetration are limited and few tools have been developed and empirically validated to directly measure toxic masculinity (Parent, Gobble, & Rochlen, 2018).

Distinguishing between various manifestations of masculinity is important for understanding the relationship between sexual violence, gender norms, and the individual. The study of masculinities posits that sexual violence is a tool for the attainment of social status, protecting the patriarchal order, and reaffirming the superiority of one group of men over another (Fahlberg & Pepper, 2016). Sexual assault victimization disproportionately involves girls and women as victims and men as perpetrators. It is well established that unequal power dynamics and social norms related to gender and sexuality impact the incidence of sexual assault. For instance, several cross-cultural studies have found that men perform masculinity though sexual violence, particularly among adolescent and young men. In a study of sexual scripts (i.e. culturally codified sequence of events leading to sexual activity) of Kenyan adolescents, Njue, Askew, and Chege (2005) found that forced sex was a common consequence of a girl's persistent refusal to engage in sexual activity for fear of exclusion, stigmatization, or rejection by peers. Male participants reported that they would be perceived as "impotent" or "not man enough" if they did not ultimately engage in sexual intercourse, forced or otherwise. Likewise, a study examining Cambodian youth and perpetration of gang rape found that participants reported that perpetration of gang rape was an affirmation of their masculinity (Wilkinson, Bearup, & Soprach, 2005). In a study of US high school males, Pascoe (2007) found that participants often felt they needed to pressure, convince, or force young women to have sex in order to prevent themselves from being harassed or emasculated by their male peers and to uphold their status as men. Sexual violence against women also asserts men's racial dominance or as a tool for combating structural subordination. For instance, Bourgois (1995) argues that sexual violence among Latinos in a New York City neighborhood is a result of the loss of normative masculine resources due to deindustrialization, decline of low-wage employment, and expansion of women's rights.

The question regarding whether hegemonic masculinity is associated with sexual violence is subject to considerable debate. Some scholars argue that due to the high rates of intimate partner violence and the low rates of women's disclosures or reporting of sexual violence, the public stature of men who engage in low-level violence against women is not diminished (Garcia-Moreno, Jansen, Ellsberg, & Watts, 2005). This may inadvertently serve to enhance men's public stature due to the perception of being in control. Other scholars, however, argue that sexual violence diminishes men's social status, particularly during the era of social media and international movements aimed at increasing awareness of gendered violence. This line of reasoning posits that hegemonic masculinity is a gender stereotype and therefore sexual violence may not necessarily be hegemonic in a particular culture (Messerschmidt, 2012). As such, the concept of hypermasculinity may be more useful as a potential risk factor for sexual assault victimization.

Hypermasculinity

The concept of hypermasculinity has been defined as the adherence to an exaggerated ideology of the prototypical male. Similar to hegemonic masculinity, hypermasculine men hold exaggerated beliefs regarding the behaviors of the ideal male. According to Mosher and Sirkin (1984), hypermasculinity is comprised of four beliefs:

1. *Insensitive attitudes towards sex and women*: such beliefs include an emphasis on the male sexual experience at the expense of the woman's sexual experience and sexual intercourse is equated with women's sexual dominance. Within this paradigm, sexual intercourse is an aggressive and depersonalized act for men that serves to exert male power and female submission (Vokey, Tefft, & Tysiaczny, 2013).
2. *Violent aggression is an acceptable expression of male dominance*: this belief reflects the attitude that violence is manly and aggression, verbal and/or physical, is an acceptable method for exerting dominance over other men and women.
3. *Danger is exciting*: Dangerous situations are perceived as opportunities to demonstrate power and dominance over men and women or the environment.
4. *Emotional self-control*: Expressing emotions is perceived as a feminine act and a sign of weakness. The suppression of emotions such as sadness, fear, or empathy is considered to be a legitimate display of male toughness.

The four domains of hypermasculinity combine to legitimize the use of violence against women and are believed to reflect gender role socialization across the lifespan, particularly during childhood. The cultural ideology of hypermasculinity is perpetuated by mass media and reinforces earlier parental socialization by normalizing and promoting hypermasculine behaviors (Vokey et al., 2013). Gender role socialization via multiple pathways engenders conformity to stereotypical masculine behaviors, particularly during adolescence and young adulthood. Traits such as aggression and toughness are highly valued and reinforced via social sanctions. Nonconformity to hypermasculine ideals is severely punished via social exclusion, rejection, and/or bullying. Males who demonstrate willingness to engage in aggressive behaviors avoid becoming the recipients of harassment (Vokey et al., 2013). Previous research with young adult males has found that hypermasculinity is associate with increased risk-taking behaviors such as large number of sexual partners and substance use (Burk, Burkhart, & Sikorski, 2004), aggression towards men who violate gender norms (Parrott & Zeichner, 2008), and aggression toward women (Seaton, 2007). High levels of hypermasculinity are associated with past sexual aggression (Gold, Fultz, Burke, Prisco, & Willett, 1992) and are significant predictors of future sexual aggression (Vaas & Gold, 1995). There is strong support in the literature for the positive association between hypermasculinity and sexual assault perpetration.

Sociocultural Correlates of Hypermasculinity

The most abundant support for the correlation between hypermasculinity and sexual aggression stems from a plethora of studies examining specific domains of hypermasculinity, such as attitudes and beliefs about sex and women. Specifically, the endorsement of:

- *Impersonal attitudes towards sex*: Men who hold more casual attitudes towards sex, such as, "love is not a necessary part of sex" are more likely to perpetrate sexual assault (White, McMullin, Swartout, Sechrist, & Gollehon, 2008). Additionally, in a sample of community men, casual attitudes towards sex were directly related to the number of sexual assaults committed (Abbey, Parkhill, BeShears, Clinton-Sherrod, & Zawacki, 2006). The link between impersonal attitudes and sexual assault victimization may be explained by increased opportunities for perpetration. For instance, men who endorse impersonal attitudes towards sex prefer to engage in casual sexual encounters, thereby preferring multiple partners. Access to a higher number of sexual partners increases the opportunities to use coercive control or aggression in order to obtain sex or desired sexual practices.

- *Traditional gender roles*: The belief that men and women should adhere to the traditional roles and behaviors dictated by societal norms has been associated with higher rates of sexual assault perpetration. For instance, the belief in traditional gender roles was found to be the only significant predictor of sexual aggression in one study, even after controlling for perceived token resistance (Loh & Gidycz, 2006). An international study examining the relationship between rape proclivity and hostile sexism (antagonistic attitudes towards women) in Zimbabwe found a significant relationship between the two constructs for acquaintance rape but not for stranger rape (Viki, Chiroro, & Abrams, 2006). The authors speculate that cultural norms regarding men and women's traditional roles in relationships may explain this finding. Men who hold more traditional beliefs about gender roles or antagonistic attitudes towards women may be more prone to express their hostility in intimate relationships where their behavior may be perceived as acceptable (Viki et al., 2006).
- *Token resistance*: Token resistance is the heteronormative belief that women initially and typically say "no" to sex when they really mean "yes" (Beres, 2010). Token resistance is perceived as a precursor to sexual interactions that needs to be overcome by persistence and coercion (Shafer, Ortiz, Thompson, & Hyemmer, 2018). Stronger beliefs about women's use of token resistance is associated with greater misperceptions about sexual consent (Shafer et al., 2018). For instance, in situations where women agreed to some sexual activity, men believed that the women also wanted to engage in sexual intercourse due to initial agreement to kiss (Osman, 2003). Men with stronger beliefs in token resistance are more likely to endorse rape myths because they rationalize the victim's actions as "wanting it" despite the lack of consent to all activities (Shafer et al., 2018).
- *Rape myths*: Rape myths refers to "attitudes and beliefs that are generally false but are widely and persistently held, and that serve to deny and justify male sexual aggression against women" (Lonsway & Fitzgerald, 1994, p. 133). Rape myths include the belief that women who dress provocatively deserve or are asking to be raped or that all women have an unconscious desire to be raped (Lonsway & Fitzgerald, 1994). A meta-analysis examining the relationship between rape myth acceptance and attitudes and behaviors found a significant association between rape myth acceptance and sexual aggression, and nonaggressive sexual behaviors, such as the use of degrading images of women and sexually promiscuous behavior (Suarez & Gadalla, 2010).

Overall, findings from extant research reveal that men who hold stronger beliefs about hypermasculinity, traditional attitudes about gender roles, and token resistance, and who are acceptant of rape myths and condone violence against women are more likely to perpetrate sexual violence and to be more tolerant of sexual assault in comparison with men who do not share these beliefs (Loh, Gidycz, Lobo, & Luthra, 2005). These beliefs and attitudes are further associated with rape culture, which refers to a setting in which sexual assault and rape are prevalent due to societal attitudes about gender and sexuality (Canan, Jozkowski, & Crawford, 2018). The measurement of gender-related attitudes and beliefs across studies may include some overlap (i.e. hostility towards women and rape myth acceptance); however, further research is needed to delineate the unique contribution of each factor to the variance in explaining the association between features of hypermasculinity sexual assault victimization.

Hypermasculinity and Sexual Assault on College Campuses

The link between domains of hypermasculinity and sexual assault perpetration has received increased attention on college campuses. This is particularly due to the staggering rates of sexual assault found in this context. For instance, 23% (or 1 in 5) of US college women have experienced rape or an attempted rape (Krebs, Lindquist, Warner, Fisher, & Martin, 2007). In one study, 63.3% of university men who self-reported acts qualifying as rape or attempted rape also admitted to committing multiple rapes (Lisak, Gardinier, Nicksa, & Cote, 2010). More than 90% of sexual assault victims on college campuses do not report the rape (Fisher, Cullen, & Turner, 2000). More than 50% of college sexual assaults occur in either August, September, October, or November (Kimble, Neacsiu, Flack, & Horner, 2008). It is hypothesized that the increased risk of unwanted sexual experiences or sexual assault during this time period may be related to the various Greek system activities held between the months of September–October (Kimble et al., 2008). Pledging (students are affiliated with the organization but not full members) for sororities or fraternities and social activities associated with pledging, such as fraternity parties, which often entail alcohol intoxication, are often held during the first few months of the first semester (Parrott & Zeichner, 2003).

The structure of organizations such as fraternities engender ideals of hypermasculinity via unquestioning loyalty, traditions, anti-female rituals, and hazing. Through the process of pledging or "rushing" a fraternity, young college males engage in practices that typically encourage alcohol misuse, substance use, competitiveness, and the sexual exploitation of women (Fabian, Toomey, Lenk, & Erikson, 2008). For instance, fraternity men have been found to have stronger beliefs in male dominance (Kalof & Cargill, 1991), greater belief in rape myths (Boeringer, 1999), and to hold more traditional attitudes towards women (Schaeffer & Nelson, 1993). Additionally, men in fraternities are more likely to be associated with the sexual objectification of women through pornography (Sanday, 1990), are more likely to display sexually degrading pictures of women (Bleecker & Murnen, 2005), and are more likely to use degrading language about women's genitals (Murnen, 2000) than nonfraternity men. Endorsement of hypermasculine values and rape-supportive beliefs translates into higher rates of sexual perpetration among fraternity members. Although across the nation fraternity members make up 25% of the undergraduate male population, they account for 46% of the perpetrators of sexual violence (Fritner & Robinson, 1993; Zernechel & Perry, 2017). In comparison with nonfraternity members, males who are part of fraternities are three times more likely to perpetrate a sexual assault (Foubert, Newberry, & Tatum, 2007).

Although the association between fraternity membership and endorsement of rape-supportive attitudes and hypermasculine values has been firmly established, the causal link continues to be debated. Some theorists posit that men who endorse hypermasculine values are attracted to all-male groups (i.e. fraternities, athletic groups) who hold similar beliefs (Kilmartin, 2000). Others suggest that sexual aggression and adherence to hypermasculinity is promoted by reinforcement and social punishment (Godenzi, Schwartz, & DeKeseredy, 2001). That is, the activities fraternities engage in facilitate the incidence of sexual assault (Murnen & Kohlman, 2007). For instance, a meta-analysis examining the relationship between sexual aggression and fraternity membership found that fraternity membership was significantly associated with hypermasculinity, rape-myth acceptance, and self-report of sexual aggression (Murnen & Kohlman, 2007). The effect size of the association was impacted by two factors:

1. Size of the school: Effect sizes were larger at smaller colleges. Murnen and Kohlman (2007) hypothesize that all-male groups at smaller schools have increased ability to define acceptable masculine behaviors and apply social sanctions for nonconformity due to fewer alternatives to socialization.

2. Age of the participants: Effect sizes were larger for studies with older participants. Murnen and Kohlman (2007) hypothesize that rape-supportive attitudes and beliefs and hypermasculinity are less well-developed when men first arrive at college and are acquired or reinforced as a function of fraternity membership.

To further elucidate potential factors that lead to the development or reinforcement of hypermasculine values, Murnen and Kohlman (2007) hypothesize that fraternity membership produces a strong group bonding, particularly for many of the fraternity members that live together. This bond intensifies the secrecy and loyalty among group members regarding their values and behaviors, such that any sexually aggressive behaviors are perceived to be private fraternity concerns and not subject to exposure to university forces. Thus, the correlation between fraternity membership and sexual assault perpetration may be a product of the various problematic practices and traditions that stem from hypermasculine values. Hypermasculinity then, may be a key factor in the development of attitudes and behaviors associated with sexual assault perpetration. Hypermasculinity can also be a primary target for interventions that aim to impact societal norms regarding masculinity and university campuses may be the ideal setting.

Evidence-Based Interventions and Best Practices

The current paradigms for sexual assault prevention focus almost exclusively on victims and teaching young women in particular to take "common sense measures" (i.e. safety planning, alcohol safety, etc.) to avoid becoming victims of sexual assault as well as bystander interventions. However, helping young women develop an awareness of potential dangers may not be sufficient to fully address a culture that promotes hypermasculine values. The concept of hypermasculinity can be incorporated into prevention efforts and intervention strategies for reducing sexual assault victimization and fostering gender equity. Hypermasculinity provides an overarching framework for understanding how gender inequality is produced and reproduced by shifting the attention to the way hypermasculinity is developed and maintained at the individual, group, and societal level (Jewkes et al., 2015). Evidence-based and comprehensive interventions for the prevention of sexual assault victimization should target female empowerment and changes in hypermasculine ideals. Due to the staggering rates of sexual assault on campus and the increased media attention to the gross mishandling of sexual assault allegations by university administrators across the US, intervention efforts should focus on changing hypermasculine ideals on college campuses. However, prevention efforts should start early, by engaging adolescent men in reflection and discussion regarding sexual assault victimization. Based on previous research, we recommend the implementation of separate gender programs that target consent and specific elements of hypermasculinity for men and alcohol use and self-defense tactics for women (please refer to Newlands & O'Donohue, 2016 for a review of interventions for women).

Assessment

Proper intervention strategies must first begin by accurate identification of men who hold hypermasculine values. Due to the dynamic nature of hypermasculinity and the presence of multiple masculinities, identifying men who are prone to perpetrate sexual assault is key. There is some disagreement regarding the most appropriate measures of hypermasculinity and the need to differentiate between men who may endorse hypermasculine values but don't commit a crime, those who are sexually aggressive, and those who are physically aggressive (Burk et al., 2004). There are several measures available for use that assess the multidimensionality of hypermasculinity:

- *Auburn Differential Masculinity Index-60* (ADMI-60; Burk et al., 2004): The ADMI is a

60-item self-report inventory of hypermasculinity that includes a total score and five subscales: hypermasculinity, sexual identity, dominance and aggression, conservative masculinity, and devaluation of emotion. Hypermasculinity and the devaluation of feminine traits are based on the concept of hypermasculinity as delineated by Mosher and Sirkin (1984). The ADMI has demonstrated good reliability ($\alpha = 0.83$) (Burk et al., 2004). A more recent factor analysis of the ADMI yielded four dimensions: sexual identity, anti-femininity, devaluation of emotion, and dominance and aggression (Corprew, Matthews, & Mitchell, 2014). Scores on these subscales produced four distinct and theoretically meaningful profiles: extreme hypermasculine (highest levels anti-feminine attitudes and devaluation of emotion within the sample), traditional hypermasculine (highest levels of dominance and aggression), traditional masculine, and nonhypermasculine (Corprew et al., 2014). The authors did not find evidence for a conservative masculinity dimension and instead indicate that the dominance and aggression subscale subsumed the prior dimension. They further argue that the hypermasculine dimension is conceptually erroneous as all of the combined domains of the scale measure the concept of hypermasculinity (Corprew et al., 2014). Findings from this study indicate that the men who produce either the extreme or traditional hypermasculine profile may have the highest risk for rape proclivity.

- *Hypermasculinity Inventory-Revised* (HMI-R; Peters, Nason, & Turner, 2007): The HMI-R is a revised version of the widely utilized Mosher and Sirkin's (1984) HMI. Research examining the psychometric properties of the original HMI yielded serious limitations, such as the use of dated words, cultural inadequacies, and forced choice format, where respondents were forced to choose between the "macho" response or the "wimpy" response (Peters et al., 2007). The revised version of the HMI is a 27-item questionnaire that assesses the three original dimensions of hypermasculinity: callous attitudes, danger, and fighting. The HMI-R demonstrated high reliability (($\alpha = 0.90$) (Peters et al., 2007).
- *Hypermasculine Values Questionnaire* (HVQ; Archer, 2010); The HVQ is a 26-item self-report questionnaire that assesses various domains of hypermasculinity, such as toughness, the need to avoid femininity, and control over women's sexuality. The HVQ has demonstrated high internal consistency ($\alpha = 0.92$) and test-retest reliability ($r = 0.91$) (Archer, 2010).

There are several other assessment questionnaires that may be equally psychometrically sound. However, an overreliance on self-report questionnaires increases the mono-method bias, where a questionnaire may be measuring part of the construct of hypermasculinity at the expense of other important facets. Recently, researchers have suggested the use of implicit association tests (McDermott, Kilmartin, McKelvey, & Kridel, 2015). Burgeoning research comparing the association between men and women's implicit tendencies to dehumanize or objectify women to their self-reported attitudes towards rape found that men were more likely to have lower response times pairing images of women with animal parts, tools, and objects (Rudman & Mescher, 2012). Men's implicit bias to dehumanize women was positively correlated with self-reported willingness to rape. Therefore, the most comprehensive assessment is one that allows for the identification of different profiles of masculinity and evaluates implicit and explicit biases against women. Understanding the various facets of hypermasculinity can lead to a greater understanding of the nuances of the development of masculine identity across the lifespan and provides opportunities for intervention and prevention.

Prevention and Intervention

Program evaluation studies indicate that the most effective sexual assault prevention efforts are conducted in separate gender groups due to the different strategies and goals for men and women's programs as well as the risk of providing inconsistent messages in a mixed-gender program (Berkowitz, 2002; Yeater & O'Donohue, 1999). Several programs aimed at reducing the incidence of sexual assault with all-male groups have been developed over the past three decades (i.e. *Men Can Stop Rape, Coaching Boys into Men, RealConsent, the Men's Project*). According to Berkowitz (2002), they share the following assumptions:

- The most effective workshops are comprised of all males, small in size, and conducted by peer educators.
- The most effective sexual prevention approach with men is to enlist them as potential women's allies instead of potential rapists.
- Men should take primary responsibility for sexual assault prevention.
- Group discussions should encourage honest disclosures regarding ideas, feelings, and beliefs and should be interactive.
- Educators should create opportunities for discussion of (mis)perceptions of men's experiences.

Although Berkowitz (2002) provides a more extensive list of critical elements of prevention programs with men (i.e. challenging rape myths and rape-supportive beliefs and attitudes, addressing role of substances, etc.), recent meta-analyses have revealed significant limitations for one or more of these recommendations. For instance, the most effective prevention programs are those that are longer, narrowly focused, delivered by experts, and target specific subpopulations of men (i.e. fraternity members) (Anderson & Whiston, 2005; Vladutiu, Martin, & Macy, 2010). Additionally, prevention programs often yield the largest improvements in attitudes and intentions that tend to decrease with time and have little impact on actual perpetration behavior (Newlands & O'Donohue, 2016). What appears to be missing from extant programs is the consideration of hypermasculinity as a multidimensional concept (as opposed to focusing on specific facets of hypermasculinity) and empirical validation. A systematic review of rape prevention programs that evaluated the studies based on 14 empirically derived criteria (i.e. effect sizes, length of follow-up, cost, replication) found only six studies that quantitatively evaluated to incidence of sexual perpetration among US college males and only three of the studies reported significant reduction in rates of perpetration (Newlands & O'Donohue, 2016; see Table 15.1 for a summary of results).

Of all programs examined in the review, the *Men's Project* appears to be the only one that addresses the impact of masculinity on sexual assault perpetration. Specifically, the *Men's Project* is a manualized intervention comprised of a 1.5-h prevention program and a 1-h booster session based on Berkowitz (1994) workshop protocol (Gidycz, Orchowski, & Berkowitz, 2011). The *Men's Project* addresses elements such as consent, dispelling rape myths, fostering an awareness and understanding of the impact of social norms and misperceptions, increasing participants' understanding of masculinity, misperceptions, attitudes, and behaviors regarding sexual assault, and traditional concepts of masculinity that are associated with rape proclivity (Gidycz et al., 2011). The *Men's Project* was found to produce significant reductions in sexual assault perpetration in male residents in freshman dorms that were assigned to the intervention compared to the control group at the 4-month follow-up assessment (1.5 vs. 6.7%, respectively) (Gidycz et al., 2011). These gains were not significant at the 7-month follow-up. The *Men's Project* demonstrates significant advantages over other prevention programs, such as multiple follow-up assessments, evaluation of social desirability, and the utilization of behavioral outcomes (Newlands & O'Donohue, 2016).

Other interventions incorporate the concept of hypermasculinity into curricula more deliberately. For instance, the *Macho Factory* is an intervention developed in Sweden for individuals aged 13–25 that is comprised of educational material and activities that focus on the prevention of sexual assault by challenging and changing social norms of masculinity (Jewkes et al., 2015). The program consists of six themes, 17

Table 15.1 Prevention programs with all-male participants

Study	Program title/ provider	N	Follow-up period	Behavioral outcomes	Effect sizes/rates of Perpetration	Limitations
Heppner, Neville, Smith, Kivlighan, and Gershuny (1999)	Not reported provider: Expert males	119	5 months	Insignificant	Not reported	Not addressed: Dosage, blindness, cost, and mechanism of change
Foubert (2000)	How to help a surveyor of sexual assault: What men can do. Provider: Peer educators	117	7 months	Insignificant	Not reported	Not addressed: Dosage, blindness, cost, mechanism of change, theoretical basis, social validity, and subject × Tx interaction
Foubert et al. (2007)	The Men's program provider: Peer educators	565	7 months	Insignificant. Men in Tx who went on to join fraternities reported significantly fewer acts of coercion at follow-up	Not reported. Rate of sexual coercion: Tx: 6%; C: 10%	Not addressed: Dosage, blindness, cost, mechanism of change, and social validity
Stephens and George (2009)	Helping victims of sexual assault provider: Male educators and videos	146	5 weeks	High-risk men in Tx were more likely to report sexually coercive behavior than high-risk controls	Tx: 82% C: 47% $d = -0.74$ 95% CI (−0.97–0.50)	Not addressed: Dosage, blindness, cost, and social validity No replication
Gidycz et al. (2011)	The Men's project provider: Males-undergraduate and doctoral students	460	7 months	Insignificant at follow-up. Significant effects were found for the Tx group at 4 months follow-up	C: 6.7%	Not addressed: Dosage, blindness, cost, mechanism of change, and social validity
Salazar, Vivolo-Kantor, Hardin, and Berkowitz (2014)	RealConsent provider: Web-based	215	6 months	Significantly less sexual violence perpetration was reported by the Tx group	Tx: 73% lower odds for perpetrating than C $d = 0.29$. AOR 0.27, 95% CI (0.11–0.70)12	Not addressed: Dosage, cost, and social validity No replication

Note: *tx* treatment; *C* control/comparison
Reproduced with permission from Newlands and O'Donohue (2016)

short films, and related exercises and is manualized (Lundqvist et al., 2010). The content of the program was explicitly based on theories of hypermasculinity and hegemonic masculinity and emphasizes that gender is learned and continuously enacted. For instance, Connell's (2005) theory of multiple masculinities was utilized to develop several association exercises in which various masculine identities are constructed (Jewkes et al., 2015). Despite its theoretical underpinnings, no studies have been located that have empirically tested the effectiveness and efficacy of the *Macho Factory*. In other words, it remains unknown whether the *Macho Factory* successfully changes attitudes and beliefs related to hypermasculinity and whether it impacts actual sexual assault perpetration.

Other international initiatives targeting the prevention of gendered violence target the concept of toxic masculinity. One such effort is the international research curriculum by *Promundo,* an international gender justice organization. The initiatives developed by *Promundo* specifically target the attitudes and behaviors of adolescent and young men (aged 15–24), have been implemented in 29 countries, and have been acknowledged by several international organizations as best practices in promoting gender equality (Abebe et al., 2018). Specifically, the initiatives include the development of the *Man Box*, a questionnaire that measures the degree to which men adhere to the tenets of toxic masculinity, and *Program H,* a sexual assault prevention program in Brazil and its U.S. adaptation, *Manhood 2.0*. *Program H* is a manualized intervention that combines group education sessions with youth activism to change stereotypical roles associated with gender and has been found to lead to lower rates of sexual harassment and violence against women, increased condom use, and improved couples communication (Abebe et al., 2018). *Manhood 2.0* involves an 18-hour curriculum implemented in six, three-hour weekly sessions and involves three main topic areas: (1) themes of gender, masculinity, and power, (2) theme of violence, and (3) sexual and reproductive health (Abebe et al., 2018). This curriculum is currently undergoing evaluation in two randomized controlled trials in Pittsburgh, Pennsylvania and Washington, D.C. The initiatives developed by *Promundo* and their U.S. partners have been found to lead to reductions in young men's reported use of violence and changes in attitudes that support gendered-violence (Abebe et al., 2018).

Despite promising evidence in several Latin American countries, the efficacy of the U.S. adaption of *Program H, Manhood 2.0,* is currently unknown. Further, no gold-standard treatments for sexual assault prevention exist due to the complex nature of sexual assault perpetration. The issue of implementing effective programs with men is further compounded by the misperception that rape prevention programs are irrelevant to some men because they do not perceive themselves as potential rapists (Scheel, Johnson, Schneider, & Smith, 2001) and they may even foster animosity towards educators as a result (Berkowitz, 2002).

As such, there is a need for the development of interventions that explicitly emphasize the impact of hypermasculinity and foster healthy perspectives on masculinity. Such interventions require a sound theoretical framework that guides the selection of treatment targets and necessary modifications, clear mechanisms of change (i.e. mediators and moderators), a manualized treatment protocol, and assessment of fidelity, acceptability, feasibility, and cost. Prevention and intervention efforts focused on hypermasculinity can be guided by Mosher and Sirkin's (1984) theory of hypermasculinity, Connell's (2005) theory of multiple masculinities, the stages of change model (individual's readiness to change and strategies for transitioning from one stage to the next), and Berkowitz' (2002) proposed critical elements of prevention programs, and can include the following components:

- Dispel rape myths and develop an accurate understanding of consent via challenging the belief in token resistance.
- Address social norms regarding the role of sexual activity in men's lives and the role of female sexual partners.

- Address male gender role socialization.
- Develop healthy attitudes regarding the expression of emotion and vulnerability.
- Understand the range of coercive behaviors employed by men (i.e. verbal pressure to actual force).
- Explore situational characteristics that facilitate sexual assault (i.e. alcohol, drugs).
- Increase empathy for victims.
- Discuss the rates of sexual perpetration against males and associated consequences in order to challenge myths that "men can't be raped."
- Discuss the role of the media in gender role socialization.
- Explore the development of different masculinities and their impacts on sexual assault perpetration.
- Discuss the role of all-male groups, such as fraternities and sports team, in developing and propagating hypermasculinity.

It is essential that interventions aimed at addressing hypermasculinity with men focus on men as allies and not place individual blame. Interventions that challenge deeply engrained practices and beliefs that maintain men's positions of power in society are likely to work slowly and require multi-level and multidisciplinary approaches. An ideal context for the implementation of such approaches is the college campus, particularly within fraternity organizations. Although Newlands and O'Donohue (2016) demonstrated that there is a paucity of evidence-based interventions that can successfully address the problem of sexual assault on college campuses, this dearth of evidence creates an impetus for the development and refinement of empirically supported strategies that target men's beliefs and values associated with hypermasculinity.

Key Gaps in the Literature

Progress in the development of interventions that target hypermasculinity as a risk factor in the perpetration of sexual assault is constrained by significant conceptual and methodological limitations. First, the prevention literature is generally limited by conceptual confusion regarding varying definitions of masculine ideals. Second, there are significant measurement issues. Third, there is a lack of sample diversity. These important limitations reveal important considerations for future research.

Conceptual Confusion

The primary cause of concern for the wider gender norms literature as it pertains to sexual assault prevention is the lack of uniformity in definitions. There are several terms that are often used interchangeably, combined, or significantly overlap in definition. For instance, there is a lack of conceptual clarity between the terms hostile masculinity, hegemonic masculinity, toxic masculinity, and hypermasculinity. *Hostile masculinity* refers to hostile, distrustful, and misogynous attitudes (i.e. rape myth acceptance, belief that all women secretly want to be raped) and emotions towards women and a desire to control and dominate women that results in sexual arousal and gratification (Malamuth, Sockloskie, Koss, & Tanaka, 1991). This has garnered significant empirical support and is a core component of the confluence model of sexual assault aggression (Malamuth et al., 1991). In regard to hegemonic masculinity, several scholars have noted differences in Connell's (2005) own conceptualization. For instance, there is significant oscillation between the term's descriptive (dominant versions of manhood), empirical (reference to an actual group of men), and mechanism (political/cultural leadership that ensure mass consent) meanings (Beasley, 2008). Connell (2005) later stated that she intended the term to be utilized as a political mechanism that legitimizes men's dominance in society and the subordination of women and that the description of hegemonic masculinity may only loosely correspond to the lives of actual men. Additional concerns include the possibility that the most dominant ideals of masculinity may not always be the most socially venerated, common, or legitimate descriptions of men's power (Beasley, 2008; Flood, 2002). The presence of several terms that may to one degree or another refer to the same attitudes and beliefs regarding women and sexuality is especially concerning. Which term is theoretically derived? Which term is most likely to fully capture the relationship between masculine ideals and sexual assault victimization? What is the conceptual/theoretical difference between hypermasculinity, hostile masculinity, and hegemonic masculinity? The lack of conceptual clarity poses significant concerns for both practical and measurement issues.

Measurement Concerns

In part related to the lack of conceptual clarity, there are significant issues with existing methods of assessment. For instance, in a narrative review of college sexual assault research, McDermott et al. (2015) found that most studies examined hostile masculinity and did so by creating a composite variable of hostile masculinity comprised of several independent questionnaires that assessed hostility toward women, attitudes condoning violence against women, adversarial sexual beliefs, and rape myth acceptance. The authors noted that this reveals significant concerns regarding the construct validity of hostile masculinity instruments. In regard to the most widely utilized measures of hypermasculinity, several researchers (see Corprew et al., 2014; Peters et al., 2007) have noted that the HMI utilized outdated language, forced choice, and wording that is likely to offend participants. Concerns with the language used in measures indicate that behaviors and experiences related to perpetration and victimization are not described in a relatable and understandable manner for a particular population (i.e. college students) and can elicit social desirability or demand characteristics (Newlands & O'Donohue, 2016). Furthermore, there is an overreliance on self-report questionnaires and a lack of consideration of the role of social desirability bias, particularly when examining hypermasculinity as it is related to sexual assault perpetration. Multi-methods of assessment should be incorporated into the measurement of hypermasculinity in order to more accurately capture the impact of gender role socialization and hypermasculinity on sexual assault aggression (i.e. implicit bias tests).

Lack of Sample Diversity

Initial definitions of the different masculinities were based on White and Eurocentric assumptions and research studies continue to utilize convenience samples that are comprised of White, middle class, college students. Less attention is dedicated to expressions of masculinity in ethnic or sexual minority men. For instance, limited research has examined the association between the hypermasculine values prevalent in White US samples and the Hispanic cultural values of *machismo*, which has been defined as the "alpha male stereotype in Latin culture and encompasses such qualities as virility, bravado, and responsibility as the decision maker of the family" (Cummings, Gonzalez- Guarda, & Sandoval, 2013, p. 167). Research indicates that machismo has been associated with an increased risk for intimate partner violence (Gonzalez-Guarda, Ortega, Vasquez, & De Santis, 2010). For instance, a literature review of 24 studies that explored male risk factors for perpetration of intimate partner violence found that 16 studies included Hispanics and machismo was a reported risk factor at both the relationship and societal level (Mancera, Dorgo, & Provencio-Vasquez, 2017). A review of empirically based prevention programs for teen dating violence found that of 10 prevention programs that targeted attitudes towards traditional gender roles only three studies targeted Hispanic youth and only one study included Hispanic gender roles as an element of the intervention (Malhotra, Gonzalez-Guarda, & Mitchell, 2015). More research is needed to explore the effects of machismo and other cultural endemics on sexual assault perpetration. Prevention and intervention efforts specific to Hispanic youth and men are also needed.

Due to the dearth of research with ethnic minorities, it can be argued that there might be a dimension of hypermasculinity that is not properly evaluated. For instance, few studies examine the interaction between cultural variables such as acculturation, immigration status, perceived racism or discrimination, and the development of hypermasculinity and sexual assault victimization. This is particularly important as some studies have found that Asian cultural values may buffer the effects of hostile masculinity on sexual assault aggression despite scoring higher on measures on hostile masculinity (McDermott et al., 2015). The examination of cultural variables is also important because the majority of men do not perpetuate sexual assault. In college samples, 68% of men who perpetrate sexual assault are repeat offenders (Zinzow & Thompson, 2015), indicating that there is a need to examine positive characteristics or values that differentiate offenders from nonoffenders.

Implications for Future Research

Hypermasculinity is a multidimensional and complex concept that may play an important role in the development of prevention and intervention programs aimed at reducing the incidence of sexual assault. The etiology of sexual assault, however, is highly complicated and likely influenced by an array of factors. The current state of the literature examining the association between hypermasculinity and sexual assault is rife with conceptual, methodological, and diversity issues and there are few evidence-based sexual assault prevention programs and even fewer all-male programs that focus on hypermasculinity. Future research should include the following considerations:

- Intervention efforts should be aimed at the individual, group, and societal levels: Particularly for universities, fraternities and sports teams are organizations that are ripe for intervention. These groups boast the highest levels of hypermasculinity and rape-supportive attitudes as well as highest rates of sexual assault perpetration.
- Interventions should go beyond educational programs and should incorporate empirically based principles of change (i.e. stages of change models).
- Prevention efforts should target adolescent males, particularly within existing infrastructures, such as youth organizations.
- The role of hypermasculinity in sexual assault perpetration should be incorporated into all-male and all-female groups, particularly because of the negative consequences for men and women.
- Extant prevention programs that focus on hypermasculinity require more rigorous empirical testing.
- In tandem with hypermasculinity, cultural identity, subgroup affiliation, and other racial experiences should be examined as they may impact the development of masculine ideals.

Although not exhaustive, it is imperative that researchers and clinicians consider psychosocial and societal factors that may impact the development and maintenance of hypermasculinity. Concerted efforts to reduce the sexual objectification of women in society, creating gender equality in academic, employment, and social relationships are necessary if the patriarchal culture that sustains these ideals of masculinity is to be changed.

Conclusion

Hypermasculinity may be an important risk factor for sexual assault victimization. Men who endorse higher hypermasculine beliefs are more likely to endorse rape-supportive attitudes, believe in token resistance, and endorse more hostile and callous attitudes toward women and sexuality. There is a need to further study hypermasculinity and to devise interventions aimed at changing misogynistic cognitions and beliefs that aid men in developing healthy masculine ideals. There is a concern that dedicating resources to men's prevention programs will divert much-needed resources from women, particularly as women are more likely to be the victims of sexual violence. However, hypermasculinity is a problem not only for women but also for men. The patriarchal system that maintains men's dominant position in power and subordinates women comes at a cost for marginalized men and to the health and quality of life for men in general. Furthermore, men's practices, beliefs, and attitudes are part of the problem that continue to maintain gender inequality and the perpetration of gendered violence and as such, should also be part of the solution. The examination of hypermasculinity provides a pathway for addressing the most harmful beliefs and practices impacting sexual assault victimization.

References

Abbey, A., Parkhill, M. R., BeShears, R., Clinton-Sherrod, A. M., & Zawacki, T. (2006). Cross-sectional predictors of sexual assault perpetration in a community sample of single African American and Caucasian men. *Aggressive Behavior, 32*(1), 54–67.

Abebe, K. Z., Jones, K. A., Culyba, A. J., Feliz, N. B., Anderson, H., Torres, I., … Miller, E. (2018). Engendering healthy masculinities to prevent sexual violence. Rationale for and design of the manhood 2.0 trial. *Contemporary Clinical Trials, 71*, 18–32. https://doi.org/10.1016/j.cct.2018.05.01

Anderson, L. A., & Whiston, S. C. (2005). Sexual assault education programs: A meta-analytic examination of their effectiveness. *Psychology Women Quarterly, 29*, 374–388.

Archer, J. (2010). Derivation and assessment of a hypermasculine values questionnaire. *British Journal of Social Psychology, 49*, 525–551.

Beasley, C. (2008). Rethinking hegemonic masculinity in a globalizing world. *Men & Masculinities, 11*(1), 86–103.

Beres, M. (2010). Sexual miscommunication? Untangling assumptions about sexual communication between casual sex partners. *Culture, Health & Sexuality, 12*, 1–14.

Berkowitz, A. D. (1994). A model acquaintance rape prevention program for men. In A. D. Berkowitz (Ed.), Men and rape: Theory, research and prevention programs in higher education (pp. 35–42). San Francisco, CA: Jossey-Bass.

Berkowitz, A. D. (2002). Fostering men's responsibility for preventing sexual assault. In P. A. Schewe (Ed.), *Preventing violence in relationships* (pp. 163–196). Washington, DC: American Psychological Association.

Bleecker, E. T., & Murnen, S. K. (2005). Fraternity membership, the display of degrading sexual images of women, and rape myth acceptance. *Sex Roles, 53*, 487–493.

Boeringer, S. B. (1999). Associations of rape-supportive attitudes with fraternal and athletic participation. *Violence Against Women, 5*, 81–90.

Bourgois, P. (1995). *In search of respect: Selling crack in el barrio*. New York: Cambridge University Press.

Breiding, M. J., Smith, S. G., Basile, K. G., Walters, M. L., Chen, J., & Merrick, M. T. (2014). Prevalence and characteristics of sexual violence, stalking, and intimate partner violence victimization: National Intimate Partner and Sexual Violence Survey, United States, 2011. *Surveillance Summaries, 63*(SS08), 1–18.

Burk, L. R., Burkhart, B. R., & Sikorski, J. F. (2004). Construction and preliminary validation of the Auburn differential masculinity inventory. *Psychology of Men & Masculinity, 5*, 4–17. https://doi.org/10.1037/1524-9220.5.1.4

Canan, S. N., Jozkowski, K. N., & Crawford, B. L. (2018). Sexual assault supportive attitudes: Rape myth acceptance and token resistance in Greek and non-Greek college students from two university samples in the United States. *Journal of Interpersonal Violence, 33*(22), 3502–3530.

Connell, R. W. (1987). *Gender and power: Society, the person and sexual politics*. Palo Alto, CA: University of California Press.

Connell, R. W. (2005). *Masculinities* (2nd ed.). Los Angeles, CA: University of California Press.

Corprew, C. S., Matthews, J. S., & Mitchell, A. D. V. (2014). Men at the crossroads: A profile analysis of hypermasculinity in emerging adulthood. *Journal of Men's Studies, 22*(2), 105–121.

Cummings, A. M., Gonzalez-Guarda, R. M., & Sandoval, M. F. (2013). Intimate partner violence in Hispanics: A review of the literature. *Journal of Family Violence, 28*(2), 153–171. https://doi.org/10.1007/s10896-012-9478-5

Fabian, L. E., Toomey, T. I., Lenk, K. M., & Erikson, D. J. (2008). Where do underage college students get alcohol? *Journal of Drug Education, 38*(1), 15–26.

Fahlberg, A., & Pepper, M. (2016). Masculinity and sexual violence: Assessing the state of the field. *Sociology Compass, 10*(8), 673–683. https://doi.org/10.1111/soc4.12397

Fisher, B., Cullen, F., & Turner, M. (2000). *The sexual victimization of college women* (NCJ 182369). National Criminal Justice Reference Service. Retrieved from https://www.ncjrs.gov/pdffiles1/nij/182369.pdf

Flood, M. (2002). Between men and masculinity: An assessment of the term "masculinity" in recent scholarship on men. In S. Pearce & V. Muller (Eds.), *Manning the next millennium: Studies in masculinities*. Perth: Black Swan.

Foubert, J. D. (2000). The longitudinal effects of a rape-prevention program on fraternity men's attitudes, behavioral intent, and behavior. *Journal of American College Health, 48*, 158–163.

Foubert, J. D., Newberry, J. T., & Tatum, J. L. (2007). Behavior differences seven months later: Effects of a rape prevention program. *NASPA Journal, 44*, 728–749.

Fritner, M. P., & Robinson, L. (1993). Acquaintance rape: The influence of alcohol, fraternity membership, and sports team membership. *Journal of Sex Education & Therapy, 19*, 272–284.

Garcia-Moreno, C., Jansen, H., Ellsberg, M., & Watts, C. (2005). *WHO Multi-Country Study on Women's Health and Domestic Violence against Women: Initial Results on Prevalence, Health Outcomes and Women's Responses*. Geneva: World Health Organization.

Gidycz, C. A., Orchowski, L. M., & Berkowitz, A. D. (2011). Preventing sexual aggression among college men: An evaluation of a social norms and bystander intervention program. *Violence Against Women, 17*, 720–742.

Godenzi, A., Schwartz, M. D., & DeKeseredy, W. S. (2001). Toward a gendered social bond/male peer support theory of university woman abuse. *Critical Criminology, 10*, 1–16.

Gold, S. R., Fultz, J., Burke, C. H., Prisco, A. G., & Willett, J. A. (1992). Vicarious emotional responses of macho college males. *Journal of Interpersonal Violence, 7*, 165–174.

Gonzalez-Guarda, R. M., Ortega, J., Vasquez, E. P., & De Santis, J. (2010). La mancha negra: Substance abuse, violence, and sexual risks among Hispanic males. *Western Journal of Nursing Research, 32*, 128–148. https://doi.org/10.1177/0193945909343594

Gramsci, A. (1971). *Selections from a prison notebook*. London: Lawrence & Wishart.

Heppner, M., Neville, H., Smith, K., Kivlighan, D., & Gershuny, B. (1999). Examining immediate and long-term efficacy of rape prevention programming with racially diverse college men. *Journal of Counselling Psychology, 46*, 16–26.

Jewkes, R., Morrell, R., Hearn, J., Lundqvist, E., Blackbeard, D., Lindegger, G., … Gottzen, L. (2015). Hegemonic masculinity: Combining theory and practice in gender interventions. *Culture. Health & Sexuality, 17*(S2), 96–111. https://doi.org/10.1080/13691058.2015.1085094

Kalof, L., & Cargill, T. (1991). Fraternity and sorority membership and gender dominance attitudes. *Sex Roles, 23*, 417–423.

Kilmartin, C. T. (2000). *The masculine self* (2nd ed.). Boston, MA: McGraw-Hill.

Kimble, M., Neacsiu, A., Flack, W. F., & Horner, J. (2008). Risk of unwanted sex for college women: Evidence for a red zone. *Journal of American College Health, 57*(3), 331–337.

Krebs, C. P., Lindquist, C., Warner, T., Fisher, B., & Martin, S. (2007). The campus sexual assault (CSA) study: Final report. National Criminal Justice Reference Service. Retrieved from http://www.ncjrs.gov/pdffiles1/nij/grants/221153.pdf

Kupers, T. A. (2005). Toxic masculinity as a barrier to mental health treatment in prison. *Journal of Clinical Psychology, 61*(6), 713–724. https://doi.org/10.1002/jclp.20105

Lisak, D., Gardinier, L., Nicksa, S. C., & Cote, A. M. (2010). False allegations of sexual assault: An analysis of ten years of reported cases. *Violence Against Women, 16*, 1318–1334. https://doi.org/10.1177/1077801210387747

Locke, B. D., & Mahalik, J. R. (2005). Examining masculinity norms, problem drinking and athletic involvement as predictors of sexual aggression in college men. *Journal of Counselling Psychology, 52*(3), 279–283. https://doi.org/10.1037/0022-0167.52.3.279

Loh, C.I., Gidycz, C.A., Lobo, T.R., & Luthra, R. (2005). A prospective analysis of sexual assault perpetration: risk factors related to perpetrator characteristics. *Journal of Interpersonal Violence, 20*(10), 1325–48.

Loh, C., & Gidycz, C. A. (2006). A prospective analysis of the relationship between childhood sexual victimization and perpetration of dating violence and sexual assault in adulthood. *Journal of Interpersonal Violence, 21*(6), 732–749.

Lonsway, K. A., & Fitzgerald, L. F. (1994). Rape myths: In review. *Psychology Women Quarterly, 18*(2), 133–164.

Lundqvist, E., Röcklinger, K., Malmberg, L., Gulbrandsen, I., Nettelbladh-Malm, C., & Söderström, D. (2010). *Machofabriken*. Malmö: Liber.

Malamuth, N. M., Sockloskie, R. J., Koss, M. P., & Tanaka, J. S. (1991). Characteristics of aggressors against women: Testing a model using a national sample of college students. *Journal of Consulting and Clinical Psychology, 59*, 670–681. https://doi.org/10.1037/0022-006x.59.5.670

Malhotra, K., Gonzalez-Guarda, R. M., & Mitchell, E. M. (2015). A review of teen dating violence prevention research: What about Hispanic youth? *Trauma, Violence, & Abuse, 16*(4), 444–465. https://doi.org/10.1177/1524838014537903

Mancera, B. M., Dorgo, S., & Provencio-Vasquez, E. (2017). Risk factors for Hispanic male intimate partner violence perpetration. *American Journal of Men's Health, 11*(4), 969–983. https://doi.org/10.1177/1557988315579196

McDermott, R. C., Kilmartin, C., McKelvey, D. K., & Kridel, M. M. (2015). College male sexual assault of women and the psychology of men: Past, present, and future directions for research. *Psychology of Men & Masculinity, 16*(4), 355–366. https://doi.org/10.1037/a0039544

Messerschmidt, J. W. (2012). Engendering gendered knowledge: Assessing the academic appropriation of hegemonic masculinity. *Men and Masculinities, 15*(1), 56–76. https://doi.org/10.1177/1097184X11428384

Mosher, D. L., & Sirkin, M. (1984). Measuring a macho personality constellation. *Journal of Research in Personality, 18*, 150–163.

Murnen, S. K. (2000). Gender and the use of sexually degrading language. *Psychology of Women Quarterly, 24*, 319–327.

Murnen, S. K., & Kohlman, M. H. (2007). Athletic participation, fraternity membership, and sexual aggression among college men: A meta-analytic review. *Sex Roles, 57*, 145–157.

Newlands, R., & O'Donohue, W. T. (2016). A critical review of sexual violence prevention on college campuses. *Acta Psychopathologica, 2*, 14. https://doi.org/10.4172/2469-6676.100040

Njue, C., Askew, I., & Chege, J. (2005). Non-consensual sexual experiences of young people in Kenya: Boys as perpetrators and victims. In S. Jejeebhoy, I. Shah, & S. Thapa (Eds.), *Sex without consent: Young people in developing countries* (pp. 139–157). London/New York: Zed Books.

Osman, S. L. (2003). Predicting men's rape perceptions based on the belief that "no" really means "yes". *Journal of Applied Social Psychology, 33*, 683–692.

Parent, M. C., Gobble, T. D., & Rochlen, A. (2018). Social media behavior, toxic masculinity, and depression. *Psychology of Men & Masculinity, 20*, 277. https://doi.org/10.1037/men0000156

Parrott, D. J., & Zeichner, A. (2003). Effects of hypermasculinity on physical aggression against women. *Psychology of Men & Masclunity, 4*(1), 70–78. https://doi.org/10.1037/1524-9220.4.1.70

Parrott, D. J., & Zeichner, A. (2008). Determinants of anger and physical aggression based on sexual orientation: An experimental examination of hypermasculinity and exposure to male gender role violations. *Archives of Sexual Behavior, 37*, 891–901. https://doi.org/10.1007/s10508-007-9194-z

Pascoe, C. J. (2007). *Dude, you're a fag: Masculinity and sexuality in high school*. Berkeley: University of California Press.

Peters, J., Nason, C., & Turner, W. M. (2007). Developing and testing of a new version of the Hypermasculinity index. *Social Work Research, 31*(3), 171–182.

Rudman, L. A., & Mescher, K. (2012). Of animals and objects: Men's implicit dehumanization of women and likelihood of sexual aggression. *Personality and Social Psychology Bulletin, 38*, 734–746. https://doi.org/10.1177/0146167212436401

Salazar, L. F., Vivolo-Kantor, A., Hardin, J., & Berkowitz, A. (2014). A web-based sexual violence bystander intervention for male college students: Randomized controlled trial. *Journal of Medical Internet Research, 16*, e203.

Sanday, P. R. (1990). *Fraternity gang rape: Sex, brotherhood, and privileges on campus*. New York: New York University Press.

Schaeffer, A. M., & Nelson, E. S. (1993). Rape-supportive attitudes: Effects of on-campus residence and education. *Journal of College Student Development, 34*, 175–179.

Scheel, E. D., Johnson, E. J., Schneider, M., & Smith, B. (2001). Making rape education meaningful for men: The case for eliminating the emphasis on men as perpetrators, protectors, or victims. *Sociological Practice, 3*, 257–278.

Seaton, G. (2007). Toward a theoretical understanding of hypermasculine coping among urban black adolescent males. *Journal of Human Behavior in the Social Environment, 15*, 367–390. https://doi.org/10.1300/J137vl5n02_21

Shafer, A., Ortiz, R. R., Thompson, B., & Hyemmer, J. (2018). The role of hypermasculinity, token resistance, rape myth, and assertive sexual consent communication among college men. *Journal of Adolescent Men, 62*(S3), S44–S50. https://doi.org/10.1016/j.jadohealth.2017.10.015

Stephens, K. A., & George, W. H. (2009). Rape prevention with college men evaluating risk status. *Journal of Interpersonal Violence, 24*, 996–1013.

Suarez, E., & Gadalla, T. M. (2010). Stop blaming the victim: A meta-analysis on rape myths. *Journal of Interpersonal Violence, 25*(11), 2010–2035.

Vaas, J., & Gold, S. (1995). Effects of feedback on emotion in hypermasculine men. *Violence and Victims, 10*, 217–226.

Viki, G., Chiroro, P., & Abrams, D. (2006). Hostile sexism, type of rape, and self-reported rape proclivity within a sample of Zimbabwean males. *Violence Against Women, 12*(8), 789–798.

Vladutiu, C. J., Martin, S. L., & Macy, R. J. (2010). College-or university-based sexual assault prevention programs: A review of program outcomes, characteristics, and recommendations. *Trauma Violence & Abuse, 12*, 67–86.

Vokey, M., Tefft, B., & Tysiaczny, C. (2013). An analysis of hypermasculinity in magazine advertisements. *Sex Roles, 68*, 562–576. https://doi.org/10.1007/s11199-013-0268-1

White, J. W., McMullin, D., Swartout, K., Sechrist, S., & Gollehon, A. (2008). Violence in intimate relationships: A conceptual and empirical examination of sexual and physical aggression. *Children and Youth Services Review, 30*(3), 338–351.

Wilkinson, D., Bearup, L. S., & Soprach, T. (2005). Youth gang rape in Phnom Penh. In S. Jejeebhoy, I. Shah, & S. Thapa (Eds.), *Sex without consent: Young people in developing countries* (pp. 158–168). London/New York: Zed Books.

Yeater, E. A., & O'Donohue, W. T. (1999). Sexual assault prevention programs: Current issues, future directions, and the potential efficacy of interventions with women. *Clinical Psychology Review, 19*(7), 739–771. https://doi.org/10.1016/S0272-7358(98)00075-0

Zernechel, A., & Perry, A. L. (2017). The final battle: Constructs of hegemonic masculinity and hypermasculinity in fraternity membership. *College Student Affairs Leadership, 4*(1).

Zinzow, H. M., & Thompson, M. (2015). Factors associated with use of verbally coercive, incapacitated, and forcible sexual assault tactics in a longitudinal study of college men. *Aggressive Behavior, 41*, 34–43.

Part IV

Victimology

The Sequelae of Sexual Assault

16

Kimberly A. Arditte Hall, Ellen T. Healy, and Tara E. Galovski

The experience of sexual assault is common, particularly for women. Whereas the modal outcome following sexual assault is acute distress followed by recovery, approximately 30 to 50% of sexual assault survivors will develop mental and/or physical health difficulties over time (Resnick, Kilpatrick, Dansky, Saunders, & Best, 1993; Rothbaum, Foa, Riggs, Murdock, & Walsh, 1992). When symptoms persist beyond the immediate aftermath of a sexual trauma, they can become chronic and debilitating. In this chapter, we provide a broad overview of the sequelae of sexual assault. First, we focus on *psychological* sequelae. Special attention is paid to the relationship between sexual assault and posttraumatic stress disorder (PTSD), though we also review associations between sexual assault and other forms of psychopathlogy, such as depressive, substance use, eating, and borderline personality disorders, as well as transdiagnostic psychological phenomena (e.g., changes to cognition and emotion that can occur even in the absence of disorder). Next, we discuss *physiological* sequelae, including tonic immobility as a frequently occurring immediate response to sexual assault and changes in autonomic nervous system activity over time. Third, we review research examining the effects of sexual assault on a variety of *physical and sexual health* problems. This section also includes a brief review of the literature on health care utilization among sexual assault survivors. Finally, we discuss the associations between sexual assault and aspects of *psychosocial functioning*, including interpersonal and occupational functioning. We conclude with a brief summary of findings, as well as directions for future research.

The views expressed in this chapter are those of the authors and do not necessarily reflect the Department of Veterans Affairs or the United States Government.

K. A. Arditte Hall (✉) · E. T. Healy · T. E. Galovski
VA National Center for PTSD, VA Boston Healthcare System, and Boston University School of Medicine, Boston, MA, USA
e-mail: kimberly.ardittehall@va.gov

Prevalence of Exposure to Sexual Assault

Exposure to traumatic events is not uncommon. Epidemiological studies estimate that approximately 50–90% of people in the United States alone are exposed to at least one traumatic event over the course of their lifetimes (Breslau et al., 1998; Kessler, 2000). Exposure in nonindustrialized and, particularly, war-torn countries is likely greater (De Jong et al., 2001; Kessler, 2000). Prevalence rates in United States studies reveal clear gender differences in overall exposure to trauma with men reporting significantly higher rates of trauma exposure than women (61% of men compared to 51% of women; Kessler, 1995). Gender differences are similar in other industrial-

W. T. O'Donohue and P. A. Schewe (eds.), *Handbook of Sexual Assault and Sexual Assault Prevention*,
https://doi.org/10.1007/978-3-030-23645-8_16

ized countries (e.g. Australia; Creamer, Burgess, & McFarlane, 2001). However, these gender differences vary according to type of traumatic event. Sexual traumas, including rape, sexual molestation, and assault, are one of the few types of trauma that are more commonly experienced by women (Resnick et al., 1993).

The most common sequela of exposure to any traumatic event is recovery. That being said, in the immediate aftermath of the trauma, elevated rates of distress (e.g. posttraumatic stress, depression) are fairly normative. For some portion of the population, distress will progress into diagnosable psychiatric conditions such as PTSD and depression. While men are more often exposed to traumatic events, women are twice as likely to develop PTSD secondary to a traumatic event and, once PTSD develops, women may be more likely to experience a chronic course of the disorder (Kessler, Sonnega, Bromet, Hughes, & Nelson, 1995). Important clinical correlates of PTSD, such as anger, guilt, negative self-worth, dissociation, somatization, health-related concerns, and poor impulse control, are also more commonly observed in women as compared to men (Olff, Langeland, Draijer, & Gersons, 2007; Tolin & Foa, 2006).

The type of trauma with the highest conditional risk of precipitating PTSD for both men and women is rape (Resnick et al., 1993), with sexual assaults accounting for approximately half of all PTSD cases in women and about one third of cases in men. Seemingly, it might be argued that women's greater exposure to sexual trauma, coupled with the higher conditional risk for PTSD after exposure to sexual trauma vs. other types of trauma, might account for the gender differences in PTSD prevalence. Breslau, Davis, Andreski, Peterson, and Schultz (1997) examined whether the excess rates of PTSD in women could be accounted for by exposure to elevated rates of childhood sexual abuse. They found that even after controlling for trauma exposure, women were more likely than men to develop PTSD. In summary, women are more likely to be sexually assaulted than men (with sexual assault constituting the type of trauma that holds the highest conditional risk for PTSD) *and* develop PTSD at twice the rate of men, *but* the higher incidence of sexual trauma does not entirely explain the gender differences observed in PTSD prevalence rates.

Trajectories of Recovery and Non-recovery Following Exposure to Trauma

Given the relative paucity of studies examining the long-term mental health trajectories of exposure to interpersonal assault broadly defined, we first look to the larger trauma literature to provide guidance in understanding the trajectories of mental health outcomes following exposure to traumatic events and predictors of poor outcomes. Long-term mental health outcomes secondary to exposure to traumatic events have been most consistently evaluated following single traumas, such as a disaster, mass casualty, or terrorist attacks (e.g., Gruebner et al., 2016), within specific populations such as combat veterans (Berntsen et al., 2012), first responders (Marchand, Nadeau, Beaulieu-Prévost, Boyer, & Martin, 2015), and war refugees (Hobfoll et al., 2009). The historical, contextual, situational, and individual variables encasing these traumatic events vary across studies with implications for the trajectories of mental health outcomes over time.

The bulk of the research focusing on pathological responses to exposure to traumatic events attends primarily to the development and maintenance of posttraumatic stress and, to a lesser extent, depression (Hobfoll et al., 2009). Studies of trajectories of mental health outcomes in individuals exposed to mass casualty, terrorism (Bonanno, 2005; Bonanno, Rennicke, & Dekel, 2005; Hobfoll et al., 2009), and natural disaster (reviewed in Norris, Byrne, Diaz, & Kaniasty, 2007) consistently show that the majority of individuals exposed to trauma do not report pathological distress, or are *resistant* and do not develop clinical levels of symptoms. Further, survivors of trauma may be classified as *resilient,* a trajectory marked by initially elevated symptomatology which decreases naturally over time and eventually returns to baseline (Bonanno, 2005;

Norris, Stevens, Pfefferbaum, Wyche, & Pfefferbaum, 2008). The resilience trajectory is the modal outcome irrespective of type of trauma (Bonanno, 2004), with the possible exception of sexual trauma (Steenkamp, Dickstein, Salters-Pedneault, Hofmann, & Litz, 2012; discussed in more detail below). However, a substantial minority of trauma survivors fares less well after exposure to trauma and are neither resistant nor resilient to poor mental health outcomes. A third trajectory, termed the *chronic distress* trajectory (Hobfoll et al., 2009), includes individuals who report significant distress immediately after exposure to the trauma and remain symptomatic over time. Finally, a fourth trajectory, also described by Hobfoll et al. (2009), and termed *delayed distress*, describes individuals who report low levels of distress in the short-term following the event, but with increasing distress over time. From a public health perspective, understanding trajectories of resilience, resistance, and distress in the aftermath of a traumatic event is important in informing both prevention and intervention strategies. Given the particularly elevated rates of PTSD among individuals exposed to sexual trauma, understanding trajectories of recovery specifically following sexual trauma is essential.

Several studies have assessed the natural course of PTSD following sexual trauma over time. The trajectories of PTSD in rape survivors (Rothbaum et al., 1992) indicate that, similar to the trajectories observed in other trauma populations, the prevalence of PTSD decreases over time for the majority of survivors. In a study assessing female rape survivors on a weekly basis for 12 weeks after the rape, investigators found that almost all the participants (94%) reported symptoms and symptom severity consistent with a diagnosis of PTSD (minus the necessary 1 month time criterion) in the week immediately following the rape. Thus, symptom expression that closely mimics a full diagnosis of PTSD is quite common in the immediate aftermath of rape. Approximately 1 month following the rape, the rates of PTSD diminished to 65% of the study respondents and, at 3 months posttrauma, PTSD remained present in 47% of the study sample. For those whose symptoms persist, the course of distress may be chronic and enduring, with significant negative physical health complications and poor functioning in major life domains over time.

Riggs, Kilpatrick, and Resnick (1992) compared subsets of individuals who had been exposed to different types of violent crimes (rape vs. aggravated assault) and considered the relationship to the assailant (stranger or husband) to a group of nonvictimized women. Perhaps not surprisingly, the results showed significantly elevated levels of distress in the women who had been victimized as compared to the women who had not. However, there were very little differences in distress in women who had been assaulted by a husband vs. someone else. Also of note, the long-term distress observed in women who suffered a nonsexual violent assault did not differ from that reported by women who had been raped. The authors interpret this departure from previous studies' findings that sexual traumas resulted in higher rates of PTSD, as compared to nonsexual, violent assaults, by noting that fear of death during the assault was significantly greater in the nonsexual assault portion of the study sample. The violence during these assaults may have been more severe than that in the larger epidemiological studies accounting for rates of PTSD that were more similar to the prevalence rates observed in the sexual trauma cohort.

More recently, Steenkamp et al. (2012) assessed the response to sexual trauma to evaluate trajectories of PTSD in an effort to compare theoretical models of response to sexual trauma with models of response to other types of trauma. They hypothesized that, unlike models of recovery following serious illness, severe injury, war-related trauma, and mass disaster, resistance and resilience trajectories would not be the modal courses of recovery following exposure to sexual trauma. As expected, few participants demonstrated resistance or resilience trajectories, and nearly all participants endorsed high levels of distress 1 month post-assault. When data were examined using latent class analysis, approximately 7% of participants demonstrated a trajectory of high and chronic PTSD symptoms, 16% of participants demonstrated a trajectory of moderate and chronic PTSD symptoms, 48% of participants demonstrated a trajectory of moderate recovery in PTSD symptoms over time, and 29% of participants demonstrated a trajectory of marked recovery in PTSD symptoms over time. The authors conclude that most survivors will experience significant PTSD symptoms in the immediate aftermath of the event with a gradual decline in PTSD symptoms over the following months. They conclude that clinical intervention may be warranted for those individuals whose symptoms persist over time as the likelihood that symptoms will remit in the absence of treatment decreases with time.

In summary, we see that the most common outcome following a traumatic event, including sexual assault, is recovery. However, in mapping observed trajectories of mental health outcomes following sexual traumas onto epidemiological studies assessing response trajectories observed in nonsexual trauma populations, the conditional risk for developing PTSD is quite high following sexual traumas specifically.

Predictors of Non-recovery Following Sexual Assault

The importance of identifying those trauma survivors who will develop persistent trauma symptoms, including but not limited to PTSD, is important because early identification may result in early intervention. Likewise, identifying predictors of poor outcomes is paramount to informing successful interventions. In other words, what precisely is preventing recovery in those individuals who go on to develop PTSD and other mental health concerns? What variables differentiate those who recover from those who do not? Understanding the factors that contribute to interruptions in recovery is critical to resolving those interruptions and resuming the process of recovery.

Early identification of those who will go on to exhibit persistent, poor outcomes is a lofty goal. The preponderance of evidence suggests that consideration of an interaction of a number of variables including acute symptoms, biology, and cognitive variables is critical for predicting who will go on to develop PTSD (Bryant, 2003). Contextual and demographic variables also likely contribute to poor outcomes, including the development of PTSD. Socioeconomic disadvantage, racial minority membership, unemployment, younger age, and lower income have consistently been identified as predictors of poor outcomes following exposures to trauma (Brewin, Andrews, & Valentine, 2000). Extensive trauma histories also were associated with posttraumatic stress symptom severity (Lowe, Galea, Uddin, & Koenen, 2014), particularly with respect to the experience of prior assaultive or interpersonal violence traumas (Goldmann et al., 2011). Perhaps not surprisingly, Lowe et al. (2014) found that chronically severe posttraumatic stress symptoms were associated with socioeconomic disadvantage and lack of social supports and resources. While the treatment of PTSD will be detailed elsewhere in this book, it is important to note that the accumulation of information regarding the sequelae of sexual assault, including prevalence rates of trauma-related disorders, the natural trajectories of these disorders, and predictors of poor outcomes, directly informs treatment of the negative outcomes resulting from this type of violence.

Psychiatric Diagnoses Following Sexual Assault

For a substantial minority of survivors of sexual trauma, the assault is related to the subsequent development of psychological dysfunction. A recent meta-analysis found that those who had experienced sexual assault reported significantly worse psychopathology than those who had not been assaulted (average Hedges' $g = 0.61$; Dworkin, Menon, Bystrynski, & Allen, 2017). Sexual assault conferred increased risk of developing a range of psychiatric diagnoses, and the risk was highest for PTSD, which is not surprising given that the experience of trauma is a criterion for the diagnosis. It is less clear whether the higher prevalence of other psychiatric conditions such as depression, substance use disorders and eating disorders are directly related to the experience of sexual trauma or are secondary to PTSD.

Posttraumatic Stress Disorder. According to the *Diagnostic and Statistical Manual of Mental Disorders, 5th Edition* (DSM-5; American Psychiatric Association [APA], 2013), PTSD is characterized by four clusters of symptoms: (1) intrusion symptoms, including recurrent distressing memories and nightmares, (2) marked avoidance of memories and reminders of the traumatic experience, (3) changes in mood and beliefs, including self-blame and exaggerated negative beliefs, and (4) increased arousal and reactivity, including hypervigilance, increased startle, and sleep disturbance. As reviewed in detail above, symptoms of PTSD are quite common in the immediate aftermath of a rape with more severe initial PTSD symptoms predicting a more chronic course of the disorder (Riggs, Rothbaum, & Foa, 1995). A large epidemiological study found that about one third of women who experienced rape or other sexual assault developed PTSD in their lifetime (Resnick et al., 1993). This is lower than the 47% rate of PTSD noted in a previous study (Rothbaum et al., 1992), though the previous sample primarily comprised women who reported the incident to police, which may indicate higher levels of life threat and injury from those who do not report their rape (Resnick et al., 1993). Women have been found to have consistently higher rates of PTSD than men, and though some hypothesize that this is due to higher rates of sexual assault in women, it does not appear that this fully explains observed gender differences in PTSD rates (Olff et al., 2007).

Depressive Disorders and Suicidality. Sexual assault is associated with increased rates of depression, and specifically with one notable symptom of depression – suicidality (Chen et al., 2010; Dworkin et al., 2017). Major depressive disorder is a common psychiatric diagnosis with higher prevalence rates occurring in young adults and females (APA, 2013). Predominant features include depressed mood, diminished interest in activities, changes in sleep, eating, and motor activity, fatigue, feelings of worthlessness, concentration problems, and suicidal thoughts. Trauma, and specifically sexual assault, is one of many etiological factors that may contribute to depression, though depression can occur in the absence of trauma. Depression and PTSD are commonly comorbid, and have some overlap in symptoms, but it is less clear whether these are distinct posttrauma phenomena. There is some support for depression as a unique construct in the aftermath of trauma for some people (O'Donnell, Creamer, & Pattison, 2004), as well as data to suggest that depression and PTSD symptoms are reflections of a common posttrauma sequela (Breslau, Davis, Peterson, & Schultz, 2000).

Survivors of sexual assault are at increased risk for suicidal ideation and for engaging in suicide attempts in their lifetime (Ullman, 2004). This relationship between trauma history and suicidality appears to be stronger for sexual assault than other types of trauma. Additionally, sexual assault is more predictive of the persistence of suicidality (Stein et al., 2010). This relationship between sexual assault and suicidal behavior applies to sexual traumas experienced in childhood through adulthood. Among adult sexual assault survivors, younger and minority women may be at higher risk of suicidal ideation; women who also had histories of childhood sexual trauma or who experienced adult assaults by multiple assailants may also be at increased risk of suicidal ideation (Ullman & Najdowski, 2009). While both PTSD and depression are associated with increased suicidal ideation, depression alone has been found to predict suicide attempts, indicating that perhaps depression confers specific risk for suicidal behavior (Ullman, 2004). Substance use disorders are also highly comorbid with depression and PTSD in survivors of sexual assault, which together increase risk of suicidal behavior.

Substance Use Disorders. The experience of rape has been associated with increased subsequent alcohol and drug use (Kilpatrick, Acierno, Resnick, Saunders, & Best, 1997), with those experiencing multiple sexual traumas reporting higher levels of problematic substance use (Walsh et al., 2014). There appears to be a relatively lower risk of developing a substance use disorder than other psychiatric disorders, such as PTSD or depression, after sexual assault, though much of the literature has examined the use of substances after sexual assault, rather than the presence of a substance use disorder per se (Dworkin et al., 2017). Additional research clarifying the nature of the relationship between sexual assault and substance use disorders is needed. When alcohol use is involved in the sexual assault, there is a higher rate of alcohol use in the years following (Kaysen, Neighbors, Martell, Fossos, & Larimer, 2006). It is hypothesized that increased alcohol use after sexual assault can function as a form of self-medication, helping the individual avoid the psychological distress resulting from the trauma (Miranda Jr., Meyerson, Long, Marx, & Simpson, 2002). Furthermore, the development of PTSD appears to mediate the relationship between rape and subsequent alcohol use (Epstein, Saunders, Kilpatrick, & Resnick, 1998).

Eating Disorders. Eating disorders may also manifest in the aftermath of a sexual trauma. There are various clinical presentations of eating disorders which include (a) anorexia nervosa, characterized by eating restriction and significantly low weight, (b) bulimia nervosa, which involves binge eating episodes and recurrent compensatory/purging behaviors, and (c) binge eating disorder, in which there are recurrent episodes of binge eating in the absence of purging behavior. Studies of both clinical and epidemiological samples demonstrate the relationship between the history of sexual assault and disordered eating across all ages (Romans, Gendall, Martin, & Mullen, 2001; Wonderlich et al., 2000; Wonderlich, Wilsnack, Wilsnack, & Harris, 1996). Childhood sexual abuse is a nonspecific risk factor for eating disorders, meaning that while it is a risk factor for disordered eating, it is also a risk factor for other psychiatric disorders as well (Brewerton, 2007). However, the association between childhood sexual abuse and eating disorder symptomatology may vary by population. For example, among male and female military veterans, a history of childhood sexual abuse was not significantly associated with eating disorder symptoms, whereas a history of military-related trauma, including potential experiences of military sexual trauma, was (Arditte Hall, Bartlett, Iverson, & Mitchell, 2017; Arditte Hall, Bartlett, Iverson, & Mitchell, 2018).

Multiple studies have found that sexual trauma histories are more commonly associated with eating disorders that involve bulimic/purging behavior rather than restricting subtypes of anorexia (Carter, Bewell, Blackwell, & Woodside, 2006). Following sexual trauma, disordered eating behaviors may serve as a form of avoidance coping that temporarily reduces trauma-related thoughts and emotions; additionally, disordered eating and associated weight changes may help sexual assault survivors to avoid unwanted attention from potential perpetrators of sexual violence (Breland, Donalson, Dinh, & Maguen, 2018). The relationship between disordered eating and sexual trauma is significantly mediated by the presence of PTSD (Holzer, Uppala, Wonderlich, Crosby, & Simonich, 2008).

Borderline Personality Disorder. Borderline personality disorder (BPD) is characterized by an enduring pattern of instability in interpersonal relationships, self-concept, and emotion regulation. Individuals with BPD endorse sexual trauma more often than those without BPD, with the rates of sexual assault among those with BPD varying widely by sample (20% to 80%; Zanarini, 1997). However, the etiology of BPD is thought to be multidimensional, so sexual assault during childhood may be a risk factor, but not the only contributing factor. For some people who develop BPD, history of sexual trauma may be a defining environmental contributing factor whereas for others, sexual trauma does not play a role. BPD may be more strongly related to sexual abuse that occurs at a young age than sexual trauma that happens when older (McLean & Gallop, 2003).

Transdiagnostic Psychological Consequences of Sexual Assault

Sexual assault survivors may experience specific psychological changes that transcend, or occur in the absence of, specific mental health diagnoses. Below, we focus on changes across three domains: sleep, cognition and emotion, and posttraumatic growth.

Sleep Difficulties. Though sleep difficulties are common among sexual assault survivors with

PTSD and depression, impairments in sleep may also occur outside the context of these diagnoses and may help to explain the association between sexual assault and mental health symptoms. A large body of literature links childhood sexual abuse to sleep difficulties in adulthood. As compared to adults without a history of childhood sexual abuse, adults with a history of childhood sexual abuse have poorer sleep quality and are more likely to experience nightmares, difficulty falling asleep, fear of sleeping, sleep paralysis, and violent behavior during sleep (for a review, see Kajeepeta, Gelaye, Jackson, & Williams, 2015). Among women with a history of childhood sexual abuse, sleep difficulties are positively associated with posttraumatic stress and depression symptom severity and may mediate the association between sexual abuse and these mental health symptoms (Noll, Trickett, Susman, & Putnam, 2006).

Relatively less work has been done to document an association between adult sexual assault and impaired sleep. As discussed by Krakow, Ulibarri, Moore, and McIver (2015), a series of papers published between 2000 and 2002 examined the presence of sleep-disordered breathing (e.g., obstructive sleep apnea; upper airway resistance syndrome) in female adult sexual assault survivors with posttraumatic stress symptoms. Findings revealed that sleep-disordered breathing was common in this population and associated with worse psychological distress. Conversely, treating sleep-disordered breathing was found to decrease PTSD symptom severity. More recently, Jenkins, Colvonen, Norman, Afari, and Allard (2015) examined insomnia in 917 male and female veterans with and without a history of military sexual trauma. Women with military sexual trauma endorsed higher rates of insomnia and more severe insomnia symptoms than women without military sexual trauma.

Cognitive and Emotional Changes. Sexual assault survivors may experience broad changes to their belief systems, self-concept, and emotions. Again, these changes may occur outside the context of specific diagnoses and/or may help to explain the associations between sexual assault, psychological symptoms, and other relevant outcomes such as engagement in mental health treatment. Several cognitive processes have been identified as increasing risk for PTSD and other mental health difficulties following an experience of sexual assault. These can include processes that occur during the assault (e.g., mental defeat, confusion, or detachment), the manner in which assault sequelae are appraised (e.g., negative appraisal of symptoms, beliefs that the individual has incurred permanent change), dysfunctional cognitive or behavioral coping strategies (e.g., avoidance, safety behaviors), and other beliefs that are affected by the assault (e.g., negative beliefs about oneself and the world; e.g., Dunmore, Clark, & Ehlers, 1999). Self-blame is an especially common negative belief among sexual assault survivors. Self-blame beliefs can be particularly pernicious because they reinforce internalized stigma, interfere with disclosure and treatment seeking behaviors, and are associated with increased likelihood for revictimization (Kennedy & Prock, 2016). Sexual assault has also been linked with rumination, or the tendency to perseverate on negative aspects of oneself, one's symptoms, or one's life experiences (Sarin & Nolen-Hoeksema, 2010; Stermac, Cabral, Clarke, & Toner, 2014). Sexual assault survivors who ruminate have been found to experience increased distress (Stermac et al., 2014) and may be more likely to engage in maladaptive strategies to cope with distress (e.g., emotional eating, use of drugs or alcohol; Sarin & Nolen-Hoeksema, 2010).

Survivors of sexual assault in childhood or adulthood may also struggle with increased shame (for a review, see Kennedy & Prock, 2016). Without intervention, experiences of shame appear to be stable over time (Feiring & Taska, 2005), and are associated with a range of negative mental health consequences (e.g., global distress, PTSD, anxiety, and depression; DeCou, Cole, Lynch, Wong, & Matthews, 2017; Willie et al., 2016). As with self-blame, shame is related to internalized stigma, decreases the likelihood of disclosure, and increases likelihood of revictimization (Kennedy & Prock, 2016). The extent to which sexual assault is associated with other emotional difficulties is less clear. There has been some evidence suggesting broad emotional impairments among individuals with a history of sexual trauma. Documented impairments include difficulty identifying and labeling one's emotions (termed *alexithymia*), nonacceptance of emotions, and ineffective use of specific emotion regulation strategies (see Ehring & Quack, 2010). However, such emotional difficulties seem to be most evident in individuals: 1) who experienced sexual trauma in early life vs. as adults and 2) who have multiple or chronic experiences of sexual trauma vs. a single incident of sexual assault (Ehring & Quack, 2010; Ullman, Peter-Hagene, & Relyea, 2014; Walsh, DiLillo, & Scalora, 2011). Thus, it should not be assumed that all individuals with a history of sexual assault will experience broad difficulties with emotional functioning.

Posttraumatic Growth. Posttraumatic growth is the extent to which a person experiences positive changes (e.g., greater appreciation for life, spiritual growth, personal strength, etc.) following a traumatic experience (Tedeschi & Calhoun, 1996). A recent review of the literature revealed a reliable association between sexual violence and posttraumatic growth (Ulloa, Guzman, Salazar, & Cala, 2016). Almost universally, people report at least small degrees of growth following sexual assault; moderate to large degrees of growth may be expected to occur in a large minority (~45%) of sexual assault survivors (Grubaugh & Resick, 2007). Several individual difference factors predict greater posttraumatic growth following sexual assault. These include demographic factors (e.g., older age, ethnic minority, less education), assault characteristics (e.g., perception of life threat during assault), post-assault factors (e.g., adaptive coping, positive social reactions from others, perceived control over recovery), and mental health treatment use (Hassija & Turchik, 2016; Ullman, 2014). Importantly, among individuals who have experienced sexual assault as children or adults, posttraumatic growth is inversely related to general distress, as well as anxiety, depression, and posttraumatic stress symptoms, suggesting that it functions as a protective factor (Frazier, Conlon, & Glaser, 2001; Stermac et al., 2014; Willie et al., 2016).

Physiological Consequences of Sexual Assault

As discussed in a recent review by Cuevas, Balbo, Duval, and Beverly (2018), there are a variety of neurobiological and physiological changes that occur during the course of a sexual assault. These changes represent the body's defense against physical threat and serve to prepare the person to fight off or flee from their perpetrator (i.e., "fight or flight" response). In addition, sexual assault survivors may experience a "freeze" response, also known as *tonic immobility*. Tonic immobility may occur after attempts to fight or escape from a predator are found to be ineffective. It is characterized in part by motor immobility, muscular rigidity, suppressed vocalization, and changes in heart rate and body temperature. Though sexual assault survivors may often be questioned about or blamed for not doing more to escape from their perpetrator, it is important to remember that tonic immobility is an involuntary physiological process that occurs in the context of extreme fear and perceived inability to escape. Tonic immobility is common among children or adults experiencing sexual assault, and is associated with subsequent PTSD symptom severity (Bovin, Jager-Hyman, Gold, Marx, & Sloan, 2008; Humphreys, Sauder, Martin, & Marx, 2010).

A large literature has documented autonomic nervous system (ANS) dysregulation, characterized by overactivation of the sympathetic nervous system and underactivation of the parasympathetic nervous system, among individuals with PTSD (for a review see, Arditte Hall, Osterberg, Orr, & Pineles, 2018), including sexual assault survivors (e.g., Orr et al., 1998; Rothbaum, Kozak, Foa, & Whitaker, 2001). In contrast, relatively little work has been done to examine the direct association between sexual assault and ANS dysregulation and existing research has produced mixed results. Some studies suggest that individuals with, vs. without, a history of sexual assault experience increased sympathetic activity and decreased parasympathetic activity in response to stress (Heim et al., 2000; Lorenz, Harte, & Meston, 2015); other studies have found evidence of blunted sympathetic activity in individuals with, vs. without, a history of sexual assault (Marx & Soler-Baillo, 2008; Soler-Baillo, Marx, & Sloan, 2005). Future research aimed at clarifying the nature of the association between sexual assault and ANS dysregulation and the factors that predict variability in ANS dysregulation among sexual assault survivors is needed.

Physical Health Consequences of Sexual Assault

Sexual assault in childhood and adulthood may increase risk for a variety of physical health problems. Individuals with a lifetime history of sexual assault report poorer general health and are at increased risk for autoimmune disorders (e.g., asthma, fibromyalgia), gastrointestinal disorders (e.g., irritable bowel syndrome), gynecological problems, pain, and poor cardiopulmonary health (for reviews, see Irish, Kobayashi, & Delahanty, 2010, Golding, 1999, and Wilson, 2010). Evidence has also been found for a "dose-response" effect; as the number of sexual assaults a person has experienced increases so too does the likelihood for experiencing specific physical health problems (Stein & Barrett-Connor, 2000; Turchik & Hassija, 2014). Although it is difficult to determine a causal connection between experiences of sexual assault and subsequent physical health problems, it has been posited that specific health risk factors may help to explain the association. In a national sample of treatment-seeking female veterans, Frayne, Skinner, Sullivan, and Freund (2003) found that obesity, smoking, problematic alcohol use, sedentary lifestyle, and a history of hysterectomy before age 40 were each more common in women with vs. without a history of military sexual trauma. Such risk factors may mediate the association between sexual assault and subsequent cardiac disease.

Sexual Functioning. Given the nature of sexual assault, it is not surprising that a several studies have been devoted to understanding its effects on sexual functioning. Sexually transmitted infection (STI) can be contracted during a sexual assault and individuals with a history of sexual assault may be at increased risk for STIs, more generally (Goyal et al., 2017; Schwarcz & Whittington, 1990). Rates of sexual dysfunction are also elevated among individuals with a history of sexual assault. Specifically, during sexual encounters, sexual assault survivors may experience decreased sexual satisfaction, pleasure, and desire, as well as increased fear and arousal (Turchik & Hassija, 2014; van Berlo & Ensink, 2000). Despite these findings, patterns of sexual activity vary considerably among individuals with a history of sexual assault. One study found that, among female rape survivors, approximately 48% indicated their sexual health behaviors became less risky post-rape, whereas 52% reported that their sexual health behaviors became moderately or substantially *more* risky post-rape (Campbell, Sefl, & Ahrens, 2004). Risky sexual behaviors can include frequent sexual activity with multiple sexual partners, infrequent condom use, and use of drugs and/or alcohol during sex. Though it is unclear why individuals with a history of sexual assault may be more likely to engage in such behaviors, insight may be gleaned from a recent study that found the association between sexual assault and condomless sex was mediated by perceptions of partners' pressure for condomless sex (Wells et al., 2016).

Health Care Utilization. Understanding patterns of health care utilization among sexual assault survivors can be complicated. Research generally indicates that rates of service utilization immediately following or within one year of a sexual assault are low (Kintzle et al., 2015; Sabrina & Ho, 2014). Among those who do seek treatment, use of medical services tends to occur before use of mental health services (within 1 month vs. more than 6 months following assault; Mengeling, Booth, Torner, & Sadler, 2015). Barriers to seeking care may include concerns that the individual's account of his/her sexual assault will not be believed or that the individual will feel blamed for what happened (Walsh, Banyard, Moynihan, Ward, & Cohn, 2010). In contrast, lifetime rates of service utilization, particularly mental health services, may be higher among individuals with vs. without a history of sexual assault. Stein et al. (2004) found that a history of sexual assault was associated with a greater number of primary care visits in the previous 6 months. Likewise, Kintzle et al. (2015) found that 86% of their sample of female veterans with a history of military sexual trauma had sought mental health counseling in the past 12 months.

Effects of Sexual Assault on Psychosocial Functioning

The experience of trauma in general, and sexual assault specifically, can affect many domains of psychosocial functioning including interpersonal and occupational arenas. In a recent review, 15–47% of adults who had histories of childhood sexual abuse were considered resilient in terms of their level of functioning, with social support from family and community resources serving as a strong protective factor (Domhardt, Munzer, Fegert, & Goldbeck, 2015). However, this finding indicates a large portion of survivors experience difficulties in various realms of functioning. Sexual abuse in childhood is a risk factor for a range of interpersonal functioning difficulties, including poorer quality of intimacy and sexual relationships, higher divorce rates, and parenting difficulties (DiLillo, 2001). Women who have experienced sexual assaults during both childhood and adulthood have been found to report more interpersonal dysfunction than women who were sexually assaulted as adults (Cloitre, Scarvalone, & Difede, 1997). PTSD appears to mediate the relationship between childhood trauma and functional impairment as an adult (Cloitre, Miranda, Stovall-McClough, & Han, 2005). Further evidence of this relationship with PTSD and functioning is the substantial improvements to diverse domains of psychosocial functioning that women experience when treated with evidence-based treatments for PTSD – both cognitive processing therapy and prolonged exposure (Galovski, Phipps, & Resick, 2005).

With respect to occupational functioning, there is evidence that sexual assaults suffered by adults can impact work-related outcomes. A case controlled analysis found that Army female service members who had administratively recorded histories of sexual assault were at increased risk of demotion and attrition from the service in the subsequent 12 months after their trauma (Rossellini et al., 2017). This is consistent with a prospective study with civilian women in which interpersonal violence including sexual assault was associated with higher rates of unemployment after the assault (Byrne, Resnick, Kilpatrick, Best, & Saunders, 1999).

Potentially Problematic Accounts of Sexual Assault Sequelae

Above, we have surveyed the most commonly occurring sexual assault sequelae. We would be remiss, however, not to mention several other potential sequelae for which there is equivocal empirical support and/or enduring controversy amongst researchers. We encourage readers interested in these topics to reference other chapters in this book, which address several of them in greater detail.

Rape trauma syndrome (RTS; Burgess & Holmstrom, 1974) is characterized by a two-phase reaction; in the *acute phase* rape survivors may experience variable emotional and somatic reactions, whereas in the *long-term reorganization* process they may demonstrate increased motor activity, experience nightmares, and develop fear and avoidance of trauma-related situations (termed traumaphobia). In a recent review, O'Donohue, Carlson, Benuto, and Bennett (2014) outlined several criticisms of the RTS model, including: its vague and imprecise definition, the lack of empirical research on its validity as a diagnosis, and its inconsistency with other conceptualizations of sexual assault-related psychopathology (e.g., acute stress reactions and PTSD). Based on these criticisms, the authors concluded that there is little evidence to date to warrant consideration of RTS in legal or clinical practice settings.

Dissociation during and after sexual assault is not uncommon. For example, among individuals with PTSD, 15% of men and 30% of women endorse high levels of dissociative symptoms

(Wolf et al., 2012). However, the emergence of dissociative disorders, and particularly dissociative identity disorder (DID) following experiences of sexual trauma remains controversial. For example, there is disagreement over the validity of DID as a diagnosis, as well as the possibility that DID reflects a more severe subtype of BPD or other personality disorders (see reviews by Brand et al., 2016 and Gillig, 2009). DID is most likely to occur following experiences of severe and chronic childhood sexual abuse and the prevalence of the disorder (~1–1.5%; APA, 2013; Brand et al., 2016) is lower than other forms of trauma-related psychopathology. Likewise, the extent to which sexual assault survivors repress trauma memories and/or experience dissociative amnesia remains controversial. One study found that memories for sexual trauma are not impaired or fragmented and, instead, are often more vivid and detailed, as compared to non-trauma-related memories (Peace, Porter, & ten Brinke, 2008). It has been posited that recovery of repressed memories is influenced by factors such as therapist suggestiveness and coverage of childhood sexual abuse in the media (Loftus, 1993). Though recovered memories are often remembered with confidence, it can difficult to determine if they are authentic. As discussed by Rydberg (2017), dissociative amnesia may involve complete loss of recall for sexual abuse, but is much more likely to involve fragmented or partial trauma memories.

Finally, there have been some efforts to link experiences of sexual trauma, particularly childhood sexual abuse, to changes to the structure or function of the brain. For example, a study by Andersen et al. (2008) provided preliminary evidence to suggest that sexual abuse occurring at different developmental stages was associated with structural brain changes (e.g., reduced hippocampal volume) in adulthood. However, other research has found that such changes are most likely to occur in individuals with a history of childhood sexual abuse and PTSD (Bremner et al., 2003). Indeed, when individuals with a history of childhood sexual abuse but without PTSD were compared against individuals without a history of childhood sexual abuse, no significant differences were found (Bremner et al., 2003). Thus, research does not currently provide clear or convincing evidence directly linking experiences of sexual trauma to specific brain changes.

Conclusion

Individuals who experience sexual assault are at increased risk for a variety of negative mental and physical health sequelae. PTSD is perhaps the most common psychiatric disorder that can develop after a sexual trauma, but a host of other disorders (e.g. depression, substance use, eating, and borderline personality disorder) can manifest independently, comorbid to PTSD, or as a result of PTSD. Other clinical correlates (e.g., sleep impairment, shame, and self-blame) are also frequently reported among individuals with a history of sexual assault, even in the absence of specific psychiatric disorders. Of note, not all of the changes experienced by sexual assault survivors are negative. For example, some individuals will experience posttraumatic growth after a sexual assault, which may be protective against chronic negative psychological sequelae.

Relatively little research has been done to examine the physiological sequelae of sexual assault and extant results are equivocal. Given that dysregulated physiology can increase risk for psychological and physical health problems over time, additional research on the psychophysiological profiles of sexual assault survivors with and without PTSD and other psychological disorders is needed. Sexual assault survivors appear to be at increased risk for a variety of physical and sexual health problems spanning numerous bodily systems. Though preliminary research indicates that some of these problems may be mediated by maladaptive health behaviors, such as smoking, alcohol use, or sedentary lifestyle, it will be important to more fully elucidate the pathways from sexual assault to poor physical health. This line of research stands to improve early detection and intervention efforts. Similarly, it is important to gain a better understanding of how sexual assault survivors utilize health services, including medical and mental health services, and to identify and reduce barriers to healthcare engagement. Finally, research links experiences of sexual assault to impairments in functioning, though again, it remains unclear whether these associations are driven by the presence of specific mental health diagnoses. Continued investigation into the sequelae of sexual assault specifically will be useful to our understanding of the effects of this unique and all too common experience.

References

American Psychiatric Association. (2013). *Diagnostic and statistical manual of mental disorders: DSM-5* (5th ed.). Washington, DC: American Psychiatric Publishing.

Andersen, S. L., Tomada, A., Vincow, E. S., Valente, E., Polcari, A., & Teicher, M. H. (2008). Preliminary evidence for sensitive periods in the effect of childhood sexual abuse on regional brain development. *The Journal of Neuropsychiatry and Clinical Neurosciences, 20*, 292–301.

Arditte Hall, K. A., Bartlett, B. A., Iverson, K. M., & Mitchell, K. S. (2018). Eating disorder symptoms in female veterans: The role of childhood, adult, and military trauma exposure. *Psychological Trauma Theory Research Practice and Policy, 10*(3), 345–351.

Arditte Hall, K. A., Bartlett, B. A., Iverson, K. M., & Mitchell, K. S. (2017). Military-related trauma is associated with eating disorder symptoms in male veterans. *International Journal of Eating Disorders, 50*, 1328–1331.

Arditte Hall, K. A., Osterberg, T. J., Orr, S. P., & Pineles, S. L. (2018). The cardiovascular consequences of autonomic nervous system dysregulation in PTSD. In G. Pinna (Ed.), *Facilitating Resilience After Trauma*. Hauppauge, NY: Nova Science Publishers, Inc.

Berntsen, D., Johannessen, K. B., Thomsen, Y. D., Bertelsen, M., Hoyle, R. H., & Rubin, D. C. (2012). Peace and war: Trajectories of posttraumatic stress disorder symptoms before, during, and after military deployment in Afghanistan. *Psychological Science, 23*(12), 1557–1565.

Bonanno, G. A. (2004). Loss, trauma, and human resilience: Have we underestimated the human capacity to thrive after extremely aversive events? *American Psychologist, 59*(1), 20–28.

Bonanno, G. A. (2005). Clarifying and extending the construct of adult resilience. *American Psychologist, 60*(3), 265–267.

Bonanno, G. A., Rennicke, C., & Dekel, S. (2005). Self-enhancement among high-exposure survivors of the September 11th terrorist attack: Resilience or social maladjustment? *Journal of Personality and Social Psychology, 88*(6), 984–998.

Bovin, M. J., Jager-Hyman, S., Gold, S. D., Marx, B. P., & Sloan, D. M. (2008). Tonic immobility mediates the influence of peritraumatic fear and perceived inescapability on posttraumatic stress symptom severity among sexual assault survivors. *Journal of Traumatic Stress, 21*(4), 402–409.

Brand, B. L., Sar, V., Stavropoulos, P., Krüger, C., Korzekwa, M., Martínez-Toboas, A., & Middleton, W. (2016). Separating fact from fiction: An empirical examination of six myths about dissociative identity disorder. *Harvard Review of Psychiatry, 24*, 257–270.

Breland, J. Y., Donalson, R., Dinh, J. V., & Maguen, S. (2018). Trauma exposure and disordered eating: A qualitative study. *Women & Health, 58*, 160–174.

Bremner, J. D., Vythilingam, M., Vermetten, E., Southwick, S. M., McGlashan, T., … Charney, D. S. (2003). MRI and PET study of deficits in hippocampal structure and function in women with childhood sexual abuse and posttraumatic stress disorder. *American Journal of Psychiatry, 160*, 924–932.

Breslau, N., Davis, G. C., Andreski, P., Peterson, E. L., & Schultz, L. R. (1997). Sex differences in posttraumatic stress disorder. *Archives of General Psychiatry, 54*(11), 1044–1048.

Breslau, N., Davis, G., C., Peterson, E., L., Schultz, L. R. (2000). A second look at the comorbidity in victims of trauma: The posttraumatic stress disorder-major depression connection. *Biological Psychiatry, 48*, 902-909.

Breslau, N., Kessler, R. C., Chilcoat, H. D., Schultz, L. R., Davis, G. C., & Andreski, P. (1998). Trauma and posttraumatic stress disorder in the community: The 1996 Detroit Area Survey of Trauma. *Archives of General Psychiatry, 55*(7), 626–632.

Brewerton, T. D. (2007). Eating Disorders, trauma, and comorbidity: Focus on PTSD. *Eating Disorders, 15*, 285–304.

Brewin, C. R., Andrews, B., & Valentine, J. D. (2000). Meta-analysis of risk factors for posttraumatic stress disorder in trauma-exposed adults. *Journal of Consulting and Clinical Psychology, 68*(5), 748–766.

Bryant, R. A. (2003). Early predictors of posttraumatic stress disorder. *Biological Psychiatry, 53*(9), 789–795.

Burgess, A. W., & Holmstrom, L. L. (1974). Rape trauma syndrome. *American Journal of Psychiatry, 131*, 980–986.

Byrne, C. A., Resnick, H. S., Kilpatrick, D. G., Best, C. L., & Saunders, B. E. (1999). The socioeconomic impact of interpersonal violence on women. *Journal of Consulting and Clinical Psychology, 67*, 362–366.

Campbell, R., Sefl, T., & Ahrens, C. E. (2004). The impact of rape on women's sexual health risk behaviors. *Health Psychology, 23*(1), 67–74.

Carter, J. C., Bewell, C., Blackwell, E., & Woodside, D. B. (2006). The impact of childhood sexual abuse on anorexia nervosa. *Child Abuse & Neglect, 30*, 257–269.

Chen, L. P., Murad, H., Paras, M. L., Colbenson, K. M., Sattler, B. S., Goranson, E. N., … Zirakzadeh, A. (2010). Sexual abuse and lifetime diagnosis of psychiatric disorders: Systematic review and meta-analysis. *Mayo Clinic Proceedings, 85*, 618–629.

Cloitre, M., Miranda, R., Stovall-McClough, K. C., & Han, H. (2005). Beyond PTSD: Emotion regulation and interpersonal problems as predictors of functional impairment in survivors of childhood abuse. *Behavior Therapy, 36*, 119–124.

Cloitre, M., Scarvalone, P., & Difede, J. (1997). Posttraumatic stress disorder, self- and interpersonal dysfunction among sexually retraumatized women. *Journal of Traumatic Stress, 10*, 437–452.

Creamer, M., Burgess, P., & McFarlane, A. C. (2001). Post-traumatic stress disorder: Findings from the Australian National Survey of Mental Health and Well-being. *Psychological Medicine, 31*(7), 1237–1247.

Cuevas, K. M., Balbo, J., Duval, K., & Beverly, E. A. (2018). Neurobiology of sexual assault and osteopathic considerations for trauma-informed care and practice. *Journal of the American Osteopathic Association, 118*(2), e2–e10.

De Jong, J. T., Komproe, I. H., Van Ommeren, M., El Masri, M., Araya, M., Khaled, N., … Somasundaram, D. (2001). Lifetime events and posttraumatic stress disorder in 4 postconflict settings. *Journal of the American Medical Association, 286*(5), 555–562.

DeCou, C. R., Cole, T. T., Lynch, S. M., Wong, M. M., & Matthews, K. C. (2017). Assault-related shame mediates the association between negative social reactions to disclosure of sexual assault and psychological distress. *Psychological Trauma Theory Research Practice and Policy, 9*(2), 166–172.

DiLillo, D. (2001). Interpersonal functioning among women reporting a history of childhood sexual abuse: Empirical findings and methodological issues. *Clinical Psychology Review, 21*, 553–576.

Domhardt, M., Munzer, A., Fegert, J. M., & Goldbeck, L. (2015). Resilience in survivors of child sexual abuse: A systematic review of the literature. *Trauma, Violence & Abuse, 16*, 476–493.

Dunmore, E., Clark, D. M., & Ehlers, A. (1999). Cognitive factors involved in the onset and maintenance of posttraumatic stress disorder (PTSD) after physical or sexual assault. *Behaviour Research and Therapy, 37*, 809–829.

Dworkin, E. R., Menon, S. V., Bystrynski, J., & Allen, N. E. (2017). Sexual assault victimization and psychopathology: A review and meta-analysis. *Clinical Psychology Review, 56*, 65–81.

Ehring, T., & Quack, D. (2010). Emotion regulation difficulties in trauma survivors: The role of trauma type and PTSD symptom severity. *Behavior Therapy, 41*, 587–598.

Epstein, J. N., Saunders, B. E., Kilpatrick, D. G., & Resnick, H. S. (1998). PTSD as a mediator between childhood rape and alcohol use in adult women. *Child Abuse & Neglect, 22*, 223–234.

Feiring, C., & Taska, L. S. (2005). The persistence of shame following sexual abuse: A longitudinal look at risk and recovery. *Child Maltreatment, 10*(4), 337–349.

Frayne, S. M., Skinner, K. M., Sullivan, L. M., & Freund, K. M. (2003). Sexual assault while in the military: Violence as a predictor of cardiac risk? *Violence and Victims, 18*(2), 219–225.

Frazier, P., Conlon, A., & Glaser, T. (2001). Positive and negative life changes following sexual assault. *Journal of Consulting and Clinical Psychology, 69*(6), 1048–1055.

Galovski, T. E., Sobel., A. A., Phipps, K. A., Resick, P. A. (2005). Trauma recovery: Beyond posttraumatic stress disorder and other axis I symptom severity. In T. A. Corales (Ed.), *Trends in posttraumatic stress disorder research* (pp. 207-227). New York: Nova Science Publishers, Inc.

Gillig, P. M. (2009). Dissociative identity disorder: A controversial diagnosis. *Psychiatry, 6*, 24–29.

Golding, J. M. (1999). Sexual-assault history and long-term physical health problems: Evidence from clinical and population epidemiology. *Current Directions in Psychological Science, 8*(6), 191–194.

Goldmann, E., Aiello, A., Uddin, M., Delva, J., Koenen, K., Gant, L. M., & Galea, S. (2011). Pervasive exposure to violence and posttraumatic stress disorder in a predominantly African American Urban Community: The Detroit Neighborhood Health Study. *Journal of Traumatic Stress, 24*(6), 747–751.

Goyal, V., Mengeling, M. A., Booth, B. M., Torner, J. C., Syrop, C. H., & Sadler, A. G. (2017). Lifetime sexual assault and sexually transmitted infections among women veterans. *Journal of Women's Health, 26*(7), 745–754.

Grubaugh, A. L., & Resick, P. A. (2007). Posttraumatic growth in treatment-seeking female assault victims. *Psychiatric Quarterly, 78*(2), 145–155.

Gruebner, O., Sykora, M., Lowe, S. R., Shankardass, K., Trinquart, L., Jackson, T., … Galea, S. (2016). Mental health surveillance after the terrorist attacks in Paris. *The Lancet, 387*(10034), 2195–2196.

Hassija, C. M., & Turchik, J. A. (2016). An examination of disclosure, mental health treatment use, and posttraumatic growth among college women who experienced sexual victimization. *Journal of Loss and Trauma, 21*(2), 124–136.

Heim, C., Newport, D. J., Heit, S., Graham, Y. P., Wilcox, M., Bonsall, R., … Nemeroff, C. B. (2000). Pituitary-adrenal and autonomic responses to stress in women after sexual and physical abuse in childhood. *Journal of the American Medical Association, 284*(5), 592–597.

Hobfoll, S. E., Palmieri, P. A., Johnson, R. J., Canetti-Nisim, D., Hall, B. J., & Galea, S. (2009). Trajectories of resilience, resistance, and distress during ongoing terrorism: The case of Jews and Arabs in Israel. *Journal of Consulting and Clinical Psychology, 77*(1), 138–148.

Holzer, S. R., Uppala, S., Wonderlich, S. A., Crosby, R. D., & Simonich, H. (2008). Mediational significance of PTSD in the relationship of sexual trauma and eating disorders. *Child Abuse & Neglect, 32*, 561–566.

Humphreys, K. L., Sauder, C. L., Martin, E. K., & Marx, B. P. (2010). Tonic immobility in childhood sexual abuse survivors and its relationship to posttraumatic stress symptomatology. *Journal of Interpersonal Violence, 25*(2), 358–373.

Irish, L., Kobayashi, I., & Delahanty, D. L. (2010). Long-term physical health consequences of childhood sexual abuse: A meta-analytic review. *Journal of Pediatric Psychology, 35*(5), 450–461.

Jenkins, M. M., Colvonen, P. J., Norman, S. B., Afari, N., & Allard, C. B. (2015). Prevalence and mental health correlates of insomnia in first-encounter veterans with and without military sexual trauma. *Sleep, 38*(10), 1547–1554.

Kajeepeta, S., Gelaye, B., Jackson, C. L., & Williams, M. A. (2015). Adverse childhood experiences are associated with adult sleep disorders: A systematic review. *Sleep Medicine, 16*(3), 320–330.

Kaysen, D., Neighbors, C., Martell, J., Fossos, N., & Larimer, M. E. (2006). Incapacitated rape and alcohol use: A prospective analysis. *Addictive Behaviors, 31*, 1820–1832.

Kennedy, A. C., & Prock, K. A. (2016). "I still feel like I am not normal": A review of the role of stigma and stigmatization among female survivors of child sexual abuse, sexual assault, and intimate partner violence. *Trauma, Violence & Abuse*, 1–16.

Kessler, R. C. (1995). The national comorbidity survey: Preliminary results and future directions. *International Journal of Methods in Psychiatric Research, 5*(2), 139–151.

Kessler, R. C. (2000). Posttraumatic stress disorder: The burden to the individual and to society. *The Journal of Clinical Psychiatry, 61*(5), 4–14.

Kessler, R. C., Sonnega, A., Bromet, E., Hughes, M., & Nelson, C. B. (1995). Posttraumatic stress disorder in the National Comorbidity Survey. *Archives of General Psychiatry, 52*(12), 1048–1060.

Kilpatrick, D. G., Acierno, R., Resnick, H. S., Saunders, B. E., & Best, C. L. (1997). A 2-year longitudinal analysis of the relationships between violent assault and substance use in women. *Journal of Consulting and Clinical Psychology, 65*, 834–847.

Kintzle, S., Schuyler, A. C., Ray-Letourneau, D., Ozuna, S. M., Munch, C., Xintarianos, E., … Castro, C. A. (2015). Sexual trauma in the military: Exploring PTSD and mental health care utilization in female veterans. *Psychological Services, 12*(4), 394–401.

Krakow, B. J., Ulibarri, V. A., Moore, B. A., & McIver, N. D. (2015). Posttraumatic stress disorder and sleep-disordered breathing: A review of comorbidity research. *Sleep Medicine Reviews, 23*, 1–9.

Loftus, E. F. (1993). The reality of repressed memories. *American Psychologist, 48*, 518–537.

Lorenz, T. K., Harte, C. B., & Meston, C. M. (2015). Changes in sympathetic nervous system activity are associated with changes in sexual wellbeing in women with a history of childhood sexual abuse. *The Journal of Sexual Medicine, 12*(7), 1545–1554.

Lowe, S. R., Galea, S., Uddin, M., & Koenen, K. C. (2014). Trajectories of posttraumatic stress among urban residents. *American Journal of Community Psychology, 53*(1-2), 159–172.

McLean, L. M., & Gallop, R. (2003). Implications of childhood sexual abuse for adult borderline personality disorder and complex posttraumatic stress disorder. *American Journal of Psychiatry, 160*, 369–371.

Mengeling, M. A., Booth, B. M., Torner, J. C., & Sadler, A. G. (2015). Post-sexual assault health care utilization among OEF/OIF servicewomen. *Medical Care, 53*(4), S136–S142.

Miranda, R., Jr., Meyerson, L. A., Long, P. J., Marx, B. P., & Simpson, S. M. (2002). Sexual assault and alcohol use: Exploring the self-medication hypothesis. *Violence and Victims, 17*, 205–217.

Marchand, A., Nadeau, C., Beaulieu-Prévost, D., Boyer, R., & Martin, M. (2015). Predictors of posttraumatic stress disorder among police officers: A prospective study. *Psychological Trauma Theory Research Practice and Policy, 7*(3), 212–221.

Marx, B. P., & Soler-Baillo, J. M. (2008). The relationship among risk recognition, autonomic and self-reported arousal, and posttraumatic stress symptomatology in acknowledged and unacknowledged victims of sexual assault. *Psychosomatic Medicine, 67*, 618–624.

Noll, J. G., Trickett, P. K., Susman, E. J., & Putnam, F. W. (2006). Sleep disturbances and childhood sexual abuse. *Journal of Pediatric Psychology, 31*(5), 469–480.

Norris, F. H., Byrne, C. M., Diaz, E., & Kaniasty, K. (2007). *Risk factors for adverse outcomes in natural and human-caused disasters: A review of the empirical literature. A national center for PTSD fact sheet. National Center for PTSD, Department of Veterans Affairs.*

Norris, F. H., Stevens, S. P., Pfefferbaum, B., Wyche, K. F., & Pfefferbaum, R. L. (2008). Community resilience as a metaphor, theory, set of capacities, and strategy for disaster readiness. *American Journal of Community Psychology, 41*(1-2), 127–150.

O'Donnell, M. L., Creamer, M., & Pattison, P. (2004). Posttraumatic stress disorder and depression following trauma: Understanding comorbidity. *The American Journal of Psychiatry, 161*, 139–1396.

O'Donohue, W., Carlson, G. C., Benuto, L. T., & Bennett, N. M. (2014). Examining the scientific validity of rape trauma syndrome. *Psychiatry, Psychology and Law, 21*, 858–876.

Olff, M., Langeland, W., Draijer, N., & Gersons, B. P. (2007). Gender differences in posttraumatic stress disorder. *Psychological Bulletin, 133*(2), 183–204.

Orr, S. P., Lasko, N. B., Metzger, L. J., Berry, N. J., Ahern, C. E., & Pitman, R. K. (1998). Psychophysiologic assessment of women with posttraumatic stress disorder resulting from childhood sexual abuse. *Journal of Consulting and Clinical Psychology, 66*(6), 906–913.

Peace, K. A., Porter, S., & ten Brinke, L. (2008). Are memories for sexually traumatic events "special"? A

within-subjects investigation of trauma and memory in a clinical sample. *Memory, 16*, 10–21.
Resnick, H. S., Kilpatrick, D. G., Dansky, B. S., Saunders, B. E., & Best, C. L. (1993). Prevalence of civilian trauma and posttraumatic stress disorder in a representative national sample of women. *Journal of Consulting and Clinical Psychology, 61*(6), 984.
Riggs, D. S., Kilpatrick, D. G., & Resnick, H. S. (1992). Long-term psychological distress associated with marital rape and aggravated assault: A comparison to other crime victims. *Journal of Family Violence, 7*(4), 283–296.
Riggs, D. S., Rothbaum, B. O., & Foa, E. B. (1995). A prospective examination of symptoms of posttraumatic stress disorder in victims of nonsexual assault. *Journal of Interpersonal Violence, 10*, 201–214.
Romans, S. E., Gendall, K. A., Martin, J. L., & Mullen, P. E. (2001). Child sexual abuse and later disordered eating: A New Zealand epidemiological study. *International Journal of Eating Disorders, 29*, 380–392.
Rossellini, A. J., Street, A. E., Ursano, R. J., Chiu, W. T., Heeringa, S. G., Monahan, J., … Kessler, R. C. (2017). Sexual assault victimization and mental health treatment, suicide attempts and career outcomes among women in the US Army. *American Journal of Public Health, 107*, 732–739.
Rothbaum, B. O., Foa, E. B., Riggs, D. S., Murdock, T., & Walsh, W. (1992). A prospective examination of posttraumatic stress disorder in rape victims. *Journal of Traumatic Stress, 5*(3), 455–475.
Rothbaum, B. O., Kozak, M. J., Foa, E. B., & Whitaker, D. J. (2001). Posttraumatic stress disorder in rape victims: Autonomic habituation to auditory stimuli. *Journal of Traumatic Stress, 14*(2), 283–293.
Rydberg, J. A. (2017). Research and clinical issues in trauma and dissociation: Ethical and logical fallacies, myths, misreports, and misrepresentations. *European Journal of Trauma & Dissociation, 1*, 89–99.
Sabrina, C., & Ho, L. Y. (2014). Campus and college victim responses to sexual assault and dating violence: Disclosure, service utilization, and service provision. *Trauma, Violence & Abuse, 15*(3), 201–226.
Sarin, S., & Nolen-Hoeksema, S. (2010). The dangers of dwelling: An examination of the relationship between rumination and consumptive coping in survivors of childhood sexual abuse. *Cognition and Emotion, 24*, 71–85.
Schwarcz, S. K., & Whittington, W. L. (1990). Sexual assault and sexually transmitted diseases: Detection and management in adults and children. *Reviews of Infectious Diseases, 12*(6), S682–S690.
Soler-Baillo, J. M., Marx, B. P., & Sloan, D. M. (2005). The psychophysiological correlates of risk recognition among victims and non-victims of sexual assault. *Behaviour Research and Therapy, 43*, 169–181.
Steenkamp, M. M., Dickstein, B. D., Salters-Pedneault, K., Hofmann, S. G., & Litz, B. T. (2012). Trajectories of PTSD symptoms following sexual assault: Is resilience the modal outcome? *Journal of Traumatic Stress, 25*(4), 469–474.
Stein, D. J., Chiu, W. T., Hwang, I., Kessler, R. C., Sampson, N., Alonso, J., … Nock, M. K. (2010). Cross-national analysis of the associations between traumatic events and suicidal behavior: Findings for the WHO world mental health surveys. *PLoS One, 5*, 1–13.
Stein, M. B., & Barrett-Connor, E. (2000). Sexual assault and physical health: Findings from a population-based study of older adults. *Psychosomatic Medicine, 62*, 838–843.
Stein, M. B., Lang, A. J., Laffaye, C., Satz, L. E., Lenox, R. J., & Dresselhaus, T. R. (2004). Relationship of sexual assault history to somatic symptoms and health anxiety in women. *General Hospital Psychiatry, 26*, 178–183.
Stermac, L., Cabral, C. M., Clarke, A. K., & Toner, B. (2014). Mediators of posttraumatic mental health in sexual assault survivors. *Journal of Aggression, Maltreatment & Trauma, 23*(3), 301–317.
Tedeschi, R. G., & Calhoun, L. G. (1996). The Posttraumatic Growth Inventory: Measuring the positive legacy of trauma. *Journal of Traumatic Stress, 9*(3), 455–471.
Tolin, D. F., & Foa, E. B. (2006). Sex differences in trauma and posttraumatic stress disorder: A quantitative review of 25 years of research. *Psychological Bulletin, 132*(6), 959–992.
Turchik, J. A., & Hassija, C. M. (2014). Female sexual victimization among college students: Assault severity, health risk behaviors, and sexual functioning. *Journal of Interpersonal Violence, 29*(13), 2439–2457.
Ullman, S. E. (2004). Sexual assault victimization and suicidal behavior in women: A review of the literature. *Aggression and Violent Behavior, 9*, 331–351.
Ullman, S. E. (2014). Correlates of posttraumatic growth in adult sexual assault victims. *Traumatology, 20*(3), 219–224.
Ullman, S. E., & Najdowski, B. A. (2009). Correlates of serious suicidal ideation and attempts in female adult sexual assault survivors. *Suicide and Life-threatening Behavior, 39*, 47–57.
Ullman, S. E., Peter-Hagene, L. C., & Relyea, M. (2014). Coping, emotion regulation, and self-blame as mediators of sexual abuse and psychological symptoms in adult sexual assault. *Journal of Child Sexual Abuse, 23*(1), 1–16.
Ulloa, E., Guzman, M. L., Salazar, M., & Cala, C. (2016). Posttraumatic growth and sexual violence: A literature review. *Journal of Aggression, Maltreatment & Trauma, 25*(3), 286–304.
van Berlo, W., & Ensink, B. (2000). Problems with sexuality after sexual assault. *Annual Review of Sex Research, 11*, 235–257.
Walsh, K., DiLillo, D., & Scalora, M. J. (2011). The cumulative impact of sexual revictimization on emotion regulation difficulties: An examination of female inmates. *Violence Against Women, 17*(8), 1103–1118.

Walsh, K., Resnick, H. S., Danielson, C. K., McCauley, J. L., Saunders, B. E., & Kilpatrick, D. G. (2014). Patterns of drug and alcohol use associated with lifetime sexual revictimization and current posttraumatic stress disorder among three national samples of adolescent, college, and household-residing women. *Addictive Behaviors, 39*, 684–689.

Walsh, W. A., Banyard, V. L., Moynihan, M. M., Ward, S., & Cohn, E. S. (2010). Disclosure and service use on a college campus after an unwanted sexual experience. *Journal of Trauma & Dissociation, 11*(2), 134–151.

Wells, B. E., Starks, T. J., Robel, E., Kelly, B. C., Parsons, J. T., & Golub, S. A. (2016). From sexual assault to sexual risk: A relational pathway? *Journal of Interpersonal Violence, 31*(20), 3377–3395.

Willie, T. C., Overstreet, N. M., Peasant, C., Kershaw, T., Sikkema, K. J., & Hansen, N. B. (2016). Anxiety and depressive symptoms among people living with HIV and childhood sexual abuse: The role of shame and posttraumatic growth. *AIDS and Behavior, 20*(8), 1609–1620.

Wilson, D. R. (2010). Health consequences of childhood sexual abuse. *Perspectives in Psychiatric Care, 46*(1), 56–64.

Wolf, E. J., Lunney, C. A., Miller, M. W., Resick, P. A., Friedman, M. J., & Schnurr, P. P. (2012). The dissociative subtype of PTSD: A replication and extension. *Depression and Anxiety, 29*, 679–688.

Wonderlich, S. A., Crosby, R. D., Mitchell, J. E., Roberts, J. A., Haseltine, B., Demuth, G., & Thompson, K. M. (2000). Relationship of childhood sexual abuse and eating disturbance in children. *Journal of the American Academy of Child and Adolescent Psychiatry, 9*, 1277–1283.

Wonderlich, S. A., Wilsnack, R. W., Wilsnack, S. C., & Harris, T. R. (1996). The relationship of childhood sexual abuse and bulimic behavior: Results of a US national survey. *American Journal of Public Health, 86*, 1082–1086.

Zanarini, M. C. (Ed.). (1997). *Role of sexual abuse in etiology of borderline personality disorder*. Washington DC: American Psychiatric Press, Inc..

Understanding PTSD and Sexual Assault

17

Emily R. Dworkin, Heidi J. Ojalehto, Charlotte D. Brill, Skye Fitzpatrick, Michele A. Bedard-Gilligan, and Debra Kaysen

Posttraumatic stress disorder (PTSD) is one of the most common mental health consequences of sexual assault (SA) (Dworkin, Menon, Bystrynski, & Allen, 2017). In this chapter, we begin by introducing the diagnosis of PTSD and reviewing prominent theories regarding how PTSD develops after SA. Then, we discuss the prevalence of PTSD after SA and factors that may increase risk. After discussing best clinical practices for assessing and treating PTSD after SA, we conclude with future directions for research, policy, and practice.

What is PTSD?

According to the Diagnostic and Statistical Manual of Mental Disorders, fifth Edition (DSM-5), PTSD involves a set of symptoms that develop in the wake of exposure to specific qualifying events, including SA (American Psychiatric Association, 2013). DSM diagnostic criteria for PTSD includes four "clusters" of symptoms experienced in reaction to traumatic events. *Reexperiencing* symptoms involve persistently reliving the SA, including nightmares, flashbacks, and intrusive memories. *Avoidance* symptoms include avoidance of trauma-related stimuli, such as situations that remind the survivor of the SA, and SA-related emotions, thoughts, and memories. *Negative changes in mood or cognition* can involve persistent negative beliefs about oneself and the world, excessively blaming oneself or others for the SA or its aftermath, persistent negative emotions, and a lack of positive emotions. *Alterations in arousal and reactivity* symptoms include problems with irritability, hypervigilance, sleep, and concentration. Such symptoms are observed in most survivors in the first weeks after SA and are considered a natural reaction to trauma (Rothbaum, Foa, Riggs, Murdock, & Walsh, 1992). Their failure to resolve within 1 month is what characterizes a pathological trauma response.

The construct of PTSD was first applied to SA when researchers and clinicians recognized that a set of symptoms observed in SA survivors, then called "rape trauma syndrome" (Burgess & Holstrom, 1974), had similarities to conditions observed in survivors of other forms of trauma, such as combat, then called "shell shock" or "combat fatigue." These syndromes were

Manuscript preparation for this article was supported by National Institute of Alcohol Abuse and Alcoholism (NIAAA) Grants T32AA007455 (PI: Larimer) and K99AA026317 (PI: Dworkin). The views expressed in this article are those of the author and do not necessarily reflect the positions or policies of the University of Washington or the NIAAA.

E. R. Dworkin (✉) · H. J. Ojalehto · C. D. Brill
S. Fitzpatrick · M. A. Bedard-Gilligan · D. Kaysen
University of Washington School of Medicine, Seattle, WA, USA
e-mail: edworkin@uw.edu

W. T. O'Donohue and P. A. Schewe (eds.), *Handbook of Sexual Assault and Sexual Assault Prevention*,
https://doi.org/10.1007/978-3-030-23645-8_17

classified as a single condition, called PTSD, in 1980 in DSM-III (American Psychiatric Association, 1980). Aspects of the diagnosis have changed since that time over the various iterations of the DSM, including what specific symptoms are included and how trauma is defined. Generally, the newest iteration of the DSM has narrowed the scope of what is included as a traumatic event and has expanded both the number of symptoms and scope of symptoms to include a wider variety of emotion changes and a stronger emphasis on cognitive changes.

Several critiques have been levied against the diagnostic construct of PTSD. Feminist scholars argue that PTSD divorces survivors' psychological suffering from the patriarchal social context that facilitated the SA (Burstow, 2005; Gilfus, 1999; Wasco, 2003). For example, self-blame cognitions are framed as arising from the trauma itself, which is argued to ignore sociocultural norms that encourage survivors to blame themselves for victimization (Wasco, 2003). In addition, some argue that the accepted construction of PTSD may not account for distinct symptom presentations among marginalized groups (Wasco, 2003). For example, Latinx and Asian Americans appear to be more likely to express distress in somatic terms, and Latinx individuals with PTSD are more likely to report auditory hallucinations than members of other ethnic groups (Pole, Gone, & Kulkarni, 2008). Understanding the cross-cultural relevance of PTSD is thus an important task for future research. Finally, there is debate regarding whether exposure to repeated, prolonged, and severe stressors can produce a variant of PTSD, termed "complex PTSD," that involves symptoms such as somatic, affective, self-perceptual, attentional, and interpersonal dysfunction (Resick et al., 2012). Complex PTSD was considered for inclusion in both the DSM-IV and DSM-5, but empirical studies suggested that there was insufficient evidence to demonstrate that complex PTSD was a distinct phenomenon from PTSD. As a result, complex PTSD is not currently recognized as a diagnostic construct by the DSM.

In addition to critiques of the diagnosis of PTSD, there are critiques regarding the types of events that are considered by the DSM to be potentially traumatic, and therefore have the potential to elicit PTSD (Brewin, Lanius, Novac, Schnyder, & Galea, 2009). Qualifying traumas are termed "criterion A" events in the DSM. In DSM-5, criterion A stipulates that the trauma must involve "exposure to actual or threatened death, serious injury, or sexual violence," and the following examples are provided of sexual violence: "forced sexual penetration, alcohol/drug-facilitated sexual penetration, abusive sexual contact, noncontact sexual abuse, sexual trafficking." Criterion A further specifies that the event must have been experienced either (1) directly, (2) through observation, (3) by learning of its occurrence to a close family member or friend, or (4) through repeated exposure to trauma details (e.g., therapists hearing extensively about client's traumas; APA, 2013, pp. 271). The inclusion of the last two forms of trauma exposure is recent, and some scholars suggest that it has resulted in an overly inclusive PTSD diagnosis that includes individuals with highly distinct symptom profiles (McNally, 2003). Alternatively, many (especially feminist scholars) have asserted that criterion A's definition of trauma is too narrow. They argue that events that do not involve threatened death, serious injury, or overt sexual violence—such as systemic marginalization, street harassment, and sexual harassment (Avina & O'Donohue, 2002; Burstow, 2005; Wasco, 2003)—have traumatic potential, although a meta-analytic review suggests that the impact of such stressors is relatively smaller than criterion A traumas (Larsen & Pacella, 2016). Moreover, feminist scholars argue that the diagnostic criteria focus too narrowly on a single, discrete event and ignore threats to survivors' wellbeing that persist after the assault has ended (e.g., victim blaming; Burstow, 2005).

How Does PTSD Develop After Sexual Assault?

Although there are multiple theories that explain the etiology of PTSD following SA and other traumas, among the most prominent are emotional processing theory (Foa & Kozak,

1986) and social-cognitive theory (Resick & Schnicke, 1992).

Emotional Processing Theory

Foa and Kozak's (1986) emotional processing theory is the theoretical foundation of Prolonged Exposure (Foa & Rothbaum, 1998), an evidence-based PTSD treatment (e.g., Powers, Halpern, Ferenschak, Gillihan, & Foa, 2010) reviewed later in this chapter. This theory builds upon Lang's (1977, 1979) concept of "fear structures," which conceptualize fear as a memory network of information about (1) a feared situation (e.g., the SA); (2) verbal, bodily, and behavioral responses to the situation (e.g., heart rate increases, running away); and (3) the interpreted meaning of the situation and one's responses (e.g., "I am in danger"). Adaptive fear structures accurately reflect reality and act as a "program" to identify and respond to dangerous situations (e.g., escaping an assault).

The fear structures underlying PTSD are thought to be pathological because they are (1) activated by nonthreatening situations and stimuli; (2) elicit verbal, bodily, and behavioral fear responses that are disproportionate to the reality of the situation; and (3) include distorted or inaccurate meanings and interpretations of the situation and one's response to it. For example, after SA, a pathological fear structure may be activated by smells or sounds that remind a survivor of a perpetrator, even though the perpetrator is not there, which result in fear-network responses (e.g., heart rate increases, urges to escape a situation) although the survivor is not in danger. The fear structure may also involve distorted interpretations about the situation (e.g., "it is never safe to be in a bar"), or responses (e.g., "I cannot cope with being reminded of my assault") (Ehlers & Clark, 2000). Pathological fear structures are resistant to change because they lead individuals to avoid trauma-related thoughts and reminders. This avoidance prevents survivors from incorporating new information into the fear structure that could correct the inaccuracies (e.g., learning that one will not be sexually assaulted every time they are in a bar). This theory suggests that SA-related PTSD treatment should involve activating fear structures and integrating corrective and realistic information into it by approaching feared stimuli, as in Prolonged Exposure treatment for PTSD (Foa & Kozak, 1986).

Social-Cognitive Theory

Social-cognitive theory of PTSD emphasizes the content of trauma-related beliefs and their associated emotions (Janoff-Bulman & Frieze, 1983; Resick, Monson, & Chard, 2016). This theory underpins Cognitive Processing Therapy (Resick & Schnicke, 1992), another leading evidence-based treatment for PTSD reviewed later.

Social-cognitive theory emphasizes schemas, which are mental frameworks that allow individuals to organize information into categories to interpret their world and predict their future (Janoff-Bulman, 1989). Experiences like SA can result in information that does not "fit" with existing positive schemas and confirms negative schemas (Resick et al., 2016). For example, a common schema prior to trauma, called the "just world belief," reflects the idea that good things happen to good people, and bad things happen to bad people. These positive schemas are incompatible with new information from a SA (e.g., "a bad thing happened to me, even though I thought I was a good person"). Therefore, survivors may change their understanding of the trauma in unhelpful and inaccurate ways to fit it into their previously held schema (e.g., their belief may change to, "this bad thing happened to me because I am a bad person"). For individuals who held negative schemas, such as "the world is dangerous," the traumatic event may confirm these schemas, holding the prior unhelpful schemas intact (Resick et al., 2016). Individuals also may modify schemas with new information as a result of the assault. This modification, if it accurately incorporates the new learning from the assault without being extreme, facilitates recovery (e.g., their belief may change to, "sometimes bad things happen even to good people"). Other individuals may modify schemas in ways that become too rigid, inaccurate, and extreme. For example, rather than updating the schema of "bad things happen to bad people" to "bad things sometimes happen even to good people," some trauma survivors may instead believe "I am never safe from bad things even if I do the right thing all the time."

Also embedded in social-cognitive theory is the transaction between trauma-related beliefs and trauma-related emotions. The theory distinguishes between *natural emotions* that occur as a direct consequence of the assault, like fear or anger from an immediate life threat, and *manufactured emotions*, which come from inaccurate, unhelpful, or extreme beliefs (e.g., shame or guilt in response to beliefs such as "I am a bad person"). Natural emotions will decrease over time on their own if experienced and expressed, but manufactured emotions change only when beliefs change. Avoidance of trauma memories, emotions, and reminders prevents opportunities to correct the problematic beliefs and experience natural emotions, so treatment requires stopping avoidance and correcting problematic beliefs (Resick et al., 2016).

How Common and Severe is PTSD After Sexual Assault?

SA is associated with high rates of PTSD relative to other traumatic events (Brewin, Andrews, & Valentine, 2000; Dworkin, Menon, et al., 2017). Recent epidemiological research found that between a quarter and a third of women who have been raped meet full criteria for a current PTSD diagnosis (Kilpatrick, Resnick, Ruggiero, Conoscenti, & McCauley, 2007). Similarly, a recent meta-analysis identified that 26% of survivors of SA met diagnostic criteria for past-year PTSD as compared to 10% of people who had not (Dworkin, in press). SA is associated with more severe PTSD as well. In a comparison of symptom severity, a randomly selected person who had experienced SA had a 69% chance of having more severe PTSD symptoms than a randomly selected person without a SA history (Dworkin, Menon, et al., 2017).

Several prospective studies show that most survivors of SA have PTSD symptoms after SA, although overall symptoms decrease over time. When removing the criterion that symptoms endure for at least 1 month, 67–94% of SA survivors evidenced sufficient symptoms to warrant a PTSD diagnosis within the first month following the rape (Frazier, 2000; Frazier, Conlon, & Glaser, 2001; Gutner, Rizvi, Monson, & Resick, 2006; Rothbaum et al., 1992; Steenkamp et al., 2012). At 3 months post-SA, 42–78% met criteria (Darves-Bornoz, Degiovanni, & Gaillard, 1998; Frazier, 2000; Gutner et al., 2006; Rothbaum et al., 1992; Steenkamp et al., 2012; Ulirsch et al., 2013), and 48–58% met criteria for PTSD by 1 year (Darves-Bornoz et al., 1998; Frazier, 2000; Frazier et al., 2001).

What Factors Increase the Likelihood of Developing PTSD After Sexual Assault?

Substantial research has examined characteristics of assaults, SA survivors, and the contexts in which they recover to understand who is most likely to develop PTSD.

Assault Characteristics

A variety of assault characteristics have been associated with the likelihood of developing PTSD and other disorders, including whether assaults involve physical injury (Bownes, O'Gorman, & Sayers, 1991; Dworkin, Menon, et al., 2017; Möller, Bäckström, Söndergaard, & Helström, 2014), force or physical violence (Brown, Testa, & Messman-Moore, 2009; Peter-Hagene & Ullman, 2015; Ullman, Townsend, Filipas, & Starzynski, 2007; Zinzow et al., 2010), a perpetrator who is a stranger (Bownes et al., 1991; Ullman, Townsend, Starzynski, & Long, 2006) or a partner (Temple, Weston, Rodriguez, & Marshall, 2007; Ullman et al., 2006), more than one perpetrator (Möller et al., 2014), distress or perceived life threat (Elklit & Christiansen, 2013; Kaysen, Rosen, Bowman, & Resick, 2010;

Ullman, Filipas, Townsend, & Starzynski, 2007), having a "freeze response" (Bovin, Jager-Hyman, Gold, Marx, & Sloan, 2008; Rizvi, Kaysen, Gutner, Griffin, & Resick, 2008; Rocha-Rego et al., 2009), and weapon use (Bownes et al., 1991; Dworkin, Menon, et al., 2017). SAs involving different types of tactics, like force, coercion, and incapacitation, do not appear to differ substantially in terms of their risk for PTSD. Varying the definition of SA to include coerced and incapacitated SA as well as completed forced SA did not significantly alter the observed relationship with psychopathology when comparing sexually assaulted to unassaulted samples in a meta-analysis (Dworkin, Menon, et al., 2017). Including attempted SAs along with completed SAs decreased the effect size of the relationship with psychopathology in this meta-analysis, but it remained statistically significant, suggesting that noncompleted SA also can lead to psychopathology. As the authors noted, conclusions that can be drawn are somewhat limited as the research is based solely on study definitions of SA. Still, these findings are compelling in suggesting that SA is highly predictive of PTSD and other forms of psychopathology, regardless of the tactics used. Of note, individual studies that have looked at severity of assault as a predictor of PTSD generally show that higher severity SAs are related to increased PTSD (Pegram & Abbey, 2016; Peter-Hagene & Ullman, 2015; Resnick et al., 1993; Ullman & Filipas, 2001). However, one study demonstrated that alcohol-involved assaults evidenced as strong a relationship with PTSD as forcible assaults over a longer-term follow-up (Peter-Hagene & Ullman, 2015), which is consistent with an epidemiological study that found PTSD associated with both forcible and incapacitated SA (Zinzow et al., 2010). Thus, the relationship between assault severity and PTSD is likely complicated by varied definitions of SA and associated individual and situational factors.

Characteristics of Survivors

Demographic factors have been explored in relation to risk of developing PTSD after SA. Across all trauma types, women are more likely to develop PTSD than men, but there do not appear to be gender differences after SA specifically. Similarly, although racial differences have been found for PTSD prevalence (Roberts, Gilman, Breslau, Breslau, & Koenen, 2011), reviews have not found racial differences in PTSD following SA (Campbell, Dworkin, & Cabral, 2009; Dworkin, Menon, et al., 2017). It is possible that the higher likelihood of developing PTSD after SA versus other forms of trauma reduces observed racial differences. With regard to sexual orientation, higher rates of PTSD have been observed among sexual minority individuals (Balsam, Rothblum, & Beauchaine, 2005; Rothman, Exner, & Baughman, 2011), but no studies to our knowledge have looked at sexual orientation as a predictor of PTSD after SA specifically. Finally, younger age predicts increased PTSD severity in assault victims, as does a history of childhood sexual abuse (CSA; Ullman, Filipas, et al., 2007; Ullman, Najdowski, & Filipas, 2009). One large study of 1769 women in the US showed increased PTSD prevalence in women assaulted before age 18 (35.3%) compared to those assaulted after 18 (30.2%; Masho & Ahmed, 2007). Experiencing multiple SAs over the lifespan also predicts PTSD severity (Ullman, 2016). Consistent with these findings, in two large meta-analyses, experiencing trauma at a younger age was a significant predictor of increased likelihood of developing PTSD (Brewin et al., 2000; Ozer, Best, Lipsey, & Weiss, 2003).

Genetic and biological factors have been proposed as determinants for post-SA adjustment including PTSD, although to our knowledge, no studies have looked specifically at genetic determinants of PTSD following SA. Results of twin and large-scale genome-wide association studies do suggest that heritability may play a significant role in the development of PTSD following trauma, particularly for women (see Yehuda et al., 2015 for a review). The hypothalamic pituitary adrenal axis and sympathetic nervous system are implicated in the stress response that occurs following trauma, and thus stress hormones (e.g., cortisol) may be affected by SA and influence the development of PTSD (Zoladz & Diamond, 2013). Studies on cortisol levels following SA show mixed findings in relationship to predicting PTSD, with some studies finding elevated cortisol levels to be related to PTSD (Resnick, Yehuda, & Acierno, 1997) and other studies finding cortisol levels to be unrelated to PTSD in those exposed to SA (Resnick, Yehuda, Pitman, & Foy, 1995). A recent review proposed the posttrauma administration of pharmacological interventions that target systems related to cortisol (e.g., glucocorticoid receptor agonists, oxytocin) to prevent PTSD (van Zuiden, Kavelaars, Geuze, Olff, & Heijnen, 2013). Others point out that ovarian hormones may influence emotional memory processing and, potentially, partially account for gender differences in PTSD (Zoladz & Diamond, 2013).

Psychophysiological indicators have also been explored as possible indicators of who is likely to develop PTSD following trauma. No psychophysiological studies to our knowledge have focused specifically on participants exposed to SA, but two studies of survivors of primarily physical assaults show that this may be an important area of exploration. Individuals with higher resting heart rate 2 weeks after assault were more likely to develop PTSD at 6 months post assault, although the observed effect size was small (Kleim, Ehlers, & Glucksman, 2007). Women with increased heart rate reactivity to assault imagery at 2 weeks post-assault were significantly more likely to develop PTSD compared to men and to women without high heart rate reactivity (Kleim, Wilhelm, Glucksman, & Ehlers, 2010). This indicates that physiological reactivity to trauma reminders—which is a symptom of PTSD if it endures for more than 1 month—may be an early indicator of the likelihood that trauma symptoms will naturally remit. A large meta-analysis on psychophysiology and PTSD showed that presence of PTSD following trauma exposure more broadly was associated with diverse psychophysiological reactions, including elevated heart rate and skin conductance at rest and in response to startle probe tasks and trauma cues (Pole, 2007).

The types of coping strategies used by survivors appear to alter the risk of PTSD following SA. Maladaptive coping strategies, typically defined as those that involve avoidance instead of approach strategies (e.g., substance use, isolation, avoidance of thoughts or feelings related to the SA, avoidance of reminders of the SA, withdrawal from social support) predict higher PTSD symptoms in SA survivors (Frazier, Mortensen, & Steward, 2005; Gutner et al., 2006; Read et al., 2013; Ullman, Relyea, Peter-Hagene, & Vasquez, 2013; Ullman, Townsend, et al., 2007). In contrast, adaptive coping strategies, such as problem-focused coping and seeking social support, have been associated with lower PTSD symptoms in survivors of SA (Frazier et al., 2005; Gutner et al., 2006; Valentiner, Foa, Riggs, & Gershuny, 1996). The context in which a coping strategy is employed may be important in determining its relationship with PTSD. For example, among college women who experienced SA, the positive effects of social support on PTSD symptoms were lower for women who were using substances to cope (Dworkin, Ojalehto, Bedard-Gilligan, Cadigan, & Kaysen, 2018). This suggests that coping strategies should not be considered in isolation.

Contextual Factors

SA occurs within a multilevel social context that influences recovery (Campbell et al., 2009). On a societal level, it is clear that there is significant stigma associated with SA, as evidenced by the pervasiveness of rape myths (e.g., the beliefs that victims are to blame for the assault and that victims lie about being sexually assaulted; Deitz, Williams, Rife, & Cantrell, 2015; Edwards, Turchik, Dardis, Reynolds, & Gidycz, 2011) and victim blaming in response to SA disclosure (Ullman, 2010). These social-context-related factors may increase self-blame and ultimately affect survivors' post-assault mental health, including PTSD (Kennedy & Prock, 2018). Indeed, most SA survivors (80% or more) choose to disclose to at least one person (Ahrens, Campbell, Ternier-Thames, Wasco, & Sefl, 2007) and often receive negative social reactions (e.g., victim blaming, taking control of survivors' decision-making, disbelief), which are associated with psychopathology (Dworkin, Brill, & Ullman, 2019; Littleton, 2010; Ullman & Peter-Hagene, 2014; Ullman, Starzynski, Long, Mason, & Long, 2008; Ullman, Townsend, et al., 2007). Preliminary evidence also suggests that SA survivors in more stigmatizing contexts, regardless of whether they disclose, have worse mental health (Dworkin, Sessarego, Pittenger, Edwards, & Banyard, 2017). The detrimental effects of stigma on survivors' current distress and trajectories of recovery are robust and warrant further research into effective interventions following SA.

What Are the Best Clinical Practices for Addressing Sexual Assault-Related PTSD?

In the past 30 years, substantial research has focused on developing effective strategies to assess, treat, and prevent the development of PTSD. We review this work next.

Assessment of Trauma Exposure and Psychopathology

It is important to assess trauma exposure broadly, rather than SA history alone, in order to create a comprehensive picture of the client's trauma history. One challenge is selecting between longer, more thorough measures of SA that use behaviorally specific definitions of traumatic events, such as the Sexual Experiences Survey (Koss et al., 2007), which are thought to more accurately capture SA exposure as compared to briefer measures which use only terms such as "rape" (Cook, Gidycz, Koss, & Murphy, 2011). There are several commonly used brief measures of broader trauma exposure, including the trauma history portion of the Posttraumatic Diagnostic Scale (Foa, Cashman, Jaycox, & Perry, 1997) and the Life Events Checklist (Weathers et al., 2013).

It is also important to systematically assess PTSD through the use of validated psychological assessments (Briere & Jordan, 2004). This can include clinical interviews like the Clinician-Administered PTSD Scale (Blake et al., 1995), or self-report measures like the Primary Care-PTSD Screen (Prins et al., 2003) or the Posttraumatic Checklist for DSM-5 (Weathers et al., 2013). These PTSD measures must be asked in reference to a specific trauma. It is important to not solely assess PTSD, though, as SA can be associated with other psychological symptoms such as depression and anxiety (Dworkin, Menon, et al., 2017).

Treating PTSD Related to Sexual Assault

The treatment of PTSD has been significantly influenced by the adoption and implementation of evidence-based practices, defined by the American Psychological Association (APA) as, "the integration of the best available research with clinical expertise in the context of patient characteristics, culture, and preferences" (APA Presidential Task Force on Evidence-Based Practice, 2006, p. 273). Based on substantial research, only cognitive behavioral therapies (CBTs) with an explicit trauma focus received strong recommendations as evidence-based practices for PTSD by the APA (APA, 2017), meaning that the treatments have been rigorously tested by independent investigators with a preponderance of studies agreeing that the treatment is efficacious (Chambless & Hollon, 1998). Broadly speaking, CBTs include cognitive components like *cognitive restructuring* (i.e., identifying and changing rigid or inaccurate beliefs) and/or behavioral components like *exposure* (i.e., systematically confronting feared and/or avoided stimuli until fear is extinguished). All major clinical practice guidelines currently recommend trauma-focused CBTs as a first-line treatment for PTSD (see Forbes et al., 2010 for a review of guidelines). A report by the Institute of Medicine (IOM), which is considered the most rigorous of the current published treatment guidelines for PTSD (Forbes et al., 2010), concluded that only exposure therapies and Cognitive Processing

Therapy specifically met the designation of "efficacious," and that other psychotherapies (e.g., eye movement desensitization and reprocessing) and pharmacotherapies (e.g., SSRIs, benzodiazapines) had insufficient evidence to determine efficacy (IOM, 2007). Meta-analyses of randomized controlled trials assessing PTSD treatments found large effect sizes for improvements in PTSD symptoms in CBTs relative to control groups, and medium effects for pharmacotherapy (Bradley, Greene, Russ, Dutra, & Westen, 2005; Watts et al., 2013). Of individuals receiving exposure therapy, 90% improved more than individuals on a waitlist, and 79% improved more than individuals receiving supportive counseling. Of those receiving combined exposure and cognitive restructuring, 93% improved more than individuals receiving no treatment, and 84% improved more than those receiving supportive counseling. This indicates that it is especially important to ensure that SA survivors with PTSD have access to trauma-focused CBTs as treatment options. Next, we describe two commonly used trauma-focused CBT treatments for PTSD—Cognitive Processing Therapy and Prolonged Exposure—both of which were developed for use with female rape victims and have an extensive evidence base for their efficacy in treating PTSD. Then, we review other treatment options.

Prolonged Exposure

Prolonged Exposure is a well-validated treatment for PTSD (Foa, Rothbaum, Riggs, & Murdock, 1991). It utilizes two forms of exposure—in vivo exposure and imaginal exposure—over 8 to 15 sessions. Through *in vivo exposure*, clients construct a list of feared or avoided, but objectively safe, stimuli that are gradually approached throughout the course of treatment. For example, a SA survivor who was assaulted at a party may avoid all parties thereafter due to the expectation that parties are dangerous or reminders of the original SA cued by the party; a natural in vivo exposure for such a client would be to attend a safe party. By approaching these situations, clients learn that the feared consequence is unlikely to happen and that they can tolerate the distress associated with the situation. Clients usually stay in exposure situations until distress decreases by at least half, or for an agreed-upon amount of time (e.g., 30 min), to allow time for new learning (i.e., that the feared situation is not actually dangerous) to occur. Through *imaginal exposure*, clients repeatedly recount the trauma memory aloud in session to the therapist for 30–45 min. Following imaginal exposure, therapists guide clients in processing their emotions and cognitions related to the traumatic event in order to promote new learning, ability to tolerate distress, and extinction of emotional responses. In a meta-analysis, Prolonged Exposure was highly effective in reducing PTSD; 86% of those receiving Prolonged Exposure experienced greater reductions in PTSD symptoms than those in a control condition (Powers et al., 2010). Prolonged Exposure was equally effective in treating SA-related PTSD as compared to PTSD due to other traumas, and treatment effects remained in follow-up assessments up to 10 years later (Resick, Williams, Suvak, Monson, & Gradus, 2012).

Cognitive Processing Therapy

Cognitive Processing Therapy is a well-validated treatment for PTSD following many kinds of trauma, including SA (Resick et al., 2016; Resick & Schnicke, 1992). It is typically delivered in 12 sessions, and involves cognitive restructuring (i.e., identifying and modifying maladaptive thoughts to develop more balanced, flexible, and adaptive beliefs) and emotional processing of trauma-related content. Initially, sessions focus on cognitive restructuring of beliefs about the traumatic event, such as self-blame or hindsight bias (e.g., "It was all my fault," "I should have prevented the assault"). Cognitive restructuring then targets beliefs about the self and others that are the result of a traumatic event in five key areas: safety (e.g., "the world is dangerous"), trust (e.g., "I can never trust anyone"), power (e.g., "I am helpless"), esteem (e.g., "all people are evil"), and intimacy (e.g., "I can't get close to other people"). Randomized clinical trials conducted with different trauma-exposed populations, including survivors of SA, show that Cognitive Processing Therapy is effective in treating PTSD and depression (Bass et al., 2013; Chard, 2005; Resick, Nishith, Weaver, Astin, & Feuer, 2002; Surís, Link-Malcolm, Chard, Ahn, & North, 2013). In these trials, effects largely endured 5 to 10 years later (Resick, Williams, et al., 2012).

Other Psychological Treatments

Several other treatments have some evidence for their effectiveness in treating PTSD. First, eye-movement desensitization and reprocessing therapy (EMDR) is a common treatment for PTSD that shows similar effects to trauma-focused CBT in research studies (Watts et al., 2013), although the quality of evidence is somewhat less strong than for CBT (IOM, 2007). EMDR involves in-session recall of the traumatic memory (as in imaginal exposure) while focusing on an external stimulus (commonly, therapist-directed lateral eye movements). The focus on an external stimulus that defines EMDR is considered by its creators to be an active ingredient of the treatment, but the absence of theoretical or empirical support for the additive benefit of this portion of the treatment (Seidler & Wagner, 2006) has led to criticisms that EMDR is a variant of exposure therapy (Rosen & Davison, 2003). Moreover, concerns have been raised about treatment fidelity in practice (Rosen, 1999), given the emphasis placed on eye movements as the active ingredient rather than exposure. As a result, the APA gave EMDR a second-strength rating, and the Australian clinical practice guidelines recommended EMDR only when in vivo exposure is additionally included (Ironson, Freund, Strauss, & Williams, 2002). Second, Narrative Exposure Therapy (NET) is an exposure-based treatment adapted from Prolonged Exposure therapy and testimony therapy that has a growing evidence base supporting its efficacy (see Robjant & Fazel, 2010 for a review). In NET, the client constructs a narrative of their life from childhood through the present moment, including traumatic events. The therapist then goes back and processes the details of those traumatic events as exposure. NET is proposed to work through habituation and through creating an integrated autobiographic memory. The APA has given NET a second strength rating, whereas other practice guidelines, like the Australian practice guidelines, group NET in with other trauma-focused CBTs. There are currently no trials of NET specifically focusing on SA survivors. Other treatments, such as Acceptance and Commitment Therapy (ACT) and mindfulness-based therapies, show initial promise in reducing PTSD in case studies and small, pilot trials (Kearney, McDermott, Malte, Martinez, & Simpson, 2013; Orsillo & Batten, 2005) but have not yet been tested in large-scale randomized controlled trials.

Preventing PTSD Related to Sexual Assault

Increasingly, efforts have been made to intervene in the aftermath of trauma exposure to prevent the development of PTSD. One type of early intervention, critical incident stress debriefing (Mitchell, 1983), involves a single psychological debriefing session for a group of trauma survivors and is typically provided 1–10 days after trauma exposure. Despite its widespread use, several meta-analyses have found that critical incident stress debriefing and other forms of psychological debriefing are ineffective in preventing PTSD and may even increase the risk of developing PTSD, perhaps by interfering with a survivor's natural recovery process (Rose, Bisson, Churchill, & Wessely, 2002; van Emmerik, Kamphuis, Hulsbosch, & Emmelkamp, 2002). Similarly, the positive-psychology-based Comprehensive Soldier Fitness program (Cornum, Matthews, & Seligman, 2011), which provides soldiers with resiliency training to buffer against the negative effects of trauma exposure, does not have empirical evidence for its efficacy (Eidelson & Soldz, 2012). However, other interventions have had more promising effects, including with SA survivors. In a review, a brief form of CBT reduced PTSD severity among individuals with acute stress disorder (Forneris et al., 2013). Similarly, a small randomized controlled trial of a video intervention that taught CBT-based strategies to SA survivors receiving a forensic medical exam was associated with significantly lower PTSD symptoms compared to treatment as usual among women who had a prior SA history (Resnick et al., 2007). A qualitative review on reducing PTSD after SA via early intervention found that perceptions of the helpfulness of early contact with responders was associated with lower PTSD severity (Dworkin & Schumacher, 2018).

Future Directions

There are several gaps in extant literature regarding the impact of SA on PTSD and how PTSD can be most effectively treated in this population. First, there is a need for longitudinal research with at-risk populations (e.g., military recruits) to understand the effects of risk factors measured before SA (e.g., personality traits, mental disorders, other traumatic life experiences) on the likelihood of developing PTSD and its trajectory. Such research could improve the ability to predict risk for PTSD. Second, more focus is needed on under-researched populations. There is a tremendous need for research on the experiences of male survivors and for members of historically marginalized groups (e.g., sexual minority populations, people of color). This work is critical to understand how the unique processes that affect these groups (e.g., stigma) interact with PTSD risk and recovery, and to inform tailored treatments for them. Third, to reduce the degree to which survivors of SA develop PTSD, early interventions delivered soon after SA should be tested and refined. Finally, given that characteristics of survivors' social contexts (e.g., social reactions to disclosure) may affect PTSD symptoms, it is important to continue to search for contextual variables that could impact symptoms.

There are also several important priorities for intervention efforts and policy to support these efforts. Given that cognitive behavioral therapies with a focus on the traumatic event have strong research evidence regarding their ability to treat PTSD and are able to do so in a short-term (e.g., 12-week) manner, it is important that these interventions be made broadly available to survivors as a first-line option. However, the vast majority of therapists and rape crisis centers do not offer these treatments, and instead commonly offer treatments of unknown efficacy (Foa, Gillihan, & Bryant, 2013), which limits survivor choice and autonomy. To address this gap between research and practice, it is critical that service providers be trained in delivering these treatments. Additionally, service provider misconceptions about these treatments that get in the way of offering such treatments should be addressed (Cook, Schnurr, & Foa, 2004; Shafran et al., 2009). From a policy perspective, increasing funding for dissemination and implementation of these treatments, including in non-US settings, is important. It is also apparent that survivors face many barriers in accessing effective treatments, including lack of access to therapists, financial barriers, and lack of knowledge about effective treatment options (Gunter & Whittal, 2010). Making treatments available via technology (e.g., apps) and remote delivery (e.g., telehealth), and addressing policy issues such as reimbursement for telepsychology and increasing health literacy, could increase access to care. Healthcare reform is also an important part of removing financial barriers to treatment access. Further, interventions that prevent PTSD are needed. PTSD prevention efforts should focus on reducing changeable risk factors, such as maladaptive coping strategies, and building protective factors. Immutable risk factors (e.g., survivor characteristics) could be used to identify individuals in need of early intervention. Efforts should also be made to improve the degree to which contexts promote recovery. This could include efforts to improve social responses to SA, by, for example, training likely disclosure recipients (e.g., college students, police officers) in avoiding negative social reactions. More broadly, social movements that aim to reduce societal stigma are a critical component of improving the climate for SA survivors.

Conclusion

It is clear that PTSD is common among SA survivors. Although there are many known risk factors for PTSD, many have yet to be identified, and intervention efforts have largely focused on treating PTSD after it has already developed rather than reducing risk factors directly. Further, although effective treatments exist, they are not widely available. As a result, there is much work left to be done to reduce the degree to which survivors of SA suffer from PTSD.

References

Ahrens, C. E., Campbell, R., Ternier-Thames, N. K., Wasco, S. M., & Sefl, T. (2007). Deciding whom to tell: Expectations and outcomes of rape survivors' first disclosures. *Psychology of Women Quarterly, 31*, 38–49.

American Psychiatric Association. (1980). *Diagnostic and statistical manual of mental disorders: DSM-III*. Washington, DC: Author.

American Psychiatric Association. (2013). *Diagnostic and statistical manual of mental disorders* (5th ed.). Washington, DC: Author.

American Psychological Association. (2017). *Clinical practice guideline for the treatment of posttraumatic stress disorder (PTSD) in adults*. Washington, DC: APA, Guideline Development Panel for the Treatment of Posttraumatic Stress Disorder in Adults.

APA Presidential Task Force on Evidence-Based Practice. (2006). Evidence-based practice in psychology. *American Psychologist, 61*(4), 271–285.

Avina, C., & O'Donohue, W. (2002). Sexual harassment and PTSD: Is sexual harrassment diagnosable trauma? *Journal of Traumatic Stress, 15*, 69–75.

Balsam, K. F., Rothblum, E. D., & Beauchaine, T. P. (2005). Victimization over the life span: A comparison of lesbian, gay, bisexual, and heterosexual siblings. *Journal of Consulting and Clinical Psychology, 73*, 477.

Bass, J. K., Annan, J., McIvor Murray, S., Kaysen, D., Griffiths, S., Cetinoglu, T., … Bolton, P. A. (2013). Controlled trial of psychotherapy for Congolese survivors of sexual violence. *New England Journal of Medicine, 368*, 2182–2191.

Blake, D. D., Weathers, F. W., Nagy, L. M., Kaloupek, D. G., Gusman, F. D., Charney, D. S., & Keane, T. M. (1995). The development of a Clinician-Administered PTSD Scale. *Journal of Traumatic Stress, 8*, 75–90.

Bovin, M. J., Jager-Hyman, S., Gold, S. D., Marx, B. P., & Sloan, D. M. (2008). Tonic immobility mediates the influence of peritraumatic fear and perceived inescapability on posttraumatic stress symptom severity among sexual assault survivors. *Journal of Traumatic Stress, 21*, 402–409.

Bownes, I. T., O'Gorman, E. C., & Sayers, A. (1991). Assault characteristics and posttraumatic stress disorder in rape victims. *Acta Psychiatrica Scandinavica, 83*, 27–30.

Bradley, R., Greene, J., Russ, E., Dutra, L., & Westen, D. (2005). A multidimensional meta-analysis of psychotherapy for PTSD. *American Journal of Psychiatry, 162*, 214–227.

Brewin, C. R., Andrews, B., & Valentine, J. D. (2000). Meta-analysis of risk factors for posttraumatic stress disorder in trauma-exposed adults. *Journal of Consulting and Clinical Psychology, 68*, 748–766.

Brewin, C. R., Lanius, R. A., Novac, A., Schnyder, U., & Galea, S. (2009). Reformulating PTSD for DSM-V: Life after criterion A. *Journal of Traumatic Stress, 22*, 366–373.

Briere, J., & Jordan, C. E. (2004). Violence against women: Outcome complexity and implications for assessment and treatment. *Journal of Interpersonal Violence, 19*, 1252–1276.

Brown, A. L., Testa, M., & Messman-Moore, T. L. (2009). Psychological consequences of sexual victimization resulting from force, incapacitation, or verbal coercion. *Violence Against Women, 15*, 898–919.

Burgess, A. W., & Holstrom, L. L. (1974). Rape trauma syndrome. *The American Journal of Psychiatry, 131*, 981–986.

Burstow, B. (2005). A critique of posttraumatic stress disorder and the DSM. *Journal of Humanistic Psychology, 45*, 429–445.

Campbell, R., Dworkin, E. R., & Cabral, G. (2009). An ecological model of the impact of sexual assault on women's mental health. *Trauma, Violence & Abuse, 10*, 225–246.

Chambless, D. L., & Hollon, S. D. (1998). Defining empirically supported therapies. *Journal of Cconsulting and Clinical Psychology, 66*, 7–18.

Chard, K. M. (2005). An evaluation of cognitive processing therapy for the treatment of posttraumatic stress disorder related to childhood sexual abuse. *Journal of Consulting and Clinical Psychology, 73*, 965–971.

Cook, J. M., Schnurr, P. P., & Foa, E. B. (2004). Bridging the gap between posttraumatic stress disorder research and clinical practice: The example of exposure therapy. *Psychotherapy: Theory, Research, Practice, Training, 41*(4), 374.

Cook, S. L., Gidycz, C. A., Koss, M. P., & Murphy, M. (2011). Emerging issues in the measurement of rape victimization. *Violence Against Women, 17*, 201–218.

Cornum, R., Matthews, M. D., & Seligman, M. E. P. (2011). Comprehensive Soldier Fitness: Building resilience in a challenging institutional context. *American Psychologist, 66*(1), 4–9. https://doi.org/10.1037/a0021420

Darves-Bornoz, J. M., Degiovanni, A., & Gaillard, P. (1998). Predictive factors of chronic post-traumatic stress disorder in rape victims. *European Psychiatry, 13*, 281–287.

Deitz, M. F., Williams, S. L., Rife, S. C., & Cantrell, P. (2015). Examining cultural, social, and self-related aspects of stigma in relation to sexual assault and trauma symptoms. *Violence Against Women, 21*, 598–615.

Dworkin, E. R. (in press). The prevalence of mental disorders in sexually assaulted versus unassaulted samples: A systematic review and meta-analysis. *Trauma, Violence and Abuse*.

Dworkin, E. R., Menon, S. V., Bystrynski, J., & Allen, N. E. (2017). Sexual assault victimization and psychopathology: A review and meta-analysis. *Clinical Psychology Review, 56*, 65–81.

Dworkin, E. R., Ojalehto, H., Bedard-Gilligan, M., Cadigan, J., & Kaysen, D. (2018). Social support predicts reductions in PTSD symptoms when substances are not used to cope: A longitudinal study of sexual assault survivors. *Journal of Affective Disorders, 229*, 135–140.

Dworkin, E. R., & Schumacher, J. A. (2018). Preventing posttraumatic stress related to sexual assault through early intervention: A systematic review. *Trauma, Violence & Abuse, 19*(4), 459–472.

Dworkin, E. R., Sessarego, S. N., Pittenger, S. L., Edwards, K. M., & Banyard, V. L. (2017). Rape myth acceptance in sexually assaulted adolescents' school contexts: Associations with depressed mood and alcohol use. *American Journal of Community Psychology, 60*, 516–526.

Dworkin, E. R., Brill, C. D., & Ullman, S. E. (2019). Social reactions to disclosure of interpersonal violence and psychopathology: A systematic review and meta-analysis. *Clinical Psychology Review, 72*, 101750.

Edwards, K. M., Turchik, J. A., Dardis, C. M., Reynolds, N., & Gidycz, C. A. (2011). Rape myths: History, individual and instiutional-level presence, and implications for change. *Sex Roles, 65*, 761–773.

Ehlers, A., & Clark, D. M. (2000). A cognitive model of posttraumatic stress disorder. *Behaviour Research and Therapy, 38*, 319–345.

Eidelson, R., & Soldz, S. (2012). *Does Comprehensive Soldier Fitness work? Research fails the test.* Retrieved from http://www.ethicalpsychology.org/Eidelson-&-Soldz-CSF_Research_Fails_the_Test.pdf

Elklit, A., & Christiansen, D. M. (2013). Risk factors for posttraumatic stress disorder in female help-seeking victims of sexual assault. *Violence and Victims, 28*, 552–568.

Foa, E., Cashman, L., Jaycox, L., & Perry, K. (1997). The validation of a self-report measure of PTSD: The Posttraumatic Diagnostic Scale. *Psychological Assessment, 9*, 445–451.

Foa, E. B., Gillihan, S. J., & Bryant, R. A. (2013). Challenges and successes in dissemination of evidence-based treatments for posttraumatic stress: Lessons learned from prolonged exposure therapy for PTSD. *Psychological Science in the Public Interest, 14*, 65–111.

Foa, E. B., & Kozak, M. J. (1986). Emotional processing of fear: Exposure to corrective information. *Psychological Bulletin, 99*, 20–35.

Foa, E. B., & Rothbaum, B. O. (1998). *Treating the trauma of rape: Cognitive– behavioral therapy for PTSD*. New York: Guilford Press.

Foa, E. B., Rothbaum, B. O., Riggs, D. S., & Murdock, T. B. (1991). Treatment of posttraumatic stress disorder in rape victims: A comparison between cognitive-behavioral procedures and counseling. *Journal of Consulting and Clinical Psychology, 59*, 715–723.

Forbes, D., Creamer, M., Bisson, J. I., Cohen, J. A., Crow, B. E., Foa, E. B., ... Ursano, R. J. (2010). A guide to guidelines for the treatment of PTSD and related conditions. *Journal of Traumatic Stress, 23*(5), 537–552.

Forneris, C. A., Gartlehner, G., Brownley, K. A., Gaynes, B. N., Sonis, J., Coker-Schwimmer, E., ... Lohr, K. N. (2013). Interventions to prevent post-traumatic stress disorder: A systematic review. *American Journal of Preventive Medicine, 44*, 635–650.

Frazier, P. A. (2000). The role of attributions and perceived control in recovery from rape. *Journal of Personal and Interpersonal Loss, 5*, 203–225.

Frazier, P. A., Conlon, A., & Glaser, T. (2001). Positive and negative life changes following sexual assault. *Journal of Consulting and Clinical Psychology, 69*, 1048–1055.

Frazier, P. A., Mortensen, H., & Steward, J. (2005). Coping strategies as mediators of the relations among perceived control and distress in sexual assault survivors. *Journal of Counseling Psychology, 52*, 267–278.

Gilfus, M. E. (1999). The price of the ticket: A survivor-centered appraisal of trauma theory. *Violence Against Women, 5*, 1238–1257.

Gunter, R. W., & Whittal, M. L. (2010). Dissemination of cognitive-behavioral treatments for anxiety disorders: Overcoming barriers and improving patient access. *Clinical Psychology Review, 30*, 194–202.

Gutner, C. A., Rizvi, S. L., Monson, C. M., & Resick, P. A. (2006). Changes in coping strategies, relationship to the perpetrator, and posttraumatic distress in female crime victims. *Journal of Traumatic Stress, 19*, 813–823.

Institute of Medicine. (2007). *Treatment of PTSD: Assessment of the evidence*. Washington, DC: National Academies Press.

Ironson, G., Freund, B., Strauss, J. L., & Williams, J. (2002). Comparison of two treatments for traumatic stress: A community-based study of EMDR and prolonged exposure. *Journal of Clinical Psychology, 58*, 113–128.

Janoff-Bulman, R. (1989). Assumptive worlds and the stress of traumatic events: Applications of the schema construct. *Social Cognition, 7*, 113–136.

Janoff-Bulman, R., & Frieze, I. H. (1983). A theoretical perspective for understanding reactions to victimization. *Journal of Social Issues, 39*, 1–17.

Kaysen, D., Rosen, G., Bowman, M., & Resick, P. A. (2010). Duration of exposure and the dose-response model of PTSD. *Journal of Interpersonal Violence, 25*, 63–74.

Kearney, D. J., McDermott, K., Malte, C., Martinez, M., & Simpson, T. L. (2013). Effects of participation in a mindfulness program for veterans with posttraumatic stress disorder: A randomized controlled pilot study. *Journal of Clinical Psychology, 69*, 14–27.

Kennedy, A. C., & Prock, K. A. (2018). "I still feel like I am not normal": A review of the role of stigma and stigmatization among female survivors of child sexual abuse, sexual assault, and intimate partner violence. Trauma, Violence, & Abuse 19(5):512–527.

Kilpatrick, D. G., Resnick, H. S., Ruggiero, K. J., Conoscenti, L. M., & McCauley, J. (2007). *Drug-facilitated, incapacitated, and forcible rape: A national study*. Charleston, SC.

Kleim, B., Ehlers, A., & Glucksman, E. (2007). Early predictors of chronic post-traumatic stress disorder in assault survivors. *Psychological Medicine, 37*, 1457–1467.

Kleim, B., Wilhelm, F. H., Glucksman, E., & Ehlers, A. (2010). Sex differences in heart rate responses to script-driven imagery soon after and risk of posttraumatic stress disorder. *Psychosomatic Medicine, 72*, 917–924.

Koss, M. P., Abbey, A., Campbell, R., Cook, S., Norris, J., Testa, M., … White, J. (2007). Revising the SES: A collaborative process to improve assessment of sexual aggression and victimization. *Psychology of Women Quarterly, 31*, 357–370.

Lang, P. J. (1977). Imagery in therapy: An information processing analysis of fear. *Behavior Therapy, 8*, 862–886.

Lang, P. J. (1979). A bio-informational theory of emotional imagery. *Psychophysiology, 16*, 495–512.

Larsen, S. E., & Pacella, M. L. (2016). Comparing the effect of DSM-congruent traumas vs. DSM-incongruent stressors on PTSD symptoms: A meta-analytic review. *Journal of Anxiety Disorders, 38*, 37–46.

Littleton, H. L. (2010). The impact of social support and negative disclosure reactions on sexual assault victims: A cross-sectional and longitudinal investigation. *Journal of Trauma & Dissociation, 11*, 210–227. https://doi.org/10.1080/15299730903502946

Masho, S. W., & Ahmed, G. (2007). Age at sexual assault and posttraumatic stress disorder among women: Prevalence, correlates, and implications for prevention. *Journal of Women's Health, 16*, 262–271. https://doi.org/10.1089/jwh.2006.M076

McNally, R. J. (2003). Progress and controversy in the study of posttraumatic stress disorder. *Annual Review of Psychology, 54*, 229–252.

Mitchell, J. T. (1983). When disaster strikes: The critical incident stress debriefing process. *Journal of Emergency Medical Services*, 36–39.

Möller, A. T., Bäckström, T., Söndergaard, H. P., & Helström, L. (2014). Identifying risk factors for PTSD in women seeking medical help after rape. *PLoS One, 9*, 1–9.

Orsillo, S. M., & Batten, S. V. (2005). Acceptance and commitment therapy in the treatment of posttraumatic stress disorder. *Behavior Modification, 29*, 95–129. https://doi.org/10.1177/0145445504270876

Ozer, E. J., Best, S. R., Lipsey, T. L., & Weiss, D. S. (2003). Predictors of posttraumatic stress disorder and symptoms in adults: A meta-analysis. *Psychological Bulletin, 129*, 52–73.

Pegram, S. E., & Abbey, A. (2016). Associations between sexual assault severity and psychological and physical health outcomes. *Journal of Interpersonal Violence*.

Peter-Hagene, L. C., & Ullman, S. E. (2015). Sexual assault-characteristics effects on PTSD and psychosocial mediators: A cluster-analysis approach to sexual assault types. *Psychological Trauma Theory Research Practice and Policy, 7*, 162–170.

Pole, N. (2007). The psychophysiology of posttraumatic stress disorder: A meta-analysis. *Psychological Bulletin, 133*, 725–746.

Pole, N., Gone, J. P., & Kulkarni, M. (2008). Posttraumatic stess disorder among ethnoracial minorities in the United States. *Clinical Psychology: Science and Practice, 15*, 35–61.

Powers, M. B., Halpern, J. M., Ferenschak, M. P., Gillihan, S. J., & Foa, E. B. (2010). A meta-analytic review of prolonged exposure for posttraumatic stress disorder. *Clinical Psychology Review, 30*, 635–641. https://doi.org/10.1016/j.cpr.2010.04.007

Prins, A., Ouimette, P., Kimerling, R., Cameron, R. P., Hugelshofer, D. S., Thrailkill, A., & Gusman, F. D. (2003). The primary care PTSD screen (PC-PTSD): Development and operating characteristics. *Primary Care Psychiatry, 9*, 9–14.

Read, J. P., Wardell, J. D., Vermont, L. N., Colder, C. R., Ouimette, P., & White, J. (2013). Transition and change: Prospective effects of posttraumatic stress on smoking trajectories in the first year of college. *Health Psychology, 32*, 757–767.

Resick, P. A., Bovin, M. J., Calloway, A. L., Dick, A. M., King, M. W., Mitchell, K. S., … Wolf, E. J. (2012). A critical evaluation of the complex PTSD literature: Implications for DSM-5. *Journal of Traumatic Stress, 25*, 241–251.

Resick, P. A., Monson, C. M., & Chard, K. M. (2016). *Cognitive processing therapy for PTSD: A comprehensive manual*. New York, NY: Guilford Publications.

Resick, P. A., Nishith, P., Weaver, T. L., Astin, M. C., & Feuer, C. A. (2002). A comparison of cognitive-processing therapy with prolonged exposure and a waiting condition for the treatment of chronic posttraumatic stress disorder in female rape victims. *Journal of Consulting and Clinical Psychology, 70*, 867–879.

Resick, P. A., & Schnicke, M. K. (1992). Cognitive processing therapy for sexual assault victims. *Journal of Consulting and Clinical Psychology, 60*, 748–756.

Resick, P. A., Williams, L. F., Suvak, M. K., Monson, C. M., & Gradus, J. L. (2012). Long-term outcomes of cognitive–behavioral treatments for posttraumatic stress disorder among female rape survivors. *Journal of Consulting and Clinical Psychology, 80*, 201–210.

Resnick, H. S., Acierno, R., Waldrop, A. E., King, L., King, D., Danielson, C., … Kilpatrick, D. G. (2007).

Randomized controlled evaluation of an early intervention to prevent post-rape psychopathology. *Behaviour Research and Therapy, 45*, 2432–2447.

Resnick, H. S., Kilpatrick, D. G., Dansky, B. S., Saunders, B. E., Best, C. L., Danksy, B. S., … Best, C. L. (1993). Prevalence of civilian trauma and posttraumatic stress disorder in a representative national sample of women. *Journal of Consulting and Clinical Psychology, 61*, 984–991.

Resnick, H. S., Yehuda, R., & Acierno, R. (1997). Acute post-rape plasma cortisol, alcohol use, and PTSD symptom profile among recent rape victims. *Annals of the New York Academy of Sciences, 821*, 433–436.

Resnick, H. S., Yehuda, R., Pitman, R. K., & Foy, D. W. (1995). Effect of previous trauma on acute plasma cortisol level following rape. *The American Journal of Psychiatry, 152*, 1675–1677.

Rizvi, S. L., Kaysen, D., Gutner, C. A., Griffin, M. G., & Resick, P. A. (2008). Beyond fear: The role of peritraumatic responses in posttraumatic stress among female crime victims. *Journal of Interpersonal Violence, 23*, 853–868.

Roberts, A., Gilman, S., Breslau, J., Breslau, N., & Koenen, K. (2011). Race/ethnic differences in exposure to traumatic events, development of post-traumatic stress disorder, and treatment- seeking for post-traumatic stress disorder in the United States. *Psychological Medicine, 41*, 71–83.

Robjant, K., & Fazel, M. (2010). The emerging evidence for narrative exposure therapy: A review. *Clinical Psychology Review, 30*, 1030–1039.

Rocha-Rego, V., Fiszman, A., Catarina, L., Marques-portella, C., Berger, W., Silva, E., … Volchan, E. (2009). Is tonic immobility the core sign among conventional peritraumatic signs and symptoms listed for PTSD? *Journal of Affective Disorders, 115*, 269–273.

Rose, S., Bisson, J., Churchill, R., & Wessely, S. (2002). Psychological debriefing for preventing post traumatic stress disorder (PTSD). *Cochrane Database of Systematic Reviews, 2*(2).

Rosen, G. M. (1999). Treatment fidelity and research on eye movement desensitization and reprocessing (EMDR). *Journal of Anxiety Disorders, 13*, 173–184.

Rosen, G. M., & Davison, G. C. (2003). Psychology should list empirically supported principles of change (ESPs) and not credential trademarked therapies or other treatment packages. *Behavior Modification, 27*, 300–312.

Rothbaum, B. O., Foa, E. B., Riggs, D. S., Murdock, T., & Walsh, W. (1992). A prospective examination of post-traumatic stress disorder in rape victims. *Journal of Traumatic Stress, 5*, 455–475.

Rothman, E. F., Exner, D., & Baughman, A. L. (2011). The prevalence of sexual assault against people who identify as gay, lesbian, or bisexual in the United States: A systematic review. *Trauma, Violence & Abuse, 12*, 55–66.

Seidler, G. H., & Wagner, F. E. (2006). Comparing the efficacy of EMDR and trauma-focused cognitive-behavioral therapy in the treatment of PTSD: A meta-analytic study. *Psychological Medicine, 36*, 1515–1522. https://doi.org/10.1017/S0033291706007963

Shafran, R., Clark, D. M., Fairburn, C. G., Arntz, A., Barlow, D. H., Ehlers, A., … Salkovskis, P. M. (2009). Mind the gap: Improving the dissemination of CBT. *Behaviour Research and Therapy, 47*(11), 902–909.

Steenkamp, M. M., Dickstein, B. D., Salters-Pedneault, K., Hofmann, S. G., Litz, B. T., & Salters-Pedneault, K. (2012). Trajectories of PTSD symptoms following sexual assault: Is resilience the modal outcome? *Journal of Traumatic Stress, 25*, 469–474.

Surís, A., Link-Malcolm, J., Chard, K., Ahn, C., & North, C. (2013). A randomized clinical trial of cognitive processing therapy for veterans with PTSD related to military sexual trauma. *Journal of Traumatic Stress, 26*, 28–37.

Temple, J. R., Weston, R., Rodriguez, B. F., & Marshall, L. L. (2007). Differing effects of partner and nonpartner sexual assault on women's mental health. *Violence Against Women, 13*, 285–297.

Ulirsch, J. C., Ballina, L. E., Soward, A. C., Rossi, C., Hauda, W., Holbrook, D., … McLean, S. A. (2013). Pain and somatic symptoms are sequelae of sexual assault: Results of a prospective longitudinal study. *European Journal of Pain, 18*, 1–8.

Ullman, S. E. (2010). *Talking about sexual assault: Society's response to survivors*. Washington, DC: American Psychological Association.

Ullman, S. E. (2016). Sexual revictimization, PTSD, and problem drinking in sexual assault survivors. *Addictive Behaviors, 53*, 7–10.

Ullman, S. E., & Filipas, H. H. (2001). Predictors of PTSD symptom severity and social reactions in sexual assault victims. *Journal of Traumatic Stress, 14*, 369–389.

Ullman, S. E., Filipas, H. H., Townsend, S. M., & Starzynski, L. L. (2007). Psychosocial correlates of PTSD symptom severity in sexual assault survivors. *Journal of Traumatic Stress, 20*, 821–831.

Ullman, S. E., Najdowski, C. J., & Filipas, H. H. (2009). Child sexual abuse, post-traumatic stress disorder, and substance use: Predictors of revictimization in adult sexual assault survivors. *Journal of Child Sexual Abuse, 18*, 367–385.

Ullman, S. E., & Peter-Hagene, L. C. (2014). Social reactions to sexual assault disclosure, coping, perceived control, and PTSD symptoms in sexual assault victims. *Journal of Community Psychology, 42*, 495–508.

Ullman, S. E., Relyea, M., Peter-Hagene, L., & Vasquez, A. L. (2013). Trauma histories, substance use coping, PTSD, and problem substance use among sexual assault victims. *Addictive Behaviors, 38*, 2219–2223.

Ullman, S. E., Starzynski, L. L., Long, S. M., Mason, G. E., & Long, L. M. (2008). Exploring the relationships of women's sexual assault disclosure, social reactions, and problem drinking. *Journal of Interpersonal Violence, 23*, 1235–1257.

Ullman, S. E., Townsend, S. M., Filipas, H. H., & Starzynski, L. L. (2007). Structural models of the relations of assault severity, social support, avoidance coping, self-blame, and PTSD among sexual assault survivors. *Psychology of Women Quarterly, 31*, 23–37.

Ullman, S. E., Townsend, S. M., Starzynski, L. L., & Long, L. M. (2006). Correlates of comorbid PTSD and polysubstance use in sexual assault victims. *Violence and Victims, 21*, 725–743.

van Emmerik, A. A., Kamphuis, J. H., Hulsbosch, A. M., & Emmelkamp, P. M. (2002). Single session debriefing after psychological trauma: A meta-analysis. *The Lancet, 360*(9335), 766–771.

van Zuiden, M., Kavelaars, A., Geuze, E., Olff, M., & Heijnen, C. J. (2013). Predicting PTSD: Pre-existing vulnerabilities in glucocorticoid-signaling and implications for preventive interventions. *Brain, Behavior, and Immunity, 30*, 12–21.

Valentiner, D. P., Foa, E. B., Riggs, D. S., & Gershuny, B. S. (1996). Coping strategies and posttraumatic stress disorder in female victims of sexual and nonsexual assault. *Journal of Abnormal Psychology, 105*, 455–458.

Wasco, S. M. (2003). Conceptualizing the harm done by rape: Applications of trauma theory to experiences of sexual assault. *Trauma, Violence & Abuse, 4*, 309–322.

Watts, B. V., Schnurr, P. P., Mayo, L., Young-Xu, Y., Weeks, W. B., & Friedman, M. J. (2013). Meta-analysis of the efficacy of treatments for posttraumatic stress disorder. *Journal of Clinical Psychiatry, 74*, e541–e550.

Weathers, F. W., Blake, D. D., Schnurr, P. P., Kaloupek, D. G., Marx, B. P., & Keane, T. M. (2013). *The Life Events Checklist for DSM-5 (LEC-5)*. Instrument available from the National Center for PTSD at www.ptsd.va.gov

Weathers, F. W., Litz, B. T., Keane, T. M., Palmieri, P. A., Marx, B. P., & Schnurr, P. P. (2013). The PTSD Checklist for DSM-5 (PCL-5). Scale available from the National Center for PTSD at www.ptsd.va.gov

Yehuda, R., Hoge, C. W., McFarlane, A. C., Vermetten, E., Lanius, R. A., Nievergelt, C. M., ... Hyman, S. E. (2015). Post-traumatic stress disorder. *Nature Reviews. Disease Primers, 1*, 1–22.

Zinzow, H. M., Resnick, H. S., McCauley, J. L., Amstadter, A. B., Ruggiero, K. J., & Kilpatrick, D. G. (2010). The role of rape tactics in risk for posttraumatic stress disorder and major depression: Results from a national sample of college women. *Depression and Anxiety, 27*, 708–715.

Zoladz, P. R., & Diamond, D. M. (2013). Current status on behavioral and biological markers of PTSD: A search for clarity in a conflicting literature. *Neuroscience & Biobehavioral Reviews, 37*, 860–895.

Blame and Shame in Sexual Assault

18

Prachi H. Bhuptani and Terri L. Messman-Moore

The victims of rape must carry their memories with them for the rest of their lives. They must not also carry the burden of silence and shame" (pg. 6).

Nancy Venable Raine (1998)

Sexual assault, including rape, is a common form of trauma experienced by women. The National Intimate Partner and Sexual Violence Survey (2015) estimates that 19.3% of women have been raped during their lifetime. Additionally, an estimated 27.3% of women have experienced other forms of unwanted sexual assault contact. The high prevalence of sexual assault is particularly concerning in light of its significant, negative impact on victim's mental health. In a meta-analysis, sexual assault was significantly associated with elevated risk in numerous domains of psychopathology, including PTSD, suicidality, obsessive-compulsive disorder, bipolar disorder, depression, anxiety, disordered eating, and substance abuse/dependence (Dworkin, Menon, Bystrynski, & Allen, 2017). In another review, 17–65% of sexual assault victims developed PTSD, 13–51% met diagnostic criteria for depression, 12–40% experienced anxiety symptoms, 13–49% developed alcohol use disorders, 28–61% developed drug use disorders, 23–44% experienced suicidal ideation, and 2–19% attempted suicide (Campbell, Dworkin, & Cabral, 2009). Indeed, research suggests that sexual assault appears to have a substantial impact on mental health compared to other types of trauma (Kelley, Weathers, McDevitt-Murphy, Eakin, & Flood, 2009). This extensive body of literature indicates sexual assault has a debilitating impact on victims. Thus, many researchers have attempted to identify mechanisms underlying risk for posttrauma psychopathology. Apart from focusing on individual characteristics (e.g., demographics, prior assault history) and sexual assault characteristics (e.g., assault severity, assailant type), researchers have increasingly adopted an ecological lens when explaining the emergence of psychopathology among victims (see Campbell et al., 2009 for a review). An ecological approach emphasizes that sexual assault and recovery is embedded in a multilevel social context, in which sexual assault is a highly stigmatized experience (Kennedy & Prock, 2016). Such stigma emerges from societal beliefs and rape myths, including that sexual assault victims are responsible for the assault itself (Edwards, Turchik, Dardis, Reynolds, & Gidycz, 2011). Indeed, individuals must recover from sexual assault surrounded by an uniquely unfavorable cultural context typified by prejudice and victim-blaming attitudes that hold victims responsible for their assault (Moor & Farchi, 2011). This is evident by the fact that no other groups of trauma victims are blamed for their ordeal as frequently as are sexual assault survivors. When

P. H. Bhuptani · T. L. Messman-Moore (✉)
Department of Psychology, Miami University, Oxford, OH, USA
e-mail: messmat@miamioh.edu

W. T. O'Donohue and P. A. Schewe (eds.), *Handbook of Sexual Assault and Sexual Assault Prevention*, https://doi.org/10.1007/978-3-030-23645-8_18

victims disclose their sexual assault to friends, family, or professionals, they often receive victim-blaming responses, which in turn are related to negative psychological outcomes such as PTSD, depression, and anxiety symptoms (Littleton, 2010; Ullman & Peter-Hagene, 2016). There is evidence victims internalize the pervasive stigma and/or blame associated with sexual assault, leading to feelings of shame and self-blame, which also contribute to psychological distress (Kennedy & Prock, 2016). Thus, one must examine the role of shame and blame when considering the emergence of psychological distress among sexual assault victims.

Chapter Overview

The current chapter focuses on the impact of sexual assault on blame and shame, as well as their impact on negative posttrauma outcomes. The concept of blame and shame will be discussed along with theories governing their study. Next, we briefly review studies investigating the relation between different types of sexual assault (i.e., child sexual abuse [CSA], adult sexual assault, and revictimization). We will then investigate how blame and shame may influence posttrauma outcomes. Finally, we will briefly review clinical interventions targeting blame and shame among sexual assault victims along with future research recommendations.

What is Blame?

In the sexual assault literature, blame is broadly conceptualized as a cognitive attribution of stigma where the fault for sexual assault is placed on the victim (Feiring, Taska, & Lewis, 1996). Blame is typically conceptualized from two perspectives: self and other. Self-blame emerges when the victim makes appraisals about the assault, including why the assault happened, and blames herself for it (Ullman, Peter-Hagene, & Relyea, 2014). Self-blame may evolve from other blame, which involves negative reactions, such as victim-blaming responses, from an individual who is told about the sexual assault by the victim (i.e., the recipient of disclosure) including family, friends, or service providers. Victim blame occurs when the disclosure recipient holds the victim, wholly or in part, responsible for their assault.

Unsurprisingly, self-blame and victim-blaming responses to sexual assault disclosure mirror beliefs found in the social context in which sexual assault occurs. Sexual assault victims are faced with a particular prejudiced ideology comprised by a set of culturally agreed upon victim-blaming attitudes that are subsumed under rape myths. Originally defined as "prejudicial, stereotyped, or false beliefs about rape, rape victims, and rapists" (Burt, 1980, p. 217), rape myths include beliefs such as "If a victim of sexual assault does not fight back, they must have wanted it," or "Wearing revealing clothing or being intoxicated means the victim is 'asking for it'." Rape myths are widely accepted, with some studies showing that more than 50% of individuals endorse some sort of rape myth (Buddie & Miller, 2001). Unfortunately, rape myth acceptance can be pervasive among formal service providers such as law enforcement, clergy, and even mental health professionals (Ullman & Filipas, 2001). One commonly held rape myth, victim blaming or victim precipitation, reflects the belief that that the victim in some way, either by her character or behavior, provoked the sexual assault. Unfortunately, victims may often internalize such victim-blaming societal attitudes (Lebowitz & Roth, 1994). Thus, while searching for an explanation for their own sexual assault experience, victims may readily turn to widely available societal rape myths for explanations, and consequently be more inclined to place blame on themselves. Similarly, when a sexual assault victim discloses their assault, the disclosure recipient's response may reflect these rape myths and involve blaming the victim for their assault. Indeed, empirical studies suggest disclosure recipients are more likely to blame the victim for their assault if they subscribe to rape myths that hold victims responsible for the assault (Frese, Moya, & Megías, 2004; Krahe, 1988).

Theories and Types of Blame

Several theoretical frameworks have been proposed to explain why individuals engage in self-blame or victim-blame. One such approach is the just-world theory (Lerner & Miller, 1978), which suggests that individuals within Western cultures maintain a belief in a just world where socially prescribed behaviors are rewarded (e.g., working hard is rewarded through financial gain). Conversely, this belief would entail that if rules are violated, individuals deserve their misfortunes (e.g., bad things happen to only bad people). Therefore, in order to maintain this "just world" belief individuals may blame the victim, argue that sexual assault is deserved or justified, or distance themselves from the victim in order to preserve the just world belief and a sense that "This cannot happen to me" (i.e., I am safe). Similarly, in response to one's own sexual assault, the victim may blame themselves to the extent they ascribe to the just world belief. Similarly, control theory (Walster, 1966) is another way of explaining blame. According to this theory, individuals may attribute the cause of trauma to themselves as a way to regain a sense of control. Consequently, individuals may blame themselves to enhance a sense of control over the future recurrence of trauma and the severity of its consequences. Further, control theory assumes self-blame is an adaptive response following trauma which leads to better recovery.

Empirical studies have examined the impact of self-blame on recovery and report mixed findings, with some studies finding self-blame leading to better recovery (e.g., Janoff-Bulman & Wortman, 1977) and others finding no impact (e.g., Ullman, 1997) or detrimental impact (e.g., Frazier & Schauben, 1994). To resolve these contradictory findings, Ronnie Janoff-Bulman (1979) developed a revised control theory incorporating aspects of just world theory, in which she distinguished between two types of self-blame: behavioral self-blame and characterological self-blame. Behavioral self-blame is defined as a cognitive attribution where the victim blames their controllable (and modifiable) behavior for the assault (e.g., "I shouldn't have walked down that dark alley alone late at night"). Consistent with control theory, behavioral self-blame was originally conceptualized as being adaptive for recovery through increasing the individual's perception of control over further victimization. In contrast, characterological self-blame was defined as a cognitive attribution where the victim blames their nonmodifiable character for the sexual assault (e.g., "It happened because I am bad person."). Additionally, Janoff-Bulman (1979) further suggested that characterological self-blame may be the more deleterious of the two forms of self-blame, and lead to poor outcomes given that character traits are construed to be more global and stable, whereas behaviors can be changed. In support of Janoff-Bulman's distinction between the two types of self-blame, a meta-analysis examining self-blame in relation to three different types of trauma (i.e., sexual assault, illness, and severe injury) showed that characterological self-blame and behavioral self-blame are distinct constructs, although both are related to poorer recovery among sexual assault victims (Frazier, 2003; Littleton & Breitkopf, 2006). Studies assessing both types of self-blame typically find stronger effects of characterological self-blame (compared to behavioral self-blame) on distress (e.g., Breitenbecher, 2006; Ullman, Filipas, Townsend, & Starzynski, 2007).

The Relation of Self-Blame and Victim-Blaming Responses

Since self-blame and victim-blame emerge within the same social context, one can expect these constructs to be related. One way these variables may be related is that victim-blaming responses can exacerbate victim self-blame. Indeed, cross-sectional studies with samples of college and community women demonstrate that negative responses to sexual assault disclosure, including victim blaming responses, lead to greater self-blame (Littleton & Breitkopf, 2006; Ullman, Townsend, Filipas, & Starzynski, 2007). Conversely, initial victim self-blame may influence the responses a victim receives from others upon sexual assault disclosure. In an experimental study of female rape counselors and undergraduate students, participants who read a fictitious victim's account of sexual assault were significantly more likely to blame the victim for the assault if the victim engaged in either characterological or behavioral self-blame than if she blamed chance for the assault (Thornton et al., 1988). More evidence for the relation between self-blame and victim-blaming responses emerges from a longitudinal study conducted with a sample of community women (Ullman & Najdowski, 2011), which assessed self-blame and responses to adult sexual assault disclosure twice, 1 year apart. Neither characterological self-blame nor behavioral self-blame prospectively predicted negative social reactions, including victim-blaming reactions from others, over the 1-year follow-up period. However, victim-blaming reactions from others led to greater characterological self-blame, but not behavioral self-blame, over the course of the study. These results suggest that victim-blaming reactions are particularly damaging as they contribute to, or exacerbate, characterological self-blame (the more deleterious form of self-blame) over time. Thus self-blame, particularly characterological self-blame, may result from of a process of internalizing victim-blaming messages received directly when survivors seek support, as well as through a less conscious, passive absorption of rape myth beliefs promulgated in society.

What is Shame?

Shame is an important affective component of stigmatization following abuse or assault (Wilson, Drozdek, & Turkovic, 2006). Some researchers described shame as "the master emotion of everyday life" and a prominent cause of psychological distress among sexual assault victims (p. 239, Scheff, 2003; Wilson et al., 2006). Lewis (1987), one of the early pioneers in the study of shame, writes "Shame is one's own vicarious experience of the other's scorn. The self- in-the eyes-of-the-other is the focus of awareness…The experience of shame often occurs in the form of imagery, of looking or being looked at. Shame may also be played out as an internal colloquy, in which the whole self is condemned" (pp. 15, 18). Brown (2006) defines shame as "An intensely painful feeling or experience of believing we are flawed and therefore unworthy of acceptance and belonging" (p. 45). Shame is, therefore, a highly aversive negative emotional response, in which the victim feels deeply unworthy, defective, and debased.

Shame is a social emotion (Hareli & Parkinson, 2008). The experience of shame is contingent upon other people's thoughts, feelings or actions, as they are experienced, anticipated, or inferred from a generalized consideration of social norms or conventions. Therefore, it exists in relation to other people and broader societal norms in general. Shame can be contrasted with guilt by its focus on the self as opposed to behavior (Brown, 2006). Shame invokes behavioral responses that focus on hiding the perceived flawed self, including withdrawal. In contrast, guilt emerges when a behavior, as opposed to the whole self, is seen as flawed or morally unacceptable—and promotes prosocial behavior aiming at making amends (Tangney & Dearing, 2002). Moreover, shame involves seeing the whole self as flawed and morally unacceptable, which can lead to self-blame (La Bash & Papa, 2014).

Child Sexual Abuse, Self-Blame, and Shame

Two influential theoretical models that examine shame and self-blame in relation to sexual abuse focus on child sexual abuse (CSA): the Traumagenic Dynamics Model and the Process Model. The Traumagenic Dynamics Model (Finkelhor & Browne, 1985) aims to explain how and why CSA leads to psychological distress, and emphasizes stigmatization as one of four traumagenic dynamics (along with betrayal, powerlessness, and traumatic sexualization) which alter victims' identity and self-worth. The authors define stigmatization as "negative connotations (e.g., badness, shame, and guilt) that are communicated to the child around the [CSA] experiences and that then become incorporated into the child's self-image" (p. 532). This suggests that within the broader societal context—including media representations, stereotypes, dominant narratives, and many other sources—a victim may learn that their experience of sexual abuse is stigmatized and blameworthy. In addition to this broader, more general stigma, a victim may also receive specific victim-blaming responses upon disclosure of CSA or sexual assault (e.g., a sexual abuse survivor as "damaged" or "spoiled goods"). Further, these stigma-laden messages are often internalized by victims and incorporated into their self-image. Consequently, self-blame and shame, stemming from the dynamic of stigmatization, lead to negative psychological outcomes.

The Process Model focuses on how stigma operates in CSA victims (Feiring et al., 1996). The central premise of the model is that CSA leads to shame, which then leads to poor adjustment. The model further posits that shame, as opposed to guilt, is the core emotion of stigmatization. Feiring et al. suggest that negative cognitive attributions, including self-blame, mediate the influence of sexual abuse on shame. Thus, both models identify shame as a common outcome of sexual violence, but differ in their explanation of the role of self-blame in internalized stigma.

To test the Process Model, Feiring (2005) conducted a 6-year longitudinal study with a diverse, low-income sample of documented CSA victims who were interviewed three times—at the time of discovery of CSA, 1 year after abuse discovery and 6 years after abuse discovery—during which two different types of shame were assessed: shame for everyday events (i.e., general shame) and abuse-specific shame. Similarly, two different forms of self-blame were assessed: general and abuse-specific. Individuals reporting high levels of assault-related shame 1 year following abuse discovery reported high levels of assault-related shame 6 years following discovery, illustrating the longstanding nature of shame in the context of sexual abuse. Another study also found gender differences in the temporal trajectory of shame and self-blame (Feiring, Taska, & Lewis, 2002), with girls reporting higher levels of general self-blame, abuse-specific self-blame, and abuse-specific shame compared to boys. Further, girls reported a steeper decline in abuse-specific shame between discovery of abuse and 1 year after discovery compared to boys. Taken together, these studies suggest shame and self-blame are common responses to CSA. However, sexual abuse in childhood, compared to adulthood, may exert a particularly negative impact on shame and self-blame. Indeed, Finkelhor and Browne (1985) suggest the Traumagenic Dynamics "alter children's cognitive and emotional orientation to the world, and create trauma by distorting children's self-concept, world view, and affective capacities" (p. 530). Therefore, CSA and stigmatization may inevitably affect such development.

A meta-analysis on self-blame after trauma, including sexual victimization experiences, highlighted that CSA victims had higher levels of self-blame compared to adult SA victims (Littleton, Magee, & Axsom, 2007). Additionally, specific CSA characteristics are thought to be uniquely related to self-blame, such as duration of CSA, type of CSA, older age of onset, and peer-perpetrated abuse (Zinzow, Seth, Jackson, Niehaus, & Fitzgerald, 2010). Although largely ignored in the literature, the association between particular CSA characteristics and shame may reveal similar patterns found for self-blame, given the conceptual and theoretical temporal precedence of self-blame in relation to shame (Feiring et al., 1996).

Adult Sexual Assault, Self-Blame, and Shame

Although potentially less formative than CSA, adult sexual assault is also associated with elevated self-blame and shame. In a community sample of female victims of adult sexual assault (Vidal & Petrak, 2007), approximately 75% endorsed assault-related shame—a widespread impact. Although any type of crime victimization can evoke shame, sexual assault generally poses a greater risk for this aversive emotion, particularly in comparison with physical assault (Felson & Paré, 2005). Moreover, when comparing the sequelae of different trauma types (e.g., adult sexual assault, physical assault, transportation accident, and illness/injury), Amstadter and Vernon (2008) found that sexual assault was associated with higher levels of shame than other traumatic events. Moreover, shame drastically increased posttrauma for those experiencing sexual assault, a pattern not found in other trauma groups, and which may be explained by the stigma inherent in *sexual* assault experiences. Sexual assault victims may receive more victim-blaming messages upon disclosure of their assault, which may contribute to shame-related appraisals of the trauma. As evident from these studies, sexual assault victims commonly experience shame and are more vulnerable to shame than other crime victims. However, longitudinal research is required to determine how shame unfolds and persists among sexual assault victims.

In addition to shame, adult sexual assault victims are particularly vulnerable to self-blame, and may experience more self-blame than individuals who experience other types of trauma. In a cross-sectional study of female community members and college students (Moor & Farchi, 2011), adult rape victims reported higher levels of self-blame than other trauma victims (e.g., combat stress, severe illness, car accidents, and loss). Moreover, in a community sample of adult sexual assault victims, higher assault severity (i.e., physical injury resulting from assault, type of coercion including force or use of a weapon, and more severe acts such as penetration) predicted less self-blame (Ullman, Townsend, et al., 2007). However, in another community sample of female rape victims, self-blame did not vary according to the coercion tactic used (McConnell, Messman-Moore, Gratz, & DiLillo, 2017). Given such mixed results, more research is needed to clarify the relation between specific assault characteristics and self-blame. Further, research on adult sexual assault has thus far ignored the relation between specific assault characteristics and shame, similar to the CSA literature. However, unlike the self-blame literature, research examining shame following adult sexual assault exists in the absence of an adequate theoretical foundation or guiding framework. Finkelhor and Browne's (1985) Traumagenic Dynamics model and Feiring's Feiring et al. (1996) process model are both situated with a developmental context examining the impact of CSA. Stigmatization arising after CSA appears to impact psychological distress by shaping victims' developing self-image, world view, and affective regulation capacity. It is unclear whether adult sexual assault may exert a similar effect, or potentially disrupt previously adaptive and healthy beliefs, as posited by the process model. Additional studies are needed to test theoretical frameworks that may explain shame in the context of adult sexual assault.

Sexual Victimization and Victim-Blame

When CSA and ASA victims disclose abuse experiences, they often receive negative responses such as victim blame and disbelief. Such responses, often called secondary rape or secondary victimization, can exacerbate psychological distress (e.g., Littleton, 2010). In a diverse community-based sample of women who had been sexually assaulted in adulthood and disclosed to at least one person (Ahrens, Cabral, & Abeling, 2009), most victims received mixed responses (i.e., positive/supportive and negative) involving at least one blaming reaction which was perceived as hurtful by the victim. Similarly, in a college sample, negative responses to CSA disclosure, including blaming responses, were common especially when CSA was perpetrated by a family member (Ullman, 2007).

Apart from focusing on the presence of blaming responses to disclosure, one study has examined how shame and victim blame are related. In a community sample, Ahrens (2006) found that victim-blaming responses to sexual assault disclosure reinforced victims' feelings of shame as well as self-blame. Such negative, blaming responses to disclosure eventually led to victims feeling silenced—preventing future disclosures to others. Thus, the negative ramifications of victim-blaming not only appear to exacerbate shame and self-blame within individuals who experience sexual assault, but the eventual silencing of victims appears to effectively prevent future disclosures, likely impeding help-seeking and recovery efforts. In addition, failure to disclose and seek protection or support may also increase vulnerability for future revictimization, a topic to which we turn next.

Revictimization, Blame, and Shame

Research discussed thus far has tended to focus solely on sexual abuse (or assault) in childhood or adulthood, despite widespread evidence that sexual violence experiences across the lifespan are linked. Women who experience CSA are at greater risk for adult sexual assault, a phenomenon called revictimization (Messman-Moore & Long, 2003; Roodman & Clum, 2001). Given the already elevated levels of shame and self-blame among individuals reporting either CSA or ASA, sexual revictimization deserves special attention as the cumulative impact of lifetime sexual violence may exacerbate shame and self-blame originating from earlier sexual abuse. Moreover, there is evidence that blame and shame may increase vulnerability for future revictimization as well.

Impact of Revictimization on Blame and Shame

The negative psychological impact of interpersonal violence, including sexual assault, is cumulative. Revictimization is associated with greater distress, including depression, posttraumatic stress, and anxiety than sexual violence in either adulthood or childhood (e.g., Messman-Moore, Long, & Siegfried, 2000). In a similar vein, revictimization is associated with elevations in self-blame and shame. Among college women, individuals with a history of CSA (i.e., revictimized women) report higher levels of self-blame and shame related to a recent sexual assault compared to those without a history of CSA (Gibson & Leitenberg, 2001). Revictimization is also associated with heightened self-blame connected to earlier CSA, including current levels of self-blame as well as memories of self-blame at the time of CSA. A cross-sectional study of female college students indicates that revictimized women report higher CSA-related self-blame than those who experienced CSA but were not later revictimized (Filipas & Ullman, 2006). These studies, however, focused solely on two incidents of sexual assault. In contrast, Aakvaag et al. (2016) examined the cumulative impact of multiple traumatic experiences on trauma-related shame within a Norwegian community sample. This study examined the differential impact of various forms of lifetime sexual violence (i.e., CSA, childhood rape, and adult sexual assault and rape) as well as other interpersonal traumas (e.g., childhood physical abuse, severe parental intimate partner violence, adult rape, adult intimate partner violence, and severe adult physical violence from a nonpartner), finding a graded (i.e., dose response) relation between number of traumatic events and trauma-related shame, suggesting that revictimization exacerbates self-blame and shame. Such findings suggest additional revictimization experiences reinforce preexisting beliefs of blameworthiness and internalized stigma among victims of sexual violence.

A longitudinal study utilizing a sample of diverse, urban women, corroborates earlier cross-sectional studies that revictimization predicts self-blame and negative responses to sexual assault disclosure, including victim blame (Ullman & Najdowski, 2011; Ullman & Peter-Hagene, 2016). In this sample revictimization was associated with initial levels of negative (e.g., blaming) responses, and prospectively predicted behavioral self-blame but not characterological self-blame. Ullman and colleagues suggest rape myths and sexual assault-related stigma appear to be conveyed to victims via negative, blaming responses, and revictimization may lead women to internalize such stigma in terms of self-blame. Beliefs that careless behavior causes rape are not uncommon among rape victims, likely because such beliefs are propagated in society through rape myths.

Blame and Shame as Risk Factors for Revictimization

In their review, Messman-Moore and Long (2003) concluded that research should adopt an ecological framework when examining pathways to revictimization, and focus on the impact of societal and cultural factors such as victim blame. Indeed, several studies demonstrate that self-blame and victim-blame play critical roles in *risk for* revictimization. Mokma, Eshelman, and Messman-Moore (2016) reported that characterological and behavioral self-blame were directly associated with sexual revictimization (i.e., forcible and substance-facilitated adult sexual assault) among CSA survivors in a cross-sectional study of college women. In addition, the relation between CSA and sexual assault was mediated by the impact of global self-blame (not CSA-specific self-blame) on posttraumatic stress and alcohol use, which in turn predicted adult sexual assault. Similarly, in another cross-sectional study of undergraduate women, self-blame mediated the relation between CSA and later sexual assault (Arata, 2000). Unfortunately, predictive interpretations regarding the role of self-blame in both studies are limited by the retrospective design. However, a prospective study which followed a sample of female college rape victims for a period of 4 months examined behavioral self-blame, characterological self-blame, and negative cognitions about the world, finding that only behavioral self-blame prospectively predicted revictimization (Miller, Markman, & Handley, 2007). Along this vein, another study followed a sample of college women who had experienced adolescent sexual assault over a period of 6 months, measuring behavioral and characterological self-blame (Katz, May, Sörensen, & DelTosta, 2010). Although neither type of self-blame directly predicted revictimization over the follow up period, behavioral self-blame predicted decreased sexual assertiveness, which in turn predicted revictimization. Taken together, these findings suggest behavioral self-blame plays a critical role in future risk for sexual revictimization.

Apart from self-blame, victim-blame also predicts revictimization. A cross-sectional study of Israeli women with a history of CSA found revictimization rates were higher among women who had received blaming responses to CSA disclosure compared to those who received supportive reactions and those who had not disclosed CSA at all (Brenner & Ben-Amitay, 2015). Further, a 12-month longitudinal study of 625 female CSA victims in a community sample indicated that of the numerous negative responses to CSA disclosure (e.g., victim-blaming responses, egocentric responses, taking control), only victim-blaming responses predicted future sexual revictimization (Mason, Ullman, Long, Long, & Starzynski, 2009). These results emphasize how victim-blaming responses are uniquely damaging, especially in the context of revictimization. Apart from actually receiving victim-blaming responses to disclosure, anticipation of these responses also appears to have a similar impact. In the longitudinal study conducted by Miller et al. (2007), most victims did not disclose their sexual assault to a formal source out of fear of receiving a blaming response (Miller, Canales, Amacker, Backstrom, & Gidycz, 2011). This fear of receiving a blaming response, or stigma threat, prospectively predicted revictimization over a 4.2-month period. Therefore, both *anticipation* of victim-blaming responses to disclosure as well as actually experiencing victim-blame predicts revictimization.

Similar to blame, shame may also contribute to risk for revictimization, although only one study to date has examined this possibility. A cross-sectional study of female college students reported that general shame mediated the relation between CSA and adult sexual assault (Kessler & Bieschke, 1999). However, as of yet there are no longitudinal studies available to corroborate this relation. Nevertheless, given high overlap between shame and blame, we may assume that shame would play a similar role in predicting revictimization. Longitudinal studies should empirically test this hypothesis, and future investigations should examine whether abuse-related shame and general shame play equal roles in predicting revictimization. Apart from focusing on blame and shame as risk factors for revictimization, we should also examine the impact of revictimization on blame and shame.

Consequences of Blame and Shame

Although victims are at a greater risk for experiencing psychological distress (e.g., Dworkin et al., 2017), sexual assault does not inevitably lead to negative psychological outcomes. Rather, shame, self-blame, and victim blame may explain negative sexual assault outcomes such as depression, PTSD, decreased self-esteem, and problematic drinking in cross-sectional studies (Ahrens, Campbell, Ternier-Thames, Wasco, & Sefl, 2007; Arata, 1999; Ullman & Filipas, 2001; Vidal & Petrak, 2007). Longitudinal designs provide stronger evidence for the contribution of shame, self-blame, and victim-blaming responses to negative outcomes. Utilizing a community sample, Ullman and Najdowski (2009) found that negative responses to CSA disclosure, including victim-blaming responses, predicted problematic drinking over the 1-year study, especially among participants who had been revictimized. Longitudinal mediation analyses suggest that both characterological self-blame and victim blame mediated the effect of assault characteristics on PTSD over 1 year (Peter-Hagene & Ullman, 2015). Another longitudinal study indicated that reductions in self-blame were associated with a decrease in PTSD over 1 year, whereas decreases in assault-related shame were linked to declines in PTSD and depression, as well as improved self-esteem (Feiring et al., 2002).

Multivariate models demonstrate how shame, self-blame and victim-blame responses may contribute to psychological distress. Among a college sample of CSA survivors, negative responses to CSA disclosure uniquely predicted increased PTSD, controlling for current self-blame and abuse severity (Ullman & Filipas, 2005). However, in a community-based sample of African-American and Latina CSA victims, there was no evidence of a direct link between victim-blaming responses and depression. Instead, depression symptoms were highest amongst those who disclosed *and* endorsed high levels of self-blame (Sciolla et al., 2011). Mediation analyses provide further evidence on how blame and shame contribute to psychological distress. Two separate studies, using community and college samples, indicated that characterological self-blame mediated the relation between negative responses to sexual assault disclosure and PTSD, as well as problematic drinking (Hassija & Gray, 2012; Sigurvinsdottir & Ullman, 2015). Similarly, DeCou, Cole, Lynch, Wong, and Matthews (2017) report that assault-related shame mediated the relation between negative responses to sexual assault disclosure and PTSD, as well as depression. However, these are cross-sectional studies. Additional longitudinal studies are needed to confirm these findings and determine how shame, self-blame, and victim-blaming responses following sexual assault contribute to negative outcomes.

Clinical Interventions

A deeply aversive experience, shame involves global attacks on the self, sometimes resulting in development of behaviors that facilitate escape from shame. Since both attributions arise in the context of a meaning-making process, and are thus malleable, targeting these variables and reducing internalized stigma will facilitate recovery among sexual assault victims. Interventions for sexual assault-related PTSD, including Cognitive Processing Therapy (CPT) and Skills Training in Affective and Interpersonal Regulation with Prolonged Exposure (STAIR-PE) examine shame and self-blame in the context of addressing maladaptive cognitions and dysfunctional schemas associated with sexual violence. Clients learn skills recognizing and challenging dysfunctional cognitions with regard to the meaning of the traumatic events for current beliefs about self and others, which included beliefs stemming from shame and self-blame. In a random clinical trial, Patricia Resick and colleagues examined whether CPT affected shame and self-blame in women with PTSD (Resick et al., 2008). Decreases in shame and self-blame occurred over the course of treatment, emphasizing the utility of CPT in treating shame and self-blame. STAIR-PE (Cloitre, Cohen, & Koenen, 2011) also targets shame among sexual violence victims. Developed for treating PTSD and depression among adult survivors of CSA, STAIR-PE is a phase-based treatment where the first phase focuses on building emotional and social competencies, including skills related to emotional awareness, emotional regulation, understanding and changing relationship patterns, and establishing agency and flexibility in interpersonal relationships. The second phase of the treatment, called Narrative Story Telling, involves emotional processing of the traumatic events in a safe and supportive environment. Shame is targeted in both phases of treatment, where clients learn how to identify and manage shame, internally as well as within their interpersonal relationships. Additionally, the second phase also involves titration of shame narratives related to the traumatic events.

Other therapies target shame without overt focus or emphasis on traumatic experiences. Compassion-focused therapy (CFT) and related approaches help reduce shame. Shame is associated with high levels of self-criticism and an inability to self-soothe and offer oneself compassion (Gilbert & Procter, 2006). Compassion-focused therapies directly challenge shame and self-criticism, and build an individual's capacity to offer kindness to themselves. In a pilot study where trauma history was not assessed, Gilbert and Proctor (Gilbert & Procter, 2006) taught compassionate mind training (CMT) to decrease shame and self-criticism. CMT includes identifying the safety strategies in self-criticism, the consequences from self-criticism, and developing compassionate images to counteract the shame and self-criticism (Gilbert & Procter, 2006). Over the course of the study, which lasted for 12 weeks, participants demonstrated a reduction in self-criticism, shame, as well as negative evaluations of themselves, which is likened to self-blame. More relevant to sexual assault, there is preliminary evidence that suggests compassion-based therapy aids in reducing assault-related shame, with subsequent decreases in PTSD symptom severity, self-blame, and improvements in self-compassion (Au et al., 2017). Similarly, Mindfulness-Based Stress Reduction (MBSR) leads to decreases in PTSD and depression symptoms through reductions in shame (as well as increases in emotional acceptance) among participants with sexual victimization experiences (Ginzburg et al., 2009; Goldsmith et al., 2014). Goldsmith and colleagues investigated the effect of an MBSR group on trauma-related shame and self-blame. The authors reported decreased shame, as well as improved PTSD and depression symptoms. Importantly, participants' self-reported duration of mindfulness practice was associated with increased acceptance and decreases in shame from pre- to post-treatment. Ginzburg and colleagues compared two group therapy formats, Trauma-Focused Group Therapy and Present-Focused Group Therapy. Improvement in PTSD symptoms for both groups were mediated by reductions in shame. These results suggest reduced shame is associated with symptom reduction (for both PTSD and depression). The group therapy format provides space for creating interpersonal connections and reducing isolation, which may lead to reductions in perceived stigmatization along with shame. Moreover, a group fosters empathy and a correcting emotional experience by shifting the social dimension of shame and sense of devaluation related to sexual abuse.

Therapists working with sexual violence survivors should be on the lookout for shame, which may manifest in various ways within a therapy session (Talbot, 1996), and may be disguised as boredom, hostility, somatization, dissociation, and substance use (all of which are shame avoidance behaviors). Other verbal, paralinguistic, and nonverbal cues assist in alerting the therapist to shame states (Herman, 2012). Words such as "ridiculous, foolish, silly, idiotic, stupid, dumb, humiliated, disrespected, helpless, weak, inept, dependent, small, inferior, unworthy, worthless, trivial, shy, vulnerable, uncomfortable, or embarrassed" can indicate feelings of shame (Herman, 2012, p. 165). Confusion of thought, hesitation, soft speech, mumbling, silences, stammering, long pauses, rapid speech, or tensely laughed words are some paralinguistic cues of shame. Nonverbal cues include hiding behaviors, such as covering all or parts of the face, gaze aversion, with eyes downcast or averted, hanging head, hunching shoulders, squirming, fidgeting, blushing, biting, or licking the lips, biting the tongue, or false smiling (Retzinger, 1995). Shame may also influence transference and counter-transference issues. In her description on therapeutic work with incest victims, Courtois (1988) indicates that the effect of shame on transference may lead to difficulties in addressing it. She suggests that incest victims may expect the therapist to feel the same contempt for clients that they feel for themselves, leading to difficulty trusting the therapist or accepting the therapist's empathy and positive regard. Shame may also affect counter-transference as therapists may avoid addressing this aversive emotion directly because of their own discomfort (Lewis, 1987).

Given that sexual assault in particular is one form of trauma associated with significantly elevated shame responses, therapists and other professionals who frequently encounter individuals exposed to sexual violence should be aware of behavioral indicators of shame and be prepared with strategies to reduce a sense of stigma and shame among their clients. If warranted, therapies such as CPT or STAIR-PE are appropriate choices to treat self-blame, shame, PTSD and depression in survivors. Group therapies such as those described here are also beneficial to address shame and self-blame among survivors given the increased sense of connection and de-stigmatization that naturally occurs through the group process (Herman, 2012).

Conclusion

Numerous studies document the ubiquitous and pernicious nature of self-blame and shame among survivors of sexual assault, rape, and child sexual abuse. Negative outcomes associated with sexual violence appear to involve internalization of assault-related stigma conveyed directly through victim blame and indirectly through societal rape myth acceptance. Research consistently demonstrates victim blame results in heightened shame, behavioral self-blame, and characterological self-blame among victims, and these attributions predict psychological distress. Interventions designed to treat PTSD, as well as those designed to directly target shame and self-blame, also appear to facilitate recovery among victims of sexual violence. Additional longitudinal studies, specifically designed to examine the development of shame and self-blame following sexual assault, are necessary to continue to clarify the proximal and directional influences of shame and self-blame in negative outcomes and recovery processes.

References

Aakvaag, H. F., Thoresen, S., Wentzel-Larsen, T., Dyb, G., Røysamb, E., & Olff, M. (2016). Broken and guilty since it happened: A population study of trauma-related shame and guilt after violence and sexual abuse. *Journal of Affective Disorders, 204*, 16–23. https://doi.org/10.1016/j.jad.2016.06.004

Ahrens, C. E. (2006). Being silenced: The impact of negative social reactions on the disclosure of rape. *American Journal of Community Psychology, 38*, 263–274. https://doi.org/10.1007/s10464-006-9069-9

Ahrens, C. E., Cabral, G., & Abeling, S. (2009). Healing or hurtful: Sexual assault survivors' interpretations of social reactions from support providers. *Psychology of Women Quarterly, 33*, 81–94. https://doi.org/10.1111/j.1471-6402.2008.01476.x

Ahrens, C. E., Campbell, R., Ternier-Thames, N. K., Wasco, S. M., & Sefl, T. (2007). Deciding whom to tell: Expectations and outcomes of rape survivors' first disclosures. *Psychology of Women Quarterly, 31*, 38–49. https://doi.org/10.1111/j.1471-6402.2007.00329.x

Amstadter, A. B., & Vernon, L. L. (2008). Emotional reactions during and after trauma: A comparison of trauma types. *Journal of Aggression, Maltreatment & Trauma, 16*, 391–408. https://doi.org/10.1080/10926770801926492

Arata, C. M. (1999). Coping with rape the roles of prior sexual abuse and attributions of blame. *Journal of Interpersonal Violence, 14*, 62–78. https://doi.org/10.1177/088626099014001004

Arata, C. M. (2000). From child victim to adult victim: A model for predicting sexual revictimization. *Child Maltreatment, 5*, 26–38. https://doi.org/10.1177/1077559500005001004

Au, T. M., Sauer-Zavala, S., King, M. W., Petrocchi, N., Barlow, D. H., & Litz, B. T. (2017). Compassion-based therapy for trauma-related shame and posttraumatic stress: Initial evaluation using a multiple baseline design. *Behavior Therapy, 48*, 207–221. https://doi.org/10.1016/j.beth.2016.11.012

Breitenbecher, K. H. (2006). The relationships among self-blame, psychological distress, and sexual victimization. *Journal of Interpersonal Violence, 21*, 597–611. https://doi.org/10.1177/0886260506286842

Brenner, I., & Ben-Amitay, G. (2015). Sexual revictimization: The impact of attachment anxiety, accumulated trauma, and response to childhood sexual abuse disclosure. *Violence and Victims, 30*, 49–66. https://doi.org/10.1891/0886-6708.vv-d-13-00098

Brown, B. (2006). Shame resilience theory: A grounded theory study on women and shame. *Families in Society, 87*, 43–52. https://doi.org/10.1606/1044-3894.3483

Buddie, A. M., & Miller, A. G. (2001). Beyond rape myths: A more complex view of perceptions of rape victims. *Sex Roles, 45*, 139–160. https://doi.org/10.1023/A:1013575209803

Bulman, R. J., & Wortman, C. B. (1977). Attributions of blame and coping in the "real world": Severe accident victims react to their lot. *Journal of Personality and Social Psychology, 35*, 351–363. https://doi.org/10.1037//0022-3514.35.5.351

Burt, M. R. (1980). Cultural myths and support for rape. *Journal of Personality and Social Psychology, 39*, 217–230. https://doi.org/10.1037/0022-3514.38.2.217

Campbell, R., Dworkin, E., & Cabral, G. (2009). An ecological model of the impact of sexual assault on women's mental health. *Trauma, Violence & Abuse, 10*, 225–246. https://doi.org/10.1177/1524838009334456

Cloitre, M., Cohen, L. R., & Koenen, K. C. (2011). *Treating survivors of childhood abuse: Psychotherapy for the interrupted life*. New York, NY: Guildford.

Courtois, C. A. (1988). *Healing the incest wound: Adult survivors in therapy*. New York: Norton.

DeCou, C. R., Cole, T. T., Lynch, S. M., Wong, M. M., & Matthews, K. C. (2017). Assault-related shame mediates the association between negative social reactions to disclosure of sexual assault and psychological distress. *Psychological Trauma Theory Research Practice and Policy, 9*, 166–172. https://doi.org/10.1037/tra0000186

Dworkin, E. R., Menon, S. V., Bystrynski, J., & Allen, N. E. (2017). Sexual assault victimization and psychopathology: A review and meta-analysis. *Clinical Psychology Review, 56*, 65–81. https://doi.org/10.1016/j.cpr.2017.06.002

Edwards, K. M., Turchik, J. A., Dardis, C. M., Reynolds, N., & Gidycz, C. A. (2011). Rape myths: History, individual and institutional-level presence, and implications for change. *Sex Roles, 65*, 761–773. https://doi.org/10.1007/s11199-011-9943-2

Feiring, C. (2005). The persistence of shame following sexual abuse: A longitudinal look at risk and recovery. *Child Maltreatment, 10*, 337–349. https://doi.org/10.1177/1077559505276686

Feiring, C., Taska, L., & Lewis, M. (1996). A process model for understanding adaptation to sexual abuse: The role of shame in defining stigmatization. *Child Abuse & Neglect, 20*, 767–782. https://doi.org/10.1016/0145-2134(96)00064-6

Feiring, C., Taska, L., & Lewis, M. (2002). Adjustment following sexual abuse discovery: The role of shame and attributional style. *Developmental Psychology, 38*, 79–92. https://doi.org/10.1037//0012-1649.38.1.79

Felson, R. B., & Paré, P. P. (2005). The reporting of domestic violence and sexual assault by nonstrangers to the police. *Journal of Marriage and Family, 67*, 597–610. https://doi.org/10.1111/j.1741-3737.2005.00156.x

Filipas, H. H., & Ullman, S. E. (2006). Child sexual abuse, coping responses, self-blame, posttraumatic stress disorder, and adult sexual revictimization. *Journal of Interpersonal Violence, 21*, 652–672. https://doi.org/10.1177/0886260506286879

Finkelhor, D., & Browne, A. (1985). The traumatic impact of child sexual abuse: A conceptualization. *American Journal of Orthopsychiatry, 55*, 530–541. https://doi.org/10.1111/j.1939-0025.1985.tb02703.x

Frazier, P. A. (2003). Perceived control and distress following sexual assault: A longitudinal test of a new model. *Journal of Personality and Social Psychology, 84*, 1257–1269. https://doi.org/10.1037/0022-3514.84.6.1257

Frazier, P. A., & Schauben, L. (1994). Causal attributions and recovery from rape and other stressful life events. *Journal of Social and Clinical Psychology, 13*, 1–14. https://doi.org/10.1521/jscp.1994.13.1.1

Frese, B., Moya, M., & Megías, J. L. (2004). Social perception of rape: How rape myth acceptance modulates the influence of situational factors. *Journal of Interpersonal Violence, 19*, 143–161. https://doi.org/10.1177/0886260503260245

Gibson, L. E., & Leitenberg, H. (2001). The impact of child sexual abuse and stigma on methods of coping with sexual assault among undergraduate women. *Child Abuse and Neglect, 25*, 1343–1361. https://doi.org/10.1016/S0145-2134(01)00279-4

Gilbert, P., & Procter, S. (2006). Compassionate mind training for people with high shame and self-criticism: Overview and pilot study of a group therapy approach. *Clinical Psychology & Psychotherapy, 13*, 353–379. https://doi.org/10.1002/cpp.507

Ginzburg, K., Butler, L. D., Giese-Davis, J., Cavanaugh, C. E., Neri, E., Koopman, C., … Spiegel, D. (2009). Shame, guilt, and posttraumatic stress disorder in adult survivors of childhood sexual abuse at risk for human immunodeficiency virus: Outcomes of a randomized clinical trial of group psychotherapy treatment. *The Journal of Nervous and Mental Disease, 197*, 536–542. https://doi.org/10.1097/NMD.0b013e3181ab2ebd

Goldsmith, R. E., Gerhart, J. I., Chesney, S. A., Burns, J. W., Kleinman, B., & Hood, M. M. (2014). Mindfulness-based stress reduction for posttraumatic stress symptoms: Building acceptance and decreasing shame. *Journal of Evidence-Based Complementary & Alternative Medicine, 19*, 227–234. https://doi.org/10.1177/2156587214533703

Hareli, S., & Parkinson, B. (2008). What's social about social emotions? *Journal for the Theory of Social Behaviour, 38*(2), 131–156. https://doi.org/10.1111/j.1468-5914.2008.00363.x

Hassija, C. M., & Gray, M. J. (2012). Negative social reactions to assault disclosure as a mediator between self-blame and posttraumatic stress symptoms among survivors of interpersonal assault. *Journal of Interpersonal Violence, 27*, 3425–3441. https://doi.org/10.1177/0886260512445379

Herman, J. L. (2012). Shattered shame states and their repair. In J. Yellin & K. White (Eds.), *Shattered states: Disorganised attachment and its repair* (pp. 157–170). London: Karnac Books Ltd.

Janoff-Bulman, R. (1979). Characterological versus behavioral self-blame: Inquiries into depression and rape. *Journal of Personality and Social Psychology, 37*, 1798–1809. https://doi.org/10.1037//0022-3514.37.10.1798

Katz, J., May, P., Sörensen, S., & DelTosta, J. (2010). Sexual revictimization during women's first year of college: Self-blame and sexual refusal assertiveness as possible mechanisms. *Journal of Interpersonal Violence, 25*, 2113–2126. https://doi.org/10.1177/0886260509354515

Kelley, L. P., Weathers, F. W., McDevitt-Murphy, M. E., Eakin, D. E., & Flood, A. M. (2009). A comparison of PTSD symptom patterns in three types of civilian trauma. *Journal of Traumatic Stress, 22*, 227–235. https://doi.org/10.1002/jts.20406

Kennedy, A. C., & Prock, K. A. (2016). "I still feel like I am not normal": A review of the role of stigma and stigmatization among female survivors of child sexual abuse, sexual assault, and intimate partner violence. *Trauma, Violence & Abuse, 19*(5), 512–527. https://doi.org/10.1177/1524838016673601

Kessler, B. L., & Bieschke, K. J. (1999). A retrospective analysis of shame, dissociation, and adult victimization in survivors of childhood sexual abuse. *Journal of Counseling Psychology, 46*, 335–341. https://doi.org/10.1037/0022-0167.46.3.335

Krahe, B. (1988). Victim and observer characteristics as determinants of responsibility attributions to victims of rape. *Journal of Applied Social Psychology, 18*, 50–58. https://doi.org/10.1111/j.1559-1816.1988.tb00004.x

La Bash, H., & Papa, A. (2014). Shame and PTSD symptoms. *Psychological Trauma Theory Research Practice and Policy, 6*, 159–166. https://doi.org/10.1037/a0032637

Lebowitz, L., & Roth, S. (1994). "I felt like a slut": The cultural context and women's response to being raped. *Journal of Traumatic Stress, 7*, 363–390. https://doi.org/10.1002/jts.2490070304

Lerner, M. J., & Miller, D. T. (1978). Just world research and the attribution process: Looking back and ahead. *Psychological Bulletin, 85*, 1030–1051. https://doi.org/10.1037/0033-2909.85.5.1030

Lewis, H. B. (1987). In H. B. Lewis (Ed.), *Shame: The "sleeper" in psychopathology*. Hillsdale, NJ: Erlbaum.

Littleton, H., & Breitkopf, C. R. (2006). Coping with the experience of rape. *Psychology of Women Quarterly, 30*, 106–116. https://doi.org/10.1111/j.1471-6402.2006.00267.x

Littleton, H. L. (2010). The impact of social support and negative disclosure reactions on sexual assault victims : A cross-sectional and longitudinal investigation. *Journal of Trauma & Dissociation, 11*, 210–227. https://doi.org/10.1080/15299730903502946

Littleton, H. L., Magee, K. T., & Axsom, D. (2007). A meta-analysis of self-attributions following three types of trauma: Sexual victimization, illness, and injury. *Journal of Applied Social Psychology, 37*, 515–538. https://doi.org/10.1111/j.1559-1816.2007.00172.x

Mason, G. E., Ullman, S., Long, S., Long, L., & Starzynski, L. (2009). Social support and risk of sexual assault revictimization. *Journal of Community Psychology, 37*, 58–72. https://doi.org/10.1002/jcop.20270

McConnell, A. A., Messman-Moore, T. L., Gratz, K. L., & DiLillo, D. (2017). Beyond the force–substance dichotomy: Examining the experience of combined and incapacitated type rapes and their relation to PTSD symptoms. *Journal of Interpersonal Violence*, 1–24. https://doi.org/10.1177/0886260517724252

Messman-Moore, T. L., & Long, P. J. (2003). The role of childhood sexual abuse sequelae in the sexual revictimization of women: An empirical review and theoretical reformulation. *Clinical Psychology Review, 23*, 537–571. https://doi.org/10.1016/S0272-7358(02)00203-9

Messman-Moore, T. L., Long, P. J., & Siegfried, N. J. (2000). The revictimization of child sexual abuse survivors: An examination of the adjustment of college women with child sexual abuse, adult sexual assault, and adult physical abuse. *Child Maltreatment, 5*, 18–27. https://doi.org/10.1177/1077559500005001003

Miller, A. K., Canales, E. J., Amacker, A. M., Backstrom, T. L., & Gidycz, C. A. (2011). Stigma-threat motivated nondisclosure of sexual assault and sexual revictimization: A prospective analysis. *Psychology of Women Quarterly, 35*, 119–128. https://doi.org/10.1177/0361684310384104

Miller, A. K., Markman, K. D., & Handley, I. M. (2007). Self-blame among sexual assault victims prospectively predicts revictimization: A perceived sociolegal context model of risk. *Basic and Applied Social Psychology, 29*, 129–136. https://doi.org/10.1080/01973530701331585

Mokma, T. R., Eshelman, L. R., & Messman-Moore, T. L. (2016). Contributions of child sexual abuse, self-blame, posttraumatic stress symptoms, and alcohol use to women's risk for forcible and substance-facilitated sexual assault. *Journal of Child Sexual Abuse, 25*, 428–448. https://doi.org/10.1080/10538712.2016.1161688

Moor, A., & Farchi, M. (2011). Is rape-related self blame distinct from other post traumatic attributions of blame? A comparison of severity and implications for treatment. *Women & Therapy, 34*, 447–460. https://doi.org/10.1080/02703149.2011.591671

Peter-Hagene, L. C., & Ullman, S. E. (2015). Sexual assault-characteristics effects on PTSD and psychosocial mediators: A cluster-analysis approach to sexual assault types. *Psychological Trauma Theory Research Practice and Policy, 7*, 162–170. https://doi.org/10.1037/a0037304

Raine, N. V. (1998). *After silence: Rape and my journey back*. New York, NY: Three Rivers Press.

Resick, P. A., Galovski, T. E., Uhlmansiek, M. O. B., Scher, C. D., Clum, G. A., & Young-Xu, Y. (2008). A randomized clinical trial to dismantle components of cognitive processing therapy for posttraumatic stress disorder in female victims of interpersonal niolence. *Journal of Consulting and Clinical Psychology, 76*, 243–258. https://doi.org/10.1037/0022-006X.76.2.243

Retzinger, S. M. (1995). Identifying shame and anger in discourse. *American Behavioral Scientist, 38*, 1104–1113. https://doi.org/10.1177/0002764295038008006

Roodman, A. A., & Clum, G. A. (2001). Revictimization rates and method variance: A meta-analysis. *Clinical Psychology Review, 21*, 183–204. https://doi.org/10.1016/S0272-7358(99)00045-8

Scheff, T. J. (2003). Shame in self and society. *Symbolic Interaction, 26*, 239–262. https://doi.org/10.1525/si.2003.26.2.239

Sciolla, A., Glover, D. A., Loeb, T. B., Zhang, M., Myers, H. F., & Wyatt, G. E. (2011). Childhood sexual abuse severity and disclosure as predictors of depression among adult African-American and Latina women. *The Journal of Nervous and Mental Disease, 199*, 471–477. https://doi.org/10.1097/NMD.0b013e31822142ac

Sigurvinsdottir, R., & Ullman, S. E. (2015). Social reactions, self-blame, and problem drinking in adult sexual assault survivors. *Psychology of Violence, 5*, 192–198. https://doi.org/10.1037/a0036316

Talbot, N. L. (1996). Women sexually abused as children: The centrality of shame issues and treatment implications. *Psychotherapy, 33*, 11–18. https://doi.org/10.1037/0033-3204.33.1.11

Tangney, J. P., & Dearing, R. L. (2002). *Shame and guilt*. New York, NY: Guildford.

Thornton, B., Ryckman, R. M., Kirchner, G., Jacobs, J., Kaczor, L., & Kuehnel, R. H. (1988). Reaction to self-attributed victim responsibility: A comparative analysis of rape crisis counselors and lay observers. *Journal of Applied Social Psychology, 18*, 409–422. https://doi.org/10.1111/j.1559-1816.1988.tb00025.x

Ullman, S. E. (1997). Attributions, world assumptions, and recovery from sexual assault. *Journal of Child Sexual Abuse, 6*, 1–19. https://doi.org/10.1300/J070v06n01_01

Ullman, S. E. (2007). Relationship to perpetrator, disclosure, social reactions, and PTSD symptoms in child sexual abuse survivors. *Journal of Child Sexual Abuse, 16*, 19–36. https://doi.org/10.1300/J070v16n01_02

Ullman, S. E., & Filipas, H. H. (2001). Predictors of PTSD symptom severity and social reactions in sexual assault victims. *Journal of Traumatic Stress, 14*, 369–389. https://doi.org/10.1023/A:1011125220522

Ullman, S. E., & Filipas, H. H. (2005). Gender differences in social reactions to abuse disclosures, post-abuse coping, and PTSD of child sexual abuse survivors. *Child Abuse & Neglect, 29*, 767–782. https://doi.org/10.1016/j.chiabu.2005.01.005

Ullman, S. E., Filipas, H. H., Townsend, S. M., & Starzynski, L. L. (2007). Psychosocial correlates of PTSD symptom severity in sexual assault survivors. *Journal of Traumatic Stress, 20*, 821–831. https://doi.org/10.1002/jts.20290

Ullman, S. E., & Najdowski, C. J. (2009). Revictimization as a moderator of psychosocial risk factors for problem drinking in female sexual assault survivors. *Journal of Studies on Alcohol and Drugs, 70*, 41–49. https://doi.org/10.15288/jsad.2009.70.41

Ullman, S. E., & Najdowski, C. J. (2011). Prospective changes in attributions of self-blame and social reactions to women's disclosures of adult sexual assault. *Journal of Interpersonal Violence, 26*, 1934–1962. https://doi.org/10.1177/0886260510372940

Ullman, S. E., & Peter-Hagene, L. C. (2016). Longitudinal relationships of social reactions, PTSD, and revictimization in sexual assault survivors. *Journal of Interpersonal Violence, 31*, 1074–1094. https://doi.org/10.1177/0886260514564069

Ullman, S. E., Peter-Hagene, L. C., & Relyea, M. (2014). Coping, emotion regulation, and self-blame as mediators of sexual abuse and psychological symptoms in adult sexual assault. *Journal of Child Sexual Abuse, 23*, 74–93. https://doi.org/10.1080/10538712.2014.864747

Ullman, S. E., Townsend, S. M., Filipas, H. H., & Starzynski, L. L. (2007). Structural models of the relations of assault severity, social support, avoidance coping, self-blame, and PTSD among sexual assault survivors. *Psychology of Women Quarterly, 31*, 23–37. https://doi.org/10.1111/j.1471-6402.2007.00328.x

Vidal, M. E., & Petrak, J. (2007). Shame and adult sexual assault: A study with a group of female survivors recruited from an East London population. *Sexual and Relationship Therapy, 22*, 159–171. https://doi.org/10.1080/14681990600784143

Walster, E. (1966). Assignment of responsibility for an accident. *Journal of Personality and Social Psychology, 3*, 73–79. https://doi.org/10.1037/h0022733

Wilson, J. P., Drozdek, B., & Turkovic, S. (2006). Posttraumatic shame and guilt. *Trauma, Violence & Abuse, 7*, 122–141. https://doi.org/10.1177/1524838005285914

Zinzow, H. M., Seth, P., Jackson, J., Niehaus, A., & Fitzgerald, M. (2010). Abuse and parental characteristics, attributions of blame, and psychological adjustment in adult survivors of child sexual abuse. *Journal of Child Sexual Abuse, 19*, 79–98. https://doi.org/10.1080/10538710903485989

Recovered Memory and Sexual Assault

19

Allie Mann and Amy E. Naugle

Introduction and Background

A true recovered memory has been defined as an event that a person experienced that they could not recall at some later time, and which later can be successfully recalled by the person (Gleaves, Smith, Butler, Spiegel, & Kihlstrom, 2010). A false recovered memory is a memory a person experiences of an event that did not occur. Definitive sorting of memories into either of these categories requires external corroboration of events in a person's life. The majority of scholarly investigation surrounding recovered memories has centered around the recovered memory of child sexual abuse (CSA) in adult survivors (Brown, 2000). This was a hotly debated topic with a substantial amount of empirical/clinical studies and scholarly reaction to reports emerging in the 1990s. In addition to discussion in scholarly communities, ideological groups dominated the popular media discussion during this time and greatly influenced public opinion on the topic. Today, it is widely accepted that both true and false memories exist in the body of recoveries of CSA memories by adults (Belli, 2012; Freyd, 1996; Pezdek & Banks, 1996).

Outside empirical and scholarly investigation of recovered CSA memories, two major ideological groups shaped public opinion of the issue in the United States. The False Memory Syndrome Foundation (FMSF) is an ideological group founded by parents who have been accused of CSA by their adult children and others whose careers were defined by defending men accused of sexually abusing children (Brown, 2000). The current activities of the still operating FMSF includes asserting the innocence of Jerry Sandusky, a convicted serial rapist and child molester who was a football coach at Pennsylvania State University (False Memory Syndrome Foundation, 2018). The FMSF holds the position that intrusive recall is the only true form of traumatic memory; that memory of traumatic events can only be characterized by continuous unwanted imagery following the trauma. They also hold the position that it is impossible for memory of sexual trauma to be forgotten and then subsequently recovered (Loftus & Ketcham, 1994). Some members of the organization have also asserted that CSA is not traumatic to children, stating that "it is not clear that fondling or even fellatio are experienced by infants and young children as assaultive" (p.403), and thus such memories could not be affected by memory disruption associated with trauma (Ceci, Huffman, Smith, & Loftus, 1994). The FMSF asserts that any individuals who claim to recover memories of CSA as adults are afflicted with a "false memory syndrome." This "syndrome" is best defined as a condition in which an individual

A. Mann · A. E. Naugle (✉)
Department of Psychology, Western Michigan University, Kalamazoo, MI, USA
e-mail: amy.naugle@wmich.edu

W. T. O'Donohue and P. A. Schewe (eds.), *Handbook of Sexual Assault and Sexual Assault Prevention*,
https://doi.org/10.1007/978-3-030-23645-8_19

is affected in their relationships and self-identity by the strong belief of a false memory (Michels, 2009), although there are no clear criteria for this "syndrome." False memory syndrome is not included in any major medical or mental health classification systems including the Diagnostic and Statistical Manual of Mental Disorders, fifth ed. (DSM-V) or the International Classification of Diseases, tenth ed. (ICD-10). Trauma researchers have concluded that the possibility of the existence of false memories does not support the existence of a "false memory syndrome," and that there is no empirical evidence of such a syndrome (Gleaves et al., 2010).

The other branch of ideological groups that emerged in the public conversation of recovered memories of CSA is the Incest Survivor Movement. This loosely organized movement has been identified as an opponent to the FMSF (Brown, 2000). While the goal of the FMSF was to advocate for those accused of perpetrating CSA by discrediting victim claims, the goal of the Incest Survivor Movement was to support survivors of CSA by believing them and connecting them to formal and informal resources including networks of other survivors and appropriate medical, psychological, and legal services. It was a grassroots movement comprised of survivors of CSA, with both continuous and recovered memories, sharing first-hand accounts of their abuse as a way to promote empowerment (Bass & Thornton, 1983; McNaron & Morgan, 1982).

Both of these factions were very influential in influencing public opinion on the topic of recovered memories as it pertains to the popular issue of the time, CSA. While both of these politically motivated branches were influenced by the science surrounding memory and trauma, most of their momentum was propelled by anecdotal reports of individuals who claim to have experienced one aspect of the recovered memory phenomenon either first- or second-hand. Alongside this hotly debated popular culture discussion, scientists who were experts in the fields of trauma and memory embarked on a rich investigation of the subject, leading to a more complete and balanced understanding of the topic adopted by the field today.

Empirical Research

An understanding of the trauma experience and traumatic memory initially arose in the field of trauma research from clinical examples of those who had experienced CSA, including those with delayed recall of memory after a period of forgetting (Herman, 1992). There is significant case study evidence of true memories of CSA recovered by adults (e.g. Schooler, Ambadar, & Bendiksen, 1997; Schooler, Bendiksen, & Ambadar, 1997; Williams, 1994, 1995), suggesting that the experience is not uncommon. Empirical evidence has moved beyond case studies and has found support for the existence of both true and false recovered memories. Much of the scholarly activity on this issue is relevant to the conversation of recovered memories of CSA.

False Memory Research

There have been many definitions of a false memory in the literature including, when recalling a list of words, the naming of a word not originally included in the list (Roediger III & McDermott, 1995), an event that has been deceptively suggested to a research participant by a person close to them (Hyman Jr., Husband, & Billings, 1995; Loftus & Pickrell, 1995; Pezdek & Roe, 1994), and a complex trauma perpetrated by a family member that has been falsely suggested to a patient in psychotherapy by a therapist (Loftus & Ketcham, 1994). A general definition of a false memory is a memory of an event that did not occur. It is accepted in the field that false memories do exist, but more uncertainty concerning the question of whether false memories of complex trauma can be adopted by an individual. It is almost impossible to design experiments that study this question directly, due to ethical constraints. Still, the field has used both clinical case studies and empirical laboratory studies to fully investigate the existence and formation of both simple and complex false memories.

One source of evidence for false recovered memories of CSA comes from clinical reports of individuals who claim to have been falsely accused of perpetrating CSA or individuals who claim to have had recovered memory of CSA that they subsequently believe to be false, known as recantors (Gleaves et al., 2010). A small number of studies investigating the experiences of recantors have been conducted (de Rivera, 1997, 2000; Gavigan, 1992; McElroy & Keck Jr., 1995; Nelson & Simpson, 1994; Pasley, 1994). These experiences are more credible than reports of those who claim to be falsely accused of CSA, due to the societal consequences for those who have been found to have perpetrated CSA and potential motivation of those accused to avoid those consequences. However, the concern with these case reports of both scenarios described above is that in most cases there is no way to determine if the recovered memory is in fact false. Even individuals with verifiable histories of abuse have alternated between believing and denying their abuse (Gleaves et al., 2010; Gleaves, 1994), so denying a memory of abuse or believing it to be false is not sufficient evidence to determine with certainty if a person has ever experienced sexual abuse. Only documented external corroboration would provide a definitive answer, which in most cases is impossible to obtain.

An additional source of evidence for false memories more generally comes from laboratory research. Lines of inquiry have included study of and positive evidence for the misinformation effect (Loftus & Palmer, 1974), failures in reality monitoring (Johnson & Raye, 1981), and false recall of word lists (Roediger III & McDermott, 1995). The misinformation effect is a phenomenon that occurs when incorrect information about an event or experience is integrated into a memory after the original event occurs, resulting in inaccurate recall of the original event. In one seminal study of the misinformation effect, Loftus, Miller, and Burns (1978) investigated how post-event information could impact later recall of the original event. Participants were shown slides of a car accident in which a stop sign was present. Then, participants were exposed to information that was either consistent with the original slides (assumed a stop sign was present), misleading about the original slides (assumed a yield sign was present), or irrelevant to the original slides. Finally, participants were asked questions about the original slides. They found that participants exposed to misleading information were more likely to incorrectly remember the original slides. This study demonstrates that post-event misinformation can negatively impact memory accuracy.

Reality monitoring consists of correct identification of information that originated externally (information individuals perceive through the senses) and information that originated internally (through thoughts, dreams, or other internal experiences). Failures in reality monitoring occur when individuals misattribute the source of information or experiences. Johnson and Raye (1981) propose a model of reality monitoring that suggests that there are differences between internal originating and external originating information, and individuals use different cues to determine what the origin of specific information or memories are. They suggest that externally originating memories might contain more sensory, semantic, or contextual details and internally originating memories might contain more details about cognitive operations. This working model has created a framework with which to start to evaluate the "reality" of memories. Deficits in reality monitoring are thought to be one way in which false memories are adopted by adults who believe to have recovered true childhood memories.

The correct recall of a word in a list has been treated as analogous to the correct recall of a memory of any length and complexity. For example, Roediger III and McDermott (1995) conducted a study attempting to make participants recall a word as a member of a list they had studied, when in fact that word was never on the original list. Participants were given a list of 12 words to study. The words on the list were related to some other word that was not included in the list. For example, the list might be comprised of words such as bed, dream, and pillow, which are all related to the word "sleep," which is not presented in the list. Results indicated that almost half the participants incorrectly recalled the related, nonpresented word as being part of the original list. This line of research indicates that individuals can be made to report things that did not happen.

Most of this laboratory research with the aim of investigating false memory as it relates to CSA involved the use of schema-consistent suggestion of neutral events in nonclinical subjects (Gleaves et al., 2010), such as lines of research that use word or picture sequence recall as an analog for memories of personal, complex experiences such as sexual abuse. Thus, lines of research that focus on narrow or brief memory impairment may not be directly applicable to more complex memories such as recovered memories of CSA. One line of inquiry with more applicability to such memories is the question of the impact of suggestibility on memory.

There are two major tests of suggestion pursued in the literature, the possibility to change a recalled memory and the possibility to encode information or events that never occurred as memories (Brown, 2000). Loftus (1979) was a leader in investigating the impact of suggestion on eyewitness memory. They found that in a number of studies a portion of participants will report a different memory of an experimental event due to experimental suggestion in a particular direction (Loftus & Davies, 1984; Loftus & Hoffman, 1989; Loftus & Loftus, 1980; Loftus, 1979, 1979). Loftus & Davies (1984) suggested in a survey of eyewitness literature that adults are able to more correctly recall events that have happened to them than are children, but children might not more susceptible to suggestion than adults. They concluded that both children and adults are vulnerable to suggestion in eyewitness scenarios. Loftus & Hoffman (1989) discusses potential sources of memory impairment including source misattribution, or confusion concerning the origin of a memory item, and asserts that this is a prominent phenomenon that occurs in the misinformation effect. They concede, however, that the mechanism of adopting the misinformation (e.g. interfering with an original memory or standing independently) is unknown. Loftus & Loftus (1980) assert that there is no such thing as permeant, unchangeable long-term memory and concludes that all memory is theoretically susceptible to post-event alteration. However, other investigations suggest that Loftus' low-stakes experimental settings might be responsible for the results. Participants in laboratory studies do not have the same emotional relationship with memories as real-world individuals who experience an event. Further, the consequences of error are more extreme in real-world contexts than in laboratory contexts. Other investigations into real forensic eyewitness situations find lower susceptibility to suggestion when the stakes are higher, as they are in real life (Yuille & Cutshall, 1989; Yuille, 1993). It is also suggested that the type of crime or event witnessed by an individual might impact their memory performance.

Ceci et al. (1994) and Ceci, Ross, and Toglia (1987) developed another line of inquiry investigating how vulnerable children are to suggestibility. In these studies, children were read either a passage about an event they are told that they have experienced but have not, or a story about an unrelated topic, and then questioned on their memory of their own lives or the presented story. The results indicate that children are vulnerable to suggestion. Ceci et al. (1994) conducted a study attempting to implant a memory of an event that can be shown to have not occurred, and to have that memory be accepted by very young children. Participants in this study were 96 preschool children of diverse sociodemographic composition. This study investigated age differences of the children and thus one group was composed of younger preschoolers aged 3–4 years and a second group was composed of older preschoolers aged 5–6 years. The children were presented with a list of events they had experienced mixed with events they had not experienced, and subsequently asked which events had actually happened to them once a week for 10 weeks. Results indicated that while children were made to adopt some memories of events that did not happen to them, the frequency of this did not increase over time. Importantly, children were overwhelmingly accurate in identifying that the real events did in fact happen to them. In this study, older children were more accurate in their memory than younger children.

Ceci, Ross, and Toglia (1987) presented several experiments examining the eyewitness memory of children, ranging throughout the experiments from preschool to early middle school age. In one experiment, children were read a story from a picture book and then asked questions that were either neutral or leading concerning the pictures accompanying the story. Results of this experiment indicated that there was no difference in memory between ages when children were asked neutral questions, but younger children were much more susceptible to suggestion in the leading question condition. However, in other experiments when conditions were altered, age differences between young and very young children disappeared. However, further studies might complicate these findings. Others have found in similar studies that fewer individuals are vulnerable to suggestion (McClouskey and Zaragoza 1985; Zaragoza, McCloskey & Jamis, 1987; Zaragoza, 1991), including suggestion with CSA overtones (Goodman, Quas, Batterman-Faunce, Riddlesberger & Kuhn, 1994; Goodman, Bottoms, Schwartz-Kenney & Rudy, 1991; Pezdek & Roe 1994), than were reported in Ceci's investigations.

Zaragoza, McCloskey, and Jamis (1987) examined the effect of post-event information on subject's memory of an event, utilizing a similar method to Ceci's memory experiments with children. Participants were undergraduate students who viewed a series of slides depicting a scene or event. Participants then read a lengthy written narrative about the slides that was either neutral (did not provide information contradicting what was viewed in the slides) or misleading (contained information contradicting what was viewed in the slides). In two experiments following this protocol, Zaragoza, McCloskey, and Jamis (1987) found no difference in recall accuracy between the neutral and mislead groups. The authors present explanations as to why their results seems so different than others who investigate misleading post-event information's effect on memory. They assert that other studies are not detecting true changes in an original memory and are failing to account for phenomenon such as forgetting, response bias, and non-encoding of original event information.

McClouskey and Zaragoza (1985) even go so far as to claim that their series of six experiments, with methods and results similar to the two Zaragoza, McCloskey, and Jamis (1987) experiments, prove that post-event misleading information has no effect on memory of the original event. They argue that while post-event information might influence response to questions about an event, actual memory of what a person experienced of an event is unchanged. This finding is important as it may demonstrate that more extreme circumstances are required to develop a true false memory. The work of McClouskey and Zaragoza (1985) and Zaragoza, McCloskey, and Jamis (1987) is likely more applicable to the issue at hand of cases of individuals who are reporting recovered memories of CSA as adults, as it investigates memory error originating in adulthood. The work of Ceci et al. (1994) and Ceci, Ross & Toglia (1987) is likely more applicable to individuals who are children reporting current or past experiences of CSA.

Pezdek and Roe (1994) investigated the resiliency of children's memory. In one experiment, a group of 4-year-old children and a group of 10-year-old children were shown a series of slides either once or twice. Following viewing of the slides, the children were read a narrative summarizing the slides that either did or did not contain misleading information about the slides. The results of this experiment indicated that "stronger" memories, or memories of events that have occurred multiple times, are resistant to suggestion regardless of age. This finding is particularly salient to individuals who are reporting CSA experiences, where children are often victimized multiple times by the same perpetrator.

A second experiment conducted by Pezdek and Roe (1994) investigated how vulnerable children are to suggestions with sexual overtones. In this experiment 10-year-old children were individually shown slides by an experimenter who throughout the activity either touched the child's shoulder, touched the child's hand, or did not touch the child. The children were later read statements that either confirmed what had actually happened in the session or presented misleading information (e.g., That the experimenter had touched the child's shoulder when the experimenter had actually touched the child's hand). The results of this experiment indicated that children did not easily adopt the suggestion. This finding suggests that it is not easy to convince a child that something happened to them that did not happen in reality. This is a distinct finding from other studies of suggestion that include suggesting a slight change in an event the individual knows to have occurred.

One study conducted by Loftus (1993) provides evidence for the possibility to implant false memories. In this study, an undergraduate research assistant experimentally convinced their younger sibling that they had been lost in a shopping mall as a child. The sibling adopted the "lost in a shopping mall" story as a memory they believed to be true. While there have been ethical criticisms of the conduct of this study, its results are applicable to the conversation of recovered memory of CSA and questions of the ability to retroactively "implant" memories of events that did not occur. Hyman, Husband, and Billings (1995) conducted a larger variation of this study in which parents of college students told their children stories of actual events that had happened to them and scattered in false suggestions, such as an experience of needing to go to the hospital due to a severe earache as a child. The results of this study reported that 20% of participants adopted the suggestion, and most participants required multiple exposures to the suggestion in order to adopt it.

Loftus's (1993) study has been questioned in terms of its applicability to CSA (Gleaves et al., 2010) due to the content of the suggested memory being relatively common and nontraumatic. Pezdek (1995) attempted to extend this line of research to suggesting a more traumatic event (a rectal enema) to research participants. This suggestion was not adopted by any participants in this study. Some have argued that Pezdek's (1995) study indicates that although it is less difficult to achieve adoption of a suggestion of neutral material (mall or earache), it is more difficult to achieve adoption via suggestion of false stories of extremely painful events that violate a person's beliefs about loved individuals (Brown, 2000), as would be the case with implanting a false memory of CSA.

For ethical reasons, it is impossible to empirically test directly if false memories of CSA can be adopted by individuals, leaving an obvious gap in the literature on this topic. The experimental research that we do have on false memory demonstrates that under some conditions individuals can report memory of events that are false or report observing things that were not observed. However, there are several limitations to the body of false memory research as it has been applied to the conversation around recovered memory and CSA. The body of research may only suggest that individuals are likely to adopt false memories in situations where the stakes are low, and the degree to which these reported errors are in fact fully adopted false memories has been questioned (Gleaves et al., 2010). The degree to which these lines of inquiry can be generalized to cases of recovered memory of CSA has been questioned as well (Butler & Speigel, 1997; Freyd & Gleaves, 1996). The research clearly suggests that memory is fallible, and that memory error could result in the adoption of a false memory of CSA is a distinct possibility.

Recovered Memory Research

There have been several names in the trauma literature for the phenomenon of recovered or delayed trauma memories including dissociative amnesia, repressed memory, and posttraumatic amnesia (Brown, 2000). A considerable number of case studies have accumulated documenting recovered memories of various traumatic experiences (Cheit, 1998; Corwin & Olafson, 1997; Freyd, 1996; Scheflin & Brown, 1996; Schooler, Beudikson & Ambadar, 1997; Williams, 1994, 1995). In a notable case study, Duggal and Strouge (1998) detail a woman who recovered memories of CSA outside of the context of therapy. In this case several sources corroborate the occurrence of the CSA, the forgetting, and the recovery event. The author interprets this case as evidence for memory loss with an explanation beyond simple childhood amnesia.

The most important and reliable case studies that have been considered on this topic are those that can be corroborated. One such notable and illustrative case study was presented by Corwin and Olafson (1997). In this case a young girl, "Jane," was videotaped reporting sexual abuse at the hands of her mother when she was 6 years old when talking to a psychologist who was investigating the custody situation of Jane. The doctor, after using the tape for teaching purposes reached out to Jane at age 17 to reattain her consent to use the tape. At that time, Jane did not remember the contents of the tape and asked to see it. Before watching it, in a videotaped conversation with the doctor, Jane recovered the memory of the abuse as a child. This case is significant because of the documentation, and the ability to compare Jane's reports both as a child and as a 17-year-old. Corwin and Olafson (1997) discuss that while Jane did not remember every event of her abuse that she reported at age 6, the events that she remembered after the recovery at age 17 were consistent with her original report. This case, while an isolated example, provides evidence that a noncontinuous memory can be an accurate memory.

Beyond individual case examples, a large-scale study of adult survivors of CSA contacted by authorities who had documented original CSA incidents provides evidence for the prevalence of forgetting CSA experiences as an adult. Williams (1994) and Williams (1995) interviewed 129 adult women (age 18–31) who had disclosed their CSA experiences to authorities as children at the initial time of their abuse. The women were asked a series of questions to determine if they recalled the abuse at the time of the interview and, if so, if there was ever a period of time where they had forgotten the abuse. Williams (1994) reported that 38% of the women in the sample did not remember their abuse at all. In this study they found that being younger at the time of the initial abuse and women who were abused by a family member (or other known person) were more likely to report not remembering the abuse. Williams (1995) reported that 16% of the women who remembered the abuse at the time of the interview had entirely forgotten the abuse at some point in the past, and therefore had recovered memories. Importantly, Williams (1995) reported that women with recovered memories, defined as women who reported a period of forgetting the memory of their abuse, were just as accurate in their memory of the abuse as women with continuous memories of their abuse. The accumulation of these larger studies along with the numerous case studies implies that forgetting experiences of CSA, and even subsequently recovering those CSA memories, might not be uncommon in the general population.

Experiences of the forgetting and ensuing recovery of trauma memories are also common in studies of clinical populations who have experienced child physical and sexual abuse (Gleaves et al., 2010; Brown, Scheflin & Whittfield, 1999), suggesting that the real-world experience of a trauma, which would be difficult to replicate in laboratory settings for ethical reasons, is the best scenario to investigate the existence and course of recovered memories. The field has certainly reached a balanced consensus on the subject of the existence of recovered memories of sexual abuse. The American Psychological Association itself put together a working group to evaluate this issue and determined that while false memories can be created through suggestion, it is also possible to recover memories of CSA as an adult (Sales, 1998). All recovered memories are not false memories, and further there is no evidence that the continuity of a memory determines its accuracy (Freyd & DePrince, 2001; Dalenberg, 1996; Pope & Brown, 1996; Scheflin & Brown, 1996; Williams, 1995). While there is strong evidence for the existence of the recovered memory phenomenon, the evidence for the process by which forgetting and recovery occurs is less complete.

There are several lines of empirical inquiry that have yielded evidence for the mechanisms that might lead to forgetting and recovering memories including: spontaneous recovery from retroactive interference (Wheeler, 1995), tip of the tongue research (Jones, 1989; Smith, 1994), blocking in implicit memory (Lustig & Hasher,

2001; Smith & Tindell, 1997), and retrieval-induced forgetting (Anderson, Bjork & Bjork, 1994). Spontaneous recovery is the improvement in memory over time without practice or additional exposure. Wheeler (1995) conducted a study in which subjects were repeatedly presented a list of pictures, tested on their initial recall of the list, and then tested again after a delay in time. The results of this study demonstrated that subjects could exhibit spontaneous recovery over time in memory of a presented list of pictures, as for several participants their memory improved on the second delayed recall test. Jones (1989) investigated the tip-of-the-tongue phenomenon, or the reported feeling of almost being able to remember something. They discussed that the tip-of-the-tongue state can lead to recall of similar memory items to the target memory item and suggested that the tip-of-the-tongue state might be caused by present events interfering with retrieval of the target memory item.

Lustig and Hasher (2001) investigated the impact of early items from a list on later items on a list when the early items were intended distractors, similar to the later items on the list. This is an investigation of the potential for proactive blocking or interference. The results indicated that the presentation of certain early list words could decrease later recall of later list words, affirming the vulnerability of memory to proactive interference. Smith and Tindell (1997) conducted a variation of Lustig and Hasher's (2001) study, with the alteration that participants were warned of the memory blocking potential and instructed to specifically only remember the words at the end of the list. Results of this study were consistent with the results of Lustig and Hasher (2001), indicating that even when individuals are aware of memory blocking risks, the effect remains essentially unchanged. Anderson, Bjork, and Bjork (1994) discuss the possibility that retrieving and recalling information from long-term memory can lead to forgetting of that information. It is hypothesized that the encoding of new information that accompanies retrieval of old information might be the culprit. In a series of experiments, Anderson, Bjork, and Bjork (1994) find that repeatedly retrieving information can decrease recall of related information, the more closely related the related cue is to the target information the more robust this impairment becomes, and that this memory impairment can be long term (stretching beyond the immediate experimental situation).

These lines of research provide evidence for the phenomenon of forgetting information, including traumatic information through a variety of hypothesized processes. However, the precise mechanisms for posttraumatic amnesia, or the process of forgetting a traumatic memory before recovery, are not understood. Little direct laboratory research on the process exists, due to the ethical constraints creating a barrier to experimentally simulating trauma. However, there are theories that might move in the direction of pointing to a cognitive mechanism of forgetting. Two theories that attempt to describe such a mechanism are Betrayal Trauma Theory (Freyd, 1996) and dissociation more broadly.

Betrayal Trauma Theory (BTT) asserts that the effects of a traumatic experience are related to the level of interpersonal or social betrayal in the trauma. In this aim, CSA is highly traumatic because it has a high level of social betrayal. Supporters of this theory argue that evolutionarily it may be adaptive to block the memory of betrayal (CSA) while the individual is still a child due to the continued dependence on caregivers for survival. There is empirical support for the prediction of BTT that abuse by family perpetrators will be forgotten more than abuse by nonfamily perpetrators of CSA (Belli, 2012; Freyd, DePrince & Zurbriggen, 2001; Freyd, Klest & DePrince, 2010; Lindblom & Gray, 2010). Similarly, it has been found that rates of forgetting do vary between trauma types (Gleaves et al., 2010, Freyd & DePrince, 2001; Elliott, 1997), suggesting that the impact trauma has on memory is related to the level of social betrayal of the trauma. BTT supposes that it is effective for a person to forget CSA trauma, especially when perpetrated by someone socially significant such as a caregiver, until the danger has passed and the individual has more autonomy. Once the individual is out of danger, likely by becoming an adult, it is no longer necessary for survival that the memory be inaccessible, and therefore the memory may become accessible again.

Dissociation has also been suggested as the mechanism accounting for posttraumatic amnesia (Yates & Nasby, 1993). Spiegel (1986) suggested that dissociation might block pain from a traumatic experience. As is also suggested in BTT, this may become maladaptive without continuing or subsequent trauma (Duggal & Stroufe, 1998), leading to a recovery. However, the exact relationship between dissociation and trauma is complex and not completely understood (Chiu, Yeh, Ross & Lin, 2012; Giesbrecht, Lynn, Lilienfeld & Merckelbach, 2008; Bremmer, 2010). It has been established in the literature that there are individual differences in trait dissociation, such that some individuals have more dissociative experiences than others even outside of the context of trauma (Freyd & DePrince, 2001; Freyd, 1996). Dissociation is thought to contribute to psychiatric disorders including PTSD (Freyd &DePrince, 2001; Bremner et al., 1992; Carlson & Putnam, 1993; Marmar et al., 1994). In fact, trait dissociation has been found to be high in trauma survivor populations (Freyd & DePrince, 2001; Bremner et al., 1992; Carlson & Putnam, 1993; Marmar et al., 1994; Putnam & Trickett, 1997).

Freyd et al. (1998) conducted a study investigating the relationship between dissociation and attention. Results of this study suggest a relationship between dissociative tendencies and selective attention. Controlled attentional abilities were disturbed in individuals with high trait dissociation, in that high dissociators performed worse on the selective attention directed task. It is important to note that these disruptions were not related to the emotional content of the situation. In other words, dissociation negatively impacted attention even when the situation was not distressing, indicating that the high impact of trait dissociation on attention is independent of context. By interfering with attention and the encoding of information, trait dissociation might be a mechanism that accounts for the forgetting or recovery of traumatic memories, or memories in general. This relationship between dissociation and attention is made more salient by other studies that have established a relationship between trauma and dissociation, such that individuals with high trait dissociation are more likely to have experienced more traumatic events (Freyd, 1996).

DePrince and Freyd (1999) conducted another relevant study investigating dissociative tendencies and memory. They found that participants with high trait dissociation, compared to participants with low trait dissociation, remembered fewer emotionally charged words and more emotionally neutral words. Trait dissociation in this way might explain posttraumatic amnesia. Further, laboratory studies have shown that dissociation does not relate to false recognition (Chiu et al., 2012; Platt, Lacey, Iobst & Finkelman, 1998; Geraerts, Smeets, Jelicic, van Heerden & Merckelbach, 2005). One study found that when recovered memories are associated with dissociative tendencies they have a corroboration rate of 86% (Chiu et al., 2012).

While most people who experience CSA do not forget the experience, the experience of forgetting and recovering true CSA memories does occur (Duggal & Strouge, 1998) and might not be uncommon (Williams, 1994, 1995). Though the occurrence of recovered memories is recognized by most trauma researchers and the APA (Sales, 1998), the mechanism for this phenomenon is not well understood. However, there is some evidence that dissociation (DePrince & Freyd, 1999) or betrayal trauma (Freyd, 1996) processes may contribute to forgetting and recovering memories of CSA.

The theory of betrayal trauma starts to move toward a mechanism that might explain why victims forget experiences of CSA, as well as explain why as an individual's environment changes they might be more inclined to recover the previously inaccessible memory. Empirical evidence of rates of forgetting supports this theory and suggests that it is on the right track. Investigation into dissociation moves even closer toward a mechanism that may account for major memory interference surrounding trauma and CSA. However, cognitive psychology does not have a more precise mechanism that accounts for the forgetting and subsequent recall of CSA that is experienced by some survivors. Further insight into the constructs and mechanisms of memory are required for a deeper understanding of recovered memory. This knowledge gap does not obscure the evidence that the phenomena of true recovered memories does exist in a minority of trauma survivors.

Treatment Implications

When considering cases of recovered memories in the context of sexual assault or CSA, there are two major considerations for practitioners: supporting survivors of trauma and not aiding in the formation of false memories. The evidence firmly supports that recovering memory of CSA is a real phenomenon, and survivors should not be denied access to care if they report this experience. There is no such thing as a false memory syndrome, and as such those who have recovered memories should receive care only for their reported trauma symptoms and not for memory problems. Whether memory of trauma is continuous or was lost and subsequently recovered, the trauma of sexual assault is linked to many physical and psychological problems that survivors may need assistance with.

It is also firmly established that memory is likely vulnerable to suggestion or other influence, and false recovered memories are also a true phenomenon. Practitioners must be mindful to not aid in the formation of false memories. The literature provides several clues as to some best practices for practitioners. There are several historical therapeutic strategies that should be avoided, and special consideration should be followed when working with children, who may be especially vulnerable to the formation of false memories. Therapist malpractice leading to the creation of false memories has resulted in lawsuits (Brown, 2000) and harm to individuals as well as families. Strategies such as hypnosis and guided recall should not be used to retrieve potential forgotten memories, and recovery of memories should not be a goal of therapy. Beyond case examples, some scholarly activity has addressed the question of what practices should be avoided by treatment providers in order to decrease the risk of aiding in the formation of false memories.

Loftus and Loftus (1980) discuss dubious methods for attempting to retrieve forgotten memories, under the assumption that memories are fixed items that exist somewhere in the mind. These methods include brain stimulations, hypnosis, and Freudian psychoanalysis. Brain stimulation techniques that were used specifically to identify memories include using electrodes to send electrical impulses directly to the cerebral cortex. Hypnosis involves encouraging individuals to enter a trance-like state before asking questions or exploring other internal experiences. Psychoanalysis involves the assumptions that client difficulties can be traced back to early childhood experiences or unresolved issues of which the client may have no memory.

All of these methods are likely to introduce suggestion into the memory and may increase the likelihood for the development of false memories. Treatment providers should avoid these methods, as well as avoiding stating recovering a forgotten memory as a treatment goal. Some clients also may seek aid in determining if a recovered memory is true or false. Research on the topic of reality monitoring might provide some assistance to this end. Johnson and Raye (1981) suggested that memories with an external origin might contain more sensory or contextual details than memories with an internal origin. However, the distinction is not an exact science and it will likely be impossible for practitioners to know for sure if a memory of abuse is true or false without external corroboration.

When working with younger children care must be taken to avoid aiding in the creation of false memories. As discussed in Ceci et al. (1994), presenting known real and known false events together might increase memory error in children. Additionally, asking children to talk about what might have happened, or some variation of asking a child to imagine if an event had happened to them, may also increase likelihood of false memory creation. This might be explained in younger children by a desire to confirm the statements of adults or authority figures, as is suggested by Ceci, Ross & Toglia (1987). These memory disturbances could result in later experiences of forgetting and recovering memories that could be difficult for children to work through and discern.

Conclusions

Despite the historical conversations surrounding recovered memory and CSA, it is without question that forgetting and recovering memories of CSA is real and experienced by adult CSA survivors. The experience might even be a relatively common occurrence. It is also true that false memories can be created through processes such as suggestion, and people can make false reports of their experiences in experimental settings. Based on this information, it is important that adults who recover memories of CSA should not be discounted. The proposed mechanisms of forgetting involved in recovered memories are not associated with decreased memory accuracy, so recovering a memory does not necessarily make it a false memory. Other memory research suggests that unlike false memories, true memories are more likely to be held with confidence and clarity (Gleaves et al., 2010; Oakes & Hyman, 2000; Pezdek & Taylor, 2000), and even if peripheral details are less accurate central details are well-maintained (Christianson, 1992). These guidelines might help to differentiate between true and false recovered memoires, but without external corroboration no memory can be definitively labeled as true or false. It is clear that memory is likely vulnerable to suggestion, so practitioners should avoid aiding in recovering memories as a treatment goal, as the possibility of creating a false memory is high if using certain therapeutic techniques. When working with individuals who have recovered memories of sexual abuse, it is most important for practitioners to prioritize the safety and care of the survivor.

References

Anderson, M. C., Bjork, R. A., & Bjork, E. L. (1994). Remembering can cause forgetting: Retrieval dynamics in long-term memory. *Journal of Experimental Psychology. Learning, Memory, and Cognition, 20*, 1063–1087.

Bass, E., & Thornton, L. (Eds.). (1983). *I never told anyone: Writing by women survivors of child sexual abuse*. New York: Harper Colophon.

Belli, R. F. (2012). *True and false recovered memories: Toward a reconciliation of the debate*. New York: Springer.

Bremmer, J. D. (2010). Cognitive processes in dissociation: Comment on Giesbbrecht et al. (2008). *Psychological Bulletin, 136*, 1–6.

Bremner, J. D., Southwick, S., Brett, E., Fontana, A., Rosenheck, R., & Charney, D. (1992). Dissociation and posttraumatic stress disorder in Vietnam combat veterans. *American Journal of Psychiatry, 149*(3), 328–332.

Brown, D., Scheflin, A. W., & Whitfield, C. L. (1999). Recovered memories: The current weight of the evidence in science and in the courts. *Journal of Psychiatry & Law, 27*, 5–156.

Brown, L. S. (2000). The controversy concerning recovered memory of traumatic events. In A. Y. Shalev, R. Yehuda, & A. C. McFarlane (Eds.), *International handbook of human response to trauma* (Springer Series on Stress and Coping). Boston, MA: Springer.

Butler, L. D., & Spiegel, D. (1997). Trauma and memory. In L. J. Dickstein, M. B. Riba, & J. M. Oldham (Eds.), *American Psychiatric Press review of psychiatry* (Vol. 16, pp. II-13–II-53). Arlington, VA: American Psychiatric Association.

Carlson, E. B., & Putnam, F. W. (1993). An update on the dissociative experiences scale. *Dissociation, 6*, 16–27.

Ceci, S. J., Huffman, M. L. C., Smith, E., & Loftus, E. F. (1994). Repeatedly thinking about a non-event; source misattributions among preschoolers. *Consciousness and Cognition, 3*, 388–407.

Ceci, S. J., Ross, D. F., & Toglia, M. P. (1987). Suggestibility of children's memory: Psycholegal implications. *Journal of Experimental Psychology, 116*, 38–49.

Cheit, R. E. (1998). Consider this, skeptics of recovered memory. *Ethics & Behavior, 8*, 141–160.

Chiu, C., Yeh, Y., Ross, C. A., Lin, S., Huang, W., & Hwu, H. (2012). Recovered memory experience in a nonclinical sample is associated with dissociation rather than with aversive experiences. *Psychiatry Research, 197*(3), 265–269.

Christianson, S. A. (1992). Emotional stress and eyewitness memory. *Psychological Bulletin, 112*, 284–309.

Corwin, D. L., & Olafson, E. (1997). Videotaped discovery of a reportedly unrecallable memory of child sexual abuse: Comparison with a childhood interview videotaped 11 years before. *Child Maltreatment, 2*, 91–112.

de Rivera, J. (1997). The construction of False Memory Syndrome: The experience of retractors. *Psychological Inquiry, 8*, 271–292.

de Rivera, J. (2000). Understanding persons who repudiate memories recovered in therapy. *Professional Psychology: Research and Practice, 31*, 378–386.

Dalenberg, C. J. (1996). Accuracy, timing and circumstances of disclosure in therapy of recovered and continuous memories of abuse. *Journal of Psychiatry and Law, 24*, 229–275.

DePrince, A. P., & Freyd, J. J. (1999). Dissociative tendencies, attention, and memory. *Psychological Science, 10*, 449–452.

Duggal, S., & Stroufe, L. A. (1998). Recovered memory of childhood sexual trauma: A documented case from a longitudinal study. *Journal of Traumatic Stress, 11*(2), 301–321.

Elliott, D. M. (1997). Traumatic events: Prevalence and delayed recall in the general population. *Journal of Consulting and Clinical Practice, 65*, 811–820.

False Memory Syndrome Foundation (2018, January 7). The Most Hated Man in America. Retrieved from http://www.fmsfonline.org/index.php?news2018update=TheMost Hated Man in America

Freyd, J. J. (1996). *Betrayal trauma theory: The logic of forgetting childhood abuse*. Cambridge, MA: Harvard University Press.

Freyd, J. J., & DePrince, A. P. (2001). Perspectives on memory for trauma and cognitive processes associated with dissociative tendencies. *Journal of Aggression, Maltreatment & Trauma, 4*(2), 137–163.

Freyd, J. J., DePrince, A. P., & Zurbriggen, E. L. (2001). Self-reported Memory for abuse depends upon victim-perpetrator relationship. *Journal of Trauma & Dissociation, 2*(3), 5–17.

Freyd, J. J., & Gleaves, D. H. (1996). Remembering words not presented in lists: Relevance to the current recovered/false memory controversy. *Journal of Experimental Psychology: Learning, Memory, and Cognition, 22*, 811–813.

Freyd, J. J., Klest, B., & DePrince, A. P. (2010). Avoiding awareness of betrayal: Comment on Lindblom and Gray (2009). *Applied Cognitive Psychology, 24*(1), 20–26.

Freyd, J. J., Martorello, S. R., Alvarado, J. S., Hayes, A. E., & Christman, J. C. (1998). Cognitive environments and dissociative tendencies: Performance on the standard Stroop task for high versus low dissociators. *Applied Cognitive Psychology, 12*, S91–S103.

Gavigan, M. (1992). False memories of childhood sexual abuse: A personal account. *Issues in Child Abuse Accusations, 4*, 246–247.

Geraerts, E., Smeets, E., Jelicic, M., van Heerden, J., & Merckelbach, H. (2005). Fantasy proneness, but not self-reported trauma is related to DRM performance of women reporting recovered memories of childhood sexual abuse. *Consciousness and Cognition, 14*, 602–612.

Giesbrecht, T., Lynn, S. J., Lilienfeld, S. O., & Merckelbach, H. (2008). Cognitive processes in dissociation: An analysis of core theoretical assumptions. *Psychological Bulletin, 134*, 617–647.

Gleaves, D. H. (1994). On the reality of repressed memories. *American Psychologist, 49*, 440–441.

Gleaves, D. H., Smith, S. M., Butler, L. D., Spiegel, D., & Kihlstrom, J. E. (2010). In B. Slife (Ed.), *Are the recovered memories of psychological trauma valid?* (16th ed.). New York, NY: McGraw-Hill.

Goodman, G. S., Bottoms, B. L., Schwartz-Kenney, B., & Rudy, L. A. (1991). Children's memory for a stressful event: Improving children's report. *Journal of Narrative and Life History, 1*, 69–99.

Goodman, G. S., Quas, J. A., Batterman-Faunce, J. M., Riddlesberger, M. M., & Kuhn, J. (1994). Predictors of accurate and inaccurate memories of traumatic events experienced in childhood. *Consciousness and Cognition, 3*, 269–294.

Herman, J. L. (1992). *Trauma and recovery*. New York: Basic Books.

Hyman, I. E., Jr., Husband, T. H., & Billings, F. J. (1995). False memories of childhood experiences. *Applied Cognitive Psychology, 9*, 181–187.

Johnson, M. K., & Raye, C. L. (1981). Reality monitoring. *Psychological Review, 88*, 67–85.

Jones, G. V. (1989). Back to Woodworth: The role of interlopers in the tip of the tongue phenomenon. *Memory & Cognition, 17*, 69–76.

Lindblom, K. M., & Gray, M. J. (2010). Relationship closeness and trauma narrative detail: A critical analysis of betrayal trauma theory. *Applied Cognitive Psychology, 24*(1), 1–19.

Loftus, E., Miller, D., & Burns, H. (1978). Semantic integration of verbal information into a visual memory. *Journal of Experimental Psychology: Human Learning and Memory, 4*(1), 19–31.

Loftus, E. F. (1979). *Eyewitness testimony*. Cambridge, MA: Harvard University Press.

Loftus, E. F. (1993). The reality of repressed memories. *American Psychologist, 48*, 518–537.

Loftus, E. F., & Davies, G. M. (1984). Distortions in the memory of children. *Journal of Social Issues, 40*, 51–67.

Loftus, E. F., & Hoffman, H. G. (1989). Misinformation and memory: The creation of new memories. *Journal of Experimental Psychology, 118*, 100–104.

Loftus, E. F., & Ketcham, K. (1994). *The myth of repressed memory: False memories and allegations of abuse*. New York: St. Martin's Press.

Loftus, E. F., & Loftus, G. (1980). On the permanence of stored information in the human brain. *American Psychologist, 35*, 409–420.

Loftus, E. F., & Palmer, J. C. (1974). Reconstruction of automobile destruction: An example of the interaction between language and memory. *Journal of Verbal Learning and Verbal Behavior, 13*, 585–589.

Loftus, E. F., & Pickrell, J. E. (1995). The formation of false memories. *Psychiatric Annals, 25*(12), 720–725.

Lustig, C., & Hasher, L. (2001). Implicit memory is vulnerable to proactive interference. *Psychological Bulletin, 127*, 618–628.

Marmar, C. R., Weiss, D. S., Schlenger, W. E., Fairbank, J. A., Jordan, B. K., Kulka, R. A., & Hough, R. L. (1994). Peritraumatic dissociation and posttraumatic stress in male Vietnam theater veterans. *American Journal of Psychiatry, 151*, 902–907.

McCloskey, M., & Zaragoza, M. A. (1985). Misleading postevent information and memory for events: Arguments and evidence against memory impairment hypotheses. *Journal of Experimental Psychology: General, 114*, 1–16.

McElroy, S. L., & Keck, P. E., Jr. (1995). The formation of false memories. *Psychiatric Annals, 25*, 720–725.

McNaron, T., & Morgan, Y. (Eds.). (1982). *Voices in the nights: Women speaking out about incest*. Minneapolis: Cleis Press.

Michels, R. (2009). Try to remember: Psychiatry's clash over meaning, memory, and mind. *American Journal of Psychiatry, 166*(6), 733–734.

Nelson, E. L., & Simpson, P. (1994). First glimpse: An initial examination of subjects who have rejected their visualizations as false memories. *Issues in Child Abuse Accusations, 6*, 123–133.

Oakes, M. A., & Hyman, I. E. (2000). The changing face of memory and self. In D. F. Bjorklund (Ed.), *False-memory creation in children and adults* (pp. 45–67). Mahwah, NJ: Erlbaum.

Pasley, L. (1994). Misplaced trust: A first-person account of how my therapist created false memories. *Skeptic, 2*, 62–67.

Pezdek, K. (1995). What types of false childhood memories are not likely to be suggestively implanted. Presented at the Annual Meeting of the Psychonomic Society, Los Angeles, CA.

Pezdek, K., & Banks, W. P. (Eds.). (1996). *The recovered memory/false memory debate*. San Diego, CA: Academic Press.

Pezdek, K., & Roe, C. (1994). Memory for childhood events: How suggestible is it? *Consciousness and Cognition, 3*, 374–387.

Pezdek, K., & Taylor, J. (2000). Discriminating between accounts of true and false events. In D. F. Bjorklund (Ed.), *False-memory creation in children and adults* (pp. 69–91). Mahwah, NJ: Erlbaum.

Platt, R. D., Lacey, S. C., Iobst, A. D., & Finkelman, D. (1998). Absorption, dissociation, and fantasy proneness as predictors of memory distortion in autobiographical and laboratory-generated memories. *Applied Cognitive Psychology, 12*, S77–S89.

Pope, K. S., & Brown, L. S. (1996). *Recovered memories of abuse: Assessment, therapy, forensics*. Washington, DC: American Psychological Association.

Putnam, F. W., & Trickett, P. K. (1997). The psychobiological effects of sexual abuse: A longitudinal study. *Annals of the New York Academy of Sciences, 821*, 150–159.

Roediger, H. L., III, & McDermott, K. B. (1995). Creating false memories: Remembering words not presented in lists. *Journal of Experimental Psychology. Learning, Memory, and Cognition, 21*, 803–814.

Sales, B. D. (1998). Final conclusions of the American Psychological Association working group on investigation of memories of childhood abuse. *Psychology, Public Policy, and Law, 4*(4), 933–940.

Scheflin, A. W., & Brown, D. (1996). Repressed memory or dissociative amnesia: What the science says. *The Journal of Psychiatry & Law, 24*, 143–188.

Schooler, J. W., Ambadar, Z., & Bendiksen, M. (1997). A cognitive corroborative case study approach for investigating discovered memories for sexual abuse. In J. D. Read & D. S. Lindsay (Eds.), *Recollections of trauma—Scientific evidence and clinical practice* (pp. 379–387). New York: Plenum Press.

Schooler, J. W., Bendiksen, M. A., & Ambadar, Z. (1997). Taking the Middle Line: Can we accommodate both fabricated and recovered memories of sexual abuse? In M. Conway (Ed.), *Recovered memories and false memories*. Oxford: Oxford University Press.

Smith, S. M. (1994). Frustrated feelings of imminence: On the tip-of-the-tongue. In J. Metcalfe & A. Shimamura (Eds.), *Metacognition: Knowing about knowing* (pp. 27–45). Cambridge, MA: MIT Press.

Smith, S. M., & Tindell, D. R. (1997). Memory blocks in word fragment completion caused by involuntary retrieval of orthographically similar primes. *Journal of Experimental Psychology. Learning, Memory, and Cognition, 23*, 355–370.

Spiegel, D. (1986). Dissociating damage. *American Journal of Clinical Hypnosis, 29*(2), 123–131.

Wheeler, M. A. (1995). Improvement in recall overtime without repeated testing: Spontaneous recovery revisited. *Journal of Experimental Psychology: Learning, Memory, and Cognition, 10*, 733–744.

Williams, L. M. (1994). Recall of childhood trauma: A prospective study of women's memories of child sexual abuse. *Journal of Consulting and Clinical Psychology, 62*(6), 1167–1176.

Williams, L. M. (1995). Recovered memories of abuse in women with documented child sexual victimization histories. *Journal of Traumatic Stress, 8*(4), 649–674.

Yates, J. L., & Nasby, W. (1993). Dissociation, affect, and network models of memory: An integrative proposal. *Journal of Traumatic Stress, 6*, 305–326.

Yuille, J. C. (1993). We must study forensic eyewitnesses to know about them. *American Psychologist, 48*, 572–573.

Yuille, J. C., & Cutshall, J. E. (1989). Analysis of the statements of victims, witnesses and suspects. In C. Yuille (Ed.), *Credibility assessment* (pp. 175–191). Norwell, MA: Kluwer Academic.

Zaragoza, M. S. (1991). Preschool children's susceptibility to memory impairment. In Doris (Ed.), *The suggestibility of children's recollections: Implications for eyewitness testimony* (pp. 27–39). Washington, DC: American Psychological Association.

Zaragoza, M. S., McCloskey, M., & Jamis, M. (1987). Misleading postevent information and the recall of the original event: Further evidence against the memory impairment hypothesis. *Journal of Experimental Psychology. Learning, Memory, and Cognition, 13*, 36–44.

Sexual Assault and Memory

20

Lori A. Zoellner, Ifrah S. Sheikh, Rosemary W. Walker, Peter Rosencrans, Natalia M. Garcia, Elizabeth H. Marks, Heidi J. Ojalehto, and Michele A. Bedard-Gilligan

We found to our great surprise ... that each individual symptom immediately and permanently disappeared when we had succeeded in bringing clearly to the light the memory of the event...when the patient had described the event in the greatest possible detail and had put the affect into words....

—Breuer & Freud, 1893–1898/1955, p. 6

Memory for a sexual assault is dynamic and reconstructive; it is not fixed or indelible. What is encoded in memory depends on a person's past, the event itself, and processing of that event. What is remembered depends on encoding of the event and the later retrieval of the event as well as related content such as previous similar experiences. Memory for a sexual assault is not like a series of photographs or a digital recording. Even if photographs or recordings were available, these would only show one perspective of what happened and not necessarily depict the perspective of the assault survivor, which depends on where his or her attention was focused and many other factors such as the role of repeated retrieval. Memory for a sexual assault and memory functioning are also directly related to persistent assault-related psychopathology such as depression and posttraumatic stress disorder (PTSD) and its treatment. Some of the best evidence-based treatments for assault-related psychopathology focus on revisiting or re-examining the memory of the event. Indeed, as seen by the quote from Breuer and Freud above, the understanding of the crucial role of memory in recovery following trauma is not a new view.

A complex, dynamic conceptualization of memory following a sexual assault requires understanding the processes involved in the strong encoding of emotional events and the physiological factors that alter this encoding. It also requires understanding the role of retrieval and re-experiencing as well as the acceptance of the fact that any form of memory is susceptible to unintentional memory distortions and actual errors. There are also general memory effects involved beyond the memory for the assault itself, including attention to threat, working memory deficits, and lack of specificity for memory of autobiographical events. Finally, memory is often the target for some of the strongest evidence-based treatments for assault-related psychopathology. These processes will be reviewed over the course of this chapter.

L. A. Zoellner (✉) · I. S. Sheikh · R. W. Walker
P. Rosencrans · N. M. Garcia · E. H. Marks
H. J. Ojalehto · M. A. Bedard-Gilligan
Department of Psychology, University of Washington, Seattle, WA, USA
e-mail: zoellner@uw.edu

W. T. O'Donohue and P. A. Schewe (eds.), *Handbook of Sexual Assault and Sexual Assault Prevention*,
https://doi.org/10.1007/978-3-030-23645-8_20

Encoding of a Sexual Assault

Enhanced memory for stressful events is a normal and, in many circumstances, an adaptive function of human cognitive functioning. By forming strong memory traces that are easily remembered and enduring of potentially life-threatening events, humans are more likely to be able to recognize and avoid similarly dangerous situations in the future (e.g., Lazarus, 1991). It is well-established that emotional arousal enhances the storage of memory (Christianson & Loftus, 1991), with numerous studies demonstrating that emotional events, both positive and negative, are recalled better than neutral events (e.g., Walker, Skowronski, & Thompson, 2003). Neurobiological theories suggest that humans are evolutionarily wired to remember emotionally arousing experiences such as sexual assault (e.g., McGaugh, 2013; Müller & Pilzecker's, 1900). HistoricallyMüller and Pilzecker's (1900) perseveration-consolidation theory of memory posited that neural processes involved in memory formation are initiated during an event, but it is the perseveration of these processes over time that leads to the consolidation of memory in long-term storage. Recent research has firmly established that lasting memories are formed through a gradual, time-dependent memory consolidation process, whereby the strength of memory may be influenced by endogenous processes such as endogenous stress hormones and neuromodulators occurring after the event (McGaugh, 2013). Importantly, this opportunity for the modulation of memory strength serves an adaptive function, allowing emotional arousal to strengthen memory for our most important experiences.

The amygdala, activated in response to an emotional stimulus, modulates activity in the hippocampus and other brain regions responsible for consolidating an experience into long-term memory (McGaugh, 2013; Phelps, Delgado, Nearing, & LeDoux, 2004). Fittingly, when a memory associated with emotion is undergoing consolidation and the amygdala is more activated, the degree of amygdala activation during encoding is positively correlated with later memory recall (e.g., McGaugh, 2004). In other words, an individual experiencing high stress or distress as an event is being encoded will likely encode a more persistent, durable memory due to greater amygdala activation modulating hippocampal encoding processes. McGaugh's (2013) modulation hypothesis posits that following an emotionally arousing experience, high levels of endogenous stress hormones and neuromodulators such as epinephrine and cortisol interact with the amygdala. The interaction between stress hormone systems and the amygdala promotes memory storage, resulting in particularly strong and long-lasting memories for important information encountered during a stressful event (e.g., McGaugh, 2013).

There is substantial evidence that glucocorticoids (e.g., cortisol, corticosterone) and the noradrenergic system (e.g., epinephrine, norepinephrine) modulate the consolidation of emotional memory following their release from the adrenal medulla (e.g., epinephrine, norepinephrine) and cortex (e.g., glucocorticoids) (e.g., de Quervain, Schwabe, & Roozendaal, 2017). The basolateral amygdala (BLA), specifically, appears critical in this modulation of memory consolidation. Infusions of β-adrenoreceptor agonists into the BLA block memory-enhancing effects of epinephrine (e.g., Liang, Juler, & McGaugh, 1986), and glucocorticoid receptor agonists administered into the BLA enhance emotional memory in a dose- and time-dependent manner (e.g., Roozendaal, Okuda, Van der Zee, & McGaugh, 2006). Critically, the memory-enhancing effects of glucocorticoids appear contingent on endogenous noradrenergic activity in the BLA (Roozendaal et al., 2006). Glucocorticoids bind to glucocorticoid receptors in noradrenergic neurons in the brainstem (e.g., Roozendaal, Quirarte, & McGaugh, 2002). This then triggers norepinephrine release in the BLA and initiates a noradrenergic cascade thought to modulate the prefrontal cortex, hippocampus, and other brain regions involved, ultimately leading to enhanced memory. The timing of glucocorticoid arousal and noradrenergic activity appears important, in that increases in cortisol levels must occur in tandem with release of noradrenaline (e.g., Joëls, Fernandez, & Roozendaal, 2011).

Numerous studies have demonstrated that increased activity in the amygdala in response to viewing emotional stimuli predicts better recall (e.g., Kensinger, Addis, & Atapattu, 2011). Experimental research has also found that inducing the release of stress hormones during a learning phase (e.g., administering shocks) and post-learning administration of stress hormones enhances memory for the learned material (e.g., Hupbach & Fieman, 2012). Taken together, the amygdala, hippocampus, and stress hormones are consistently implicated as neurobiological processes associated with enhanced memory for emotional events, ensuring that highly emotional experiences such as sexual assault will be retained in memory.

Physiological responses and memory. Beside the release of endogenous stress hormones, immediate physiological responses to sexual assault may include sexual arousal or responses to physical or biological insult, including head injuries resulting in loss of consciousness or loss of oxygen (e.g., strangulation), as well as intoxication by drugs (e.g., rohypnol) or alcohol. These factors influence what a person initially encodes and therefore stores in their memory of the assault, with the potential for enhancing or impairing effects depending on the characteristics of the assault and the nature of the physiological responses.

Some may experience unwanted sexual arousal (e.g., lubrication, orgasm) in response to sexual stimulation that occurs during the assault (e.g., Levin & van Berlo, 2004). These responses are understood not as an indication of consent or enjoyment of the assault, but rather as an automatic physical response to sexual stimulation. In one small unpublished study of sexual assault survivors, 21% reported some form of physical response; and, of these women, a substantial number of the rapists attempted to produce sexual arousal (see Levin & van Berlo, 2004). Laboratory studies of the effects of sexual arousal on memory encoding have been mixed, with some finding that exposure to sexual stimuli impaired memory functioning (e.g., Laier, Schulte, & Brand, 2013), and others finding enhanced memory for sexually arousing stimuli (e.g., Wright Jr & Adams, 1999). However, these studies differ dramatically from an actual sexual assault by presenting sexually arousing stimuli to consenting participants with no substantial threat to life or well-being present. Further, it is not clear whether the observed effects were attributable to sexual stimulation as opposed to the broader cognitive, emotional, and physical aspects of sexual arousal.

Any biological insult or injury during a sexual assault that results in loss of consciousness will prevent the encoding of events during the period of unconsciousness, as an unconscious individual cannot attend to details in their environment. For example, a survivor who is choked by an assailant to the point of unconsciousness will not encode, and thus will be unable to recall, any information about events that occurred during the period of unconsciousness. In the case of head injuries that do not result in loss of consciousness, the presence and magnitude of impairments in memory storage depends on the extent to which the head injury damaged parts of the brain involved in memory encoding such as the temporal lobe (McGaugh, 2013).

Alcohol intoxication also affects consciousness and arousal. In general, alcohol has been shown to impair the formation of long-term memories, following a dose-response curve (e.g., White, 2003). However, studies of individuals who consumed alcohol during the encoding of a hypothetical sexual assault scenario have found that, although they remembered fewer overall details, they did not differ from alcohol-free controls in their ability to accurately recall key aspects of the scenario, including the perpetrator's identity (Flowe, Takarangi, Humphries, & Write, 2016). In line with McGaugh's (2013) modulation hypothesis, it may be that intoxication at the time of an assault may impair encoding of fewer peripheral details of the assault (e.g., objects within the room where they assault occurred), but central details of the assault, such the perpetrator's general description, may be encoded.

Strong memory storage of sexual assaults may put individuals at risk for developing chronic, trauma-related difficulties such as PTSD. Indeed, trauma severity and higher levels of physiological arousal in the immediate aftermath of a trauma have been shown to modestly predict who will develop PTSD (e.g., Bryant, Harvey, Guthrie, & Moulds, 2000; Ozer, Best, Lipsey, & Weiss, 2003) and physiological arousal has been shown to play a significant role in the link between stress hormones and emotional memory, particularly in individuals with PTSD (e.g., Nicholson, Bryant, & Felmingham, 2014). However, characteristics of the trauma and the intensity of physiological responding to the trauma do not fully explain who will develop PTSD, suggesting memory storage strength is not the only factor influencing risk of PTSD.

Allocation of attention and memory. Attention plays a fundamental role during a sexual assault in terms of influencing what is encoded and then remembered. In general, attending to something enhances the likelihood of it being encoded in memory and retrievable later (Chun & Turke-Browne, 2007). What is attended to can be narrowed in on small details or can be broader in scope, open to taking in a range of information. During traumatic events, attention is thought to narrow to the most threatening aspects of the encounter. Loftus (1979) coined the term "weapon focus" to account for the narrowing of attention to the most salient features of the environment to the exclusion of other details. Consistently, as the most central features become the focus of attention, these details are best remembered; on the other hand, encoding and later recalling more peripheral details can be hindered (e.g., Christianson & Loftus, 1991).

One theory of weapon focus emphasizes the role of stress and arousal during emotional events, which may narrow overall attentional processing, restricting attention to central aspects of the event at the expense of peripheral events (Christianson & Loftus, 1991). Consistent with this hypothesis, in a meta-analytic review of the weapon focus literature, Steblay (1992) found larger effect sizes in studies that reported higher levels of autonomic arousal. Alternatively, details that stand out or are unusual or unexpected may call for increased attention and subsequent better memory recall (e.g., Loftus & Mackworth, 1978; Pickel, 1998); conversely, details that appear in context that would be expected are not as well recalled (e.g., Pickel, 1999). Thus, attentional focus during a sexual assault will determine what is encoded for later memory storage and the weapon focus effect may help explain why survivors of sexual assault report that they do not remember some of the more tangential details but clearly remember the more salient, unexpected, or anxiety-eliciting features of the event.

Event processing and memory. The way that a sexual assault is encoded and processed may also affect later retrieval of the memory, with potential implications for post-trauma adjustment. Encoding and storage of autobiographical events occurs through associating the event with semantically and temporally related experiences, placing the event within a broader autobiographical memory base (Roediger, 1990). For example, a general category may be sexual experiences, which includes specific life events, shared and unique event characteristics, and general sexual knowledge. This associative, conceptual processing facilitates intentional retrieval by increasing the number of meaningful associations by which to retrieve the memory through higher-order, meaning-based strategies (Roediger, 1990). However, during a traumatic event, individuals may engage in data-driven processing, that is, focused on perceptual and sensory elements, resulting in poorly elaborated, perceptual memory traces. These perceptual memory traces (e.g., the smell of the perpetrator's breath) are thought to lack the conceptual detail necessary to integrate the memory within autobiographical memory, resulting in impaired intentional retrieval of some aspects of the event and also increasing the chance that trauma-related cues will trigger the memory, leading to increased experiencing of intrusive symptoms (e.g., Ehlers & Clark, 2000).

Memory Phenomena After Sexual Assault

Intrusive memories. It is not uncommon for sexual assault survivors to have intrusive memories, defined as intense, brief, and vivid often image-based recollections of a specific autobiographical event (Brewin, Gregory, Lipton, & Burgess, 2010) that typically emerge involuntarily, "out of the blue," and include strong sensory components (Ehlers, Hackmann, & Michael, 2004). For instance, intrusions for a sexual assault survivor may include images of the perpetrator's face, body odor, smells, sounds, or the feeling of having hands placed over their eyes. Intrusive memories can be triggered by a range of internal and external stimuli, such as physical bodily sensations, objects, or situations, and lack of awareness of triggering cues can sometimes make intrusive memories seem to pop up out the blue (e.g., Ehlers et al., 2004).

The mere presence of intrusive memories is not considered pathological. In fact, intrusive memories are common immediately after sexual assault and typically decline in frequency and intensity over time (Rothbaum et al., 1992). For some individuals, these intrusive memories persist (reliving: 45.4%; flashbacks: 46.2%) and contribute to significant distress and functional impairment (PTSD: 47%; Rothbaum et al., 1992). Trauma survivors with PTSD report a distinct "here and now quality" of their trauma memories and associated emotional response compared to those without PTSD (e.g., Kleim, Graham, Bryant, & Ehlers, 2013). Sexual assault tactics may also influence intrusions, with forcible rape associated with highest risk for developing PTSD and depression after assault, and incapacitated rape (e.g., lack of consciousness/awareness or ability to control behavior) associated with lower likelihood of remembering the event well (e.g., Zinzow et al., 2010). Intrusive memories can have downstream effects, increasing guilt or shame about the assault, low self-esteem, or a sense of loss of control, which interferes with functioning in work and interpersonal relationships, including loss of interest or avoidance of sex (e.g., Jaycox, Zoellner, & Foa, 2002).

There are various theories that seek to account for the development and persistence of intrusive memories. Dual representation theory (e.g., Brewin et al., 2010) posits that poor integration between contextual representations of memory ("C-reps") and sensory representations of memory ("S-reps") make individuals vulnerable to involuntary retrieval via intrusive re-experiencing. Similarly, Ehler's cognitive theory (e.g., 2000) posits that sensory-perceptual encoding of the trauma in the absence of conceptual organization leads individuals to have fragmented sensory details (e.g., images of the perpetrator's face) that are poorly integrated within a larger autobiographical memory context and highly susceptible to popping up as involuntary intrusions. A dynamic retrieval model of intrusions (Marks, Franklin, & Zoellner, 2018) emphasizes the role of retrieval processes in the pathological persistence of trauma-related intrusions. This model argues that the process of re-experiencing itself alters retrieval processes, such that distress caused by the unwanted memories actually increases retrieval strength, creating a vicious cycle where distressing memories become more and more vulnerable to involuntary retrieval over time, and, conversely, decreasing distress associated with intrusive memories decreases the retrieval strength of these unwanted memory traces.

Although intrusive re-experiencing is a common phenomenon across all kinds of traumatic events, some studies suggest that sexual assault survivors in particular are at risk for higher-re-experiencing symptoms (Kelley, Weathers, McDevitt-Murphy, Eakin, & Flood, 2009). A systematic review of predictors of intrusions found that higher pre-existing anxiety and depression, and tendencies towards negative appraisals increased risk for intrusions, and data-driven processing (bottom-up processing focused on perceptual and sensory elements) predicted higher intrusions (Marks et al., 2018). Further, post-event negative appraisals (e.g., I should have been able to stop the rape) predicted higher intrusions, whereas conceptual processing (top-down processing focusing on meaning) predicted lower intrusions (Marks et al., 2018). Clinically, this suggests that directly targeting post-event negative appraisals and encouraging contextual processing that focuses on making meaning from the event may decrease risk for persistent and distressing intrusive memories of the trauma.

Many sexual assault survivors, like most trauma survivors, will go to great lengths to avoid or push away intrusive memories of the trauma, using cognitive strategies such as suppression, defined as intentionally stopping thoughts, and rumination, defined as focusing on distress in a passive, repetitive manner. These post-event strategies are commonly believed to increase risk for intrusive memories, though evidence is mixed. Some have found that instructions to "not to think about" being sexually assaulted increased the likelihood of generating assault-related thoughts (e.g., Shipherd & Beck, 1999); whereas other have not (e.g., Rosenthal & Follette, 2007). Notably, poorer executive functioning was found to moderate the effect of these strategies (e.g., suppression, negative dwelling, self-punishment) on subsequent intrusions (Bomyea & Lang, 2016). In other words, higher cognitive capacity may mitigate the otherwise detrimental effect of these thought regulation strategies.

Fragmented memories. Several theories posit that fragmented and disorganized recall of traumatic events is a crucial causal mechanism for PTSD. Typically, narrative fragmentation and disorganization refer to abnormalities of sequence, coherence, and content when intentionally recalling a detailed trauma memory (e.g., van der Kolk, 1987). According to these theories, trauma memories are uniquely encoded and processed in autobiographical memory, separated from the overall memory network, and are thus difficult to recall intentionally. Similarly, related memory theories (e.g., Ehlers et al., 2004; Ehlers & Clark, 2000) argue that PTSD results from incomplete processing and a memory representation dominated by perceptual details and lacking meaning and self-referential perspective (i.e., "inability to establish a self-referential perspective while experiencing the trauma that can be integrated into the continuum of other autobiographic memories in time." p. 330; Ehlers & Clark, 2000). Dissociation, typically including phenomena such as depersonalization, derealization, and emotional numbing, during the traumatic event may be one process that interferes with encoding of the full trauma memory, resulting in a trauma memory representation that is experienced as vivid flashbacks and intrusive images but is unable to be recalled in a cohesive and organized way (e.g., Brewin, Dalgleish, & Joseph, 1996; Ehlers et al., 2004). These theories are consistent in suggesting that integrating and organizing the traumatic memory is necessary for recovery from PTSD.

Research evaluating fragmentation theories is generally mixed. Although dissociation is reported by survivors of both adult (e.g., Dancu, Riggs, Hearst-Ikeda, Shoyer, & Foa, 1996) and childhood sexual abuse (e.g., Draijer & Langeland, 1999), an extensive review of the literature found that dissociation was related to perceived trauma narrative fragmentation, but not actual fragmented recall (Bedard-Gilligan & Zoellner, 2012). Existing studies in diverse trauma-exposed samples do not robustly support narrative fragmentation as predictive of PTSD or uniquely related to trauma narratives compared to other narrative types (Crespo & Fernandez-Lansac, 2016). In assault survivors, specifically, two studies have shown a prospective relationship between higher trauma narrative fragmentation and development of PTSD symptoms (Amir, Stafford, Freshman, & Foa, 1998; Halligan, Michael, Clark, & Ehlers, 2003). However, in adult survivors of childhood sexual abuse (Greenhoot, Sun, Bunnell, & Lindboe, 2013), although deficits in organization were related to increased PTSD and depression, other narrative elements such as positive aspects of the narrative were more strongly related. Across studies, coding measures vary widely both in their methods (e.g., linguistic coding, rater coding) and their definitions of fragmentation. Further, self-report and objective coding measures of fragmentation often do not converge (e.g., Bedard-Gilligan & Zoellner, 2012) and may be measuring distinct constructs. Conclusions that can be drawn are also limited by not controlling for factors such as verbal ability and distress during narrative recall that may cause narratives to appear fragmented or disorganized (Gray, Pumphrey, & Lombardo, 2003).

Importantly, studies that have explored memory fragmentation as a mechanism underlying reduction of PTSD symptoms during treatment have produced mixed findings and have not shown robust changes with fragmentation following PTSD treatment (e.g., Kindt et al., 2007; Moulds & Bryant, 2005; van Minnen, Wessel, Dijkstra, & Roelofs, 2002). One of the largest and most empirically rigorous studies to date that included sexual assault survivors did not find changes in fragmentation, measured with both self-report and objective measures, to be related to either treatment response or treatment type (psychotherapy vs. pharmacotherapy), arguing against the notion that trauma memories need to become less fragmented and more organized for symptom recovery following trauma (Bedard-Gilligan, Zoellner, & Feeny, 2017). Taken together, treatment studies do not consistently suggest fragmentation as a crucial mechanism of recovery from PTSD.

Memory amnesia and forgetting. Due to the emphasis on trauma memories as separated from an individual's overall memory system, fragmentation theories are often utilized to explain the occurrence of traumatic amnesia, or the complete inability to recall a traumatic event for significant periods of time, even when the memory was encoded and in the absence of physical explanations for forgetting (e.g., blackout, head injury). Much of the research in this area has examined forgetting in adult survivors of childhood sexual abuse (Scheflin & Brown, 1996), although at least one study has looked at those who have experienced adult sexual assault (Mechanic, Resick, & Griffin, 1998), demonstrating that self-reported deficits in memory were more commonly reported immediately 2 weeks after assault but decreased by 3 months.

The phenomenon termed "motivated forgetting" posits that it can be adaptive and functional for individuals to forget aversive experiences, including sexual assault. It has been argued that individuals, particularly those with a history of trauma exposure or dissocation, are prone to forget traumatic experiences, especially those involving betrayal by a close or trusted person, out of a wish to avoid or repress painful memories and emotions (e.g., Freyd, 1994). Research exploring this phenomenon is decidedly more mixed, with two studies by DePrince and Freyd (2001, 2004) finding that, following instructions to remember words, those higher in trait dissociation recalled fewer trauma words and more neutral words during a divided attention task, while those lower in trait dissociation displayed the opposite pattern of remembering more trauma and fewer neutral words. Of note, a replication of this study found no significant interaction effect for trait dissociation and word type (neutral, trauma) under conditions of divided attention (Devilly et al., 2007). In addition, several other studies using directed forgetting paradigms have not found consistent differences in directed forgetting for those with varying levels of trauma exposure and dissociation (e.g., McNally, Metzger, Lasko, Clancy, & Pitman, 1998; Patihis & Place, 2018). When manipulating dissociation, the standard directed forgetting effect also disappears, arguing that the impact of dissociation may be more on encoding or impairing repeated reheresal than on forgetting per se (Zoellner, Sacks, & Foa, 2003). Interestingly, studies done by Moulds and colleagues have demonstrated increased directed forgetting of trauma-related words in survivors with acute stress disorder in the acute phase following trauma exposure compared to those without acute stress disorder (Moulds & Bryant, 2005), although this enhanced forgetting effect disappeared after 1 year (Moulds & Bryant, 2008), suggesting that the effects are temporary and do not persist over the period of natural recovery where chronic, persistent PTSD emerges (typically 1–3 months post trauma). Collectively, there is little empirical evidence to support the notion of motivated forgetting as a process that is predicted by trauma exposure or dissocation.

Still, although most trauma victims report remembering traumatic experiences, a significant minority will report amnesia for all or parts of the traumatic experience (Loftus, Garry, & Feldman, 1994; Wolf et al., 2012, 2017). For example, 14.3% of a national sample of trauma exposed veterans reported an inability to recall important details about the traumatic event (Wolf et al., 2017). However, it is worth noting that much of what is termed "traumatic amnesia" may actually be better accounted for by mechanisms such as normal forgetting, nondisclosure, incomplete encoding of the memory, and infantile amnesia (i.e., expected lack of memory before age three; e.g., McNally, 2005). Thus, the issue of amnesia and sexual abuse or assault remains contentious. At the very least, limitations of memory and its reconstructive nature must be considered in regard to expected recall of sexual assault and abuse.

False memories. In the 1990s, memories of sexual abuse recovered in psychotherapy sparked a divisive debate in the field of psychology regarding the validity of recovered memories, referred to as the "memory wars" (Crews, 1995). Proponents of the validity of recovered memory argued that dissociation at the time of the traumatic event leads to traumatic amnesia, resulting in loss of memory which may later be recovered (e.g., Dalenberg, 2006). Others argued that suggestive therapeutic techniques fostered the development of false memories, given memory fallibility (e.g., Lindsay & Read, 1994). Today, many scholars express skepticism about the validity of recovered memories (Patihis, Lilienfeld, Ho, & Loftus, 2014).

Memory is not thought to involve perfect recollection of past events, but rather a flexible, reconstructive process that is prone to error (Brewer, 1986). These errors range from a failure to recall certain aspects of an event (i.e., errors of omission) to the recall of inaccurate information (i.e., errors of commission) or even entirely false autobiographical memories, as in the case of implanted memories of childhood sexual abuse (Hyman & Loftus, 1998; Loftus, 2003). Across studies, a significant minority (30.5% false memory rate) of individuals can indeed come to remember events that never happened (Scoboria et al., 2017).

Evidence from false memory research carries important implications for the accuracy of memory for traumatic events; namely, while high emotion has been shown to enhance memory, it does not inoculate the memory from distortion or forgetting (Laney & Loftus, 2010). Certainly, memories for traumatic events are also subjective to forgetting and contain errors and distortions, as demonstrated by significant instability in the consistency of retrospective reports for childhood sexual abuse (e.g., Fergusson, Horwood, & Woodward, 2000; Ghetti et al., 2006). Trauma-exposed individuals, particularly those who go on to develop PTSD, may be especially vulnerable to laboratory-induced false memories, as evidenced by higher incidences of commission errors (Vasterling, Brailey, Constans, & Sutker, 1998) and higher susceptibility to false memories for previously unpresented words (e.g., Zoellner, Foa, Brigidi, & Przeworski, 2000). However, van Giezen, Arensman, Spinhoven, and Wolters (2005) conducted a review of longitudinal studies examining autobiographical memory for traumatic events specifically and found that traumatic events tend to be remembered with more consistency than non-traumatic events. Furthermore, higher severity traumas and interpersonal traumas, such as sexual assault, were more consistently remembered. Notably, they also found that memory for traumatic events was subject to memory inflation, or the tendency to provide more details at later time points. This tendency may be a result of improved memory with repeated recall but may also be a result of PTSD, as higher PTSD symptoms have been linked to increased memory inflation (e.g., Giosan, Malta, Jayasinghe, Spielman, & Difede, 2009).

The relationship between confidence in memory and accuracy of memory is complex. A recent series of studies demonstrated that more confidence is related to more accuracy, except in recognition tasks in which the stimuli presented highly resemble (but are not the same) as the experienced stimuli; in these situations, high confidence in memory is not correlated with accuracy (DeSoto & Roediger III, 2014; Roediger III & DeSoto, 2014). In eye-witness testimony, findings support the notion that low confidence predicts low accuracy and high confidence predicts high accuracy if confidence is assessed at the time of the initial identification and not weeks, months, or even years later (Wixted, Mickes, Clark, Gronlund, & Roediger III, 2015).

Taken together, research on the role of emotion in memory and evidence from the false memory literature suggest that while highly emotional events like sexual assault tend to be remembered better than non-emotional events, traumatic experiences are also subject to memory distortion and forgetting, consistent with a reconstructive view of memory. Notably, an event being strongly encoded and susceptible to errors are not incompatible, especially when considering that any memory for an event is reconstructed and reconstruction is a complex retrieval process integrating many pieces of information and reliant on current and past cognitive functioning.

Memory Corollaries Associated with Sexual Assault or Related Psychopathology

There are also more general memory functioning impairments commonly observed in sexual assault survivors, particularly for those with related psychopathology, such as PTSD.

Working memory. Working memory capacity (WMC) refers to the amount of information an individual can hold in working memory at one time (Diamond, 2013) and is typically measured by tasks requiring a person to hold distinct pieces of information in mind while simultaneously manipulating the information. Individuals with PTSD exhibit deficits in working memory capacity that do not seem to be accounted for by trauma exposure alone (e.g., Morey et al., 2009) and deficits in the related capacity of verbal memory (e.g., memory for words on a word list read out loud; Gilbertson et al., 2006). Further, structural and functional impairments in brain regions implicated in WMC, such as decreased hippocampal volume (e.g., Karl et al., 2006) and decreased activation in the dorsolateral prefrontal cortex (e.g., Morey et al., 2009), have been seen in individuals with PTSD as compared to trauma-exposed controls. Although there is a clear association between PTSD and WMC deficits, it is not clear whether these deficits reflect a pre-trauma risk factor or are a consequence of the disorder. Some well-done studies argue for a pre-existing vulnerability factor (e.g., Gilbertson et al., 2006), yet improvement of PTSD symptoms is also associated with increases in WMC (e.g., Mozzambani et al., 2017) and increases in hippocampal volume (e.g., Bremner, Elzinga, Schmahl, & Vermetten, 2007).

Attentional focus toward threat. After sexual assault, there are shifts in attentional processes with the development of trauma-related psychopathology. Individuals with anxiety show attentional biases towards threat, defined as differential allocation of attention towards threat relative to neutral stimuli, including an attentional bias towards trauma-related stimuli in PTSD (e.g., Lee & Lee, 2012). In addition to enhanced threat detection, individuals with PTSD may also experience increased difficulty disengaging from trauma-related stimuli (e.g., Pineles, Shipherd, Mostoufi, Abramovitz, & Yovel, 2009). Both attentional bias towards trauma-related cues and difficulty disengaging from trauma-related stimuli may alter retrieval of information.

Despite attentional biases towards trauma-related information, individuals with PTSD do not consistently show better memory recall of trauma-related information compared to those who are trauma-exposed but without PTSD or those without a history of trauma (e.g., McNally et al., 1998). This paradox may be explained by the vigilant-avoidance hypothesis where, after initial attention towards threat, individuals with anxiety subsequently direct attention away from threat (Mogg, Bradley, Miles, & Dixon, 2004). This attention away may, in turn, interfere with detailed processing, elaboration, and encoding of information. In individuals with PTSD, some studies are consistent with this vigilance-avoidance hypothesis (e.g., Adenauer et al., 2010) while others only find attention towards threat (e.g., Kimble, Fleming, Bandy, Kim, & Zambetti, 2010). Finally, these processes have implications for the maintenance of PTSD after sexual assault given that quick avoidance of trauma reminders may impede emotional or more elaborative processing, important for inhibitory learning and the reduction of fear (e.g., Craske, Treanor, Conway, Zbozinek, & Vervliet, 2014).

Interpretation bias. Following sexual assault, information processing biases towards trauma-related information may cause individuals to feel as if they are in a state of current threat, influencing the trajectory of recovery following trauma (e.g., Dalgleish, 2004; Ehlers & Clark, 2000). Selective attention to threat may lead to disruptions in subsequent processing stages, resulting in interpretive biases (White, Suway, Pine, Bar-Haim, & Fox, 2011). Interpretation bias, or the tendency to interpret novel information from the environment as threatening, often occurs after individuals have been sexually assaulted. For example, Elwood, Williams, Olatunji, and Lohr (2007) rated the threatening film clips as more predictable and as more quickly increasing in risk than those who had not been assaulted. These biases may be even more pronounced among individuals who go on to develop psychopathology, with higher threat-related interpretation bias among individuals with PTSD (e.g., Amir, Elias, Klumpp, & Przeworski, 2003).

Autobiographical memory. Autobiographical memory refers to individual person's recollections of his or her life (Williams, Conway, & Cohen, 2007). These memories can be specific to a particular moment and context or more general autobiographical memories referring to events with similar characteristics or events over an extended period of time (e.g., going out with friends on my 21st birthday versus birthday parties I have had). Notably, when instructed to recall specific memories, individuals with PTSD tend to narrate general memories of events, termed overgeneral memory, even with repeated instruction or prompting in relation to a positive and negative cue word (e.g., happy, hurt), including those with PTSD after sexual assault; this deficit is also seen with individuals with major depressive disorder and may be an effect of psychopathology or trauma exposure (Barry, Lenaert, Hermans, Raes, & Griffith, 2018; Moore & Zoellner, 2007).

Overgeneral memory following sexual assault and related psychopathology may serve to reduce or dampen the emotional focus and allow avoidance of specific memories. The CaRFAX model (Williams, 2006) argues that cues capture cognitive resources through the activation of ruminative, repetitive thinking and truncates the search for specific autobiographical memories both through reduced executive capacity and functional avoidance of emotional material. Reduced autobiographical memory specificity has also been presented as an affect-regulating strategy and as avoidant coping style (e.g., Herman, Ostrander, Mueller, & Figueiredo, 2005), serving as a protective mechanism that buffers the emotional pain associated with traumatic experiences and may reflect a learned memory retrieval blocking (Williams, 2006). Overgeneral memory functioning has been linked to impaired problem solving (Williams, 2006) and delayed recovery from affective disorder episodes (Serrano, Latorre, Gatz, & Montanes, 2004).

Implications for Treatment of Sexual Assault-Related Psychopathology

Of the empirically-supported treatments for PTSD (Cusack et al., 2016), both prolonged exposure (PE; Foa, Rothbaum, Riggs, & Murdock, 1991) and cognitive processing therapy (CPT; Resick & Schnicke, 1992) were both developed for addressing psychopathology following sexual assault. These and other empirically-supported psychotherapies such as narrative exposure therapy (NET; e.g., Neuner, Schauer, Klaschik, Karunakara, & Elbert, 2004) and trauma-focused cognitive behavioral therapy in children (TF-CBT; e.g., Cohen, Deblinger, Mannarino, & Steer, 2004) include an explicit focus on the memory for the traumatic event. These interventions can be more broadly understood within a network model of memory, where trauma memories fit into an overarching schema, defined as a packet of information associated with a specific concept (e.g., walking the dog, dangerous men, rape). These associations affect memory, providing filters that drive subsequent retrieval (e.g., Norman, Newman, & Detre, 2007). Specifically, the more meaningfully-related pieces of information are to one another and grouped together during repeated memory retrieval, the better new information can be retrieved. This refers to what is termed elaborative processing.

One candidate for shifting and elaborating the meaning of the memory for the traumatic event may be negative beliefs about one's self, others, and the world. Indeed, in PTSD treatment, meaning changes differentially underlie symptom changes in exposure therapy compared to pharmacotherapy (e.g., Cooper, Zoellner, Roy-Byrne, Mavissakalian, & Feeny, 2017). This is also consistent with an inhibitory learning approach.

With new inhibitory learning, new meanings among associations are created that alter future retrieval, inhibiting associations that inappropriately signal threat and instead promoting new, more flexible or ambiguous meaning associations that are linked with more adaptive responses (Craske et al., 2014). Thus, across psychotherapies, a common hypothesized mechanism involves creating new meaning via effortful retrieval as a way to shape future, adaptive memory retrieval and reduce trauma-related psychopathology. For example, in prolonged exposure therapy, when a sexual assault survivor repeatedly revisits the memory of the rape via imaginal exposure, she may come to alter her beliefs that "I should have prevented the rape; I'm such a weak person" as she recalls details of the perpetrator's hand on her throat, feeling short of breath, his verbal threats of killing her, and how she thought he really could kill her. Her new associative meanings may be something akin to, "I did what I needed to do to survive; if I didn't acquiesce, I would have been killed." This may help explain the process observed by Breuer and Freud; adaptive memory retrieval can facilitate recovery.

Limitations of Understanding Memory for Sexual Assault

Obviously, from a legal perspective, there is a push to "know the truth." Historical and current failures to believe the memories of sexual assault survivors make many reticent to come forward. Recognizing that memories are complex and dynamic, include gaps and sometimes errors, ought not be used against sexual assault survivors, but instead provide a general framework for understanding the range of sexual assault memories. This ought to allow for a more flexible understanding of the range sexual assault memories can take and reduce inaccurate, misguided judgments about what "ought to be remembered."

Acknowledgment This chapter was funded in part by NIH grants R34DA040034 (Bedard-Gilligan, PI) and R34MH112756 (Zoellner, PI).

References

Adenauer, H., Pinösch, S., Catani, C., Gola, H., Keil, J., Kibler, J., & Neuner, F. (2010). Early processing of threat cues in posttraumatic stress disorder – evidence for a cortical vigilance-avoidance reaction. *Biological Psychiatry, 68*(5), 451–458. https://doi.org/10.1016/j.biopsych.2010.05.015

Amir, N., Elias, J., Klumpp, H., & Przeworski, A. (2003). Attentional bias to threat in social phobia: Facilitated processing of threat or difficulty disengaging attention from threat? *Behaviour Research and Therapy, 41*(11), 1325–1335. https://doi.org/10.1016/S0005-7967(03)00039-1

Amir, N., Stafford, J., Freshman, M. S., & Foa, E. B. (1998). Relationship between trauma narratives and trauma pathology. *Journal of Traumatic Stress, 11*(2), 385–392. https://doi.org/10.1023/A:1024415523495

Barry, T. J., Lenaert, B., Hermans, D., Raes, F., & Griffith, J. W. (2018). Meta-analysis of the association between autobiographical memory specificity and exposure to trauma. *Journal of Traumatic Stress, 31*(1), 35–46. https://doi.org/10.1002/jts.22263

Bedard-Gilligan, M., & Zoellner, L. A. (2012). Dissociation and memory fragmentation in posttraumatic stress disorder: An evaluation of the dissociative encoding hypothesis. *Memory, 20*(3), 277–299. https://doi.org/10.1080/09658211.2012.655747

Bedard-Gilligan, M., Zoellner, L. A., & Feeny, N. C. (2017). Is trauma memory special? Trauma narrative fragmentation in PTSD: Effects of treatment and response. *Clinical Psychological Science, 5*(2), 212–225. https://doi.org/10.1177/2167702616676581

Bomyea, J., & Lang, A. J. (2016). Accounting for intrusive thoughts in PTSD: Contributions of cognitive control and deliberate regulation strategies. *Journal of Affective Disorders, 192*(1), 184–190. https://doi.org/10.1016/j.jad.2015.12.021

Bremner, J. D., Elzinga, B., Schmahl, C., & Vermetten, E. (2007). Structural and functional plasticity of the human brain in posttraumatic stress disorder. *Progress in Brain Research, 167*(1), 171–186. https://doi.org/10.1016/S0079-6123(07)67012-5

Breuer, J., & Freud, S. (1955). Studies on hysteria 1895 Standard Edition 2 London.

Brewer, W. F. (1986). What is autobiographical memory? In D. C. Rubin (Ed.), Autobiographical memory (pp. 25–49). New York, NY, US: Cambridge University Press.

Brewin, C. R., Dalgleish, T., & Joseph, S. (1996). A dual representation theory of posttraumatic stress disorder. *Psychological Review, 103*(4), 670–686. https://doi.org/10.1037/0033-295X.103.4.670

Brewin, C. R., Gregory, J. D., Lipton, M., & Burgess, N. (2010). Intrusive images in psychological disorders: Characteristics, neural mechanisms, and treatment implications. *Psychological Review, 117*(1), 210–232. https://doi.org/10.1037/a0018113

Bryant, R. A., Harvey, A. G., Guthrie, R. M., & Moulds, M. L. (2000). A prospective study of psychophysiological arousal, acute stress disorder, and posttraumatic stress disorder. *Journal of Abnormal Psychology, 109*(2), 341–344. https://doi.org/10.1037/0021-843X.109.2.341

Christianson, S. Å., & Loftus, E. F. (1991). Remembering emotional events: The fate of detailed information. *Cognition and Emotion, 5*(2), 91–108. https://doi.org/10.1080/02699939108411027

Chun, M. M., & Turke-Browne, N. B. (2007). Interactions between attention and memory. *Current Opinion in Neurobiology, 17*(2), 177–194. https://doi.org/10.1016/j.conb.2007.03.005

Cohen, J. A., Deblinger, E., Mannarino, A. P., & Steer, R. A. (2004). A multisite, randomized controlled trial for children with sexual abuse–related PTSD symptoms. *Journal of the American Academy of Child & Adolescent Psychiatry, 43*(4), 393–402. https://doi.org/10.1097/00004583-200404000-00005

Cooper, A. A., Zoellner, L. A., Roy-Byrne, P., Mavissakalian, M. R., & Feeny, N. C. (2017). Do changes in trauma-related beliefs predict PTSD symptom improvement in prolonged exposure and sertraline? *Journal of Consulting and Clinical Psychology, 85*(9), 873–882. https://doi.org/10.1037/ccp0000220.

Craske, M. G., Treanor, M., Conway, C. C., Zbozinek, T., & Vervliet, B. (2014). Maximizing exposure therapy: An inhibitory learning approach. *Behaviour Research and Therapy, 58*(1), 10–23. https://doi.org/10.1016/j.brat.2014.04.006

Crespo, M., & Fernández-Lansac, V. (2016). Memory and narrative of traumatic events: A literature review. *Psychological Trauma: Theory, Research, Practice, and Policy, 8*(2), 149. https://doi.org/10.1037/tra0000041.

Crews, F. C. (Ed.). (1995). *The memory wars: Freud's legacy in dispute*. New York, NY: New York Review of Books.

Dalenberg, C. (2006). Recovered memory and the Daubert criteria: Recovered memory as professionally tested, peer reviewed, and accepted in the relevant scientific community. *Trauma, Violence & Abuse, 7*(4), 274–310. https://doi.org/10.1177/1524838006294572

Dalgleish, T. (2004). Cognitive approaches to posttraumatic stress disorder: The evolution of multirepresentational theorizing. *Psychological Bulletin, 130*(2), 228–260. https://doi.org/10.1037/0033-2909.130.2.228.

Dancu, C. V., Riggs, D. S., Hearst-Ikeda, D., Shoyer, B. G., & Foa, E. B. (1996). Dissociative experiences and posttraumatic stress disorder among female victims of criminal assault and rape. *Journal of Traumatic Stress, 9*(2), 253–267. https://doi.org/10.1007/BF02110659

de Quervain, D., Schwabe, L., & Roozendaal, B. (2017). Stress, glucocorticoids and memory: Implications for treating fear-related disorders. *Nature Reviews Neuroscience, 18*(1), 7–19.

DePrince, A. P., & Freyd, J. J. (2001). Memory and dissociative tendencies: The roles of attentional context and word meaning in a directed forgetting task. *Journal of Trauma & Dissociation, 2*(2), 67–82. https://doi.org/10.1300/J229v02n02_06.

DePrince, A. P., & Freyd, J. J. (2004). Forgetting trauma stimuli. *Psychological Science, 15*(7), 488–492. https://doi.org/10.1111/j.0956-7976.2004.00706.x

DeSoto, K. A., & Roediger, H. L., III. (2014). Positive and negative correlations between confidence and accuracy for the same events in recognition of categorized lists. *Psychological Science, 25*(3), 781–788. https://doi.org/10.1177/0956797613516149

Devilly, G. J., Ciorciari, J., Piesse, A., Sherwell, S., Zammit, S., Cook, F., & Turton, C. (2007). Dissociative tendencies and memory performance on directed-forgetting tasks. *Psychological Science, 18*(3), 212–217. https://doi.org/10.1111/j.1467-9280.2007.01875

Diamond. A. (2013) Executive Functions. *Annual Review of Psychology, 64*(1), 135–168. https://doi.org/10.1146/annurev-psych-113011-143750

Draijer, N., & Langeland, W. (1999). Childhood trauma and perceived parental dysfunction in the etiology of dissociative symptoms in psychiatric inpatients. *American Journal of Psychiatry, 156*(3), 379–385. https://doi.org/10.1176/ajp.156.3.379

Ehlers, A., & Clark, D. M. (2000). A cognitive model of posttraumatic stress disorder. *Behaviour Research and Therapy, 38*(4), 319–345. https://doi.org/10.1016/S0005-7967(99)00123-0

Ehlers, A., Hackmann, A., & Michael, T. (2004). Intrusive re-experiencing in post-traumatic stress disorder: Phenomenology, theory, and therapy. *Memory, 12*(4), 403–415. https://doi.org/10.1080/09658210444000025

Elwood, L. S., Williams, N. L., Olatunji, B. O., & Lohr, J. M. (2007). Interpretation biases in victims and non-victims of interpersonal trauma and their relation to symptom development. *Journal of Anxiety Disorders, 21*(4), 554–567. https://doi.org/10.1016/j.janxdis.2006.08.006

Fergusson, D. M., Horwood, L. J., & Woodward, L. J. (2000). The stability of child abuse reports: A longitudinal study of the reporting behaviour of young adults. *Psychological Medicine, 30*(3), 529–544. https://doi.org/10.1017/S0033291799002111

Flowe, H. D., Takarangi, M. K. T., Humphries, J. E., & Write, D. S. (2016). Alcohol and remembering a hypothetical sexual assault: Can people who were under the influence of alcohol during the event provide accurate testimony? *Memory, 24*(8), 1042–1061. https://doi.org/10.1080/09658211.2015.1064536

Foa, E. B., Rothbaum, B. O., Riggs, D. S., & Murdock, T. B. (1991). Treatment of posttraumatic stress disorder in rape victims: A comparison between cognitive-behavioral procedures and counseling. *Journal of Consulting and Clinical Psychology, 59*(5), 715. https://doi.org/10.1037/0022-006X.59.5.715

Freyd, J. J. (1994). Betrayal trauma: Traumatic amnesia as an adaptive response to childhood abuse. *Ethics & Behavior, 4*(4), 307–329. https://doi.org/10.1207/s15327019eb0404_1

Ghetti, S., Edelstein, R. S., Goodman, G. S., Cordòn, I. M., Quas, J. A., Alexander, K. W., … Jones, D. P. (2006). What can subjective forgetting tell us about memory for childhood trauma? *Memory & Cognition, 34*(5), 1011–1025.

Gilbertson, M. W., Paulus, L. A., Williston, S. K., Gurvits, T. V., Lasko, N. B., Pitman, R. K., & Orr, S. P. (2006). Neurocognitive function in monozygotic twins discordant for combat exposure: Relationship to posttraumatic stress disorder. *Journal of Abnormal Psychology, 115*(3), 484–495. https://doi.org/10.1037/0021-843X.115.3.484

Giosan, C., Malta, L., Jayasinghe, N., Spielman, L., & Difede, J. (2009). Relationships between memory inconsistency for traumatic events following 9/11 and PTSD in disaster restoration workers. *Journal of Anxiety Disorders, 23*(4), 557–561. https://doi.org/10.1016/j.janxdis.2008.11.004.

Gray, M. J., Pumphrey, J. E., & Lombardo, T. W. (2003). The relationship between dispositional pessimistic attributional style versus trauma-specific attributions and PTSD symptoms. *Journal of Anxiety Disorders, 17*(3), 289–303. https://doi.org/10.1016/S0887-6185(02)00205-0

Greenhoot, A. F., Sun, S., Bunnell, S. L., & Lindboe, K. (2013). Making sense of traumatic memories: Memory qualities and psychological symptoms in emerging adults with and without abuse histories. *Memory, 21*(1), 125–142. https://doi.org/10.1080/09658211.2012.712975.

Halligan, S. L., Michael, T., Clark, D. M., & Ehlers, A. (2003). Posttraumatic stress disorder following assault: The role of cognitive processing, trauma memory, and appraisals. *Journal of Consulting and Clinical Psychology, 71*(3), 419–431. https://doi.org/10.1037/0022-006X.71.3.419

Herman, J. P., Ostrander, M. M., Mueller, N. K., & Figueiredo, H. (2005). Limbic system mechanisms of stress regulation: Hypothalamo-pituitary-adrenocortical axis. *Progress in Neuro-Psychopharmacology and Biological Psychiatry, 29*(8), 1201–1213. https://doi.org/10.1016/j.pnpbp.2005.08.006

Hupbach, A., & Fieman, R. (2012). Moderate stress enhances immediate and delayed retrieval of educationally relevant material in healthy young men. *Behavioral Neuroscience, 126*(6), 819. https://doi.org/10.1037/bne0000152

Hyman, I. E., Jr., & Loftus, E. F. (1998). Errors in autobiographical memory. *Clinical Psychology Review, 18*(8), 933–947. https://doi.org/10.1016/S0272-7358(98)00041-5

Jaycox, L. H., Zoellner, L., & Foa, E. B. (2002). Cognitive–behavior therapy for PTSD in rape survivors. *Journal of Clinical Psychology, 58*(8), 891–906. https://doi.org/10.1002/jclp.10065

Joëls, M., Fernandez, G., & Roozendaal, B. (2011). Stress and emotional memory: A matter of timing. *Trends in Cognitive Sciences, 15*(6), 280–288. https://doi.org/10.1016/j.tics.2011.04.004

Karl, A., Schaefer, M., Malta, L. S., Dörfel, D., Rohleder, N., & Werner, A. (2006). A meta-analysis of structural brain abnormalities in PTSD. *Neuroscience & Biobehavioral Reviews, 30*(7), 1004–1031. https://doi.org/10.1016/j.neubiorev.2006.03.004

Kelley, L. P., Weathers, F. W., McDevitt-Murphy, M. E., Eakin, D. E., & Flood, A. M. (2009). A comparison of PTSD symptom patterns in three types of civilian trauma. *Journal of Traumatic Stress, 22*(3), 227–235. https://doi.org/10.1002/jts.20406

Kensinger, E. A., Addis, D. R., & Atapattu, R. K. (2011). Amygdala activity at encoding corresponds with memory vividness and with memory for select episodic details. *Neuropsychologia, 49*(4), 663–673. https://doi.org/10.1016/j.neuropsychologia.2011.01.017

Kimble, M. O., Fleming, K., Bandy, C., Kim, J., & Zambetti, A. (2010). Eye tracking and visual attention to threatening stimuli in veterans of the Iraq war. *Journal of Anxiety Disorders, 24*(3), 293–299. https://doi.org/10.1016/j.janxdis.2009.12.006

Kindt, M., Buck, N., Arntz, A., & Soeter, M. (2007). Perceptual and conceptual processing as predictors of treatment outcome in PTSD. *Journal of Behavior Therapy and Experimental Psychiatry, 38*(4), 491–506. https://doi.org/10.1016/j.jbtep.2007.10.002

Kleim, B., Graham, B., Bryant, R. A., & Ehlers, A. (2013). Capturing intrusive re-experiencing in trauma survivors' daily lives using ecological momentary assessment. *Journal of Abnormal Psychology, 122*(4), 998–1009. https://doi.org/10.1037/a0034957

Laier, C., Schulte, F. P., & Brand, M. (2013). Pornographic picture processing interferes with working memory performance. *Journal of Sex Research, 50*(7), 642–652. https://doi.org/10.1080/00224499.2012.716873

Laney, C., & Loftus, E. F. (2010). False memory. In J. M. Brown & E. A. Campbell (Eds.), *The Cambridge handbook of forensic psychology* (pp. 187–194). New York, NY: Cambridge University Press. https://doi.org/10.1017/CBO9780511730290.023

Lazarus, R. S. (1991). Progress on a cognitive-motivational-relational theory of emotion. *American Psychologist, 46*(8), 819–834. https://doi.org/10.1037/0003-066X.46.8.819

Lee, J.-H., & Lee, J.-A. (2012). Attentional bias to violent images in survivors of dating violence. *Cognition and Emotion, 26*(6), 1124–1133. https://doi.org/10.1080/02699931.2011.638906

Levin, R. J., & van Berlo, W. (2004). Sexual arousal and orgasm in subjects who experience forced or non-consensual sexual stimulation–a review. *Journal of Clinical Forensic Medicine, 11*(2), 82–88. https://doi.org/10.1016/j.jcfm.2003.10.008

Liang, K. C., Juler, R. G., & McGaugh, J. L. (1986). Modulating effects of posttraining epinephrine on memory: Involvement of the amygdala noradrenergic system. *Brain Research, 368*(1), 125–133. https://doi.org/10.1016/0006-8993(86)91049-8

Lindsay, D. S., & Read, J. D. (1994). Psychotherapy and memories of childhood sexual abuse: A cognitive perspective. *Applied Cognitive Psychology, 8*(4), 281–338. https://doi.org/10.1002/acp.1780

Loftus, E. F. (1979). *Eyewitness testimony*. Cambridge, MA: Harvard University Press.

Loftus, E. F. (2003). Make-believe memories. *American Psychologist, 58*(11), 867–873. https://doi.org/10.1037/0003-066X.58.11.867

Loftus, E. F., Garry, M., & Feldman, J. (1994). Forgetting sexual trauma: What does it mean when 38% forget? *Journal of Consulting and Clinical Psychology, 62*(6), 1177–1181. https://doi.org/10.1037/0022-006X.62.6.1177

Loftus, G. R., & Mackworth, N. H. (1978). Cognitive determinants of fixation location during picture viewing. *Journal of Experimental Psychology: Human Perception and Performance, 4*(4), 565–572. https://doi.org/10.1037/0096-1523.4.4.565

Marks, E. H., Franklin, A. R., & Zoellner, L. A. (2018). Can't get it out of my mind: A systematic review of predictors of intrusive memories of distressing events. *Psychological Bulletin, 144*(6), 584–640. https://doi.org/10.1037/bul0000132

McGaugh, J. L. (2004). Memory reconsolidation hypothesis revived but restrained: Theoretical comment on Biedenkapp and Rudy (2004). *Behavioral Neuroscience, 118*(5), 1140–1142. https://doi.org/10.1037/0735-7044.118.5.1140

McGaugh, J. L. (2013). Making lasting memories: Remembering the significant. *Proceedings of the National Academy of Sciences, 110*(2), 10402–10407. https://doi.org/10.1073/pnas.1301209110

McNally, R. J. (2005). Debunking myths about trauma and memory. *The Canadian Journal of Psychiatry, 50*(13), 817–822. https://doi.org/10.1177/070674370505001302

McNally, R. J., Metzger, L. J., Lasko, N. B., Clancy, S. A., & Pitman, R. K. (1998). Directed forgetting of trauma cues in adult survivors of childhood sexual abuse with and without posttraumatic stress disorder. *Journal of Abnormal Psychology, 107*(4), 596–601. https://doi.org/10.1037/0021-843X.107.4.596

Mechanic, M. B., Resick, P. A., & Griffin, M. G. (1998). A comparison of normal forgetting, psychopathology, and information-processing models of reported amnesia for recent sexual trauma. *Journal of Consulting and Clinical Psychology, 66*(6), 948–957. https://doi.org/10.1037/0022-006X.66.6.948

Mogg, K., Bradley, B., Miles, F., & Dixon, R. (2004). Brief report time course for attentional bias for threat scenes: Testing the vigilance-avoidance hypothesis. *Cognition and Emotion, 18*(5), 689–700. https://doi.org/10.1080/02699930341000158

Moore, S. A., & Zoellner, L. A. (2007). Overgeneral autobiographical memory and traumatic events: An evaluative review. *Psychological Bulletin, 133*(3), 419–437.https://doi.org/10.1037/0033-2909.133.3.419

Morey, R. A., Dolcos, F., Petty, C. M., Cooper, D. A., Hayes, J. P., LaBar, K. S., & McCarthy, G. (2009). The role of trauma-related distractors on neural systems for working memory and emotion processing in posttraumatic stress disorder. *Journal of Psychiatric Research, 43*(8), 809–817. https://doi.org/10.1016/j.jpsychires.2008.10.014

Moulds, M. L., & Bryant, R. A. (2005). Traumatic memories in acute stress disorder: An analysis of narratives before and after treatment. *Clinical Psychologist, 9*(1), 10–14. https://doi.org/10.1080/13284200500116971

Moulds, M. L., & Bryant, R. A. (2008). Avoidant encoding in acute stress disorder: A prospective study. *Depression and Anxiety, 25*(12), E195–E198. https://doi.org/10.1002/da.20368

Mozzambani, A. C., Fuso, S. F., Malta, S. M., Ribeiro, R. L., Pupo, M. C., Flaks, M. K., & Mello, M. F. (2017). Long-term follow-up of attentional and executive functions of PTSD patients. *Psychology & Neuroscience, 10*(2), 215–224. https://doi.org/10.1037/pne0000088

Müller, G. E., & Pilzecker, A. (1900). *Experimentelle beiträge zur lehre vom gedächtniss*. Leipzig: JA Barth.

Neuner, F., Schauer, M., Klaschik, C., Karunakara, U., & Elbert, T. (2004). A comparison of narrative exposure therapy, supportive counseling, and psychoeducation for treating posttraumatic stress disorder in an African refugee settlement. *Journal of Consulting and Clinical Psychology, 72*(4), 579–587. https://doi.org/10.1037/0022-006X.72.4.579

Nicholson, E. L., Bryant, R. A., & Felmingham, K. L. (2014). Interaction of noradrenaline and cortisol predicts negative intrusive memories in posttraumatic stress disorder. *Neurobiology of Learning and Memory, 112*, 204–211. https://doi.org/10.1016/j.nlm.2013.11.018

Norman, K. A., Newman, E. L., & Detre, G. (2007). A neural network model of retrieval-induced forgetting. *Psychological Review, 114*(4), 887–953. https://doi.org/10.1037/0033-295X.114.4.887

Ozer, E. J., Best, S. R., Lipsey, T. L., & Weiss, D. S. (2003). Predictors of posttraumatic stress disorder and symptoms in adults: *A meta-analysis. Psychological Bulletin, 129*(1), 52–73. https://doi.org/10.1037/0033-2909.129.1.52.

Patihis, L., Lilienfeld, S. O., Ho, L., & Loftus, E. (2014). Unconscious repressed memory is scientifically questionable. *Psychological Science, 25*(10), 1967–1968. https://doi.org/10.1177/0956797614547365

Patihis, L., & Place, P. J. (2018). Weak evidence for increased motivated forgetting of trauma-related words in dissociated or traumatised individuals in a directed forgetting experiment. *Memory, 26*(5), 619–633. https://doi.org/10.1080/09658211.2017.1387666

Phelps, E. A., Delgado, M. R., Nearing, K. I., & LeDoux, J. E. (2004). Extinction learning in humans: Role of the amygdala and vmPFC. *Neuron, 43*(6), 897–905. https://doi.org/10.1016/j.neuron.2004.08.042Get

Pickel, K. L. (1998). Unusualness and threat as possible causes of "weapon focus". *Memory, 6*(3), 277–295. https://doi.org/10.1080/741942361

Pickel, K. L. (1999). The influence of context on the "weapon focus" effect. *Law and Human Behavior, 23*(3), 299–311. https://doi.org/10.1023/A:1022356431375

Pineles, S. L., Shipherd, J. C., Mostoufi, S. M., Abramovitz, S. M., & Yovel, I. (2009). Attentional biases in PTSD: More evidence for interference. *Behavior Research and Therapy, 47*(12), 1050–1057. https://doi.org/10.1016/j.brat.2009.08.001

Resick, P. A., & Schnicke, M. K. (1992). Cognitive processing therapy for sexual assault victims. *Journal of Consulting and Clinical Psychology, 60*(5), 748. https://doi.org/10.1037/0022-006X.60.5.748

Roediger, H. L. (1990). Implicit memory: Retention without remembering. *American Psychologist, 45*(9), 1043–1056. https://doi.org/10.1037/0003-066X.45.9.1043

Roediger, H. L., III, & DeSoto, K. A. (2014). Confidence and memory: *Assessing positive and negative correlations. Memory, 22*(1), 76–91. https://doi.org/10.1080/09658211.2013.795974

Roozendaal, B., Okuda, S., Van der Zee, E. A., & McGaugh, J. L. (2006). Glucocorticoid enhancement of memory requires arousal-induced noradrenergic activation in the basolateral amygdala. *Proceedings of the National Academy of Sciences, 103*(17), 6741–6746. https://doi.org/10.1073/pnas.0601874103

Roozendaal, B., Quirarte, G. L., & McGaugh, J. L. (2002). Glucocorticoids interact with the basolateral amygdala β-adrenoceptor–cAMP/cAMP/PKA system in influencing memory consolidation. *European Journal of Neuroscience, 15*(3), 553–560. https://doi.org/10.1046/j.0953-816x.2001.01876.x

Rosenthal, M. Z., & Follette, V. M. (2007). The effects of sexual assault-related intrusion suppression in the laboratory and natural environment. *Behaviour Research and Therapy, 45*(1), 73–87. https://doi.org/10.1016/j.brat.2006.01.013

Rothbaum, B. O., Foa, E. B., Riggs, D. S., Murdock, T., & Walsh, W. (1992). A prospective examination of post-traumatic stress disorder in rape victims. *Journal of Traumatic Stress, 5*(3), 455–475. https://doi.org/10.1002/jts.2490050309.

Scheflin, A. W., & Brown, D. (1996). Repressed memory or dissociative amnesia: What the science says. *Journal of Psychiatry & Law, 24*(2), 143–188. https://doi.org/10.1177/009318539602400203

Scoboria, A., Wade, K. A., Lindsay, D. S., Azad, T., Strange, D., Ost, J., & Hyman, I. E. (2017). A mega-analysis of memory reports from eight peer-reviewed false memory implantation studies. *Memory, 25*(2), 146–163. https://doi.org/10.1080/09658211.2016.1260747.

Serrano, J. P., Latorre, J. M., Gatz, M., & Montanes, J. (2004). Life review therapy using autobiographical retrieval practice for older adults with depressive symptomatology. *Psychology and Aging, 19*(2), 272–277. https://doi.org/10.1037/0882-7974.19.2.272

Shipherd, J. C., & Beck, J. G. (1999). The effects of suppressing trauma-related thoughts on women with rape-related posttraumatic stress disorder. *Behaviour Research and Therapy, 37*(2), 99–112. https://doi.org/10.1016/S0005-7967(98)00136-3

Steblay, N. M. (1992). A meta-analytic review of the weapon focus effect. *Law and Human Behavior, 16*(4), 413–424. https://doi.org/10.1007/BF02352267

van der Kolk, B. A. (1987). *Psychological trauma*. Washington, DC: American Psychiatric Press.

van Giezen, A. E., Arensman, E., Spinhoven, P., & Wolters, G. (2005). Consistency of memory for emotionally arousing events: A review of prospective and experimental studies. *Clinical Psychology Review, 25*(7), 935–953. https://doi.org/10.1016/j.cpr.2005.04.011

van Minnen, A., Wessel, I., Dijkstra, T., & Roelofs, K. (2002). Changes in PTSD patients' narratives during prolonged exposure therapy: A replication and extension. *Journal of Traumatic Stress, 15*(3), 255–258. https://doi.org/10.1023/A:1015263513654

Vasterling, J. J., Brailey, K., Constans, J. I., & Sutker, P. B. (1998). Attention and memory dysfunction in posttraumatic stress disorder. *Neuropsychology, 12*(1), 125–133. dio: https://doi.org/10.1037/0894-4105.12.1.125

Walker, W. R., Skowronski, J. J., & Thompson, C. P. (2003). Life is pleasant-and memory helps to keep it that way! *Review of General Psychology, 7*(2), 203–210. https://doi.org/10.1037/1089-2680.7.2.203

White, A. M. (2003). What happened? Alcohol, memory blackouts, and the brain. *Alcohol Research and Health, 27*(2), 186–196.

White, L. K., Suway, J. G., Pine, D. S., Bar-Haim, Y., & Fox, N. A. (2011). Cascading effects: The influence of attention bias to threat on the interpretation of ambiguous information. *Behaviour Research and Therapy, 49*(4), 244-251. dio: https://doi.org/10.1016/j.brat.2011.01.004

Williams, H. L., Conway, M. A., & Cohen, G. (2007). Autobiographical memory. In G. Cohen & M. A. Conway (Eds.), *Memory in the real world* (3rd ed.). London: Psychology Press.

Williams, J. M. G. (2006). Capture and rumination, functional avoidance, and executive control (CaRFAX): Three processes that underlie overgeneral memory. *Cognition and Emotion, 20*(3-4), 548-568. dio: https://doi.org/10.1080/02699930500450465

Wixted, J. T., Mickes, L., Clark, S. E., Gronlund, S. D., & Roediger, H. L., III. (2015). Initial eyewitness confidence reliably predicts eyewitness identification accuracy. *American Psychologist, 70*(6), 515–526. https://doi.org/10.1037/a0039510

Wolf, E. J., Miller, M. W., Reardon, A. F., Ryabchenko, K. A., Castillo, D., & Freund, R. (2012). A latent class analysis of dissociation and posttraumatic stress disorder: Evidence for a dissociative subtype. *Archives of General Psychiatry, 69*(7), 698–705. https://doi.org/10.1001/archgenpsychiatry.2011.1574

Wolf, E. J., Mitchell, K. S., Sadeh, N., Hein, C., Fuhrman, I., Pietrzak, R. H., & Miller, M. W. (2017). The

Dissociative Subtype of PTSD Scale: Initial evaluation in a national sample of trauma-exposed veterans. *Assessment, 24*(4), 503–516. https://doi.org/10.1177/1073191115615212

Wright, L. W., Jr., & Adams, H. E. (1999). The effects of stimuli that vary in erotic content on cognitive processes. *Journal of Sex Research, 36*(2), 145–151. https://doi.org/10.1080/00224499909551979

Zinzow, H. M., Resnick, H. S., McCauley, J. L., Amstadter, A. B., Ruggiero, K. J., & Kilpatrick, D. G. (2010). The role of rape tactics in risk for posttraumatic stress disorder and major depression: Results from a national sample of college women. *Depression and Anxiety, 27*(8), 708-715. dio: https://doi.org/10.1002/da.20719

Zoellner, L. A., Foa, E. B., Brigidi, B. D., & Przeworski, A. (2000). Are trauma victims susceptible to "false memories"? *Journal of Abnormal Psychology, 109*(3), 517–524. dio: https://doi.org/10.1037/0021-843X.109.3.517

Zoellner, L. A., Sacks, M. B., & Foa, E. B. (2003). Directed forgetting following mood induction in chronic posttraumatic stress disorder patients. *Journal of Abnormal Psychology, 112*(3), 508–514. https://doi.org/10.1037/0021-843X.112.3.508

The Impact of Sexual Assault on Sexual Function: Strategies for Treatment and Prevention

21

Catalina Vechiu

Sexual victimization is a pervasive problem associated with immediate and long-term psychopathology and sexual health impairment. The impact of sexual assault on mental health has been extensively examined. Findings indicate that women who experience sexual assault are more likely to use illicit drugs, report symptoms of anxiety, depression, or posttraumatic stress disorder (PTSD), and interpersonal difficulties in comparison to the general population (Briere & Jordan, 2004; Tolin & Foa, 2006). Ample evidence indicate that sexual victimization is also associated with negative sexual health outcomes including orgasm difficulties, inhibited arousal or desire, fear of sex, negative attitudes about sex, and engaging in risky sexual behaviors (Leonard & Follette, 2002; Lutfey, Link, Litman, Rosen, & McKinlay, 2008; Rellini & Meston, 2007). Although there is little disagreement that sexual assault is associated with negative mental health sequelae, the treatment of sexual dysfunction is subject to considerable debate. Evidence-based treatments for trauma-related sequelae have been extensively examined, and variations of cognitive behavioral therapy (CBT) have been demonstrated to successfully treat commonly experienced trauma-related psychopathology (i.e. depression, anxiety, and PTSD; Resick, Nishith, Weaver, Astin, & Feuer, 2002). There is a dearth of research on protocols assessing and treating female sexual functioning following experiences of sexual victimization. As such, the aim of this chapter is to identify the key findings and gaps in the literature regarding the treatment and prevention of sexual dysfunction and discuss strategies for intervention. The chapter will begin with a brief overview of the prevalence rates of sexual assault and sexual dysfunction disorders, followed by an examination of evidence-based treatments of sexual dysfunction including best practices for assessment and intervention.

Definitions and Prevalence

Prevalence of Sexual Assault

Epidemiological studies indicate that exposure to traumatic events may vary dramatically based on gender. The pattern of findings indicates that men broadly have a higher risk of exposure to traumatic events and that the overall rate of trauma exposure does not appear to be higher among women (Breslau, Davis, Andreski, & Peterson, 1991; Creamer, Burgess, & McFarlane, 2001). Despite lower exposure to traumatic events, women have a higher likelihood of experiencing certain trauma types. For instance, in a national sample of U.S. adults the overall prevalence rate for sexual assault victimization was 29.7%, but 42.4% of women reported a history of sexual assault in comparison to 15.8% of men (Kilpatrick et al., 2013). Data from the National Intimate Partner and Sexual Violence Survey found that an

C. Vechiu (✉)
University of Nevada, Reno, Reno, NV, USA

W. T. O'Donohue and P. A. Schewe (eds.), *Handbook of Sexual Assault and Sexual Assault Prevention*,
https://doi.org/10.1007/978-3-030-23645-8_21

estimated 19.3% of women and 1.7% of men were raped during their lifetime and an estimated 1.6% of women reported being raped in the 12 months preceding the survey (Breiding et al., 2014). Consistent with the findings from Kilpatrick et al. (2013), an estimated 43.9% of women and 23.4% of men reported experiencing other forms of sexual violence during their lifetimes, including unwanted sexual contact, noncontact unwanted sexual experiences, sexual coercion, and being made to penetrate (Breiding et al., 2014). These findings are consistent with previous studies indicating that women are more likely to experience interpersonal assaults, such as sexual abuse in childhood or adulthood and rape (i.e. Breslau, Davis, Andreski, Peterson, & Schultz, 1997; Kessler, Sonnega, Bromet, Hughes, & Nelson, 1995). For these reasons, the focus of this chapter is on the experiences of sexual assault and sexual dysfunction for women.

Prevalence of Sexual Dysfunction

Sexual dysfunction is a major health concern in the general population and associated with impaired quality of life, diminished satisfaction with one's sexual life, and personal and/or relationship difficulties. In the Diagnostic and Statistics Manual of Mental Disorders (DSM-5), sexual dysfunctions "are typically characterized by a clinically significant disturbance in a person's ability to respond sexually or to experience sexual pleasure" (American Psychiatric Association [APA], 2013, p. 423). For women, there are currently three sexual dysfunctions:

1. **Female orgasmic disorder**: Presence of one or both of the following: delay, infrequency, or absence of orgasm, and/or reduced intensity of orgasm present 75–100% of the time.
2. **Female sexual interest/arousal disorder**: New category that represents the combination of sexual desire and arousal disorders diagnosed by the decrease or absence of three of the following: sexual activity, sexual interest, erotic thoughts or fantasies, initiation of sexual activity or responsiveness to a partner's attempts, sexual excitement, response to sexual cues, and genital and nongenital sensations during sexual activity.
3. **Genito-pelvic pain/penetration disorder**: New category that represents the merging of dyspareunia and vaginismus and diagnosed by the persistence and recurrence of one or more of the following difficulties: vaginal penetration, marked vulvovaginal or pelvic pain during penetration or attempt at penetration, fear or anxiety about pain in anticipation of, during, or after penetration, and tightening or tensing of pelvic floor muscles during attempted penetration (APA, 2013).

Sexual dysfunction is highly prevalent, with data from the 1992 National Health and Social Life Survey in the United States estimating that 43% of women experience sexual dysfunction (Laumann, Paik, & Rosen, 1999), with 37.7% of women reporting low sexual desire, 25.3% report low arousal, and 21.1% reporting difficulties with orgasm (Shifren, Monz, Russo, Segreti, & Johannes, 2008). In studies examining DSM-IV female sexual dysfunction disorders, estimates of dysfunction are highest for orgasmic disorder (4–7% in the general population and 5–42% in primary care settings) and sexual interest/arousal disorders (6–46% in the general population), followed by dyspareunia (now genito-pelvic pain penetration disorder; 3–18% in the general population and 3–46% in primary care settings) and vaginismus (now genito-pelvic pain penetration disorder; 0.5–1% in the general population and up to 30% in primary care settings) (APA, 2000; Frank, Mistretta, & Will, 2008; Simons & Carey, 2001). Despite findings that the rate of sexual dysfunction increases with age and tends to be highest around middle age, younger women also experience high rates of sexual dysfunction. In a study examining rates of sexual dysfunction in a sample of women age 18–39, Laumann et al. (1999) found that 18% of women reported experiencing pain during sexual intercourse, 27% of women reported an inability to achieve orgasm, and 32% reported an absence of sexual interest.

Epidemiological studies examining the prevalence rates of sexual dysfunction in women with a history of sexual trauma have found that 60% of women with a history of sexual assault or rape report a sexual dysfunction (Öberg, Fugl-Meyer, & Fugl-Meyer, 2004). Victims of rape during childhood report problems with desire and arousal (Van Berlo & Ensink, 2000), vaginismus, and orgasm problems (Lutfey et al., 2008). Women with a history of childhood sexual abuse (CSA) experience sexual difficulties that may persist for several years, such as orgasm problems, painful intercourse, sexual dissatisfaction, and a lack of sexual interest and arousal (Loeb et al., 2002; Najman, Dunne, Purdie, Boyle, & Coxeter, 2005). The experience of rape in adulthood doubles the risk of developing sexual difficulties (Letourneau, Resnick, Kilpatrick, Saunders, & Best, 1996; Lutfey et al., 2008), and one of the most consistent findings is that the ability to achieve orgasm is significantly impaired in women with a history of sexual assault. For instance, in a nationally representative sample of Swedish women two-thirds of those sexually abused reported at least one sexual dysfunction, and all types of sexual abuse (i.e. vaginal penetration, genital manipulation, etc.) except abusive cunnilingus were associated with lower levels of achieving orgasm (Öberg, Fugl-Meyer, & Fugl-Meyer, 2002). Additionally, 81% of the women who reported being abused several times had one or more sexual dysfunctions in comparison to 54% of women who reported being abused one time (Öberg et al., 2002). Women who were sexually abused also reported lower levels of sexual satisfaction in comparison with nonabused women (Öberg et al., 2002).

Comorbid Sexual Dysfunction and Psychopathology

Women who have experienced sexual assault report higher rates of lifetime anxiety and mood disorders (Iverson et al., 2013), are twice as likely to experience a major depressive episode following assault (Hedtke et al., 2008), and three times more likely to have PTSD (Hedtke et al., 2008) in comparison with those without such experiences. Symptoms of depression and PTSD are often comorbid and may include a high degree of overlap (Gros, Price, Magruder, & Frueh, 2012). Despite the well-documented consequences of sexual victimization, data on direct associations between victimization and sexual functioning are mixed. Specifically, the degree to which psychopathology (i.e. depression and PTSD) influences the relationship between sexual victimization and sexual functioning is subject to debate. For instance, Rellini and Meston (2007) found that women with a history of CSA were more likely to be depressed in comparison to a sample of nonabused women. In a similar sample, Meston, Rellini, and Heiman (2006) found an inverse relationship between passionate/romantic sexual self-schemas and negative sexual affect during sexual arousal, which was independent from symptoms of depression. Lutfey et al. (2008) found that a history of adult sexual abuse was significantly and positively associated with sexual dysfunction even after controlling for depression. However, it is unclear whether depression is an outcome to sexual dysfunction or a contributor, particularly as symptoms of depression are independently associated with sexual functioning (Kashdan et al., 2011). One longitudinal study with women who reported a history of sexual assault victimization found that the interaction of depressive symptoms with lifetime assault severity predicted pain experienced during sex over 1 year (Neilson, Norris, Bryan, & Stapenbeck, 2017). Women who were victimized during the follow-up assessment periods reported less sexual enjoyment and satisfaction and more sexual pain, indicating that the acute period following assault is associated with more severe symptomatology (Neilson et al., 2017).

Furthermore, PTSD has been found to act as a moderating factor in the development of sexual difficulties in women with trauma histories even after controlling for depression (Letourneau et al., 1996). One study found that women with a history of sexual assault who reported having PTSD were four times more likely to report sexual difficulties in comparison with women with a history of nonsexual trauma (Haase, Boos, Schönfeld, & Hoyer, 2009). Another study with female veterans found that women were more likely to have a sexual dysfunction if they had PTSD in comparison with women without PTSD (Breyer et al., 2016). Studies that examine the relationship of sexual victimization with trauma and PTSD typically evaluate this relationship using PTSD severity (Blais, Geiser, & Cruz, 2018). Examining this association with symptom clusters may provide a more nuanced understanding of the mechanisms involved. One such study found that symptoms of hyperarousal and numbing were the most closely associated with impaired sexual functioning (Schnurr et al., 2009). A more recent study with female veterans who experienced military sexual trauma found that negative alterations in cognitions and mood, anhedonia, and dysphoric arousal symptom clusters fully mediated the association between assault with sexual satisfaction and function (Blais et al., 2018). These results indicate that PTSD may function as an important mediator variable. The frequent comorbidity and significant symptom overlap between depression and PTSD may make it difficult to delineate the effects of each disorder on sexual functioning, particularly because both appear to uniquely impact the relationship between sexual abuse and sexual functioning (Letourneau et al., 1996).

Evidence-Based Treatments and Best Practices

Survivors of sexual assault often face multiple challenges that are not adequately addressed by the "gold standard" treatments for trauma-related distress. Specifically, trauma responses can generalize beyond specific triggers to impair sexual functioning, where women may experience negative cognitions and beliefs regarding sexual relationships, desired sexual activities, self-esteem regarding their sexuality, and appropriate and healthy sexual behavior and intimacy. Impairments in these domains may not be adequately captured by PTSD diagnostic criteria and may therefore warrant a multi-pronged approach to treatment. There are empirically based treatments for trauma-related distress, particularly PTSD, but few empirically validated treatments for sexual dysfunction (see O'Donohue, Dopke, & Swingen, 1997 and O'Donohue, Swingen, Dopke, & Regev, 1999 for a review) and even fewer treatments that specifically target comorbid PTSD and sexual dysfunction. For this reason, we propose the use of exposure therapy (i.e. Prolonged Exposure, Cognitive Processing Therapy) provided concurrently with traditional treatment components of sex therapy (i.e. sensate focused exercises and mindfulness).

Assessment

A comprehensive assessment should be conducted in order to formulate a treatment plan. Wincze and Weisberg (2015) suggest conducting an evaluation over one to three sessions depending on the severity of the presenting problems and partner involvement. The first session can be conducted with a partner, if available and interested, the second session is often conducted with the client alone, and the third session serves as an opportunity to present an initial case formulation and outline for treatment. During the assessment phase, the following domains should be evaluated:

- **Psychosexual/psychosocial history**: Including experiences of sexual trauma or abuse, personal, family, and cultural beliefs about sexuality, psychological and interpersonal factors, history of psychological distress, partner attitudes and beliefs, patient's self-esteem and coping skills.
- **Sexual history**: Including sexual activity, practices, experiences, problems and satisfaction, positive and negative sexual relationships.
- **Medical history**: Including the use of medications and substances, past or present sexually transmitted infections (STIs), reproductive, menstrual and obstetric histories as well as an evaluation of childhood/adolescence surgeries,

disease, medical care, and how they experienced secondary sex changes.
- **Self-report questionnaires**: Brief measures, such as the Female Sexual Functioning Inventory (FSFI; Rosen et al., 2000), Sexual Functioning Questionnaire (SFQ; Quirk et al., 2002), and daily diaries and sexual encounter logs such as the Sexual Encounter Profile for Women, can be administered regularly for the assessment of sexual problems.

A comprehensive psychosocial/psychosexual history can aid the clinician in developing a case formulation for trauma-related distress such as PTSD and sexual dysfunction. Discussions about sexuality, particularly after sexual assault, can often be uncomfortable for both the client and the clinician. This can impact the client's willingness to discuss sexual health concerns and the type of information the client is willing to disclose during assessment and therapy. Several models for facilitating a conversation regarding sexual concerns, building rapport, and engendering client comfort have been developed. One of the most widely researched approaches is the Extended Permission giving, Limited Information, Specific Suggestions, and Intensive Therapy (EX-PLISSIT; Davis & Taylor, 2006; see Table 21.1) model and will be discussed in detail next.

EX-PLISSIT Model

The EX-PLISSIT model is an extension of the widely used PLISSIT (Permission, Limited Information, Specific Suggestions, Intensive Therapy) model that is utilized by clinicians as both a facilitator of conversations regarding the sexual healthcare needs of clients as well as a foundation for the treatment of sexual dysfunctions (Annon, 1976). A core feature of the extended model is permission-giving at each stage of the model. An additional feature is reflection, during which time the clinician surveys his or her own attitudes about the client and his or her dysfunction and how this may impact the care the clinician provides (Taylor & Davis, 2006). A third element is review, during which time the clinician seeks the client's perspective on their sexual health concerns during the current session and at future visits (Taylor & Davis, 2006).

Permission-giving. The first level of the EX-PLISSIT model involves giving clients permission to voice concerns regarding their sexual health by broaching the subject first. Clients are often embarrassed or uncomfortable raising the topic of sexual difficulties and by giving clients permission to openly discuss their concerns clinicians have the opportunity to normalize sexuality. During this stage, clinicians should explicitly invite the client to express any concerns by asking direct questions. It is also important to remember that hesitation on the part of the client may not necessarily reflect an unwillingness to discuss sexual health concerns. It might be helpful to ask questions such as "Would you like to talk about this further?" to gauge the client's level of comfort and willingness to discuss sexual health (Taylor & Davis, 2006). Permission to discuss sexual health issues should not only be given once; further permission-giving is necessary to inform the client that they may discuss their sexual health worries at any stage or session.

Limited Information. The second level of the EX-PLISSIT model necessitates further permission-giving because the client may not feel at ease to disclose all of their sexual concerns. Thus, the information the clinician provides should be relevant to the sexual topics the client chooses to discuss. This stage highlights the clinician's role as a source of information and it is an optimal opportunity for providing limited factual information, clarifying misinformation, and discussing common sexual myths. The clinician can provide this information via different modalities and can direct client to websites, books, or brochures that normalize any sexual health concerns that the client may have.

Specific Suggestions. At this level, information gathered from the comprehensive assessment of the client's sexual health concerns is incorporated into individualized specific suggestions that address concerns beyond sexual behavior. This includes a problem-solving approach that requires

Table 21.1 EX-PLISSIT model of initiating discussion of sexual dysfunctions

Level	Scope	Examples
Permission-giving	Give permission for the client to comfortably discuss their sexual health/dysfunction concerns in a nonjudgmental and relaxed environment	"Clients who have experienced sexual assault often experience sexual difficulties. What has been your experience?" "How satisfied are you with your current sexual relationships?" "Many clients find that they often experience changes in their sexual satisfaction/desire/interest. Is it okay if we discuss this?"
Limited Information	Provide accurate information, correct misconceptions, and normalize the client's experiences	"This brochure provides information on some of the common side effects of [medication] including some information on sexual activity. Once you've read it, let's discuss some of your questions at your next session"
Specific suggestions	Make specific suggestions for the patient's particular concern by adopting a problem-solving approach	"How would you and your partner feel about incorporating other sexual activities to help you reconnect?" "To address the issue of [concern], let's consider a few activities that you can still safely enjoy until you recover. What can you focus on?"
Intensive therapy	Identify further resources for the elicited concerns and provide specialist referrals	"Some clients find it helpful to talk to someone who has experience in this area. Are you interested in getting more support for the issues we've discussed?" Some clients with a history of trauma and PTSD can benefit from therapy for sexual concerns. I'd like to tell you about the options available for treatment "There are a number of websites/books that some of my clients with similar concerns have found helpful. Are you interested in that information?"
Review	Seek the client's perspective	"Are there any other concerns/things that you might think of?" "How useful was the brochure I gave you in answering some of your questions about sexual activity?" "What might your partner think/feel about this?" "At your last session, we discussed [concern] and you mentioned [client issue]. How has this been since we last talked?"
Reflect	Challenge own assumptions and develop knowledge informally or through supervision with peers	"Which conversations make me feel uncomfortable or embarrassed?" "When was the last time a patient expressed concerns with their sexual life?"

Adapted from Taylor and Davis (2007)

more knowledge and experience in the domain of sexual dysfunction. Permission-giving should also occur at this stage, particularly to encourage clients to express concerns regarding the suggestions made by the clinician. It is possible that the client may not find them relevant or is uncomfortable incorporating the recommendations; giving clients permission at this stage facilitates an open dialogue and helps the client and the clinician implement a problem-solving approach to the client's concerns.

Intensive Therapy. The final level includes referral to specialized interventions, which can include both psychological and medical assessment and treatment. Within the context of psychosocial treatment, this phase of assessment can consist of providing the client with a case conceptualization and rationale for treatment. If during the evaluation it is determined that the client is experiencing PTSD, this level may be utilized as an opportunity to discuss PE as a first-line intervention followed by traditional sex therapy.

The EX-PLISSIT model provides standardization to the discussion of sexual dysfunction and enables clinicians to incorporate the elements of permission-giving at each level, reflection, and review in order to initiate an open dialogue with clients to identify and address their individual needs. This framework, however, does not necessitate a sequential progression through the different levels. Instead, the model allows clinicians to recognize that they may not necessarily function at all levels in all situations confidently or competently. For instance, if the clinician is faced with an issue that may not fall within their scope of practice after giving the client initial Permission, the clinician can refer the client to another practitioner (Taylor & Davis, 2006).

Treatment Approaches

The most recent clinical practice guidelines from the American Psychological Association (APA, 2017) strongly recommend the use of cognitive behavioral therapy (CBT), cognitive processing therapy (CPT), and Prolonged Exposure (PE) as first-line interventions for PTSD. A meta-analysis on the effectiveness of psychotherapy for PTSD found that on average, 50–70% of patients who complete these treatments no longer met diagnostic criteria for PTSD (Bradley, Greene, Russ, Dutra, & Western, 2005). Cognitive behavioral therapy for trauma includes a broad class of therapies unified by a shared emphasis on the relationship among thoughts, emotions, and behaviors. Cognitive Processing Therapy and PE are variants of CBT, although there are conceptual differences regarding the theory of mechanisms of change (i.e. PE highlights the role of a maladaptive learning process in the development of PTSD). All variants of cognitive theory view the appraisal of a traumatic event as integral to the development and maintenance of PTSD (Lancaster, Teeters, Gros, & Back, 2016). What follows is a brief description of PE (for a detailed review see McLean & Foa, 2011) and CPT (for a detailed review see Lancaster, et al., 2016).

Prolonged Exposure consists of 8–15 weekly or biweekly sessions that are approximately 60–90 min in duration focused on gradual and systematic exposure to trauma-related memories, situations, and feelings. The PE protocol is manualized and includes psychoeducation (PTSD symptoms and factors that maintain PTSD, treatment rationale), breathing retraining, in vivo exercises (confronting people, places, and things that serve as trauma reminders and triggers), imaginal exposures (revisiting the trauma memory and emotionally engaging with the content), and emotional processing (open-ended discussion about the experiences of the exposures). PE has amassed the greatest amount of empirical support across various populations with PTSD and other comorbid conditions (Zayfert & Black Becker, 2007). In a review of the existing evidence for PE, McLean and Foa (2011) report that 25 randomized controlled trials have been conducted that indicate that PE is effective in reducing PTSD symptomatology. PE has consistently been found to be effective for acute and chronic PTSD (Bryant, Sackville, Dang, Moulds, & Guthrie, 1999; Foa, Keane, Friedman, & Cohen, 2009). A meta-analysis found large effect sizes of PE at post-treatment, and medium to large effects at follow-up time points in comparison to control groups (Powers et al., 2010).

Cognitive processing therapy is a variant of CBT that focuses on a client's trauma-related cognitions and their subsequent impact on emotions and behaviors. CPT consists of cognitive therapy (assimilated-distorted beliefs such as denial and self-blame) and exposure elements (clients write detailed accounts of the most traumatic incident that they read to the therapist and themselves) (Resick & Schnicke, 1993). The aim of CPT is to identify and restructure maladaptive cognitions in order to reduce PTSD symptoms. CPT is typically delivered over 12 weekly sessions, which are approximately 50 min in duration, that place more emphasis on the role of maladaptive cognitions in maintaining PTSD. In a systematic review of the literature, there was moderate strength of evidence of a medium to large magnitude benefit of CPT for PSTD symptom reduction, loss of PTSD diagnosis and reduction of comorbid depression (APA, 2017). In an RCT comparing CPT and PE in a sample of rape victims, results indicate that CPT was as successful as PE in treating PTSD and depression but was superior in remediating guilt cognitions (Resick et al., 2002).

For couples, Cognitive Behavioral Conjoint Therapy for PTSD (CBCT) may be another efficacious option. CBCT is an evidence-based intervention that targets PTSD and intimate relationship functioning (Monson & Fredman, 2012). It consists of 15 treatment sessions scheduled for 75 min each. CBCT is organized into three phases (Brown-Bowers, Fredman, Wanklyn, & Monson, 2012):

- Phase I: Focus is on providing psychoeducation and teaching couples conflict management skills
- Phase II: Focus is on behavioral methods of addressing avoidance and couples engage in approaching feared situations
- Phase III: Focus is on trauma-specific appraisals and maladaptive conditions that maintain PTSD and relationship difficulties

CBCT effectively addresses concerns with sexual health and intimacy and symptoms of PTSD, while enlisting the client's partner in treatment. This is particularly important as partners may assume a nonsexualized role and engage in accommodative behaviors that can facilitate avoidance of sexual behavior (Brown-Bowers et al., 2012; Yehuda, Lehrner, & Rosenbaum, 2015). Partners may also experience their own psychological distress that can contribute to problems with emotional and physical intimacy. A study examining CBCT for PTSD with community participants revealed large pre- to posttreatment improvements in clients' and their partners' ratings of clients' PTSD symptoms (Monson et al., 2011). An earlier version of CBCT with Vietnam combat veterans and their wives found that veterans reported moderate improvements in their PTSD symptoms and large improvements in their depression symptoms (Monson, Schnurr, Stevens, & Guthrie, 2004). Wives reported large improvements in their own relationship satisfaction (Brown-Bowers et al., 2012). Although the extant literature for the effectiveness of CBCT is not extensive, it holds promise, particularly as it fills an existing treatment gap.

Treatment for sexual dysfunctions can be undertaken concurrently with stable treatment for PTSD. Sex therapy is often the treatment of choice and is a derivative of the intensive and daily specialized sex therapy initially developed by Masters and Johnson (1970), which targeted the alleviation of performance anxiety and improvement of sexual pleasure (Vechiu & O'Donohue, 2018). Sex therapies can include sexual skills training (SST), comprised of sensate focused exercises focused on improving sexual skills; or orgasm consistency training (OCT) and systematic desensitization (SD) if the sexual dysfunction is specific to achieving orgasm or genito-pelvic pain during intercourse or attempted intercourse respectively (Vechiu & O'Donohue, 2018). The common factor of most specialized sex therapies is the emphasis on sensate focused exercises, such as nongenital touching, genital touching, mutual touching, and sensual intercourse.

Unfortunately, survivors of sexual trauma may find traditional sex therapy challenging due to the overt focus on improvement of sexual pleasure. Sexual arousal or pleasure can trigger intrusive thoughts, flashbacks, dissociation, or feelings of guilt and shame, particularly if survivors experienced signs of physiological arousal or orgasm despite the lack of consent. This physiological response is often difficult for survivors to cope with, and they may engage in avoidance of sexual activity due to feelings of shame or self-blame. Furthermore, specialized sex therapy was initially based on the sexual response model developed by Masters and Johnson (1962) and assumes a linear progression from arousal to orgasm as the outcome of sexual activity. Traditional sex therapies may not be well tolerated by survivors of sexual trauma as they may need to relearn healthy sexual intimacy and relearn to tolerate and enjoy their own bodily responses to sexual stimuli instead of avoiding them. With orgasm as the epitome of "normal" sexual response, survivors of sexual trauma may experience further shame and guilt if unable to achieve orgasm.

As such, alternative approaches may include a sex-positive framework, which promotes positive regard for sexuality and intimacy, encourages openness regarding discussions of sexuality, and emphasizes boundaries, safety, and pleasure (Baggett et al., 2017). This may be particularly important for survivors of sexual assault because they have the opportunity to reclaim their healthy sexuality following the unsafe and boundary-violating experience of sexual trauma (Baggett et al., 2017). Within this framework, clinicians model the acceptance of healthy sexuality. This can aid clients in developing healthy romantic relationships that lead to improved enjoyment sexual intimacy. Sex-positive approaches can be implemented from a CBT framework. Specific components of sex-positive approaches can include:

- *Psychoeducation about sex and sexuality*: An important feature of psychoeducation is dispelling common myths about optimal sexual functioning, such as "Women always have an orgasm" or "Sex must be spontaneous" or "Sexual intercourse always leads to an orgasm" (Bitzer & Brandenburg, 2009). Other important features include the physiology of arousal and the association between PTSD symptoms, or the fight or flight response and inhibition of sexual arousal. Providing education about how these factors can alter an individual's quality of sexual experiences may be necessary based on the client's sexual problems and current life stressors.
- *Skill-building exercises*: Sensate focused exercises begin with clothed and nongenital touching but may also begin with self-stimulation if a partner is not present. These exercises can decrease sex-related anxiety and avoidance by emphasizing sensations instead of performance via gradual behavioral exposure to sexual stimuli (Wincze & Weisberg, 2015). The goal of sensate focused exercises is to reduce any expectations or pressure to engage in penetrative sex or achieve orgasm. Instead, the aim is to increase the focus on sensuality and the client's sensory experience.
- *Mindfulness and guided meditation exercises:* Mindfulness exercises can teach clients to tolerate their bodies' physiological responses and trauma-related emotions thereby creating a new and positive association with pleasure. Cultivating a mindfulness practice can teach clients to develop nonjudgmental awareness of their thoughts, recognize that they're just thoughts, and purposefully redirect their attention to physical sensations (Stephenson & Kerth, 2017). Mindfulness can be utilized as a stand-alone treatment separate from traditional sex therapies or specific mindfulness exercises and relaxation training can be incorporated into treatment along with sensate focused exercises. One important benefit of mindfulness-based therapies (MBT) is that it can be used by clients who do not have partners. In a study examining the effects of group CBT in comparison with group MBT for women with histories of CSA and sexual dysfunction, Brotto, Seal, and Rellini (2012) found that women in the MBT condition reported increased subjective sexual arousal to an erotic film relative to women in the CBT condition. Although the women in the MBT condition did not report an increase in genital sexual arousal, the authors hypothesize that the mindfulness training might have aided the participants in fully attending to the sexual stimulus of the erotic film in the present moment and disconnect from negative cognitions (Brotto et al., 2012). A meta-analysis of MBT for female sexual dysfunction found moderate effect sizes for MBTs in comparison to waitlist control groups (Stephenson & Kerth, 2017).

Combining trauma-focused and traditional modalities of sex therapy can create a treatment plan that addresses all of the client's needs, alleviates or reduces symptoms of PTSD, engenders comfort and confidence in the client's sexuality, and improves negative cognitions regarding sexual beliefs.

Key Gaps in the Literature

Despite the high prevalence of sexual dysfunction among women of all ages, sexual dysfunction is poorly understood and rarely recognized. The under-detection of sexual difficulties is even more prevalent for women who have experienced rape or sexual assault. There are several key gaps in the literature that prevent adequate identification of female sexual dysfunction, assessment, and treatment with women with trauma histories: (1) theoretical confusion, (2) measurement concerns, and (3) few evidence-based therapies.

Theoretical Confusion

One of the most widely acknowledged criticisms regarding extant definitions of female sexual functioning centers around the initial diagnostic and classification system that was developed based on the four-phase model of sexual response delineated by Masters and Johnson (1962). This model assumed that both women and men experience a linear progression from excitement, plateau, orgasm, to resolution (Kammerer-Doak & Rogers, 2008; Masters & Johnson, 1962). While Masters and Johnson's work revolutionized the study of sexual science, recent research indicates that the original model may not adequately explain female sexuality. Basson (2001) proposed that the sexual response of women is better conceptualized as circular and not linear. This sexual response model indicate that female sexual functioning consists of multiple biopsychosocial (cognitive, affective, physiological, and behavioral) processes that interact to shape women's responses to sexual stimuli (Basson, 2001). In this model, sexual response is significantly affected by women's satisfaction with the relationship, self-image, and previous negative sexual experiences (Basson, 2001). Basson (2001) notes that women may not experience spontaneous desire; rather, they are approached and sexually stimulated by their partners, which leads to arousal and desire. The goal of sexual activity is not necessarily orgasm, but rather personal satisfaction, which can manifest as emotional satisfaction (i.e. feeling of intimacy with one's partner) and/or physical satisfaction (i.e. orgasm) (Basson, 2001). Previous negative or positive sexual experiences impact women's responses to sexual stimuli and levels of sexual functioning. As such, sexual assault or rape may function as a risk factor for female sexual dysfunction. This model more adequately captures the intricacies of the female sexual cycle, to include both social and psychological features, such as physical and emotional satisfaction, sexual desire, and emotional intimacy (Basson, 2001).

Although Basson's model is widely accepted within the study of the human sexual response, the initial overreliance on Masters and Johnson's four-phase sexual response model placed undue attention on sexual performance. Some researchers argue that this has created an unrealistic and nonrepresentative standard, where a majority of women report some sexual concerns (Moynihan & Cassels, 2005). If 43% of US women aged 18–59 (Laumann et al., 1999) report a sexual dysfunction, does this actually conflate the perceived problem or is it a variation of the norm? Does this lead women to have greater expectations for their sexual functioning that is not within the norm? Problematic female sexual functioning is difficult to quantify, and emotional health and personal relationship factors are often much more relevant to a client's well-being than the ability to achieve orgasm.

Measurement Concerns

Although female sexual dysfunction is highly prevalent, there are few empirically validated and brief standardized protocols for the assessment of sexual dysfunction particularly for women with comorbid PTSD. Currently, two diagnostic interviews are currently available for use, the DeRogatis Interview for Sexual Functioning (DISF; DeRogatis, 1996) and the Women's Sexual Interest Diagnostic Interview (WSID; DeRogatis et al., 2010). The DISF is a 26-item measure of sexual function across five domains: sexual arousal, sexual behavior/experience, orgasm, sexual cognition/fantasy, and sexual drive/relationship. The

DISF is available as a semi-structured interview that takes approximately 15 min to administer and a self-report questionnaire. Both versions have demonstrated good psychometric properties, although it appears that norms for women with sexual dysfunction are currently not available. The WSID only assesses hypoactive sexual desire disorder (HSDD) in postmenopausal women.

One available self-report instrument that is comprehensive is the DeRogatis Sexual Function Inventory (DSFI; DeRogatis & Mellisaratos, 1979), which consists of 254 items across 10 dimensions that are related to sexual functioning, such as gender role definition, body image, sexual satisfaction, fantasies, psychological symptoms, and attitudes. The DSFI has demonstrated strong psychometric properties and is multidimensional in nature. Due to its length and complexity, the DSFI may not be feasible for administration in most clinical settings, particularly as initial evaluations include a battery of assessments. The relative drawbacks of the DISF and the DSFI are that they are proprietary, which necessitates purchase. Few other alternatives have been identified.

As a result, there is an overreliance on self-report measures. Several validated self-report questionnaires are available for assessing female sexual dysfunction but a protocol for practicing clinicians who are not trained in female sexual dysfunction is highly needed. With the exception of the DSFI, most existing self-report questionnaires fail to assess psychosocial factors that may impact sexual functioning, particularly for women who have experienced traumatic events. Other salient factors that may be relevant to treatment include the onset and duration of the sexual difficulties and the context in which they occur; whether symptoms predate the traumatic event, whether they occur with a specific partner or in a particular setting, whether symptoms are global, or whether some sexual activities serve as triggers for trauma-related memories, thoughts, or feelings. Most questionnaires focus on current sexual experiences and fail to examine sexual dysfunction if the respondent does not engage in sexual activities during the time of assessment.

Few Evidence-Based Therapies

At present, concerns with sexual satisfaction and function are not part of standard screening for general mental health, PTSD, or trauma. This may be partly due to PTSD diagnostic criteria lacking reference to sexual problems. As a result, sexual problems are not incorporated into standardized PTSD assessments (O'Driscoll & Flanagan, 2016). Additionally, some women who have experienced sexual victimization may abstain from sexual activity. Therefore, a different assessment approach may be necessary to identify and treat women who do not engage in sexual activity but are experiencing impairment in sexual health. Proper identification of women who have sexual dysfunctions and comorbid PTSD or depression is necessary for treatment.

Further complicating the treatment of comorbid sexual dysfunction and common trauma-related distress is the lack of clarity regarding the sequence of treatment. Should symptoms of depression or PTSD be targeted first or is an integrated approach more appropriate? This is particularly important as PE and CBT do not specifically target changes in women's intimate and personal relationships, sexual expression, or sexual difficulties that can manifest following sexual assault. When sexual dysfunction is identified, it may not be prioritized by the client or clinician as a primary symptom for intervention. Some researchers argue that sexual dysfunction may resolve following successful psychological treatment for PTSD (Schnurr et al., 2009), but a recent meta-analysis found that treatment for PTSD had little effect on sexual problems (O'Driscoll & Flanagan, 2016). Transdiagnostic assessments and intervention options could provide additional approaches for the treatment of sexual dysfunction following sexual assault.

Implications for Future Research

The sexual functioning of women is a dynamic and complex interplay of psychological, biological, and sociocultural factors. For women who have experienced sexual assault victimization, sexual difficulties may develop through differential pathways. One potential mechanism is the function of PTSD as a mediator. However, the current state of the literature examining the association between sexual assault and sexual dysfunction is rife with theoretical and measurement issues. There are few evidence-based treatments that effectively target symptoms of PTSD and depression with sexual dysfunction. Future research should include the following considerations:

- *Indicators of sexual health*: More research is needed to identify models of positive sexual health for women. For instance, current models define female sexual health as a lack of sexual risk factors (Lustig, 2012). However, sexual health is not simply the absence of negative consequences; it consists of behavioral, emotional, and cognitive aspects of sexuality. Domains to be evaluated can include dating/romantic (i.e. ability to negotiate and obtain intimacy in relationships, leaving abusive relationships, condom/contraceptive use), social (i.e. social support), individual (i.e. being comfortable with one's sexuality, resisting objectifying sex, positive experiences of sexual desire, behavior, and experiences without guilt), and sociocultural (i.e. access to and ability to utilize reproductive healthcare, education regarding positive sexual health; Lustig, 2012).
- *Mechanisms of action:* Researchers have proposed several contributing factors to the development of sexual dysfunction in women who have experienced sexual assault: feelings of shame and guilt, sexual self-schema, low body image and self-esteem, cognitions associated with sexuality, and activation of the sympathetic nervous system (Pulverman, Kilimnik, & Meston, 2017). Unfortunately, studies examining these factors have yielded inconsistent results due to the complex nature of sexual assault (Pulverman et al., 2017). More research is needed to identify which mechanisms are most relevant for treatment.
- *Cultural attitudes about sex*: Myths regarding ideal sexual relationships may have a negative impact on sexual functioning and satisfaction. For instance, the concept of *marianismo* in Hispanic American females is rooted in Catholicism and places Latina females in roles of passivity, caretaking, self-sacrifice, honor, and sexual morality (Heinemann, Atallah, & Rosenbaum, 2016). Additionally, certain practices, such as "dry sex" observed in some parts of Asia, Latin America, and Sub-Saharan Africa impact the presentation of sexual dysfunction. Evaluating cultural beliefs, attitudes, and expectations may identify sources of anxiety that can be addressed in treatment. Clinicians can evaluate these beliefs by following the guidelines proposed by the International Consultation on Sexual Medicine: (1) awareness of differences, (2) knowledge of the client's culture, (3) distinguishing between pathology and culture, and (4) use of a culturally appropriate therapy (Heinemann et al., 2016). Furthermore, sex positivity (sex is viewed as more than a purely procreative act) and sex negativity (sex is viewed as fundamentally procreative) are also predictive of sexual functioning (Atallah et al., 2016).
- *Anchors of sexual satisfaction*: Many of the standardized measures assessing sexual function and dysfunction in women incorporate one item that assesses global satisfaction with one's sexual life. This practice may be problematic because women's perceptions of low, high, and everything in between is not comprehensively assessed. What counts as low and high sexual satisfaction? It is important to understand how item responses relate to the sociocultural context of women.

Although not exhaustive, it is imperative that researchers and clinicians consider psychosocial factors that may impact sexual functioning and utilize this understanding to develop evidence-based assessment and intervention protocols.

Conclusion

Sexual dysfunction is a complex and highly prevalent class of disorders with multiple etiologies, maintaining factors, and pathways to care. Sexual functioning is further complicated by interpersonal and psychological factors, such as sexual assault victimization and subsequent development of trauma-related distress such as PTSD. Due to the complexity of sexual dysfunction and comorbid PTSD, there are few evidence-based assessment and intervention protocols for survivors of sexual assault. Although psychological interventions for PTSD and sexual dysfunctions are separately available, a unified treatment plan is needed. This chapter has provided suggestions for assessment and treatment of sexual dysfunction for women who have been sexually victimized. The integration of trauma and sex-focused therapy may be a useful way of identifying and targeting the factors that shape the thresholds for survivors' experiences of sexual dissatisfaction and dysfunction.

References

American Psychiatric Association. (2000). Diagnostic and statistical manual of mental disorders, (4 th ed., text revision). Washington, DC: American Psychiatric.

American Psychiatric Association. (2013). *DSM-5: Diagnostic and statistical manual for mental disorders* (5th ed.). Washington, DC: American Psychiatric Press.

American Psychological Association. (2017). Clinical practice guideline for the treatment of posttraumatic stress disorder (PTSD) in adults. Retrieved from http://www.apa.org/about/offices/directorates/guidelines/ptsd.pdf

Annon, J. (1976). The PLISSIT Model: A proposed conceptual scheme for the behavioural treatment of sexual problems. *Journal of Sex Education Therapy, 2*(1), 1–15.

Atallah, S., Johnson-Agbakwu, C., Rosenbaum, T., Abdo, C., Byers, E. S., Graham, C., ... Brotto, L. (2016). Ethical and sociocultural aspects of sexual function and dysfunction in both sexes. *The Journal of Sexual Medicine, 13*, 591–606.

Baggett, L. R., Eisen, E., Gonzalez-Rivas, S., Olson, L. A., Cameron, R. P., & Mona, L. R. (2017). Sex-positive assessment and treatment among female trauma survivors. *Journal of Clinical Psychology, 73*(8), 965–974. https://doi.org/10.1002/jclp.22510

Basson, R. (2001). Female sexual response: The role of drugs in the management of sexual dysfunction. *Obstetrics and Gynecology, 98*, 350–353.

Bitzer, J., & Brandenburg, U. (2009). Psychotherapeutic interventions for female sexual dysfunction. *Maturitas, 63*, 16–163.

Blais, R. K., Geiser, C., & Cruz, R. A. (2018). Specific PTSD symptom clusters mediate the association of military sexual trauma severity and satisfaction in female service members/veterans. *Journal of Affective Disorders, 238*(1), 680–688.

Bradley, R., Greene, J., Russ, E., Dutra, L., & Western, D. (2005). A multidimensional meta-analysis of psychotherapy for PTSD. *American Journal of Psychiatry, 162*(2), 214–227.

Breiding, M. J., Smith, S. G., Basile, K. G., Walters, M. L., Chen, J., & Merrick, M. T. (2014). Prevalence and characteristics of sexual violence, stalking, and intimate partner violence victimization: National Intimate Partner and Sexual Violence Survey, United States, 2011. *Surveillance Summaries, 63*(SS08), 1–18.

Breslau, N., Davis, G. C., Andreski, P., & Peterson, E. L. (1991). Traumatic events and posttraumatic stress disorder in an urban population of young adults. *Archives of General Psychiatry, 48*, 216–222.

Breslau, N., Davis, G. C., Andreski, P., Peterson, E. L., & Schultz, L. R. (1997). Sex differences in posttraumatic stress disorder. *Archives of General Psychiatry, 54*, 1044–1048.

Breyer, B. N., Fang, S. C., Seal, K. H., Ranganathan, G., Marx, P., Keane, T. M., & Rosen, R. C. (2016). Sexual health in male and female Iraq and Afghanistan U.S. war veterans with and without PTSD: Findings from the VALOR cohort. *Journal of Traumatic Stress, 29*, 229–236. https://doi.org/10.1002/jts.22097

Briere, J., & Jordan, C. (2004). Violence against women: Outcome complexity and implications for assessment and treatment. *Journal of Interpersonal Violence, 19*, 1252–1276.

Brotto, L. A., Seal, B. N., & Rellini, A. (2012). Pilot study of a brief cognitive behavioral versus mindfulness-based intervention for women with sexual distress and a history of childhood sexual abuse. *Journal of Sex & Marital Therapy, 38*, 1–27.

Brown-Bowers, A., Fredman, S. J., Wanklyn, S. G., & Monson, C. M. (2012). Cognitive-behavioral conjoint therapy for posttraumatic stress disorder: Application to a couple's shared traumatic experience. *Journal of Clinical Psychology, 68*(5), 536–547.

Bryant, R., Sackville, T., Dang, S., Moulds, M., & Guthrie, R. (1999). Treating acute stress disorder: An evaluation of cognitive behavior therapy and supporting counseling techniques. *American Journal of Psychiatry, 156*(11), 1780–1786.

Creamer, M., Burgess, P., & McFarlane, A. C. (2001). Post-traumatic stress disorder: Findings from the Australian National Survey of Mental Health and Wellbeing. *Psychological Medicine, 31*, 1237–1247.

Davis, S.M., & Taylor, B. (2006). From PLISSIT to Ex-PLISSIT. In: Davis, S. (ed.) Rehabilitation: The

Use of Theories and Models in Practice. pp. 101–129. Edinburgh: Churchill Livingstone.

DeRogatis, L. R. (1996). *DeRogatis interview for sexual functioning (DISF/DISF-SR): Preliminary scoring, procedures & administration manual*. Baltimore, MD: Clinical Psychometric Research.

DeRogatis, L. R., Allgood, A., Auerbach, P., Eubank, D., Greist, J., Bharmal, M., … Guo, Y. (2010). Validation of a women's sexual interest diagnostic interview-short form (WSID-SF) and a daily log of sexual activities (DLSA) in postmenopausal women with hypoactive sexual desire disorder. *The Journal of Sexual Medicine, 7*(2), 917–927. https://doi.org/10.1111/j.1743-6109.2009.01528.x

DeRogatis, L. R., & Mellisaratos, N. (1979). The DSFI: A multidimensional measure of sexual functioning. *Journal of Sex & Marital Therapy, 5*, 244–281.

Foa, E. B., Keane, T., Friedman, M., & Cohen, J. (2009). *Effective Treatments for PTSD: Practice Guidelines from the International Society for Traumatic Stress Studies*. New York: Guilford Press.

Frank, J. E., Mistretta, P., & Will, J. (2008). Diagnosis and treatment of female sexual dysfunction. *American Family Physician, 77*(5), 635–642.

Gros, D. F., Price, M., Magruder, K. M., & Frueh, B. C. (2012). Symptom overlap in posttraumatic stress disorder and major depression. *Psychiatry Research, 196*(2–3), 267–270. https://doi.org/10.1016/j.psychres.2011.10.022

Haase, A., Boos, A., Schönfeld, S., & Hoyer, J. (2009). Sexual dysfunctions and sexual satisfaction in female PTSD patients. *Verhaltenstherapie, 19*, 161–167. https://doi.org/10.1159/000228725

Hedtke, K. A., Ruggerio, K. J., Fitzgerald, M. M., Zinzow, H. M., Saunders, B. E., Resnick, H. S., & Kilpatrick, D. G. (2008). A longitudinal investigation of interpersonal violence in relation to mental health and substance use. *Journal of Consulting and Clinical Psychology, 76*, 633–647. https://doi.org/10.1037/0022-006X.76.4.633

Heinemann, J., Atallah, S., & Rosenbaum, T. (2016). The impact of culture and ethnicity on sexuality and sexual functioning. *Current Sexual Health Reports, 8*, 144–150.

Iverson, K. M., McLaughlin, K. A., Gerber, M. R., Dick, A., Smith, B. N., Bell, M. E., … & Mitchell, K. S. (2013). Exposure to interpersonal violence and its associations with psychiatric morbidity in a U.S. national sample: A gender comparison. *Psychological Violence, 3*(3), 273–287.

Kammerer-Doak, D., & Rogers, R. G. (2008). Female sexual function and dysfunction. *Obstetrics & Gynecology Clinics of North America, 35*(2), 169–183. https://doi.org/10.1016/j.ogc.2008.03.006

Kashdan, T. B., Adams, L., Savostyanova, A., Ferssizidis, P., McKnight, P. E., & Nezlek, J. B. (2011). Effects of social anxiety and depressive symptoms on the frequency and quality of sexual activity: A daily process approach. *Behaviour Research and Therapy, 49*, 352–360. https://doi.org/10.1016/j.brat.2011.03.004

Kessler, R. C., Sonnega, A., Bromet, E., Hughes, M., & Nelson, C. B. (1995). Posttraumatic stress disorder in the National Comorbidity Survey. *Archives of General Psychiatry, 52*, 1048–1060. https://doi.org/10.1001/archpsyc.1995.03950240066012

Kilpatrick, D. G., Resnick, H. S., Milanak, M. E., Miller, M. W., Keyes, K. M., & Friedman, M. J. (2013). National estimates of exposure to traumatic events and PTSD prevalence using DSM-IV and DSM-5 criteria. *Journal of Traumatic Stress, 26*, 537–547. https://doi.org/10.1002/jts.21848

Lancaster, C. L., Teeters, J. B., Gros, D. F., & Back, S. E. (2016). Posttraumatic stress disorder: Overview of evidence-based assessment and treatment. *Journal of Clinical Medicine, 5*(11), 105–118.

Laumann, E. O., Paik, A., & Rosen, R. (1999). Sexual dysfunction in the United States: Prevalence and predictors. *JAMA, 281*, 537–544.

Leonard, L. M., & Follette, V. M. (2002). Sexual functioning in women reporting a history of child sexual abuse: Review of the empirical literature and clinical implications. *Annual Review of Sex Research, 13*, 346–388.

Letourneau, E. J., Resnick, H. S., Kilpatrick, D. G., Saunders, B. E., & Best, C. L. (1996). Comorbidity of sexual problems and posttraumatic stress disorder in female crime victims. *Behavior Therapy, 27*(3), 321–336.

Loeb, T. B., Williams, J. K., Carmona, J. V., Rivkin, I., Wyatt, G. E., Chin, D., & Asuan-O'Brien, A. (2002). Child sexual abuse: Associations with the sexual functioning of adolescents and adults. *Annual Review of Sex Research, 13*, 307–345.

Lustig, K. (2012). Objectification theory and sexual health among women. *Graduate Doctoral Dissertations*.

Lutfey, K. E., Link, C. L., Litman, H. J., Rosen, R. C., & McKinlay, J. B. (2008). An examination of the association of abuse (physical, sexual, or emotional) and female sexual dysfunction: Results from the Boston Area Community Health Survey. *Fertility and Sterility, 90*, 957–964.

Masters, W. H., & Johnson, V. E. (1962). The sexual response cycle of the human female. III. The clitoris: Anatomic and clinical consideration. *Western Journal of Surgery, Obstetrics, Gynecology, 70*, 248–257.

Masters, W. H., & Johnson, V. E. (1970). *Human sexual inadequacy*. New York: Bantam Books.

McLean, C. P., & Foa, E. B. (2011). Prolonged exposure therapy for post-traumatic stress disorder: A review of evidence and dissemination. *Expert Review of Neurotherapeutics, 11*(8), 1151–1163.

Meston, C. M., Rellini, A. H., & Heiman, J. R. (2006). Women's history of sexual abuse, their sexuality, and sexual self-schemas. *Journal of Consulting and Clinical Psychology, 74*, 229–236.

Monson, C. M., & Fredman, S. J. (2012). *Cognitive-behavioral conjoint therapy for PTSD: Harnessing the healing power of relationships*. New York: Guilford Press.

Monson, C. M., Fredman, S. J., Adair, K. C., Stevens, S. P., Resick, P. A., Schnurr, P. P., … Macdonald, A. (2011). Cognitive-behavioral conjoint therapy for PTSD: Pilot results from a community sample. *Journal of Traumatic Stress, 24*, 97–101. https://doi.org/10.1002/jts.20604

Monson, C. M., Schnurr, P. P., Stevens, S. P., & Guthrie, K. A. (2004). Cognitive-behavioral couple's treatment for posttraumatic stress disorder: Initial findings. *Journal of Traumatic Stress, 17*, 341–344. https://doi.org/10.1023/B:JOTS.0000038483.69570.5b

Moynihan, R., & Cassels, A. (2005). *Selling sickness: How drug companies are turning us all into patients*. Crows Nest: Allen & Unwin.

Najman, J. M., Dunne, M. P., Purdie, D. M., Boyle, F. M., & Coxeter, P. D. (2005). Sexual abuse in childhood and sexual dysfunction in adulthood: An Australian population-based study. *Archives of Sexual Behavior, 34*, 517–526.

Neilson, E. C., Norris, J., Bryan, A. E. B., & Stapenbeck, C. A. (2017). Sexual assault severity and depressive symptoms as longitudinal predictors of the quality of women's sexual experiences. *Journal of Sex & Marital Therapy, 43*(5), 4630478. https://doi.org/10.1080/0092623X.2016.1208127

O'Donohue, W. T., Dopke, C. A., & Swingen, D. N. (1997). Psychotherapy for female sexual dysfunction: A review. *Clinical Psychology Review, 17*(5), 537–566.

O'Donohue, W. T., Swingen, D. N., Dopke, C. A., & Regev, L. G. (1999). Psychotherapy for male sexual dysfunction: A review. *Clinical Psychology Review, 19*(5), 591–630. https://doi.org/10.1016/S0272-7358(98)00063-4

O'Driscoll, C., & Flanagan, E. (2016). Sexual problems and post-traumatic stress disorder following sexual trauma: A meta-analytic review. *Psychology and Psychotherapy: Theory, Research and Practice, 89*, 351–367.

Öberg, K., Fugl-Meyer, A. R., & Fugl-Meyer, K. S. (2004). On categorization and quantification of women's sexual dysfunctions: An epidemiological approach. *International Journal of Impotence Research, 16*, 261–269.

Öberg, K., Fugl-Meyer, K. S., & Fugl-Meyer, A. R. (2002). On sexual well-being in sexually abused Swedish women: Epidemiological aspects. *Sexual and Relationship Therapy, 17*(4), 329–341. https://doi.org/10.1080/14681990210000017182

Powers, M. B., Halpern, J. M., Ferenschak, M. P., Gillihan, S. J., & Foa, E. B. (2010). A meta-analytic review of prolonged exposure for posttraumatic stress disorder. *Clinical Psychology Review, 30*(6), 635–641. https://doi.org/10.1016/j.cpr.2010.04.007

Pulverman, C. S., Kilimnik, C. D., & Meston, C. M. (2017). The impact of childhood sexual abuse on women's sexual health: A comprehensive review. *Sexual Medicine Reviews, 6*, 188–200.

Quirk, F. H., Heiman, J. R., Rosen, R. C., Laan, E., Smith, M. D., & Boolell, M. (2002). Development of a sexual function questionnaire for clinical trials of female sexual dysfunction. *Journal of Women's Health & Gender-Based Medicine, 11*(3), 277–289. https://doi.org/10.1089/152460902753668475

Rellini, A. H., & Meston, C. M. (2007). Sexual desire and linguistic analysis: A comparison of sexually-abused and non-abused women. *Archives of Sexual Behavior, 36*, 67–77.

Resick, P. A., Nishith, P., Weaver, T. L., Astin, M. C., & Feuer, C. A. (2002). A comparison of cognitive-processing therapy with prolonged exposure and a waiting condition for the treatment of chronic posttruamtic stress disorder in female rape victims. *Journal of Consulting and Clinical Psychology, 70*(4), 867–879.

Resick, P. A., & Schnicke, M. K. (1993). *Cognitive processing therapy for rape victims: A treatment manual*. Newbury Park, CA: Sage.

Rosen, R.C., Brown, C., Heiman, J., Leiblum, S., Meston, C., Shabsigh, R., … D'Agostino, R. (2000). The female sexual function index (FSFI): A multidimensional self-report instrument for the assessment of female sexual function. *Journal of Sex & Marriage Therapy, 26*, 191–120.

Schnurr, P. P., Lunney, C. A., Forshay, E., Thurston, V. L., Chow, B. K., Resick, P. A., & Foa, E. B. (2009). Sexual function outcomes in women treated for posttraumatic stress disorder. *Journal of Women's Health, 18*, 1549–1557. https://doi.org/10.1089/jwh.2008.1165.

Shifren, J. L., Monz, B., Russo, P. A., Segreti, A., & Johannes, C. B. (2008). Sexual problems and distress in United States women: Prevalence and correlates. *Obstetrics & Gynecology, 112*(5), 970–978. https://doi.org/10.1097/AOG.0b013e3181898cdb.

Simons, J. S., & Carey, M. P. (2001). Prevalence of sexual dysfunctions: Results from a decade of research. *Archives of Sexual Behavavior, 30*(2), 177–219.

Stephenson, K. R., & Kerth, J. (2017). Effects of mindfulness-based therapies for female sexual dysfunction: A meta-analytic review. *The Journal of Sex Research, 54*(7), 1–18.

Taylor, B., & Davis, S. (2006). Using the Extended PLISSIT model to address sexual healthcare needs. *Nursing Standard, 21*(11), 35–40.

Taylor, B., & Davis, S. M. (2007). The Extended PLISSIT Model for addressing the sexual wellbeing of individuals with an acquired disability or chronic illness. *Sexuality and Disability, 25*(3), 135–139.

Tolin, D., & Foa, E. (2006). Sex differences in trauma and posttraumatic stress disorder: A quantitative review of 25 years of research. *Psychological Bulletin, 132*, 959–992.

Van Berlo, W., & Ensink, B. (2000). Problems with sexuality after sexual assault. *Annual Review of Sex Research, 11*, 235–257.

Vechiu, C., & O'Donohue, W. T. (2018). *Sexual dysfunction*. In A. Maragakis & W. T. O'Donohue (Eds.), *Principle-based stepped care and brief psychotherapy for integrated care settings* (pp. 389–398). Switzerland: Springer.

Wincze, J. P., & Weisberg, R. B. (2015). *Sexual dysfunction: A guide for assessment and treatment* (3rd ed.). New York: Guilford Press.

Yehuda, R., Lehrner, A., & Rosenbaum, T. Y. (2015). PTSD and sexual dysfunction in men and women. *The Journal of Sexual Medicine, 12*, 1107–1119. https://doi.org/10.1111/jsm.12856.

Zayfert, C., & Black Becker, C. (2007). Cognitive behavioral therapy for PTSD: Overview and empirical foundation. In C. Zayfert & C. Black Blecker (Eds.), *Cognitive behavioral therapy for PTSD: A case formulation approach* (pp. 1–8). New York, NY: Guilford Publications.

Impulsivity and Sexual Assault

22

Brittney M. Holcomb, Colin T. Mahoney, and Steven R. Lawyer

Introduction

The processes that underlie sexual assault perpetration and victimization are varied and complex, but impulsivity is one factor related to both perpetrators and survivors. Impulsivity is generally described by a range of disadvantageous or potentially harmful behaviors, while impulsive sexual decision-making refers to patterns of choices surrounding sexual behaviors with little regard for or forethought of the potential for negative consequences. Impulsivity broadly presents as a factor associated with perpetration of sexual assault. Conversely, impulsive sexual decision-making appears to be a consequence of sexual assault for some survivors.

Impulsivity

Impulsivity is not a well-defined construct, yet it is well researched. Impulsivity frequently is used to describe the way we make behavioral choices and traits we may have. These descriptions include (but are not limited to) a diminished ability to delay gratification, acting without forethought or sufficient forethought of consequences, disinhibition or lack of self-discipline, self-reported diminished abilities to self-regulate (i.e., impulsiveness as a personality trait), and inordinate sensation seeking (Costa & McCrae, 1992; de Wit, 2008; MacKillop et al., 2016; Odum, 2011; Weafer, Baggott, & de Wit, 2013; Whiteside & Lynam, 2001). Several models and hypotheses have been formulated to understand impulsivity, finding some unique facets of impulsivity and some construct overlap. Much of the extant research, when taken together, suggests that impulsivity is composed of three main facets: impulsive choice, impulsive action, and impulsive personality traits (MacKillop et al., 2016).

Impulsive choice reflects a tendency to devalue rewards based upon a temporal delay in receiving the reward (i.e., delay discounting or delay of gratification; Ainslie, 1975; Logue & King, 1991; Schneider & Lysgaard, 1953). Delay discounting is a measurable behavioral phenomenon, often used to assess impulsive choice by a task involving a series of choices between two rewards (one available immediately or a larger reward available after a delay). Individual patterns of delay discounting are typically measured by establishing the subjective value of a large amount of money across a series of delays (e.g., the immediate subjective value of $100 in a day, a week, a month; Rachlin, Raineri, & Cross, 1991) but can also be determined for other nonmonetary

B. M. Holcomb · S. R. Lawyer (✉)
Idaho State University, Pocatello, ID, USA
e-mail: lawystev@isu.edu

C. T. Mahoney
National Center for PTSD, VA Boston Healthcare System, Boston, MA, USA

W. T. O'Donohue and P. A. Schewe (eds.), *Handbook of Sexual Assault and Sexual Assault Prevention*,
https://doi.org/10.1007/978-3-030-23645-8_22

outcomes as well such as food, substance use, and sexual outcomes (e.g., Johnson & Bruner, 2012; Lawyer, 2008; Lawyer & Schoepflin, 2013; Lawyer, Williams, Prihodova, Rollins, & Lester, 2010; Odum & Rainaud, 2003; Rasmussen, Lawyer, & Reilly, 2010). Lower subjective values of delayed outcomes are indicated by a steeper "rate" of delay discounting, suggesting a pattern of preference for smaller-sooner outcomes over larger-delayed outcomes, indicative of difficulty with delaying gratification.

Impulsive action accounts for an inability to inhibit a motor response when it would be otherwise beneficial or necessary (e.g., Fillmore & Weafer, 2013; Rosvold, Mirsky, Sarason, Bransome, & Beck; 1956). There are several laboratory tasks used to measure impulsive action, such as the Go/No-go Task (GNG), the Stop Signal Task (SST; Fillmore & Weafer, 2013), and the Continuous Performance Test (CPT; Rosvold, Mirsky, Sarason, Bransome, & Beck; 1956). These tasks all require the examinee to respond to a specific cue (e.g., visual stimulus such as an arrow pointing one way or the other) by either inhibiting a prepotent motor response (e.g., mouse click, button click) or engaging in the said motor response, depending upon the stimulus. Impulsive action is indicated when an individual makes a motor response when otherwise instructed to inhibit that action.

Impulsive personality traits refer to patterns of thoughts, feelings, and behaviors related to one's ability to self-regulate behavior (e.g., Patton, Stanford, & Barratt 1995; Whiteside, Lynam, Miller, & Reynolds 2005). These traits are frequently measured by self- and other-report questionnaires that sample a range of qualities. The NEO-Personality Inventory-Revised assesses neuroticism, extraversion, openness, agreeableness, and conscientiousness, and includes several traits (including impulsivity) within these main categories (Costa & McCrae, 1992). A measure that is more focused upon impulsivity is the Barratt Impulsiveness Scale (BIS; Patton et al., 1995). Within this scale, there are three subtypes of impulsiveness, including attentional, motor, and nonplanning impulsivity. Attentional impulsivity refers to the inability to sustain attention to a task, which includes the subjectively rated difficulty of doing so and interfering thoughts that may occur while trying to concentrate. Motor impulsivity suggests a tendency to act in a disinhibited fashion. Nonplanning impulsivity reflects a lack of ability to plan and dedicate adequate time to contemplate a decision, as well as avoidance of or displeasure in challenging mental tasks. Together, impulsivity is a complex construct, wrought with vague description or conflicting definitions amongst researchers, but it is certainly related to a variety of problematic outcomes.

Impulsivity and Perpetrators of Sexual Assault

Sexual Assault Perpetration and Impulsive Choice

Sexual assault perpetration is one such issue related to impulsivity. Impulsive choice differentiated offenders (sexual and nonsexual) from nonoffenders by using a delay discounting measure such that offenders more greatly devalued hypothetical monetary rewards due to delay in their receipt, as compared to nonoffenders (Arantes, Berg, Lawlor, & Grace, 2013; Hanoch, Rolison, & Gummerum, 2013). In other words, offenders demonstrated greater impulsive choice tendencies regarding financial gain. Conversely, delay discounting of hypothetical money did not differentiate juvenile offenders and nonoffenders (Wilson & Daly, 2006). Of note, the impulsive choice literature (in relation to sexual perpetration) mainly utilizes sex offender populations, rather than a more representative sample of perpetrators. Incarcerated sexual offenders overrepresent perpetrators in other sexual assault research, as most assaults are never reported and therefore most perpetrators are community members (Ingemann-Hansen, Brink, Sabroe, Sorensen, & Charles, 2008).

In one study of college men, those who self-reported having perpetrated sexual assault by use of verbal coercion demonstrated significantly greater impulsive choice for sexual outcomes but not monetary outcomes, as compared to men who denied perpetration (Emond, Gagnon, Nolet, Cyr, & Rouleau, 2017). This implies that college perpetrators of sexual assault demonstrate domain-specific discounting for sexual outcomes. In other words, these perpetrators did not exhibit broad impulsive choice across a variety of situations, but rather were specifically impulsive when faced with sexual decision-making tasks.

Sexual Assault Perpetration and Impulsive Action. Some mixed evidence suggests that incarcerated adult sexual offenders evidence more impulsivity than pedophilic perpetrators on measures of impulsive action of prepotent motor responses (Carvalho & Nobre, 2012; Joyal, Beaulieu-Plante, & de Chanterac, 2014). This suggests that pedophiles have more self-control over their overt behaviors, whereas perpetrators of sexual violence against adults struggle more with disinhibition of their behaviors. However, Kalal (2000) found that self-reported impulsive action related to lack of motor control did not differentiate pedophilic offenders from nonsexual violent offenders nor those of a community sample, and Snowden, Smith, and Gray (2017) found that impulsive motor actions did not differentiate a sexual and nonsexual offender sample from a community sample. These mixed findings indicate a clear need for further research regarding impulsive action among sexual assault perpetrator groups, as well as a need to study impulsive sexual actions.

Sexual Assault Perpetration and Impulsive Traits. Those who have perpetrated sexual assault against women typically endorse various contributing factors, including antisocial (i.e., psychopathic) traits, difficulty incorporating societal and legal behavioral expectations, authority problems, family conflicts, underachievement, and impulsivity (DeGue & DiLillo, 2004; Giotakos, Markianos, Vaidakis, & Christodoulou, 2003; Hoertel, Le Strat, Schuster, & Limosin, 2012; Kosson, Kelly, & White, 1997; Mouilso, Calhoun, & Rosenbloom, 2016; Zawacki, Abbey, Buck, McAuslan, & Clinton-Sherrod, 2003). Impulsivity is frequently combined with other behavioral patterns or traits to form the construct of psychopathy or antisocial personality (Guay, Ruscio, Knight, & Hare, 2007; Hare, 2003; Lewing, 2006), which complicates understanding the unique influence of impulsivity on perpetration. For example, those meeting criteria for attention-deficit/hyperactivity disorder (ADHD) and conduct disorder (CD; a disorder characterized by antisocial behaviors) are significantly more likely to employ physical and sexual aggression in relationships (Theriault & Holmberg, 2001). However, when Theriault and Holmberg (2001) accounted for impulsive action (in this case, verbal disinhibition), ADHD and CD were no longer significant predictors of aggression.

Zinzow and Thompson (2015a) found that college men who perpetrated sexual assault reported more impulsivity and engagement in risky behaviors, such as high-risk drinking, drug use, and having a higher number of sexual partners than nonperpetrating controls. Furthermore, men who admitted perpetrating multiple sexual assaults scored significantly higher on measures of antisocial personality traits (e.g., low empathy, impulsivity, superficial charm, pervasive anger) and sexually aggressive beliefs, as compared to single offenders. Those men admitting to more severe tactics of sexual assault, such as physical force, also reported significantly more antisocial personality traits and sexually aggressive beliefs as compared to those who used verbal coercion and nonperpetrators (Zinzow & Thompson, 2015b). Within another college sample, impulsive and antisocial traits distinguished perpetrators of sexual assault from nonperpetrators (Mouilso & Calhoun, 2013).

However, some researchers report weak relationships between impulsivity traits and sexual assault. Voller and Long (2010) measured personality differences, using the NEO-PI-R (Costa & McCrae, 1992) between college men, who were divided into three groups based on perpetration status, specifically perpetrators of rape, sexual assault perpetrators, and nonperpetrators. Perpetrators of rape endorsed significantly different personality traits than sexual assault perpetrators, who were actually more similar to nonperpetrators. Rape perpetrators scored significantly lower on agreeableness, extraversion, and conscientiousness, and scored higher on neuroticism than non-perpetrators. Contrary to other findings, rape perpetrators did not significantly differ from other groups on impulse control or self-discipline. Voller and Long (2010) hypothesized that these groups did not differ from each other on measures of impulsivity because the sample group consisted of college men, who may have better impulse control and have therefore not been arrested for their sexual aggression (as compared to incarcerated offenders).

Wegner, Pierce, and Abbey (2014) sampled a community group of single, socioeconomically and racially diverse young men who had reported perpetrating at least one act of sexual aggression. The findings indicated that perpetrators who had a consensual sexual encounter with their victim(s) before the assault(s) reported greater traits of impulsivity related to lack of forethought and sensation seeking, as compared to perpetrators who assaulted their victim(s) first. The clinical significance of this finding may be questionable, as the perpetrator group with higher impulsivity had mean ratings indicative of indifference (i.e., far closer to "neutral" ratings than ratings of agreement with traits measured). This sample was a subset from a larger study, which included nonperpetrators as well (Abbey, Jacques-Tiura, & LeBreton, 2011). Abbey et al. (2011) found a significant relationship between perpetration of sexual aggression and traits of impulsivity, but this relationship was indirect and better explained by hostile masculinity (i.e., dominating, aggressive attitudes toward women) and heavy alcohol consumption.

Variability of Impulsivity and Perpetration. Impulsivity is likely not a rigid or single-faceted trait with a stable relationship with sexual assault perpetration. Various types of impulsivity (e.g., inattentiveness, behavioral impulsivity, nonplanning) are positively correlated with problem sexual behaviors in a young adult community sample, including preoccupation with sexuality or being sexually active, inability to control repetitive sexual fantasies, inability to control sexual urges, and out-of-control repetitive sexual behavior (Leppink, Chamberlain, Redden, & Grant, 2016). Thompson, Kingree, Zinzow, and Swartout (2015) sampled university men's beliefs about rape, frequency of sexual aggression, impulsivity, and sexual compulsivity. The authors found that various types of sexual aggression styles emerged over the men's four years in college, including consistently low sexual aggression, decreasing sexual aggression, increasing sexual aggression, and consistently high sexual aggression. These participants' self-reported impulsive actions (e.g., acting before stopping and thinking) were positively correlated to the men's reported changes in sexual aggression (i.e., the group that reported engaging in decreasing levels of sexual aggression also reported less impulsivity over time). The authors hypothesize that intervention efforts targeted at risk behaviors, such as reducing impulsivity, may reduce perpetration of sexual aggression.

Impulsivity and Survivors of Sexual Assault

Sexual Assault and Coping. Sexual assault survivors sometimes engage in strategies, such as avoidant coping, in attempts to manage overwhelming distress. Avoidant coping strategies are used to relieve distress without confronting the origin of the distress itself (Ullman, Peter-Hagene, & Relyea, 2014) and increase risk of developing posttraumatic psychopathology following exposure to a trauma (e.g., Benotsch et al., 2000; Mellman, David, Bustamante, Fins, & Esposito, 2001). In particular, for survivors of interpersonal violence, avoidant coping significantly predicts posttraumatic stress disorder (PTSD) symptoms at two different time points, the first within a month of the index trauma and the second at follow-up one year later (Krause, Kaltman, Goodman, & Dutton, 2008). Thus, avoidant coping behavior is typically viewed as maladaptive, as it increases vulnerability for developing long-term psychological distress. One common maladaptive coping behavior following sexual trauma is impulsive sexual decision-making (i.e., risky sexual behavior).

Risky Sexual Behavior. Risky sexual behavior is relatively common from adolescence to adulthood. The CDC (2015) found that, among high school students, 41% have experienced sexual intercourse and 30% have had sexual intercourse in the previous 3 months; 43% reported that they did not use condoms during the last time and 21% drank alcohol or used drugs before having sexual intercourse. Risky sexual behavior can include increased promiscuity, sexual intercourse without a condom, and early sexual activity (Beadnell et al., 2005; Levy, Sherritt, Gabrielli, Shrier, & Knight, 2009). These behaviors increase risk for negative health outcomes, such as sexually transmitted infections (STIs), HIV/AIDS, and unexpected pregnancy (e.g., Bryan, Schmiege, & Magnan, 2012).

Risky Sexual Behavior and Sexual Victimization. In the case of sexual victimization, traumatic experiences can have varying effects on survivors' decision-making tendencies in future sexual situations. The role of childhood sexual trauma is particularly important, as childhood sexual abuse (CSA) predicts the likelihood of engaging in sexual activity on the first date or with a stranger (Molitor, Ruiz, Klausner, & McFarland, 2000; Walker et al., 1999). Women with a history of CSA and/or adolescent sexual victimization also have a higher number of consensual sexual partners, reduced use of condoms during intercourse, a higher incidence of sexual intercourse with strangers, increased pregnancies during adolescence, higher rates of sexually transmitted infections including HIV, are more likely to be a younger age at the time of first consensual sexual intercourse, and have higher rates of sexual assault after the age of 16 years (e.g., Elze, Auslander, McMillen, Edmond, & Thompson, 2001; Fergusson, Horwood, & Lynskey, 1997; Rodriguez-Srednicki, 2001; Siegel & Williams, 2003) than women without CSA histories.

Adult sexual trauma is related also to risky sexual behavior in women. Multiple assaults are associated with higher levels of risk behaviors than single assaults, and risky behavior is highest in sexual and physical assault groups in comparison to nonvictim groups with sexual traumatization as the only significant predictor of risky sexual behavior (Davis, Combs-Lane, & Jackson, 2002). Furthermore, Green et al. (2005) found that female college students exposed to a single sexual assault incident tend to report significantly more risky sexual behavior than those who have experienced no trauma, a physical trauma, or a noninterpersonal trauma (i.e., traumatic loss). Violent sexual assault for females in adolescence or adulthood also is significantly associated with anticipation of a higher negative reaction from sexual partners if the victim refuses unprotected sex (Masters et al., 2014).

Risky sexual behavior also occurs following sexual trauma exposure in men. For example, several studies indicate that sexually abused men exhibit increased levels of hypersexuality, prostitution, reduced use of condoms during sexual intercourse, and high numbers of consensual sexual partners (e.g., DiIorio, Hartwell, & Hansen, 2002; O'Leary, Purcell, Remien, & Gomez, 2003; Paul, Catania, Pollack, & Stall, 2001) relative to nonassaulted men. Sexually traumatized men are also more likely than men without a history of sexual trauma to have higher rates of STIs, multiple sexual partners, and higher rates of partner pregnancy (Jinich et al., 1998; Lodico & DiClemente, 1994; Raj, Silverman, & Amaro, 2000) than men without a history of sexual trauma.

Characteristics of the trauma are important to consider as well in men, with greater frequency of CSA associated with higher rates of risky sexual behavior (Paul et al., 2001), and higher coercion during CSA related to elevated rates of risky sexual behavior and HIV diagnosis (Jinich et al., 1998). The relationship between CSA and risky sexual behavior is mediated by a higher incidence of sexual intercourse with strangers, frequent drug use during sexual intercourse, and recently having an abusive partner (Paul et al., 2001). Also, in comparison to adolescent females with a history of CSA, adolescent males are more likely to have higher numbers of consensual sexual partners and engage in sexual intercourse that results in pregnancy (Raj et al., 2000).

Risky Sexual Behavior as Avoidant Coping. Polusny and Follette (1995) theorize that risky sexual behavior may be a form of avoidant coping in which behavioral strategies are used to avoid and/or reduce negative internal emotional experiences following trauma, including reexperiencing and numbing PTSD symptoms. Emotional avoidance is a process that entails disproportionately high negative evaluations of unpleasant internal experiences (e.g., intrusive thoughts, dissociative flashbacks), an unwillingness to endure these experiences, and efforts to reduce, control, numb, or escape from them (Polusny & Follette, 1995).

Risky sexual behavior can also be understood as avoidant coping perpetuated by the temporary alleviation or suppression of aversive posttraumatic distress and subsequent relief (Polusny & Follette, 1995). These behaviors can also be described as tension-reduction behaviors in that they soothe, distract, and/or reduce debilitating negative emotionality associated with the traumatic event (Briere, 1992, 2001). Thus, risky sexual behavior may be a behavioral avoidant coping strategy that is negatively reinforced by the short-term reduction of distress despite long-term posttraumatic difficulties and increased risk of revictimization (e.g., Livingston, Testa, & VanZile-Tamsen, 2007) and/or other negative health outcomes, such as unwanted pregnancy or sexually transmitted infections (e.g., Bryan et al., 2012).

Risky Sexual Behavior and Impulsivity. Risky sexual behavior following sexual trauma may be mediated by a variety of different factors, including condom use self-efficacy (Thompson, Potter, Sanderson, & Maibach, 1997), sexual assertiveness (Morokoff et al., 1997), and/or self-esteem (Low, Jones, MacLeod, Power, & Duggan, 2000). However, one aspect of risky sexual behavior that has received relatively little study is the influence of impulsivity on these health-related decisions for sexual trauma survivors, which may be vitally relevant to understanding risky sexual behavior (Hoyle, Fejfar, & Miller, 2000). Measures of impulsive choice may be a potential avenue of exploration to determine how state and trait impulsivity influence risky sexual behavior for this clinical population. Considering delay discounting (i.e., a behavioral measure of impulsivity) is associated with sexual risk taking, such as unsafe sexual activity, sexual infidelity, and infrequent condom use (e.g., Daugherty & Brase, 2010; Johnson & Bruner, 2012; Lawyer & Mahoney, 2017), measures of impulsive choice may be essential in elucidating this relationship.

Impulsivity and Discounting for Sexual Activity. Sexual decision-making and risk-taking can be measured with behavioral measures of impulsive choice. Steep rates of discounting for sexual activity would indicate that an individual prefers small amounts of sexual activity over longer—and perhaps more pleasurable—sexual activity at a later date. For instance, these discounting procedures are composed of questions such as "which do you prefer, 3 min of sexual activity right now or 10 min of sexual activity in 1 week?" Delay discounting can be influenced by the nature of the commodity (i.e., domain specificity), with evidence that individuals exhibit higher rates of discounting for sexual activity than money (e.g., Jarmolowicz, Bickel, & Gatchalian, 2013). Higher rates of sexual, but not monetary, discounting are associated with HIV sexual risk behavior and sexual promiscuity (Jarmolowicz, Lemley, Asmussen, & Reed, 2015; Johnson & Bruner, 2012). Lawyer and Schoepflin (2013) have also found varying effects of domain specificity, with sexual activity discounting predicting sexual excitability, but not nonsexual outcomes or sexual inhibition. The relationship between delay discounting and risky sexual behavior has received relatively minimal empirical focus to date. However, examining impulsive choice patterns that are contingent upon the commodity (i.e., sexual activity) is important to accurately reflect sexual trauma survivors' engagement in impulsive behavior within the context of sexual health.

For example, Johnson and Bruner (2012) developed and established a discounting procedure with clinical implications for risky sexual behavior. Cocaine-dependent participants indicated their likelihood of having immediate unprotected sex (i.e., without a condom right now) or delayed protected sex (e.g., with a condom in 3 h) with specific photographed individuals judged to be sexually desirable when no condom was available right away. Participants demonstrated significantly greater discounting (i.e., preference for unprotected sex right now) for partners considered to be the most sexually desirable or least likely to have an STI versus those found least sexually attractive or most likely to have an STI (Johnson & Bruner, 2012). Risk of STI and/or unwanted pregnancy may be more indicative of risky healthy behaviors within the context of sexual activity. Thus, this discounting procedure could be particularly relevant for elucidating how moment-to-moment cognitive, emotional, and physiological experiences and processes can affect the use of risky sexual behavior as an avoidant coping mechanism for sexual trauma survivors in a controlled, laboratory setting.

The mechanisms that underlie the relationship between impulsivity and sexual risk-taking behavior following sexual trauma remain unclear. Impulsivity is a multidimensional construct that includes a range of disparate individual difference factors that remain relatively stable. For instance, impulsivity is at times behaviorally characterized as a deficit in inhibitory control (Logan, Cowan, & Davis, 1984), an insensitivity to delayed consequences (e.g., Madden & Bickel, 2010), and a tendency toward risk-taking (Green & Myerson, 2013). In addition, insensitivity to risky or punishing outcomes (e.g., STIs, unwanted pregnancies) can be measured with a variety of laboratory measures including the probability discounting task (Green & Myerson, 2013). This task is similar to the delay discounting task, except that individuals choose between a series of relatively small but certain outcomes and a larger but probabilistic outcome. Higher subjective values of probabilistic outcomes are indicated by a shallower 'rate' of probability discounting, suggesting a pattern of preference for larger/uncertain outcomes over smaller/certain outcomes, indicative of a tendency toward engaging in risk-taking.

Although several studies have assessed impulsive or risky sexual behavior using self-report measures (e.g., Turchik & Garske, 2009), behavioral measures of impulsivity-related constructs explain unique variance in negative health-related behaviors such as alcohol use and associated problems above and beyond self-report measures of impulsivity (e.g., Fernie, Cole, Goudie, & Field, 2010). Therefore, the use of behavioral/laboratory measures of impulsivity may be essential to understanding risky sexual behavior following sexual trauma. In particular, delay discounting and probability discounting, but not response inhibition, are significantly associated with risky sexual behavior in young adults (Lawyer & Mahoney, 2017). The robustness of these relationships between impulsivity and risky sexual behavior suggests that traumatic sexual experiences may increase generalized impulsivity, resulting in a higher likelihood to engage in risky sexual behavior. Indeed, Moore et al. (2017) found that impulsivity was significantly related to risky sexual behavior with sexual potentially traumatic events significantly mediating this relationship. Furthermore, some research suggests that sexually abusive experiences may precede damaged cognitive mechanisms such as reduced self-esteem and reality testing strategies that increase the likelihood of risky sexual behaviors (e.g., inaccurately evaluating risk, having multiple sexual partners, reduced condom use; Zurbriggen & Freyd, 2004), further implicating decision-making processes. More substantial behavioral research in controlled settings to corroborate these self-report findings is unequivocally necessary to understand the function of these behaviors.

Conclusions and Future Directions

Impulsivity and Perpetration. With regard to the role of impulsiveness in sexual assault perpetration, findings are complicated and it may be that certain types of impulsivity are uniquely related to particular sexual assault perpetration. Research suggests that impulsivity is associated with more severe perpetration (Yeater, Lenberg, & Bryan, 2012) and recidivism (Thompson et al., 2015; Waite et al., 2005). Other findings indicate that impulsivity is indirectly related to perpetration and better accounted for by other factors, such as substance abuse and/or hostile masculinity (e.g., Abbey et al., 2002; Abbey et al., 2011; Baltieri & de Andrade, 2008), or not related at all in the case of some highly deviant perpetrators (Beauregard

& Leclerc, 2007; Carvalho & Nobre, 2012; Giotakos et al., 2003; Joyal et al., 2014). Given these conflicting findings, there is more to investigate within the relationship between indicators of impulsivity and perpetration of sexual assault.

Future research involving sexual assault perpetration and impulsivity should utilize an operational definition of the type of impulsivity of interest. MacKillop et al. (2016) provide some guidance with their categorization of impulsive choice, action, and personality traits that may be useful for researchers. Research should expand to also include impulsivity specifically related to sexual assault behaviors. Studies would benefit from specifying the type of perpetration assessed, as well as inclusion of a variety of perpetrator groups. Groups might include juvenile and adult perpetrators of juveniles, children, and adults, as well as incarcerated, community, and college samples. Types of sexual assault (e.g., groping, attempted rape, rape) could be another useful categorization to help understand differential relationships with impulsivity. Specification and measurement of impulsivity, perpetration, and assault type will hopefully clarify the complex relationship between these factors. Once these relationships are better understood, research may shift focus onto intervention efforts, as there is very limited extant empirical literature on impulsivity intervention and sexual assault prevention.

Impulsivity and Victimization. The limited research on the interconnections between sexual trauma, impulsivity, and sexual risk behaviors allows relatively few substantive statements, but points to a rich opportunity for researchers. Future research should compare risky sexual behavior within clinical samples of sexually traumatized individuals formally diagnosed with PTSD from sexual trauma exposure, individuals with a history of sexual trauma and subclinical PTSD symptoms, individuals with no sexual trauma history (but other forms of trauma exposure), and individuals with no trauma history. Furthermore, beyond using behavioral measures of impulsivity, future studies could be strengthened with psychophysiological measures of anxious arousal such as measures of skin conductance, systolic and diastolic blood pressures, heart rate activity, and facial electromyography often used with individuals with PTSD (Pole, 2007) to corroborate self-reported emotional distress and its influence on risky sexual behavior.

Considering the potential for negative health sequelae of risky sexual behavior (e.g., sex with HIV-positive individuals or intravenous drug users, unprotected sex, multiple sex partners) including STIs and unwanted pregnancy (Zietsch, Verweij, Bailey, Wright, & Martin, 2010), as well as the increased risk of revictimization for sexually traumatized individuals (e.g., Messman-Moore, Walsh, & DiLillo, 2010), it is imperative to elucidate underlying factors that drive relationships between CSA/sexual assault, impulsivity, and risky sexual behavior. Prospective studies to establish temporality/causality with randomly selected community and clinical samples that examine a wide range of factors, including state and trait impulsivity, that may underlie the relationship between sexual trauma and risky sexual behavior is highly warranted in the effort to engage in primary, secondary, and tertiary prevention of both sexual victimization and the path to revictimization.

References

Abbey, A., Jacques-Tiura, A. J., & LeBreton, J. M. (2011). Risk factors for sexual aggression in young men: An expansion of the confluence model. *Aggressive Behavior, 37*(5), 450–464. https://doi.org/10.1002/ab.20399

Abbey, A., Zawacki, T., Buck, P. O., Testa, M., Parks, K., Norris, J., … Martell, J. (2002). How does alcohol contribute to sexual assault? Explanations from laboratory and survey data. *Alcoholism: Clinical and Experimental Research, 26*(4), 575–581. https://doi.org/10.1111/j.1530-0277.2002.tb02576.x

Ainslie, G. (1975). Specious reward: A behavioral theory of impulsiveness and impulse control. *Psychological Bulletin, 82*(4), 463–496.

Arantes, J., Berg, M. E., Lawlor, D., & Grace, R. C. (2013). Offenders have higher delay- discounting rates than non-offenders after controlling for differences in drug and alcohol abuse. *Legal and Criminological Psychology, 18*(2), 240–253. https://doi.org/10.1111/j.2044-8333.2012.02052.x

Baltieri, D. A., & de Andrade, A. G. (2008). Drug consumption among sexual offenders against females. *International Journal of Offender Therapy and Comparative Criminology, 52*(1), 62–80. https://doi.org/10.1177/0306624X07299345

Beadnell, B., Morrison, D. M., Wilsdon, A., Wells, E. A., Murowchick, E., Hoppe, M., … Nahom, D. (2005). Condom use, frequency of sex, and number of partners: Multidimensional characterization of adolescent sexual risk-taking. *The Journal of Sex Research, 42*, 192–202.

Beauregard, E., & Leclerc, B. (2007). An application of the rational choice approach to the offending process of sex offenders: A closer look at the decision-making. *Sexual Abuse: Journal of Research and Treatment, 19*(2), 115–133. https://doi.org/10.1177/107906320701900204

Benotsch, E. G., Brailey, K., Vasterling, J. J., Uddo, M. M., Constans, J. I., & Sutker, P. B. (2000). War zone stress, personal and environmental resources, and PTSD symptoms in gulf war veterans: A longitudinal perspective. *Journal of Abnormal Psychology, 109*, 205–213.

Briere, J. (1992). *Child abuse trauma: Theory and treatment of the lasting effects*. Newbury Park, CA: Sage.

Briere, J. (2001). Treating adult survivors of severe childhood abuse and neglect: Further development of an integrative model. In J. E. B. Myers, L. Berliner, J. Briere, C. T. Hendrix, T. Reid, & C. Jenny (Eds.), *The APSAC handbook on child maltreatment* (2nd ed., pp. 175–203). Newbury Park, CA: Sage.

Bryan, A. D., Schmiege, S. J., & Magnan, R. E. (2012). Marijuana use and risky sexual behavior among high-risk adolescents: Trajectories, risk factors, and event-level relationships. *Developmental Psychology, 48*, 1429–1442.

Carvalho, J., & Nobre, P. (2012). Dynamic factors of sexual aggression: The role of affect and impulsiveness. *Criminal Justice and Behavior, 40*(4), 376–387. https://doi.org/10.1177/0093854812451682

Centers for Disease Control and Prevention. Fact sheets on STDs. (2015). Retrieved from https://www.cdc.gov/healthyyouth/sexualbehaviors/

Costa, P. T., & McCrae, R. R. (1992). Normal personality assessment in clinical practice: The NEO Personality Inventory. *Psychological Assessment, 4*(1), 5–13. https://doi.org/10.1037/1040-3590.4.1.5

Davis, J. L., Combs-Lane, A. M., & Jackson, T. L. (2002). Risky behaviors associated with interpersonal victimization: Comparisons based on type, number, and characteristics of assault incidents. *Journal of Interpersonal Violence, 17*, 611–629.

Daugherty, J. R., & Brase, G. L. (2010). Taking time to be healthy: Predicting health behaviors with delay discounting and time perspective. *Personality and Individual Differences, 48*, 202–207.

de Wit, H. (2008). Impulsivity as a determinant and consequence of drug use: A review of underlying processes. *Addiction Biology, 14*(1), 22–31. https://doi.org/10.1111/j.1369-1600.2008.00129.x

DeGue, S., & DiLillo, D. (2004). Understanding perpetrators of nonphysical sexual coercion: Characteristics of those who Cross the line. *Violence and Victims, 19*(6), 673–688. https://doi.org/10.1891/vivi.19.6.673.66345

DiIorio, C., Hartwell, T., & Hansen, N. (2002). Childhood sexual abuse and risk behaviors among men at high risk for HIV infection. *American Journal of Public Health, 92*(2), 214–219.

Elze, D. E., Auslander, W., McMillen, C., Edmond, T., & Thompson, R. (2001). Untangling the impact of sexual abuse on HIV risk behaviors among youth in foster care. *AIDS Education and Prevention, 13*(4), 377–389.

Emond, F. C., Gagnon, J., Nolet, K., Cyr, G., & Rouleau, J. (2017). What money can't buy: Different patterns in decision making about sex and money predict past sexual coercion perpetration. *Archives of Sexual Behavior, 47*, 429. https://doi.org/10.1007/s10508-017-1116-0

Fergusson, D. M., Horwood, L. J., & Lynskey, M. T. (1997). Childhood sexual abuse, adolescent sexual behaviors and sexual revictimization. *Child Abuse and Neglect, 21*, 789–803.

Fernie, G., Cole, J. C., Goudie, A. J., & Field, M. (2010). Risk-taking but not response inhibition or delay discounting predict alcohol consumption in social drinkers. *Drug & Alcohol Dependence, 112*, 54–61.

Fillmore, M. T., & Weafer, J. (2013). Behavioral inhibition and addiction. In J. MacKillop, H. de Wit, J. MacKillop, & H. O. de Wit (Eds.), *The Wiley-Blackwell handbook of addiction psychopharmacology* (pp. 135–164). Malden, MA: John Wiley & Sons. https://doi.org/10.1002/9781118384404.ch6

Giotakos, O., Markianos, M., Vaidakis, N., & Christodoulou, G. N. (2003). Aggression, impulsivity, plasma sex hormones, and biogenic amine turnover in a forensic population of rapists. *Journal of Sex and Marital Therapy, 29*(3), 215–225. https://doi.org/10.1080/00926230390155113

Green, B. L., Krupnick, J. L., Stockton, P., Goodman, L., Corcoran, C., & Petty, R. (2005). Effects of adolescent trauma exposure on risky behavior in college women. *Psychiatry, 68*, 363–378.

Green, L., & Myerson, J. (2013). How many impulsivities? A discounting perspective. *Journal of the Experimental Analysis of Behavior, 99*, 3–13.

Guay, J. P., Ruscio, J., Knight, R. A., & Hare, R. D. (2007). A taxometric analysis of the latent structure of psychopathy: Evidence for dimensionality. *Journal of Abnormal Psychology, 116*, 701–716. https://doi.org/10.1037/0021-843X.116.4.701

Hanoch, Y., Rolison, J., & Gummerum, M. (2013). Good things come to those who wait: Time discounting differences between adult offenders and nonoffenders. *Personality and Individual Differences, 54*(1), 128–132. https://doi.org/10.1016/j.paid.2012.08.025

Hare, R. D. (2003). *The Hare psychopathy checklist-revised* (2nd ed.). Toronto, ON: Multi-Health Systems.

Hollander, E., & Rosen, J. (2000). Impulsivity. *Journal of Psychopharmacology, 14*(2,Suppl1), S39–S44. https://doi.org/10.1177/02698811000142S106

Hoyle, R. H., Fejfar, M. C., & Miller, J. D. (2000). Personality and sexual risk taking: A quantitative review. *Journal of Personality, 68*, 1203–1231.

Ingemann-Hansen, O., Brink, O., Sabroe, S., Sørensen, V., & Charles, A. V. (2008). Legal aspects of sexual violence—Does forensic evidence make a difference? *Forensic Science International, 180*(2–3), 98–104.

Jarmolowicz, D. P., Bickel, W. K., & Gatchalian, K. M. (2013). Alcohol-dependent individuals discount sex at higher rates than controls. *Drug & Alcohol Dependence, 131*, 320–323.

Jarmolowicz, D. P., Lemley, S. M., Asmussen, L., & Reed, D. D. (2015). Mr. right versus Mr. right now: A discounting-based approach to promiscuity. *Behavioural Processes, 115*, 117–122.

Jinich, S., Paul, J. P., Stall, R., Acree, M., Kegeles, S., Hoff, C., & Coates, T. J. (1998). Childhood sexual abuse and HIV risk-taking behavior among gay and bisexual men. *AIDS and Behavior, 2*, 41–51.

Johnson, M. W., & Bruner, N. R. (2012). The sexual discounting task: HIV risk behavior and the discounting of delayed sexual rewards in cocaine dependence. *Drug and Alcohol Dependence, 123*, 15–21.

Joyal, C. C., Beaulieu-Plante, J., & de Chanterac, A. (2014). The neuropsychology of sex offenders: A meta-analysis. *Sexual Abuse: A Journal of Research and Treatment, 26*(2), 149–177. https://doi.org/10.1177/1079063213482842

Kalal, D. M. (2000, February). Impulsivity in pedophilic sexual offenders. Dissertation Abstracts International: Section B: The Sciences and Engineering. ProQuest Information & Learning.

Leppink, E. W., Chamberlain, S. R., Redden, S. A., & Grant, J. E. (2016). Problematic sexual behavior in young adults: Associations across clinical, behavioral, and neurocognitive variables. *Psychiatry Research, 246*, 230–235. https://doi.org/10.1016/j.psychres.2016.09.044

Lewing, C. A. (2006). Psychopathy as a moderator of the relationship between psychological reactance and sexual assault acceptance and perpetration among incarcerated and non-incarcerated males. Dissertation Abstracts International: Section B: The Sciences and Engineering. ProQuest Information & Learning. Retrieved from http://libpublic3.library.isu.edu/login?url=http://search.ebscohost.com/login.aspx?direct=true&db=psyh&AN=2006-99016-171&site=ehost-live&scope=site

Logue, A. N., & King, G. R. (1991). Self-control and impulsiveness in adult humans when food is the reinforcer. *Appetite, 17*, 105–120.

Kosson, D. S., Kelly, J. C., & White, J. W. (1997). Psychopathy-related traits predict self- reported sexual aggression among college men. *Journal of Interpersonal Violence, 12*(2), 241–254. https://doi.org/10.1177/088626097012002006

Krause, E. D., Kaltman, S., Goodman, L. A., & Dutton, M. A. (2008). Avoidant coping and PTSD symptoms related to domestic violence exposure: A longitudinal study. *Journal of Traumatic Stress, 21*, 83–90.

Lawyer, S. R. (2008). Probability and delay discounting of erotic stimuli. *Behavioural Processes, 79*(1), 36–42. https://doi.org/10.1016/j.beproc.2008.04.009lawyer

Lawyer, S. R., & Mahoney, C. T. (2017). Delay discounting and probability discounting, but not response inhibition, are associated with sexual risk taking in adults. *The Journal of Sex Research*, 1–8.

Lawyer, S. R., & Schoepflin, F. J. (2013). Predicting domain-specific outcomes using delay and probability discounting for sexual versus monetary outcomes. *Behavioural Processes, 96*, 71–78.

Lawyer, S. R., Williams, S. A., Prihodova, T., Rollins, J. D., & Lester, A. C. (2010). Probability and delay discounting of hypothetical sexual outcomes. *Behavioural Processes, 84*, 687–692.

Levy, S., Sherritt, L., Gabrielli, J., Shrier, L. A., & Knight, J. R. (2009). Screening adolescents for substance use-related high-risk sexual behaviors. *Journal of Adolescent Health, 45*, 473–477.

Livingston, J. A., Testa, M., & VanZile-Tamsen, C. (2007). The reciprocal relationship between sexual victimization and sexual assertiveness. *Violence Against Women, 13*, 298–313.

Lodico, M. A., & DiClemente, R. J. (1994). The association between childhood sexual abuse and prevalence of HIV-related risk behaviors. *Clinical Pediatrics, 33*, 498–502.

Logan, G. D., Cowan, W. B., & Davis, K. A. (1984). On the ability to inhibit simple and choice reaction time responses: A model and a method. *Journal of Experimental Psychology: Human Perception and Performance, 10*, 276.

Low, G., Jones, D., MacLeod, A., Power, M., & Duggan, C. (2000). Childhood trauma, dissociation and self-harming behaviour: A pilot study. *Psychology and Psychotherapy: Theory, Research and Practice, 73*, 269–278.

MacKillop, J., Weafer, J., Gray, J. C., Oshri, A., Palmer, A., & de Wit, H. (2016). The latent structure of impulsivity: Impulsive choice, impulsive action, and impulsive personality traits. *Psychopharmacology, 233*, 3361. https://doi.org/10.1007/s00213-016-4372-0

Madden, G. J., & Bickel, W. K. (2010). *Impulsivity: The behavioral and neurological science of discounting*. Washington, DC: American Psychological Association.

Masters, N. T., George, W. H., Davis, K. C., Norris, J., Heiman, J. R., Jacques-Tiura, A. J., … Stappenbeck, C. A. (2014). Women's unprotected sex intentions: Roles of sexual victimization, intoxication, and partner perception. *Journal of Sex Research, 51*(5), 586–598.

Mellman, T. A., David, D., Bustamante, V., Fins, A. I., & Esposito, K. (2001). Predictors of post-traumatic stress disorder following severe injury. *Depression and Anxiety, 14*, 226–231.

Messman-Moore, T. L., Walsh, K., & DiLillo, D. (2010). Emotion dysregulation and risky sexual behavior in revictimization. *Child Abuse & Neglect, 34*, 967–976.

Molitor, F., Ruiz, J. D., Klausner, J. D., & McFarland, W. (2000). History of forced sex in association with drug use and sexual HIV risk behaviors, infection with STD's and diagnostic medical care. *Journal of Interpersonal Violence, 15*, 262–278.

Moore, A. A., Overstreet, C., Kendler, K. S., Dick, D. M., Adkins, A., & Amstadter, A. B. (2017). Potentially traumatic events, personality, and risky sexual behavior in undergraduate college students. *Psychological Trauma Theory Research Practice and Policy, 9*, 105.

Morokoff, P. J., Quina, K., Harlow, L. L., Whitmire, L., Grimley, D. M., Gibson, P. R., & Burkholder, G. J. (1997). Sexual assertiveness scale (SAS) for women: Development and validation. *Journal of Personality and Social Psychology, 73*, 790–804.

Mouilso, E. R., & Calhoun, K. S. (2013). The role of rape myth acceptance and psychopathy in sexual assault perpetration. *Journal of Aggression, Maltreatment & Trauma, 22*(2), 159–174. https://doi.org/10.1080/10926771.2013.743937. http://libpublic3.library.isu.edu/login?url=http://search.ebscohost.com/login.aspx?direct=true&db=psyh&AN=2000-95004-522&site=ehost-live&scope=site

Mouilso, E. R., Calhoun, K. S., & Rosenbloom, T. G. (2016). Impulsivity and sexual assault in college men. In R. D. Maiuro (Ed.), *Perspectives on college sexual assault: Perpetrator, victim, and bystander* (pp. 137–150). New York, NY: Springer Publishing.

Odum, A. L. (2011). Delay discounting: Trait variable? *Behavioural Processes, 87*(1), 1–9. https://doi.org/10.1016/j.beproc.2011.02.007

Odum, A. L., & Rainaud, C. P. (2003). Discounting of delayed hypothetical money, alcohol, and food. *Behavioural Processes, 64*, 305–313.

O'Leary, A., Purcell, D., Remien, R. H., & Gomez, C. (2003). Childhood sexual abuse and sexual transmission risk behaviour among HIV-positive men who have sex with men. *AIDS Care, 15*(1), 17–26. https://doi.org/10.1080/0954012021000039725

Patton, J. H., Stanford, M. S., & Barratt, E. S. (1995). Factor structure of the Barratt impulsiveness scale. *Journal of Clinical Psychology, 51*, 768–774.

Pole, N. (2007). The psychophysiology of posttraumatic stress disorder: A meta-analysis. *Psychological Bulletin, 133*, 725.

Polusny, M. A., & Follette, V. M. (1995). Long-term correlates of child sexual abuse: Theory and review of the empirical literature. *Applied and Preventive Psychology, 4*, 143–166.

Paul, J. P., Catania, J., Pollack, L., & Stall, R. (2001). Understanding childhood sexual abuse as a predictor of sexual risk-taking among men who have sex with men: The Urban Men's Health Study. *Child Abuse and Neglect, 25*, 557–584.

Rachlin, H., Raineri, A., & Cross, D. (1991). Subjective probability and delay. *Journal of the Experimental Analysis of Behavior, 55*(2), 233–244.

Raj, A., Silverman, J. G., & Amaro, H. (2000). The relationship between sexual abuse and sexual risk among high school students: Findings from the 1997 Massachusetts youth risk behavior survey. *Maternal and Child Health Journal, 4*, 125–134.

Rasmussen, E., Lawyer, S. R., & Reilly, W. (2010). Percent body fat is related to delay and probability discounting for food in humans. *Behavioural Processes, 83*, 23–30.

Rodriguez-Srednicki, O. (2001). Childhood sexual abuse, dissociation, and adult self-destructive behavior. *Journal of Child Sexual Abuse, 10*, 75–89.

Rosvold, H. E., Mirsky, A. F., Sarason, I., Bransome, E. J., & Beck, L. H. (1956). A continuous performance test of brain damage. *Journal of Consulting Psychology, 20*(5), 343–350. https://doi.org/10.1037/h0043220

Schneider, L., & Lysgaard, S. (1953). The deferred gratification pattern: A preliminary study. *American Sociological Review, 18*, 142–149.

Siegel, J. A., & Williams, L. M. (2003). Risk factors for sexual victimization of women: Results from a prospective study. *Violence Against Women, 9*, 902–930.

Snowden, R. J., Smith, C., & Gray, N. S. (2017). Risk taking and the triarchic model of psychopathy. *Journal of Clinical and Experimental Neuropsychology, 39*(10), 988–1001.

Theriault, S. W., & Holmberg, D. (2001). Impulsive, but violent? Are components of the attention deficit-hyperactivity syndrome associated with aggression in relationships? *Violence Against Women, 7*(12), 1464–1489. https://doi.org/10.1177/10778010122183946

Thompson, M. P., Kingree, J. B., Zinzow, H., & Swartout, K. (2015). Time-varying risk factors and sexual aggression perpetration among male college students. *Journal of Adolescent Health, 57*(6), 637–642. https://doi.org/10.1016/j.jadohealth.2015.08.015

Thompson, N. J., Potter, J. S., Sanderson, C. A., & Maibach, E. W. (1997). The relationship of sexual abuse and HIV risk behaviors among heterosexual adult female STD patients. *Child Abuse & Neglect, 21*, 149–156.

Turchik, J. A., & Garske, J. P. (2009). Measurement of sexual risk taking among college students. *Archives of Sexual Behavior, 38*, 936–948.

Ullman, S. E., Peter-Hagene, L. C., & Relyea, M. (2014). Coping, emotion regulation, and self-blame as mediators of sexual abuse and psychological symptoms in adult sexual assault. *Journal of Child Sexual Abuse, 23*, 74–93.

Voller, E. K., & Long, P. J. (2010). Sexual assault and rape perpetration by college men: The role of the big five personality traits. *Journal of Interpersonal Violence, 25*(3), 457–480. https://doi.org/10.1177/0886260509334390

Waite, D., Keller, A., McGarvey, E. L., Wieckowski, E., Pinkerton, R., & Brown, G. L. (2005). Juvenile sex offender re-arrest rates for sexual, violent nonsexual and property crimes: A 10-year follow-up. *Sexual Abuse: Journal of Research and Treatment, 17*(3), 313–331. https://doi.org/10.1177/107906320501700305

Walker, E. A., Gelfand, A., Katon, W. J., Koss, M. P., Von Korff, M., Bernstein, D., & Russo, J. (1999). Adult health status of women with histories of childhood abuse and neglect. *American Journal of Medicine, 107*, 332–339.

Weafer, J., Baggott, M. J., & de Wit, H. (2013). Test–retest reliability of behavioral measures of impulsive choice, impulsive action, and inattention. *Experimental and Clinical Psychopharmacology, 21*(6), 475–481. https://doi.org/10.1037/a0033659

Wegner, R., Pierce, J., & Abbey, A. (2014). Relationship type and sexual precedence: Their associations with characteristics of sexual assault perpetrators and incidents. *Violence Against Women, 20*(11), 1360–1382. https://doi.org/10.1177/1077801214552856

Whiteside, S. P., & Lynam, D. R. (2001). The five factor model and impulsivity: Using a structural model of personality to understand impulsivity. *Personality and Individual Differences, 30*(4), 669–689. https://doi.org/10.1016/S0191-8869(00)00064-7

Whiteside, S. P., Lynam, D. R., Miller, J. D., & Reynolds, S. K. (2005). Validation of the UPPS impulsive behaviour scale: A four-factor model of impulsivity. *European Journal of Personality, 19*(7), 559–574. https://doi.org/10.1002/per.556

Wilson, M., & Daly, M. (2006). Are juvenile offenders extreme future discounters? *Psychological Science, 17*, 989–994.

Yeater, E. A., Lenberg, K. L., & Bryan, A. D. (2012). Predictors of sexual aggression among male juvenile offenders. *Journal of Interpersonal Violence, 27*(7), 1242–1258. https://doi.org/10.1177/0886260511425243

Zawacki, T., Abbey, A., Buck, P. O., McAuslan, P., & Clinton-Sherrod, A. M. (2003). Perpetrators of alcohol-involved sexual assaults: How do they differ from other sexual assault perpetrators and nonperpetrators? *Aggressive Behavior, 29*(4), 366–380.

Zietsch, B. P., Verweij, K. J. H., Bailey, J. M., Wright, M. J., & Martin, N. G. (2010). Genetic and environmental influences on risky sexual behaviour and its relationship with personality. *Behavior Genetics, 40*, 12.

Zinzow, H. M., & Thompson, M. (2015a). A longitudinal study of risk factors for repeated sexual coercion and assault in U.S. college men. *Archives of Sexual Behavior, 44*(1), 213–222.

Zinzow, H. M., & Thompson, M. (2015b). Factors associated with use of verbally coercive, incapacitated, and forcible sexual assault tactics in a longitudinal study of college men. *Aggressive Behavior, 41*(1), 34–43.

Zurbriggen, E. L., & Freyd, J. J. (2004). The link between child sexual abuse and risky sexual behavior: The role of dissociative tendencies, information-processing effects, and consensual sex decision mechanisms. In L. J. Koenig, L. S. Doll, A. O'Leary, & W. Pequenat (Eds.), *From child sexual abuse to adult sexual risk: Trauma, revictimization, and intervention* (pp. 135–157). Washington, DC: American Psychological Association.

Part V

Prevention and Intervention

Theories of Sexual Violence Prevention

23

Sarah McMahon, Leila Wood, and Julia Cusano

Prevention means addressing a problem before it happens. It can most generally be defined as "a systematic process that promotes healthy environments and behaviors and reduces the likelihood or frequency of an incident, injury, or condition occurring" (Cohen, Davis, & Mikkelsen, 2000, p. 1). In the field of sexual violence, prevention means creating healthy, safe environments and fostering attitudes, behaviors, and norms that will not endorse sexual violence, therefore hindering the perpetration of sexually violent acts before these happen. The identification of sexual violence as a problem and the concept of sexual violence *prevention* gained prominence alongside increased attention on private and community experiences of violence borne from the civil rights, LGBT rights and women's movements of the 1960s and 1970s (Danis & Bhandari, 2010). From these social justice movements, interventions aimed at supporting survivors of sexual violence grew from both grassroots and professional models. Sexual violence intervention work was later bolstered by seminal studies establishing the scope of the problem in communities (for example, see Tjaden & Thoennes, 2006) and on college campuses (for example, see Koss, Gidycz, & Wisniewski, 1987; Krebs, Lindquist, Berzofsky, Shook-Sa, & Peterson, 2016). Empirical evidence about the extent and impact of sexual violence led to a call from service providers, law enforcement, activists, and researchers to do something to prevent future violence from occurring.

Prevention efforts are typically primary, secondary, or tertiary. Primary prevention of sexual violence means preventing a first incident from occurring (Lundgren & Amin, 2015). Primary prevention efforts address reducing or removing risk factors for violence victimization and perpetration (Chamberlain, 2008). Secondary prevention efforts, such as those that prevent re-victimization, stop subsequent acts of violence. Tertiary prevention involves interventions such as counseling and medical support (Carlson et al., 2015). As Cohen and Swift (1999) articulated, primary prevention typically occurs at six different levels (1). Individual knowledge and skills, (2). Community involvement, (3). Educating providers, (4). Fostering coalitions, (5). Change organizational practices, and (6). Change policy and legislation. An activity at any level is an intervention, but strategies that incorporate different levels together are comprehensive.

Many theoretical frameworks and perspectives are used to shape prevention strategies to address sexual violence from a variety of

S. McMahon (✉) · J. Cusano
School of Social Work, Rutgers University, New Brunswick, NJ, USA
e-mail: smcmahon@ssw.rutgers.edu

L. Wood
School of Social Work, University of Texas, Austin, Austin, TX, USA

W. T. O'Donohue and P. A. Schewe (eds.), *Handbook of Sexual Assault and Sexual Assault Prevention*,
https://doi.org/10.1007/978-3-030-23645-8_23

disciplines, including public health, psychology, sociology, criminal justice, social work, and health sciences and medicine. Sexual violence prevention efforts are often based on theories used to explain why sexual violence happens. Previous research has established several individual risk factors that increase risk for sexual violence perpetration, including history of child victimization, insecure attachment, alcohol use, personality, adolescent delinquency, past aggressive behavior, participation in hook-up culture, sexism, and hostile/toxic gender beliefs (Abbey, Parkhill, Beshears, Monique Clinton-Sherrod, & Zawacki, 2006; Casey & Lindhorst, 2009; McDermott, Kilmartin, McKelvey, & Kridel, 2015; Sutton & Simons, 2015). In addition, peer networks have been found to impact perpetration (Abbey et al., 2006; Schwartz, DeKeseredy, Tait, & Alvi, 2001; Swartout, 2013). However, individual and peer risk factors alone do not explain the full cause of sexual assault, so community and societal factors merit consideration (Casey & Lindhorst, 2009). Some researchers present a confluence model of perpetration, in which pathways formed by either childhood experiences, personality, and toxic masculinity or gender role socialization, delinquency, or risk-taking intersect to increase motivation, predisposition, and opportunity to perpetrate (Malamuth, Heavey, & Linz, 1996). This chapter critically reviews a number of theories that support and influence sexual violence prevention work, but first examines how prevention efforts and corresponding theories evolved over the past few decades.

Evolution of Sexual Violence Prevention Efforts and Theories

Early sexual violence prevention efforts tended to focus on the ways that potential victims could protect themselves, or risk reduction approaches. Women were encouraged to take self-defense classes, travel in groups, carry mace, and avoid walking alone at night (Sochting, Fairbrother, & Koch, 2004). While some risk reduction approaches are still advocated to help promote safety and a sense of empowerment, the concept of prevention today is primarily focused on the actions of potential perpetrators and examining the root causes of sexual violence. The modern sexual violence prevention approach comes from a union between the public health field and the violence against women movement (Cook-Craig et al., 2014). Funding from the 1994 Violence Against Women Act (VAWA) allocated resources to the Centers for Disease Control and Prevention's Division of Violence Prevention for prevention programming (DeGue et al., 2012). Efforts from the CDC and other researchers helped to shape a broader lens of sexual violence informed not just by a criminal justice but a public health lens, with a focus on primary prevention and efforts across the social ecology (DeGue et al., 2012). The public health approach involves four critical steps: (1). Data collection to understand the extent of sexual violence; (2). Data collection to understand risk and protective factors for sexual violence perpetration and victimization; (3). Development of data- and evidence-driven approaches for sexual violence prevention across the lifespan; and (4). Dissemination, testing, and adaptation of approaches to sexual violence prevention (Chamberlain, 2008; DeGue et al., 2012). Another key aspect of the public health approach is their reliance on ecological frameworks.

Ecological Framework for Sexual Violence Prevention

There is increasing recognition over recent years that effective prevention needs to address not only individual actions but also the environment in which the individual interacts with others. This approach is rooted in an ecological systems framework originally developed by Bronfenbrenner (1979), who posited that behavior is a result of interactions between individuals and their social environments in four nested environmental systems. These systems include personal history/ontogenetic, which are the individual's experiences and development; the microsystem, which represents the immediate environment of the individual, such as the family, peer group, or place of employment; the exosystem, which contains external environmental settings including social institutions and structures; and the macrosystem, which represents the larger cultural attitudes, views and context. A fifth level of the ecological model is the mesosystem, which consists of interactions between the microsystems such as between family and work (Bronfenbrenner, 1977).

In addition to its application to understanding the etiology of violence, the ecological framework has also been proposed to illuminate a comprehensive approach to violence prevention. The CDC has adapted this model to explain the etiology of violence as multilayered, including the individual, group, community, and societal levels, thereby offering multiple points of prevention (Dills, Fowler, & Payne, 2016). The ecological model has been proposed as a useful framework specifically for the prevention of sexual violence in recent years (Banyard, 2011; Casey & Lindhorst, 2009; Dills et al., 2016; Townsend & Campbell, 2007). Within the context of sexual violence prevention, there has been an emphasis in research and practice on changing individual-level attitudes and behaviors, which is viewed as inadequate (Banyard, 2011). The ecological model addresses the multilevel, complex nature of sexual violence and accounts for multiple causes of the problem and therefore offers multiple levels of prevention (Dills et al., 2016). Prevention programming is most effective when it is rooted in theory (Banyard, 2014). The ecological framework is a useful tool to map different types of sexual violence prevention theories, including individual behavior change theories, peer and community-level theories, and societal/community-level prevention theories.

Individual-Level Theories of Sexual Violence Prevention

The majority of theories put forth to support sexual violence prevention address the individual level of the social ecology. Theories on this level typically emphasize why individuals may perpetrate sexual violence and/or why individuals may help to prevent sexual violence. Individual-level theories focus on the mechanisms related to changing individual attitudes and behaviors related to sexual violence and come from a variety of disciplines. These include Social Learning Theory, Theories of Reasoned Action and Planned Behavior, Elaboration Likelihood Model, and the Transtheoretical Model of Change.

Social Learning Theory

A theory of individual behavior change is Social Learning Theory (SLT). SLT dates back to the late 1800s primarily building off of the work of the study of "the social self," or the examination of person and environmental interactions (Lanier, Elliott, Martin, & Kapadia, 1998). The central principle of SLT is that human behavior is learned rather than innate (Bandura, 1969). SLT asserts that behavior is contingent upon socio-environmental influences, a process referred to as reciprocal determinism (Bandura, 1969). Reciprocal determinism views behavior not as a passive process, as was conceptualized in prior theories of operant learning, but rather as a dynamic process occurring as a result of relationships between the person, environment, individuals, particularly peers, and past behavior.

The core constructs of SLT focus on the influence of external factors in relationship to behavioral response patterns, seen predominantly within the concept of vicarious learning, or modeling (Wareham, Paquette Boots, & Jorge, 2012). SLT has been used as a framework for examining environmental and peer influences within the context of several problematic behaviors, including alcohol use, aggression and intimate partner violence (Durkin, Wolfe, & Clark, 2005). Researchers that have applied SLT in an attempt to explain the perpetration of intimate partner violence suggest that individuals learn to be violent towards their partners by observing both the behaviors of people who are important in their lives, which primarily include parents and peers, and the positive consequences of these observed behaviors (Arriaga & Foshee, 2004; Bandura, 1986). For college populations specifically, when examining the peer influence, research demonstrates that the perception that male peers are sexually aggressive toward a female partner has been found to increase the likelihood of self-reported forced sex behaviors (Wareham et al., 2012). Such findings highlight the association between sexually aggressive behaviors and peers' attitudes toward both women and sex.

When applying SLT to sexual violence prevention programs, the goal of interventions is to reduce rape myths among participants as a means to promote individuals' active bystander behaviors. Rape myths are "attitudes and beliefs that are generally false but are widely and persistently held, and they serve to deny and justify male sexual aggression against women" (Lonsway & Fitzgerald, 1994, p. 134). Research on bystander behaviors in the college population suggests that students often consider their peers' attitudes towards sexual violence when deciding whether to intervene in a potential incident of sexual violence as well as in the degree to which they believe sexually aggressive behaviors are acceptable themselves (Swartout, 2013).

A large number of interventions have employed core constructs of SLT, particularly the core component of self-efficacy (Hawkins, Clarke, & Seeley, 1993). Self-efficacy, a core component of SLT, may be defined as one's belief in their own ability to organize and execute a specific course of action that is required to manage prospective situations (Bandura, 1986). More recently violence prevention programs have transitioned to utilizing multiple components of SLT, including expectations, emotional coping, behavioral capability i.e., knowledge and skill to perform a specific behavior, and self-control (Hawkins et al., 1993). Sexual violence prevention programs based on SLT have incorporated interactive components into intervention programs, such as a video clips or live peer student theater performances, that portray the events leading up to a potential incident of sexual violence as a method for changing attitudes about sexual violence and promoting bystander behaviors (Lanier et al., 1998; McMahon, Postmus, Warrener, & Koenick, 2014). While a number of sexual violence prevention programs use elements of SLT, there has yet to be any explicit testing of the theory application.

Theory of Reasoned Action and Theory of Planned Behavior

TRA asserts that behavior intention is the best predictor of behavior, especially when salient beliefs exist that a behavior will produce a desired outcome. Behavior intention stems from attitudes about the behavior, and perceived social and subjective norms about the behavior (Fishbein & Ajzen, 1975). In short, behavior intention is a function of attitude about the behavior, perception of what others think about the behavior, and the subsequent decision balance of the two (Meyer, Roberto, Boster, & Roberto, 2004). Theory of reasoned action suggests that behavior intention (belief-intention) predicts actual behavior (belief-behavior). However, environmental restraints and conditions may limit the belief-intention and belief-behavior relationships (Nabi, Southwell, & Hornik, 2002). TRA, with its focus on cognition, is applied to violence prevention primarily to determine motivations to avoid violent behaviors (Meyer et al., 2004). As an extension of TRA, theory of planned behavior (TPB) asserts that behavior is predicted by intention and perceived behavioral control, which is the extent to which resources and options are available to use said behaviors (Ajzen, 1991; Muñoz-Silva, Sánchez-García, Nunes, & Martins, 2007).

The TRA and TPB have been applied to bystander intervention, with research demonstrating that participation in bystander education program results in positive outcomes related to TRA and TPB including increased behavioral intent to intervene in prosocial ways, increased efficacy, and increased perceptions of the positive outcomes related to intervening (Banyard, Moynihan, & Crossman, 2009;

Peterson et al., 2016). In their review of 12 bystander intervention program studies, Katz and Moore (2013) found moderate effects on efficacy to intervene and intentions to help, two key components of TRA and TPB. They found smaller but still significant effects on actual bystander behavior. While these results are promising, more explicit testing of the theory applied to bystander intervention is needed, especially to test the link between behavioral intent and actual behavior. In addition, further work is needed to understand the applicability of TRA and TPB to different modalities of sexual assault prevention other than bystander intervention.

Elaboration Likelihood Model

The Elaboration Likelihood Model (ELM) was developed in the 1970s by social psychologists, Cacioppo and Perry, and suggests two routes of attitudinal change: (1). The peripheral route which consists of passive processing of information that is secondary to the main content of a message and (2). The central route which consists of thoughtful consideration of ideas and content of the message (Petty & Cacioppo, 1986). According to ELM, people process information differently depending on their level of engagement with the material, which affects both the retention of information as well as subsequent attitude and behavior change. When people do not feel personally invested in information presented to them or lack the motivation to hear such information, they are more likely to focus their attention on peripheral cues, such as qualities related to the presenter or the room (Heppner et al., 1995; Petty & Cacioppo, 1986). These peripheral cues become more important than the content of the material presented to them. Attitudinal changes resulting from the peripheral route are therefore less likely to be maintained over time (Heppner et al., 1995). However, when participants have a high level of engagement in material and are motivated to hear key messages of a program, participants are more likely to focus their attention on the information or the intervention itself and the information is processed centrally (Heppner et al., 1995). According to ELM, centrally processed information is key to sustained attitude change over time. Therefore, intervention programs designed to result in attitude and behavior changes are more likely to be successful when they elicit central route processing.

Several violence prevention programs have adopted ELM as a theoretical model, and have demonstrated efficacy, specifically for all-male peer education prevention programs (Katz, Heisterkamp, & Fleming, 2011). All-male prevention programs utilizing ELM as a theoretical framework take a unique approach by treating men as potential sources of help rather than as potential perpetrators in order to reduce participant defensiveness to the program and increase openness and motivation (Foubert & Marriott, 1997). Programs typically include educational components, such as basic sexual violence information and statistics, conversations regarding societal norms, as well as development of skills for how to identify sexual violence and safely intervene, all while utilizing a nonconfrontational tone. Foubert and McEwen (1998) found that when applying ELM to an all-male peer education type of programming, the more motivated participants were to understand the material, the less they endorsed rape myths and the less they reported intent to engage in sexually coercive behaviors.

Further, Heppner et al. (1995) utilized an evaluation tool intended to assess whether central processing is related to knowledge and behavioral intent in the months following the administration of an all-male prevention program. Results suggested that information processed centrally was associated with greater change in knowledge about sexual violence and behavioral intent months following administration of the program (Heppner et al., 1995). These findings demonstrate that all-male programs utilizing ELM have great potential for prevention of sexual violence as they seem to lower participants' levels of defensiveness, and increase levels of motivation and engagement affecting cognitive processing and attitude change.

The Transtheoretical Model of Change

Developed by Prochaska, DiClemente, and colleagues in the late 1970s, the Transtheoretical Model of Change (TTM), asserts that behavior change is a dynamic process in which individuals progress through a series of stages. TTM borrows principles and processes of change from a multitude of theories of intervention, which specifically include the integration of Freudian, Skinnerian, and Rogerian traditions in TTM's conceptualization of several processes of change which include consciousness raising contingency management and helping relationships (Prochaska et al., 1994). TTM concentrates on five stages, which refer to individuals' readiness to change a particular behavior. People begin in the precontemplation stage, not intending to take action in the near future (Prochaska, 2013). Individuals in this stage may be uninformed that there is a problem or lack the tools necessary to change. People then move to contemplation, where they are intending to change (Prochaska, 2013). A cost benefit analysis may occur in the contemplation stage in which the pros and cons of helping are weighed. People progress to the preparation stage, actively planning to take action in the immediate future; then move to action, in which observable behavior change occurs (Banyard, Eckstein, & Moynihan, 2010; Prochaska, 2013). Lastly, in the maintenance stage, people are working to prevent relapse, but do not apply change processes as frequently as those in the action stage. While TTM uses a temporal dimension, progression through the stages often does not occur linearly, but cyclically (Prochaska, 2013).

In order to progress from stage to stage, experiential techniques or strategies are utilized, referred to as processes of change. Some processes of change utilized in prevention programming include consciousness raising which may be defined as providing participants with knowledge and facts regarding the issue, dramatic relief defined as methods for appealing to participants' emotions in relation to the issue, self-evaluation, and counter-conditioning. These processes are essential for intervention programs as they serve as variables that can be manipulated in order to assist peoples' progression through the stages of change (Banyard et al., 2010; Prochaska, 2013). Therefore, intervention programs that tailor methods to participants' specific stage may yield more successful behavioral outcomes. In addition to the stages and processes of change, TTM integrates decisional balance, weighing the pros and cons of changing, as well as self-efficacy, the confidence that one can change and prevent relapse (Prochaska, 2013; Prochaska et al., 1994).

TTM has been broadly applied to interventions targeting many adverse health and mental health behaviors, including smoking, substance abuse, anxiety and depression, bullying, delinquency, and preventative medicine (Prochaska et al., 1994). After finding consistent outcomes across such applications, TTM offers a framework for changing behaviors through a series of stages and processes of change that lend themselves to the successful implementation of violence prevention programs. TTM has been expanded to child maltreatment and intimate partner violence interventions (Brown, 1997), including, more recently, bystander prevention programming to prevent sexual violence. Bystander prevention programming focuses on individual change by increasing community members' receptiveness to prevention messages and education. Bystander prevention programs apply many of the core strategies of TTM in order to enable participants to move through the stages of change, ultimately decreasing rape supportive attitudes, and replacing them with an increased willingness to act as prosocial bystanders (Banyard et al., 2010).

As an example of how TTM is utilized in bystander prevention programming is the *Bringing in the Bystander Program.* The program utilizes multiple processes of change, including *consciousness raising* to first provide education to participants regarding the problem of intimate partner violence and the potential impact of bystanders (Banyard et al., 2010). Once participants understand that intimate partner violence is a pervasive problem within their community, the program then facilitates conversations with participants in order to identify any possible maladaptive strategies utilized in past situations, a process of change referred to as self-evaluation. Throughout this evaluative process, participants also learn safe and effective strategies to intervene to replace maladaptive, unsafe strategies, referred to as counter-conditioning (Banyard et al., 2010). The bystander prevention program then engages in reinforcement management to increase the likelihood that participants will utilize the new intervention strategies (Banyard et al., 2010). There are multiple, rigorous evaluations of the Bringing in the Bystander program that demonstrates its effectiveness with increasing students' bystander intervention (Banyard et al., 2018; Banyard, Moynihan, & Plante; Peterson et al., 2016)

While TTM offers a framework for facilitating behavioral change through the utilization of processes intended to help individuals' progression through a series of stages, the model is not without criticism. Although not specifically related to sexual violence programming, researchers have argued that in general the model's stages are arbitrarily determined and based on the notion that individuals are not influenced by reward, punishment, and associative learning and how these systems contribute to the maintenance of problematic behaviors (Shaffer, 2013). Further work is needed to address these gaps and to test the application of the model to sexual violence prevention efforts.

Peer- and Community-Level Sexual Violence Prevention Theories

While it is important to understand what motivates individuals to engage in behaviors related to personal and social change aimed at sexual violence prevention, there is growing recognition that a focus on the individual level alone is insufficient. Increasingly, peer- and community-level settings for change have been recognized as especially salient to address relational and environmental factors that contribute to sexual violence perpetration and prevalence. A number of sexual violence prevention theories addressing these peer and community contexts provide a foundation for understanding how change can occur at this level, including social norms and male peer support theories; diffusion of innovations and popular opinion leader theories; and the community readiness model.

Social Norms and Male Peer Support Theories

"Social norms" are often referred to as an important factor in sexual violence prevention work (Banyard, Moynihan, & Plante, 2007; Berkowitz, 2003). Social norms theories are rooted in the idea that people behave according to the way they perceive others to behave, including their peers and wider society (Dardis, Murphy, Bill, & Gidycz, 2016; Perkins, 2003). In particular, the perceptions of others' approval or disapproval of certain behaviors can impact how someone acts (Berkowitz, 2003; Haines, 2009). Social norms theories explain that often, individuals misperceive what their peers are doing or would do in a given situation. This typically involves an overestimation of risky behaviors (e.g. alcohol use or abusive behavior), called *false consensus*, and an underestimation of protective or prosocial behaviors (e.g. willingness to intervene in an abusive situation), called *pluralistic ignorance* (Berkowitz, 2010). Because of these misperceptions, individuals may feel pressure to adopt the over-perceived, unhealthy behavior or to avoid the healthy, pro-social behavior (Haines, Perkins, Rice, & Barker, 2005).

Males may have particular pressure to rely on their perceptions of social norms in relationship to sexual violence and aggression. Rooted in social norm theory, male peer support theory suggests that men who receive social support for violence against women may be more likely to engage in acts of violence (Schwartz & DeKeseredy, 2008). The association between men who report acts of sexual violence and interaction with sexually aggressive peers has been supported by a number of studies (Abbey & McAuslan, 2004; Schwartz et al., 2001; Schwartz & Nogrady, 1996; Thompson, Swartout, & Koss,

2013; Zinzow & Thompson, 2015). Recently, Dardis et al. (2016) found that perpetrators of sexual assault were more likely than other men to overestimate their peers' sexually aggressive attitudes and behaviors. Some researchers argue that male peer support for sexual aggression is particularly salient in certain subgroups where highly masculine norms prevail (Schwartz & DeKeseredy, 1997). Certain all-male subcultures, including fraternities, athletics, and the military, have been identified as potential "rape prone cultures," where group beliefs and norms contribute to the creation of an atmosphere that tolerates or even promotes violence against women (Sanday, 1996; Schwartz & DeKeseredy, 1997).

Based on this body of work, a number of sexual violence prevention efforts are targeted to work specifically with men to challenge gender norms that promote dominance and instead, cultivate avenues for healthy masculinity (Carlson, Casey, Edelson, Tolman, Walsh & Kimball; Casey & Ohler, 2012).Social norms and male peer support theories can serve to promote harmful behavior such as sexual aggression but can also be utilized in positive ways for health promotion. The idea of male peer support has been extended to examining men's willingness to intervene as prosocial bystanders in situations involving sexual violence. Research indicates that men's willingness to intervene in positive, prosocial ways is heavily influenced by the perceptions of other men's willingness to intervene (Brown & Messman-Moore, 2010; Casey, 2010; Fabiano, Perkins, Berkowitz, Linkenbach, & Stark, 2003; Gidycz, Orchowski, & Berkowitz, 2011). As a result, many colleges and universities are implementing bystander education programs to encourage prosocial intervention and also to change norms around sexual violence (Gidycz et al., 2011; Katz & Moore, 2013). In addition, social norms marketing campaigns have been introduced as a way to model prosocial bystander behaviors (Potter, 2012), and found to be particularly effective for men who are less likely to engage in bystander intervention (Mabry & Turner, 2016). Recent work by Moynihan et al. (2015) and Banyard et al. (2018) demonstrates that combining social marketing strategies with an in-person bystander intervention education program) sustains better outcomes over time than either one of the strategies alone. Further work is needed to understand how the combination of prevention strategies may work.

Diffusion of Innovations and Popular Opinion Leader Strategies

Increasingly, sexual violence prevention programs are relying on peer educators and student leaders to help create change on campus. In addition to building upon social norms theories, there are communications theories that support this work. For example, Diffusion of Innovation theories are used to support community-level social change efforts to change norms and behaviors related to sexual violence. Based on the work of Everett Rogers (1983), this theory is used to explain how ideas (or "innovations") are transmitted and accepted by communities. Diffusion is the process by which the innovation is introduced and over time, communicated within people's social networks (Rogers, 2003). Many times diffusion is unsuccessful and the ideas are not adopted. However, over time and through "waves of innovations," diffusion can create change within society (Dearing & Cox, 2018, 184).

One of the factors that can drive whether diffusion is successful is the role of the opinion leaders in sharing the message (Rogers, 2003). These opinion leaders are influential members of the community and social networks. Once informed about the idea, opinion leaders are able to transmit and communicate the information they have learned to others in their community. Because they are regarded as leaders in their communities or networks, they are theorized to have the ability to influence the perceptions of others and can help facilitate adoption of the idea. Using opinion leaders is regarded as an important social change strategy because it involves community members and thus can be tailored to meet the needs of that particular group. The concept of opinion leaders has been infused into a number of different prevention fields, including safe sex practices to prevent HIV

(Kelly, 2004; Theall, Fleckman, & Jacobs, 2015). More recently, the theory has been applied to sexual violence prevention through bystander intervention. Diffusion of innovations has been used to explain how peer educators are able to create social change on issues of sexual violence within the general college campus community, and has been used as a pillar of bystander intervention programs (Coker et al., 2015; McMahon et al., 2014). For example, the Green Dot bystander intervention program trains popular opinion leaders based on the notion that trained students will diffuse the information learned through their own networks (Coker et al., 2015). Rigorous evaluation has demonstrated not only that Green Dot is effective in impacting individual students' bystander beliefs and actions, but also that those campuses where Green Dot takes place have less victimization and perpetration of sexual violence (Coker et al., 2016, Coker et al., 2015).

Community Readiness Model

Another theoretical perspective used to help frame sexual violence prevention efforts beyond the individual level is the Community Readiness Model (CRM), which is an extension of the transtheoretical model (Prochaska et al., 1994; Prochaska & DiClemente, 1984). The model purports that the level of a community's readiness to address a particular issue is an essential component of creating social change. The CRM includes nine stages of community readiness to engage in addressing a particular issue, ranging from "no awareness" to "high level of community ownership" (Plested, Edwards, & Jumper-Thurman, 2006). There are also six dimensions of community readiness, including existing community efforts, community knowledge of efforts, leadership, community climate, community knowledge about the issue, and resources related to the issue. Intervention efforts based on the CRM are designed to help communities increase their readiness and strengthen the various dimensions.

The CRM has been applied to other issues such as substance abuse, but has more recently been applied to address sexual violence and intimate partner violence (see Edwards, Littleton, Sylaska, Crossman, & Craig, 2016; Edwards, Moynihan, Rodenhizer-Stämpfli, Demers, & Banyard, 2015). Edwards et al. (2016) have developed a measure to help campus communities assess their readiness to engage around issues of sexual violence and IPV, which can be used to monitor progress towards increasing their efforts to address these issues over time. They propose modifications to the CRM to include three stages of community readiness: denial (e.g. while some community members recognize the issue as a concern, there is little awareness that is happening locally); initiation (e.g., the community has enough information to begin taking action); and sustainability (e.g. efforts are in place and community members are aware of them and support their expansion). They also identify two dimensions of community readiness when applied to campuses: leadership (to what extent community leaders are concerned with the issues), and resources available to address the issues (time, money, people, space). Edwards and her team (2016) have called for future research to continue to test the application of the CRM to issues of sexual violence and intimate partner violence. They called for larger, national samples of college campuses to help validate the tool they developed to see if their application of CRM to the campus context is indeed a good fit.

Cultural/Societal-Level Theories

As noted, the majority of sexual violence prevention theories focus on the individual level, which explains how to prevent a person from perpetrating sexual violence and typically emphasize mechanisms for changing attitudes and behaviors. Community/peer theories are emerging and often work on environmental norms that support violence and try to replace them with more healthy messages about relationships and gender norms. At the societal level of the ecology, the focus is on systematic issues that pervade our culture. There are fewer theories available to explain social change at this level, but both feminist and intersectional perspectives provide frameworks at this level.

Feminist and Intersectional Perspectives

Feminist theories are broadly applied in the prevention of sexual violence, largely bolstered by the overwhelming evidence of disproportionate experiences and impact of sexual violence on girls, women, and gender nonbinary people (Black et al., 2011; Cantor et al., 2015; Krebs et al., 2016). In general, feminist theories look at gender oppression and strategies for change and empowerment (DeKeseredy, 2011; Nichols, 2014). Some feminist theories look at patriarchy as the source of victimization, while most include other determinants alongside social and familial patriarchy, such as capitalism, classism and racism (DeKeseredy, 2011). Violence researchers have conceptualized gender inequity to be a root cause of sexual violence at the population level (Lundgren & Amin, 2015), supporting feminist perspectives on prevention. Strict gender roles hurt women and men, and endorse men's violence against women (Carlson et al., 2015). Perpetrators describe justifications for their behaviors by use of sexual scripts, victim blaming, sexism, biological essentialist, objectification, and sociosexuality, perspectives that suggest feminist and social justice perspectives of sexual violence are rooted in some etiological evidence (Hipp et al., 2017). Prevention approaches rooted in feminist theories seek to address underlying gender-based hostility, misconceptions, roles and inequities that allow sexual violence to occur, often without consequence. An extension of feminist perspectives on the prevention of sexual violence is to address and counter "rape culture." Rape culture refers to the norms and beliefs where violence is sexual, and male sexual aggression is routine. In rape culture, women experience threatened and real violence along a continuum from harassment to assault (Rentschler, 2014). Traditional sexual violence prevention and education implicitly promoted rape culture. For example, Bedera and Nordmeyer (2015) analyzed rape prevention tips from 40 college websites. The analysis found that most resources directed at women are in the form of risk reduction and convey four themes: There are no safe places for women; women should not trust anyone; women should avoid being alone; and women are vulnerable. Messages like these confirm the influence of rape culture on programming and messaging. Recent prevention efforts have used feminist theories to counter rape culture narratives, in recognition of past narratives.

Feminist approaches to preventing sexual violence focus on the deconstruction of gender roles that promote rape culture, the empowerment of women and girls, equality among all genders, and promotion of positive masculinity. Positive masculinity rejects hegemonic sexism and is inclusive in nature, focusing on strengths and empowerment, and awareness of the impact of traditional gender roles (Claussen, 2017). Many prevention strategies aimed at preventing sexual violence address issues of gender roles and equality, either explicitly or implicitly. Approaches that address social norms, like bystander intervention and men's involvement, challenge underlying assumptions and behaviors that promote a culture in support of sexual violence (Basile et al., 2016). Programs that address women's economic empowerment, job training, and social status can prevent sexual violence by reducing risk factors (Basile et al., 2016). Many educational programs aimed at middle schools and high schools, such as *Safe Dates*, address gender roles as part of the curriculum (Basile et al., 2016). McCaughey and Cermele (2017) advocate for the use of self-defensive training as a potentially feminist approach to prevention of sexual violence. A way to address rape culture is social media, in particular, "feminist response-ability" which is the use of social media to counter messages of rape culture and support survivors of violence (Rentschler, 2014).

Prevention strategies have grown from feminism models to incorporate more of an intersectional social justice perspective. An intersectional perspective takes into account multiple identity positions and forms of oppression when considering a social problem (Crenshaw, 1991; Danis &

Bhandari, 2010). An example of this approach can be found in the explicit social justice framework that guides the Mentors in Violence Prevention (MVP) program (Katz et al., 2011). The MVP program, which engages participants, in particular men, uses the strategies from anti-racism movements to engage bystanders to address issues around gender, sexual orientation and racism that support a culture of power-based violence (Katz et al., 2011).

Next Steps for Sexual Violence Prevention Theoretical Work

As discussed, a number of theoretical perspectives are currently found in the research to support sexual violence prevention efforts. Some are focused on preventing an individual from perpetrating sexual violence while other theories explore how to change peer and social culture to great environments where sexual violence is not tolerated. There is no "one" theory that is all encompassing and therefore there are calls to use multiple theories to support comprehensive sexual violence efforts (Banyard, 2014). For example, the Rape Prevention and Education (RPE) program, created by the Centers for Disease Control and Prevention, draws upon multiple theories across the social ecology including individual-level theories and societal-level change theories. Their model encourages practitioners to use theory-driven strategies and to address not only individual-level change but also community change (Cox, Lang, Townsend, & Campbell, 2010). Another example of a collection of theories is the feminist version of routine activities theory. Routine activities theory posits that the amount and location of a crime depends on the presence of likely offenders, the absence of effective guardians, and the availability of suitable targets. In the feminist modification, motivation to perpetrate is explained by presence of male peer groups that promote harmful gender norms, along with structural gendered oppression and heavy substance use. These motivations create likely offenders (Schwartz et al., 2001). Further work is needed to conceptualize how to best integrate theories in a way that will provide a solid foundation to guide comprehensive sexual violence prevention efforts. There are a few key areas for improvement of the use of theory in sexual violence prevention work. Past sexual violence prevention work has been criticized for lacking theoretical support (Banyard, 2014), although this may be changing.

In addition to the need for prevention programs to be theoretically driven and for research and evaluation to explicitly cite theory, there is a need to test the actual application of theory to practice to assess the fit. While a number of theories are available and have been used to help formulate prevention programs, the testing of the actual theoretical constructs as applied to sexual violence is limited. We may find that the theory does not fully apply or applies for certain populations.

An example of the type of theory-testing work needed is the work that Banyard and her colleagues (2010) have engaged in on testing the application of the Transtheoretical Model of Change (TTM). To measure and assess the application of TTM as part of an evaluation of the *Bringing in the Bystander* program, Banyard et al. (2010) utilized self-report questionnaires to determine individuals' particular stage-of-change prior to participation in the program, how participation in the program impacted self-reported stage, and the relationship between stage-of-change on behavior and attitude outcomes. Findings revealed that individuals' self-reported stage, or readiness to change prior to participating in the program, impacted their endorsement of rape-supportive attitudes and willingness to engage as a bystander following the program and that participants who went through the program demonstrated movement in their readiness for change (Banyard et al., 2010). Edwards et al. (2015) also provide a model for testing theory with their work on applying the Community Readiness Model to campus communities. They adapted the model to fit the context of campus sexual assault and dating violence, and then tested the construct through an examination of the factor structure of the "Campus Community Readiness to Engage" measure.

In addition to strengthening the role of theory in driving the creation of programs, and the need to evaluate the fit of the actual theory in sexual violence prevention contexts, there is also a need for continued theory-building. As demonstrated in this review, the majority of theories used in sexual violence prevention literature focus on individual-level behavior change. In line with an ecological approach, further work is needed to explore peer-, community-, and societal-level change theories and their connections with individual theories and with each other. Further work can also continue to explore how various theories may work together to provide an optimal foundation for prevention efforts. Most of the testing of sexual violence prevention strategies and theories have been conducted on teens and college aged students. Teen and emerging adulthood is a key developmental time for prevention (Lundgren & Amin, 2015), but more information is needed about theories that can guide prevention among children and adults. There is a need for research to explore the lifespan to determine if various approaches and theories are more salient based on developmental and life stages.

Sexual violence is a complex problem with individual and community causes that merit a robust response. Theory influences not only how we understand the causes of sexual violence, but also how individuals, groups, and communities can approach prevention. Theories have been developed across the social ecology from both individualist and societal perspectives—the person and the political—to guide the creation and implementation of prevention models primarily at the adolescent and emerging adulthood stage. More evaluation is needed to test the efficacy of prevention models built in individual and hybrid theoretical approaches.

References

Abbey, A., & McAuslan, P. (2004). A longitudinal examination of male college students' perpetration of sexual assault. *Journal of Consulting and Clinical Psychology, 72*(5), 747.

Abbey, A., Parkhill, M. R., Beshears, R., Monique Clinton-Sherrod, A., & Zawacki, T. (2006). Cross-sectional predictors of sexual assault perpetration in a community sample of single African American and Caucasian men. *Aggressive Behavior, 32*, 54–67.

Ajzen, I. (1991). The theory of planned behavior. *Organizational Behavior and Human Decision Processes, 50*, 179–211.

Arriaga, X. B., & Foshee, V. A. (2004). Adolescent dating violence: Do adolescents follow in their friends' or their parents' footsteps. *Journal of Interpersonal Violence, 19*(2), 162–184.

Bandura, A. (1969). *Social-learning theory of identificatory processes. Handbook of socialization theory and research* (Vol. 213, p. 262).

Bandura, A. (1986). *The social foundations of thought and action: A social cognitive theory*. Eagleton Cliffs, NJ: Prentice Hall.

Banyard, V. L. (2011). Who will help prevent sexual violence: Creating an ecological model of bystander intervention. *Psychology of Violence, 1*(3), 216.

Banyard, V. L. (2014). Improving college campus–based prevention of violence against women: A strategic plan for research built on multipronged practices and policies. *Trauma, Violence & Abuse, 15*(4), 339–351.

Banyard, V. L., Eckstein, R. P., & Moynihan, M. M. (2010). Sexual violence prevention: The role of stages of change. *Journal of Interpersonal Violence, 25*, 111–135.

Banyard, V. L., Moynihan, M. M., & Crossman, M. T. (2009). Reducing sexual violence on campus: The role of student leaders as empowered bystanders. *Journal of College Student Development, 50*(4), 446–457.

Banyard, V. L., Moynihan, M. M., & Plante, E. G. (2007). Sexual violence prevention through bystander education: An experimental evaluation. *Journal of Community Psychology, 35*(4), 463–481.

Banyard, V. L., Potter, S. J., Cares, A. C., Williams, L. M., Moynihan, M. M., & Stapleton, J. G. (2018). Multiple sexual violence prevention tools: Doses and boosters. *Journal of Aggression, Conflict and Peace Research, 10*(2), 145–155. https://doi.org/10.1108/JACPR-05-2017-0287

Basile, K. C., DeGue, S., Jones, K., Freire, K., Dills, J., Smith, S. G., & Raiford, J. L. (2016). *STOP SV: A technical package to prevent sexual violence*. Atlanta, GA: National Center for Injury Prevention and Control, Centers for Disease Control and Prevention.

Bedera, N., & Nordmeyer, K. (2015). "Never Go Out Alone": An analysis of college rape prevention tips. *Sexuality and Culture, 19*(3), 533–542.

Berkowitz, A. D. (2003). *Applications of social norms theory to other health and social justice issues. The social norms approach to preventing school and college age substance abuse: A handbook for educators, counselors, and clinicians* (pp. 259–279). San Francisco, CA: Jossey-Bass.

Berkowitz, A. D. (2010). Fostering healthy norms to prevent violence and abuse: The social norms approach. In K. Kaufman (Ed.), *The prevention of sexual violence: A practitioner's sourcebook* (pp. 147–171). Holyoke, MA: NEARI Press.

Black, M.C., Basile, K.C., Breiding, M.J., Smith, S.G., Walters, M.L., Merrick, M.T., ... & Stevens, M.R. (2011). The National Intimate Partner and Sexual Violence Survey (NISVS): 2010 Summary Report. Atlanta, GA: National Center for Injury Prevention and Control, Centers for Disease Control and Prevention.

Bronfenbrenner, U. (1977). Toward an experimental ecology of human development. *American Psychologist, 32*(7), 513.

Bronfenbrenner, U. (1979). The ecology of human development. Harvard university press.

Brown, A. L., & Messman-Moore, T. L. (2010). Personal and perceived peer attitudes supporting sexual aggression as predictors of male college students' willingness to intervene against sexual aggression. *Journal of Interpersonal Violence, 25*(3), 503–517.

Brown, J. (1997). Working toward freedom from violence. *Violence Against Women, 3*, 5–26.

Cantor, D., Fisher, B., Chibnall, S., Townsend, R., Lee, H., Bruce, C., & Thomas, G. (2015). *Report on the AAU campus climate survey on sexual assault and sexual misconduct.* Retrieved from https://ias.virginia.edu/sites/ias.virginia.edu/files/University%20of%20Virginia_2015_climate_final_report.pdf

Carlson, J., Casey, E., Edleson, J. L., Tolman, R. M., Walsh, T. B., & Kimball, E. (2015). Strategies to Engage Men and Boys in Violence Prevention: A Global Organizational Perspective. *Violence Against Women, 21*(1), 1406–1425.

Casey, E. (2010). Strategies for engaging men as anti-violence allies: Implications for ally movements. *Advances in Social Work, 11*(2), 267–282.

Casey, E. A., & Lindhorst, T. P. (2009). Toward a multi-level, ecological approach to the primary prevention of sexual assault: Prevention in peer and community contexts. *Trauma, Violence & Abuse, 10*(2), 91–114.

Casey, E. A., & Ohler, K. (2012). Being a positive bystander: Male antiviolence allies' experiences of "stepping up". *Journal of Interpersonal Violence, 27*(1), 62–83.

Chamberlain, L. (2008). A prevention primer for domestic violence: Terminology, tools, and the public health approach. *VAWnet: The National Online Resource Center on Violence Against Women (March).*

Claussen, C. (2017). The WiseGuyz program: Sexual health education as a pathway to supporting changes in endorsement of traditional masculinity ideologies. *Journal of Men's Studies, 25*(2), 150–167.

Cohen, L., Davis, R., & Mikkelsen, L.(2000). *Comprehensive prevention: Improving health outcomes through practice.* The Prevention Institute. Retrieved from http://old.preventioninstitute.org/minorityhealth.html

Cohen, L., & Swift, S. (1999). The spectrum of prevention: Developing a comprehensive approach to injury prevention. *Injury Prevention, 5*(3), 203–207.

Coker, A. L., Fisher, B. S., Bush, H. M., Swan, S. C., Williams, C. M., Clear, E. R., & DeGue, S. (2015). Evaluation of the Green Dot bystander intervention to reduce interpersonal violence among college students across three campuses. *Violence Against Women, 21*(12), 1507–1527.

Coker, A. L., Bush, H. M., Fisher, B. S., Swan, S. C., Williams, C. M., Clear, E. R., & DeGue, S. (2016). Multi-college bystander intervention evaluation for violence prevention. *American journal of preventive medicine, 50*(3), 295–302.

Cook-Craig, P. G., Millspaugh, P. H., Recktenwald, E. A., Kelly, N. C., Hegge, L. M., Coker, A. L., & Pletcher, T. S. (2014). From Empower to Green Dot: Successful strategies and lessons learned in developing comprehensive sexual violence primary prevention programming. *Violence Against Women, 20*(10), 1162–1178.

Cox, P. J., Lang, K. S., Townsend, S. M., & Campbell, R. (2010). The rape prevention and education (RPE) theory model of community change: Connecting individual and social change. *Journal of Family Social Work, 13*, 297–312.

Crenshaw, K. (1991). Mapping the margins: Intersectionality, identity politics, and violence against women of color. *Stanford Law Review, 43*(6), 1241–1299.

Danis, F. S., & Bhandari, S. (2010). Understanding domestic violence: A primer. In L. L. Lockhart & F. S. Danis (Eds.), *Domestic violence: Intersectionality and culturally competent practice* (pp. 29–66). New York, NY: Columbia University Press.

Dardis, C. M., Murphy, M. J., Bill, A. C., & Gidycz, C. A. (2016). An investigation of the tenets of social norms theory as they relate to sexually aggressive attitudes and sexual assault perpetration: A comparison of men and their friends. *Psychology of Violence, 6*(1), 163–171.

Dearing, J. W., & Cox, J. G. (2018). Diffusion of Innovations theory, principles, and practice. *Health Affairs, 37*(2), 183–190.

DeGue, S., Simon, T. R., Basile, K. C., Yee, S. L., Lang, K. W., & Spivak, H. (2012). Moving forward by looking back: Reflecting on a decade of CDC's work in sexual violence prevention, 2000–2010. *Journal of Women's Health, 21*(12), 1211–1218.

DeKeseredy, W. S. (2011). Feminist contributions to understanding woman abuse: Myths, controversies, and realities. *Aggression and Violent Behavior, 16*, 297–302.

Dills, J., Fowler, D., & Payne, G. (2016). Sexual Violence on Campus: Strategies for Prevention. Retrieved from https://www.cdc.gov/violenceprevention/pdf/campussvprevention.pdf

Durkin, K. F., Wolfe, T. W., & Clark, G. A. (2005). College students and binge drinking: An evaluation of social learning theory. *Sociological Spectrum, 25*(3), 255–272.

Edwards, K. M., Littleton, H. L., Sylaska, K. M., Crossman, A. L., & Craig, M. (2016). College campus community readiness to address intimate partner violence among LGBTQ+ young adults: A conceptual and empirical examination. *American Journal of Community Psychology, 58*(1-2), 16–26.

Edwards, K. M., Moynihan, M. M., Rodenhizer-Stämpfli, K. A., Demers, J. M., & Banyard, V. L. (2015). Campus community readiness to engage measure: Its utility for campus violence prevention initiatives—preliminary psychometrics. *Violence and Gender, 2*(4), 214–224.

Fabiano, P. M., Perkins, H. W., Berkowitz, A., Linkenbach, J., & Stark, C. (2003). Engaging men as social justice allies in ending violence against women: Evidence for a social norms approach. *Journal of American College Health, 52*(3), 105–112.

Fishbein, M., & Ajzen, I. (1975). *Belief, attitude, intention, and behavior: An introduction to theory and research.* Reading, MA: Addison-Wesley.

Foubert, J. D., & Marriott, K. A. (1997). Effects of a sexual assault peer education program on men's belief in rape myths. *Sex Roles, 36*(3-4), 259–268.

Foubert, J. D., & McEwen, J. (1998). An all-male rape prevention peer education program: Decreasing fraternity men's behavioral intent to rape. *Journal of College Student Development, 39*(6), 548–556.

Gidycz, C. A., Orchowski, L. M., & Berkowitz, A. D. (2011). Preventing sexual aggression among college men: An evaluation of a social norms and bystander intervention program. *Violence Against Women, 17*(6), 720–742.

Haines, M. P. (2009). *Best practices: Social Norms.* National Social Norms Resource Center. Retrieved from http://wch.uhs.wisc.edu/13-Eval/Tools/Resources/Social%20Norms.pdf

Haines, M. P., Perkins, H. W., Rice, R. M. & Barker, G. (2005). *A guide to marketing social norms for health promotion in schools and communities.* National Social Norms Resource Center. Reftrieved from http://www.socialnormsresources.org/pdf/Guidebook2.pdf

Hawkins, W. E., Clarke, G. N., & Seeley, J. R. (1993). Application of social learning theory to the primary prevention of depression in adolescents. *Health Values: The Journal of Health Behavior, Education & Promotion, 17*(6), 31–39.

Heppner, M. J., Good, G. E., Hillenbrand-Gunn, T. L., Hawkins, A. K., Hacquard, L. L., Nichols, R. K., … Brock, K. J. (1995). Examining sex differences in altering attitudes about rape: A test of the Elaboration Likelihood Model. *Journal of Counseling & Development, 73*(6), 640–647.

Hipp, T. N., Bellis, A. L., Goodnight, B. L., Brennan, C. L., Swartout, K. M., & Cook, S. L. (2017). Justifying sexual assault: Anonymous perpetrators speak out online. *Psychology of Violence, 17*(6), 684–702.

Katz, J., Heisterkamp, H. A., & Fleming, W. M. (2011). The social justice roots of the mentors in violence prevention model and its application in a high school setting. *Violence Against Women, 17*(6), 684–702.

Katz, J., & Moore, J. (2013). Bystander education training for campus sexual assault prevention: An initial meta-analysis. *Violence and Victims, 28*(6), 1054–1067.

Kelly, J. (2004). Popular opinion leaders and HIV prevention peer education: Resolving discrepent findings, and the implications for the development of effective community programs. *AIDS Care, 16*, 139–150.

Koss, M. P., Gidycz, C. A., & Wisniewski, N. (1987). The scope of rape: Incidence and prevalence of sexual aggression and victimization in a national sample of higher education students. *Journal of Counseling and Clinical Psychology, 55*(2), 162–170.

Krebs, C., Lindquist, C., Berzofsky, M., Shook-Sa, B., & Peterson, K. (2016). *Campus Climate Survey Validation Study: Final Technical Report.* Research Triangle Park, NC: RTI International.

Lanier, C. A., Elliott, M. N., Martin, D. W., & Kapadia, A. (1998). Evaluation of an intervention to change attitudes toward date rape. *Journal of American College Health, 46*(4), 177–180.

Lonsway, K. A., & Fitzgerald, L. F. (1994). Rape myths: In review. *Psychology of Women Quarterly, 18*(2), 133–164. https://doi.org/10.1111/j.1471-6402.1994.tb00448.x

Lundgren, R., & Amin, A. (2015). Addressing intimate partner violence and sexual violence among adolescents: Emerging evidence of effectiveness. *Journal of Adolescent Health, 56*(1), S42–S50.

Mabry, A., & Turner, M. M. (2016). Do sexual assault bystander interventions change men's intentions? Applying the theory of normative social behavior to predicting bystander outcomes. *Journal of Health Communication, 21*, 276–292.

Malamuth, N. M., Heavey, C. L., & Linz, D. (1996). The Confluence Model of sexual aggression. *Journal of Offender Rehabilitation*, 13–37.

McCaughey, M., & Cermele, J. (2017). Changing the hidden curriculum of campus rape prevention and education: Women's self-defense as a key protective factor for a public health model of prevention. *Trauma, Violence & Abuse, 18*(3), 287–302.

McDermott, R. C., Kilmartin, C., McKelvey, D. K., & Kridel, M. M. (2015). College male sexual assault of women and the psychology of men: Past, present, and future directions for research. *Psychology of Men & Masculinity, 16*(4), 355–366. https://doi.org/10.1037/a0039544

McMahon, S., Postmus, J. L., Warrener, C., & Koenick, R. A. (2014). Utilizing peer education theater for the primary prevention of sexual violence on college campuses. *Journal of College Student Development, 55*(1), 78–85.

Meyer, G., Roberto, A. J., Boster, F. J., & Roberto, H. L. (2004). Assessing the Get Real about Violence curriculum: Process and outcomes evaluation results and implications. *Health Communication, 16*(4), 451–474.

Moynihan, M. M., Banyard, V. L., Cares, A. C., Potter, S. J., Williams, L. M., & Stapleton, J. G. (2015). Encouraging responses in sexual and relationship violence prevention: What program effects remain 1 year later? *Journal of Interpersonal Violence, 30*(1), 110–132.

Muñoz-Silva, A., Sánchez-García, M., Nunes, C., & Martins, A. (2007). Gender differences in condom use prediction with theory of reasoned action and planned behaviour: The role of self-efficacy and control. *AIDS Care - Psychological and Socio-Medical Aspects of AIDS/HIV, 19*(9), 1177–1181.

Nabi, R. L., Southwell, B., & Hornik, R. (2002). Predicting intentions versus predicting behaviors: Domestic violence prevention from a theory of reasoned action perspective. *Health Communication, 14*(4), 429–449.

Nichols, A. J. (2014). *Feminist advocacy: Gendered organizations in community-based responses to domestic violence*. Lanham, MD: Lexington Books.

Perkins, H. W. (2003). *The social norms approach to preventing school and college age substance abuse: A handbook for educators, counselors, and clinicians*. San Francisco, CA: Jossey-Bass.

Peterson, K., Sharps, P., Banyard, V., Powers, R. A., Kaukinen, C., Gross, D., … Campbell, J. (2016). An evaluation of two dating violence prevention programs on a college campus. *Journal of Interpersonal Violence, 33*(23), 3630–3655. https://doi.org/10.1177/0886260516636069

Petty, R. E., & Cacioppo, J. T. (1986). The elaboration likelihood model of persuasion. In D. Bar-Tal, C. F. Graumann, A. W. Kruglanski, & W. Stroebe (Eds.), *Communication and persuasion* (pp. 1–24). New York: Springer.

Plested, B. A., Edwards, R. W., & Jumper-Thurman, P. (2006). *Community readiness: A handbook for successful change*. Fort Collins, CO: Tri-Ethnic Center for Prevention Research.

Potter, S. J. (2012). Using a multimedia social marketing campaign to increase active bystander on the college campus. *Journal of American College Health, 60*(4), 282–295.

Prochaska, J. O. (2013). Transtheoretical model of behavior change. In M. D. Gellman & J. R. Turner (Eds.), *Encyclopedia of behavioral medicine* (pp. 1997–2000). New York: Springer.

Prochaska, J. O., & DiClemente, C. C. (1984). Self change processes, self efficacy and decisional balance across five stages of smoking cessation. *Progress in Clinical and Biological Research, 156*, 131–140.

Prochaska, J. O., Velicer, W. F., Rossi, J. S., Goldstein, M. G., Marcus, B. H., Rakowski, W., … Rossi, S. R. (1994). Stages of change and decisional balance for 12 problem behaviors. *Health Psychology, 13*(1), 39.

Rentschler, C. A. (2014). Rape culture and the feminist politics of social media. *Girlhood Studies, 7*(1), 65–82.

Rogers, E. M. (2003). *Diffusion of innovations*. New York: Free Press.

Rogers, E. M., & Williams, D. (1983). Diffusion of. Innovations (Glencoe, IL: The Free Press, 1962).

Sanday, P. (1996). Rape-prone versus rape-free campus cultures. *Violence Against Women, 2*(2), 191–208.

Schwartz, M. D., & DeKeseredy, W. S. (1997). *Sexual assault on the college campus: The role of male peer support*. Thousand Oaks, CA: SAGE.

Schwartz, M. D., & DeKeseredy, W. S. (2008). Interpersonal violence against women: The role of men. *Journal of Contemporary Criminal Justice, 24*(2), 178–185.

Schwartz, M. D., DeKeseredy, W. S., Tait, D., & Alvi, S. (2001). Male peer support and a feminist routing activities theory: Understanding sexual assault on the college campus. *Justice Quarterly, 18*(3), 623–649.

Schwartz, M. D., & Nogrady, C. A. (1996). Fraternity membership, rape myths, and sexual aggression on a college campus. *Violence Against Women, 2*(2), 148–162.

Shaffer, J. A. (2013). Stages-of-change model. In M. D. Gellman & J. R. Turner (Eds.), *Encyclopedia of behavioral medicine*. New York, NY: Springer.

Sochting, I., Fairbrother, N., & Koch, W. J. (2004). Sexual assault of women: Prevention efforts and risk factors. *Violence Against Women, 10*, 73–93.

Sutton, T. E., & Simons, L. G. (2015). Sexual assault among college students: Family of origin hostility, attachment, and the hook-up culture as risk factors. *Journal of Child and Family Studies, 24*, 2827–2840.

Swartout, K. M. (2013). The company they keep: How peer networks influence male sexual aggression. *Psychology of Violence, 3*(2), 157–171.

Theall, K. P., Fleckman, J., & Jacobs, M. (2015). Impact of a community popular opinion leader intervention among African American adults in a Southeastern United States community. *AIDS Education and Prevention, 27*(3), 275–288.

Thompson, M. P., Swartout, K. M., & Koss, M. P. (2013). Trajectories and predictors of sexually aggressive behaviors during emerging adulthood. *Psychology of Violence, 3*(3), 247.

Tjaden, P. G., & Thoennes, N. (2006). *Extent, nature, and consequences of rape victimization: Findings from the National Violence Against Women Survey*. Washington, DC: U.S. Department of Justice, National Institutions of Justice. Retrieved from https://www.ncjrs.gov/pdffiles1/nij/210346.pdf

Townsend, S. M., & Campbell, R. (2007). Homogeneity in community-based rape prevention programs: Empirical evidence of institutional isomorphism. *Journal of Community Psychology, 35*(3), 367–382.

Wareham, J., Paquette Boots, D., & Jorge, C. (2012). Social learning theory and intimate Violence among men participating in a family violence intervention program. *Journal of Crime and Justice, 32*, 93–124. https://doi.org/10.1080/0735648X.2009.9721263

Zinzow, H. M., & Thompson, M. (2015). A longitudinal study of risk factors for repeated sexual coercion and assault in US college men. *Archives of Sexual Behavior, 44*(1), 213–222.

24 Definition, Communication, and Interpretation of Sexual Consent

Emily F. Wood, Kristina J. Rikkonen, and Deborah Davis

Saifullah Khan, a Yale student who was accused of sexual assault and suspended from the university in 2015 was found not guilty by a criminal court in early 2018. Khan was accused of sexually assaulting a fellow Yale student after a Halloween Party. The accuser alleged that as she and Khan walked back to her dorm room she slipped in and out of consciousness and he sexually assaulted her (Wang & Weinstock, 2018). Khan claimed that the accuser invited him back to her dorm room and took off her clothes. At the trial, Khan's layer asked the accuser if she flirted with Khan, how much she drank, and why she did not wear a more modest Halloween costume (Wang & Weinstock, 2018). As in most cases of alleged sexual assault, jurors had to rely on "he said she said" accounts to determine what happened. To further complicate matters, both the accuser and accused were intoxicated, as is common in sexual assault cases. Although Khan was found not guilty in a criminal court where guilt must be proven "beyond reasonable doubt," he could still face a judiciary hearing at the university, which relies on a preponderance of the evidence standard and a "yes means yes" definition of consent. Stories like this one highlight the complexities of defining and interpreting what constitutes consent socially and under different laws and policies.

Universities, the judiciary, and society are under pressure to address instances of alleged sexual assault. As a result, the issue of sexual consent has received attention from educators, the media, and policy makers. When an alleged sexual assault occurs between acquaintances, most parties agree that sexual contact occurred but disagree about whether it was consensual. Despite inconsistent and ambiguous definitions, consent is the central issue for determination of whether a sexual assault occurred. Reflecting the complexity of the concept, however, there are many definitions of sexual consent, across contexts ranging from specifications in legal statutes to university policies to concepts prevalent in popular culture. Even when definitions of consent are established in the form of statutes or policies, these generally include little to no specification of what words or behaviors constitute consent (see DeMatteo, Galloway, Arnold, & Patel, 2015 for review). Furthermore, legal definitions of consent do not always match those of an average person.

These factors can make it difficult to determine whether consent was obtained or a sexual assault occurred. In the remainder of this chapter we first broadly outline formal definitions of sexual assault and consent, including federal and state legal statutes, campus policies, military rules, and academic definitions. We then present research on how consent is communicated and

E. F. Wood · K. J. Rikkonen
University of Nevada, Reno,
Reno, NV, USA
D. Davis (✉)
Department of Psychology/296,
University of Nevada, Reno, Reno, NV, USA
e-mail: debdavis@unr.edu

W. T. O'Donohue and P. A. Schewe (eds.), *Handbook of Sexual Assault and Sexual Assault Prevention*,
https://doi.org/10.1007/978-3-030-23645-8_24

interpreted, including instances when men and women interpret behaviors differently. In this context, we discuss factors inherent to the parties, their relationship, and/or their condition at the time of the encounter that can affect perceptions of consent. Finally, we note that formal definitions of consent do not always align with the average person's conceptualization of consent and the problems this may pose.

Formal Definitions of Consent

Definitions of sexual consent vary widely. In the United States, there are distinctive state and federal laws. In the realm of higher education, each university or college composes its own policies regarding sexual conduct and consent, with certain exceptions. In the military, there are overarching definitions of sexual consent and assault that apply to each branch of the military. Definitions (or lack of definitions) of consent in each of those domains will be examined broadly. Additionally, we explore the impact of ingestion of intoxicants or narcotics on ability to consent to a sexual act and its link to legal definitions of sexual assault and sexual consent.

Federal Statutes

At the federal level, the statute defining and delineating sexual assault contains no actual definition for sexual consent. In fact, the word *consent* does not appear in the federal statutes describing the two major classes of sexual assault (18 U.S.C. § 2241, 2018; 18 U.S.C. § 2242, 2018). Instead, the federal statutes describe the elements of "aggravated sexual assault" and "sexual abuse" as involving sexual assault inflicted with the use of force, threat, or fear, or inflicted in situations in which the victim is mentally or physically incapacitated (18 U.S.C. § 2241, 2018; 18 U.S.C. § 2242, 2018). Neither consent nor nonconsent is explicitly considered a relevant element in these statutes or other related sexual assault statutes.

Furthermore, only one federal statute addresses the involvement of alcohol or other drugs, which merely pertains to forced intoxication (18 U.S.C. § 2241, 2018). That is, sexual assault is considered aggravated if, prior to the assault, the assailant administers a drug, intoxicant, or other substance to the victim—without the victim's knowledge or consent—in order to impair the victim. Additional references to mental or physical incapacitation in other federal statutes require the victim to be incapable of understanding the nature of the situation or physically unable to refuse participation in the sexual act (18 U.S.C. § 2242, 2018). The impact of willingly ingested intoxicants or narcotics is unclear, as is the threshold at which an individual becomes incapable of understanding and willingly participating in the sexual act. Thus, the federal statutes regarding sexual assault do not provide language regarding consent to engage in a sexual act or whether voluntary intoxication nullifies consent. This is problematic in that many cases of alleged sexual assault involve one or both people being intoxicated (see below sections for further discussion of alcohol and consent).

State Statutes

Each state has latitude to create its own laws regarding sexual assault and sexual consent, and the result is heterogeneity among states. Only nine state statutes provide an explicit definition of consent to participate in a sexual act (California, Colorado, Florida, Illinois, Minnesota, Montana, Vermont, Washington, Wisconsin).[1] Another 11 states provide a definition for *lack* of consent or contexts/behaviors *without* consent (Alabama, Alaska, Arizona, Delaware, Kentucky, Louisiana, Nebraska, New York, Texas, Utah, West Virginia).[2]

[1] Cal. Penal Code § 261.6; Colo. Rev. Stat. § 18-3-401; Fla. Stat. § 794.011; 720 Ill. Comp. Stat. 5/11-1.70; Minn. Stat. § 609.341; Mont. Code Ann. § 45-5-501; Vt. Stat. Ann. tit. 13, § 3251; Wash. Rev. Code § 9A.44.010; Wis. Stat. § 940.225.

[2] Ala. Code § 13A-6-70; Alaska Stat. § 11.41.470; Ariz. Rev. Stat. § 13-1401; Del. Code Ann. tit. 11, § 761; Ky. Rev. Stat. Ann. § 510.020; La. Stat. Ann. § 14:42; Neb. Rev. Stat. § 28-318; N.Y. Penal Law § 130.05; Tex. Penal Code Ann. § 22.011; Utah Code Ann. § 76-5-406; W. Va.

The remaining 30 states do not provide any consent definition whatsoever.[3]

Standard language for a legal definition of consent includes a provision of voluntary action and knowledge of the possible act. For example, Florida's definition reads: "'Consent' means intelligent, knowing, and voluntary consent and does not include coerced submission. 'Consent' shall not be deemed or construed to mean the failure by the alleged victim to offer physical resistance to the offender" (Fla. Stat. § 794.011, 2017).

Of the nine states with definitions of consent, five require affirmative consent (Minnesota, Montana, Vermont, Washington, and Wisconsin).[4] Standard language for an affirmative consent definition contains explicit reference to words or actions expressing permission and willingness to participate in the sexual act by both persons engaging in the act. For example, Wisconsin's sexual assault statute provides the following affirmative consent definition: "'Consent,' as used in this section, means words or overt actions by a person who is competent to give informed consent indicating a freely given agreement to have sexual intercourse or sexual contact" (Wis. Stat. § 940.225, 2018). Such definitions go beyond the standard consent definition by stating that a mere absence of "no" does not constitute consent; rather, the individual must in some way overtly display his or her permission to engage in the act, whether through actions or words. This follows the "yes means yes" standard, whereas nonaffirmative consent conceptions follow the "no means no" standard.

In the states lacking a specific legal definition of consent, consent or lack of consent is instead implied through the language of which elements constitute a sexual assault. For example, Maine's statute states that "gross sexual assault" occurs if a person engages in a sexual act with another person by forcing or compelling the victim, with a person who has a mental disability,[5] or with a person unconscious or physically incapable of resisting the perpetrator (M.R.S.A. 17-A, § 253, 2017). Thus, the will or consent of the victim is inferred rather than explicitly defined.

State statutes addressing the impact of intoxicants and narcotics on consent are equally varied. The majority are unclear in describing the impact of such substances, especially when ingested voluntarily. Only eight states (Arizona, Iowa, Kansas, Maryland, Montana, South Dakota, Washington, and Wisconsin) provide explicit language stating that an individual may be incapable of consent due to the impact of intoxicants or narcotics, which may cause impairment in functioning or judgment.[6] Still others are unclear as to whether intoxication itself negates consent, or whether intoxication negates consent *only* when that intoxication prevents an individual from resisting an attack (e.g., California and Idaho; Cal. Penal Code § 261; Idaho Code § 18-6101).

Code § 61-8B-2.

[3] Ark. Code Ann. § 5-14-103; Ark. Code Ann. § 5-14-125; Conn. Gen. Stat. § 53a-70; Conn. Gen. Stat. § 53a-71; Ga. Code Ann. § 16-6-1; Haw. Rev. Stat. § 707-730; Idaho Code § 18-6101; Ind. Code § 35-42-4-1; Iowa Code § 709.1; Iowa Code § 709.5; Kan. Stat. Ann. § 21-5503; Me. Stat. tit. 17-A, § 253; Md. Code Ann., Crim. Law § 3-303; Md. Code Ann., Crim. Law § 3-304; Mass. Gen. Laws Ann. ch. 265, § 22; Mich. Comp. Laws § 750.520b; Miss. Code Ann. § 97-3-95; Mo. Rev. Stat. § 566.030; Nev. Rev. Stat. § 200.366; N.H. Rev. Stat. Ann § 632-A:2; N.J. Stat. Ann. § 2C:14-2; N.M. Stat. Ann. § 30-9-11; N.C. Gen. Stat. § 14-27.21; N.C. Gen. Stat. § 14-27.22; N.D. Cent. Code § 12.1-20-03; Ohio Rev. Code Ann. § 2907.02; Okla. Stat. tit. 21, § 1111; Or. Rev. Stat. § 163.375; 18 Pa. Cons. Stat. § 3121; 11 R.I. Gen. Laws § 11-37-2; S.C. Code Ann. § 16-3-652; S.D. Codified Laws § 22-22-1; Tenn. Code Ann. § 39-13-503; Va. Code Ann. § 18.2-61; Wyo. Stat. Ann. § 6-2-302.

[4] Minn. Stat. § 609.341; Mont. Code Ann. § 45-5-501; Vt. Stat. Ann. tit. 13, § 3251; Wash. Rev. Code § 9A.44.010; Wis. Stat. § 940.225.

[5] Those with mental disabilities are presumed unable to consent because consent is assumed to require the knowing, rational and voluntary decision to engage in the activity. The "knowing" part of this entails the ability to understand the nature of the sexual act and its potential consequences (such as pregnancy and others; *State vs. Mosbrucker*, 758 N.W.2d 663 (ND; 2008)). If mental disability is sufficient, it can undermine such understanding.

[6] Ariz. Rev. Stat. § 13-1401; Iowa Code § 709.1A; Kan. Stat. Ann. § 21-5503; Md. Code Ann., Crim. Law § 3-301; Mont. Code Ann. § 45-2-101; S.D. Codified Laws § 22-22-1; Wash. Rev. Code § 9A.44.010; Wis. Stat. § 940.225.

A further 27 states make mention of intoxicants, but only contain a provision negating consent *if the victim was forcibly intoxicated.*[7] New Jersey's statute states that mental incapacitation (which negates consent) means, "that condition in which a person is rendered temporarily incapable of understanding or controlling his conduct due to the influence of a narcotic, anesthetic, intoxicant, or other substance *administered to that person without his prior knowledge or consent"* (N.J. Stat. Ann. § 2C:14-2, 2014; N.J. Stat. Ann. § 2C:14-1, 2012; emphasis not in original). As such, these state statutes do not address contexts in which victims of assault had knowingly and voluntarily consumed intoxicants. It should be noted that some state statutes address voluntary alcohol consumption with lesser charges, such as in Louisiana, where the charge drops from second-degree rape to third-degree rape if the intoxication was not forced (La. Stat. Ann. § 14:43). Another subset of states provides that mental incapacitation negates ability to consent, but does not include intoxication by alcohol or narcotics as an element of incapacitation (e.g., Missouri & Virginia; Mo. Rev. Stat. § 566.030; Va. Code Ann. § 18.2-61). As such, the majority of statutes do not provide clear guidance for courts on how to interpret issues of assault involving intoxication.

University and College Campuses

Federal Statutes. Historically, federal regulations regarding sexual conduct codes were quite lenient. However, with the passing of the Violence Against Women Reauthorization Act (VAWA) of 2013, federal mandates now exist for all institutions of higher education regarding sexual assault policies (34 C.F.R. § 668.46). Specifically, the statute now requires universities and colleges to provide students and employees with security awareness programs, including a definition of sexual consent. The definition itself is not mandated, with institutions retaining autonomy in the construction of these definitions.

State Statutes. In a fashion similar to the U.S. state governments, universities and colleges have free reign to compose sexual conduct codes and define sexual consent (34 C.F.R. § 668.46). As such, institutions may also determine whether affirmative consent will be a component of sexual interactions. However, there are now two notable exceptions: California and New York are the first and only states to enact legislation mandating all institutions receiving state funds to incorporate affirmative consent definitions into their sexual conduct codes, with some individual universities doing the same ("Yes Means Yes," n.d.). California led with the Donahoe Higher Education Act (Cal. Educ. Code § 67386), imposing a detailed affirmative consent standard in determining whether all parties consented to sexual activity. New York followed suit a year later with a successful "enough is enough" campaign, imposing a mandate which must be adopted by all institutions receiving government funding (N.Y. Educ. Law § 6441, 2015).

A number of individual institutions have also voluntarily enacted sexual conduct codes including an affirmative consent definition. Yale University's Title IX policy, for example, states that, "[c]onsent cannot be inferred from the absence of a 'no;' a clear 'yes,' verbal or otherwise, is necessary. Consent to some sexual acts does not constitute consent to others, nor does past consent to a given act constitute present or future consent. Consent must be ongoing throughout a sexual encounter and can be revoked at any time." (Yale Sexual Misconduct Policies and Related Definitions, 2018). Although such universities and colleges remain the minority, and there is no clear consensus regarding the definition of consent, each institution now has some sort of definition at minimum due to VAWA.

[7] Ala. Code § 13A-6-60; Colo. Rev. Stat. § 18-3-402; Conn. Gen. Stat. § 53a-65; Del. Code Ann. tit. 11, § 761; Fla. Stat. § 794.011; Haw. Rev. Stat. § 707-700; Ind. Code § 35-42-4-1; Ky. Rev. Stat. Ann. § 510.010; La. Stat. Ann. § 14:42.1; Mich. Comp. Laws § 750.520a; Minn. Stat. § 609.341; Miss. Code Ann. § 97-3-97; N.H. Rev. Stat. Ann § 632-A:2; N.J. Stat. Ann. § 2C:14-1; N.Y. Penal Law § 130.00; N.C. Gen. Stat. § 14-27.20; N.D. Cent. Code § 12.1-20-03; Ohio Rev. Code Ann. § 2907.02; Okla. Stat. tit. 21, § 1111; 18 Pa. Cons. Stat. § 3121; 11 R.I. Gen. Laws § 11-37-1; S.C. Code Ann. § 16-3-652; Tenn. Code Ann. § 39-13-501; Tex. Penal Code Ann. § 22.011; Utah Code Ann. § 76-5-406; W. Va. Code § 61-8B-1; Wyo. Stat. Ann. § 6-2-303.

Military

As in broader society, the military offers conflicting legal definitions. Although there is one overarching definition of sexual assault, each state military code also contains its own definition. Only the federal statute will be discussed here. Different from general civilian federal standards, the military code has a detailed definition for consent, including factors that constitute consent as well as provisions for elements that negate consent. According to the Uniform Code of Military Justice, consent "means a freely given agreement to the conduct at issue by a competent person" (10 U.S.C. § 920). Factors which negate consent include expression of lack of consent, force, threat, incompetence, and unconsciousness. Lack of verbal or physical resistance resulting from fear or force, the dress of the victim, and any prior or current relationships do not equate to consent. That is, a person cannot assume that another person consents when that other is frightened into silence, and a person cannot infer consent on the basis of another's clothing. The latter is rarely found in state statutes (e.g., Montana; Mont. Code Ann. § 45-5-501), and federal statutes do not address clothing at all. This code also states that a person cannot assume consent from a spouse, intimate partner, or ex, similar to some state statutes (e.g., Colorado; Colo. Rev. Stat. § 18-3-401).

Further, the military code provides for both involuntary and voluntary intoxication on behalf of the victim of sexual assault, though the implication differs depending on whether the intoxication is voluntary or involuntary. In the case of involuntary intoxication, in which an assailant administers an intoxicant or narcotic to the victim "without the knowledge or consent of that person" (10 U.S.C. § 920(a)(5)), the assailant has committed "rape." In the case of voluntary intoxication, in which an assailant engages in a sexual act with an individual incapable of consenting due to impairment by an intoxicant or narcotic which "reasonably should be known by the person" (10 U.S.C. § 920(b)(3)(a)), the assailant has committed the lesser offense of "sexual assault." While the statute is clear that certain levels of intoxication negate consent, it does not state dosages or levels of intoxication at which it is acceptable versus unacceptable to engage in a sexual act.

Scholars

Legal and social science scholars have offered more varied and nuanced definitions of consent. Most suggest that consent can be conveyed through both verbal and nonverbal means, varying in their level of explicitness. Consent can be explicitly agreeing to something in the form of verbal affirmative consent or implied based on an individual's behaviors. Consent as an act refers to explicitly agreeing to something (e.g., "I will have sex with you"). Explicit consent is not usually used during sexual encounters and instead partners usually rely on indirect indications of willingness, referred to as implied or inferred consent. Implied consent is conveyed by behaviors or cues that a partner interprets as willingness to have sex. However, because interpretations of behaviors can vary between observers, implied consent is inherently more ambiguous than explicit consent (see Muehlenhard, Humphreys, Jozkowski, & Peterson, 2016 for review). A particularly nuanced review of issues surrounding sexual consent is offered by Wertheimer (2003), who reviews varying conceptual definitions of consent as well as the many ways in which circumstances such as power and relationship dynamics and incapacities in addition to alcohol can negate the ability to consent (see also West, 2008).

An additional aspect of consent is the question of which sexual behaviors and actions individuals are actually consenting to, made equivocal by the variation among statutes and policies. University policies appear to contain the most consensus; consent definitions instituted in California universities, New York universities, and Yale University maintain that sexual consent is an ongoing process, and "consent to some sexual acts does not constitute consent to others," (Yale Sexual Misconduct Policies and Related Definitions, 2018). State statutes are more divided, with most states lacking a definition of consent, as delineated above. This lack of definition inherently precludes any possible specification for how consent is construed throughout a sexual encounter. Of the five state statutes including an affirmative consent definition, only Minnesota's statute specifies that consent indicates an "agreement to perform a particular sexual act with the actor," (Minn. Stat. § 609.341). The remaining four state statutes include a vague statement that consent is an agreement to have "sexual intercourse or sexual contact" with an actor, neglecting to identify whether consent to one sexual act equates to consent to another (Wash. Rev. Code § 9A.44.010). The four state statutes containing nonaffirmative definitions of consent do not address this issue. The military's definition of consent arguably contains the most ambiguous identification of the sexual behaviors a person might be sanctioning, for consent is defined as "agreement to *the conduct at issue* by a competent person," (10 U.S.C. § 920, emphasis not in original). Last, federal statutes do not provide a consent definition, precluding any consideration for the behaviors and actions a person might be consenting to during a sexual encounter.

In sum, although statutes, policies, and scholars' conceptualizations exist that define sexual assault, and in some cases consent, these are quite basic and difficult to apply in practice. Formal definitions of consent are often unclear, ambiguous, and inconsistent across jurisdictions or contexts, often misunderstood, and not uniformly applied in practice (see above discussion and Rerick, Livingston & Davis, this volume). They may use the word consent or related words, but offer little detail of what the concept of consent means and little to no concrete guidance on how to judge whether a person has consented, or the range of behaviors they have consented to. In reality, the concept of consent is complex, may be interpreted in terms of a wide variety of feelings and behaviors, and is not universally defined across jurisdictions or understood uniformly by those who must apply it. Though seemingly clearer, even the "yes means yes" standard that is increasingly common in universities can be subject to ambiguity and disagreement in its application. This ambiguity of definitions and application of the concept of consent makes cases of alleged sexual assault adjudicated in courts, universities, or the military particularly difficult to assess. To understand how such assessments are made in practice, it is useful to have some information about what a reasonable person infers as being indicative of willingness to have sex. The next section of the chapter discusses research investigating how laypersons communicate and interpret consent. It also highlights gender differences in these processes. In this context we discuss difficulties created by some inconsistencies between the way consent is communicated in practice and the way it tends to be interpreted by potential sexual partners and lay jurors (see also Rerick, Livingston, & Davis, this volume regarding jury reactions).

Communicating Consent

As the preceding discussion has begun to develop, consent is an exceedingly complex concept. Existing legal, organizational, and research definitions barely scratch the surface of the complexities of the concept. Even if, for example, one says "Yes, I definitely want to have sex with you," is this truly consent if the initiator has sufficient power over the respondent? That is, other aspects of the situation and relationship between partners can have profound effects on the implications of one's statements and behaviors for sexual consent. Here we cannot explore all complexities of the concept of consent or its application. We refer the reader to the most thorough exploration of the concept of which we are aware (Wertheimer, 2003). Below we restrict our discussion to research addressing women's reports of how they convey consent or nonconsent, versus men's perceptions of the implications of women's behaviors for sexual consent.

Mechanisms of Consent Communications

As a starting point, it is worth discussing three general mechanisms through which consent or nonconsent is commonly conveyed before turning to specific behaviors. These three mechanisms fall into the conceptual category of "implied consent," or consent that "is indirectly given and usually indicated by a sign, an action or inaction, or a silence that creates a reasonable presumption that an acquiescence of the will has been given" (Block, 2004, p. 51). Specifically, research has indicated that, in practice, though explicit verbal communications may be as common as other mechanisms for communication of nonconsent (e.g., Marcantonio, Jozkowski, & Lo, 2018), consent is most often communicated passively (e.g., not resisting a partner's advances), indirectly (e.g., dressing sexily), and often nonverbally (e.g., undressing oneself or one's partner, touching; Beres, 2007; Davis & Villalobos, 2014; Hickman & Muehlenhard, 1999; Jozkowski, 2013; Jozkowski, Sanders, Peterson, Dennis, & Reece, 2014; Jozkowski & Wiersma, 2015; Villalobos, Davis, & Leo, 2016). These less than explicit means of communication provide a challenge of interpretation for those involved in sexual situations as well as for those who later judge them.

Passivity as a Primary Mechanism of Consent

A number of studies, even of recent vintage, have indicated that failure to resist through behavior or failure to say no are the most frequently used (or among the top) strategies for indicating consent among both homosexual and heterosexual couples, and among both males and females (Burkett & Hamilton, 2012; Byers, 1980; Fantasia, 2011; Hall, 1998; Hickman & Muehlenhard, 1999; Jozkowski, Sanders, et al., 2014; Jozkowski & Wiersma, 2015; Lim & Roloff, 1999; O'Sullivan & Byers, 1992; Perper & Weis, 1987; Beres, Herold, & Maitland, 2004). Sexual scripts common in our culture cast the man as the initiator of sex and the woman as the gatekeeper. As such, she is expected to actively resist unwanted advances (e.g., Jozkowski & Peterson, 2013; Wiederman, 2005). Belief in such scripts would encourage interpretation of failure to verbally or physically resist as indicating consent. However, it is clear that a person may fail to resist for a variety of reasons other than desire to have sex: such as fear of the initiator or freezing in fear, power imbalance, lack of social skills, inability to choose a response quickly enough to avoid sexual engagement, and others. It is for such reasons that many legal standards for consent specify that failure to resist cannot be taken as consent (see above).

Sexual Consent Communications Tend to be Indirect and Often Nonverbal

Although people tend to agree that direct verbal consent communications are the easiest to interpret, research has generally indicated that nonverbal communications are most frequently used to convey and interpret (non) consent (see Muehlenhard et al., 2016 for review) unless a partner explicitly asks about willingness (Jozkowski, 2011; Jozkowski & Peterson, 2013): and even when verbal communications are used, they tend to be indirect, taking the form of hints or innuendos rather than directly stating desires or intent (Hickman & Muehlenhard, 1999; Lee & Pinker, 2010). Explicit verbal consent is more likely in first-time encounters: and for the most intimate, novel (e.g., bondage and dominance), or deviant acts, or when necessary (such as negotiating use of a condom), and at the beginning of sexual encounters more so than as the sexual interaction proceeds. Moreover, despite affirmative consent policies, many regard verbal consent as unnecessary, unnatural, and as interfering with the mood and rhythm of the sexual encounter (see Muehlenhard et al., 2016 for review). These authors note, however, that explicit forms of initiation, and especially refusal, of sexual encounters may become more likely if indirect means are initially unsuccessful.

Individuals are also more likely to rely on nonverbal cues to gauge a partner's willingness to engage in sexual activities, with men being more likely than women to rely on nonverbal cues from their partner (Jozkowski, Peterson, Sanders, Dennis, & Reece, 2014). Qualitative research has also found that participants report "just knowing" when someone is interested or consenting to sexual activity and deem explicit verbal consent unnecessary when interpreting consent (Beres, 2010; Jozkowski & Hunt, 2014).

Though less clear, and therefore posing greater risk of misunderstanding, communicating (non)consent via nonverbal, indirect, and passive messages can minimize other social risks: such as embarrassment of the self or one's partner, damage to the relationship, rejection, and others. In their theory of the "strategic speaker," for example, Lee and Pinker (2010) suggested that we are generally likely to use indirect communications to convey messages involving social risks such as embarrassment or rejection: and particularly in circumstances where the communication could suggest a significant change in the nature of the relationship between the actor and recipient (such as change from platonic to sexual), or when the message might entail potentially embarrassing (e.g., a sexual suggestion that might be rebuffed) or illegal (e.g., suggestion to engage in theft) messages. Because they can be interpreted in more than one way, indirect communications provide plausible deniability of the intended meaning, and provide potential protection against embarrassment or other unwanted social or legal consequences.

While much indirect communication is likely to be understood as intended, its inherent ambiguity in meaning can nevertheless result in significant miscommunication (Abbey, 1991). Misinterpretation of these indirect and often nonverbal cues has the potential to result in unwanted sexual acts, though without the perpetrator's awareness that they were unwanted. A number of qualitative studies have found that this is recognized, in that participants express that anything other than a direct "no" has the potential for miscommunication (e.g., Burkett & Hamilton, 2012; Starfelt, Young, Palk, & White, 2015).

Misinterpretation of Indirect Communications in Sexual Situations

As Davis and colleagues have reviewed (Davis & Loftus, 2016; Davis & Villalobos, 2014; Villalobos et al., 2016), indirect communications in potentially sexual situations can increase the risk of misunderstanding for several reasons.

Social Norms. First are social norms supporting behavioral patterns that may promote misunderstanding. For example, socialization of women to be indirect and submissive with men (e.g., Jordan, 2005) can encourage use of less assertive indirect means of communicating nonconsent, even in the presence of very strong feelings against sexual engagement that might otherwise result in explicit refusal. At minimum, this could lead men to underestimate the intensity of actual nonconsent or to misinterpret the meaning as consent instead.

Misleading Sexual Scripts. Second are sexual scripts promoting misperception of sexual consent. Some directly suggest misinterpretation of sexual communications, as they include beliefs about the meaning of behaviors that are mistaken. As noted above, sexual scripts casting men as the initiator and women as the active gatekeeper for sexual activity promote interpretation of passivity as consent. Perhaps most widely known among specific misleading sexual scripts is the "token resistance" script suggesting that a person will initially refuse sexual advances even when actually desiring to engage in sexual activities (see Muehlenhard, 2011 for review). Many males believe women engage in such "token resistance," one-third to one-half of women report doing so (Muehlenhard & Hollabaugh, 1988; Sprecher, Hatfield, Cortese, Potapova, & Levitskaya, 1994), and males do so at similar rates (Muehlenhard & Rogers, 1998). The token resistance script and the widespread actual practice by both sexes complicates interpretation of even explicit refusals, and likely does so even more for those that are indirect.

Third, "Rape Myth Acceptance" (RMA: see Chapter this volume) entails a number of rape-supportive beliefs concerning the meaning of female behaviors, and those high in RMA have been shown to more likely read sexual intent into female behaviors, as well as to render perpetrator-supportive judgments in mock jury studies (see Rerick, Livingston & Davis, this volume).

A fourth common category of sexual scripts is those involving alcohol and sexual intentions. Studies of "alcohol expectancies" have generally shown, for example, that people expect that alcohol promotes sexual arousal and desire (see Davis & Loftus, 2004 for review), and those who use alcohol are perceived as more sexually willing (see Davis & Loftus, 2004; Farris, Treat, Viken, & McFall, 2008; Lindren, Parkhill, George, & Hendershot, 2008; Wood & Davis, 2017 for reviews). Those with strong "alcohol expectancies" suggesting that alcohol promotes sexual desire are particularly likely to perceive inebriated females as more sexually aroused and willing (Abbey, Buck, Zawacki, & Saenz, 2003; George, Cue, Lopez, Crowe, & Norris, 1995). However, as with indirect indicators of consent generally, alcohol use has multiple determinants and therefore multiple meanings: arguably, most having nothing to do with sexual intentions (such as stress or anxiety reduction, compliance with social pressures, and others).

The Problem of Multiple Meaning. Many behaviors are more likely to occur in potential sexual situations *and* those same behaviors are more likely to occur in other situations involving positive reactions to another. These are thus associated with multiple meanings related to feelings and intentions toward others: including, but not limited to, potential sexual partners. As Villalobos and colleagues (2016) note, many behaviors that are more likely to occur when one is sexually willing are also more likely to occur when one likes the other person in other ways (e.g., expressions of liking or affection, various forms of touch, willingness to do other things together), or when one is generally interested in the conversation (e.g., smiling, expressing interest in a person's statements, excited demeanor, intimate disclosures), or when one just wants to appear attractive and sexy or to compete favorably with attractive same sex others (wearing perfume, or scanty, sexy or provocative grooming, or attire), among others.

As Davis and Loftus (6; see also Greer & Buss, 1994) noted, many behaviors are actually more likely performed when one is sexually willing and thus are legitimately probative of sexual intentions. Nevertheless, no behavior definitively indicates sexual consent. All, however, are subject to multiple meanings. These three facts make interpretation of sexual intentions difficult and error prone: particularly given the tendency for consent communications to occur via hints, innuendo, tentative attempts, and nonverbal and/or indirect means.

The Problem of Motivated Perception. Even with no motivational influence to bias one's judgment, the potential to misinterpret indirect communications as reflecting sexual willingness is significant when in potentially sexual situations. However, such tendencies can be magnified by desires to have sex, to believe oneself sexually attractive, and/or to believe the specific person one wants to have sex with also wants the same. Indeed, regardless of gender, perceivers tend to project their own sexual and relationship desires onto those with whom they are interacting (e.g., Henningsen & Henningsen, 2010). Additionally, both men and women with generally high interest in short-term and casual sexual relationships are more likely to "overperceive" sexual intentions in others (Howell, Etchells, & Penton-Voak, 2012).

One of the most important motivators, however, is sexual arousal itself (e.g., Stephan, Berscheid, & Walter, 1971). Several studies have found an association between self-reported sexual arousal and perceptions of the degree to which women's behaviors reflect willingness to have sex (Bouffard & Miller, 2014; Livingston, Rerick, & Davis, 2018; Rerick, Livingston, & Davis, 2019). Rerick and colleagues (2019) also showed that manipulated sexual arousal among males increases perceptions that specific female behaviors reflect sexual intentions, particularly among single participants.

Intertwined with motivation is the issue of influences of emotion on perception. Some emotions entail specific motivations: such as fear-escape. But strong emotions also tend to impair executive functions, narrow attention to emotion relevant information, and to result in interpretations of incoming information as consistent with the emotion (see Davis & Loftus, 2016): such as when a male's positive emotions may lead him to exaggerate the extent to which the woman is indicating consent or a female's negative emotions may lead her to exaggerate the extent to which the male is coercive.

Enter Alcohol! Alcohol use by one or both parties is common in cases of sexual assault (Abbey, 2002, 2011). There is evidence to suggest that sexual miscommunication might be more likely under these circumstances. This can be understood in part through application of Steele and Josephs' (1990) work on "alcohol myopia." The theory asserts that alcohol narrows attention to immediate concerns and salient, impulse-consistent cues at the expense of attention to other potentially inhibitory cues relevant to the salient impulse. Consistent with this, Abbey and colleagues (Abbey, 2011; Abbey, McAuslan, & Ross, 1998) suggested the link between alcohol and sexual violence is in part a function of alcohol's promotion of errors in men's perception of women's sexual intentions.

Indeed, alcohol seems to impair recognition of nonconsent by men (e.g., Abbey, 2011; Abbey, Zawacki, & Buck, 2005; Gross, Bennett, Sloan, Marx, & Juergens, 2001; Marx, Gross, & Adams, 1999; Marx, Gross, & Juergens, 1997). Moreover, intoxicated men perceive women as more sexually aroused than unintoxicated men, generally perceive women's behaviors as more reflective of sexual intentions (e.g., Abbey et al., 2005; Abbey, Zawacki, & McAuslan, 2000; Davis et al., 2012; Farris, Treat, & Viken, 2010), and perceive their own and others' sexual aggression as more appropriate (e.g., Johnson, Noel, & Sutter-Hernandez, 2000; Norris & Kerr, 1993). Alcohol facilitates misperception more among men high in rape-supportive attitudes (e.g., Benbouriche, Teste, Guay, & Lavole, 2018). Notably, motivational biases, alcohol, and other influences can operate more strongly to influence interpretation of ambiguous communications, as is the case for indirect and many nonverbal messages.

Inexperience. Young people typically do not enter their sexually active years with extensive understanding of sexual communications and interactions, as reflected in many comedic portrayals of youthful interpretations of behaviors and intentions of the opposite sex. Such inexperience, combined with hormones, sexual motivation, and often alcohol, provides a toxic recipe for misunderstanding.

Notably, the issues with indirect communication covered in the preceding sections are problematic even under many affirmative consent standards. For example, recent California legislation (California Senate Bill SB-967, 2014), like many affirmative consent definitions, states what is *not* consent more explicitly (lack of protest or resistance, silence, existence of dating relationships, fact of past sexual activities) than what is ("affirmative, conscious, and voluntary agreement to engage in sexual activity"). This is also characteristic of many "no means no" standards. This suggests that those operating under affirmative consent and other standards may accept usage of any number of indirect verbal and nonverbal indicators of consent subject to multiple meanings and potential misinterpretation.

Gender Differences in Communication and Interpretation of Consent

Gender and Modes of Consent Communication

Some research has found gender differences in how consent is communicated. Men are more likely than women to use nonverbal cues to indicate consent and look for nonverbal cues from their partner to assess consent (Jozkowski, Peterson, et al., 2014). Men are more likely to communicate their consent by using initiating behavior such as taking off their clothes, and women are more likely to communicate their consent by engaging in passive behaviors such as not resisting when a partner attempts intercourse (Jozkowski, Sanders, et al., 2014; Jozkowski & Wiersma, 2015). Men are also more likely than women to use aggressive means to communicate their consent (e.g., to just do the activity without asking or being asked: Jozkowski & Peterson, 2013), and to view consent as a single event rather than an ongoing process (Humphreys, 2004).

In addition to the question of the general mechanisms of consent communications, research has addressed the related issue of the specifics of consent communications: both how (non)consent is conveyed and how it is interpreted. To address this question, we consider two lines of research, the first on the question of whether men generally tend to accurately perceive the meaning of women's behaviors, the second on the degree to which women report that specific behaviors reflect consent versus the degree to which men interpret them to do so.

The Question of the "Overperception Bias"

Research spanning decades has addressed the issue of whether men tend to perceive that women's behaviors reflect sexual intentions more strongly than women perceive or intend them to. The bulk of this research for many years indicated that, indeed, men "overperceive" sexual interest and intentions in women's behaviors: though much of this research has suffered from methodological flaws (see Farris et al., 2008 for review). Presumably, men who overperceive sexual willingness will appear more confident (and hence more attractive), will more likely have sex, and therefore will more likely reproduce and propagate their genes (see Haselton & Buss, 2000; Murray, Murphy, von Hippel, Trivers, & Haselton, 2017). However, rather than male overestimation of sexual intent or consent, the observed difference might be an instance of either actor–observer differences in perceptions (that actors see more reasons for their behaviors than observers); female underreporting of their sexual interest/intentions, research method artifacts, or some combination of these.

In a series of studies by Perilloux & Kurzban (2014), for example, the authors found that sex differences in reports of implied consent were significant when women were asked how likely they were to want sex themselves if they engaged in each of 15 behaviors. However, when asked either of two questions about women in general rather than about themselves (either what women in general *would say* about how likely they wanted sex given the behaviors, or how likely women in general *actually wanted* sex given the behavior) these differences disappeared and women read just as much sexual interest in other women's behaviors as men did.

The authors also found that both men and women thought women in general were less likely to *say* that the behaviors meant they wanted sex than to report that the behaviors indicated they *actually wanted* sex. Though potentially indicating that women underreport sexual interest, this finding cannot support anything other than the perception on the part of both sexes that this is what women do (see also Murray et al., 2017 for discussion of methodological issues compromising interpretation of Perilloux & Kurzban's (2014) findings regarding underreporting). However, subsequent research (Engeler & Raghubir, 2018) indicates that both men and women tend to underreport their own sexual intentions, partially explaining findings that each sex tends to overestimate sexual intentions of the other. However, even when accounting for women's underreporting of their own sexual intention, men still tend to overestimate women's sexual intentions: but at lower rates (Engeler & Raghubir, 2018). Each of these studies employed the same 15 behaviors originally used by Haselton and Buss (2000). However, they were unrepresentative of the full range of consent-related behaviors.

Several additional recent studies have failed to find overperception of sexual interest by men. For example, Treat, Church, & Viken, 2017 had men and women judge cues of sexual interest in photographed women. There were no overall sex differences, though men and women differed somewhat in which cues they responded to (Treat et al., 2017; see also Fisher & Walters, 2003).

Davis and colleagues (Davis, Follette, & Merlino, 1999; Wood & Davis, 2016, 2017) investigated gender differences in perceptions of up to 95 behaviors, using questions designed to be more analogous to legal concepts of the "probative" versus "definitive" value of evidence. Probative evidence is probabilistically associated with the conclusion (i.e., the conclusion is more likely given the evidence), whereas definitive evidence assures the conclusion is true (i.e., the conclusion is certain given the evidence). The authors asked males and females two questions regarding specific female behaviors. Females were asked whether they are generally 1 (much less likely) to 4 (equally likely) to 7 (much more likely to perform the behavior) when willing to have intercourse): and, secondly, whether they performed the behavior if, and only if, willing to have intercourse, sometimes performed it when not willing, or often performed it when not willing. In the two later studies, women were asked to answer these questions either regarding their own behavior or regarding the behavior of women in general on a five-point scale. Men were asked to answer regarding the behavior of women in general.

Results for specific behaviors are discussed in the sections to come. Here, we wish to note that results did not generally support the notion of the "overperception bias." For example, Davis et al. (1999) found very small, but statistically significant mean differences in ratings of probativeness across 73 behaviors between men (3.06/7) and women (2.99/7); as well as in the percent of men (59.6%) versus women (53.3%) who rated the behavior as more likely to occur when the woman is willing to have sex. Nevertheless, like many studies, the results indicated a lot of agreement between sexes, in that correlations between male and female ratings of probativeness ranged from 0.964 to 0.965 for mean ratings on the 7-point scale, ranked mean ratings of specific behaviors, and percent of respondents who rated the behavior as more likely to occur when the women was willing to have intercourse (above 4/7).

Results more strongly contradicted the overperception hypothesis for the index of definitiveness. The correlation between the percent of men and women who indicated the behavior is performed if and only if the woman is willing to have intercourse, across 73 behaviors was 0.85. However, the percent of respondents who indicated the behaviors were definitive averaged 25.7% for women, versus 18.3% for men. Overall, men and women agreed on the behaviors most strongly associated with consent, though men were more conservative in reading definite willingness into women's behaviors!

Wood and Davis (2016, 2017) replicated and expanded these findings to include more behaviors, reflecting emerging behaviors such as sexting, for example (Wood & Davis, 2016), and to specifically address behaviors related to alcohol use (Wood & Davis, 2017). In their first study, Wood and Davis (2016) found that, across 95 behaviors, men's average ratings of probativeness were slightly (but significantly) lower (2.3/5) than those of women rating themselves (2.53/5), but the percent of men and women who rated the behaviors as more likely to occur when the woman was willing to have sex did not differ (2.3 average across the 95 behaviors for each). As in the previous study, more women rated their own behaviors as definitive than did men: again indicating that men were more conservative in interpreting behaviors as definitely indicating sexual consent than women were in reporting that their own behaviors did so.

In a second study, Wood and Davis (2016) replicated this again with 48 of the original 95 behaviors and additionally asked women to answer either regarding their own behavior or the behaviors of "women in general." Across the 48 behaviors, average probativeness ratings for men (2.36/5) were more similar to those of women answering about other women (2.33/5) than those of women answering about themselves (2.64/5). The same was true of definitiveness: in that across behaviors the average percent reporting that women performed the behaviors only when willing to have sex was lower for both male (23.2%) and female (18.5%) observers reporting on "women in general" than for women reporting for themselves (34.6%).

Only results from the Wood and Davis (2017) study of behaviors involving alcohol indicated that males generally viewed use of alcohol across a number of situations as more indicative of sexual willingness than women themselves. In this case males' average ratings of probativeness were higher than those of women. But in contrast to the other studies, a higher percent of males reporting on females than females reporting on themselves indicated that the behaviors were performed only when the woman was willing to have sex. However, like the Wood and Davis (2016) second study, women and men who were judging behaviors of "women in general" did not differ significantly from one another.

Together, available evidence does not support the idea that there is substantial disagreement between men and women on either what behaviors reflect consent or how strongly they do so. Men and women describe the same consent and refusal cues in response to open ended questions (e.g., Beres, 2010), and when rating the implications of various behaviors for consent, even statistically significant differences tend to be small, and correspondence between which cues are seen as most significant is high. In three of the Davis and colleagues studies (Davis et al., 1999; Wood & Davis, 2016) men read less, rather than more, definite intent into women's behaviors than women reported for themselves. Moreover, men and women report that they believe they are not miscommunicating and share an understanding of consent (Jozkowski & Hunt, 2014). Finally, when women judge the import of other women's behaviors, they do not differ from men.

It is important to note, however, that most studies of gender differences in interpretation of consent cues are decontextualized. Many ask participants the meaning of various behaviors in the abstract, unsituated in specific social contexts. And, with few exceptions, research participants are not in the physical and psychological context of most negotiations of real life sex (such as alcohol, power differentials, sexual arousal, and others). As our previous discussion of effects of alcohol and sexual arousal and those in later sections regarding such factors as power or relationship dynamics make clear, contextual factors can magnify the difference between the actual versus perceived implications of behavior for sexual consent.

Also with few exceptions (such as Wood & Davis, 2017), research has investigated perceptions of single behaviors, rather than combinations of behaviors. It remains unknown whether gender differences might be either magnified or further reduced when multiple consent cues combine.

The Role of Specific Behaviors in Communicating and Interpreting Consent

Other research has investigated what specific behaviors women use to communicate their willingness to engage in sex. The most extensive of these is the previously described studies of Davis and colleagues.

As discussed earlier, the authors asked respondents to indicate whether they are less likely, equally likely, or more likely to perform specific behaviors when willing to have sex (than not willing): and to indicate whether they performed each behavior only when willing to have sex, versus sometimes or often when not willing (Davis et al., 1999; Wood & Davis, 2016, 2017). Three studies involved 48, 73, and 95 behaviors and the third included 28 behaviors specifically involving drugs or alcohol (Wood & Davis, 2017). The Davis et al., 1999 and Wood and Davis (2016) studies did not specify the relationship context of the behaviors, while the alcohol study specified behaviors either at a party with no date, with a person met that day, or with a date with whom they have not yet had sex.

The specifics of data for each behavior are beyond our ability to convey here. But there are several takeaways from this set of studies and the broader literature on the topic.

1. *No Behaviors Were Viewed by all Members of Either Gender as Either Probative or Definitive.* As noted earlier, one of the problems with interpreting sexual consent communications is that most behaviors have multiple meanings, and can be performed in circumstances other than those involving intentions to have sex. Reflecting this, no behavior in any of our stud-

ies was rated as either probative or definitive by all members of either gender. That is, of the behaviors asked about in this study there was not a single behavior that was universally agreed upon as being indicative of willingness to have intercourse. Even for such seemingly indicative behaviors as performing or receiving oral sex or taking off clothes, 30–40% of females indicated they performed the behaviors when not willing to have sex, and 40–65% of men indicated that women did so. Moreover, for these same behaviors, while the vast majority of each gender viewed them as probative, 3–4% of males and 3–15% of females did not. However, we did not ask about explicit verbal statements indicating consent.

2. *All Behaviors Were Reported and Viewed as More Probative than Definitive.* As with the above examples, the percent of males and females who self-reported or viewed the behaviors as probative was much higher than those who self-reported or viewed them as definitive. Generally, these differences were greater for males than for females. Males appear to be generally cautious in drawing definite inferences of sexual intent from women's behaviors, even though they do see them as cues predicting greater likelihood of sexual intentions.

   Generally, the results indicate that there are in fact multiple meanings and reasons for all behaviors, and circumstances in which they may be performed without sexual intent (as indicated by the fact that some females report that they perform the behavior in question when not willing to have sex). These are also perceived by observers, in that for both males and females reporting on the meaning of the behavior for women in general, some report that the behavior is performed when the woman is not willing to have sex.

3. *Some Behaviors Decried as Inappropriate Cues for Determination of Sexual Intentions Are Actually Probative for Women Generally, and Definitive for Many.* Many have suggested that much of the information about women's behaviors that has been presented in rape trials is irrelevant to whether sex was voluntary. Although assessment of these behaviors in their research was decontextualized with respect to relationship and other situational variables, the data from the Davis and colleagues studies indicate that many such behaviors are actually probative of sexual willingness. For example, Davis et al. (1999) found that two-thirds or more of women indicated that they were more likely to engage in behaviors such as wearing see-through fabric, wearing no bra or underpants, wearing a blouse or dress that shows cleavage, dressing very sexily or sexually provocatively, showing as much skin as possible, and others when willing to have intercourse than when not willing. For some of these behaviors more than half of women indicated that they perform the behavior only when willing to have sex. For others, such as dressing sexily, fewer than 20% did so.

   Notably, these authors also found that both number of previous sexual partners and self-rated sexual experience (also decried as inappropriate evidence) were predictive of self-reported likelihood of having sex with partners on first and later dates.

4. *Some Behaviors Were Actually, or Perceived as, Most Indicative of Sexual Intentions.* Behaviors considered most probative and most definitive by males and females alike mostly concerned preliminary sexual behaviors: such as taking off one's clothes, touching or allowing touch of intimate body parts (particularly bare), performing or receiving oral sex, making out without clothes, or doing nothing when the male attempts intercourse. Also high in these indices were signals of availability, such as wearing no underpants or bra, sexting naked pictures of oneself, or wearing sexy or provocative clothing (though clothing was rated as less indicative of sexual intentions in the 2016 studies than the 1999 study).

   These results are consistent with those of other studies assessing implications of behavior for sexual consent. For example, using a measure more akin to "definitiveness" a survey of a representative national random sample of 1023 college students or recent graduates conducted by the Washington Post and the Kaiser Family Foundation in 2015 found that 47% and 40% of participants agreed that a person taking off their own clothes or getting a condom establishes consent for more sexual activity. Fewer, 22% and 18%, agreed that engaging in foreplay such as kissing or touching and not saying "no" establishes consent for more sexual activity. In all cases more men felt these behaviors indicated consent than women. A number of studies have found similar results, indicating that college students tend to agree that consent to a number of activities, such as kissing or going home with a date, implies consent to other sexual acts (Jozkowski & Peterson, 2013).

Other behaviors often featured in rape trials entail the woman's willingness to be in circumstances that might put her at risk, such as going somewhere to be alone or voluntary impairment through drugs or alcohol. Alcohol and drug use was self-reported and viewed as probative by roughly two-thirds of both sexes, and as definitive by a quarter or more (Wood & Davis, 2017; see more detailed discussion of alcohol below). Such behaviors as going to his or her residence to be alone, leaving a party to be alone, or going into a bedroom were viewed as probative but as less definitive for males than self-reported for females.

Also featured in rape trials are behaviors reflecting the female's liking or interest in the man: such as sitting close, smiling a lot or laughing at his jokes, complimenting him frequently, or looking into his eyes. Such behaviors were generally self-reported and viewed as probative by half or more of participants, but were seen as definitive by 20% or less.

Finally, the topics of discussion by the female might be considered important. Talking about sexual topics was self-reported and rated as probative by 43% -75% across studies, and as definitive by 23% or less. Likewise, disclosing personal information or talking about intimate topics were self-reported and seen as probative by 40–79% of males and females (more so by males), but as definitive by 22% or fewer (less so by males).

In sum, most behaviors were seen as probative by at least a significant minority and often a large majority of males, and were actually probative for slightly lower proportions of females. In contrast, few behaviors were seen as definitive by a large majority of males or were actually definitive for the majority of females. Moreover, they were seen as less definitive by males than females reported for themselves. Overall, for most behaviors discussed here the results suggest it is reasonable for observers to use them as cues associated with sexual willingness, but unreasonable to conclude with certainty that they indicate consent.

5. *For Some Behaviors the Odds of Miscommunication of Sexual Consent are High.*

Despite research indicating general agreement between men and women on cues indicating consent, evidence indicates that some behaviors are more likely to be misconstrued than others. Davis and colleagues (1999; Wood & Davis, 2016, 2017) calculated a "rape seed" index based on their measure of the actual and perceived definitiveness of specific behaviors; The index consisted of the odds of pairing a man who believed the specific behavior definitively indicates sexual willingness (i.e., who believes women would engage in the behavior if, and only if, the women are willing to have intercourse) with a woman who sometimes or often performs the behavior when not willing. This was calculated by multiplying the proportion of women for whom the behavior was not definitive and the proportion of men who believed it was. By definition, couples are most likely to miscommunicate based on these behaviors when the rapeseed index is high. Some of the highest rapeseed values were obtained for alcohol or drug consumption under various circumstances (see section on alcohol below).

Behaviors that yielded rapeseed indices of 10% or higher in both studies (Davis et al., 1999; Wood & Davis, 2016) included those from each of the categories discussed above.

These included preliminary sexual behaviors such as undressing, letting him touch (or touching his) genitals, breasts, or thigh through clothes or bare, or making out with or without clothes; dressing sexily or provocatively; and talking about intimate or sexual topics. Ironically, performing or receiving oral sex, which one might naturally assume to clearly indicate consent for intercourse, yielded substantial rapeseed indices in both studies (0.18; 0.17 for receiving and 0.19, 0.16 for performing). Whereas these behaviors are seen as highly probative and often definitive by men, many women indicate participation in these activities when they are not willing to have intercourse (40% and 38% for performing oral sex; and 33% and 33% for receiving oral sex). This is likely one among other sexual behaviors that women might do *instead* of intercourse that might be interpreted as consent for intercourse.

Overall, 31 of 95 behaviors from the Wood and Davis (2016) study and 34 of 73 behaviors from the Davis and colleagues study (1999) yielded rapeseed indices greater than 10%. Some ranged over 20%. While these numbers may seem small, they indicate that there are many behaviors for which 10% to 27% of couples (or as many as roughly 1 in four) will include a male who believes the behavior equals consent and the female may do it whether she consents to sex or not.

Alcohol is Special. Alcohol use has been of considerable interest to sexuality researchers for a variety of reasons. For sexual assault researchers it has been of particular interest due to the pervasive involvement of alcohol use by one or both parties involved in cases of disputed sexual assault (Abbey, 2002; Muehlenhard et al., 2016). In most cases the consumption of alcohol or other intoxicants is voluntary and not forced. Though researchers have addressed a wide variety of issues concerning effects of alcohol on sexual encounters (e.g., George & Stoner, 2000), the issue of alcohol's effects regarding consent is arguably most relevant to litigation of sexual assault claims, in that many laws and policies explicitly state that someone who is incapacitated by alcohol or drugs cannot give consent. These laws create difficulties in application, however (see Davis & Loftus, 2004, 2016). For example, there is no clear metric to judge whether someone is too incapacitated to give consent (e.g., number of drinks, BAC, behaviors indicative of intoxication). Further, it is unclear what metric should be used to determine if the alleged perpetrator should have known that the complainant was incapacitated. In addition to the logistical challenges of determining if someone is too intoxicated to consent, most relevant to our current discussion is the issue of how alcohol relates to actual sexual willingness versus how alcohol use is interpreted to reflect sexual willingness.

Davis and Loftus (2004) argued that there are many inconsistencies between the law and psychology of voluntary intoxication and sexual intent. They presented evidence that alcohol use (1) enhances subjective arousal/enjoyment of sex, (2) is often used for the specific purpose of enhancing sexual pleasure or reducing inhibitions, (3) makes it more difficult to suppress sexual arousal, and (4) promotes interest in erotica. Additionally, men and women (5) expect to become aroused when using alcohol (and relatedly use alcohol to promote sexual interest in potential partners), (6) perceive others who consume alcohol as more sexually aroused, willing to consent, and easy to seduce, (7) are slower to recognize nonconsent if the woman is intoxicated, (8) deliberately use alcohol to avoid responsibility for undesirable sexual behaviors (another reflection of the expectation that alcohol promotes sexual interest), and (9) are actually more likely to engage in voluntary sexual activities. Moreover, Davis and Loftus reviewed substantial research literature indicating that alleged victims who were intoxicated are perceived as less credible (see also Livingston, Rerick, & Davis, this volume). Finally, Davis and Loftus (2004) reviewed evidence of widespread awareness of the link between alcohol use and sexual assault, awareness that has only increased among college students as sexual assault prevention programs and other educational programs have emphasized the link.

Davis & Loftus argued that the widespread use of alcohol to promote sexual interest and enjoyment suggests that women's choice to use alcohol when with men or a specific man is actually probative of sexual intentions: that is, that women are more likely to use alcohol around men when willing to have sex. More generally, they argued that legal attempts to suppress alcohol use in sexual contexts directly contradicts widespread behavioral tendencies; and attempts to reverse judgments that intoxicated women are more likely to have consented to conform to the law that intoxicated women cannot consent will be difficult, at the least.

The previously referenced study by Wood and Davis (2017) indicated both that women are more likely to use alcohol in a variety of contexts when willing to have sex, *and* that both men and women believe this. At the same time, this study revealed stronger and more dangerous discrepancies between women's actual intentions and men's perceptions of them.

The authors asked respondents to rate 30 behaviors, of which 24 involved the use of alcohol or drugs. They also included combined behaviors or situations, such as leaving a party with a man met that day while intoxicated or spending the night with a date one has not yet had sex with while severely (moderately, or not intoxicated), and others.

For women, some of the behaviors involving alcohol that were the most probative and definitive of sexual intent were becoming moderately intoxicated in a private location with a date she has not yet had sex with (54% and 23% probative and definitive respectively) and becoming moderately intoxicated at a party with a date she has not yet had sex with (35% and 10%). A number of other behaviors coupled with being intoxicated produced even higher probative and definitive values reported by women. For example, 67% and 31% of women surveyed indicated that being moderately to severely intoxicated and touching a date she has not yet had sex with under his clothes was probative and definitive of their sexual intent. 58% and 32% of women reported that being moderately to severely intoxicated and leaving a party to spend the night with a person they just met that day was probative and definitive of their sexual intent. Thus, the majority of women indicated they were actually more likely to perform many behaviors involving alcohol when willing to have intercourse, and substantial minority engaged in such behaviors *only* when willing. This pattern was accurately perceived by others.

Across 24 behaviors involving intoxication, the majority of both men (56.6%) and women reporting perceptions of women in general (56.3%) believed the behaviors to be more likely among sexually willing women: and a substantial minority of women (41.3%) reported that this was actually true for them.

Across behaviors involving intoxication, the percent of respondents who indicated the behaviors were definitive were also higher for men (27.3%) and women answering about women in general (26.9%) than for women answering about themselves (16.3%). Notably, both perceived probativeness and perceived definitiveness of alcohol-related behaviors were significantly higher than the actual probativeness or definitiveness reported by women for themselves. This stands in stark contrast to the previous two studies in which perceived probativeness differed slightly between men and women, but men viewed the behaviors as *less*, rather than more definitive than women. The general willingness of men (and women judging other women's behavior rather than their own) to view intoxication itself as indicative of sexual availability (in this study and others) suggests significant potential for juries to ignore laws regarding intoxication and consent in favor of their own intuitive assumptions.

Perhaps most disturbingly, larger rapeseed values were obtained for several behaviors involving alcohol than for any other types of behaviors across the three studies, and overall the average rapeseed values were higher than for the previous studies. The largest rapeseed values were obtained for behaviors such as getting intoxicated in a private location with a person she just met that day (0.323) or with a date (0.303), when severely intoxicated leaving a party with a person she just met (0.282), and getting severely intoxicated at a party when she doesn't have a date with her (0.221). These values indicate that as many as roughly a third of randomly paired couples will consist of a woman who may become intoxicated with no sexual intentions with a man who believes that intoxication definitively indicates consent, perhaps explaining in part the substantial proportion of sexual assaults involving alcohol.

Conclusions

Our review has shown that while men and women tend to communicate and interpret sexual intentions similarly, based on comparable cues, it has also shown there are some behaviors that are particularly prone to misinterpretation by male and female observers. It is important for future research to continue to identify which specific behaviors are most subject to misinterpretation, and to begin to incorporate relevant training into sexual assault prevention and other relevant educational programs.

The research reviewed in this chapter also indicates a disconnect between law and social policy and the actual ways in which participants describe communicating and interpreting consent (see also Beres, 2014). This was shown clearly with respect to affirmative consent policies, for example. Policies requiring that consent be communicated explicitly and verbally are inconsistent with sexual norms and scripts, and the pervasive tendency to communicate sexual intentions indirectly and nonverbally. Although requiring affirmative consent might be popular from a policy standpoint, there is strong evidence that it is not the way the majority of young people communicate and interpret consent in practice. This does not mean that affirmative consent cannot be a healthy and productive way to negotiate sexual encounters but simply indicates that changing laws or policies is not enough to change engrained sexual norms (e.g., Humphreys & Herold, 2003).

As did Davis and Loftus in 2004, we also highlighted inconsistencies between the law and psychology of voluntary intoxication and sexual intentions. We began the process of exploring the actual implications of women's alcohol use for sexual willingness, as well as further developed how use of alcohol in various circumstances is perceived. But while much research has indicated that intoxicated women are viewed as more sexually willing and are judged as more culpable in sexual assault scenarios, much less is known about the actual relationship between women's choices to use alcohol and sexual intentions. This is an area that can benefit from much future research. We also know little about the circumstances in which alcohol use is viewed as most linked to sexual intentions, most inappropriate, or both; and the implications of these factors for judgments of sexual assault claims.

Perhaps our most glaring lack of coverage, as well as that of the general empirical literature on sexual consent, concerns the context of sexual consent interactions. In part, this concerns how *combinations* of various consent behaviors are related to actual and perceived consent. Most research reported here asked respondents to rate the significance of individual behaviors for consent, though Wood and Davis (2017) did include some combinations of behaviors. Overall, we currently have very little evidence regarding sets of behaviors.

This lack also concerns other contextual issues, such as the relationship context of behaviors (new versus existing, prior sex versus not, power imbalances, and so on), as well as situational contexts (such as public settings versus private).

Some research has addressed relationship contexts, as does the law. Some formal definitions of consent specify that the existence of a dating relationship or past sexual encounters does not indicate consent (e.g., California SB

967). Currently, a minority of states include language in their sexual consent statutes denouncing relationship history as establishing consent. For example, Minnesota's sexual assault statute asserts that "[c]onsent does not mean the existence of a prior or current social relationship between the actor and the complainant" (Minn. Stat. § 609.341(4)(a)). Whereas other states, such as California, limit the language to dating or marital relationships in maligning history as equating to consent, Minnesota's statute moves further by precluding *any* social relationship as justification or proxy for consent.

Nevertheless, though not yet well developed, there is some social science literature addressing how consent is negotiated or viewed in different relationship contexts. For example, Humphreys (2007) found that the more intense and involved a relationship became, the more sexual activity was expected by perceivers, and the less explicit consent was required by perceivers. This difference emerged for couples presented as dating for a mere 3 months, despite only having a few sexual encounters during that time period. In nearly every situation, a newer relationship necessitated explicit sexual consent more often than a seasoned relationship (Humphreys, 2007). Consent is more likely to be communicated the first time partners have sex but is less likely to be communicated in subsequent sexual encounters (Humphreys & Herold, 2007).

Research has also identified differences between relationship types in how consent scenarios are viewed. For example, individuals are more likely to support rape myths when the assailant is the victim's husband (Ferro, Cermele, & Saltzman, 2008). Additionally, the exact same scenarios were less likely to be labeled rape by participants when the length of the relationship in the scenarios increased (Humphreys, 2007). In essence, relationship history yields consequences for issues of consent (Rebeiz & Harb, 2010; see Livingston et al., this volume for review of relationship effects on rape perceptions).

Research on such issues is thus far rare, however, and given that the law has deemed relationship context to be irrelevant in some respects, it is important to test this assumption. Most research to date has investigated two issues: whether consent is communicated at all in various stages of the relationship, and how consent is judged by observers in different relationship types (see Livingston, Rerick & Davis, this volume on this issue). But we could not locate studies investigating *how* consent tends to be conveyed and interpreted by participants in different relationship contexts: or how observers interpret specific consent-related behaviors differently in different relationship contexts (with the exception of Wood & Davis, 2017: where this was not the main focus). We hope future researchers will tackle these issues in more depth. The import of relationship specific consent communication patterns may, like alcohol, be yet another area in which the law is inconsistent with patterns of behavior and judgment.

Another area in need of more research is that of the impact of power dynamics on consent communication and interpretation. Definitions of consent often specify that consent to participate in a sexual act must be freely given and willing (e.g., Hickman & Muehlenhard, 1999). Yet, in certain power-imbalanced relationships, consent is impossible due to the coercive implications or potential retaliatory ramifications for rejecting the sexual advances of a person in a higher status position. In many states, disparate power or positional authority are assumed to make it impossible to give consent. In Montana, the victim of a sexual assault is incapable of providing consent if the victim is incarcerated in a correctional facility, receiving services from a youth care facility, or admitted to a mental health facility, and the assailant is an employee, contractor, or volunteer in any of those domains (45-5-501, MCA). This is standard language for most state statutes. However, numerous additional relationships contain inherent power imbalances, such as professor–student, employer–employee, coach–athlete, clergyman–parishioner, etc.

With such intrinsic imbalances, it would appear logical to address issues of consent both legally and psychologically. However, most state statutes do not address such relationships, and social science research in this sphere is sparse. Singling out the professor–student relationship, research has found that faculty members and students alike perceive a professor to be acting unethically by engaging in sexual activity with a student, but consent was not considered a relevant factor (Paludi, 1996). Thus, though power and authority differentials distinctly shape perceptions of sexual activity, more attention is required by legal and social pundits to parse out the implications for sexual consent. Research is needed to address the same issues that have been the focus of this chapter: How is consent communicated and perceived by those inside the relationship? and How is consent to sexual interactions in these various contexts judged by observers?

Other important issues were also left unaddressed. For example, we barely touched on individual differences in communication and interpretation of consent: and evidence exists regarding such issues. Incorrectly judging signals of sexual interest seems to be related to a history of sexual coercion, for example (Farris, Viken, Treat, & McFall, 2006). And, other individual differences in the tendency to overperceive sexual intentions have been identified (for review, see Wegner & Abbey, 2016).

In sum, though we have learned a great deal about consent communications and sources of misunderstanding, much remains to be done: particularly regarding the more complicated issues of how behaviors combine to indicate consent; how consent is communicated and judged in various kinds of relationship contexts; as well as with more diverse participants (such as the mentally impaired and LGBTQ individuals). Such research can and should inform both social policy and the law.

Research findings on sexual consent communications could profitably be more fully incorporated into sexual assault education programs. Though such programs commonly include discussion of consent statutes and campus regulations, including implications of alcohol use, little detail is typically offered regarding the specific landmines of consent communications. That is, little information covered in this chapter is commonly included. Given that significant potential for misunderstanding of sexual intentions exists, and that this is particularly true for some behaviors, discussion of these issues might encourage greater conservatism in reading sexual intentions into behaviors; and perhaps encourage use of more explicit verbal communications that are less likely to be misinterpreted. Some encouragement in this regard was provided by Treat et al. (2017), who showed that explicit instruction regarding the meaning of female cues led participants to focus more on appropriate versus inappropriate cues of consent. Moreover, even though rape-supportive attitudes were associated with greater deficits in understanding cues of consent, instruction improved judgments of those high and low in such attitudes.

References

34 C.F.R. (2018). § 668.46.

18 U.S.C. (2018). § 2242.

10 U.S.C. (2018). § 920.

18 U.S.C. (2018). § 2241.

Abbey, A. (1991). Misperception as an antecedent of acquaintance rape: A consequence of ambiguity in communication between men and women. In A. Parrot & L. Bechhofer (Eds.), *Acquaintance rape: The hidden crime* (pp. 96–111). New York: John Wiley.

Abbey, A. (2002). Alcohol-related sexual assault: A common problem among college students. *Journal of Studies on Alcohol, 14*(Suppl. 14), 118–128. https://doi.org/10.15288/jsas.2002.s14.118

Abbey, A. (2011). Alcohol's role in sexual violence perpetration: Theoretical explanations, existing evidence and future directions. *Drug and Alcohol Review, 30*, 481–489. https://doi.org/10.1111/j.1465-3362.2011.00296.x

Abbey, A., Buck, P. O., Zawacki, T., & Saenz, C. (2003). Alcohol's effects on perceptions of a potential date rape. *Journal of Studies on Alcohol, 64*, 669–677. https://doi.org/10.15288/jsa.2003.64.669

Abbey, A., McAuslan, P., & Ross, L. T. (1998). Sexual assault perpetration by college men: The role of alcohol, misperception of sexual intent, and sexual beliefs and experiences. *Journal of Social and Clinical Psychology, 17*(2), 167–195. https://doi.org/10.1521/jscp.1998.17.2.167

Abbey, A., Zawacki, T., & Buck, P. O. (2005). The effects of past sexual assault perpetration and alcohol consumption on men's reactions to mixed signals. *Journal of Social and Clinical Psychology, 25*, 129–155. https://doi.org/10.1521/jscp.24.2.129.62273

Abbey, A., Zawacki, T., & McAuslan, P. (2000). Alcohol's effects on sexual perception. *Journal of Studies on Alcohol and Drugs, 61*, 688–697. https://doi.org/10.15288/jsa.2000.61.688

Benbouriche, M., Teste, B., Guay, J.-P., & Lavole, M. E. (2018). The role of rape-supportive attitudes, alcohol, and sexual arousal in sexual misperception: An experimental study. *Journal of Sex Research, 56*(6), 766–777. https://doi.org/10.1080/00224499.2018.1496221

Beres, M. A. (2007). "Spontaneous" sexual consent: An analysis of sexual consent literature. *Feminism and Psychology, 17*, 93–108. https://doi.org/10.1177/0959353507072914

Beres, M. A. (2010). Sexual miscommunication? Untangling assumptions about sexual communication between casual sex partners. *Culture, Health, and Sexuality, 12*, 1–14. https://doi.org/10.1080/13691050903075226

Beres, M. A. (2014). Rethinking the concept of consent for anti-sexual violence activism and education. *Feminism and Psychology, 24*, 373–389. https://doi.org/10.1177/0959353514539652

Beres, M. A., Herold, E., & Maitland, S. B. (2004). Sexual consent behaviors in same-sex relationships. *Archives of Sexual Behavior, 33*, 475–486. https://doi.org/10.1023/B:ASEB.0000037428.41757.10

Block, M. (2004). Consent. In M. D. Smith (Ed.), *Encyclopedia of rape* (pp. 51–52). Westport, CT: Greenwood Press.

Bouffard, J. A., & Miller, H. A. (2014). The role of sexual arousal and overperception of sexual intent within the decision to engage in sexual coercion. *Journal of Interpersonal Violence, 29*(11), 1967–1986. https://doi.org/10.1177/0886260513515950

Burkett, M., & Hamilton, K. (2012). Postfeminist sexual agency: Young women's negotiations of sexual consent. *Sexualities, 15*, 815–833. https://doi.org/10.1177/1363460712454076

Byers, E. S. (1980). Female communication of consent and nonconsent to sexual intercourse. *Journal of the New Brunswick Psychological Association, 5*, 12–18.

Cal. Educ. Code. (2015). § 67386.

Davis, D., Follette, W. C., & Merlino, M. L. (1999). Seeds of rape: Female behavior is probative for females, definitive for males. In *Psychological expertise and criminal justice* (pp. 101–140). Washington, DC: American Psychological Association.

Davis, D., & Loftus, E. F. (2004). What's good for the goose cooks the gander: Inconsistencies between the law and psychology of voluntary intoxication and sexual assault. In W. T. O'Donohue & E. Levensky (Eds.), *Handbook of forensic psychology* (pp. 997–1032). New York: Elsevier Academic Press.

Davis, D., & Loftus, E. F. (2016). Remembering disputed sexual encounters: A new frontier for witness memory research. *Journal of Criminal Law and Criminology (Invited Contribution), 105*(4), 811–851.

Davis, D., & Villalobos, J. G. (2014). Language and the law: Illustrations from cases of disputed sexual consent. In T. Holtgraves (Ed.), *Handbook of Language and Social Psychology*. Oxford: Oxford University Press.

Davis, K. C., Schraufnagel, T. J., Jacques-Tiura, A. J., Norris, J., George, W. H., & Kiekel, P. A. (2012). Childhood sexual abuse and acute alcohol effects on men's sexual aggression intentions. *Psychology of Violence, 2*, 179–193. https://doi.org/10.1037/a0027185

DeMatteo, D., Galloway, M., Arnold, S., & Patel, U. (2015). Sexual assault on college campuses: A 50-state survey of criminal sexual assault statutes and their relevance to campus sexual assault. *Psychology, Public Policy, and Law, 21*(3), 227–238.

Engeler, I., & Raghubir, P. (2018). Decomposing the cross-sex misprediction bias of dating behaviors: Do men overestimate or women underreport their sexual intentions? *Journal of Personality and Social Psychology, 114*, 95–100. https://doi.org/10.1037/pspi0000105

Fantasia, H. C. (2011). Really not even a decision any more: Late adolescent narratives of implied sexual consent. *Journal of Forensic Nursing, 7*, 120–129.

Farris, C., Treat, T. A., & Viken, R. J. (2010). Alcohol alters men's perceptual and decisional processing of women's sexual interest. *Journal of Abnormal Psychology, 119*(2), 427–432. https://doi.org/10.1037/a0019343

Farris, C., Treat, T. A., Viken, R. J., & McFall, R. M. (2008). Sexual coercion and the misperception of sexual intent. *Clinical Psychology Review, 28*, 48–66. https://doi.org/10.1016/j.cpr.2007.03.002

Farris, C., Viken, R. J., Treat, T. A., & McFall, R. M. (2006). Heterosocial perceptual organization: Application of the choice model to sexual coercion. *Psychological Science, 17*, 861–875. http://dx.doi.org.unr.idm.oclc.org/10.1111/j.1467-9280.2006.01796.x

Ferro, C., Cermele, J., & Saltzman, A. (2008). Current perceptions of marital rape: Some good and not-so-good news. *Journal of Interpersonal Violence, 23*(6), 764–779. https://doi.org/10.1177/0886260507313947

Fisher, T. D., & Walters, A. S. (2003). Variables in addition to gender that help to explain differences in perceived sexual interest. *Psychology of Men and Masculinity, 4*, 154–162.

Fla. Stat. (2017). § 794.011.

George, W. H., Cue, K. L., Lopez, P. A., Crowe, L. C., & Norris, J. (1995). Self-reported alcohol expectancies and postdrinking sexual inferences about women. *Journal of Applied Social Psychology, 25*, 164–186. https://doi.org/10.1111/j.1559-1816.1995.tb01589.x

George, W. H., & Stoner, S. A. (2000). Understanding acute alcohol effects on sexual behavior. In J. R. Heiman & C. M. Davis (Eds.), *Annual review of sex research* (Vol. 11, pp. 92–124). Allentown, PA: The Society for the Scientific Study of Sexuality.

Greer, A. E., & Buss, D. M. (1994). Tactics for promoting sexual encounters. *Journal of Sex Research, 31*, 185–201.

Gross, A. M., Bennett, T., Sloan, L., Marx, B. P., & Juergens, J. (2001). The impact of alcohol and alcohol expectancies on male perception of female sexual arousal in a date rape analog. *Experimental and*

Clinical Psychopharmacology, 9, 380–388. https://doi.org/10.1037/1064-1297.9.4.380

Hall, D. S. (1998). Consent for sexual behavior in a college student population. *Electronic Journal of Human Sexuality, 1*. Retrieved from http://www.ejhs.org/volume1/consent1.htm

Haselton, M. G., & Buss, D. M. (2000). Error management theory: A new perspective on biases in cross-sex mind reading. *Journal of Personality and Social Psychology, 78*, 81–91. https://doi.org/10.1037/0022-3514.78.1.81

Henningsen, D., & Henningsen, M. (2010). Testing error management theory: Exploring the commitment skepticism bias and the sexual overperception bias. *Human Communication Research, 36*(4), 618–634. https://doi.org/10.1111/j.1468-2958.2010.01391.x

Hickman, S. E., & Muehlenhard, C. L. (1999). "By the semi-mystical appearance of a condom": How young women and men communicate sexual consent in heterosexual situations. *Journal of Sex Research, 36*, 258–272. https://doi.org/10.1080/00224499909551996

Howell, E. C., Etchells, P. J., & Penton-Voak, I. S. (2012). The sexual overperception bias is associated with sociosexuality. *Personality and Individual Differences, 53*, 1012–1016.

Humphreys, T. (2004). Understanding sexual consent: An empirical investigation of the normative script for young heterosexual adults. In M. Cowling & P. Reynolds (Eds.), *Making sense of sexual consent* (pp. 209–225). Burlington, VT: Ashgate.

Humphreys, T. (2007). Perceptions of sexual consent: The impact of relationship history and gender. *Journal of Sex Research, 44*(4), 307–315.

Humphreys, T., & Herold, E. (2003). Should universities and colleges mandate sexual behavior? Student perceptions of Antioch College's consent policy. *Journal of Psychology and Human Sexuality, 15*, 35–51. https://doi.org/10.1300/J056v15n01_04

Humphreys, T., & Herold, E. (2007). Sexual consent in heterosexual relationships: Development of a new measure. *Sex Roles, 57*, 305–315. https://doi.org/10.1007/s11199-007-9264-7

Johnson, J. D., Noel, N. E., & Sutter-Hernandez, J. (2000). Alcohol and male acceptance of sexual aggression: The role of perceptual ambiguity. *Journal of Applied Social Psychology, 30*, 1186–1200. https://doi.org/10.1111/j.1559-1816.2000.tb02516.x

Jordan, J. (2005). What Would MacGyver Do?: The meaning(s) of resistance and survival. *Violence Against Women, 11*(4), 531–559. https://doi.org/10.1177/1077801204273299

Jozkowski, K. N. (2011). *Measuring internal and external conceptualizations of sexual consent: A mixed-methods exploration of sexual consent.* Doctoral dissertation. Retrieved from ProQuest Dissertations and Theses database. (UMI No. 3466353).

Jozkowski, K. N. (2013). The influence of consent on college students' perceptions of the quality of sexual intercourse at last event. *International Journal of Sexual Health, 25*, 260–272. https://doi.org/10.1080/19317611.2013.799626

Jozkowski, K. N., & Hunt, M. (2014). "Who wants a quitter? … So you just keep trying": How college students' perceptions of sex ual consent privilege men. Paper presented at the Annual Meeting of the Society for the Scientific Study of Sexuality, Omaha, NE

Jozkowski, K. N., & Peterson, Z. D. (2013). College students and sexual consent: Unique insights. *Journal of Sex Research, 50*, 517–523. https://doi.org/10.1080/00224499.2012.700739

Jozkowski, K. N., Peterson, Z. D., Sanders, S. A., Dennis, B., & Reece, M. (2014). Gender differences in heterosexual college students' conceptualizations and indicators of sexual consent: Implications for contemporary sexual assault prevention education. *Journal of Sex Research, 51*, 904–916. https://doi.org/10.1080/00224499.2013.792326

Jozkowski, K. N., Sanders, S., Peterson, Z. D., Dennis, B., & Reece, M. (2014). Consenting to sexual activity: The development and psychometric assessment of dual measures of consent. *Archives of Sexual Behavior, 43*, 437–450. https://doi.org/10.1007/s10508-013-0225-7

Jozkowski, K. N., & Wiersma, J. D. (2015). Does drinking alcohol prior to sexual activity influence college students' consent? *International Journal of Sexual Health, 27*, 156–174. https://doi.org/10.1080/19317611.2014.951505

Lee, J. J., & Pinker, S. (2010). Rationales for indirect speech: The theory of the strategic speaker. *Psychological Review, 117*, 785–807.

Lim, G. Y., & Roloff, M. E. (1999). Attributing sexual consent. *Journal of Applied Communication Research, 27*, 1–23.

Lindren, K. P., Parkhill, M. R., George, W. H., & Hendershot, C. S. (2008). Gender differences in perceptions of sexual intent: a qualitative review and integration. *Psychology of Women Qarterly, 32*, 423–439.

Livingston, T. N., Rerick, P. O., & Davis, D. (2018, March). *Sexual arousal predicts men's perceptions of women's sexual intent.* Poster presented at the annual meeting of the American Psychology-Law Society, Memphis, TN.

Marcantonio, T. L., Jozkowski, K. N., & Lo, W.-J. (2018). Beyond "just saying no": A preliminary evaluation of strategies college students use to refuse sexual activity. *Archives of Sexual Behavior, 47*, 341–351. https://doi.org/10.1007/s10508-017-1130-2

Marx, B. P., Gross, A. M., & Adams, H. E. (1999). The effect of alcohol on the responses of sexually coercive and noncoercive men to an experimental rape analogue. *Sexual Abuse: A Journal of Research and Treatment, 11*, 131–145. https://doi.org/10.1007/BF02658843

Marx, B. P., Gross, A. M., & Juergens, J. P. (1997). The effects of alcohol consumption and expectancies in an experimental date rape analogue. *Journal of Psychopathology and Behavioral Assessment, 19*, 281–302. https://doi.org/10.1007/BF02229022

Me. Rev. Stat. Ann. (2017). tit 17-A, § 253.

Muehlenhard, C. L. (2011). Examining stereotypes about token resistance to sex. *Psychology of Women Quarterly, 35*, 676–683.

Muehlenhard, C. L., & Hollabaugh, L. C. (1988). So women sometimes say no when they mean yes? The prevalence and correlates of women's token resistance to sex. *Journal of Personality and Social Psychology, 54*, 872–879.

Muehlenhard, C. L., Humphreys, T. P., Jozkowski, K. N., & Peterson, Z. D. (2016). The complexities of sexual consent among college students: A conceptual and empirical review. *The Journal of Sex Research, 53*(4–5), 457–487. https://doi.org/10.1080/00224499.2016.1146651

Muehlenhard, C. L., & Rogers, C. S. (1998). Token resistance to sex: New perspectives on an old stereotype. *Psychology of Women Quarterly, 33*, 443–463.

Murray, D. R., Murphy, S. C., von Hippel, W., Trivers, R., & Haselton, M. G. (2017). A preregistered study of competing predictions suggests that men do overestimate women's sexual intent. *Psychological Science, 28*, 253–255. https://doi.org/10.1177/0956797616675474

N.J. Stat. Ann. (2012) § 2C:14–1.

N.J. Stat. Ann. (2014). § 2C:14–2.

N.Y. Educ. Law (2015). § 6441.

Norris, J., & Kerr, K. L. (1993). Alcohol and violent pornography: Responses to permissive and nonpermissive cues. *Journal of Studies on Alcohol*, (11), 118–127. https://doi.org/10.15288/jsas.1993.s11.118

O'Sullivan, L. F., & Byers, E. (1992). College students' incorporation of initiator and restrictor roles in sexual dating interactions. *Journal of Sex Research, 29*, 435–446.

Paludi, M. A. (1996). *Sexual Harassment on College Campuses : Abusing the Ivory Power*. Albany, NY: State University of New York Press.

Perilloux, C., & Kurzban, R. (2014). Do men overperceive women's sexual interest? *Psychological Science, 26*, 70–77. https://doi.org/10.1177/0956797614555727

Rebeiz, M. J., & Harb, C. (2010). Perceptions of rape and attitudes toward women in a sample of Lebanese students. *Journal of Interpersonal Violence, 25*, 735–752. https://doi.org/10.1177/0886260509334410

Perper, T., & Weis, D. L. (1987). Proceptive and rejective strategies of U. S. and Canadian college women. *Journal of Sex Research, 23*, 455–480.

Rerick, P. O., Livingston, T. N., & Davis, D. (in press). Rape and the jury. In W. O. O'Donohue & P. Schewe (Eds.), *Handbook of sexual assault and sexual assault prevention*. New York, NY: Springer.

Rerick, P. O., Livingston, T. N.,& Davis, D. (2019, March). *The effect of men's sexual arousal on perceptions of women's sexual willingness*. Paper presented at the annual meeting of the American Psychology-Law Society, Portland, OR.

S.B. 967, 2014 Cal. Leg., 2013-2014 Reg. Sess. (Cal. 2014).

Sprecher, S., Hatfield, E., Cortese, A., Potapova, E., & Levitskaya, A. (1994). Token resistance to sexual intercourse and consent to unwanted intercourse: College students' dating experiences in three countries. *Journal of Sex Research, 31*, 125–132.

Starfelt, L. C., Young, R., Palk, G., & White, K. M. (2015). A qualitative exploration of young Australian adults' understandings of and explanations for alcohol-involved rape. *Psychiatry, Psychology and Law, 22*, 337–354. https://doi.org/10.1080/13218719.2014.945639

Steele, C. M., & Josephs, R. A. (1990). Alcohol myopia: Its prized and dangerous effects. *American Psychologist, 45*, 921–933. https://doi.org/10.1037/0003-066X.45.8.921

Stephan, W., Berscheid, E., & Walster, E. (1971). Sexual arousal and heterosexual perception. *Journal of Personality and Social Psychology, 20*, 93–101. https://doi.org/10.1037/h0031943

Treat, T. A., Church, E. K., & Viken, R. J. (2017). Effects of gender, rape-supportive attitudes, and explicit instruction on perceptions of women's momentary sexual interest. *Psychonomic Bulletin & Review, 24*, 979–986. https://doi.org/10.3758/s13423-016-1176-5

Villalobos, J. G., Davis, D., & Leo, R. A. (2016). His story, her story: Sexual miscommunication, motivated remembering, and intoxication as pathways to honest false testimony regarding sexual consent. In R. Burnett (Ed.), *Vilified: Wrongful allegations of person abuse*. Oxford: Oxford University Press.

Wang, V., & Weinstock, C. (2018). Yale Student Found Not Guilty in Rape Trial, *New York Times*.

Wegner, R., & Abbey, A. (2016). Individual differences in men's misperception of women's sexual intent: Application and extension of the confluence model. *Personality and Individual Differences, 94*, 16–20. https://doi.org/10.1016/j.paid.2015.12.027

Wertheimer, A. (2003). *Consent to sexual relations*. Cambridge: Cambridge University Press.

West, R. (2008). Sex, law, and consent. In A. Wertheimer & W. Miller (Eds.), *The ethics of consent: Theory and practice*. Retrieved from http://scholarship.law.georgetown.edu/cgi/viewcontent.cgi?article=1073&context=fwps_papers

Wiederman, M. W. (2005). The gendered nature of sexual scripts. *Family Journal, 13*, 496–502. https://doi.org/10.1177/1066480705278729

Wis. Stat. (2018). § 940.225.

Wood, E. F, & Davis, D. (2016). Perceived and actual probative and definitive value of sexual behaviors in college students: Which behaviors have most potential for miscommunication? *Society for Personality and Social Psychology*. (January).

Wood, E. F., & Davis, D. (2017). Perceived versus actual links between intoxication and sexual availability. *American Psychology Law Society*. (March).

Yale Sexual Misconduct Policies and Related Definitions. (2018). Retrieved from https://smr.yale.edu/find-policies-information/yale-sexual-misconduct-policies-and-related-definitions

History and Theoretical Understanding of Bystander Intervention

25

Laurel Mazar

Introduction

Bystander intervention is a broad phrase used to describe the action (or lack of) in an emergency when the bystander is not initially involved. Bystander intervention is encouraged as a prevention tool for health complications (helping if someone has a heart attack), bullying, sexual and interpersonal violence, drunk driving (friends don't let friends drive drunk), and terrorism on transit (if you see something, say something). Interventions can include doing nothing, involving someone else (police, bartender, friends, other bystanders), or getting physically involved (administering CPR, stepping in between people fighting). Over the last couple of decades, bystander intervention training has been used as a tool for preventing sexual violence. This chapter briefly addresses prevention efforts that have paved the way for bystander intervention, discusses the efficacy and limitations of bystander intervention, and gives recommendations for moving bystander intervention training programs forward.

L. Mazar (✉)
Criminology, Law and Justice,
University of Illinois at Chicago, Chicago, IL, USA
e-mail: lmazar2@uic.edu

How Did We Get Here?

Rape prevention has a history that spans decades and some programs have been more successful than others. This section briefly examines prevention efforts that have led the field towards bystander intervention. While their research was not specific to sexual violence prevention, it is important to discuss the origins of the theory of bystander intervention. Latane and Darley (1970) were the first researchers to examine bystanders. Their research was prompted by the violent homicide of Kitty Genovese. Kitty was stabbed multiple times in the courtyard of her apartment building in Brooklyn and it took a half hour for her assailant to kill her. Multiple neighbors watched the incident unfold and none of them acted to help. Kitty Genovese's murder was one of several similar stories preceding work by Latane and Darley which piqued their curiosity for why people witnessing a person in an emergency do not intervene to help. They offer a theoretical model for why people intervene or not. There are five different cognitive elements a bystander passes through when deciding whether to intervene. These elements are: noticing a victim or situation, interpreting the situation as an emergency, assuming responsibility to help, having knowledge on how to help in that situation, and then acting to help (Latane & Darley, 1970).

W. T. O'Donohue and P. A. Schewe (eds.), *Handbook of Sexual Assault and Sexual Assault Prevention*,
https://doi.org/10.1007/978-3-030-23645-8_25

One theme among many prevention efforts is altering people's social norms. One way to alter these norms is by examining attitudes and beliefs and then providing education and examples as to why some of these attitudes and beliefs are problematic and contribute to the norms that allow sexual violence to continue.

As men are overwhelmingly the perpetrators of sexual violence, logic suggests the power lies within them to stop engaging in this violence. One way in which prevention has targeted men is by addressing the peer level of the social-ecology. College men tend to care a great deal about what their peers think, so changing values and norms of peers may lead to behavior change among men (Fabiano et al., 2003; Schwartz, DeKeseredy, Tait, & Alvi, 2001). Some prevention programs encourage men to address their peers' language (Barone et al., 2007; McMahon, 2010). In a program called *The Men's Project*, men engaged with each other by dissecting gender roles and examining sexist language and rape myths in culture. *The Men's Project* is a program which uses the ecological model by identifying and addressing risk factors at all four levels of the social-ecology. At the individual level, *The Men's Project* dealt with rape myths and facts; the peer level taught men how to support a survivor and bystander intervention techniques; the community level looked at supportive environments; and the society level discussed privilege, gender socialization, identity intersection, and politics of oppression (Barone et al., 2007). *The Men's Project* is conducted in 2-hour sessions over 10 weeks.

Barone et al. (2007) conducted focus groups to evaluate the program's impact. Men reported observing change in peer behavior after challenging their sexist language. The men who were involved came to recognize how sexism and gender roles are very much ingrained in society. However, through speaking up (when they felt comfortable to do so), they noticed their peers began to change the language they used when describing women (Barone et al., 2007). The men who participated in this group were able to demonstrate that others' behaviors can be changed through peer influence. They recognized the importance of their role in changing attitudes which led to behavioral change.

Fabiano et al. (2003) suggest that changing culture is an enormous task as "patriarchy and hypermasculine gender roles are deeply ingrained in individuals, families, social customs, laws, institutions…virtually every facet of living" (p. 106). They suggest utilizing a social norms approach as this has found some success in reducing college drinking, which they argue is another culturally entrenched phenomenon. They were interested in discovering how students' actual norms compared with perceived norms about consent and bystander intervention. They found men's perceived norms did not match with men's actual norms regarding sexual behavior and encouraged prevention experts to engage in social norms approaches. By getting men's perceived norms in closer alignment with actual norms, Fabiano et al. argue more men will become involved as social justice allies.

Piccigallo, Lilley, and Miller (2012) conducted in-depth interviews with men who were involved in an all-male rape prevention campus group. Interested in the pathways by which these men came to be involved with these groups, the researchers conducted interviews to understand the decisions behind joining these groups. One of the main findings was most of the men had a personal connection to the issue of sexual violence against women which led to their group membership (Piccigallo et al., 2012). However, as argued by these authors, researchers and program creators must find a way to garner men's interest in the issue without an established personal connection to it: the more men with personal connections to the issue means there is more sexual violence occurring to the women in these men's lives.

Changing values towards safety and respect and engaging men in this change is an essential step in decreasing campus sexual assault (Fabiano et al., 2003). Gidycz, Orchowski, and Berkowitz (2011) conducted an evaluation of a program which combined bystander intervention approaches with social norms approaches. Follow-ups were conducted 4 months and 7 months after the program ended. They found men were less likely to intervene against sexually aggressive peers if they believed there was an absence of support from their friends. Similar to Fabiano et al. (2003), these researchers argued for a large-scale change of campus community norms. They state: "it may be necessary for the campus culture to provide continuous reinforcement of prosocial norms" (Gidycz et al., 2011, p. 735). If the campus culture values prosocial norms, males who are a part of this culture will value these norms, and peers will feel supported in situations which require intervention.

Providing education to increase knowledge about sexual violence, encouraging people to recognize the role their attitudes and beliefs play in perpetuating sexual violence, and making sexual violence *everyone's* issue all contributed to the development and use of bystander intervention as a sexual violence prevention tool.

Where Are We Now?

The Bystander Decision-Making Process

Bystander intervention encourages people to be prosocial and prevent a negative event from happening. These events can range from harassment, crude jokes, threats of violence, and acts of violence. Despite whether someone intervenes, they are making a choice. There are three main categories of choices in bystander intervention; being a prosocial bystander, intervening in a further negative way, or choosing not to act. Beginning to seek out answers as to why people make any of these choices and the pathways which led them to those choices will be an important part of the development of bystander intervention prevention techniques. Researchers are beginning to answer these questions but there are many different situations and people interacting in terms of intervention behavior, which makes answering these questions complicated. Noticing a victim or situation and interpreting the situation as an emergency are the first two cognitive stages someone goes through when deciding whether to intervene. Some people may not intervene because they fail to recognize and/or interpret the situation as an incident needing their help. There are reasons at each of Latane & Darley's five theoretical stages why someone may fail to intervene.

Fabiano et al. (2003) make suggestions for prevention educators in best utilizing a social norms approach. The authors suggest engaging men as allies and to stop "defining male culture as rape culture" (p. 110). Making these cultures synonymous causes men to be disengaged from rape prevention messages. Recognizing not all men are perpetrators of sexual violence may help nonperpetrators become active helpers in stopping the violence. Banyard et al. (2004) argue that participants in prevention programs may feel they are being addressed in a role they do not connect to: specifically women as victim and men as perpetrator. Being cast in these roles can cause individuals to tune out prevention messages because of a lack of identification with this role. Women often do not view themselves as potential victims. Men specifically tune out prevention information delivered in this fashion because they perceive it as being negative towards themselves. Schewe (2008) found that addressing people as potential bystanders, instead of dichotomizing them into victim/perpetrator roles was more effective than other types of prevention interventions.

As previously mentioned, bystanders must notice a victim and recognize the situation as an emergency (Latane & Darley, 1970). This can hinder the likelihood of intervening in situations of sexual violence because of a cultural tendency to blame the victim. Unfortunately blaming a rape victim is commonplace. Burn (2009) found when potential interveners engaged in victim blaming attitudes, they were less likely to intervene. This was found to be a stronger issue for men than women. Because of the strength victim blaming has in our society, bystander intervention prevention education efforts will need to include elements dispelling victim blaming. These efforts need to spread messages that regardless of the victim's characteristics and actions, sexual assault is always the fault of the person committing the assault (Burn, 2009). Illuminating sources of victim bias should allow possible interveners to more easily recognize a potentially risky situation and thereby increase their likelihood of intervening.

Belief in rape myths influences intervention behavior. One study found rape myths specific to victim blaming correlated positively with a lack of perceived need for intervention (McMahon, 2010). Further, regardless of the specific type of myth, higher rates of any rape myth acceptance led to lower rates of intentions to intervene, therefore sexual assault prevention educators must continue to include rape myths in their curricula. McMahon (2010) found further support which showed students are more likely to intervene in situations of blatant sexual violence, such as an actual assault, rather than intervening when another person makes a sexist joke or uses sexist language. While students are more likely to intervene in blatant sexually violent situations, increasing student awareness of the spectrum of sexual violence and how it all contributes to rape may help encourage students to also intervene in cases of sexist jokes or language.

Banyard et al. (2004) believe bystander intervention can help facilitate new norms, both at the individual and community level, which will better set up communities for intervening in sexual violence. They believe bystander intervention can model prosocial bystander behavior as well as teach bystanders valuable skills. By not labeling individuals as perpetrators or victims, but as bystanders, friends, witnesses, or allies, it places the onus of responsibility on all parties who are willing and able to help. Lastly, when looking at ecological theory, the authors posit if community-level norms are shifted in this way, then societal-level norms will eventually begin to reflect those of the community (Banyard et al., 2004). By empowering all individuals to be active bystanders, the more community members become involved in the fight against sexual violence. This empowerment will hopefully lead to prevention efforts resting on everyone's shoulders.

Casey and Ohler (2012) gathered a group of male participants who were involved with groups committed to ending violence against women. Through conversations with these men, they found only about a quarter of their participants reported intervening every time they were "confronted with exploitive, offensive, or inappropriate behavior by other men" (p. 77). They were surprised that even men who were actively engaged and trained in techniques to address behavior on the sexual violence spectrum still sometimes had difficulty in confronting others' use of sexist language, jokes, or coercive/forceful behavior. Some of the men reported difficulty intervening because of a norm in male culture to not interfere with another male's sexual exploits (i.e., cock-blocking). These men's willingness to intervene was affected by their perceived relationship and status to the offender as well as their perceived norms of group members in the area at the time of the offending situation (Casey & Ohler, 2012). While there are individual men trying to help end violence against women through addressing their peer groups, challenges still exist even to those who are trained in intervention techniques. This finding suggests the need for more work at addressing the community and society levels of the social-ecology. Men may become more comfortable with intervening as societal norms change.

When Bystander Intervention Works

Shifting the prevention focus to engaging all community members to be prosocial bystanders has had some positive evaluation results. There is a myriad of bystander training programs, some with more evaluation research than others. One of these programs is *Bringing in the Bystander®* (BITB). BITB is offered as either a one- or multisession training which includes prevalence, causes, and consequences of sexual violence and discussions and role playing surrounding prosocial bystander behavior and safe intervention techniques. Banyard, Moynihan, and Crossman (2009) evaluated the BITB program and found it to be successful at changing beliefs about bystander behavior and increasing behavioral intention to intervene among student leaders, who are already more engaged in helping other students than their nonleader peers. A different evaluation of this same program found post-tests given anywhere from 2 to 12 months after participation continued to yield results which showed attitude and behavior changes (Banyard, Moynihan, & Plante, 2007). The long-term positive change in attitudes and behaviors is significant because many evaluation studies show these changes directly after program participation, but rarely are attitudes and behaviors tested with any amount of time passing in between the program and the post-test.

In another evaluation, Cares et al. (2015) looked at BITB on two separate college campuses; one rural with most students residing on campus and the other urban with a mix of residential and commuter students. Testing this program between two different college populations was important because often campuses want a prevention program which is not expensive, does not take a long time, and applies to diverse settings and students. Despite some differences between genders and campuses, the researchers were able to demonstrate through pre- and post-tests as well as a 12 month follow-up that "initial changes in attitude lasted at least as long as twelve months post program" (Cares et al., 2015, p.180).

BITB has been widely evaluated. Moynihan et al., (2015) conducted an evaluation of BITB and the Know Your Power® social marketing campaign. Utilizing separate campuses, researchers tested the effectiveness of BITB by using Know Your Power® as a control. Both campuses were exposed to the Know Your Power® campaign and one campus participated in BITB training. While both the treatment and control groups had a decrease in reported bystander behavior after 1 year, those who also received the in-person BITB program and the social marketing campaign reported higher levels of bystander behavior after 1 year. Further, students who reported low opportunity for interventions on pre-test measures, reported an increase in helping strangers at the 1 year follow-up, leading the authors to believe that the in-person training potentially increased students' awareness and identification of intervention opportunities (Moynihan et al., 2015).

Green Dot is a bystander training method used on college campuses. Green Dot attempts to decrease barriers to engaging in bystander behaviors and teaches students to select an intervention they feel safe to carry out. One evaluation of Green Dot comes from the University of Kentucky (Coker et al., 2011). Green Dot consists of a motivational speech encouraging students to connect with the issue of sexual violence and present intervention as something manageable for students to do. Green Dot then trains smaller student groups to recognize risky situations and implement bystander behavior. Green Dot encourages diffusion of behaviors using peer opinion leaders (POL). POLs were recruited from many different student subgroups to increase student exposure to the trained POLs. Green Dot is different than BITB because it teaches students to look for "high-risk potential perpetrator behavior" as opposed to identifying victims. Students who only participated in the motivational speech reported more active bystander behaviors than students who received neither of the Green Dot components. Participating in both the motivational speech and the specialized training resulted in the most reported intervention behaviors as well as the lowest rates of rape myth acceptance (Coker et al., 2011).

Evaluations of these programs found both intent to intervene and actual intervention behavior increased and there was a decrease in attitudes which have been linked to low intervention intention such as rape myth acceptance. Further, most of the evaluations of these programs were able to conduct follow-ups after lengths of time had passed and found that intervention intentions and behaviors were still greater than prior to training.

When Bystander Intervention Does Not Work

Several limitations hinder the ability of bystander intervention to prevent sexual violence. One of these limitations involves social norms. An infrequently addressed limitation of bystander intervention is that it involves conflicting social norms. Bystander intervention encourages prosocial behavior such as helping others' in need and intervening with peers' inappropriate language. However, this is in direct conflict with the social norm of minding one's own business. Further, there is a social norm among men to not interfere with other men's sexual activity. In the moment where intervention occurs, the issue requiring intervention must be so great as to overcome the norm to not interfere too much with others' personal matters. This may be the reason behind why students are much more likely to intervene in situations of sexual assault than with peers' sexually problematic language. Further, if sexual violence is occurring between people in a relationship, bystanders may feel less responsibility for intervention because of a norm to respect others' privacy (Banyard, 2011).

A second limitation is that sexual violence is often committed in isolation. The very definition of isolation is a lack of bystanders. Therefore, bystander intervention training must focus on teaching people to recognize potentially violent situations before the victim is isolated. Lastly, situations where interventions could occur are very specific and full of nuanced details specific to each scenario. Developing measures to attempt to gauge all the different contexts under which someone chooses (or not) to intervene would be a daunting task. Using interviews with students would allow researchers to determine commonalities among all the different types of situations college students could find themselves in as potential interveners. Such research could help to create measures that could give more insight into situationally specific barriers and facilitators of bystander intervention.

Where Are We Going?

Over 20 years have passed since Schewe and O'Donohue (1993) reviewed rape prevention programs and determined prevention programming suffers from a lack of knowledge about the cause(s) of rape. Unfortunately, this is still the case for many sexual violence prevention programs. In her CDC report to the White House Task Force to Protect Students from Sexual Assault, DeGue (2014) states one best practice for sexual assault prevention is to be strongly based in theory. Until recently, sexual assault prevention has not had a strong base in any theory of sexual violence; likely caused by a limited understanding of the etiology of rape.

Training and education surrounding consent has become more predominant in the prevention landscape, but few theories argue that rape is caused because of a misunderstanding of consent. Further, much programming has focused on rape myths and traditional gender roles; and while feminist theory speaks to both, the larger context of feminist theory points to many different etiologies for rape. McPhail (2015) argues that while feminist theory is widely believed to only deal with power and control, this ignores other feminist theorizing of rape. While power and control can certainly be pointed to as a motive for rape in society (i.e. rape culture) and for individuals (man wants to be dominant over woman), this explanation alone does not count for the sexual nature of rape, the intersectionality of rape and other forms of oppression, and motivations in which men are attempting to demonstrate masculinity (McPhail, 2015). Moreover, feminist scholars discuss the importance of examining gender-based violence through a lens of intersectionality. Kimberle Crenshaw argues that race and gender cannot be viewed as mutually exclusive (Crenshaw, 1997). Angela Davis has argued that attempting to eliminate rape by only examining it as a gender issue and ignoring the role race and sexuality play will result in failure (Davis, 1990). Most prevention programming lacks an intersectionality lens and thereby neglects recognizing the complex ways in which gender, race, sexual orientation, and disability status interacts with and upon potential perpetrators, victims, and bystanders.

While Latane and Darley (1970) outlined a theory of bystander intervention, their theory accounts for the steps someone takes in the intervention decision-making process and is not specific to violence prevention. Banyard (2011) and McMahon (2015) have conceptually addressed this need for a more thorough and comprehensive theoretical approach to bystander intervention, however these pieces focus on increasing prevention efforts to community and society contexts of the social ecology, rather than developing a prevention-based theoretical model. One theory which may help bridge the gap between the social ecological model and bystander intervention that has some empirical support is routine activities theory. This theory could possibly adequately address the need for bystander intervention training. Indeed, sexual violence has all three elements of routine activities: motivated offenders, suitable targets, and lack of capable guardianship. Bystander intervention training could increase the amount of capable guardianship, thereby resulting in prevention as all three elements of routine activities theory would no longer be met (Cohen & Felson, 1979). Further, increasing capable guardianship effectively applies to the peer and community contexts of the social ecology; which has been called for by multiple scholars (Banyard, 2011; DeGue, 2014; McMahon, 2015). Prosocial bystanders and capable guardians should be considered synonymous terms.

Lack of capable guardianship can refer to several elements when viewed in the context of sexual violence. It could be a lack of bystanders to intervene or victim incapacitation. Schwartz and Pitts (1995) argue that there are an increased number of likely-or motivated-offenders on college campuses due to all male peer groups who encourage sexual abuse of women, such as fraternities and athletic teams. When looking at victims, specifically women, Schwartz & Pitts (1995) discuss suitable targets. They argue the college environment is one which encourages alcohol consumption, thereby making women who voluntarily drink large amounts of alcohol "suitable" for sexual victimization. Lastly, college campuses specifically can be lacking in capable guardianship, the third element of routine activities theory. Traditionally, campus administration does not take sexually violent crimes seriously and offenders receive little to no punishment for their actions (Schwartz & Pitts, 1995). Coupled with all male campus groups who are supportive of sexual violence towards women, the pool of guardians who are likely to intervene becomes even shallower.

Schwartz, DeKeseredy, Tait, and Alvi (2001) take capable guardianship one step further. Using the idea of rape culture from feminist theory, they argue North America has a culture which supports male sexual violence and allows for women to internalize an expectation for sexual violence and to believe they deserve what happened to them. This internalized expectation and belief of deservingness work together to decrease effective guardianship from society as a whole (Schwartz et al., 2001). A culture which supports male sexual violence not only decreases effective guardianship, but likely increases motivated offending. When sexually violent crimes are not prosecuted, not heavily punished, and victims are blamed or not believed, this may lead to offenders perceiving a lack of societal concern for this type of crime and increase motivation to commit sexual violence because the perceived risk is less than the perceived reward.

Theoretical models regarding how people view victims and offenders of sexual violence could further aid in the development of a specific prevention approach through bystander intervention theory. The *ideal victim* is a concept in which society believes some people are more deserving of victim status or than others. People who appear weak and attempt to defend themselves from an attacker are more likely to be given a victim status. Christie (1986) further discusses how the concept of ideal victims creates *ideal offenders*. Ideal offenders are explicitly dangerous and bring about visions of scary strangers lurking in shadows. Criminologists know that these rigid and explicit definitions of victims and offenders are simply not reality. Those who study sexual violence recognize how these notions affect all aspects of this crime. Rape victims can be blamed and seen as less of a victim because of previous sexual encounters, what they were wearing, or what activities they were engaged in prior to being raped. On the contrary, men of higher status who commit rape are rarely viewed as offenders; or men are not viewed as able to be victims of rape.

Two theories which hail from psychology which could be beneficial to include in a larger theory of prevention through bystander intervention are self-categorization theory and theories surrounding implicit bias (Turner, Hogg, Oakes, Reicher, & Wetherell, 1987; Greenwald & Krieger, 2006). Self-categorization theory looks at how people classify themselves in relation to different groups. Levine, Cassidy, Brazier, and Reicher (2002) found bystanders are more likely to intervene when victims are in-group members. They argued that recognition of common group membership can increase helping. Further empirical support for self-categorization theory showed categorical relation to others affected whether people viewed situations relevant to themselves (Levine, et al., 2002). If self-categorization can provide some explanation for the bystander intent to intervene with a victim, it may also provide some level of explanation for if a bystander does not intervene because of who the perpetrator is. Examining the relationship between helping behavior and identification with victim or perpetrator "may deepen our understanding of and strengthen our predictions about bystander behavior" (Levine et al., 2002, p. 1461).

Self-categorization theory may be able to provide some explanation for implicit bias. As constructs, implicit bias refers to our individual psychology and self-categorization refers to our collective psychologies. These collective psychologies are what we use to define ourselves relationally to groups similar and different from ourselves (Reynolds, Turner, Haslam, & Ryan, 2001). Combining self-categorization theory with implicit bias may hold a key into unlocking how people identify and how those identifications help or hinder bystander intervention behaviors. The ability to better predict bystander behavior will lead to more specific and tailored training programs. If people are more likely to help those with whom they identify (or, conversely, less likely to help those with whom they do not identify), program developers must figure out a way to address this subconscious identification with others. This could potentially be done by strongly encouraging situational awareness, using examples to increase empathy for all types of victims, or even including implicit association tests and education about how self-categorization may affect decision-making during bystander training to increase participant awareness of this possibility.

Theories about implicit bias suggest that people do not always have control over their perceptions, judgments, and impressions (Greenwald & Krieger, 2006). Implicit biases are based on discriminatory attitudes or stereotypes. Empirical testing of theories of implicit bias comes from the Implicit Association Test (IAT) and other computer-generated tests. Analysis of results from the IAT show that two-thirds of people show preference for whichever group is the advantaged group for that test (i.e., black vs. white or young vs. old; Greenwald & Krieger, 2006). Interestingly, those groups which are typically disadvantaged mirror these preferences, often preferring the dominant group and not the group to which they belong (Jolls & Sunstein, 2006).

Implicit bias and ideal victim/offender bias may play a role in whether someone notices a situation as worthy of intervention or classifies a situation as an emergency which requires them to act in some way. If, due to some subconscious bias, whether that be related to race, gender, or what a victim or perpetrator is *supposed* to look/act like (or a combination of these), a bystander does not perceive a person to be a victim, they will not take any action to intervene. Implicit bias is believed to be automatic, such that people have no time to engage in advance cognitive processes in situations of quick decision-making (Jolls & Sunstein, 2006). This ties in with the theoretical argument that the literature and prevention efforts neglect how racism, gender, and violence are linked.

Using theories from multiple disciplines to assess barriers behind intervention behavior is a big step in the right direction towards improving bystander intervention training. Researchers and prevention educators must continue to examine the varying reasons why people do and do not intervene with a specific focus on the role of the intersectionality of race, class, gender identity, ability, and sexual orientation. Identifying how our bias and self-categorization into varying groups affects our perceptions of other people and the role this plays in whether we believe someone to be a victim or an offender will be tantamount in prevention programs which encourage prosocial bystander behavior in situations of sexual violence.

For example, practitioners need to be aware of how intersecting roles affect not only intervention behavior but also the earliest stages in the intervention decision-making process. Men are rarely viewed as potential victims; white women are more likely to be viewed as victims than women of color; women of color are more likely to blamed for their victimization (Katz, Merrilees, Hoxmeier, & Motisi, 2017). Addressing these issues and encouraging training participants to recognize their own internal bias and how bias may contribute to their own intervention decision-making should improve the efficacy of bystander intervention sexual assault prevention programs.

References

Banyard, V. L. (2011). Who will help prevent sexual violence: Creating an ecological model of bystander intervention. *Psychology of Violence, 1*(3), 216–229.

Banyard, V. L., Moynihan, M. M., & Crossman, M. T. (2009). Reducing sexual violence on campus: The role of student leaders as empowered bystanders. *Journal of College Student Development, 50*(4), 446–457.

Banyard, V. L., Moynihan, M. M., & Plante, E. G. (2007). Sexual violence prevention through bystander education: An experimental evaluation. *Journal of Community Psychology, 35*(4), 463–481.

Banyard, V. L., Plante, E. G., & Moynihan, M. M. (2004). Bystander education: Bringing a broader community perspective to sexual violence prevention. *Journal of Community Psychology, 32*(1), 61–79.

Barone, R. P., Wolgemuth, J. R., & Linder, C. (2007). Preventing sexual assault through engaging college men. *Journal of College Student Development, 48*(5), 585–594.

Burn, S. (2009). A situational model of sexual assault prevention through bystander intervention. *Sex Roles, 60*(11), 779–792.

Cares, A., Banyard, V., Moynihan, M., Williams, L., Potter, S., & Stapleton, J. (2015). Changing attitudes about being a bystander to violence: Translating an in-person sexual violence prevention program to a new campus. *Violence Against Women, 21*(2), 165–187.

Casey, E. A., & Ohler, K. (2012). Being a positive bystander: Male antiviolence allies' experiences of "stepping up". *Journal of Interpersonal Violence, 27*(1), 62–83.

Christie, N. (1986). The ideal victim. In E. A. Fatah (Ed.), *From crime policy to victim policy; reinventing the justice system* (pp. 17–30). New York, NY: St. Martin's Press.

Cohen, L., & Felson, M. (1979). Social changes and crime rate trends: A routine activities approach. *American Sociological Review, 44*(4), 588–608.

Coker, A. L., Cook-Craig, P. G., Williams, C. M., Fisher, B. S., Clear, E. R., Garcia, L. S., & Hegge, L. M. (2011). Evaluation of Green Dot: An active bystander intervention to reduce sexual violence on college campuses. *Violence Against Women, 17*(6), 777–796.

Crenshaw, K. W. (1997). Beyond racism and misogyny: Black feminism and 2 Live Crew. In D. T. Meyers (Ed.), *Feminist social thought: A reader* (pp. 246–263). New York, NY: Routledge.

Davis, A. Y. (1990). *Women, culture & politics*. New York, NY: Vintage.

DeGue, S. (2014). Preventing sexual violence on college campuses: Lessons from research and practice. Retrieved from https://www.notalone.gov/assets/evidence-based-strategies-for-the-prevention-of-sv-perpetration.pdf. Accessed on 2.16.2018.

Fabiano, P. M., Perkins, H. W., Berkowitz, A., Linkenbach, J., & Stark, C. (2003). Engaging men as social justice allies in ending violence against women: Evidence for a social norms approach. *Journal of American College Health, 52*(3), 105–112.

Gidycz, C. A., Orchowski, L. M., & Berkowitz, A. D. (2011). Preventing sexual aggression among college men: An evaluation of a social norms and bystander intervention program. *Violence Against Women, 17*(6), 720–742.

Greenwald, A. G., & Krieger, L. H. (2006). Implicit bias: Scientific foundations. *California Law Review, 94*(4), 945–967.

Jolls, C., & Sunstein, C. R. (2006). The law of implicit bias. *California Law Review, 94*(4), 969–996.

Katz, J., Merrilees, C., Hoxmeier, J. C., & Motisi, M. (2017). White female bystanders' responses to a black woman at risk for incapacitated sexual assault. *Psychology of Women Quarterly, 41*(2), 273–285.

Latane, B., & Darley, J. M. (1970). *The unresponsive bystander: Why doesn't he help?* New York, NY: Meredith Corporation.

Levine, M., Cassidy, C., Brazier, G., & Reicher, S. (2002). Self-categorization and bystander non intervention: Two experimental studies. *Journal of Applied Social Psychology, 32*(7), 1452–1463.

McMahon, S. (2010). Rape myth beliefs and bystander attitudes among incoming college students. *Journal of American College Health, 59*(1), 3–11.

McMahon, S. (2015). Call for research on bystander intervention to prevent sexual violence: The role of campus environments. *American Journal of Community Psychology, 55*(3/4), 472–489.

McPhail, B. (2015). Feminist framework plus: Knitting feminist theories of rape etiology into a comprehensive model. *Trauma, Violence, and Abuse, 7*(3), 314–329.

Moynihan, M. M., Banyard, V. L., Cares, A. C., Potter, S. J., Williams, L. M., & Stapleton, J. G. (2015). Encouraging responses in sexual and relationship violence prevention: What program effects remain 1 year later? *Journal of Interpersonal Violence, 30*(1), 110–132.

Piccigallo, J. R., Lilley, T. G., & Miller, S. L. (2012). "It's cool to care about sexual violence" men's experiences with sexual assault prevention. *Men and Masculinities, 15*(5), 507–525.

Reynolds, K. J., Turner, J. C., Haslam, S. A., & Ryan, M. K. (2001). The role of personality and group factors in explaining prejudice. *Journal of Experimental Social Psychology, 37*(5), 427–434.

Schewe, P. A. (2008). Interventions to prevent sexual violence. In L. S. Doll, S. E. Bonzo, D. A. Sleet, & J. A. Mercy (Eds.), *Handbook of injury and violence prevention*. Boston, MA: Springer.

Schewe, P. A., & O'Donohue, W. (1993). Rape prevention: Methodological problems and new directions. *Clinical Psychology Review, 13*(7), 667–682.

Schwartz, M., & Pitts, V. (1995). Toward a feminist routine activities approach to explaining sexual assault. *Justice Quarterly, 12*(1), 10–31.

Schwartz, M. D., DeKeseredy, W. S., Tait, D., & Alvi, S. (2001). Male peer support and a feminist routing activities theory: Understanding sexual assault on the college campus. *Justice Quarterly, 18*(3), 623–649.

Turner, J. C., Hogg, M. A., Oakes, P. J., Reicher, S. D., & Wetherell, M. S. (1987). *Rediscovering the social group: A self-categorization theory*. Oxford: Basil Blackwell.

Bystander Program Effectiveness: A Review of the Evidence in Educational Settings (2007–2018)

26

Samuel C. Bell, Ann L. Coker, and Emily R. Clear

Introduction

Bystander Intervention as a method for preventing the epidemic of various forms of violence (particularly sexual violence) has been conceptualized since the late 1960s (Latané & Rodin, 1969). The concept of bystander intervention involves teaching bystanders how to intervene in situations that involve sexual violence and other potentially dangerous situations with the hope of preventing harm and/or defusing the situation. The bystander model gives community members a specific role, including interrupting situations that could lead to assault before the assault occurs, defusing an ongoing hostile situation, particularly when vulnerable parties are involved, and having the ability and necessary skills to be an effective ally and advocate to survivors of violence.

In the relatively recent past, bystander intervention programs have begun taking shape and being implemented in populations at especially high risk for rates of partner and sexual violence. These populations include high school students, college students, student-athletes, members of Greek life and other fraternal organizations, and community leaders. Research suggests that bystander intervention may be effective at grade levels as low as middle school (Midgett, Doumas, Sears, Lunquist, & Hausheer, 2015). Studies have shown that the rates of intimate partner, dating, and sexual violence are particularly high in teenagers and young adults (Williams et al., 2014). Additionally, college campuses have shown particularly high rates of sexual violence (Banyard, Moynihan, & Crossman, 2009). Thus, many of the bystander intervention efforts are designed with young adults in mind.

Bystander intervention programs tend to have similar structures, although the content and presentation in each may vary from program to program. Many bystander intervention programs involve intense training of an educator, advocate, or facilitator whose job will be to ultimately disperse and lead the program for a given population. Following this training, the facilitator will often enter an environment and engage with a population, implementing the program itself. These programs tend to be in-person, often involving one lengthened session or multiple, shorter sessions. Prior to beginning the session, the study population often completes a baseline survey to gauge their awareness of, and responsiveness to the concept of bystander intervention. Following this survey, the facilitator presents a portion of the program to the population. The method of this presentation, as you will later see, is ripe for

S. C. Bell · A. L. Coker (✉)
Office of Research Integrity, University of Kentucky, Lexington, KY, USA
e-mail: scbe223@uky.edu; ann.coker@uky.edu

E. R. Clear
College of Public Health, University of Kentucky, Lexington, KY, USA
e-mail: emily.clear@uky.edu

W. T. O'Donohue and P. A. Schewe (eds.), *Handbook of Sexual Assault and Sexual Assault Prevention*,
https://doi.org/10.1007/978-3-030-23645-8_26

debate as to the most effective means. However, following the presentation of the content, the study population typically completes a post-test to see if attitudes or awareness rates (among other variables) have changed. Subsequently, the population is often asked to take a follow-up survey or engage in a focus group discussion at some later point, often 3 months following the completion of the training. The idea behind the follow-up is to examine how bystander behaviors may have changed in the time following the training.

A minority of programs eschew this format altogether and instead utilize some form of electronic intervention, primarily involving social media or web-based training. These interventions will be included in the following evaluation as well.

The purpose of this chapter is to identify some of the currently studied intervention efforts, their effectiveness, strengths, and weaknesses of the programs, and finally best practices going forward. Of note, the programs addressed in this chapter specifically focus on the issue of violence prevention. Other forms of bystander intervention programs exist for various public health issues (e.g., alcohol/drug use), but those are outside the scope of this work.

The programs that are the focus of this chapter are divided into the following categories: (1) in-person programs and (2) technologic programs. An in-person program refers to the category of bystander intervention programs that take place in a traditional "in-class" setting where an instructor follows a curriculum when speaking to a group of program participants. The method of delivery may vary (for example, student-led presentation versus participation in a skit or performance-like setting). A technologic program refers to a bystander intervention program that is primarily disseminated through technologic means such as web-based surveys, web-based interventions, and web-based models.

Past Work

This review relies a great deal on a previous review completed by Storer and colleagues (Storer, Casey, & Herrenkohl, 2016). In that work, the authors included 15 evaluations of 9 programs for review (Storer et al., 2016). Some of the programs previously addressed have undergone greater analysis in the time since Storer's review was published. The previously analyzed studies took place between 2007 and 2015. Storer et al. (2016) sought to address four distinct variables across the 15 evaluations: (1) increased utilization of bystander behaviors, (2) increased willingness to intervene, (3) increased confidence to intervene, and (4) decreased rape myth acceptance. Storer et al. (2016) showed that the vast majority of the studies analyzed prompted increased willingness to intervene and increased confidence to intervene in potentially dangerous scenarios. However, results were mixed as to the effectiveness of bystander intervention programs on rape myth acceptance and increased utilization of bystander behaviors (Storer et al., 2016).

Bringing in the Bystander (BiTB)

The first program that is evaluated in this chapter is also perhaps the most widely studied. *Bringing in the Bystander* (BiTB) is an intervention developed by the Prevention Innovations Research Center at the University of New Hampshire. The goal of the program is to help students, faculty, staff, and community members identify behaviors on a continuum of violence, develop empathy for those who have experienced violence, practice safe and appropriate intervention skills, and commit to intervene before, during, and after an incident of sexual abuse, relationship violence, and/or stalking (Banyard, Eckstein, & Moynihan, 2010). *Bringing in the Bystander* is designed to be presented either as a 90-min program, or in a more comprehensive two-session program totaling 4.5 h (Storer et al., 2016). The content of the program covers basic information about prevalence, causes, and consequences of sexual and relationship violence (Banyard et al., 2010). Additionally, *Bringing in the Bystander* attempts to address the problem of rape myth acceptance and to prevent sexually coercive behavior from occurring.

The framework of this program seeks to introduce participants to the notion of bystander intervention gradually by having participants discuss their own ideas about community, who bystanders are, and when they have been helped or chose to help those in difficult situations (Moynihan, Banyard, Arnold, Eckstein, & Stapleton, 2010). Participants then engage in discourse regarding things that make it easier and more difficult to intervene, followed by a discussion between the facilitator and the participants about defining the problem of sexual violence, in addition to defining the concepts of sexual violence and rape themselves. This program, perhaps more than others, stresses the need for bystander personal safety, providing each participant with a list of support resources at the outset of the training. Finally, the program utilizes active learning by practicing simulated bystander scenarios focused on skill building. At conclusion, the facilitator reads a bystander pledge aloud and asks the participants to sign, stating they will intervene in potentially dangerous scenarios. The participants are allowed and encouraged to take a copy of the pledge home with them.

Bringing in the Bystander has been thoroughly evaluated among several populations, with relatively positive results across the board for certain variables. In particular, Bringing in the Bystander has shown effective at improving bystander efficacy and decreasing rape myth acceptance (Banyard, Moynihan, & Plante, 2007; Banyard et al., 2009; Cares et al., 2015; See also Table 26.1). Initial studies address the use of Bringing in the Bystander in resident halls, sororities, and college athletes. Additionally, studies have attempted to identify a wide range of outcomes, including confidence and willingness to engage in bystander intervention, awareness of bystander intervention, perceived efficacy of bystander intervention, rape myth and rape-positive language acceptance, and both negative and positive bystander intervention actions (self-reported). To date there has been no evaluation of the effectiveness of BiTB to reduce violence over time, relative to a control group, nor compared to those receiving other training.

Green Dot

Another intensively studied bystander intervention methodology is *Green Dot*. *Green Dot* was initially developed in 2006 to engage students in actions to reduce sexual violence (Cook-Craig et al., 2014). *Green Dot* is a traditional, curriculum-based, instructor/peer group bystander intervention strategy. *Green Dot* curriculum stresses the three D's: Direct, Delegate, and Distract, each of which signify a potential method or intervening in a situation that could lead to sexual assault or other violence. *Green Dot* involves two primary components. First, *Green Dot* instructors give a motivational speech, traditionally designed for an introductory college population. Second, more intensive training takes place, using video and role play exercises designed to allow participants to practice using bystander intervention techniques among peers. The purpose of the program is to generate positive bystander intervention techniques to create a more engaged and educated community.

Green Dot has shown effectiveness to reduce violence acceptance in both college and high school samples (Coker, Bush, Brancato, Clear, & Recktenwald, 2018; Coker et al., 2011). Importantly for establishing a link between bystander intervention training and violence prevention, *Green Dot* has been associated with a reduction in sexual violence victimization and both sexual harassment victimization and perpetration rates in one college campus with *Green Dot* relative to two with no bystander programming (Coker et al., 2015, 2016). In a large cluster-based randomized controlled trial over 5 years, high schools randomized to *Green Dot* experienced a 20% reduction in sexual violence and harassment perpetration and victimization events over time and with complete program implementation relative to schools not receiving *Green Dot* (Cares et al., 2017) Additional research on the effectiveness of *Green Dot* is needed by other investigators and comparing *Green Dot* training effectiveness relative to other bystander programs.

Table 26.1 Summary of 12 bystander programs (publications between 2007 and 2018) with bystander, violence acceptance and violence frequency findings

Bystander program (modality)	First author, year	Population	Sample size	Study design	↑ Bystander behaviors?	↑ Bystander efficacy, attitudes, readiness to act?	↓ Rape myth acceptance?	↓ SV/SH?
Bringing in the bystander (In-person)	Banyard et al. (2007)	College	363 post, 284 @ 2, 140 @ 4, 83 @ 12 mon	Experimental	Yes, short term @ 2, 4 $^{p<0.001}$ not 12 months	Yes ↑ bystander efficacy $^{p<0.01}$ & ↑ bystander attitudes $_{p<0.01}$ over time	Yes, ↓ RMA over time $^{p<0.01}$	NA
As above	Banyard et al. (2009)	College	196 leaders	Pre-post (no control)	NA	Yes, ↑ confidence in engaging bystander behaviors $^{p<0.001}$ and willingness to help $_{p<0.001}$	Yes, ↓ RMA over time $^{p<0.001}$	NA
As above	Moynihan et al. (2010)	College, athletes	53 I vs. 86 C; *n* = 98 @ 2 mon. fup	Experimental	NA	Yes, ↑ bystander efficacy $^{p<0.001}$ and intent $^{p<0.001}$	No difference in RMA over time	NA
As above	Moynihan et al. (2015)	College 1st yr.; 2 campuses	948 pre; 346 @ 12 mon fup	Experimental BITB + KYP vs. KYP only	Yes, ↑ bystander behaviors at 12 mon. $^{p=0.001}$	NA	NA	NA
As above	Cares et al. (2015)	College, 1st year; 2 campuses	1246 pre, 607 @ post, 346 @ 12 mon fup	Experimental	NA	Yes, ↑ bystander efficacy at 12 mon. $_{p<0.01}$	Yes, ↓ RMA up to 12 mon. $_{p<0.001}$	NA
Know your power (In-person; social media)	Potter et al. (2009)	College students	372 total; 291 saw posters	Cross-sectional	NA	Yes, seeing posters ≥1 day at higher action stage $^{(p<0.05)}$	NA	NA
Coaching boys into men (In-person)	Miller et al. (2012)	High school, male athletes	*n* = 2006 @ pre, 1798 @ 3 mon fup	RCT	Yes, ↑ positive intervention $^{p<0.001}$	Yes, ↑ intention to intervene $^{p<0.05}$	No difference in gender attitudes (RMA not measured)	No difference in abuse perpetration
As above	Miller et al. (2013)	High school, male athletes	1513 @ 12 mon fup	RCT	Yes, ↓ in NEGATIVE bystander behaviors $_{p<0.001;}$ no difference in positive bystander behaviors	No difference in intention to intervene	"	Yes, ↓ in DV perpetration $_{p<0.01}$

As above	Jaime et al. (2016)	High school, male athletes	148 @ 3 mon fup	Experimental., Randomized Advocate vs. Coach, school level	NA	No difference intention to bystand	"	No difference in DV perpetration
Green dot (In-person)	Coker et al. (2011)	College students; one university	2504; 1203 trained vs. 1301 no training	Cross-sectional	Yes, ↑ bystander behaviors in past yr. POL > speech > no training $^{p<0.001}$	NA	Yes, ↓ RMA in POL vs. no training $^{p<0.01}$; no difference for speech only	NA
As above	Cares et al. (2015)	College students; 3 campuses	2768 @ Intervention and 4258 @ Control campuses	Cross-sectional	NA	NA	NA	Yes, ↓ SVV events $^{p=.03}$ in I vs. C campuses; no difference for SVP. ↓ SHV & SHP $^{p<0.0001}$
As above	Coker et al. (2016)	College 1st-year students; 3 campuses	2979 @ Intervention and 4,132 @ Control campuses	Cross-sectional over 4 yrs	NA	NA	NA	Yes, ↓ SVV in I vs. C campuses $^{p<0.0001}$; No diff for SVP; ↓ SHV $^{p=0.05}$; ↓ SHP $^{p<0.0001}$
As above	Coker et al. (2017), Coker et al. (2018)	High school students	47,311 @ Intervention and 42,396 @ Control schools	RCT, randomized at school-level, 5 yr. fup	NA	NA	Yes, ↓ RMA CxT $^{p=0.0004}$	Yes, ↓ SVP, SVV, SHV & SHP; CxT $^{p<0.001}$
HAVEN—(Online)	Zapp et al. (2018)	College 1st yr. students	167,242 students from 80 colleges	Pre-post (no control)	NA	Yes, ↑ bystander ability and intent (68%, large to medium effect size)	Little effect on RMA (30%, small effect size)	NA
InterACT (In-person; theater)	Ahrens et al. (2011)	College students	355 @ 3 mon fup	Pre-post training (at 3 mon)	NA	Yes, ↑ likelihood of bystanding $^{p<0.05}$	NA	NA

(continued)

Table 26.1 (continued)

Bystander program (modality)	First author, year	Population	Sample size	Study design	↑ Bystander behaviors?	↑ Bystander efficacy, attitudes, readiness to act?	↓ Rape myth acceptance?	↓ SV/SH?
Men's project (In-person)	Gidycz et al. (2011)	College, 1st year male students	635 pre, 529 @ 4 and 494 @ 7 mon fup	RCT Randomized at dorm level	No difference in prosocial bystander behaviors over time	NA	No difference in RMA or negative attitudes toward women CxT	Yes, ↓ sexual aggression CxT $p<0.001$ @ 4, not 7 months
Men's program (In-person)	Langhinrichsen-Rohling et al. (2011)	College, 1st year male students	179; 85 I and 94 C	Pre-post surveys (not randomized)	NA	Yes, ↑ bystander efficacy $p<0.001$ & willingness to intervene $p<0.001$	Yes, ↓ RMA in intervention over time $p<0.001$ but not in control	NA
Women's program (In-person)	Foubert et al. (2010)	College, primarily 1st year female	189 I vs. 90 C	Pre-post; Randomized	NA	Yes, ↑ bystander efficacy I vs. C post-test $p<0.001$; not at pre-test. Same for willingness to help	Yes, ↓ IRMA in I vs. C at post-test $p<0.001$ but not at pre test	NA
Mentors in violence prevention (In-person)	Katz et al. (2011)	High school students	755 MVP School; 825 non-MVP school	Cross-sectional	NA	Yes, ↑ willingness to "Take Action Aggressive" scores highest in I vs. C $p<0.0001$; No difference for "Take Action Less Aggressive" scores	Yes, Perceived wrong scores highest in I vs. C schools $p<0.001$	NA
One Act (In-person with Online comparison)	Alegria-Flores et al. (2017)	College students; 1 campus	594 One Act vs. 336 Haven	Pre-post surveys (not randomized); One Act vs. HAVEN	No difference in bystander behaviors	Yes, ↑ bystander confidence $p<0.001$ & willingness to help $p<0.05$ in One Act vs. Haven	No difference Date Rape attitudes, One Act vs. Haven	NA
RealConsent (Online)	Salazar et al. (2014)	College men	743; pre-post to 6 mon fup	RCT: RealConsent vs. general health promotion program	Yes, ↑ intervene more often, IvC $p=0.04$	Yes, ↑ intentions to intervene $(P=0.04)$, more positive outcome expectancies for intervening $P<0.001$	Yes, ↓ RMA $P<0.001$, date rape attitudes $P<0.001$, greater empathy for rape victims $P<0.001$; CxT	Yes, ↓ SVP $P=0.04$ CxT

SCREAM theater (In-person; theater)	McMahon, Allen, et al. (2014)	College, 1st year, 1 campus	2465; 693 completed fup	Pre-post (no control)	NA	Yes, ↑ bystander attitudes over time $p < 0.001$	Yes, ↓ RMA over time $p < 0.001$	NA
TakeCARE (Online via videos)	Sargent et al. (2017)	66 high school classrooms diverse	1295; 463 TakeCARE vs. 458 attention control	RCT, classroom randomized Fup to 3 mon	Yes, ↑ engaging in helpful bystander behaviors CxT $p = 0.005$	NA	NA	NA
Summary								
12 programs	23 publications	17 college; 6 high school setting		11 experimental design	7/9 publications (5/7 programs) ↑ bystander behaviors	14/16 publications (9/10 programs) ↑ bystander efficacy or intentions	10/17 publications (7/11 programs) ↓ in violence acceptance	4/6 publications (4/4 program) ↓ in SV/SH/DV

Abbreviations: *BITB* bringing in the bystander, *C* comparison or control, *CxT* condition × time (interaction), *DV* dating violence, *Fup* follow-up, *I* (bystander program) intervention, *KYP* know your power, *Mon* months, *MVP* mentoring in violence prevention, *NA* not accessed, *RMA* rape myth acceptance (scale score), *SHV/SVP* sexual harassment victimization/sexual harassment perpetration, *SVV/SVP* sexual violence victimization/sexual violence perpetration, *Yrs* years

Coaching Boys into Men (CBIM)

Another program that has been highly tested in various populations and age ranges is *Coaching Boys into Men* (CBIM). CBIM was created in 2001 as a Public Service Announcement and ad campaign with the goal of increasing awareness of domestic and relationship violence, focused specifically on the mentoring relationship between athletic coaches and their student-athletes. The program ultimately grew into a large-scale violence prevention curriculum designed to be delivered to athletic teams at the high school and college level. The program concentrated its focus on male student athletes due to the perceived higher rates of violence against women perpetrated by male athletes, and due to the perceived leadership ability inherent in athletes compared to their nonathlete peers (Jaime et al., 2016). The program is designed to be led by coaches who receive a 60-min training to introduce the *coaches kit*, which serves as the program's toolbox for implementing the program to the athletic teams. The coaches accept the responsibility of leading 11 brief (15 min), weekly discussions with their team on the topics of respect, violence awareness, and violence prevention (Miller et al., 2012). The developers of CBIM hoped that a coach-led discussion would allow student-athletes to be more forthcoming with their attitudes towards violence perpetration, and that implementation of the program in a team environment, with a mentor-coach present, would allow for each member to hold one another accountable for their attitudes and actions towards the prevention of violence. The effectiveness of this "coach-led" concept is still debated, with one study showing little to no change in participant attitudes or behavior when the program was implemented by a coach as opposed to being implemented by a CBIM expert (Jaime et al., 2016). Additional research is needed to investigate the effectiveness of CBIM relative to other bystander-based intervention programming and, like Green Dot, by other investigators to establish repeatability of findings.

Mentors in Violence Prevention (MVP)

Mentors in Violence Prevention (MVP), is one of the first bystander intervention programs to be developed, beginning implementation in 1993 (Katz, Heisterkamp, & Fleming, 2011). MVP is unusual in that it has been designed for implementation in various settings, rather than the high school or college-aged populations; however, the primary evaluation of the program was conducted in a high school population (Katz et al., 2011). MVP was initially designed to focus exclusively on men, with a greater focus on both sexes as the program evolved. MVP utilizes the student mentor model to engage other students, with the intent that student leaders (mentors) would drive increased positive bystander behavior over time (Katz et al., 2011). The construct of the program focuses on the group discussion dynamic which is so prevalent in many other bystander intervention programs. However, as mentioned above, these groups are led by students, rather than an outside instructor. One primary study addressing the effectiveness of MVP can be found in this analysis. The results of this analysis show initial effectiveness at reducing rape myth acceptance and improving potential bystander attitudes and confidence levels (Katz et al., 2011; see Table 26.1). Additional research is needed to investigate this program's impact on changing bystander behaviors and its ability to reduce violence perpetration among those trained and within the social networks of those receiving training.

The Women's Program

The Women's Program (also known as the *Women's Program: Helping Friends Avoid Rape and Empowering Survivors to Recover*) is a bystander intervention program designed for college-aged women. This differs from many of the other programs we analyzed due to its female-specific focus; contrasted with other programs which focus specifically on men or among mixed-sex populations. The *Women's Program* was designed to increase women's bystander efficacy and their willingness to intervene in settings where sexual assault or other violent acts could occur (Foubert, Langhinrichsen-Rohling, Brasfield, & Hill, 2010). The program consists of several components, including definitions of various topics related to sexual assault and consent, a video interview from a convicted rapist, and a discussion between instructor and audience about lessons and takeaways learned from said video. Additionally, presenters identified ideas for intervention in dangerous situations, and ideas for supporting someone who experienced sexual assault. The *Women's Program* is entirely in-person, and to date, one comprehensive evaluation exists. The results of this study show overall decreases in rape myth acceptance and some indication of improved bystander efficacy and confidence levels (Foubert et al., 2010).

The Men's Program

The Men's Program is a traditional, in-person bystander intervention program which was designed as a companion to the aforementioned *Women's Program*. The focus of the *Men's Program* is the prevention of sexual violence perpetration through the implementation of a "male on male empathy component" (Storer et al., 2016). In contrast to the *Women's Program*, the *Men's Program* is delivered by a male instructor to an all-male audience. Similar to the *Women's Program*, the *Men's Program* contains a video component; however, the *Men's Program* video details a situation of male on male sexual assault, in addition to the more traditional group discussion and role-playing format followed by many other intervention programs. Additionally, the *Men's Program* stresses ways that men can respond more effectively to help women who have been victims of sexual assault (Langhinrichsen-Rohling, Foubert, Brasfield, Hill, & Shelley-Tremblay, 2011). Several evaluations of the *Men's Program* exist, one of which can be found in this analysis. This evaluation showed a decrease in rape myth acceptance in addition to an increase in bystander's willingness to intervene, as well as an increase in bystander efficacy overall (Langhinrichsen-Rohling et al., 2011). Similar to MVP, additional evaluation research is needed for both the *Women's* and *Men's Programs* to determine program impact on changing bystander behaviors and violence rates relative to those receiving no bystander training or those receiving training from other bystander programs.

The Men's Project

The *Men's Project* is an intensive in-person bystander intervention program designed to allow men the opportunity to "vent" about their experiences as men on college campuses (Gidycz, Orchowski, & Berkowitz, 2011). The program incorporates discussions on the prevention of sexual assault, affirmative consent, debunking rape myths, and a presentation on male discomfort with inappropriate behavior and language of other men (Gidycz et al., 2011). Similar to the *Men's Program*, the *Men's Project* is designed around the concept of masculinity and critiques of the gender-role script, allowing for suggestions of positive alternatives from other participants (Gidycz et al., 2011). Additionally, the concept of peer influence plays a large role in the implementation of the *Men's Project*, with the hope of encouraging positive bystander behavior among the majority to change the negative behaviors of the contrasting minority. Somewhat unlike other programs we have addressed, the *Men's Project* contains a booster session 4 months after the initial intervention (Gidycz et al., 2011). Several studies have evaluated the effectiveness of the *Men's Project*, one of which is addressed here. This evaluation showed no significant change in rape myth acceptance or bystander behavior. The *Men's Project* was among the first to show a decrease in sexual aggression levels; however this effect was only apparent for a short time following the implementation of the program (Gidycz et al., 2011; see Table 26.1). Going forward, the *Men's Project* should be evaluated against other bystander intervention programs with violence reduction as the primary outcome.

One Act

Developed by students, staff, and faculty at the University of North Carolina, *One Act's* bystander intervention model puts a spin on the traditional concept of a bystander intervention program. This program builds off other bystander intervention programs previously discussed (Green Dot, BiTB) by using a community-based framework in which all participants can contribute to preventing sexual violence. Much like *Green Dot* or BiTB, *One Act* places students within a workshop setting with an instructor (usually a graduate assistant) and peer educators. The program is administered in a four-hour session and includes awareness training, empathy building, and role play. The ultimate goals of *One Act* are to dispel rape myths, increase confidence and willingness to be a bystander, and to increase bystander activity by participants (Alegria-Flores, Raker, Pleasants, Weaver, & Weinberger, 2017).

One Act is somewhat different from other classroom/workshop-based methods in terms of cost. While not the easiest to implement given the length and nature of presentation, the One Act curriculum is publicly available for free. This is in stark contrast to many other bystander intervention methods which often provide a "tool kit" (CBIM), or other pre-prepared curricula that must be purchased before being implemented into a population. The cost savings make *One Act* unique in the field of bystander intervention, and thus ripe for future evaluation as to the effectiveness of the training. Due to the program's infancy, there have been few studies evaluating the efficacy of the program. One such study, addressed here, shows a positive effect of *One Act* Training on bystander confidence and willingness to intervene. However, this study showed no change for Rape Myth Acceptance scores and bystander behaviors (Alegria-Flores et al., 2017; see Table 26.1). The authors' comparison of *One Act* with *HAVEN*, an online training program with bystander intervention elements, is an important contribution as few evaluations to date have directly compared bystander programs. [The pros and cons of *HAVEN* will be addressed in a subsequent section.]

Students Challenging Realities and Educating Against Myths (SCREAM) Theater

Another example of an atypical method of bystander intervention is *SCREAM Theater*. *SCREAM Theater* replaces the instructor/pupil, classroom dynamic in favor of an interactive theater program designed to increase knowledge of, and participation in bystander intervention (McMahon, Postmus, Warrener, & Koenick, 2014). The overall target of the intervention is the prevention of sexual violence. *SCREAM Theater* uses theater-style presentation based on evidence supporting the use of interactive means of communication as an effective avenue of delivery for health-related messages (McMahon et al., 2014).

SCREAM Theater can be implemented as one longer session, or as a three-session program (McMahon et al., 2015). The one-session method involves a 75-min skit followed by a shorter question and answer session between participants and audience members. The three-session program includes the aforementioned skit, coupled with two follow-up skill building and brainstorming sessions, allowing for a more in-depth discussion about specific issues the participants experience in their current environment. The majority of studies focused on *SCREAM Theater* have been completed in the university environment among incoming students (McMahon, Allen, et al., 2014; McMahon et al., 2015).

SCREAM Theater analyses have provided positive signs overall. Prior studies have shown significant improvements in intent to engage in bystander behavior and decreased levels of rape myth acceptance (McMahon, Allen, et al., 2014). However, the one versus three-session question is still unanswered. One study indicates that the longer, one-session intervention is at least equally beneficial, while another supports previous findings that additional education results in more positive bystander growth (McMahon et al., 2015). It should be noted that the latter study did not find significantly more bystander behaviors in the group participating in the three-session program (McMahon, Allen, et al., 2014). *SCREAM Theater*, being a relatively new intervention strategy, needs additional study before making any definitive conclusions about the efficacy, but initial results look promising for several of the more widely-studied measures surrounding bystander intervention (see Table 26.1).

InterACT

InterACT Sexual Assault Prevention is a bystander intervention program designed at increasing the social consciousness of participants and influencing attitudes towards bystander intervention as a possibility. Somewhat like *SCREAM Theater*, *InterACT* is a role-playing intervention, with the caveat that *InterACT* is completely unscripted, allowing for, and even encouraging, a substantial amount of improvisation among participants (Storer et al., 2016). The intervention is conducted in two phases: (1) audience members watch performances by trained instructors depicting a variety of behaviors designed to replicate situations where bystander behaviors could be utilized, and (2) audience members subsequently make suggestions for possible actions that could be taken to rectify the situation. One novel component of *InterACT* is the program's engagement of participants by allowing them to act out various scenarios on the stage before the audience (Ahrens, Rich, & Ullman, 2011). One comprehensive evaluation has been conducted on the effectiveness of *InterACT* in a college-aged population, the results of which can be found in Table 26.1. The aforementioned study used surveying to determine whether students who participated in *InterACT* would increase their self-reported likelihood of engaging in bystander intervention over time. Results of this study indicate that participants exhibited a higher likelihood of intervening following participation in *InterACT* (Ahrens et al., 2011). Additional evaluation is needed to determine whether the benefits of *InterACT* participation extend beyond self-reports and appear in reduced levels of violence victimization and perpetration.

Take Care

Take Care is somewhat atypical from other bystander intervention programs in that it involves the use of an online component. Proponents of online intervention strategies cite many potential pros of shifting away, at least partially, from in-class, instructor led curricula. Included among the potential benefits of online intervention are cost-effectiveness, ease of implementation, ability to reach larger population segments, including participants traditionally thought of as difficult to reach, and rapidity of completion compared to in-person trainings (Kleinsasser, Jouriles, McDonald, & Rosenfield, 2015). Additionally, online intervention strategies may bolster participants' feelings that responses will remain confidential, lessening a potential fear of being open and honest in an intervention alongside one's peers. Finally, online interventions have proven effective in combating other societal health problems such as problem drinking (Donovan et al., 2015).

In addition to the novel nature of delivery, the makeup of *Take Care* is somewhat different from other bystander intervention methods we have analyzed. Initially, *Take Care* is delivered individually to students (Kleinsasser et al., 2015). This is opposed to more traditional bystander intervention programs which tend to focus on the grouping of students around a leader/instructor. Additionally, *Take Care* is much shorter in length than many other forms of bystander intervention. *Take Care* can be completed in one 20-min session. Finally, the brevity of the format allows for more targeted outcomes and results. One study used *Take Care* to analyze specific bystander behaviors towards friends, in part due to the perceived influences of one's peers on an individual's behavior (Kleinsasser et al., 2015). This stands in direct opposition to many prior studies which look to a broader spectrum of outcomes (ex: encouraging students to speak out against sexual assault across a college campus) (Kleinsasser et al., 2015).

Take Care is presented via a presentation-design website with three short videos designed to present potential strategies of intervention when one is placed in a situation with the potential of sexual violence (Sargent, Jouriles, Rosenfield, & McDonald, 2017). The intervention focuses on the phrase "Take Care," particularly using the word "care" to summarize how bystander behaviors can focus on "taking care" (Kleinsasser et al., 2015).

C = Show **compassion** for victims or potential victims of sexual assault.
A = Pay **attention** to the situation and whether it could be risky.
R = Take **responsibility** for acting to reduce risk or aid a victim.
E = Take **effective** action.

The intervention concludes by encouraging diligent bystander behavior, again particularly as it pertains to one's friends and acquaintances. The creators of the intervention model focused on the prevalence of sexual assault among acquaintances, believing an educated population to be more effective at curbing the spread of sexual violence in the friend/acquaintance relationship dynamic (Sargent et al., 2017). While evaluation data is limited, *Take Care* has initially proven effective at increasing levels of positive bystander activity. One study showed that the average difference in helpful bystander behavior between students viewing *Take Care* and a control population was equivalent to 0.56 situations per student, translating to 560 additional bystander behaviors among the surveyed population (Sargent et al., 2017). Additional research is needed to investigate the effectiveness of *Take Care* relative to other bystander-based online programs, where outcomes are expanded to include violence, and by other investigators to establish repeatability of findings.

Real Consent

Real Consent is another bystander intervention program hosted entirely online, with a focus of increasing prosocial intervening behaviors that reduce risk for sexual violence and preventing sexually violent behaviors towards women (Salazar, Vivolo-Kantor, Hardin, & Berkowitz, 2014). *Real Consent* consists of six 30-min modules, with various segments within each module. The program includes a web-interactivity element, and episodes of a "serial drama" aimed at modeling behaviors such as intervening in potentially dangerous situations, communication between sexual partners, and obtaining effective and affirmative consent (Salazar et al., 2014). *Real Consent* differs from other bystander program interventions in that it allows for participants to complete the intervention at their own pace (although the intervention recommends completion within 3 weeks). Only one study analyzing *Real Consent* was available at the time of this publication. The results of this evaluation are overwhelmingly positive, with *Real Consent* participants showing increases in bystander confidence levels, increased levels of bystander activity and involvement, decreased rape myth acceptance scores, and lower overall levels of sexual violence and harassment following training (Salazar et al., 2014). Additional analyses to determine repeatability of findings and relative to other promising online bystander-based programs are recommended.

Haven

One of the more well-known online intervention programs is *Haven*. *Haven* is an online course focused on increasing education, awareness, and empowerment to act. Somewhat different from other programs discussed, *Haven* incorporates a discussion about alcohol and the impact alcohol plays on sexual violence. As one might imagine, *Haven* is frequently offered to college-aged participants, often as part of an orientation or introductory program. It should be noted however, that *Haven* content can be altered for older populations, including graduate students, faculty, and staff (cultureofrespect.org, 2016).

Haven is presented through a series of videos, hosted entirely within an online platform. *Haven* is made up of two sessions, the first being approximately 45 min and a second "booster" session lasting approximately 15 min. One recently published evaluation is addressed in this work (Zapp, Buelow, Soutiea, Berkowitz, & DeJong, 2018), in addition to the study by Alegria-Flores and colleagues which focuses on *Haven* as a contrast with another bystander intervention program, One Act, in an effort to compare the effectiveness of the two programs on a similar population (2017). The study conducted by Zapp et al. showed positive increases in bystander confidence levels and for willingness to intervene. However, the same evaluation showed little effect on Rape Myth Acceptance (Zapp et al., 2018). The study conducted by Alegria-Flores showed a moderate improvement in bystander confidence levels for *Haven* participants. When compared with One Act training however, *Haven* was generally less effective at encouraging improved bystander attitudes and increased confidence to intervene.

Like many other online programs, *Haven* is consistently praised for its content delivery and ease of implementation. While overall cost of implementation is not publicly available, *Haven* nonetheless is able to reach large populations and provide consistent program materials in a relatively noninvasive setting (cultureofrespect.org).

Know Your Power

Know Your Power is completely novel in comparison to other bystander intervention programs discussed here. The primary reason for this novelty is the method of distribution. *Know Your Power* utilizes various forms of media, making it somewhat similar to other online programs discussed here. However, *Know Your Power* contains no models similar to *Real Consent* or *Haven*. Instead, *Know Your Power* can be more accurately categorized as a media marketing campaign designed to increase awareness of sexual violence, and to increase the level of bystander behavior focused on reducing the spread of sexual violence (Potter, Moynihan, Stapleton, & Banyard, 2009). Various methods of implementation exist for *Know Your Power*, including a poster campaign like the one present in the study evaluated here which sought to measure changes in attitudes towards sexual violence based on viewing *Know Your* Power posters. Results of this study show that the attitudes of those viewing the poster campaign exhibited higher levels of bystander confidence (Potter et al., 2009). Additionally, more frequent exposure to the program's posters resulted in higher action-stage scale scores compared to those who reported having not seen the poster campaign (Potter et al., 2009).

Methods

Our methods for conducting this evaluation began with an assessment of the previously mentioned review by Storer et al. (2016). We sought to update this review using recently published studies evaluating bystander intervention programs and their overall effectiveness. In order to be included in this review, we set certain exclusion criteria. We excluded qualitative studies, as our focus was primarily on reporting defined figures from program evaluations. Additionally, we excluded two studies on account of their sample size falling below 100 participants. We felt the small sample size could produce results that did not represent the overall effectiveness of a program. We also excluded studies focused on the effects of dating violence, gender-based violence, partner violence, or some combination of the above because the outcome focus of the current review is sexual violence. Finally, we attempted to avoid duplicating the excellent work done by Storer et al. (2016) while still relying on that review as a baseline for our analysis.

Inclusion criteria for this analysis included: (1) studies evaluating an established bystander intervention program, (2) bystander intervention programs focused on a reduction in the spread of sexual violence, (3) the study must have been previously peer reviewed, and (4) published in English. Additionally, to be included in this analysis, at least one of the following outcome measures (preferably multiple) was required and measured before and after program implementation: sexual violence or rape myth acceptance scores, willingness or intent to intervene as an active bystander, active or engaged bystander behaviors, and sexual violence victimization or perpetration experiences training.

Results

Twenty-three publications, representing 12 programs, were selected for this review. The publications' methods and findings are summarized in Table 26.1. Nine of the 12 programs are designed as in-person group setting training programs; 3 (TakeCARE, Haven, RealConsent) were designed to be provided to students using a web-based approach. Approximately half of the studies used an experimental design (11/23 publications; 6/12 programs). Four sets of outcomes were explored for this review. Bystander programming has been hypothesized to (1) increase (prosocial or engaged) bystander behaviors, (2) increase bystander efficacy, intentions to intervene as a bystander, (3) reduce violence acceptance typically measured as rape myth or date rape acceptance, and (4) reduce sexual violence (SV) or sexual harassment (SH) victimization (v) and/or perpetration (p).

An increase in bystander behaviors was noted for seven of nine publications (5 of 7 programs). Among the seven publications based on findings from experimentally designed studies to address bystander behaviors, the majority (86%; 6/7) found bystander training to be associated with an increase in bystander behaviors typically in the short versus longer time frame. Six of seven (86%) experimental studies to address bystander behaviors found that training increased these behaviors while one of two nonexperimental studies found the same pattern.

The question of whether bystander intervention programs actually increase active bystander behavior long-term is still unanswered. For those studies that were analyzed in this review, none showed a significant increase in the amount of bystander behaviors long-term, with many declining to near baseline levels on follow-up. A similar, unclear trend can be seen in the review completed by Storer et al. (2016) where 4 long-term studies showed an increase in bystander behavior, 2 showed no increase, and 3 showed mixed results. It should be noted that two programs (*The Men's Project, The Men's Program*) identified by Storer to have increased bystander activity had no peer reviewed evaluations to analyze in the time since that review's publication. Nonetheless, the reasons behind this failure to increase long-term bystander behavior are unclear. In Elias-Lambert and Black's evaluation of *Bringing in the Bystander*, the authors note that the lack of increased bystander activity is "surprising" (Elias-Lambert & Black, 2016). There, the authors attribute this finding to the novelty of bystander intervention programs designed to reduce sexual violence, stating that the message may be something participants are not used to hearing, thus requiring longer, more intensive interventions (Elias-Lambert & Black, 2016). This proposed reasoning seems to contrast with findings from others that rape myth acceptance scores consistently decrease with implementation across multiple programs. Perhaps the explanation for "surprising" findings may be that changing bystander actions based in part on the frequency of intervention opportunities (potentially violent events observed by the trained student) may be more difficult to achieve than inspiring a change of attitudes. Currently evaluated bystander intervention programs do a good job changing the notion of violence acceptance. However, changing bystander actions and ultimately violence rates within a community may require changes in training, with a particular emphasis on skill-building focused on changing students' efficacy to take action, especially when particularly violent events are observed.

Measures of self-perceived bystander efficacy or intentions to actively engage others or otherwise intervene were included for 16 of the 23 publications (10 of the 12 programs). The majority of publications (14/16; 88%) and programs (9/10; 90%) noted intervention training to be associated with increases in bystander intentions or efficacy in the shorter term (≤6 months). All eight of the nonexperimental studies to address bystander intentions or efficacy found an increased associated with program training while 75%, 6 of 8, of the experimental studies found this association.

These summarized findings suggest that bystander intervention programs tend succeed when attempting to improve confidence levels about potentially becoming an active bystander. Of the studies that sought to explore the levels of confidence among bystander intervention participants, only Coaching Boys into Men showed anything other than uniformly positive results. In fact, CBIM showed positive effects in participant confidence shortly after the culmination of the program. However, this number declined back to baseline in a later follow-up. The improvement in confidence cannot be tied to one particular aspect of a bystander intervention program, yet successful programs incorporate role-play into the program curriculum. Given the age of the target populations, this training may be the first time students have been in a situation when a bystander intervention could be useful. Being able to "practice" what one would do in such a situation could boost confidence levels should that person be placed into a real life situation where intervention becomes necessary. Feeling unequipped to help in a situation is not only relevant in bystander education, but is also a major barrier to intervening in real life (Banyard, 2015). Additionally, peer influences may impact confidence when intervening in a potentially dangerous situation; this experience may in turn instill confidence in another person witnessing these actions (Banyard, 2015). Trained students and those witnessing effective interventions may find it easier to engage in active bystanding when they see others model these behaviors (Banyard, 2015).

Findings regarding whether bystander programs change violence acceptance are more mixed. The majority of reviewed publications (n = 17) and programs (n = 11) addressed program-associated changes in violence acceptance, typically measured using a rape myth acceptance scale. A more modest majority of publications (10/17; 59%) and programs (7/11; 64%) that addressed this outcome did find that bystander programs were associated with reductions in violence acceptance scores over time.

The ultimate measure of a violence prevention program's effectiveness is reducing violence used (perpetration) or experienced (victimization). However, sufficient post-intervention implementation time is required to begin to see changes in violence rates among those receiving training and for those within the social network of trained students. The latter group may be the more likely beneficiary of an engaged bystander program because effective bystander actions will likely reduce violence risk for those whom the trained students know or with whom the student has contact. Further, a reduction in violence perpetration may be a more salient outcome indicating bystander program efficacy than violence victimization. Eight reviewed publications representing four programs had data to address these outcomes. Findings from six of eight publications and all four of the programs indicate that bystander programs reduced sexual violence perpetration (or victimization) over time. Violence perpetration was often measured through self-reporting in combination with an analysis of school records detailing reported violence (Coker et al., 2017). While additional research is needed to determine the exact effects bystander intervention programs play on overall violence rates by type of violence, sexual coercion rates have shown impressive declines, possibly mitigated by length of program (Gidycz et al., 2011; Salazar et al., 2014).

Suggestions for Future Research

The results of this analysis suggest three primary avenues ripe for future research. The first of these is a comparison of program length and number of sessions to determine overall effectiveness over time, with an emphasis on programs with multiple "dose" iterations. Jouriles, Krauss, Vu, Banyard, and McDonald (2018) have contributed a great deal to a similar body of research, focused on program duration and effectiveness. The results of their work show that individual program length (ex: 20 min vs. 40 min, etc.) is directly correlated with larger effects on attitudes and beliefs, but the same result cannot be shown for behavior (Jouriles et al., 2018). However, there is still progress to be made in determining whether an implementation over a period of time (ex: CBIM intervention spread over 11 weeks) encourages longstanding change in bystander behavior.

Several of the bystander intervention programs analyzed featured models with varying lengths. For example, *Bringing in the Bystander* can be offered in either a 90 min model or a longer, more intensive 4.5 h model. Similarly, *SCREAM Theater* can be offered in a one-dose format, or in three doses. Given the mixed findings on the number of program sessions or doses needed to establish program effectiveness, additional research is needed to determine the minimum program dose needed to reach the desired effect across intermediate outcomes such as changes in violence acceptance and bystander behaviors and for the ultimate outcome of reducing violence rates. With additional programs offering multiple variations in length and number of sessions, studies are needed to determine the best use of intervention time in a way that the most participants are impacted in a wide-reaching, longitudinal manner.

A second suggestion for future research falls in the evaluation of program type. As was previously mentioned, online intervention models are becoming increasingly popular with the rise of programs such as *Take Care*. The initial outcomes appear positive, but the methodology is still nascent compared to the in-person bystander intervention model. As such, future evaluations should address the effectiveness of online intervention compared to in-person intervention, accounting for factors such as cost of implementation and ability to reach the largest pool of participants, in addition to the traditionally studied effectiveness of the models. If online intervention can be proven to be as effective as in-person intervention, institutions may be able to reach increasing numbers of participants in an effective manner, resulting in a larger, more educated population overall. Additionally, due to the (traditionally) decreased cost of online interventions, institutions may be able to reduce expenses, allowing for other methods of support (rape crisis programs, survivor support systems, etc.) to be more effectively funded.

Finally, the effect of bystander intervention at younger ages should be increasingly investigated. As mentioned above, there is some evidence of bystander intervention programs being implemented to participants prior to reaching the traditional, high-school age level during which bystander intervention programs are so prevalent (Midgett et al., 2015). An increased application of bystander intervention to younger participants may allow for earlier intervention with an emphasis on education and potential actions that can be taken in the future. Additionally, adapting bystander intervention to younger populations could increase the level of peer support and peer influence in potentially dangerous situations that may arise as a population ages. Given the malleability of the adolescent mind, interventions at younger ages could prove incredibly effective at curbing the spread of sexual violence before it begins.

Conclusion

In less than a decade, evidence for the promise of engaged or active bystander intervention programming to address the epidemic of sexual violence has emerged (Degue et al., 2014; Storer et al., 2016). The majority of studies find that bystander programs reduce sexual violence acceptance and increase willingness and intentions to actively engage in violence prevention actions. Additional rigorously controlled research is needed to determine the effectiveness of programs to increase positive bystander behaviors and to reduce sexual violence and sexual harassment rates over time and among those exposed to bystander programming. Measuring bystander behaviors is not straightforward. The opportunity to be an effective bystander is dependent on (1) the frequency (and severity) of violence within one's peer network, (2) one's ability to recognize a violence intervention opportunity, (3) one's confidence and skill in effectively intervening before (proactive bystander) or after (reactive bystander) a violent event, and *for evaluation purposes* (4) one's ability to recall and report bystander behaviors. Given these contingencies in bystander measurement, additional attention to advancements in measurement of bystander behaviors and perceived effectiveness is suggested. Because the Clery Act recommends bystander training on all campuses receiving Title IX funding, comparative effectiveness research is needed to determine the more effective elements of bystander training needed to reduce sexual violence. Such research needs to be rigorous, sufficiently powered, and should include measures of sexual violence perpetration and victimization as the ultimate outcomes toward the goal of reducing the epidemic of sexual violence and its trauma-associated mental and physical health consequences.

References

Ahrens, C. E., Rich, M. D., & Ullman, J. B. (2011). Rehearsing for real life: The impact of the InterACT sexual assault prevention program on self-reported likelihood of engaging in bystander interventions. *Violence Against Women, 17*(6), 760–776. https://doi.org/10.1177/1077801211410212

Alegria-Flores, K., Raker, K., Pleasants, R. K., Weaver, M. A., & Weinberger, M. (2017). Preventing interpersonal violence on college campuses: The effect of one act training on bystander intervention. *Journal of Interpersonal Violence, 32*(7), 1103–1126. https://doi.org/10.1177/0886260515587666

Banyard, V. L. (2015). *Toward the next generation of bystander prevention of sexual and relationship violence: Action coils to engage communities* (Springer Briefs in Criminology). Cham: Springer. https://doi.org/10.1007/978-3-319-23171-6

Banyard, V. L., Eckstein, R. P., & Moynihan, M. M. (2010). Sexual violence prevention: The role of stages of change. *Journal of Interpersonal Violence, 25*(1), 111–135. https://doi.org/10.1177/0886260508329123

Banyard, V. L., Moynihan, M. M., & Crossman, M. T. (2009). Reducing sexual violence on campus: The role of student leaders as empowered bystanders. *Journal of College Student Development, 50*(4), 446–457. https://doi.org/10.1353/csd.0.0083

Banyard, V. L., Moynihan, M. M., & Plante, E. G. (2007). Sexual violence prevention through bystander education: An experimental evaluation. *Journal of Community Psychology, 35*(4), 463–481. https://doi.org/10.1002/jcop.20159

Cares, A. C., Banyard, V. L., Moynihan, M. M., Williams, L. M., Potter, S. J., & Stapleton, J. G. (2015). Changing attitudes about being a bystander to violence: Translating an in-person sexual violence prevention program to a new campus. *Violence Against Women, 21*(2), 165–187. https://doi.org/10.1177/1077801214564681

Coker, A. L., Bush, H. M., Brancato, C. J., Clear, E. R., & Recktenwald, E. A. (2018). Bystander program effectiveness to reduce violence acceptance: RCT in high schools. *Journal of Family Violence. 02 April, 2018*, 1–12. https://doi.org/10.1007/s10896-018-9961-8

Coker, A. L., Bush, H. M., Cook-Craig, P. G., DeGue, S. A., Clear, E. R., Brancato, C. J., … Recktenwald, E. A. (2017). RCT testing bystander effectiveness to reduce violence. *American Journal of Preventive Medicine, 52*(5), 566–578. https://doi.org/10.1016/j.amepre.2017.01.020

Coker, A. L., Bush, H. M., Fisher, B. S., Swan, S. C., Williams, C. M., Clear, E. R., & DeGue, S. (2016). Multi-college bystander intervention evaluation for violence prevention. *American Journal of Preventive Medicine, 50*(3), 295–302. https://doi.org/10.1016/j.amepre.2015.08.034

Coker, A. L., Cook-Craig, P. G., Williams, C. M., Fisher, B. S., Clear, E. R., Garcia, L. S., & Hegge, L. M. (2011). Evaluation of Green dot: An active bystander intervention to reduce sexual violence on college campuses. *Violence Against Women, 17*(6), 777–796. https://doi.org/10.1177/1077801211410264

Coker, A. L., Fisher, B. S., Bush, H. M., Swan, S. C., Williams, C. M., Clear, E. R., & DeGue, S. (2015). Evaluation of the Green dot bystander intervention to reduce interpersonal violence among college students across three campuses. *Violence Against Women, 21*(12), 1507–1527. https://doi.org/10.1177/1077801214545284

Cook-Craig, P. G., Millspaugh, P. H., Recktenwald, E. A., Kelly, N. C., Hegge, L. M., Coker, A. L., & Pletcher, T. S. (2014). From empower to Green dot: Successful strategies and lessons learned in developing comprehensive sexual violence primary prevention programming. *Violence Against Women, 20*(10), 1162–1178. https://doi.org/10.1177/1077801214551286

Cultureofrespect.org. (2016). Cultureofrespect.org.

DeGue, S., Valle, L. A., Holt, M. K., Massetti, G. M., Matjasko, J. L., & Tharp, A. T. (2014). A systematic review of primary prevention strategies for sexual violence perpetration. *Aggression and Violent Behavior, 19*(4), 346–362. https://doi.org/10.1016/j.avb.2014.05.004

Donovan, E., Mahapatra, P. D., Green, T. C., Chiauzzi, E., McHugh, K., & Hemm, A. (2015). Efficacy of an online intervention to reduce alcohol-related risks among community college students. *Addiction Research & Theory, 23*(5), 437–447. https://doi.org/10.3109/16066359.2015.1043625

Elias-Lambert, N., & Black, B. M. (2016). Bystander sexual violence prevention program: Outcomes for high and low risk university men. *Journal of Interpersonal Violence, 31*(19), 3211–3235. https://doi.org/10.1177/0886260515584346

Foubert, J. D., Langhinrichsen-Rohling, J., Brasfield, H., & Hill, B. (2010). Effects of a rape awareness program on college women: Increasing bystander efficacy and willingness to intervene. *Journal of Community Psychology, 38*(7), 813–827. https://doi.org/10.1002/jcop.20397

Gidycz, C. A., Orchowski, L. M., & Berkowitz, A. D. (2011). Preventing sexual aggression among college men: An evaluation of a social norms and bystander intervention program. *Violence Against Women, 17*(6), 720–742. https://doi.org/10.1177/1077801211409727

Jaime, M. D., Stocking, M., Freire, K., Perkinson, L., Ciaravino, S., & Miller, E. (2016). Using a domestic and sexual violence prevention advocate to implement a dating violence prevention program with athletes. *Health Education Research, 31*(6), 679–696. https://doi.org/10.1093/her/cyw045

Jouriles, E. N., Krauss, A., Vu, N. L., Banyard, V. L., & McDonald, R. (2018). Bystander programs addressing sexual violence on college campuses: A systematic review and meta-analysis of program outcomes and delivery methods. *Journal of American College Health, 09 March, 2018*, 1–10. https://doi.org/10.1080/07448481.2018.1431906

Katz, J., Heisterkamp, H. A., & Fleming, W. M. (2011). The social justice roots of the mentors in violence prevention model and its application in a high school setting. *Violence Against Women, 17*(6), 684–702. https://doi.org/10.1177/1077801211409725

Kleinsasser, A., Jouriles, E. N., McDonald, R., & Rosenfield, D. (2015). An online bystander Intervetion program for the prevention of sexual violence. *Psychology of Violence, 5*(3), 227–235. https://doi.org/10.1037/a0037393

Langhinrichsen-Rohling, J., Foubert, J. D., Brasfield, H. M., Hill, B., & Shelley-Tremblay, S. (2011). The Men's program: Does it impact college Men's self-reported bystander efficacy and willingness to intervene? *Violence Against Women, 17*(6), 743–759. https://doi.org/10.1177/1077801211409728

Latané, B., & Rodin, J. (1969). A lady in distress: Inhibiting effects of friends and strangers on bystander intervention. *Journal of Experimental Social Psychology, 5*, 189–202.

McMahon, S., Allen, C. T., Postmus, J. L., McMahon, S. M., Peterson, N. A., & Hoffman, M. L. (2014). Measuring bystander attitudes and behavior to prevent sexual violence. *Journal of American College Health, 62*(1), 58–66. https://doi.org/10.1080/07448481.2013.849258

McMahon, S., Postmus, J. L., Warrener, C., & Koenick, R. A. (2014). Utilizing peer education theater for the primary prevention of sexual violence on college campuses. *Journal of College Student Development, 55*(1), 78–85. https://doi.org/10.1353/csd.2014.0001

McMahon, S., Winter, S. C., Palmer, J. E., Postmus, J. L., Peterson, N. A., Zucker, S., & Koenick, R. (2015). A randomized controlled trial of a multi-dose bystander intervention program using peer education theater. *Heather Education Research, 30*(4), 554–568. https://doi.org/10.1093/her/cyv022

Midgett, A., Doumas, D., Sears, D., Lunquist, A., & Hausheer, R. (2015). A bystander bullying Psychoeducation program with middle school students: A preliminary report. *The Progessional Counselor, 5*(4), 486–500. https://doi.org/10.15241/am.5.4.486

Miller, E., Tancredi, D. J., McCauley, H. L., Decker, M. R., Virata, M. C. D., Anderson, H. A., … Silverman, J. G. (2013). One-year follow-up of a coach-delivered dating violence prevention program: A cluster randomized controlled trial. *American Journal of Preventive Medicine, 45*(1), 108–112. https://doi.org/10.1016/j.amepre.2013.03.007

Miller, E., Tancredi, D. J., McCauley, H. L., Decker, M. R., Virata, M. D., Anderson, H. A., … Silverman, J. G. (2012). "coaching boys into men": A cluster-randomized controlled trial of a dating violence prevention program. *Journal of Adolescent Health, 51*(5), 431–438. https://doi.org/10.1016/j.jadohealth.2012.01.018

Moynihan, M. M., Banyard, V. L., Arnold, J. S., Eckstein, R. P., & Stapleton, J. G. (2010). Engaging intercollegiate athletes in preventing and intervening in sexual and intimate partner violence. *Journal of American College Health, 59*(3), 197–204. https://doi.org/10.1080/07448481.2010.502195

Moynihan, M. M., Banyard, V. L., Cares, A. C., Potter, S. J., Williams, L. M., & Stapleton, J. G. (2015). Encouraging responses in sexual and relationship violence prevention: What program effects remain 1 year later. *Journal of Interpersonal Violence, 30*(1), 110–132. https://doi.org/10.1177/0886260514532719

Potter, S. J., Moynihan, M. M., Stapleton, J. G., & Banyard, V. L. (2009). Empowering bystanders to prevent campus violence against women. *Violence Against Women, 15*(1), 106–121. https://doi.org/10.1177/1077801208327482

Salazar, L. F., Vivolo-Kantor, A., Hardin, J., & Berkowitz, A. (2014). A web-based sexual violence bystander intervention for male college students: Randomized controlled trial. *Journal of Medical Internet Research, 16*(9), e203. https://doi.org/10.2196/jmir.3426

Sargent, K. S., Jouriles, E. N., Rosenfield, D., & McDonald, R. (2017). A high school-based evaluation of TakeCARE, a video bystander program to prevent adolescent relationship violence. *Journal of Youth and Adolescence, 46*(3), 633–643. https://doi.org/10.1007/s10964-016-0622-z

Storer, H. L., Casey, E., & Herrenkohl, T. (2016). Efficacy of bystander programs to prevent dating abuse among youth and young adults: A review of the literature. *Trauma, Violence, and Abuse, 17*(3), 256–269. https://doi.org/10.1177/1524838015584361

Williams, C. M., Cook-Craig, P. G., Bush, H. M., Clear, E. R., Lewis, A. M., Garcia, L. S., … Fisher, B. S. (2014). Victimization and perpetration of unwanted sexual activities among high school students: Frequency and correlates. *Violence Against Women, 20*(10), 1239–1257. https://doi.org/10.1177/1077801214551575

Zapp, D., Buelow, R., Soutiea, L., Berkowitz, A., & DeJong, W. (2018). Exploring the potential campus-level impact of online universal sexual assault prevention education. *Journal of Interpersonal Violence, 26*, 1–22. https://doi.org/10.1177/0886260518762449

The Use of Humor as an Effective Tool in Sexual Violence Prevention Education

27

Gail Stern

"You may have the facts, but you can't tell me how to feel".

—Male Lyft driver speaking to the author, on the subject of false reports of rape.

As a sexual assault prevention educator for over 25 years, I can say confidently that nearly all of the conversations I have had about rape (whether formal or informal) have been emotionally fraught. The very nature of the topic seems to implicate my listeners—whether students at college orientation or my seatmate on a plane—as either a potential offender or victim. As a result, the stakes for each conversation feel very high. It is less a debate over facts than a fierce protection of identity, and the traditional skill-set of a sexual assault prevention teacher or trainer is ill suited for the intensity of this educational task. This chapter identifies a novel way to have this critical, educational discussion: the use of humor to reduce the emotional and cognitive resistance to the subject of rape. As unlikely a pairing of subject matter and pedagogical style it may be, my research and professional experience shows how well-trained teachers, with a strongly formulated theoretical foundation in both the sexual violence prevention literature and in comedy, have incorporated the use of humor as a key pedagogical strategy in educating about rape.

I strongly believe in this nontraditional approach to sexual violence prevention education for two key reasons. In addition to my aforementioned decades in this field, I have also worked as a stand-up and improvisational comedian. I have utilized my comedy experience to craft presentations for community members, university students, military audiences, and law enforcement professionals. I have found no quicker way to build connections with audiences and translate information into ways in which they can truly hear it, than the tactical, thoughtful use of humor. I have applied my know-how to co-developing the rape prevention program, *Sex Signals* (http://www.catharsisproductions.com/programs/sex-signals). This program is presented nearly 2000 times each year for military and civilian audiences and has reached over 1 million people since 2000. This program is delivered by a cadre of educators that receives extensive training in subject matter related to sexual violence, as well as how to use humor strategically with their audiences. These experiences contributed to my desire to conduct the research upon which this chapter is based. While my dissertation study in the field of Curriculum and Instruction focused on a range of applications for the use of humor, this chapter focuses solely on its strategic importance for sexual assault prevention educators in managing the emotional and cognitive resistance of their audiences. While our programs' use of humor has not been studied as an isolated factor in contributing to positive outcomes, the data from Catharsis Productions' five-year relationship with Naval Training Center-Great Lakes is very promising.

G. Stern (✉)
Catharsis Productions, Chicago, IL, USA
e-mail: gail@catharsisproductions.com

W. T. O'Donohue and P. A. Schewe (eds.), *Handbook of Sexual Assault and Sexual Assault Prevention*,
https://doi.org/10.1007/978-3-030-23645-8_27

> As congressional staff and policymakers on Capitol Hill often say, "metrics matter", and according to the Navy's Sexual Assault Prevention and Response Office; Catharsis Production's program has, for example, contributed to a 73 percent reduction in anonymous reports of sexual assault at Great Lakes Naval Base north of Chicago. (Neiweem, 2017).

As I mentioned in my introduction, conversations about sexual violence are emotionally charged. With the aid of the Internet, we are able to "listen" in on the thoughts and even dialogues of some men processing their confusion in real time. In a reddit thread from November 2017 labeled "reactions to metoo," redditors wrestled with the issue while responding to an original post that stated;

> What I'm learning from all of this is that before you even get to the rape part of it, it doesn't take much to be a sexual predator when the norms are structured this way. Maybe it's because I never get laid and I always seem to ask women out the wrong way, but I can never tell the difference between flirtatious shyness and being too scared or passive to give a hard, affirmative no. I've wound up on the bad end of a woman's anger too many times when I've tried flirting with them and I'm wondering what I'm doing wrong.

The dialogue that followed further illustrated the confusion other individuals felt when confronting the issue:

> JackBinimbul
> 17 points·7 months ago
> At the end of the day, the fact that most women *feel* sexually pressured is a problem. But I'd argue that a huge number of men do as well and in many cases, the other person meant no harm. That doesn't mean that we shouldn't analyze why so many women consistently report these feelings or the environments that make them feel this way. But lets not start calling normal, respectful men "sexual predators", mmkay?
> Xzillerationer
> 11 points·7 months ago
> I understand where he's coming from, though. That's how he *perceives* it. If you don't have any experience in that field, it's really, really easy to be super insecure about where that "line" is and be so afraid of crossing it you never go near it in fear of being labelled a sexual predator.
> JackBinimbul
> 8 points·7 months ago
> I could see that mind frame, I suppose. But it's really concerning that someone would feel this way. That's a long path of self flagellation, shame and isolation. I really hope that we can find a middle ground.
> Xzillerationer
> 9 points·7 months ago
> I agree. It's really indicative about not enough resources for men telling them what's okay, only a huge amount telling them what's *not* okay. While we shouldn't reduce the amount telling us what's not okay, we really should have some resources telling men what's okay to do, how to ask someone out on a date, etc. etc. (redditors et al., 2017).

The dialogue above illustrates how conflicted our culture can be about acts of rape and sexual harassment—particularly when the perpetrator is not a stranger to the victim—and how defensive (and fearful) many still are about admitting those crimes exist, and whether or not they have ever accidentally crossed the line themselves. The comments are also indicative of the increasing need for better, clearer dialogue as to what "unwanted sexual contact" of any kind means, and what it means to hold individuals accountable for their actions. We will not be able to be effective preventionists if we fail to address the emotional context for the content we cover.

Identifying the Role(s) of Humor

Theories about the role and impact of humor cross academic disciplines, but I argue that those most relevant to increasing educator effectiveness come from the domains of education, persuasion, and psychology. While none of the research cited speaks directly to the use of humor to respond to issues of sexual violence, much can be extrapolated from what it does say about humor's usefulness in and outside of the traditional classroom setting.

Twentieth century scholarship on the physiological effects of laughter has shown that the cliché is true: Laughter is the "best medicine," in that it reduces anxiety and stress, and that those able to laugh at themselves are emotionally healthy people (Askenasy, 1987; Piddington, 1963; Szabo, 2003; Wrench & McCroskey, 2001). The benefit of tension reduction is confirmed by education researchers who have documented the increased effectiveness of teachers who use humor in the classroom. Citing the ability of teachers to create more positive learning environments for students, students report that when their teachers use humor that tension is decreased, which makes it easier for them to participate in class. As a result, students retain more content, and are more likely to use the information outside of the classroom (Nussbaum, 1992; White, 2001). This is particularly relevant to sexual assault prevention education; the discussion is successful when more students participate, and more students participate when the teacher is perceived as less judgmental (Hess, 2004).

The concept of identification encapsulates several effects of humor, including providing the relief of discomfort or tension. Theorists argue that tension is relieved through the use of humor as the audience identifies with the person using it, reducing the gap that exists between them. Speaker and audience are felt to occupy the same dialogic footing, and intimacy is deepened (Meyer, 2000). The relief theory of humor assumes that in part, people laugh when they perceive that tension has been reduced (Berlyne, 1972; Morreall, 1983; Shurcliff, 1968; as cited in Meyer, 2000), or when they are expressing relief at having consciously or subconsciously overcome a sociocultural inhibition (Freud, 1960; Schaeffer, 1981, as cited in Meyer, 2000). This is critical if a teacher is to have a candid conversation about any issue, let alone the "taboo topics" related to sex, gender, and sexual violence where there is often a sense that being honest about one's beliefs is forbidden.

Humor also plays a key role in the students feeling immediacy from their instructors. Teacher immediacy has been defined as,

> …those nonverbal behaviors that reduce physical and/or psychological distance between teachers and students (Andersen, 1979, p. 543).

Importantly, students who perceive greater immediacy from their teachers have been shown to take more risks in class, believing that they will not receive extreme punishment if they misspeak, or make other kinds of mistakes (Tauber & Mester, 1994; Rosiek, 2003). There is educational research that shows humor's role in decreasing anxiety and stress in the receiver (see Korobkin, 1988; Kher, Molstad, & Donahue, 1999; Szabo, 2003). With respect to teaching taboo topics, reducing apprehension is a key objective if one is to engage students in a candid discussion. When there is a reduction of stress, the learning environment becomes a safer one, increasing the teacher's ability to construct more positive frameworks for discussion about the volatile issue. Rosiek asserts that learning is an emotional experience, as it goes beyond the mere comprehension of abstract content; it is fundamentally about how the student locates herself in relation to new ideas. He stated,

> It involves surprise, revelation, delight, and sometimes outrage. It requires the cultivation of felt appreciations. It sometimes involves risking exposure, humiliation, or changes in beliefs that give us comfort. When education has happened well, we do not simply emerge knowing the world; we also come to love, resent, endure, care, and be thrilled about things in ways we did not before. (Rosiek, 2003, p. 399).

It follows that students will learn more from teachers who are better able to frame the issues being studied in ways that take into account students' potentially heightened emotional reactions to material (Vangelisti, Daly, & Friedrich, 1999). It is significant that studies of receiver apprehension, "the fear of misinterpreting, inadequately processing, and/or not being able to adjust psychologically to messages sent by others," (Chesbro & McCroskey, 2001, p. 59) have shown it to be a significant obstacle in student learning. Researchers found that apprehensive receivers actually listen in different ways from those who don't experience this condition. Wheeless, Preiss, and Gayle (1997) describe three theories about the causes and origins of receiver apprehension:

> The first holds that receiver apprehension occurs as a situational fear of encountering new information. The second explanation relates to an individual's ability to assimilate (McReynolds, 1976) incoming information in terms of that individual's cognitive complexity (Beatty, 2009; Beatty & Payne, 1981). Individuals with less cognitive complexity are likely to have greater difficulty assimilating incoming information, and therefore are likely to be

> apprehensive receivers. A third component of receiver apprehension is based on the use of interpretive schemes or strategic repertoires to respond to incoming messages (Delia, O'Keefe, & O'Keefe, 1982). Thus, a lack of schemata to process messages may lead a receiver to experience apprehension out of a fear of misinterpreting or inadequately processing messages. (Cited in Chesebro & McCroskey, 1998, p. 446).

In the same research study, they determined that teachers who were able to show greater immediacy with students, as well as an ability to clarify the material, were best able to reduce receiver apprehension (Chesebro & McCroskey, 1998, p. 446). This finding is reinforced by the results of a 2004 study of 124 undergraduates and three instructors from the disciplines of biology, educational psychology, and theatre, respectively. When researchers Torok, McMorris, and Lin asked participants about potential outcomes of using humor in the classroom, students responded that humor had the power to increase teachers' likeability, enhance their understanding of the course material, lower classroom tension, increase student attentiveness, and boost the class' morale (Torok, McMoris, & Lin, 2004).

Research in the realm of psychology confirms that it is psychologically and emotionally difficult for many people to have their beliefs, whether about the world or themselves, challenged. While the psychology literature uses the word "patient," both in the individual and group settings, an argument can be made that some of the same principles may apply to students experiencing sexual assault prevention education.

In Killinger's article, *Humor in Psychotherapy: A Shift to a New Perspective*, she stated,

> Humor seems best described as an interactive personal experience that occurs between client and therapist. Its potential lies in its utilization as a tool to enable people to view their problems from a new perspective. As Rosenheim (1974) suggests, humor serves to broaden clients' self-awareness by improving their ability to view themselves and others more objectively and to develop fuller affective reactions… The element of surprise in humor, coupled with its unpremeditated quality, encourages a progressive shift in focus. This shift may then serve to unlock or loosen the rigid, repetitive view that individuals often hold regarding their particular situation. (Killinger, 1987, p. 30).

Similarly, Farrelly and Brandsma (1974) argued,

> Humor is compelling and influential. It has impact. It changes people's minds. We suspect its compelling quality comes from the deeply paradoxical nature of our existence; people are more suggestible and compliant during the orgasm of laughter. (as cited in Farrelly & Lynch, 1987, p. 89).

A March 2011 article in *Mother Jones* Magazine featured research that drew additional important connections between emotion and cognition, citing the theory of "motivated reasoning,"

> The theory of motivated reasoning builds on a key insight of modern neuroscience (Damasio, 1994). Reasoning is actually suffused with emotion (or what researchers often call "affect"). Not only are the two inseparable, but our positive or negative feelings about people, things, and ideas arise much more rapidly than our conscious thoughts, in a matter of milliseconds—fast enough to detect with an EEG device, but long before we're aware of it. That shouldn't be surprising: Evolution required us to react very quickly to stimuli in our environment. It's a "basic human survival skill," explains political scientist Arthur Lupia of the University of Michigan. We push threatening information away; we pull friendly information close. We apply fight-or-flight reflexes not only to predators, but to data itself. (Mooney, 2011. *Mother Jones*. Retrieved from http://motherjones.com/politics/2011/03/denial-science-chris-mooney).

This may help explain some of the reasons individuals resist the data with regard to rape. Kahan (2007) finds that while presenting information directly can result in a "backfire" effect, that one can be more successful presenting the evidence in "a context that doesn't trigger a defensive, emotional reaction" (Mooney, 2011). As has already been established, humor, when used effectively, can help build a context that can minimize the defensiveness of the subject matter.

Recent research has focused on the effects of humor incorporated into a persuasive health message, specifically on individuals high in masculinity. Conway & Dubé (2016) evaluated the use of humor in persuasion on threatening topics. They stated,

> For high-masculinity individuals, there are many features of humor appeals that are congruent with their distress-avoidant response to threat. According to theories of humor (Speck, 1991; Wyer & Collins, 1992), most humor appeals involve incongruency, bringing together frames that one would not normally expect. Incongruency is resolved by reinterpreting the original frames, diminishing the value or importance of the inferred features of one or more referents (Wyer & Collins, 1992). In this manner, there is an arousal-safety process (Speck, 1991) whereby a threat is identified followed by some playful safety signal. The playful reaction to threat and the diminishment of importance arising from the humoristic resolution of the appeal's incongruency are consistent in affective tone with a distress schema that encompasses distress avoidance as a response to threat. Research supports the view that humor may serve to avoid distress (p. 865).

Their studies found that in fact, both men and women scoring high in masculinity demonstrated an increased intention to adopt the behaviors promoted—sunscreen application and condom use, respectively—when humor was incorporated into the messaging (Conway & Dubé, 2016). The use of humor helped diminish the threat the content posed to the receiver and removed it as an obstacle to behavioral change.

The aforementioned research highlights the emotional component of cognition; if the individual is not emotionally ready to receive the new ideas, or fearful of what those ideas represent, they will not be able to process them intellectually. In the context of sexual assault prevention education, this is especially critical. Much of the material may be perceived as inherently confrontational; as demonstrated earlier by the online conversation between redditors, this topic has many men worried about how their past and future behaviors might be labeled as illegal and wrong. Preventionists must build a closeness with their students while still providing enough distance between them and the subject matter so that effective information processing is possible. This challenging objective can be achieved through the intentional use of humor.

Carlson asserted that the comic frame provided enough distance for the audience to both see the fool and the fool's mistakes, and then later see the ways in which they have been and could be that same fool (Smith & Voth, 2002). In this way the teacher using humor to teach about social-justice issues both can issue the harsh truths while being perceived as more nonthreatening had they done so without humor. There is a sense that the audience doesn't feel judged or defensive, and that all present are there to confront some greater human frailty.

This is a necessary condition for students in the classroom when challenged about their beliefs; there may be realizations they want to come to, but no one has given them the safe space to figure it out. Humor may not only allow faces to be saved but also give students permission to admit a different view into their conceptualization of an issue. In writing about the usefulness of sophistic humor, humor that posits the incongruous to make a point, Wright (2000) argues, "Psychological barriers to social change represent rhetorical challenges. The critic hoping to contribute to social change must uncover discursive strategies for overcoming psychological barriers. Ideally, those strategies must be teachable to students or clients for academic critics to make positive contributions to the public sphere" (2000, p. 57). In this way, a nonstranger rape prevention educator can address an audience's indirect or direct endorsement of rape myths and rape culture in ways that are not only less-threatening but also induce recognition—an "aha" moment—in their audience.

When Humor Is Applied to Sexual Assault Prevention Education

My dissertation research in Curriculum and Instruction focused on the ways in which a cadre of 17 educators from my own company, Catharsis Productions, conceptualized the ways in which they strategically utilized humor in teaching our nonstranger rape prevention program, *Sex Signals*. *Sex Signals* is primarily scripted to ensure the consistency of the educational content. The content is driven by best practices in the sexual assault prevention field and is updated based on the latest peer-reviewed research on sexual violence. While humorous moments are written into the program, much of the comedy comes from what the individual educators contribute not only to their "scripted" characters but also to the improvisational components and in the facilitated discussions with the audience. For my dissertation study, I conducted one- to two-hour interviews of each educator, in an effort to both identify consistent applications of humor as well as illustrate the broad range of tactics utilized. I have included the following examples of my findings to provide the reader with a clearer sense of the role humor plays in the prevention educator toolkit.

The educators conceptualized their primary use of humor, by an almost 2–1 margin, as the decreasing of emotional resistance, i.e., the audience's emotional reaction to the subject matter, as opposed to its use in responding to cognitive resistance, i.e., the actual substance of arguments related to their understanding of rape. This was not because they determined that cognitive resistance was of secondary importance, but that the educators identified that unless the significant emotional resistance was reduced, that none of the ideas would permeate and affect the consciousness of their audience/class. Furthermore, they identified the role of humor in making them likable as a key advantage in getting tough ideas across. This is consistent with the research on the function of humor as a component of immediacy (Witt, Wheeless, & Allen, 2004). As teachers, they felt the scripted curriculum, for the most part, carried the content of their ideas, and that it was their role to ensure that content got through. While they didn't use the phrase, "I use humor to establish immediacy with my audiences," I believe the substance of their statements establishes that as their objective.

The presenters identified key ways in which the curriculum enabled them to decrease the emotional resistance of their audiences. It provided multiple opportunities early on to challenge audience perceptions as to the nature and tone of the program, using humor to both recalibrate expectations and engender trust.

The very beginning of *Sex Signals* is structured to provide as many low-cost opportunities for the audience to interact with the educators. The intent is that these moments will set the tone for the program, specifically that the students will play an active role in the dialogue and that they will not be shamed for participating. One of those first opportunities is an improvised scene, which is consistently the source of the first big laughs the educators receive while delivering the program. It is often the point where most of our educators feel they can really establish a positive connection with the audience. This requires the male educator ask the audience members for "pick-up lines," in order for him to begin improvising a scene where his character meets the female educator's character, for the first time. This give-and-take between educator and audience establishes a positive back-and-forth relationship between educator, audience, and the material itself. Throughout that first scene, each educator turns out to the audience to ask for suggestions for further actions. These actions reinforce the symbiotic role the audience is being asked to play with the educators, as well as the program itself. There is a sense of excitement that they are being involved in the creation of something *new*. This is distinctive from the prepackaged lectures they may have received on this and other subjects and creates a sense that anything could happen. In Scotty's words,

> When I get that pickup line from them and they see me, like saying things based on the things that they've said as opposed to something… like a script, and they know, like, "Oh wow, this guy's making things up, this guy must have just made up that joke. That's awesome. I like people that make things up." And I think that's when we got them. Jokes that apply to them based on the things that they're giving me, and that real audience interaction.

What Scotty is identifying when he says his audiences, "like people that make things up," he is drawing an explicit contrast to scripted, planned, dry content to in-the-moment, improvised interaction. This improvised moment is consistent with his analysis that audiences like "jokes that apply to them based on the things that they're giving me"—as a way of meeting his audience where they are. The modality (improvised interaction) coupled with the use of humor, helps create the sense that the audience and educator are forging a relationship, not participating in an artificial, scripted process. Furthermore, Scotty believes that "we get them" by engaging the audience as partners in the act of creation, in essence, bringing them into an authentic relationship with the presenters. In addition, Scotty is identifying the importance of the specificity of the jokes used, and how they connect him to his audience. Pre affirmed the importance of specificity during his interview, describing his experience in getting a pick up line at MIT:

P: One of the audience members said, "If you were F of X, I wish I could be F primed of X so I could be tangent to your curves." And I said, "Great!" For the uninitiated, that's a calculus joke. I turned to the actress and said that exact line, and her response was something along the lines of, "Why would you say that?" And I said, "Well, baby, with asymptotes like that, how could I not?" This comment was met with thunderous laughter and I was nearly crowned King of the Nerds... who knew we were a monarchy?

Q: What's an asymptote?

P: An asymptote is a vertical line to which a curve constantly gets closer to it but never actually touches. But I knew with that kind of a crowd, that kind of humor would build huge credibility with me versus a crowd who self-identify as being less academic and more athletic where I'll throw in the Sports Center theme or mock the Cowboys for being terrible. So I guess I do adjust my humor to try and match the crowd.

Pre identifies that it is not merely the act of incorporating the audience's suggestion that fosters engagement, but being able to use it to communicate his knowledge of who they are. His ability to amplify their pick up line with his own addition cemented his identity as someone his audience could relate to and see themselves in. While not all presenters can be as successful as Pre in succinctly communicating their identification with their audience, it is a useful example of how a presenter conceptualizes their humor engagement tactics at the beginning of the program, based on his assumptions about the nature of his audience. Furthermore, Pre's choice of "asymptote," a "vertical line to which a curve constantly gets closer to it but never actually touches" manages to insert the idea that while the initiator of the pick-up line may want to be close to the female character, there will not be physical contact. He is able to both mimic a stereotypical oafish male approach while not co-signing on the potentially misogynist messaging. While it is possible that some might still interpret Pre's response as reinforcing the very objectifying behavior the program is designed to challenge, I would argue that at this point in the program, the male educator is embodying those attitudes in order to ultimately interrogate them later on.

While Pre's connection with his MIT audience was improvised in the moment, *Sex Signals* has been adapted for a range of audiences, including the Greek, Athletic, and Military communities. It is also informally adapted for religious institutions asking for a more conservative approach. These institutions frequently request that the program deemphasize any message that could be perceived as endorsing sex before marriage; alcohol use; or condom use. In these latter cases, the language of the script is altered to remove as many of those references as possible, but the educator is trusted to adjust the humor they use in whatever situation arises.

James was very conscious of his word choice, and how that affected his use of humor in front of conservative audiences. For example, in the 2010 version of *Sex Signals,* the first two-thirds of the script built to a serious third act, known as the "David Parker Scene." The scene focused on a college student accused of rape, and the male educator is interviewed as that character, not only by the female educator but also by the audience. James understood the need to adjust the character of "David Parker" while being interviewed. He stated,

> Comedy has to be more of a reflection of what they may have seen or heard. [*Laughs.*] Okay, like with [the] David Parker [character]. If they ask me a question, "Did I use a condom?" with a conservative school or with a school that's a little more sheltered, I can simply say, "No, I didn't use a condom, you know, condoms are stupid." So, like, they might laugh at that and be affected in a big way. Ha! 'Cause he is saying the word *condom*, you know. [*Laughs.*] They may not talk about condoms as often.

> But with a not so conservative school, they're not gonna laugh at the word condom, so I have to reflect more of what *they* heard. The word condom is what they heard during an afterschool special program, like… maybe I have to use the word rubber, to reflect how they really talk or what they heard in the streets. So I would say, "No I didn't use a rubber," or "I didn't strap up, no." It would have to be more of a reflection of how they speak which is sometimes more graphic.

James has identified the need for appropriate word choice in maintaining the relationship with his audience—it is essential to both his persona, and his character's credibility. He is also making a connection to the importance of the audience laughing and being affected—if he uses the word "condom" in front of a jaded crowd, they will tune him out because they identify his approach as one for middle school children. He has to toughen his language so he doesn't become lumped in with the "afterschool special" approach. He assesses that the laugh is important—they must be shocked by the directness and confidence of the David Parker character in order for him to be real to them. In this sense, their laugh demonstrates that his objective has been achieved.

On the other hand, he must take care not to push too hard with the more conservative schools. Their laugh on the word "condom" is an indicator of their nervousness about talking about sexuality in general, and if he becomes too explicit, he may shut them down and damage the relationship. His observation, "Comedy has to be more of a reflection of what they may have seen or heard" does not apply only to conservative audiences, but to each audience to whom the program is presented. However, in this context, James' sensitivity to his audience shows a specific respect and compassion for their lived experience.

Second, the curriculum scaffolded the concepts related to coercion and rape in alignment with the level of emotional intimacy present between the presenters and the audience. This was achieved not only through the cloaking of serious concepts in exaggerated, satirical scenes but also through the careful cultivation of relatable personas that the audience trusted and identified with. This enabled the presenters to effectively manage their relationship with the audience; several identified the ways in which they determined that the relationship was in jeopardy, and how they used humor to remedy the situation.

Once again, the "David Parker Scene" requires the educators to adjust their approach based on their judgment of the emotional state of their audience. This is due to the fact that this scene marks a stark tonal change in the program, which can rattle most audiences. The program that had once been more raucous and funny has become serious very quickly, and throughout the dialogue, the presenters have to stay connected to the audience's reactions in that moment. In our first interview, Leah shared:

> So how I know it's tense is it quite literally makes me tense. I will find myself on stage feeling the nerves and the anxiety and the physical, muscular tension of the audience. It's almost as if everyone in the room just tightens up. And… or not even in the entire room, in a segment over here or a group over there. In my perception it's… it's almost a color, I mean, it's almost something that I can see happen in a group.

Leah was able to identify via her own physical reaction that the mood of her audience had changed. The type of scenario she described during her initial interview manifested during her presentation, which I viewed. In that case, the tension occurred right at the beginning of facilitation, during a sequence that clearly identified the David Parker scene as one depicting a rape, not a misunderstanding.

To provide a degree of standardization to facilitation, the presenters follow a thematic outline. In this outline, the next step is for the presenter to ask the audience members about what they may have still found confusing about the scene itself. This sequence is intended to give the audience permission to ask questions, and express disbelief that the David Parker scene depicted a rape. From that discussion, the presenters are able to counter false information, debunk myths, and challenge the audience to rethink their conceptualizations of positive and negative sexual behavior. But Leah sensed that based on what she was getting from the audience, entering into that section was premature. During the post-program interview with Leah and her partner James, they described what they identified as happening, and how they responded.

L: Well, [what] I've done before is to follow-up there and say, like, "Look, okay, is anybody freaking out?" But then I feed directly into the sort of next bullet point for all of us of "Let's talk about some of the things in the scene particularly that were confusing or that didn't mirror what you think of when you think of rape." And this is the first time that I went into the show analogy from it.

Q: Why did you do that?

L: I think part of it might have been because we had that back and forth with this crowd, because they were a little rowdy, 'cause they were engaged throughout. I think maybe it was I was trying to bolster us against the potential for that show that I think all of us hate to have where we have a great crowd, and they're rowdy and they're lively and they're fun, and then we get into facilitation and they *die*.

J: Yeah.

L: And then you're stuck there kind of lecturing and, like, getting one word answers, and it just feels like you lost a friend. You're like, "Wait, we were so. .. things were going so well." I was hoping to prevent that loss of their, of their affection and attention and trust.

J: I was glad you did that 'cause I ended with something very serious, and I was like, serious. And then you're like, "Does anyone think we're being really serious right now?" You know, and I thought it addressed right where they were. They were in that moment, like, "Wow, this is really serious now." And then you addressed that. And I thought it just worked.

Very quickly, Leah made the decision to acknowledge the tension of the audience before moving directly into asking them questions they may have been too frozen to answer. Importantly, she named her feeling as "if I've lost a friend" and identified her intention to "prevent the loss of their affection and attention and trust." As referenced in the previous chapter on using humor to maintain relationships, Leah used humor to address the sense of violation she perceived the audience was feeling, and in doing so, repaired and maintained that critical relationship. She refers to using the "Show Analogy" to do this, an argument incorporated into nearly every presentation of Sex Signals but traditionally utilized later on in facilitation. The "Show Analogy" compares the structure and methodology of Sex Signals to what a nonstranger rape scenario might look like. The 2009 Sex Signals Facilitation Manual lists its components as follows:

- Did it catch anyone off guard during the show, when you were laughing and having a good time, and then all of a sudden, she/I said that line, "I didn't really rape that girl," and it got really serious?
- Was anyone like, "What the fuck, what just happened?
- The show is designed that way for a reason, to show what it might be like in a nonstranger rape situation.
- You're having a good time, you're sharing, you're feeling listened to, and then all of a sudden it changes, just like that, and you never saw it coming.

During the presentation I viewed, Leah followed the components nearly word-for-word, using the analogy to provide tension release. Consistently, audiences laugh hard when the presenter says, "What the *fuck*, what just happened?" and they did so when Leah delivered that line. Part of this may be due to what was noted in a previous chapter, that the word "fuck" is unexpected in a program about sexual violence prevention, and its shock value precipitates the strong laugh. But more than that, that line gives permission for the audience to release the tension that has been built up over the David Parker scene, and perhaps even more importantly, identify it as their reaction to the sharp turn in the program so that they can process what they're experiencing. In this manner, the presenter is both addressing the emotional reaction of the audience while drawing an explicit connection to the reality of nonstranger rape: Many victims were having a wonderful time until they experienced what Lisak (2008) refers to as their "Hitchcock moment." They didn't "see it coming" either. While Leah and other presenters may have memorized that analogy and used it before, it was Leah's instincts as an experienced teacher that led her to use it in a different way, at a different time, because she identified that the audience needed to process their emotional reaction immediately.

In addition to defusing what could be characterized as a more silent resistance, presenters need to be able to manage their room when the resistance becomes loud, vocal, and endangers the positive dialogue they are trying to foster. The presenters must be able to make distinctions between genuinely confused audience members and those who are deliberately trying to undermine the process with vicious comments. This is very difficult, as sometimes the confused individual can sound like a mean one, and the decisions made by the presenters as to how to respond can either restore trust and order to the conversation, or create a hostile, chilled atmosphere if they respond too harshly. Chuck shared the following example of dealing with what he believed to be a more malicious audience member. Notably, the interaction he described took place at the very beginning of the program, when he asked for a pick-up line for the first improvised scene. He stated,

C: We did have a certain audience where a small section of them were being incredibly insensitive.
Q: What were they doing?
C: They would say things like… oh, well, give us a pickup line, and the pickup line was—he shouted it out. We obviously didn't use it. But, "Don't turn this rape into a murder."
Q: Whoa!
C: Now, there's a lot of ways to go with that. But it was probably a group of three or four that were kind of being just that—
Q: Out of a crowd of how big?
C: Maybe 250. They were vocal, but they were so localized.Ithinkifitwereadifferenttypeofcrowd—
Q: Like what?
C: If they had been a little bit… if the crowd itself, if the whole crowd had been a little less vocal in general, it would have been a lot easier to just call them out and say, "You know what? Don't ever say that again, period." We had a very vocal crowd, so when he said that, there was that kind of communal disgust that was vocalized, like, "Seriously? That's disgusting." You can hear them saying that. And being able to use that crowd to point out how allows me to not give them personally the attention that they're looking for.

And I think my only response was, "Dude, you're going to *jail*." [*Laughs.*] And they [audience] were right back with me. And then I think I went back to the audience and was like, "Anybody have a legit pickup line that's, you know, not *criminal*?" And so we kept going through. He was kind of isolated on his own with his three dudes from his unit.

Chuck illustrates very clearly the importance of ascertaining whether the "heckler" in the audience is representative of the whole, or an isolated element. By listening carefully, he determined that in that situation, the heckler was part of a vocal minority, and that the rest of the audience was against him. He then used the joke, "Dude, you're going to *jail*," to both isolate the heckler, showing him how the rest of the audience was on Chuck's side, not his. When the audience laughed, not only was the tension defused, and they were "right back" with Chuck, but also they clearly communicated that they are *not* with the heckler, as well. He has successfully calmed their reaction. Furthermore, Chuck's joke about the audience member going to jail, and his follow-up joke, "Anybody have a legit pickup line that's. .. not *criminal*?" also transmitted the clear message that the actions condoned in the joke are not socially acceptable, and illegal. Paul analyzed this type of situation well when he said,

> Well, the ability to make an audience laugh, especially when someone has said something that you can sense a good portion of the room finds offensive or objectionable is incredibly powerful. I mean, being able to say something which alleviates the kind of tension that's introduced when one audience member says something a lot of people

know is wrong, but they don't quite have the language to point to it as being wrong, there's just something in their gut that says that's not right, and you have the gift of being able to say that's not right with a joke.

Again, not all audience members are vocal because they are trying to be disruptive. Often they escalate because they are becoming emotional while genuinely trying to process the new, challenging information. Zelda had this example:

Z: There was one recent show where we got to the facilitation and we were getting a lot of contention. And there was this one guy that was just going on and on, and a lot of the people in the audience were just going on and on, and this one guy was standing up and wanting to be heard and saying his thing. And again, this is me trying to find agreement. But I just said, "Wow! I bet you never thought you would be this passionate about sexual assault! This is *awesome!*" [*Laughs.*]

Q: [*Laughs.*] What did he do?

Z: He didn't know what to do. He was like, "Ah! Ah! Yeah!" Sat back down and then we talked about… it was me cutting him off because he was just going to keep just going. But he stopped and went, "Ah!" And then we got to talk about what he had brought up.

Zelda described what on the surface is a positive situation: audiences actively engaged in the discussion about rape. However, when an active discussion gets out of hand, resulting in participants actually standing up in their seats and yelling at the presenters, there can be no genuine dialogue. Zelda's approach in this scenario was reflective of her overall philosophy of "finding agreement" as opposed to engaging in arguments: she met the audience member where he was and matched him in energy. Her humor was gentle, and not mocking: "Wow! I bet you never thought you would be this passionate about sexual assault! This is *awesome*!" Her positivity and calling out the incongruity of his passion for a subject he may have dreaded talking about, reframed a potentially confrontational situation into an opportunity for him to calm down, and for the group reflect on the substance of his argument. Moreover, her use of humor communicated affection and respect for that audience member, reinforcing the positive tone Zelda strives for in her presentations.

And sometimes, the audience is just so rowdy, that genuine discussion has been rendered impossible. The presenters are put in an awkward position of needing to exercise control and restore order, and yet not look like "the enforcer" or worse, that lecturer the audience may have been expecting. Anita shared an example of how her partner used humor to successfully respond to a very noisy crowd:

A: [*Laughs.*] We were in a community college in Memphis, Tennessee. [*Laughs.*] I'm sorry, I'm just laughing 'cause it was… I didn't expect him to say this. [*Laughs.*] And everybody was just talking, "*Oh, no-no-no-no-no-no*!" And we had been constantly like, "Okay, okay, calm down, calm down." My partner was like, "Black people. We are not a television set." [*Laughs.*] Which I loved all day. He was also Black, so it was okay. [*Laughs.*]

Q: That is not something that a White person should *ever* say.

A: [*Laughs.*] Right. It's like, not everybody could say that, hm-mm. [*Laughs.*] That wouldn't have been… that wouldn't have been wise.

This is a wonderful example of how Anita's partner used an example of in-group humor to connect with their audience. The simple joke cut through the noise and according to Anita, the unifying laugh actually had the effect of calming the audience down so that she and her partner could continue. It is important to note Anita's assessment, that the reason her partner was able to do this was because he was of the same race as the audience. Had he not been, his use of humor clearly would have been offensive and potentially disruptive.

In each of these examples, the presenters were very tuned in to the emotional state of both their audience as a whole, individual group members, and in Chuck's example, conscious of the disconnect between a few audience members and the majority of the audience itself. Each presenter displayed quick thinking and acted on the operating principle that tension of any kind must be addressed immediately and identified explicitly before the entire audience can move on to have a productive discussion. In Chuck's example, a small group of audience members and one individual in particular could have changed the tone of the entire program had he not emphatically stepped in and clarified that theirs was a minority view. He also demonstrated confidence, and I believe this relaxed his audience as they were reassured that he was in control of his room. In each example, the presenters determined that tension must be addressed before any learning could occur.

Presenters were very consistent in their analysis of when humor failed. With regard to its role in facilitation, they criticized it as a poor strategy when it was disconnected to not only the curricular objective but also the strongest idea within that objective. They shared that it was critical to understand the arguments in order to choose which joke or humorous analogy to support them. Failing to do so would result in an arbitrary or forced placement of the joke, which could either undercut the argument itself, or derail the conversation. Critically, they were in complete agreement that humor should never be used to make fun of victims, perpetrators, or rape itself. While it might be obvious as to why it would be wrong to make fun of rape or victims, they also understood that making fun of the rapist ran the risk of minimizing the impact of their actions by making them appear stupid, or silly.

Leah shared an example of the use of humor directly undermining an argument. In an effort to show the extreme insensitivity of the character of David Parker, who notices that Amy is lying still beneath him while he penetrates her, some of her partners have used humor in a way she disagreed with:

> [When] we're discussing the fact that the survivor in our story says "stop" and then just goes still, a few people [presenters] would physicalize that and say something like, "Yeah, they just lay there," and make kind of like a floppy, limp sort of big body. movement and occasionally say things like, you know, "If that happened, you'd be like, can I check your pulse?" And that was something that could sound, to a victim who had possibly frozen, like what they did was wrong, or like their reaction was less valid. It sounds like it's making fun of the behavior, not making fun of the response to the behavior, which is what we would intend to do, the fact that it is aberrant not to respond if your partner stops moving.

In Leah's example, it appears that her partners were genuinely intending to highlight the callousness of the offender, David Parker, as opposed to his victim, Amy. But by making a joke out of her body movement, and giving the rapist the "punch line" of "Can I check your pulse?" the victim is turned into the butt of the joke, her rape is minimized, and the rapist is made more of a comic hero than the villain he is. Again, while I believe the presenters in question had good intentions, this use of humor violates what I call the fundamental principles of using humor to address this topic: 1. Never make fun of rape. 2. Never make fun of the victim. 3. Never make fun of the rapist. Humor should never minimize the act itself, or its human casualty, and making fun of the rapist does just what Leah's example shows: it minimizes the brutal actions of a criminal and turns them into a joke.

Educators also stated that using humor at the expense of a vulnerable group could also undermine not only the content of the program but also potentially reinforce negative attitudes toward that vulnerable group. While this was sometimes a component of the original scripted program (and then revised to reflect more thoughtful practice), it was often a moment that an educator had improvised during one presentation, which became incorporated into their permanent performance repertoire.

This was true of a joke that was part of one of the semi-improvised parts of the program, the section of the show where the presenters solicited stereotypes of "what it means to be a woman" and "what it means to be a man" from the audience. The joke was intended to illustrate a parody of hypermasculinity, but it could also be read as a joke about domestic violence. Christian shared,

> When creating the male stereotype [the educator] would get these huge things from the audience, like

"What does it mean [to be a stereotypical man]? "We're big, we're manly, we're blah-blah-blah." And he would do this thing that he would do in almost every show where he's like, "And do we take charge? Yeah, we take charge. When I say I'm gonna pick you up at 8, I'm gonna pick you up at 8."

And he would literally pretend as though he physically picks up somebody, that I think is very funny, but then he would pretend to throw the person and yell, "Get in the truck!" And, like, throw the woman into the truck. That would usually elicit a huge response because it's so over the top and absurd, but at the same time, as far as I was concerned, it was contributing to this notion of domestic violence as being funny. So, when we asked him to drop it, I think it was difficult for him for him to pull back from that because it was such a big laugh.

This is a strong example of how a joke that gets an enormous, positive response must be cut when it is seen to undercut not even the messages of our program, but the principles connected to that program. Again, if the presenters were merely comedians, and they worked merely in service of the laughs and their own egos, the joke could have stayed in their "act." As teachers, and representatives of a social-justice program, however, they do not have that option.

In Leah's view, the most significant lines cut were not even jokes, per se. The lines received laughs though, and the presenters determined that they were not for the right reason. Leah said the lines,

came across as slightly homophobic, that were jokes about, like, "We've got an exercise for you. Everybody grab a buddy." "Or like we're gonna talk about sex, everybody grab a buddy." And when our audiences are largely male or simply because of the distribution of people in the audience, that would often lead to two guys sitting next to each other, and it sort of gives a lot of fuel to the potential for a homophobic moment.

Leah is referring primarily to presentations delivered to military audiences, and as our interview took place prior to the lifting of "Don't Ask, Don't Tell," any jokes that implied that two men sitting next to each other were homosexual, or that there were even homosexuals in the room, became very loaded. The laughter would have contributed to a sense of danger for gay and lesbian servicemen and undermined the safe environment the presenters and the program strive to create.

They also identified the danger of being greedy for the laughs; sometimes the need to get "high" off of the approval of the audience superseded the objectives of the program, and most of the presenters spoke of their ongoing challenge in not succumbing to that temptation.

Anyone who has told a joke and gotten a laugh can testify to the emotional rush one receives. For many performers, getting a laugh can be described as getting a high. I know from over 25 years of performance and teaching that getting a big laugh can become addictive. The presenters of Sex Signals felt similarly. Chuck and I spoke about this during our interview:

C: If we lose track of when the humor is either building the argument or sharpening the argument or tailoring the argument in some way, if we lose track of that sometimes we run the risk of making jokes to make jokes.

Q: So you can distract them from your point, is what you're saying?

C: Mm-hmm. And it's an easy trap to fall into when they're laughing.

Q: Why is that easy?

C: Because laughter is awesome.

Q: What does it feel like when you've got a room laughing with you like that?

C: I mean, it's… I mean, it's addictive, it's infectious. It makes you feel like you are doing the right thing. You're validated. All of your work is validated. I mean, that feeling is like second to none. Like 400 people, especially when you have, like, four, five hundred people who you know didn't want to see the show. You knew they didn't want to see the show, and it's brutal in the beginning. They're, you know, ah-ah-ah, just looking all over the place, they're texting. And [then] 20 minutes into the show, they are just guffawing and rolling and screaming and shouting and yelling. It's an amazing feeling.

Chuck very explicitly described the high of making an audience laugh, and in particular, an audience that hadn't wanted to be there in the first place. He is also cognizant of the danger inherent in that high: The use of humor becomes all about maintaining it, as opposed to supporting and advancing key arguments. As a result, the arguments lose their focus, and the presenters could lose time to cover important content.

What came through clearly in the data, both in the scripts that I analyzed and in the interviews that I conducted, is that the curriculum and the presenters are inextricably linked to one another. In a way, they are a team, in that one could not function without the other. I would argue that this is essential for the success of all sexual assault prevention curriculum—while the tool is only as effective as the one that wields it, it is necessary to equip our educators with the best tools possible.

In 2015, the National Sexual Violence Resource Center (NSVRC) reviewed the latest research on perpetrators of rape (Tharp, et.al., 2015). This was significant, as the thinking on sex offenders was driven primarily by the research conducted by Lisak and Miller (2002), and to a lesser extent, McWhorter, Stander, Merrill, Thomsen, & Milner, 2009. Their research found that while 6% of the men surveyed had committed rape, 4% of those who did were responsible for the vast majority of rapes—on average, one rapist committed an average of six rapes. This very clearly positioned the prevention education response away from engaging potential rapists—if they were serial predators, they would be unlikely to receive educational messages.

The new wave of studies showed a very different picture. Swartout and colleagues (2015) found that roughly 13% of college men had perpetrated a completed rape in their lifetime, with 5% reporting they had raped prior to entering college, and 11% reporting having raped during college. Significantly, 75% of the men in this study reported having raped *only once*. The NSVRC report also added another cautionary note: studies that focus solely on completed rapes miss the wide range of maladaptive behaviors, including attempted rape, sexual abuse, and the use of coercion to obtain sex.

> In fact, Zinzow and Thompson (2014) found high rates of repeated perpetration when the full range of sexually violent behaviors—unwanted sexual contact to completed rape—were analyzed together, meaning that many men (68% of offenders) consistently use coercive sexual tactics over time, but only 12–22% of repeat offenders perpetrated rape at each time point, meaning that repeat offenders perpetrated other forms of sexual violence over time and periodically perpetrated rape. Of note, these findings are based upon the same data set Swartout and colleagues (2015) used to fit their confirmatory model, providing further evidence that behavior other than rape constituted much of the repeated sexual violence (Tharp, et.al, 2015, p. 6).

This new understanding must play a role in adjusting and expanding our messaging on sexual violence prevention. As a practitioner, I appreciate the bystander intervention approach as a means of addressing the issues related to sexual violence somewhat indirectly; audiences are framed as potential heroes, not as potential rapists or victims. And while it can allow for an explicit interrogation of the cultural norms that undergird a rape culture, it does not directly address the ways in which the one-time offender may use coercion or even the mere opportunity to commit sexual violence. While bystander intervention doesn't explicitly frame potential offenders as serial predators, there is an implicit message that we are asking the good people to stop the bad people. The new research argues that sometimes it is the good people who are sometimes the bad people, and that requires a more specific kind of messaging. While the bystander intervention approach gives a kind of "identity protection" to the audience, reducing their resistance to the content because they are not directly implicated in it, the new messaging will be much more challenging. It will have to navigate the tension between giving permission to the audience to be confused about their own current and past behavior, while holding them unambiguously accountable for it.

While it is not possible to sample every audience member that experiences "Sex Signals," or any of our other programs, for that matter, both our formal data collection and informal feedback speak to the positive role humor plays in reaching our audience. In 2017, following a significant script update, students who viewed *Sex Signals* during their college orientation were invited to give feedback regarding the program via the

Catharsis Productions' Facebook page in exchange for Catharsis "swag" (i.e., temporary tattoos and stickers featuring consent and bystander intervention-related graphics). While they were likely motivated in part by the promise of freebies, the detail and nature of their comments speak consistently and clearly to the strategies utilized by our program and educators. An unedited, representative sample of the comments from the Fall Orientation 2017 (Ramirez, J., 2017) is below:

- You guys recently performed at my university, West Georgia. I know you guys came the year before but I had missed the show so I made sure to make this year. The thought that really caught my attention was about how we normalized creeping for all genders and sexualities. It never really has been brought up that way to me, so I did not think anything of it prior. You definitely made me think, why and how we can confront them, and tell them they are wrong. It's not something that will change overnight but I strongly believe I can help make it less of a normality if it's starts with us. What you guys are do is important, critical, and cool.
- Hello! I am a freshmen at Eckerd college and I just watched a presentation from you and am totally in love with what you do! Thank you so much for all you do! The thing I loved the most was how the entire presentation was humorous, even when talking about very serious subjects. It was engaging every second of the way and at no point was offensive or uncomfortable.
- Honestly, I just saw this at carthage, and it was the best sex ed. thing I've EVER experienced. My high school health teacher was woke but not this woke. I loved it. I LOVE all the intersectionality and the recognition of privilege and all that stuff. It was fun, it was real, it was entertaining. Thank you guys so much.
- Thank you so much for the program you put on tonight at IU Southeast! It was both incredibly informative and tons of fun!! Thank you for starting a discussion that is often times hard to approach, while making us laugh the whole time and showing us that hard topics don't have to be avoided!! I LOVED how it was interactive when you guys had us hold up the stop signs or asked us for the pick up lines. It kept us engaged and felt like we were active participants instead of just an audience!
- Hi! I was just at the presentation you just did and I just wanted to say I absolutely LOVED it. These are issues that I'm super passionate about. You made it funny so we stayed attentive, but you also didn't sugar coat anything. It was an incredible presentation and I would watch it again. Thank you so much for coming and for doing what y'all do! You really do make a difference. You guys had chemistry on stage which made it better, rather than it being awkward (even during the uncomfortable parts). I wouldn't have changed a thing about it.
- My school and I had really enjoyed the presentation and talks today. I go to Lourdes University and am so happy that I attended. Not exactly what I had expected to hear. I am glad to hear about what to do instead of being told to ignore it and not get involved. You guys know college and high school students better than our teachers did. Everything I was too scared to say, got answered. Thank you!
- I really liked how interactive it was. Like my boyfriend goes to MCAD and he told me his sex talk was this super cheesy video, that was partially animated because "art kids" I guess. But I bragged about how we were able to be actively apart of the conversation which made it easier to want to listen—MSMU.
- Hey I just saw your set and I really liked it, it was funny but it was also super real and I appreciated that. I liked most that y'all weren't afraid to cuss or address real issues that others are too scared to talk about Thank you for coming to coe!
- Hey! I am Nicole from SMSU! I saw your show for the second time on August 19th. Last year I saw the show and as a freshman, I had never seen adults talk about sex, consent, and parties so openly. Now, as a second year student something different stood out to me. Part of the show talked about how women and men have certain stereotypes and standards we should live up to. One line was about how women who have sex are called sluts, and women who don't have sex are still called sluts. I thought this was terrible, but very true. I remember being called a slut in middle school after I had my first kiss!! Thanks again

for coming and educating us about consent! I love your show and what your company stands for.

- I'm currently a first year at Denison University. I just watched a program of yours earlier today and it was phenomenal. I want to thank you for raising awareness of such an important topic in today's society and you have resonated a message that will remind college students at Denison to take care of themselves and others. It's the perfect balance of humor and seriousness that made this program so amazing to watch, and I'm sure it'll leave a lasting impact. Thanks again!
- I did not expect such an educational and entertaining performance. They were able to balance a serious tone with one that kept the audience engaged. They also covered a ton of controversial topics, yet were able to take control of the situation and drive it towards where it needed to go. I also would like to say the improv was marvelous and outstanding. I thoroughly enjoyed going and would like to thank you for taking time to talk to students!!!
- Thank you so much for your presentation today at Tulane! I found it very educational and really comfortably funny. As a survivor, I felt that the presenters were very nice, educated, and pro-victim.
- Hi, you came to Augustana today. I just wanted to say that I am so thankful for what you said and did! It was amazing and educational and so important! Thank you so much!!! I loved that we were treated like adults and that the speakers could be comedic without being offensive or insensitive. They constantly reminded us how serious the issue was but still made us laugh.
- Thank you so much for speaking today at Central! It was super great hearing about sex or better yet warning signs for on campus and at parties. I think the most I took away from it was not just what was said (especially how it was discussed about being a woman in today's world) but listening to how others responded in the crowd. I felt safer knowing that the people I'll be living with are on the same page as me.

These responses reinforce the fact that humor, when used intentionally and strategically, can help achieve critical educational objectives. The students' comments demonstrate that the serious messages about the nature of rape, victimization, corrosive cultural norms, and the need to intervene were not lost in a sea of jokes. The comments demonstrated an appreciation for the candor and "realness" of the material, and of how safe they felt having such important conversations. Once again, however, this reflects the prowess of Catharsis Productions' educators, and of the comprehensive training and coaching they receive. This is in no way to suggest that anyone using humor would be as consistent or as successful as well-trained educators.

The field of sexual assault prevention education faces genuine challenges, among them the need to be able to convince our audiences that our messages matter. This is especially difficult when those messages, and their messengers, are alternately perceived as boring, irrelevant, and even, threatening. This is where the strategic use of humor becomes even more crucial for effective programming. When used specifically to frame challenging ideas, situate the presenter as a friendly partner in the dialogue, and manage the emotional reactions caused by the nature of the content, humor can provide a crucial catalytic effect to the learning process. Being funny is not the objective; using humor to support critical, challenging messaging in order to reduce sexual violence, is.

References

Andersen, J. F. (1979). Teacher immediacy as a predictor of teaching effectiveness. *Annals of the International Communication Association, 3*(1), 543–559.

Askenasy, J. J. (1987). The functions and dysfunctions of laughter. *Journal of General Psychology, 114*(4), 317–334.

Beatty, M. J., & Payne, S. K. (1981). Receiver apprehension and cognitive complexity. *Western Journal of Speech Communication, 44*, 363–369.

Beatty, M. J. (2009). Receiver apprehension as a function of cognitive backlog. *Western Journal of Speech Communication, 45*(3), 277–281.

Berlyne, D. E. (1972). Humor and its kin. In J. H. Goldstein & P. E. McGhee (Eds.), *The psychology of humor* (pp. 43–60). New York, NY: Academic Press.

Chesebro, J. L., & McCroskey, J. C. (1998). The relationship of teacher clarity and teacher immediacy with students' experiences of state receiver apprehension. *Communication Quarterly, 46*(4), 446–464.

Chesebro, J. L., & McCroskey, J. C. (2001, January). The relationship of teacher clarity and immediacy with student state receiver apprehension, affect, and cognitive learning. *Communication Education, 50*(1), 59–68.

Conway, M., & Dubé, L. (2016). Humor in persuasion on threatening topics: Effectiveness is a function of audience sex role orientation. *Personality and Social Psychology Bulletin, 28*(7), 863–873.

Damasio, A. R. (1994). Descartes' error and the future of human life. *Scientific American, 271*(4), 144–144.

Delia, J. G., O'Keefe, B. J., & O'Keefe, D. J. (1982). The constructivist approach to communication. In F. E. Dance (Ed.), *Human communication theory: Comparative essays*. New York, NY: Harper & Row.

Farrelly, F., Brandsma, J. M., & McMahon, I. (1974). *Provocative therapy*. Shields Publishing Company.

Farrelly, F., & Lynch, M. (1987). Humor in provocative therapy. In W. F. Fry & W. A. Salameh (Eds.), *Handbook of humor and psychotherapy: Advances in the clinical use of humor* (pp. 81–106). Sarasota, FL: Professional Resource Press.

Freud, S. (1960). *Jokes and their relation to the unconscious*. New York: Norton.

Hess, D. E. (2004). Discussion in social studies: Is it worth the trouble? *Social Education, 68*(2), 151–155.

Kahan, D. M., Braman, D., Slovic, P., Gastil, J., & Cohen, G. L. (2007). The second national risk and culture study: Making sense of—and making progress in - the American culture war of fact. *SSRN Electronic Journal*.

Kher, N., Molstad, S., & Donahue, R. (1999). Using humor in the college classroom to enhance teaching effectiveness in "dread courses". *College Student Journal, 33*(3), 400–406.

Killinger, B. (1987). Humor in psychotherapy: A shift to a new perspective. In W. F. Fry & W. A. Salameh (Eds.), *Handbook of humor and psychotherapy: Advances in the clinical use of humor* (pp. 21–40). Sarasota, FL: Professional Resource Press.

Korobkin, D. (1988). Humor in the classroom: Considerations and strategies. *College Teaching, 36*(4), 154–158.

Lisak, D., & Miller, P. M. (2002). Repeat rape and multiple offending among undetected rapists. *Violence and Victims, 17*(1), 73–84.

Lisak, D. (2008). *Understanding the predatory nature of sexual violence.* From http://www.wcsap.org/sites/www.wcsap.org/files/uploads/webinars/SV%20on%20Campus/UnderstandingthePredatoryNatureofSexualViolence.pdf

McReynolds, P. (1976). Assimilation and anxiety. In M. Zuckerman & C. D. Spielberger (Eds.), *Emotions and anxiety: New concepts, methods, and applications* (pp. 35–86). New York, NY: Wiley.

McWhorter, S. K., Stander, V. A., Merrill, L. L., Thomsen, C. J., & Milner, J. S. (2009). Reports of rape perpetration by newly enlisted male navy personnel. *Violence and Victims, 24*, 204–218.

Meyer, J. C. (2000). Humor as a double-edged sword: Four functions of humor in communication. *Communication Theory, 10*(3), 310–331.

Mooney, C. (2011, May/June). The science of why we don't believe science how our brains fool us on climate, creationism, and the vaccine-autism link. Mother Jones. Retrieved from http://motherjones.com/politics/2011/03/denial-science-chris-mooney

Morreall, J. (1983). *Taking laughter seriously*. Albany: State University of New York.

Neiweem, C. (2017, July 9). *Sexual assault in the military is more than a political problem.* Retrieved from https://thehill.com/blogs/pundits-blog/the-military/323197-sexual-assault-in-the-military-is-more-than-a-politicalproblem

Nussbaum, J. F. (1992). Communicator style and teacher influence. In V. P. Richmond & J. C. McCroskey (Eds.), *Power in the classroom: Communication, control, and concern* (pp. 145–157). Hillsdale, NJ: Lawrence Erlbaum.

Piddington, R. (1963). *The psychology of laughter: A study in social adaptation* (2nd ed.). New York, NY: Gamut Press.

Ramirez, J. (2017). 2017 fall orientation Facebook comments. Internal Catharsis productions report: Unpublished.

Redditors. et al. (2017). Reactions to me too. *r/Menslib.* https://www.reddit.com/r/MensLib/comments/772tml/reactions_to_metoo/

Rosenheim, E. (1974). Humor in psychotherapy: An interactive experience. *American Journal of Psychotherapy, 28*(4), 584–591.

Rosiek, J. (2003). Emotional scaffolding: An exploration of the teacher knowledge at the intersection of student emotion and the subject matter. *Journal of Teacher Education, 54*, 399–412.

Schaeffer, N. (1981). *The art of laughter*. New York: Columbia University Press.

Shurcliff, A. (1968). Judged humor, arousal, and the relief theory. *Journal of Personality and Social Psychology, 8*(4, Pt.1), 360–363.

Smith, C., & Voth, B. (2002). The role of humor in political argument: How "strategery" and "lockboxes" changed a political campaign. *Argumentation and Advocacy, 39*(2), 110–129.

Speck, P. S. (1991). The humorous message taxonomy: A framework for the study of humorous ads. In J. H. Leigh & C. R. Martin (Eds.), *Current issues and research in advertising* (Vol. 13, pp. 1–44). Ann Arbor: University of Michigan.

Swartout, K. M., Koss, M. P., White, J. W., Thompson, M. P., Abbey, A., & Bellis, A. L. (2015). A trajectory analysis of the campus serial rapist assumption. *JAMA Pediatrics*. available online ahead of publication.

Szabo, A. (2003). The acute effects of humor and exercise on mood and anxiety. *Journal of Leisure Research, 35*(2), 152–162.

Tauber, R. T., & Mester, C. S. (1994). *Acting lessons for teachers: Using performance skills in the classroom.* Westport, CT: Praeger.

Tharp, A. T., Swartout, K., Koss, M. P., DeGue, S., Basile, K. C., White, J., … Thompson, M. (2015). *Key findings: Rethinking serial perpetration*. Harrisburg, PA: National Sexual Violence Resource Center; available online at www.nsvrc.org.

Torok, S. E., McMoris, R. F., & Lin, W. C. (2004). Is humor an appreciated teaching tool? Perceptions of professors' teaching styles and use of humor. *College Teaching, 52*, 14–20.

Vangelisti, A. L., Daly, J. A., & Friedrich, G. W. (Eds.). (1999). *Teaching communication: Theory, research, and methods* (2nd ed.). Mahwah, NJ: Lawrence Erlbaum.

Wheeless, L. R., Preiss, R. W., & Gayle, B. M. (1997). Receiver apprehension, informational receptivity, and cognitive processing. In *Avoiding communication: Shyness, reticence, and communication apprehension* (pp. 151–187).

White, G. W. (2001). Teachers' report of how they used humor with students perceived use of such humor. *Education, 122*(2), 337–347.

Witt, P. L., Wheeless, L. R., & Allen, M. (2004). A meta-analytical review of the relationship between teacher immediacy and student learning. *Communication Monographs, 71*(2), 184–207.

Wrench, J. S., & McCroskey, J. C. (2001). A temperamental understanding of humor communication and exhilaratability. *Communication Quarterly, 49*(2), 142–159.

Wright, M. H. (2000). Sophistic humor and social change: Overcoming identification with the aggressor. *Journal for the Psychoanalysis of Culture and Society, 5*, 57–64.

Wyer, R. S., & Collins, J. E. (1992). A theory of humor elicitation. *Psychological Review, 99*, 663–688.

Zinzow, H., & Thompson, M. (2014). A longitudinal study of risk factors for repeated sexual coercion and assault in U.S. college men. *Archives of Sexual Behavior, 44*. https://doi.org/10.1007/s10508-013-0243-5

Mindfulness and Sexual Violence 28

Daniel R. Szoke and Holly Hazlett-Stevens

Mindfulness, a purposeful and present-moment awareness, appears to ameliorate symptoms of posttraumatic stress disorder (PTSD) and depression faced by survivors of trauma (Hilton et al., 2017). Mindfulness-based interventions developed in the late 1970s, and mindfulness meditation has been around for more than 2500 years, yet these practices only recently have been implemented as a clinical treatment for sexual assault survivors. Increased attitudes of acceptance of the present moment and self-compassion may help decrease the avoidance, hyperarousal, and occurrence of negative thoughts associated with PTSD. Mindfulness-based interventions therefore are an effective adjunct (Kimbrough, Magyari, Langenberg, Chesney, & Berman, 2010), or possibly stand-alone (Kelly & Garland, 2016), treatment for survivors of sexual violence; however, much of the available outcome research has not specifically targeted this particular clinical population.

Mindfulness-based interventions are beneficial in the treatment of trauma for a variety of reasons. Mindfulness treatment components can augment the effectiveness of exposure-based interventions (Follette, Palm, & Pearson, 2006). Indeed, one specific treatment protocol that combined mindfulness practices with exposure therapy for survivors of trauma showed promising results that included a reduction in PTSD symptoms (King et al., 2016). In addition, mindfulness practices can provide naturalistic exposure to trauma-related memories and physiological experiences in the course of the practice, eventually leading to an overall decrease in negative emotions and cognitions (Brown, Ryan, & Creswell, 2007; Hölzel et al., 2011). This raises the possibility that mindfulness-based interventions can benefit trauma survivors in isolation without added imaginal or in vivo exposure.

Our chapter reviews the emerging research literature examining the effectiveness of mindfulness-based interventions for survivors of sexual violence. We first explore the roots of mindfulness practices and describe the development of mindfulness-based interventions in Western medicine and psychology. Next, we outline the theories that support implementing mindfulness-based interventions with survivors of trauma and review the evidence supporting this clinical approach. We then will report results from a literature search that identified investigations testing the effects of mindfulness-based interventions on survivors of intimate partner violence (IPV) and survivors of childhood sexual abuse specifically. Finally, we describe research conducted in areas concerning mindfulness and sexual violence prevention, perpetration, and advocacy work. While preliminary, our inquiry

D. R. Szoke
University of Nevada, Reno, Reno, NV, USA

H. Hazlett-Stevens (✉)
Department of Psychology/298,
University of Nevada, Reno, Reno, NV, USA
e-mail: hhazlett@unr.edu

W. T. O'Donohue and P. A. Schewe (eds.), *Handbook of Sexual Assault and Sexual Assault Prevention*,
https://doi.org/10.1007/978-3-030-23645-8_28

reveals that mindfulness can offer a powerful treatment option for survivors of sexual violence and can even assist prevention efforts. In addition to PTSD and depression, survivors of sexual violence often face self-blame and lower self-worth. Mindfulness-based interventions teach participants self-acceptance and self-compassion, which are likely beneficial for survivors of sexual violence.

What Is Mindfulness?

Mindfulness involves a practice of purposeful, nonjudgmental, moment-to-moment awareness (Kabat-Zinn, 2013). Contrary to common belief, mindfulness meditation is not an attempt to "empty the mind," or an attempt to prevent new thoughts from forming. Mindfulness meditation involves cultivating awareness to what is actually occurring in the present moment. When the mind wanders, the meditator merely notices that the mind has left present-time direct experience and gently guides attention back. Specific formal practices appear particularly conducive to cultivating mindful awareness, including siting meditation and yoga movement (Kabat-Zinn, 2013).

The term "mindfulness" originates from Buddhist traditions. More than 2500 years ago in present-day Nepal, the Buddha provided oral teachings detailing how he found freedom from suffering. Historical accounts state that just after reaching enlightenment underneath the Bodhi Tree, the Buddha's first sermon detailed the Four Noble Truths (Van Gordon, Shonin, Griffiths, & Singh, 2015). These truths are summarized briefly as follows: (1) Life is full of suffering, (2) suffering is caused by craving, (3) the end of craving brings about the end of suffering, and (4) the Eight-Fold Path offers a way to decrease, and possibly end, suffering. In Buddhist traditions, mindfulness involves becoming aware of the cycle of suffering detailed by the Four Noble Truths. A mindful practitioner brings attention to the suffering of the body, mind, feelings, and external phenomena and accepts that suffering is a natural part of life yet also simply a conception of the mind (Van Gordon et al., 2015).

In 1975, Buddhist meditation practitioners Sharon Salzberg, Joseph Goldstein, and Jack Kornfield founded the Insight Meditation Society to import the meditative practices of Buddhism to the West (Fronsdal, 1998). Specifically, Kornfield stated that the group intended to "offer the powerful practices of insight mediation ... as simply as possible without the complications of rituals, robes, chanting, and the whole religious tradition." (Fronsdal, 1998, p. 167). This intention to teach the essence of mindfulness practices while leaving the cultural trappings behind is reflected in the development of Western mindfulness-based interventions.

Mindfulness-Based Interventions

Jon Kabat-Zinn introduced Mindfulness-Based Stress Reduction (MBSR) in 1979 as a public health education course delivered in a medical setting for patients coping with chronic pain and illness (Kabat-Zinn, 2013). This 2-month program was housed inside the Medical School at the University of Massachusetts. MBSR soon became popular with hospital staff including doctors and nurses looking to alleviate their own stress. In turn, more patients were referred by staff to Kabat-Zinn's program (Kabat-Zinn, 2013). Recently, the University of Massachusetts Medical School announced the creation of the first ever "Division of Mindfulness," which will focus on the integration of mindfulness practices into medical care (Agsar, 2017).

MBSR patients meet weekly for eight two-and-a-half-hour group sessions as well as a full-day retreat. Throughout the 2-month period, participants learn about mindfulness and the practices that help cultivate present moment awareness. This involves didactic portions, formal practice of meditation and yoga, and group discussions about experiences with the practice. Instructors assign 45-min daily practice as homework for participants. In the final sessions, participants discuss tactics for keeping mindfulness in their lives following the intervention.

Kabat-Zinn (2013) suggested that MBSR does not eliminate stressful circumstances or internal stressors, but instead shifts participants' perception of stress. More recently, studies support the claim that one's perception of stress impacts physiological and cognitive responses to stress (Jamieson, Nock, & Mendes, 2012; Keller et al., 2012). Those with more optimistic attributions towards stress respond better both psychologically and physiologically (Seligman, 1998). With awareness skills, participants can notice their automatic negative response to stress and instead respond skillfully. MBSR provides both the skills to recognize the physiological and cognitive experience of stress and the skills necessary to select an appropriate response in the moment (Kabat-Zinn, 2013).

MBSR has proven effective in reducing anxiety and depression amongst various medical and psychiatric patient groups across multiple studies. A meta-analysis of 20 studies showed depression reduction effect size of $g = 0.49$ and anxiety reduction of $g = 0.55$ (Hofmann, Sawyer, Witt, & Oh, 2010). Medium effect sizes generally falling in the 0.5–0.6 range were replicated in similar meta-analyses conducted with patients reporting a wide variety of medical and mental health conditions, including a systematic review of randomized controlled trials of MBSR (e.g., de Vibe, Bjørndal, Tipton, Hammerstrøm, & Kowalski, 2012). Large mindfulness-based intervention effect sizes were found among patients diagnosed with anxiety or mood disorders (Hedges g of 0.97 for improving anxiety symptoms and 0.95 for improving mood symptoms; Hofmann et al., 2010), demonstrating clinical effects comparable to cognitive–behavioral interventions that consistently produce medium to large effects sizes in research (Hofmann, Asnaani, Vonk, Sawyer, & Fang, 2012). MBSR currently appears as an intervention evaluated in comparative effectiveness research studies within the Substance and Mental Health Services Administration (SAMHSA) National Registry of Evidence-based Programs and Practices (NREPP).

Clinical psychology researchers Zindel Segal, Mark Williams, and John Teasdale saw an opportunity to integrate the original MBSR protocol with cognitive therapy to treat depression (Segal, Williams, & Teasdale, 2013). They identified cognitive patterns specific to recurrent depression and applied principles of mindfulness as a means of relating skillfully to negative thoughts. Mindfulness-Based Cognitive Therapy (MBCT) aims to prevent relapse among patients who have experienced previous episodes of depression. MBCT guides participants to develop a new relationship to their thoughts and feelings, a relationship of acceptance instead of usual attempts at avoidance that are ultimately unsuccessful (Segal et al., 2013). This clinical protocol retained much of the format of MBSR, including the 8-week group session structure, the format devoted to teaching and practicing formal mindfulness meditation and movement, and daily home practice assignments. MBCT includes a similar introduction and explanation of mindfulness but provides specific psychoeducation about the negative cycles of depression not found in the MBSR curriculum (Segal et al., 2013). MBCT participants learn to recognize cognitive patterns that lead to a familiar downward spiral of thoughts and feelings. Many of those who suffer from depression eventually return to these negative thought patterns after remission of symptoms. Instead of targeting the symptoms of depression directly, MBCT aims to help participants notice and then disengage from rumination and automatic thoughts rather than regarding such thoughts as facts and believing them. This is one reason that MBCT has been considered especially successful in treating recurrent depression.

MBCT significantly reduces risk of depressive relapse over treatment as usual (TAU) from 78% to between 20% and 50% (Ma & Teasdale, 2004; Teasdale et al., 2000). A later systematic review consistently found that those who participated in MBCT plus treatment as usual had a 39% decrease in risk of depression recurrence compared to those receiving treatment as usual on its own (Galante, Iribarren, & Pearce, 2013). MBCT also may be an effective treatment option for some anxiety disorders, particularly generalized anxiety disorder and social anxiety disorder (see Segal et al., 2013, for a review).

In addition to MBCT, clinicians have created mindfulness-based interventions tailored to other client populations. For example, clinicians have designed mindfulness-based relapse prevention for substance use disorder (Witkiewitz & Marlatt, 2004), mindfulness-based therapy for insomnia (Heidenreich, Tuin, Pflug, Michal, & Michalak, 2006), mindfulness-based eating awareness therapy (Kristeller, Baer, & Quillian-Wolever, 2006), and MBSR for trauma (Magyari, 2015).

Mindfulness and Trauma

Although mindfulness-based interventions have effectively reduced stress, anxiety, and depression across many clinical trials, their implementation with survivors of trauma is nascent. Early concerns that mindfulness meditation could be contraindicated for clients with trauma histories included claims that mindfulness training could exacerbate PTSD symptoms (Germer, 2005; Lustyk, Chawla, Nolan, & Marlatt, 2009), similar to findings that critical incident stress debriefing as an early intervention does not prevent PTSD and sometimes makes its occurrence more likely (Ehlers & Clark, 2003). Early MBSR treatment manuals recommended against enrolling patients diagnosed with current PTSD out of concern that the practice may trigger overwhelming trauma-related symptoms (e.g., Santorelli & Kabat-Zinn, 2009). However, these clinical concerns were not accompanied by research documenting such adverse effects of mindfulness-based interventions for trauma survivors. Of the five studies that measured iatrogenic effects of conducting a mindfulness-based treatment on survivors of trauma, none found any negative outcomes (Bormann, Thorp, Wetherell, Golshan, & Lang, 2013; Kearney, Mcdermott, Malte, Martinez, & Simpson, 2013; Mitchell et al., 2014; Niles et al., 2012; Polusny et al., 2015), (see Hilton et al., 2017, for a complete review).

In contrast, psychological theories of trauma suggested that mindfulness could serve an important role in treating symptoms of posttraumatic stress disorder. When survivors of trauma have intrusive thoughts about their trauma, they attempt to avoid these memories. Yet, when people deliberately attempt to suppress difficult thoughts, they become paradoxically more likely to think about the very subject they are aiming to avoid (Wegner, 1997). Follette et al. (2006) described such attempted suppression of trauma-related thoughts as avoidance behaviors resulting from an inability to stay present, reflecting a deficit in the precise skill that mindfulness meditation builds. Teaching trauma survivor clients to cultivate mindfulness could help them become aware of current thoughts and feelings without trying to avoid such experiences when they naturally arise. For this reason, Follette et al. argued that increasing clients' capacity for mindful awareness could reduce such covert avoidance attempts and therefore make exposure-based treatment more successful.

Preliminary evidence for a new intervention, Mindfulness-Based Exposure Therapy (MBET), offers potential support for this theory. King et al. (2016) created MBET at the Ann Arbor VA after first testing the effectiveness of MBCT for veterans with PTSD. Their original study (King et al., 2013) compared MBCT to Present-Centered Group Therapy as the treatment as usual condition. Present-Centered Group Therapy does not involve sharing details of one's traumatic experience, but instead offers a supportive atmosphere to deal with current issues and learn more adaptive coping skills. Results showed that both therapies brought about a statistically significant reduction of PTSD symptoms, but reductions were not significantly different between treatments. Noting that mindfulness was as effective on its own as group therapy, researchers questioned whether a combination of mindfulness and exposure therapy would be able to bring about a more significant decrease in symptoms.

MBET is a 16-week program that teaches participants mindfulness and self-compassion techniques similar to those found in MBCT, offers psychoeducation about the effects of trauma, and implements in vivo exposure derived from Prolonged Exposure Therapy (King et al., 2016). In a trial with combat veterans suffering from PTSD, participants were informed beforehand that any exposure would be to situations that they currently avoid that are objectively safe (not to memories of trauma as conducted in Prolonged Exposure Therapy). The intervention was separated into four modules on the following focal points:

1. Psychoeducation about PTSD and relaxation
2. In vivo exposure and mindfulness of the breath and body
3. In vivo exposure and mindfulness of emotions
4. Training of self-compassion

MBET showed a significant reduction in Clinically Administered PTSD Scale scores. Additionally, in functional magnetic resonance imaging (fMRI) scans, MBET participants showed an increase in connectivity between the default mode network (DMN)—a large-scale network of interacting brain regions associated with self-reference and mind-wandering (Kiviniemi, Kantola, Jauhiainen, Hyvärinen, & Tervonen, 2003)—and regions of the brain involved in executive control. King and colleagues proposed that this increase may provide a physiological basis for participants' increased ability to freely choose the subject of their attention. Furthermore, they suggested that this new attentional control could be related to engaging, rather than avoiding, trauma memories, which in turn allows for successful healing (King et al., 2016), consistent with the theoretical claim of Follette et al. (2006). MBET was created for and tested with combat veterans. It is unclear whether these positive findings would generalize to survivors of sexual violence.

Other studies have examined the effects of adding mind–body interventions such as mantram repetition, yoga, and MBSR to treatment as usual (TAU). The addition of mantram repetition, a technique from transcendental meditation, to TAU showed significantly stronger reductions in PTSD symptoms and quality-of-life ratings compared to TAU on its own (Bormann et al., 2013). Importantly, this study was conducted with survivors of combat-related trauma, and therefore, results should be interpreted with caution in the context of survivors of sexual violence.

Studies testing the effects of adding yoga to TAU yield promising results. One study found a statistically significant difference in the reduction of PTSD symptoms compared to a waitlist group (Jindani, Turner, & Khalsa, 2015). Another study found a statistically significant reduction in PTSD symptoms when adding yoga to supportive psychotherapy compared to adding a women's health education course to supportive psychotherapy (van der Kolk et al., 2014). In this study, both groups improved mid-treatment, but the health education group's benefits disappeared posttreatment. Both groups of researchers hypothesized that yoga practice would ameliorate PTSD symptoms of avoidance through increased interoceptive awareness of fear responses. With mindful awareness, practitioners are encouraged to experience bodily sensations instead of attempting to escape or ignore them. van der Kolk and colleagues studied female survivors of violence but did not indicate what types of traumatic violence the participants had experienced. Jindani and colleagues are one of the few groups of researchers who described the type of trauma each participant had experienced. In this study, 13 of the 80 participants self-reported an experience with sexual abuse or sexual assault.

MBSR was examined as an adjunct to TAU for survivors of trauma as well, again with conflicting results. One study found statistically significant reductions in PTSD when adding MBSR to TAU (Kearney et al., 2013). Another study yielded nonsignificant results that favored MBSR plus TAU over TAU on its own (Polusny et al., 2015). A third study found that adding MBSR to TAU produced weaker treatment effects than TAU on its own (Niles et al., 2012). All three studies examined combat-associated trauma, and therefore again should be applied to survivors of sexual violence with caution.

However, when comparing TAU to TAU plus an adjunct intervention, it is not surprising to find that the more comprehensive treatment tends to outperform the other. This calls into question the effectiveness of mindfulness treatments on their own. Banks, Newman, and Saleem (2015) conducted a review of studies comparing mindfulness-based intervention groups to controls. Across 12 studies, reviewers found that mindfulness-based treatments show promise as a treatment for symptoms of PTSD, especially avoidance symptoms, adding that results should be interpreted with caution due to methodological issues in the studies included (Banks et al., 2015). Additionally, only one study specifically applied a mindfulness-based treatment to survivors of sexual abuse.

Mindfulness may work well as a stand-alone treatment because the practice itself leads to exposure to thoughts (Brown et al., 2007; Hölzel et al., 2011). If survivors of trauma with PTSD become more aware of their present moment experience, a natural exposure to trauma memories and interoceptive experiences can occur, facilitating change. However, no studies have yet explored the relationship between mindfulness practice and naturalistic exposure. Additionally, the grounding component of mindfulness could help alleviate the physiological arousal symptoms related to PTSD (Kelly & Garland, 2016; Lang et al., 2012). This combination of natural exposure and grounding may explain the utility of mindfulness treatments for survivors of trauma without an added exposure treatment.

Lang et al. (2012) noted that both patients and clinicians are currently dissatisfied with the treatment options for PTSD. High dropout rates on the part of clients and discomfort on the part of clinicians lead to a need for alternatives (Becker, Zayfert, & Anderson, 2004; Schottenbauer, Glass, Arnkoff, Tendick, & Gray, 2008). They discussed several explanations as to why mindfulness may lead to a decrease in symptoms of PTSD, and therefore provide a viable alternative to currently available treatments. Lang and colleagues suggested that mindfulness builds an ability to shift the subject of one's attention willfully, a more adaptive cognitive style, and a nonjudgmental stance. First, they posited that a volitional shift in attention allows patients to reduce reexperiencing symptoms and attentional bias toward reminders of trauma. Second, a present-focused cognitive style may reduce symptoms of worry and rumination associated with negative affect. Finally, Lang and colleagues argued that a nonjudgmental stance can lead to less frequent mislabeling of neutral stimuli as dangerous. In turn, they suggested that those with a nonjudgmental mindset will be more willing to approach (and be exposed to) fear provoking stimuli.

A meta-analysis conducted by Hopwood and Schutte (2017) examined 18 studies that compared a mindfulness-based intervention to a waitlist control for the treatment of PTSD. The studies included a total of 21 samples. Participants among the samples were provided MBSR, yoga interventions, or mindfulness interventions specifically tailored to trauma. Compared to waitlist control groups, mindfulness interventions showed a significant reduction in symptoms of PTSD, with an overall mean weighted effect size of $g = -0.44$. Moderator analysis revealed a significant negative relationship between the decrease in PTSD symptoms and the duration of the intervention, such that longer interventions predicted lower levels of PTSD in response to mindfulness interventions. Gender, age, the number of weeks between the end of the intervention and follow-up assessment, and the effect size of mindfulness were not significant predictors of PTSD in response to mindfulness treatments in the moderation analysis. Ten of the 18 studies examined veteran populations. Only one study explicitly tested survivors of sexual violence, which is described in more detail below.

Gallegos, Crean, Pigeon, and Heffner (2017) conducted a similar meta-analysis on the practice of mediation and yoga for symptoms of PTSD. Authors included a total of 19 randomized control trials, some with inactive and some with active controls, many of which overlap with the previous meta-analysis. Mindfulness meditation and yoga interventions achieved an effect size of $g = -0.39$, outperforming their comparison active and nonactive controls in the reduction of PTSD symptoms. All but four studies were conducted with veterans, and none of the studies specifically mentioned including survivors of sexual violence.

Both of these meta-analyses reported small to medium effect sizes of mindfulness interventions compared to control groups, indicating that practicing mindfulness ameliorates symptoms of PTSD. This provides support for the theory that the practice of mindfulness can have an impact on symptoms without added exposure therapy. However, these results do not indicate any specific mechanisms that explain how mindfulness treatment leads to improvements for survivors of trauma.

Survivors of sexual violence often encounter self-blame and lower self-worth following their assault, which may implicate mindfulness interventions as an appropriate treatment. However, of the handful of studies that examined nonveteran populations, even fewer reported the number of survivors of sexual violence included in the study. None went on to describe how survivors of sexual violence fared in the intervention compared to survivors of other types of trauma. In response to this dearth of information, we searched for studies that specifically describe the effects of mindfulness-based interventions on survivors of sexual violence.

Mindfulness for Survivors of Sexual Violence

Although only recently studied, mindfulness may have a positive impact on survivors of sexual violence. Survivors of sexual violence have higher rates of PTSD than survivors of other types of trauma (Norris, 1992). High rates of co-occurring depression can make the treatment of survivors of sexual violence even more complex (Koss, Bailey, Yuan, Herrera, & Lichter, 2003). Furthermore, the all-too-common incidence of blame from formal responders like doctors and police officers, as well as informal responders such as family and friends, increases the likelihood of negative mental health outcomes (Ullman, 1996a, 1996b). It has been suggested that self-blame may mediate the relationship between experiences with sexual violence and depression (Frazier, 1991). Mindfulness-based treatments have been proven effective in reducing rates of PTSD and depression, and additionally emphasize a component of self-compassion that could be particularly helpful to survivors of sexual violence (Hofmann et al., 2010; Neff, 2003; Tesh, Learman, & Pulliam, 2015). Therefore, although barely studied in the literature, mindfulness interventions may be specifically well suited to the unique needs of survivors of sexual violence and sexual abuse.

On the other hand, the inherent interoceptive exposure of bringing one's attention to the body in mindfulness-based interventions could pose a challenge for survivors of sexual violence. Whether sitting for formal meditation or practicing yoga, participants are asked to bring attention to present somatic experience inside their bodies. This experience could provide a healthy exposure to sensations that give rise to traumatic memories, but if participants have not yet learned how to relate to such thoughts skillfully, iatrogenic effects could result. No study has addressed this concern with survivors of sexual violence. Clinicians should exercise caution in the implementation of mindfulness-based interventions, specifically in early sessions where survivors may not yet have the necessary skills to confront triggering bodily sensations.

To determine what research has been conducted on the subject of mindfulness for survivors of sexual violence, we searched PsychInfo, Google Scholar, ProQuest Dissertations and Theses Global, and PubMed. The search results required that titles and/or abstracts included one or more of the following: "mindfulness," "mindfulness-based," "intervention," "MBSR," "MBCT," "mindfulness-based stress reduction," and "mindfulness-based cognitive therapy"; and one or more of the following: "sexual violence," "sexual abuse," and "rape." Studies had also had to be written in English. After identifying studies, meta-analyses, and dissertations that appeared relevant, we searched the full text of each article to determine whether or not that investigation tested a mindfulness-based intervention or the effects of mindfulness practice on survivors of sexual or intimate partner violence. Four articles reflecting three clinical investigations were identified.

The first such investigation implemented MBSR with survivors of childhood sexual abuse in an open trial and then followed up with participants two and a half years later (Earley et al., 2014; Kimbrough et al., 2010). The second study tested the effects of mindfulness meditation on its own for survivors of intimate partner violence (IPV) in an open trial (Centeno, 2013). The final study tested the effectiveness of a modified version of MBSR titled Trauma-Informed Mindfulness-Based Stress Reduction (TI-MBSR) on survivors of childhood sexual and physical abuse and/or IPV in adulthood in a randomized control trial (Kelly & Garland, 2016). No studies have examined the effectiveness of mindfulness-based interventions exclusively on survivors of

Table 28.1 Results from studies including survivors of sexual violence

Study	Participants (*N*)	Intervention	Measures	Results
Kimbrough et al. (2010)	Survivors of childhood sexual abuse (23)	Modified MBSR + concurrent psychotherapy	BDI-II BSI PCL MAAS	Decrease* Decrease* Decrease* Increase*
Earley et al. (2014)	Survivors of childhood sexual abuse (19)	Modified MBSR	BDI-II BSI PCL MAAS	Decrease* Decrease* Decrease* Increase*
Kelly and Garland (2016)	Survivors of IPV (19 intervention, 20 waitlist)	TI-MBSR	BDI-II PCL-C	Decrease* Decrease*
Centeno (2013)	Survivors of IPV (10)	Mindfulness meditation practice	PCL-C PSS-10	Decrease* Decrease*

Note: *BDI-II* Beck Depression Inventory II, *BSI* Brief Symptom Inventory (used to assess anxiety), *PCL/PCL-C* Posttraumatic Checklist/Posttraumatic Checklist—Civilian, *MAAS* Mindful Awareness Attention Scale, *PSS-10* Perceived Stress Scale—10
*$p < 0.05$

adult sexual violence. Results from these studies are presented in Table 28.1.

Kimbrough et al. (2010) identified MBSR as a possible treatment of depression and PTSD symptoms in survivors of childhood sexual abuse. Their rationale partly was grounded in the theories mentioned earlier, but they also noted that MBSR could be a cost-effective intervention due to its group format. Twenty-seven participants started the treatment, across three cohorts of 7–11 participants each. Four participants left before completing all eight sessions. Participants' depression was measured using the Beck Depression Inventory—II (BDI-II). Their PTSD symptoms were measured with the PTSD Symptoms Checklist (PCL). Participants' anxiety was measured using the Brief Symptom Inventory (BSI), and their mindful awareness was measured with the Mindful Attentional Awareness Scale (MAAS). Measures were collected at baseline, 4 weeks into treatment, upon completion of the MBSR program, and at a 24-week follow-up.

Kimbrough and colleagues made a few important changes to the MBSR protocol in this study. First, participants received three booster sessions after completing the treatment over the course of 3 months. Second, researchers described a change in the language they used during experiential exercises designed to remind participants that it was their own personal choice when to withdraw from any meditation experience. They reported that this is a safety precaution also used in MBCT and Dialectical Behavior Therapy. Finally, they encouraged participants to be aware of their positive growth, a practice they ascribed to positive psychology. Because this was a pilot of MBSR with this population, the researchers also required participants to enroll in concurrent psychotherapy.

Participants showed statistically significant decreases in depression, anxiety, and PTSD following the MBSR intervention, and maintained a statistically significant difference from baseline at the 24-week follow-up. Scores on the mindful awareness measure increased and stayed significantly increased from baseline at the 24-week follow-up (Kimbrough et al., 2010). Average depression scores at pretest fell in the moderate range of depression and fell into the minimal depression range after completing MBSR. At the 24-week follow-up, depression scores rose slightly, but the average still fell in the minimal depression range. Average PTSD scores at pretest were above the clinical cutoff for PTSD, but fell below the cutoff at posttest and follow-up. These findings strongly support the feasibility of MBSR as an adjunct treatment for treating the common symptoms of survivors of childhood sexual abuse.

The researchers involved in this project also conducted a two-and-a-half-year follow-up with the same group of survivors. Seventy-three percent of the original participants, or 19 survivors, responded to the same four surveys conducted in the first study (BDI-II, PCL, BSI, and MAAS). Two and a half years after participating in the MBSR program, this group continued to show statistically significantly lower symptomology and higher mindful awareness (Earley et al., 2014). Specifically, participants' average depression symptoms remained in the minimal range and average PTSD symptoms fell below the clinical cutoff. This longevity of treatment effectiveness provides strong support for the use of mindfulness-based interventions as an adjunct treatment for this population.

Kelly and Garland (2016) created and tested an alternate version of MBSR specifically for survivors of trauma, known as Trauma-Informed Mindfulness-Based Stress Reduction (TI-MBSR). This version of the program leaves intact all of the MBSR curriculum while adding in psychoeducation about psychological, neurophysiological, and relational effects of trauma. Kelly and Garland added the education component because an "understanding of reactions and experience is associated with increased self-efficacy and decreased self-blame related to survival behaviors and reactions" (Kelly, 2014, p. 38). In addition, TI-MBSR integrates strategies to help survivors regulate physiological arousal, borrowed from other trauma-informed therapies (Kelly & Garland, 2016). The specific additions to traditional MBSR modules were as follows:

- Session 1: Teaching neurophysiology of trauma, including a rationale for using mindfulness skills as a coping mechanism
- Session 2: Discussion of reactivity as related to survival of trauma and symptoms as adaptations; discussion of fight, flight, or freeze response; discussion of attempts to cope with symptoms that followed the traumatic experience; teaching to recognize physiological symptoms of trauma reactivity
- Session 3: Teaching to recognize one's individual bodily reactions to triggers and how to regulate through mindfulness techniques; teaching to recognize thought suppression and avoidance
- Session 4: Discussion of common patterns of relating to others; discuss the "trauma triangle" (roles of victim, victimizer, and bystander)
- Session 5: Review information from sessions 2 and 4
- Session 7: Discussion of how mindfulness relates to parenting and how to bring mindfulness into relationships with children
- (For more detail, see Table 1 in Kelly & Garland, 2016).

TI-MBSR was tested with a group of survivors of childhood sexual abuse, childhood physical abuse, and/or adult intimate partner violence (Kelly & Garland, 2016). The CDC estimates that 25% of survivors of IPV have experienced sexual assault (Black et al., 2011). Thus, although their sample was not limited to survivors of sexual violence, it is likely that such survivors were well represented within this sample. Research on the effects of mindfulness treatments exclusively for survivors of sexual assault remains scarce. Nevertheless, the following results from this TI-MBSR investigation should be interpreted with caution in their application to survivors of sexual assault.

Kelly and Garland (2016) measured 20 female survivors of IPV and childhood abuse before and after completing the TI-MBSR training. A waitlist group of 19 female survivors completed identical measures in the same 8-week interval. Participants were randomly assigned to either the TI-MBSR group or the waitlist group. Both groups reported a significant decrease in depression (BDI-II) and PTSD (PCL-C) over time. The TI-MBSR group showed a significantly greater reduction of depression and PTSD symptoms when compared to the waitlist group. Additionally, 80% of those in the TI-MBSR group fell below the clinical cutoff for PTSD postintervention compared to only 20% of participants in the waitlist group. Average depression scores of those in the TI-MBSR group fell from moderate to minimal. Those who spent more time meditating at home between sessions perceived the treatment as more effective. Time spent doing homework was negatively correlated with symptoms of depression. This study established the feasibility of TI-MBSR for female survivors of IPV and childhood abuse. Researchers note that survivors could have also been participating in concurrent psychotherapy, but it was not specifically measured in this study. It is unclear whether the improvements made in the TI-MBSR group can be attributed solely to participation in the intervention.

A final study tested the effects of mindfulness meditation over a 6-week course. In this study, 10 survivors of IPV were selected to participate, all of whom had received a previous diagnosis of PTSD. Participants attended two weekly guided meditation sessions. Additionally, each survivor was assigned an individualized amount of at-home meditation practice based on their previous experience. Beginners started with shorter times than those with any meditation experience. Each participant's duration of meditation stepped up incrementally over 6 weeks. Survivors showed a significant decrease in PTSD symptoms (PCL-C) and levels perceived stress (PSS-10). Nine of the ten survivors met criteria for PTSD at the beginning of the study. Only two participants continued to meet criteria after completing the 6-week practice of meditation (Centeno, 2013). While other studies have implemented manualized treatments for survivors of trauma, this study suggests that mindfulness meditation on its own could be helpful for survivors of trauma. Three of the participants were receiving concurrent psychotherapy. For these participants, the cause of positive treatment outcomes is especially blurred.

In summary, mindfulness-based interventions have shown preliminary benefits for survivors of trauma. Across multiple studies, PTSD and depression symptoms decreased in response to mindfulness training. However, most studies used small samples to pilot the intervention and no studies have isolated the benefits of mindfulness-based treatments for survivors of nonchildhood sexual violence. Mindfulness-based Exposure Therapy has been successfully piloted with veterans and Trauma-Informed Mindfulness-based Stress Reduction has shown to benefit survivors of IPV/childhood abuse. It is unclear to what extent survivors of nonchildhood sexual violence specifically may benefit from mindfulness-based interventions, whether mindfulness would be best delivered with an adjunct exposure treatment for such survivors, or if mindfulness meditation can stand on its own as an effective intervention.

Mindfulness and Self-Compassion as Protective Factors

Self-compassion is a practice from Buddhist traditions that has been integrated into mindfulness trainings, including MBSR, MBCT, and MBET. Kristen Neff (2003) described self-compassion as three interacting parts of a whole. The first piece is self-kindness, which involves providing oneself the same benevolence and goodwill that one commonly provides to others. The second piece is known as common humanity, which is the recognition that all humans experience suffering; survivors are not isolated in their experience of pain. The final piece is a mindful relationship to experiences of suffering. A mindful relationship is one where painful experiences are neither avoided nor overindulged, simply recognized as part of the present moment (Neff, 2003).

Self-compassion has been theorized to play an important role in mental health outcomes in survivors of trauma (Seligowski, Miron, & Orcutt, 2014; Tesh et al., 2015; Thompson & Waltz, 2008). As survivors of trauma experience pain, self-compassion could be an effective coping strategy. In a study with a trauma population, self-compassion predicted lower PTSD avoidance symptoms (Thompson & Waltz, 2008). A second study examined survivors of trauma to create a structural equation model in order to explore the relationship between self-compassion, psychological flexibility, psychological health, and PTSD symptoms. Self-compassion was a positive predictor of overall psychological health, while psychological flexibility was the only significant predictor of PTSD symptoms (Seligowski et al., 2014). More research is needed to understand the exact role of self-compassion for survivors of sexual violence, but results indicate that self-compassion is related to better outcomes for survivors.

A review of articles concerning the relationship between mindfulness and resiliency in the face of trauma concluded that those with higher mindfulness and acceptance tend to have better psychological adjustment following experiences with trauma (Thompson, Arnkoff, & Glass, 2011). These authors considered their findings preliminary evidence to support including mindfulness training in PTSD prevention programs. Another study found that certain facets of mindfulness, including describing, acting with awareness, and nonjudging, partially mediated the relationship between traumatic experiences and PTSD symptoms (Boughner, Thornley, Kharlas, & Frewen, 2016).

Additionally, mindfulness has been linked to posttraumatic growth (PTG) in those who practice mindfulness through meditation, yoga, or tai chi. Those who reported that they did not practice mindful activities did not have a significant relationship between mindfulness and PTG (Hanley, Peterson, Canto, & Garland, 2015). Mindfulness must be practiced to have an association with PTG. If practicing mindfulness and trait mindfulness are in fact protective factors against PTSD, increasing access to mindfulness trainings could be critical for vulnerable populations.

Mindfulness and Prevention of Sexual Violence

Preliminary studies have examined the role that mindfulness might play in the prevention of sexual violence. Because of its association with both emotion and behavior regulation (Brown et al., 2007; Hölzel et al., 2011), mindfulness has been examined as a possible protective factor against sexual violence perpetration (Gallagher, Hudepohl, & Parrott, 2010; Ramirez et al., 2017). Higher mindfulness is related to lower aggression in both correlation and experimental analyses (Borders, Earleywine, & Jajodia, 2010; Heppner et al., 2008).

One study examined the relationship between trait mindfulness (measured with the Five Facet Mindfulness Questionnaire—15) and perpetration of sexual coercion and aggression within a sample of 665 young adults. The results showed that higher mindfulness was significantly related to lower likelihood of perpetration (Ramirez et al., 2017). These authors suggested that mindfulness could be a useful tool in the prevention of sexual violence. This research team is currently developing and measuring the effectiveness of a mindfulness-based intervention that addresses alcohol misuse and dating violence perpetration (Q. Ngo, personal communication, April 15, 2018).

Mindfulness for Clinicians and Advocates

Victim advocates and clinicians who work with survivors of sexual violence provide vital support while exposing themselves to the possibility of experiencing trauma symptoms as a result of their work, known as secondary traumatic stress (Dworkin, Sorell, & Allen, 2016). Estimates of secondary traumatic stress in those who work with the traumatized range from 60% to 65% (Figley, 2002). Burnout is also common in the field of trauma advocacy. In interviews, advocates identified that burnout affects the quality of the service that they can provide and their own levels of secondary traumatization (Ullman & Townsend, 2007).

No research has been published concerning the implementation of mindfulness interventions for advocates in rape crisis centers. However, among advocates at a grief and bereavement center, high dispositional mindfulness predicted lower burnout and secondary traumatic stress across the agency (Thieleman & Cacciatore, 2014). Qualitative data from mental health professionals who practice mindfulness and have worked extensively with survivors of trauma identified mindfulness as a key self-care mechanism (Schafer, 2016). Additionally, when compared to Cognitive Behavioral Stress Management, a Yoga-Based Stress Management course resulted in better mental health outcomes and lower secondary traumatic stress over time for frontline mental health advocates (Riley et al., 2017). The implication from these findings is that mindfulness skills may benefit sexual assault victim advocates, clinicians, and others who serve survivors of sexual violence.

Mindfulness and Cultural Considerations

Little research has examined cultural considerations in mindfulness-based interventions. Preliminary research demonstrated that MBSR was successfully delivered in Spanish in inner-city programs serving largely Latino patients with additional adaptations such as flexible scheduling, providing transportation and child care, reminder calls before initial sessions, and refraining from the use of the word *yoga* when referring to mindful movement practices (Roth & Creaser, 1997; Roth & Robbins, 2004).

Mindfulness and Client Acceptability

Additional research exploring client or patient acceptability of mindfulness-based interventions is sorely needed as well. Although mindfulness-based intervention practices are presented in a secular fashion, unfavorable perceptions or misconceptions about meditation and yoga might prevent many Americans from participating in this form of intervention. Future research that identifies how the initial description of mindfulness-based interventions and the instructor's presentation of mindfulness practices impact client or patient acceptability could help clinicians address this particular barrier to access.

Summary and Future Directions

Survivors of intimate partner violence have seen significant reductions in PTSD and depression upon completion of a trauma-informed mindfulness intervention (Kelly & Garland, 2016), as well as lower stress when practicing mindfulness meditation (Centeno, 2013). Additionally, mindfulness interventions combined with treatment as usual have shown reductions in symptoms of PTSD and depression in survivors of childhood sexual abuse, with gains that are maintained at a two-and-a-half-year follow-up (Earley et al., 2014; Kimbrough et al., 2010). These promising studies provide preliminary evidence for the benefits of mindfulness practice for survivors of sexual violence.

Survivors of sexual violence could benefit from mindfulness-based interventions for a variety of reasons. Some theories postulate that a practice of mindfulness facilitates the success of exposure-based treatments (Follette et al., 2006). Mindfulness-Based Exposure Therapy outcome data lends empirical support to this theory, as mindfulness practice combined with in vivo exposure successfully reduced PTSD symptoms in veteran populations (King et al., 2016). Other studies have shown that adding mindfulness practices to treatment as usual for survivors of trauma significantly outperforms the treatment as usual on its own (Bormann et al., 2013; Kearney et al., 2013; Polusny et al., 2015; van der Kolk et al., 2014). All of this together provides an indication that adding mindfulness to a treatment plan strengthens the gains that survivors can make in therapy.

Other theories imply that mindfulness leads to a natural exposure to trauma memories and physiological arousal, which in turn alleviates PTSD symptoms (Brown et al., 2007; Hölzel et al., 2011). Kelly and Garland (2016), creators of Trauma-Informed Mindfulness-Based Stress Reduction, also theorized that the grounding component of mindfulness practice could assist survivors in settling symptoms of physiological hyperarousal. While Follette et al. (2006) argued that mindfulness could make structured exposure therapy more effective, this alternative theoretical position claims that mindfulness practice itself provides sufficient naturalistic exposure. Therefore, it might not be necessary to add additional in vivo or imaginal exposure treatment components to mindfulness-based interventions for survivors. Reviews of studies that compared mindfulness-based treatments to control groups concluded that mindfulness treatments show promise in the treatment of PTSD, especially avoidance symptoms (Banks et al., 2015; Hopwood & Schutte, 2017).

Survivors of sexual violence face high rates of PTSD and depression; mindfulness interventions are effective in treating both. Mindfulness practice reduced symptoms of PTSD and depression in survivors of childhood sexual abuse, and these gains were maintained at a two-and-a-half-year follow-up (Earley et al., 2014; Kimbrough et al., 2010). Survivors of intimate partner violence have seen significant reductions in PTSD and depression upon completion of Trauma-Informed Mindfulness-Based Stress Reduction (Kelly & Garland, 2016), and reductions of trauma and stress when practicing mindfulness meditation (Centeno, 2013).

Additionally, the self-blame commonly experienced by survivors of sexual violence could be reduced with self-compassion components of mindfulness (Tesh et al., 2015). MBSR increased self-compassion among nondistressed samples (e.g., Birnie, Speca, & Carlson, 2010), and self-compassion is negatively related to PTSD symptoms and positively related to psychological health in survivors of trauma (Seligowski et al., 2014; Thompson & Waltz, 2008). Mindfulness more broadly is associated with better psychological adjustment after trauma (Thompson et al., 2011). Also, those who practice mindfulness show a significant relationship between their level of trait mindfulness and posttraumatic growth following trauma (Hanley et al., 2015).

Mindfulness may also be a useful tool in the sexual violence prevention movement. Mindfulness is negatively related to aggression and positively related to emotion and behavior regulation (Brown et al., 2007; Gallagher et al., 2010; Hölzel et al., 2011; Ramirez et al., 2017). Burgeoning research shows that mindfulness is also negatively related to sexual assault perpetration (Ramirez et al., 2017). However, no causal relationships have been established to date.

Future studies examining the effects of mindfulness-based interventions on adult survivors of sexual violence clearly are warranted. Sufficient research conducted with survivors of general trauma, childhood sexual abuse, and IPV exists to justify future clinical trials that target this specific population. Such future research would help determine whether mindfulness-based interventions are likely to benefit survivors of sexual violence. Furthermore, randomized controlled comparative trials could help determine whether or not mindfulness practice provides an adequate level of exposure on its own, without additional treatment components. Comparing a treatment that adds in vivo exposure to mindfulness treatment (MBET) with a treatment that relies solely on mindfulness training (MBSR/TI-MBSR) would address this particular empirical question. Future outcome research conducted with survivors of sexual violence should include measures of mindfulness, self-compassion, trauma symptoms, depression symptoms, posttraumatic growth, and psychological health, as all of these variables in combination could help address how mindfulness-based interventions work.

More research is needed to determine whether mindfulness protects against PTSD and/or perpetration of sexual violence. If mindfulness protects against PTSD, populations at high risk of experiencing trauma could be offered mindfulness training as a preventive measure. At the same time, if perpetration could be reduced through mindfulness interventions, communities could attack the problem from both sides with the same tool. Mindfulness could offer a pathway to less perpetration, lower likelihood of PTSD, and higher availability of effective treatments for survivors.

Finally, clinicians and advocates who work with survivors of trauma may benefit from mindfulness practice themselves. Advocate self-care is essential to protect against burnout, high stress, and symptoms of secondary traumatic stress. Mindfulness can offer both awareness of a lack of self-care and a means to correct for this deficiency. Less secondary traumatic stress and burnout will allow advocates to provide better services to an increased number of survivors over longer periods of time. With the knowledge that survivors who access rape crisis services experience less distress posttrauma (Campbell, Dworkin, & Cabral, 2009), assisting advocates and clinicians could have a significant ripple effect on many survivors for years to come.

References

Agsar, W. (2017, December 14). *Major Medical School Announces First Dedicated Mindfulness Division*. Retrieved from http://www.tricycle.org

Banks, K., Newman, E., & Saleem, J. (2015). An overview of the research on mindfulness-based interventions for treating symptoms of posttraumatic stress disorder: A systematic review. *Journal of Clinical Psychology, 71*(10), 935–963. https://doi.org/10.1002/jclp.22200

Becker, C. B., Zayfert, C., & Anderson, E. (2004). A survey of psychologists' attitudes towards and utilization of exposure therapy for PTSD. *Behaviour Research and Therapy, 42*, 277–292. https://doi.org/10.1016/S0005-7967(03)00138-4

Birnie, K., Speca, M., & Carlson, L. E. (2010). Exploring self-compassion and empathy in the context of mindfulness-based stress reduction (MBSR). *Stress and Health, 26*(5), 359–371.

Black, M. C., Basile, K. C., Breiding, M. J., Smith, S. G., Walters, M. L., Merrick, M. T., … Stevens, M. R. (2011). *National intimate partner and sexual violence survey: 2010 summary report*. Atlanta, GA.

Borders, A., Earleywine, M., & Jajodia, A. (2010). Could mindfulness decrease anger, hostility, and aggression by decreasing rumination? *Aggressive Behavior, 36*(1), 28–44. https://doi.org/10.1002/ab.20327

Bormann, J. E., Thorp, S. R., Wetherell, J. L., Golshan, S., & Lang, A. J. (2013). Meditation-based mantram intervention for veterans with posttraumatic stress disorder: A randomized trial. *Psychological Trauma Theory Research Practice and Policy, 5*(3), 259–267. https://doi.org/10.1037/a0027522

Boughner, E., Thornley, E., Kharlas, D., & Frewen, P. (2016). Mindfulness-related traits partially mediate the association between lifetime and childhood trauma exposure and PTSD and dissociative symptoms in a community sample assessed online. *Mindfulness, 7*, 672–679. https://doi.org/10.1007/s12671-016-0502-3

Brown, K. W., Ryan, R. M., & Creswell, J. D. (2007). Mindfulness: Theoretical foundations and evidence for its salutary effects. *Psychological Inquiry, 18*(4), 211–237. https://doi.org/10.1080/10478400701598298

Campbell, R., Dworkin, E., & Cabral, G. (2009). An ecological model of the impact of sexual assault on women's mental health. *Trauma, Violence & Abuse, 10*(3), 225–246.

Centeno, E. (2013). Mindfulness meditation and its effects on survivors of intimate partner violence.

de Vibe, M., Bjørndal, A., Tipton, E., Hammerstrøm, K., & Kowalski, K. (2012). Mindfulness-based stress reduction (MBSR) for improving health, quality of life, and social functioning in adults. *Campbell Systematic Reviews, 2012*(3). https://doi.org/10.4073/csr.2012.3

Dworkin, E. R., Sorell, N. R., & Allen, N. E. (2016). Individual-and setting-level correlates of secondary traumatic stress in rape crisis center staff. *Journal of Interpersonal Violence, 31*(4), 743–752. https://doi.org/10.1177/0886260514556111

Earley, M. D., Chesney, M. A., Frye, J., Greene, P. A., Berman, B., & Kimbrough, E. (2014). Mindfulness intervention for child abuse survivors: A 2.5-year follow-up. *Journal of Clinical Psychology, 70*(10), 1–9. https://doi.org/10.1002/jclp.22102

Ehlers, A., & Clark, D. (2003). Early psychological interventions for adult survivors of trauma: A review. *Biological Psychiatry, 53*(9), 817–826.

Figley, C. R. (2002). Compassion fatigue: Psychotherapists' chronic lack of self-care. *Psychotherapy in Practice, 58*, 1433–1441.

Follette, V., Palm, K. M., & Pearson, A. N. (2006). Mindfulness and trauma: Implications for treatment. *Journal of Rational-Emotive & Cognitive-Behavior Therapy, 24*(1), 45–61. https://doi.org/10.1007/s10942-006-0025-2

Frazier, P. A. (1991). Self-blame as a mediator of postrape depressive symptoms. *Journal of Social and Clinical Psychology, 10*(1), 47–57. https://doi.org/10.1521/jscp.1991.10.1.47

Fronsdal, G. (1998). Insight meditation in the United States: Life, liberty, and the pursuit of happiness. In C. S. Perbish & K. K. Tanaka (Eds.), *The faces of Buddhism in America* (pp. 164–180). Oakland, CA: University of California Press.

Galante, J., Iribarren, S. J., & Pearce, P. F. (2013). Effects of mindfulness-based cognitive therapy on mental disorders: A systematic review and meta-analysis of randomized controlled trials. *Journal of Research in Nursing, 18*(2), 133–155.

Gallagher, K. E., Hudepohl, A. D., & Parrott, D. J. (2010). Power of being present: The role of mindfulness on the relation between men's alcohol use and sexual aggression toward intimate partners. *Aggressive Behavior, 36*(6), 405–413. https://doi.org/10.1002/ab.20351

Gallegos, A. M., Crean, H. F., Pigeon, W. R., & Heffner, K. L. (2017). Meditation and yoga for posttraumatic stress disorder: A meta-analytic review of randomized controlled trials. *Clinical Psychology Review, 58*, 115–124. https://doi.org/10.1016/j.cpr.2017.10.004

Germer, C. (2005). Teaching mindfulness in therapy. In *Mindfulness and psychotherapy, 2nd ed.* (pp. 113–129). https://doi.org/10.1007/978-1-4614-3033-9

Hanley, A. W., Peterson, G. W., Canto, A. I., & Garland, E. L. (2015). The relationship between mindfulness and posttraumatic growth with respect to contemplative practice engagement. *Mindfulness, 6*(3), 654–662. https://doi.org/10.1007/s12671-014-0302-6

Heidenreich, T., Tuin, I., Pflug, B., Michal, M., & Michalak, J. (2006). Mindfulness-based cognitive therapy for persistent insomnia: A pilot study. *Psychotherapy and Psychosomatics, 75*, 188–189. https://doi.org/10.1159/000091778

Heppner, W. L., Kernis, M. H., Lakey, C. E., Campbell, W. K., Goldman, B. M., Davis, P. J., & Cascio, E. V. (2008). Mindfulness as a means of reducing aggressive behavior: Dispositional and situational evidence. *Aggressive Behavior, 34*, 486–496. https://doi.org/10.1002/ab.20258

Hilton, L., Maher, A. R., Colaiaco, B., Apaydin, E., Sorbero, M. E., Booth, M., … Hempel, S. (2017). Meditation for posttraumatic stress: Systematic review and meta-analysis. *Psychological Trauma Theory Research Practice and Policy, 9*(4), 453–460. https://doi.org/10.1037/tra0000180

Hofmann, S. G., Asnaani, A., Vonk, I. J. J., Sawyer, A. T., & Fang, A. (2012). The efficacy of cognitive behavioral therapy: A review of meta-analyses. *Cognitive Therapy and Research, 36*, 427–440. https://doi.org/10.1007/s10608-012-9476-1

Hofmann, S. G., Sawyer, A. T., Witt, A. A., & Oh, D. (2010). The effect of mindfulness-based therapy on anxiety and expression: A meta-analytic review. *Journal of Consulting and Clinical Psychology, 78*(2), 169–183. https://doi.org/10.1037/a0018555

Hölzel, B. K., Lazar, S. W., Gard, T., Schuman-Olivier, Z., Vago, D. R., & Ott, U. (2011). How does mindfulness meditation work? Proposing mechanisms of action from a conceptual and neural perspective. *Perspectives on Psychological Science, 6*(6), 537–559. https://doi.org/10.1177/1745691611419671

Hopwood, T. L., & Schutte, N. S. (2017). A meta-analytic investigation of the impact of mindfulness-based interventions on post traumatic stress. *Clinical Psychology Review, 57*, 12–20. https://doi.org/10.1016/j.cpr.2017.08.002

Jamieson, J. P., Nock, M. K., & Mendes, W. B. (2012). Mind over matter: Reappraising arousal improves cardiovascular and cognitive responses to stress. *Journal of Experimental Psychology: General, 141*(3), 417–422. https://doi.org/10.1037/a0025719

Jindani, F., Turner, N., & Khalsa, S. B. (2015). A yoga intervention for posttraumatic stress: A preliminary randomized control trial. *Evidence-based Complementary and Alternative Medicine*, 1–8. https://doi.org/10.1155/2015/351746

Kabat-Zinn, J. (2013). *Full catastrophe living: Using the wisdom of your body and mind to face stress, pain, and illness*. New York, NY: Bantam Books.

Kearney, D. J., Mcdermott, K., Malte, C., Martinez, M., & Simpson, T. L. (2013). Effects of participation in a mindfulness program for veterans with posttraumatic stress disorder: A randomized controlled pilot study. *Journal of Clinical Psychology, 69*(1), 14–27. https://doi.org/10.1002/jclp.21911

Keller, A., Litzelman, K., Wisk, L. E., Maddox, T., Cheng, E. R., Creswell, P. D., & Witt, W. P. (2012). Does the Perception that Stress Affects Health Matter? The Association with Health and Mortality. *Health Psychology: Official Journal of the Division of Health Psychology, American Psychological Association, 31*(5), 677–684. https://doi.org/10.1037/a0026743

Kelly, A. (2014). Trauma-informed mindfulness-based stress reduction: Development of a model and an application with a sample of women who have survived interpersonal trauma.

Kelly, A., & Garland, E. L. (2016). Trauma-informed mindfulness-based stress reduction for female survivors of interpersonal violence: Results from a stage I RCT. *Journal of Clinical Psychology, 72*(4), 311–328. https://doi.org/10.1002/jclp.22273

Kimbrough, E., Magyari, T., Langenberg, P., Chesney, M., & Berman, B. (2010). Mindfulness intervention for child abuse survivors. *Journal of Clinical Psychology, 66*(1), 17–33. https://doi.org/10.1002/jclp.20624

King, A. P., Block, S. R., Sripada, R. K., Rauch, S., Giardino, N., Favorite, T., … Liberzon, I. (2016). Altered default mode network (DMN) resting state functional connectivity following a mindfulness-based exposure therapy for posttraumatic stress disorder (PTSD) in combat veterans of Afghanistan and Iraq. *Depression and Anxiety, 33*(4), 289–299. https://doi.org/10.1002/da.22481

King, A. P., Erickson, T. M., Giardino, N. D., Favorite, T., Rauch, S. A. M., Robinson, E., … Liberzon, I. (2013). A pilot study of group mindfulness-based cognitive therapy (MBCT) for combat veterans with posttraumatic stress disorder (PTSD). *Depression and Anxiety, 30*(7), 638–645. https://doi.org/10.1002/da.22104

Kiviniemi, V., Kantola, J., Jauhiainen, J., Hyvärinen, A., & Tervonen, O. (2003). Independent component analysis of nondeterministic fMRI signal sources. *NeuroImage, 19*, 253–260. https://doi.org/10.1016/S1053-8119(03)00097-1

Koss, M. P., Bailey, J. A., Yuan, N. P., Herrera, V. M., & Lichter, E. L. (2003). Depression and PTSD in survivors of male violence: Research and training initiatives to facilitate recovery. *Psychology of Women Quarterly, 27*(2), 130–142. https://doi.org/10.1111/1471-6402.00093

Kristeller, J. L., Baer, R. A., & Quillian-Wolever, R. (2006). Mindfulness-based approaches to eating disorders. In R. A. Baer (Ed.), *Mindfulness-based treatment approaches: Clinician's guide to evidence base and applications* (pp. 75–91). San Diego, CA: Elsevier Academic Press. https://doi.org/10.1016/B978-012088519-0/50005-8

Lang, A. J., Strauss, J. L., Bomyea, J., Bormann, J. E., Hickman, S. D., Good, R. C., & Essex, M. (2012). The theoretical and empirical basis for meditation as an intervention for PTSD. *Behavior Modification, 36*(6), 759–786. https://doi.org/10.1177/0145445512441200

Lustyk, M. K., Chawla, N., Nolan, R., & Marlatt, G. A. (2009). Mindfulness meditation research: Issues of participant screening, safety procedures, and researcher training. *Advances in Mind-Body Medicine, 24*(1), 20–30.

Ma, S. H., & Teasdale, J. D. (2004). Mindfulness-based cognitive therapy for depression: Replication and exploration of differential relapse prevention effects. *Journal of Consulting and Clinical Psychology, 72*, 31–40. https://doi.org/10.1037/0022-006X.72.1.31

Magyari, T. (2015). Teaching mindfulness-based stress reduction and mindfulness to women with complex trauma. In V. M. Follette, J. Briere, D. Rozelle, J. W. Hopper, & D. I. Rome (Eds.), *Mindfulness-oriented interventions for trauma: Integrating contemplative practices* (pp. 140–156). New York, NY: Guilford Press.

Mitchell, K. S., Dick, A. M., DiMartino, D. M., Smith, B. N., Niles, B., Koenen, K. C., & Street, A. (2014). A pilot study of a randomized controlled trial of yoga as an intervention for PTSD symptoms in women. *Journal of Traumatic Stress, 27*, 121–128.

Neff, K. (2003). Self-compassion: An alternative conceptualization of a healthy attitude toward oneself. *Self and Identity, 2*(2), 85–101. https://doi.org/10.1080/15298860309032

Niles, B. L., Klunk-Gillis, J., Ryngala, D. J., Silberbogen, A. K., Paysnick, A., & Wolf, E. J. (2012). Comparing mindfulness and psychoeducation treatments for combat-related PTSD using a telehealth approach. *Psychological Trauma Theory Research Practice and Policy, 4*(5). https://doi.org/10.1037/a0026161

Norris, F. H. (1992). Epidemiology of trauma: Frequency and impact of different potentially traumatic events on different demographic groups. *Journal of Consulting and Clinical Psychology, 60*(3), 409–418. https://doi.org/10.1037/0022-006X.60.3.409

Polusny, M. A., Erbes, C. R., Thuras, P., Moran, A., Lamberty, G. J., Collins, R. C., … Lim, K. O. (2015). Mindfulness-based stress reduction for posttraumatic stress disorder among veterans a randomized clinical trial. *JAMA : The Journal of the American Medical Association, 314*(5), 456–465. https://doi.org/10.1001/jama.2015.8361

Ramirez, J., Ngo, Q., Walton, M., Chermack, S., Stein, S., & Cunningham, R. (2017). The role of mindfulness in physical dating violence, injuring a partner and psychological dating violence. *Injury Prevention*.

Riley, K. E., Park, C. L., Wilson, A., Sabo, A. N., Antoni, M. H., Braun, T. D., … Cope, S. (2017). Improving physical and mental health in frontline mental health care providers: Yoga-based stress management versus cognitive behavioral stress management. *Journal of Workplace Behavioral Health, 32*(1), 26–48. https://doi.org/10.1080/15555240.2016.1261254

Roth, B., & Creaser, T. (1997). Mindfulness meditation-based stress reduction: Experience with a bilingual inner-city program. *The Nurse Practitioner, 22*, 150–e176.

Roth, B., & Robbins, D. (2004). Mindfulness-based stress reduction and health-related quality of life: Findings from a bilingual inner-city patient population. *Psychosomatic Medicine, 66*, 113–123.

Santorelli, S. F., & Kabat-Zinn, J. (2009). Mindfulness-based stress reduction (MBSR) professional education and training: MBSR curriculum and supporting materials. *University of Massachusetts Medical School, Center for Mindfulness in Medicine, Health Care, and Society.*

Schafer, C. (2016). The lived experience of mental health professionals who practice mindfulness and work with trauma survivors.

Schottenbauer, M. A., Glass, C. R., Arnkoff, D. B., Tendick, V., & Gray, S. H. (2008). Nonresponse and dropout rates in outcome studies on PTSD: Review and Methodological Considerations. *Psychiatry: Interpersonal and Biological Processes, 71*(2), 134–168. https://doi.org/10.1521/psyc.2008.71.2.134

Segal, Z. V., Williams, J. M. G., & Teasdale, J. D. (2013). *Mindfulness-based cognitive therapy for depression* (2nd ed.). New York, NY: Guilford Press.

Seligman, M. E. P. (1998). *Learned optimism* (2nd ed.). New York, NY: Simon & Schuster.

Seligowski, A. V., Miron, L. R., & Orcutt, H. K. (2014). Relations among self-compassion, PTSD symptoms, and psychological health in a trauma-exposed sample. *Mindfulness, 6*(5), 1033–1041. https://doi.org/10.1007/s12671-014-0351-x

Teasdale, J. D., Segal, Z. V., Williams, J. M., Ridgeway, V. A., Soulsby, J. M., & Lau, M. A. (2000). Prevention of relapse/recurrence in major depression by mindfulness-based cognitive therapy. *Journal of Consulting and Clinical Psychology, 68*, 615–623. https://doi.org/10.1037/0022-006X.68.4.615

Tesh, M., Learman, J., & Pulliam, R. M. (2015). Mindful self-compassion strategies for survivors of intimate partner abuse. *Mindfulness, 6*(2), 192–201. https://doi.org/10.1007/s12671-013-0244-4

Thieleman, K., & Cacciatore, J. (2014). Witness to suffering: Mindfulness and compassion fatigue among traumatic bereavement volunteers and Professionals. *Social Work (United States), 59*(1), 34–41. https://doi.org/10.1093/sw/swt044

Thompson, B. L., & Waltz, J. (2008). Self-compassion and PTSD symptom severity. *Journal of Traumatic Stress, 21*(6), 556–558. https://doi.org/10.1002/jts.20374

Thompson, R. W., Arnkoff, D. B., & Glass, C. R. (2011). Conceptualizing mindfulness and acceptance as components of psychological resilience to trauma. *Trauma, Violence & Abuse, 12*(4), 220–235. https://doi.org/10.1177/1524838011416375

Ullman, S. E. (1996a). Do social reactions to sexual assault victims vary by support provider? *Violence and Victims, 11*(2), 143–157.

Ullman, S. E. (1996b). Social reactions, coping strategies, and self-blame attributions in adjustment to sexual assault. *Psychology of Women Quarterly, 20*, 505–526.

Ullman, S. E., & Townsend, S. M. (2007). Barriers to working with sexual assault survivors: A qualitative study of rape crisis center workers. *Violence Against Women, 13*(4), 412–443.

van der Kolk, B. A., Stone, L., West, J., Rhodes, A., Emerson, D., Suvak, M., & Spinazzola, J. (2014). Yoga as an adjunctive treatment for posttraumatic stress disorder: A randomized controlled trial. *Journal of Clinical Psychiatry, 75*(6), 3559–e565. https://doi.org/10.4088/JCP.13m08561

Van Gordon, W., Shonin, E., Griffiths, M. D., & Singh, N. N. (2015). Mindfulness and the four noble truths. In E. Shonin, W. Van Gordon, & N. N. Singh (Eds.), *Buddhist foundations of mindfulness* (pp. 9–27). Switzerland: Springer International Publishing.

Wegner, D. M. (1997). When the antidote is the poison: Ironic mental control processes. *Psychological Science, 8*(3), 148–150.

Witkiewitz, K., & Marlatt, G. A. (2004). Relapse prevention for alcohol and drug problems: That was Zen, this is Tao. *American Psychologist, 59*, 224–235. https://doi.org/10.1037/0003-066X.59.4.224

Treating the Adult Sexual Assault Victim: Evidence-Based Assessment and Treatment

29

Nykia R. Leach and Lindsay M. Orchowski

Introduction

In their seminal publication within the *American Journal of Psychiatry*, Burgess and Holmstrom (1974) characterized rape as an experience that can be disruptive to a person's physical, emotional, cognitive, and interpersonal functioning. Since Burgess and Holmstrom's (1974) early description of "Rape Trauma Syndrome," research has accumulated to document a range of presentations of mental distress and physical injury among survivors of sexual violence. Specifically, whereas the adverse health effects of sexual assault are dynamic and heterogeneous, survivors of sexual violence may experience psychological distress such as posttraumatic stress, anxiety, substance use and depressive disorders (Acierno, Resnick, & Kilpatrick, 1997; Foa & Riggs, 1993; Thompson et al., 2003; Ullman & Brecklin, 2003), reproductive health consequences (Mason & Lodrick, 2013), and a range of physical injuries and health care concerns (Koss, Woodruff, & Koss, 1991). Survivors of sexual assault also often display high levels of self-blame and guilt (Nishith, Nixon, & Resick, 2005) and often have a slower rate of recovery compared to individuals who experience nonsexual forms of trauma (Foa, 1997; Gilboa-Schechtman & Foa, 2001). Of note, psychological outcomes following sexual violence vary considerably, potentially as a result of psychological well-being prior to the attack. Women with severe/serious mental illness (SMI) also experience high rates of sexual violence compared to individuals without SMI (Goodman, Rosenberg, Mueser, & Drake, 1997; Harris & Landis, 2016; Van Deinse, Macy, Cuddeback, & Allman, 2018). Furthermore, a recent study examining sexual violence among college women documented that pre-existing mental health symptoms were exacerbated following sexual violence (Bonomi, Nichols, Kammes, & Green, 2018). Furthermore, compared to women who have never been sexually assaulted, survivors of this type of crime are at an increased risk of being victimized again in the future (Daigle, Fisher, & Cullen, 2008). Women who have previously experienced sexual assault during their lifetime report higher levels of psychological symptomatology compared to those who experience a single experience of victimization (Cohen & Roth, 1987; Lau & Kristensen, 2010; Shin et al.,

N. R. Leach
Department of Psychiatry, Rhode Island Hospital, Providence, RI, USA

School of Public Health, Brown University, Providence, RI, USA

L. M. Orchowski (✉)
Department of Psychiatry, Rhode Island Hospital, Providence, RI, USA

Department of Psychiatry and Human Behavior, Alpert Medical School of Brown University, Providence, RI, USA
e-mail: Lindsay_orchowski@brown.edu

W. T. O'Donohue and P. A. Schewe (eds.), *Handbook of Sexual Assault and Sexual Assault Prevention*,
https://doi.org/10.1007/978-3-030-23645-8_29

2017; Walsh et al., 2012). These findings underscore the importance of developing and testing psychological treatments to ameliorate the aftereffects of sexual trauma, as well as the importance of utilizing a variety of assessment strategies when evaluating and exploring potential treatments.

Purpose of the Present Chapter

This chapter explores the efficacy of psychological and medical treatments for adult survivors of sexual violence. We begin by examining recommendations for clinical responses to victims who access healthcare in a hospital setting immediately after an assault. When discussing medical treatments for individuals who experience sexual violence, we use the term "victim-patient," as the identities of the victim and patient often coincide within a clinical context (Mulla, 2014). Subsequently, we explore both short-term and long-term approaches for ameliorating the aftereffects of trauma and prevent health complications in the future. These treatments include forms of postexposure prophylaxis (PEP) treatments to decrease risk of sexually transmitted infections and diseases (STIs/STDs) as well as evidence-based options for both short-term and long-term psychological care. We conclude with discussing future directions in treatments for adult survivors of sexual trauma.

Acute Care: Immediate Treatments for Sexual Assault

According to Linden (2011), approximately 17–43% of adults who experience sexual violence seek medical treatment following an assault. Estimates vary based on the sample studied. According to Zinzow and her colleagues (2012), less than one in four women seek medical treatment following sexual assault. Most often, individuals who seek medical treatment following sexual violence do so in the emergency department (Hovelson, Scheiman, & Pearlman, 2016), often because they are in physical need of medical attention and must be treated for injury or would like to have a forensic (i.e., "rape-kit") examination performed for evidence collection purposes (Campbell, 2005; see Curoso this volume). Rape kits are commonly performed by trained sexual assault nurse examiners (SANE), forensic nurse examiner (FNE), and/or another *clinical member* of a sexual assault response team (SART) (Linden, 2011). SANE and FNE practitioners receive crime-specific certifications available through the International Association of Forensic Nurses, which strives to ensure that victim-patients receive qualified and interdisciplinary care in a trauma-informed manner (International Association of Forensic Nurses [IAFN], 2017). Upon meeting requirements of the International Association of Forensic Nurses' requirements, SANE certifications are available to anyone who has two or more years of experience in critical/emergency care or maternal/child health (Sexual Assault Nurse Examiners, 2017). Those involved in the larger network of a victim-centered SART team can include general health professionals, members of law enforcement, individuals with legal expertise, clinical advocates from local rape crisis centers, as well as social workers. SART programs and related certification-specific roles are increasingly being adopted by emergency departments across the United States because of evidence suggesting that they are associated with improvements in medical treatment guidelines-related compliances, the quality of evidence collection, and successful prosecutions compared to routine care (Campbell, Patterson, & Lichty, 2005; Riviello & Rozzi, 2013). In fact, as of 2014, there were 700 SANE/FNE programs in the United States and Canada (Draughon, Anderson, Hansen, & Sheridan, 2014).

Treatment Protocols

The protocol for acute treatment of victim-patients of sexual trauma developed by the Department of Justice's Office on Violence Against Women (2013) is endorsed by the International Association of Forensic Nursing. The general guidelines to be followed when treating an adult victim-patient in the emergency department are as follows: (1) evaluate for traumatic physical injuries; (2) offer post-exposure prophylaxis (PEP) for sexually transmitted infections (STIs), pregnancy, and sometimes human immunodeficiency virus (HIV); (3) collaborate with internal and external entities to provide emotional support while in the hospital; (4) offer to perform evidence collection using a preassembled "rape-kit"; (5) offer to call the police if they would like to report the crime; (6) and coordinate safe, tangible plans for discharge (e.g., treatment plans, referrals, physical/psychological follow-ups) (Linden, 2011). As long as the victim-patient is conscious, informed consent should be obtained before treating any injuries or proceeding with evidence collection (Riviello & Rozzi, 2013). Despite these recommendations, procedures often vary from hospital to hospital. For instance, religiously affiliated institutions may not offer certain recommended treatments (i.e., emergency contraception) (Campbell et al., 2006).

Treatment of Injuries

Victim-patients who present to the emergency department often require treatment for minor injuries such as cuts and scratches, or more major injuries resulting from attempted strangulation, forced penetration, and blunt force trauma (e.g., injury to the head, face torso, limbs; Sugar, Fine, & Eckert, 2004). Other common conditions that warrant treatment include defense injuries; lacerations, abrasions, or bruises on the hands, arms, or thighs (Bowyer & Dalton, 1997). Tears or abrasions to posterior fourchette, labia minora and fossa navivularis abrasions, and hymen tearings are common locations for genital injury (Sommers, 2007). Importantly, a lack of identifiable genital or anal injury does not mean that a sexual assault did not occur (Linden, 2011). The age of the victim-patient, heteronormative virginal status, degree of resistance, the number of assailants, and time between assault and treatment can impact whether or not vaginal injury can be detected (McGregor, Le, Marion, & Wiebe, 1999).

Due to the particularly violating context in which injuries resulting from sexual assault are obtained, a higher level of sensitivity is necessary when interacting with the victim-patient during the process of treatment and evidence collection (IAFN, 2017). Trauma-informed care and practice (TICP) most appropriately aligns with the recommended victim-centered approach (Harris & Fallot, 2001; Substance Abuse and Mental Health Services Administration [SAMHSA], 2014). Towards the goal of allowing survivors to rebuild a sense of control and empowerment, TICP is a strength-based framework that realizes the multifarious impacts of traumatic lived-experiences, emphasizing physical, psychological, and emotional safety for both providers and their respective patients as they respond to the survivor's needs (SAMHSA, 2014). For example, it is suggested that the victim-patient interact with as few clinicians as possible while in the emergency department so that higher levels of comfort, stability, and privacy can be obtained alongside the development of a rapport with the health professional involved (World Health Organization [WHO], 2003).

Postexposure Prophylaxis

A common concern among victim-patients presenting in the emergency department is risk for sexually transmitted infections (STIs) and diseases (STDs). The Centers for Disease Control and Prevention (CDC) recommends that all victim-patients be offered post-exposure prophylaxis (PEP) treatments for STI/STD while in the emergency department (Riviello & Rozzi, 2013). PEP consists of defensive or protective actions that can be taken by victim-patients with the help of medical professionals to reduce likelihood of infection and disease. All patients can be offered post exposure prophylaxis *treatments* for STIs while in the emergency department. Risk for gonorrhea, chlamydia, and trichomoniasis can be addressed through antibiotics. Whereas syphilis is less prevalent, risk for contracting this infection can be addressed through common prophylaxis drug treatment for gonorrhea (i.e., ceftrioxone, cefixime, or azithromycin). A hepatitis B vaccination can also be administered if the victim-patient has not already received one (Linden, 2011). Women are also at risk for contracting human papillomavirus (HPV). Accordingly, the CDC recommends offering the HPV vaccine to anyone who is 26 years of age or younger (Markowitz et al., 2014). Furthermore, a tetanus booster is suggested if the case indicates applicability (Workowski & Berman, 2010). Of note, whereas some experts argue that STI *testing* should be offered in a noncritical care setting unless relevant symptoms are clinically identified, others suggest that all victim-patients should receive initial laboratory testing for gonorrhea, chlamydia, trichomoniasis, syphilis, HIV, and hepatitis B when presenting in the emergency department, particularly if prophylactic treatment is declined (see Hovelson et al., 2016).

Although there is a low risk (5%) of pregnancy due to a vaginally penetrative sexual assault, emergency contraception is recommended as a single dose in the emergency department (Luce, Schrager, & Gilchrist, 2010). Ulipristal (Ella) and levonorgestrel (Plan B) should be offered within 72 h of the assault for optimal efficacy in preventing conception. Women with a body mass index (BMI) score of 25 or higher are at a greater risk of becoming pregnant using these emergency contraceptive methods than those with lower BMI scores, as they are not as effective in those with a higher BMI score (Batur, Kransdorf, & Casey, 2016). Thus, more effective alternative for women with a BMI score of 25 or higher is an intrauterine copper contraceptive (Batur et al., 2016). It is important to consider, however, that an intrauterine device may be a particularly invasive option for pregnancy prevention among a recent victim of sexual trauma.

Risk for contracting human immunodeficiency virus (HIV) is also a common concern following sexual assault. The estimated risk of HIV infection or transmission is 1–2 cases per 100,000 vaginal assaults and 2–3 cases per 10,000 anal assaults (Linden, 2011). According to guidelines from the CDC (CDC, 2016), nonoccupation postexposure prophylaxis (nPEP) treatment should be offered within 72 h postassault in cases where an HIV-positive status of the perpetrator is known. While fairly costly ($600–$1200), nPEP is only a fraction of the financial burden that a lifetime's worth of CDC-recommended pharmacological HIV/AIDS treatments are estimated to be ($223,000; Draughon, 2012). Of note, explicit guidance on how to treat a victim-patient who *does not know* the HIV status of the person who assaulted them (which is often the case) is lacking. Rather, judgments on the provision of nPEP are currently made on a case-by-case basis when taking patient preference, the nature of the assault, and an estimated risk of infection from the perpetrator into account (Draughon, 2012). The National Clinicians Post-Exposure Prophylaxis Hotline may also be consulted for guidance on the provision of HIV nPEP (Clinician Consultation Center, 2018).

Notably, compliance with administering HIV nPEP to survivors of sexual violence varies across SANE/FNE programs. Specifically, a recent survey of SANE/FNE professionals regarding the state of HIV nPEP practices found that these services are inconsistently offered across SANE/FNE programs, with medical costs, patient follow-up issues, and pre-/postcounseling being cited as the most common barriers to administration (Draughon et al., 2014; Scannell, MacDonald, Berger, & Boyer, 2018). The immediate short-term use of antiretroviral therapy after exposure (or potential exposure) is notably time and energy intensive and consequently, victim-patients are prone to lack of follow-up and poor completion rates (18–33% success) after the sexual assault (Linden, Oldeg, Mehta, McCabe, & LaBelle, 2005). However, nonadherence to the 1–2 times/day 28 day-long regimen may result in the development of a drug-resistant HIV strain (Linden, 2011).

Forensic "Rape Kit" Exams

Following the presentation of various PEP treatments, clinicians should offer the option to undergo a forensic examination (i.e., "rape kit") for the purpose of collecting evidence (American College of Emergency Physicians, 2014). The decision on whether or not to have evidence collected is dependent on the victim-patient preference. Following guidelines for trauma-informed care, an individual's decision to decline a rape kit examination should not be challenged by the provider or any law enforcement representatives that may be present.

The specific components of evidence-collection and history-taking generally follow the same protocol, but can vary depending on local and state legal requirements (United States Department of Justice, 2013). SART programs, as well as other clinical respondent groups, should use preassembled rape kits (Hovelson et al., 2016). The process of collecting both an account of the assault and physical evidence to support the statement (i.e., DNA) can take upwards of 6 h. As such, the trajectory and process should be clearly outlined to the victim-patient, so that they clearly understand what exactly will happen during each of the 17 steps of the examination. These steps, generated by Linden (2011), include the following: (1) obtain consent and complete relevant forms; (2) administer control swabs (with the use of sterile water); (3) toxicologic testing within 72 h (indications include period of unconsciousness, lack of motor control, etc.); (4) obtain blood sample or saliva for victims DNA; (5) garner oral swabs and smears if <24 h since oral penetration; (6) obtain fingernail scrapings (if patient scratched assailant or has debris under nail); (7) collect foreign-material (i.e., collect debris that falls as patient takes clothes off); (8) collect clothing (e.g., underwear, ripped or torn clothing worn during assault) and examine full body for injuries or secretions (document on forms and take pictures, if appropriate); (9) if bite marks are present, swab lightly with two moist swabs; (10) conduct head-hair combings; (11) document pubic-hair combings; (12) obtain vaginal swabs and smears; (13) obtain anorectal swabs and smears (if <24 h since penetration); (15) obtain additional swabs (i.e., swabs from any areas of possibly dried semen or secretions) or saliva collection; and (16) finalize forms from step 1 and seal envelopes and sexual assault kit. In addition to the initial agreement to participate, informed consent is required at every step of the examination, and providers should reiterate that they can opt out of any step or the entire proceeding process at any time. The pace at which evidence is collected should also be determined by the victim-patient and can change upon their request (United States Department of Justice, 2013). Notwithstanding, the unfortunate reality is that most rape-kits go untested and most are not prosecuted by the criminal justice system (Campbell, Feeney, Fehler-Cabral, Shaw, & Horsford, 2017).

Psychological Care During Emergency Room Visits

While in the emergency department, victim-patients may also be offered psychological care. Advocates from local rape crisis centers are called to meet the victim-patient at the hospital and stay with them until discharge. Hospital social workers are also often involved in these efforts. Victim-patients may also be encouraged to utilize services offered by the local rape crisis center and to follow up with their primary care provider. Appropriate referrals can also be determined and provided (ACEP, 2014). On-site counselors or psychologists may also initiate brief cognitive–behavioral therapy (bCBT) intended to facilitate healing. For example, one study found that using this immediate therapy (within 8 h postassault) is effective in reducing both PTSD and anxiety following sexual trauma (Foa, Zoellner, & Feeny, 2006). Specifically, women in the trial (90 female recent survivors of sexual assault [$n = 57$] and nonsexual assault [$n = 33$]) who were treated with bCBT including orientation, skill-focusing, and relapse prevention-related components, recovered faster (e.g., PTSD and general anxiety) than women in supportive counseling (SC) over a 3-month follow-up (Foa et al., 2006).

While in the emergency room, individuals who experience sexual trauma may also be provided with psychoeducational materials or videos designed to educate victim-patients on what to expect during and after a rape kit. In one study, the 18-min medical examination preparation and psychoeducation-focused video was implemented to prevent/reduce rates of pre-examination anxiety, as well as rates of postassault substance abuse among sexual assault survivors (Resnick et al., 2007). Data suggested that over a 6-month follow-up period, individuals who viewed the video reported lower levels PTSD symptoms (Resnick, Acierno, Amstadter, Self-Brown, & Kilpatrick, 2007). Viewing the 18-min medical examination preparation video was also successful in reducing pre-examination anxiety among participants.

With the goal of improving postassault outcomes, other studies have evaluated whether videos can be useful in educating survivors on what to expect following an assault. For example, Walsh et al. (2017) examined whether a brief video intervention for recent sexual assault victims—entitled Prevention of Post-Rape Stress [PPRS]—was associated with reduced alcohol and marijuana use when delivered in an emergency department. Follow-up data were collected over the course of a 6-month follow-up, and PPRS was compared to treatment as usual, as well as an active control condition, entitled Pleasant Imagery and Relaxation Instruction (PIRI). When compared to treatment as usual, the PPRS video resulted in less frequent alcohol use 6 months following sexual assault among participants who reporting binge drinking prior to the assault as well as minority women. When compared to treatment as usual, the PPRS video was also associated with lower rates of marijuana use at the first follow-up assessment among women who reported not using marijuana prior to the assault.

Of note, psychoeducational videos are not uniformly administered as a method for enhancing psychological outcomes among victim-patients presenting for care in the emergency department. However, the dissemination of such psychoeducational videos, as well as program-specific (e.g., SANE/SART) implementation (e.g., cost, staffing) could be relatively simple. Given that preliminary evidence suggests that the use of psychoeducational videos in acute care settings may mitigate adverse mental health outcomes, further research is warranted to explore avenues for uptake and dissemination of this treatment approach.

Brief Behavioral Intervention Procedure (BBIP) is another acute prophylactic treatment used to prevent chronic psychological outcomes postassault. Administered days/weeks posttrauma, BBIP is a 4- to 6-h treatment that also involves psychoeducation, as well as coping skills training and imaginal re-exposure. Only a limited number of studies have examined BBIP use in sexual assault cases (Foa, Hearst-Ikeda, & Perry, 1995; Veronen & Kilpatrick, 1983). As indicated in Vickerman and Margolin's (2009) review of the literature, research findings assessing the efficacy of BBIP in promoting mental health outcomes among sexual assault survivors have been inconclusive, and studies assessing BBIP currently lack methodological soundness (e.g., lacking a control group) and utilize a range of follow-up periods.

Long-Term Care: Treating Sexual Trauma and Its Sequelae

Burgess and Holmstrom (1974) utilized the Crisis Theory Model to describe how sexual trauma results in externally imposed psychological disequilibrium in a person who is confronted with a seemingly inescapable problem that cannot be solved using traditional problem-solving resources. Early approaches to working with survivors of sexual violence employed by rape advocacy organizations were often informed by the Crisis Theory Model (see Koss & Harvey, 1987). Later, researchers and practitioners started to explore how evidence-based cognitive–behavioral therapies (CBTs) used for anxiety diagnoses could be adapted for the purpose of treating sexual assault survivors (see Foa & Rothbaum, 2001). CBT-based treatment approaches, as well as other promising models, are described below.

Stress Inoculation Therapy

Stress Inoculation Therapy, which can be utilized in group settings, places an intense focus on creating a toolbox of coping skills for clients to assess in the literature (Meichenbaum, 2007). Components include an interview phase (e.g., psychological testing, reading, self-monitoring), the normalization of fear and avoidance behaviors, skill acquisition including in vivo exposure to target rape-related phobias, and concludes with the practice of skill applications using role-playing, imagery, modeling, controlled breathing, and muscle relaxation (Veronen & Kilpatrick, 1983). Studies have found that for both individual and group therapy, individuals treated with SIT reported pre-/postimprovements in PTSD, hostility, tension, assertiveness, self-concept, and self-esteem as well as improvements in depression, fear, and anxiety (Foa, Rothbaum, Riggs, & Murdock, 1991; Resick, Jordan, Girelli, Hutter, & Marhoefer-Dvorak, 1988; Veronen & Kilpatrick, 1982, 1983).

Prolonged Exposure

Prolonged Exposure (PE) is consistently regarded as an efficacious treatment for PTSD (Foa, Keane, & Friedman, 2000). Whereas PE is utilized to treat PTSD resulting from various forms of trauma (see Eftekhari, Stines, & Zoellner, 2006), PE has also specifically been utilized to address rape-related PTSD (Foa et al., 1991). Numerous theories have been proposed to explain the mechanisms through which PE leads to reductions in trauma symptoms (Bouton, 1988, 1991; Brewin, 1996, 2001; Ehlers & Clark, 2000; Foa & Kozak, 1986). Broadly, PE uses imaginal and in vivo "flooding" techniques to treat anxiety and PTSD, with the goal of allowing survivors of trauma to construct a more organized trauma story through guidance on how to take control over how they understand and process their sexual assault (see Peterson, Foa, & Riggs, 2011). Treatment providers ask the survivor to essentially relive the sexual assault scene and describe it aloud as they reimagine the experience using present tense and vivid detail in their description (Jaycox, Zoellner, & Foa, 2002). PE also incorporates cognitive and coping skill components in order to correct faculty stimulus responses so that new meaning can be made of traumatic memories. Homework assignments sometimes include listening to the audio recording outside of the counseling appointment. To date, several studies have examined the efficacy of PE in ameliorating psychological distress among survivors. Studies support the efficacy of PE for reducing PTSD among trauma survivors in general (Foa et al., 2005; Rothbaum, Meadows, Resick, & Foy, 2000), as well as survivors of sexual assault in particular (Foa et al., 1991, 1999, 2005; Foa, Molnar, & Cashman, 1995; Foa & Rauch, 2004; Resick, Nishith, Weaver, Astin, & Feuer, 2002; Rothbaum et al., 2000).

Cognitive Processing Therapy

Cognitive processing therapy (CPT) was designed specifically for the treatment of psychological distress among survivors of sexual trauma (Resick & Schnicke, 1993). Drawing upon emotion processing theory (Foa & Kozak, 1986), CPT aims to successfully integrate trauma into preexisting schemas and allow patients to overcome previously unsuccessful attempts to accommodate personal trauma-related information. Psychoeducation, exposure, and cognitive techniques are primary treatment components.

CPT can be conducted with individuals or groups and has been manualized so that therapists can practice the treatment in a systematic manner. Specifically, CPT is typically a 12-step process that aids survivors in learning how to challenge and modify unhelpful beliefs related to their trauma experience (see Westwell, 1998; Wilson & Jones, 2010). The treatment process begins with writing assignments in which clients detail what the assault means to them. The therapist then facilitates a review of what these thoughts mean to the survivor. Then, after addressing their beliefs and perceptions of the trauma's unique implications on their life, the therapist engages the survivor in a discussion about safety, trust, intimacy, power/control, and esteem (Resick & Schnicke, 1993).

Several studies have evaluated the efficacy of CPT in promoting positive mental health outcomes among survivors of sexual assault. Specifically, CPT has been shown to improve PTSD, depression, guilt, hopelessness, self-blame, and social adjustment outcomes pre-/postintervention (Iverson, King, Cunningham, &

Resick, 2015; Resick et al., 2002; Sobel, Resick, & Rabalais, 2009;). CPT is effective in treating PTSD alongside various comorbid diagnoses (i.e., guilt's manifestation as a major depressive disorder) among sexual assault survivors (Chard, Resick, & Wertz, 1999; Nishith et al., 2005). Of note, cognitive–behavioral treatments—such as CPT—are also commonly utilized as evidence-based treatments for both depression and anxiety (see Hofmann, Asnaani, Vonk, Sawyer, & Fang, 2012, for a review), as well as substance abuse (McHugh, Hearon, & Otto, 2010).

Several studies have compared the efficacy of CPT and PE (Bedard-Gilligan et al., 2016; Nishith, Resick, & Griffin, 2002; Resick et al., 2002; Resick, Williams, Suvak, Monson, & Gradus, 2012; Wachen, Jimenez, Resick, & Patricia, 2014). Across these studies, data suggest that CPT and PE are relatively comparable in treating PTSD among rape survivors. For example, in a sample of 154 rape victims who received CPT or PE and were assessed pretreatment as well as posttreatment (9 months and 5–10 years), findings suggested that for PTSD both therapies have the potential to positively influence functioning outcomes long-term (Wachen et al., 2014).

Eye Movement Desensitization Reprocessing

Eye movement desensitization reprocessing (EMDR) is also grounded in exposure techniques (Shapiro & Solomon, 1995). Incorporating cognitive and exposure treatment practices, EMDR requires the survivor to describe the assault scene while the therapist moves their finger back and forth across the patient's line of vision. It is hypothesized that this dual-attention focused therapy facilitates trauma memory processing through the use of an internal and external stimulus (Posmontier, Dovydaitis, & Lipman, 2010). Studies have concluded that EMDR resulted in improvements in PTSD, depression, anxiety, and dissociation (Leiner, Kearns, Jackson, Astin, & Rothbaum, 2012; Lindsay, 1996; Regehr, Alaggia, Dennis, Pitts, & Saini, 2013). Whereas EMDR is also cited as a psychotherapeutic intervention by the American Psychological Association (2017) for treating clients with PTSD, there is continued debate regarding EMDR's mechanisms of action. For example, it is not known if the finger eye movement component is necessary as the trauma memory exposure itself may be the source of postmental health outcomes (Rothbaum, 1997). For example, one study found that when treating PTSD in adult female rape victims ($n = 74$), PE and EMDR did not differ in outcomes between baseline and 6-month follow-up (Rothbaum, Astin, & Marsteller, 2005).

Supportive Counseling

Supportive counseling (SC) is widely used in counseling settings (Artime & Buchholz, 2016; Vickerman & Margolin, 2009). Providing general unconditional support, supportive counseling relies on active listening, validation, and positive regard to facilitate positive health outcomes for survivors (Foa et al., 2006). The supportive counseling process is not manualized. SC's fluidity makes it possible for survivors to identify specific topics that they want to address and work through with their mental health professional. Specific treatment targets may not surface. While some studies have shown pre-/postimprovements in PTSD, anxiety, and fear (and sometimes depression), SC is still an underexplored treatment option. Comparative studies have concluded, however, that cognitive behavioral therapies are generally more effective than SC in reducing psychological sequelae (Foa et al., 2006; Foa & Rothbaum, 2001; Resick et al., 1988).

Solution-Focused Therapy

Solution-focused therapy (SFT) is another option for long-term psychological care of sexual assault survivors seeking treatment (Tambling, 2012). Brief in length and dependent on goal-set targets, SFT works to add or remove a behavioral component of a problem interaction (Iveson, 2002). Amplifying the presence of solutions and the ability to develop tangible coping skills, the therapy parallels Buddhist mantra: acknowledging the past without letting it dictate the future or present (O'Hanlon, 1999). SFT's practices broadly aim to produce posttraumatic growth (e.g., better sense of self, life philosophy, relationships, spirituality; Frazier, Conlon, & Glaser, 2001; Tedeshi & Calhoun, 2004). Given the potential for sexual violence to influence a relationship (see Miller, Williams, & Bernstein, 1982), treatment may also focus on immediate sexual dysfunctions, impairments, and dissatisfactions, including reproductive pain, fear of sexual activity, arousal disorders, and inhibited sexual desires (see Becker, Skinner, Abel, & Cichon, 1984). Whereas numerous studies document the effectiveness of SFT in general (for reviews, see Corcoran & Pillai, 2009; Gingerich & Peterson, 2013; Kim, 2008), research is lacking to substantiate SFT as an approach to improving psychological outcomes among sexual assault survivors in particular.

Dialectical Behavioral Therapy

Dialectical behavior therapy (DBT) (Linehan, 1993) was originally manualized for treating patients diagnosed with borderline personality disorder (BPD) and involves the following four simultaneously functioning components: (1) individual therapy; (2) group therapy; (3) phone coaching; and (4) therapist consultation teams (see Landes, Garovoy, & Burkman, 2013). Treatment focuses on emotion regulation, as well as interpersonal, behavioral, cognitive, and self-regulation skills. While the body of research is small, the current literature suggests that DBT may be uniquely suited to address the dynamic psychosocial challenges postchildhood sexual abuse (for a review, see Decker & Naugle, 2008). Research is needed, however, to explore the efficacy of DBT for adult survivors of sexual trauma, specifically. Instead, some suggest that DBT skills-training may be useful to help survivors of sexual trauma cope with the distress that may be associated with participating in exposure therapy (Becker & Zayfert, 2001; Melia & Wagner, 2000; Wagner & Linehan, 2006).

Skills Training in Affective and Interpersonal Regulation (STAIR) Narrative Therapy

Skills Training in Affective and Interpersonal Regulation (STAIR) Narrative Therapy (Cloitre, Cohen, & Koenen, 2006) requires the patients to "tell their story" as a form of therapy. STAIR Narrative Therapy is a CBT approach comprised of two phases occurring over the course of sixteen 60-min sessions: (1) training in emotion regulation and interpersonal skills (8 sessions) and (2) additional skills training and prolonged imaginal exposure. Notably, this combination therapy in which skills-based intervention precedes trauma-focused work has been cited as a promising option when treating veterans who have experienced trauma (Cloitre, Jackson, & Schmidt, 2016). STAIR Narrative Therapy, however, has not been specifically evaluated as an approach for treating the sequelae of sexual victimization in adulthood.

Future Directions

Given the growth in evidence-based treatments for adult survivors of sexual trauma, researchers and health professionals now have numerous options for attending to the needs of survivors through the use of evidence-based treatments. While some care practices for adult survivors of sexual assault have been consistently evidenced as effective in treating specific diagnoses (particularly PTSD), the literature continues to highlight areas in which further research should be conducted. Below, we delineate gaps and limitations related to sexual violence research and the clinical practices/protocols.

Future Directions in Acute Care of Victim-Patients

Within an emergency department, clinicians who serve as members of an SART team must often act not only as healthcare providers, but also as agents of the justice system (Draughton, 2012; Mulla, 2014). In addition to caring for the victim-patient's health, SART teams and other comparable acute care collaborations not only are responsible for treating injury and providing PEP treatments, but also must also complete an array of forensic tasks. As this unique treatment process is not included in general medical training, some emergency medical providers may be unprepared to navigate the medical and legal issues that arise in the case of a sexual assault victim (Draughon, 2012). Emergency room providers are often the first people that survivors encounter postassault, it is critical that no blame should be imposed upon the victim-patient seeking care. Linden (2011) suggests that explicitly telling the victim-patient that they are not to blame, no matter what occurred prior to the sexual assault, can be useful to efforts to dispel or address feelings of guilt or embarrassment. To date, research has yet to explore how the personal attitudes and training of medical providers influence the quality of care provided to survivors of sexual violence in the emergency department. Acceptance of rape myths can impact how a person responds (i.e., positive social reaction/negative social reaction) to a survivor of sexual assault (Paul, Gray, Elhai, & Davis, 2009), and it would be valuable for researchers to explore how ascription to stereotypes regarding rape influences care among emergency department healthcare providers in the United States. Although false reports of rape are quite rare (Lisak, Gardinier, Nicksa, & Cote, 2010), it is feasible that some providers who hold a high level of ascription to rape myths may assume that a survivor is falsely reporting a rape, which may bias their clinical care. Given that responses to disclosure of sexual violence can influence the healing process following an assault (Orchowski & Gidycz, 2015), it is possible that training designed to promote positive responses to sexual assault disclosure within medical settings could be useful in supporting healing among survivors.

Hospital-specific policy makers may also consider how clinically induced distress may be mitigated through trauma-informed policies pertaining to the care of sexual assault survivors. For example, hospitals are often not equipped with enough gynecological beds, improvising through the use of bedpans to raise the buttocks for a pelvic examination (Girardin, 2017). The combination of creating physical spaces, as well as teams of certified health professionals (i.e., SART programs and SANE/SFE trainings) dedicated to treating sexual assault patients, may help to minimize these sorts of discomforts experienced in the hospital setting.

Work is also needed to disseminate policy and standards of care set by public health governing bodies to emergency department providers. For example, despite the CDC (2016) recommendations for providing HIV nPEP to victim-patients in the emergency department, there is a current lack of consensus regarding the circumstances under which HIV nPEP should be offered (Linden, 2011). Recent studies of SANE/FNE programs also suggest that HIV-related services are inconsistently provided to victim-patients in hospital settings (Scannell et al., 2018).

Future Directions in Psychological Treatments for Adult Survivors of Sexual Violence

There are also several limitations to current evaluations of long-term clinical treatments for sexual assault survivors. For example, more rigorous randomized control trials are needed to improve the depth of understanding of treatments that work for treating sexual assault survivors with multiple intersecting minority identities (see Regehr et al., 2013). Absent in the literature are treatments that have been evidenced as effective in treating sexual assault symptoms among men, women of color, the homeless, those physically or mentally disabled, incarcerated persons, members of the LGBT+ community, or racial and ethnic minorities. A better understanding of how intersectional identities may impact sexual assault-induced sequelae is necessary in ensuring that clinicians are able to provide the most helpful care to patients, regardless of sociodemographic characteristics (Regehr et al., 2013; Sigurvinsdottir & Ullman, 2016). For example, it may be helpful to investigate why those with lower education levels, those who are younger in age, and those who have higher initial levels of angers tend to drop out of CPT and PE treatments more than their counterparts so to improve their ability to successfully complete the clinical process (Rizvi, Vogt, & Resick, 2009). Moreover, one study concluded that individual characteristics of patients affect their likelihood of completing a treatment (Keefe et al., 2018). Therefore, moderators such as childhood physical abuse, current relationship conflict, anger, and racial minority status should be considered when clinicians develop tailored treatment plans for their patients.

In addition, there is currently little research examining how best to treat the aftereffects of sexual violence among women with serious mental illness (SMI). Often, individuals diagnosed with psychosis or other forms of SMI are excluded from participating in randomized clinical trials evaluating the efficacy of clinical practices, leaving the suitability of most treatments untested among those with SMI (Goodman et al., 1997). As a result, there is currently an absence of clear, evidence-based treatment guidelines for addressing sexual trauma among individuals with SMI (see Mueser, Rosenberg, Goodman, & Trumbetta, 2002). Moving forward, research is needed to understand how treatment interventions may warrant adaptation to meet the specific needs of women with SMI who experience sexual violence (see Harris & Landis, 2016).

A noteworthy gap between research and practice concerns the use of supportive counseling as a psychotherapeutic technique. Cognitive behavioral therapies (e.g., CPT, PE, EMDR) have been manualized and are frequently examined in randomized controlled trials that highlight their effectiveness in treating sequelae (Regehr et al., 2013; Resnick, Acierno, Waldrop, et al., 2007). Nonetheless, a majority of therapists choose supportive counseling as their preferred treatment for survivors of sexual assault, especially in college counseling settings (Artime & Buchholz, 2016). The disparity between knowledge of evidence-based treatments—such as PE and CPT—and practitioners' day-to-day use of supportive therapies may be influenced by ethical concerns regarding exposure practices (see Olatunji, Deacon, & Abramowitz, 2009). To bridge the gap between research and practice, more information is needed as to why—despite evidence-based recommendations—supportive counseling continues to be widely utilized.

Conclusion

Whether providing acute care in an emergency department or treating the long-term adverse health effects of sexual assault through psychological intervention, professionals involved in sexual violence cases face the unique challenge of creating a safe and patient-centered space for those adults who have experienced intimate trauma. Although sexual violence prevention scholars are working to reduce the frequency of these types of violations in the United States, it is the responsibility of healthcare professionals to provide effective, trauma-informed care and treatment for survivors, and also work to enhance these practices for those who may experience harm in the future. It is our hope that this chapter provided insight into the types of evidence-based treatments both available and recommended to clinicians with a balanced discussion of limitations as well as opportunities for research, with the goal of enhancing care for adult victims of sexual trauma.

Acknowledgment *Disclosure Statement:* The authors declare that they have no relevant material financial interests related to the research outlined in this chapter. Further, this chapter has not been submitted to any research journal or other publication site.

References

Acierno, R., Resnick, H., & Kilpatrick, D. (1997). Health impact of interpersonal violence 1: Prevalence rates, case identification, and risk factors for sexual assault, physical assault, and domestic violence in men and women. *Behavioral Medicine, 23*, 53–64.

American College of Emergency Physicians. (2014). Management of the patient with the complaint of sexual assault. Retrieved from https://www.acep.org/Clinical%2D%2D-Practice-Management/Management-of-the-Patient-with-the-Complaint-of-Sexual-Assault/#sm.001vlaqcr16o7e3hssx1wz1onyes9

American Psychiatric Association. (2017). *Clinical practice guideline for the treatment of PTSD*. Washington, DC: Guideline Development Panel for the Treatment of Posttraumatic Stress Disorder in Adults.

Artime, T. M., & Buchholz, K. R. (2016). Treatment for sexual assault survivors at university counseling centers. *Journal of College Student Psychotherapy, 30*, 252–261. https://doi.org/10.1080/87568225.2016.1219610

Batur, P., Kransdorf, L. N., & Casey, P. M. (2016). Emergency contraception. *Mayo Clinic Proceedings, 91*, 802–807. https://doi.org/10.1016/j.mayocp.2016.02.018

Becker, C. B., & Zayfert, C. (2001). Integrating DBT-based techniques and concepts to facilitate exposure treatment for PTSD. *Cognitive and Behavioral Practice, 8*, 107–122.

Becker, J. V., Skinner, L. J., Abel, G. G., & Cichon, J. (1984). Time limited therapy with sexually dysfunctional sexually assaulted women. *Journal of Social Work & Human Sexuality, 3*, 97–115. https://doi.org/10.1300/J291v03n01_08

Bedard-Gilligan, M., Marks, E., Graham, B., Garcia, N., Jerud, A., & Zoellner, L. (2016). Prolonged exposure and cognitive processing therapy for military sexual trauma-related posttraumatic stress disorder. In L. S. Katz (Ed.), *Treating military sexual trauma* (pp. 135–153). New York: Springer Publishing Company.

Bonomi, A., Nichols, E., Kammes, R., & Green, T. (2018). Sexual violence and intimate partner violence in college women with a mental health and/or behavior disability. *Journal of Women's Health, 27*, 359–368. https://doi.org/10.1089/jwh.2016.6279

Bouton, M. E. (1988). Context and ambiguity in the extinction of emotional learning. Implications for exposure therapy. *Behavior Research and Therapy, 26*, 137–149.

Bouton, M. E. (1991). A contextual analysis of fear extinction. In P. R. Martin (Ed.), *Handbook of behavior therapy and psychological science: An integrative approach* (pp. 435–453). New York: Pergamon General Psychology Series.

Bowyer, L., & Dalton, M. E. (1997). Female victims of rape and their genital injuries. *BJOG: An International Journal of Obstetrics & Gynaecology, 104*, 617–620. https://doi.org/10.1111/j.1471-0528.1997.tb11543.x

Brewin, C. R. (1996). Cognitive processing of adverse experiences. *International Review of Psychiatry, 8*, 333–339.

Brewin, C. R. (2001). A cognitive neuroscience account of posttraumatic stress disorder and its treatment. *Behaviour Research and Therapy, 39*, 373–393.

Burgess, A. W., & Holmstrom, L. L. (1974). Rape trauma syndrome. *American Journal of Psychiatry, 131*, 981–986. https://doi.org/10.1176/ajp.131.9.981

Campbell, R. (2005). What really happened? A validation study of rape survivors' help-seeking experiences with the legal and medical systems. *Violence and Victims, 20*, 55–68.

Campbell, R., Feeney, H., Fehler-Cabral, G., Shaw, J., & Horsford, S. (2017). The national problem of untested sexual assault kits (SAKs): Scope, causes, and future directions for research, policy, and practice. *Trauma, Violence & Abuse, 18*, 363–376. https://doi.org/10.1177/1524838015622436

Campbell, R., Patterson, D., & Lichty, L. F. (2005). The effectiveness of sexual assault nurse examiner (SANE) programs: A review of psychological, medical, legal, and community outcomes. *Trauma, Violence & Abuse, 6*, 313–329. https://doi.org/10.1177/1524838005280328

Campbell, R., Townsend, S. M., Long, S. M., Kinnison, K. E., Pulley, E. M., Adames, S. B., & Wasco, S. M. (2006). Responding to sexual assault victims' medical and emotional needs: A national study of the services provided by SANE programs. *Research in Nursing & Health, 29*, 384–398. https://doi.org/10.1002/nur.20137

Center for Disease Control and Prevention, U.S. Department of Health and Human Services. (2016). *Updated guidelines for antiretroviral post-exposure pophylaxis after sexual, injection drug use, or other nonoccupational exposure to HIV— United States, 2016*. Atlanta, GA: CDC.

Chard, K. M., Resick, P. A., & Wertz, J. J. (1999). Group treatment of sexual assault survivors. In B. H. Young & D. D. Blake (Eds.), *Group treatments for post-traumatic stress disorder* (pp. 35–50). Burlington, MA: Taylor & Francis.

Clinician Consultation Center. (2018). PEP: Post-Exposure Prophylaxis. Retrieved from http://nccc.ucsf.edu/clinician-consultation/pep-post-exposure-prophylaxis/

Cloitre, M., Cohen, L. R., & Koenen, K. C. (2006). *Treating the trauma of childhood abuse: Therapy for the interrupted life*. New York: Guilford.

Cloitre, M., Jackson, C., & Schmidt, J. A. (2016). STAIR for strengthening social support and relationships among veterans with military sexual trauma and PTSD. *Military Medicine, 181*, e183–e187. https://doi.org/10.7205/MILMED-D-15-00209

Cohen, L. J., & Roth, S. (1987). The psychological aftermath or rape: Long-term effects and individual differences in recovery. *Journal of Social and Clinical Psychology, 5*, 525–534. https://doi.org/10.1521/jscp.1987.5.4.525

Corcoran, J., & Pillai, V. (2009). A review of the research on solution-focused therapy. *British Journal of Social*

Work, 39, 234–242. https://doi.org/10.1093/bjsw/bcm098

Daigle, L. E., Fisher, B. S., & Cullen, F. T. (2008). The violent and sexual victimization of college women: Is repeat victimization a problem? *Journal of Interpersonal Violence, 23*, 1296–1313. https://doi.org/10.1177/0886260508314293

Decker, S. E., & Naugle, A. E. (2008). DBT for sexual abuse survivors: Current status and future directions. *The Journal of Behavior Analysis of Offender and Victim Treatment and Prevention, 1*, 52–68. https://doi.org/10.1037/h0100456

Draughon, J. E. (2012). Sexual assault injuries and increased risk of HIV transmission. *Advanced Emergency Nursing Journal, 34*, 82–87. https://doi.org/10.1097/TME.0b013e3182439e1a

Draughon, J. E., Anderson, J. C., Hansen, B. R., & Sheridan, D. J. (2014). Sexual assault program HIV non-occupational post-exposure prophylaxis practices: A survey of sexual assault and forensic nurse examiner program coordinators. *The Journal of the Association of Nurses in AIDS Care: JANAC, 25*, S90–S100. https://doi.org/10.1016/j.jana.2013.07.001

Eftekhari, A., Stines, L. R., & Zoellner, L. A. (2006). Do you need to talk about it? Prolonged exposure for the treatment of chronic PTSD. *The Behavior Analyst Today, 7*, 70–83.

Ehlers, A., & Clark, D. M. (2000). A cognitive model of posttraumatic stress disorder. *Behaviour Research and Therapy, 38*, 219–345.

Foa, E. B. (1997). Trauma and women: Course, predictors, and treatment. *The Journal of Clinical Psychiatry, 58*, 25–28.

Foa, E. B., Dancu, C. V., Hembree, E. A., Jaycox, L. H., Meadows, E. A., & Street, G. P. (1999). A comparison of exposure therapy, stress inoculation training, and their combination for reducing posttraumatic stress disorder in female assault victims. *Journal of Consulting and Clinical Psychology, 67*, 194–200.

Foa, E. B., Hearst-Ikeda, D., & Perry, K. J. (1995). Evaluation of a brief cognitive-behavioral program for the prevention of chronic PTSD in recent assault victims. *Journal of Consulting and Clinical Psychology, 63*, 948–955. https://doi.org/10.1037/0022-006X.63.6.948

Foa, E. B., Hembree, E. A., Cahill, S. P., Rauch, S. A. M., Riggs, D. S., Feeny, N. C., & Yadin, E. (2005). Randomized trial of prolonged exposure for posttraumatic stress disorder with and without cognitive restructuring: Outcome at academic and community clinics. *Journal of Consulting and Clinical Psychology, 73*, 953–964. https://doi.org/10.1037/0022-006X.73.5.953

Foa, E. B., Keane, T. M., & Friedman, M. J. (2000). *Effective treatments for PTSD: Practice guidelines from the International Society for Traumatic Stress Studies*. New York: Guilford Press.

Foa, E. B., & Kozak, M. J. (1986). Emotional processing of fear: Exposure to corrective information. *Psychological Bulletin, 99*, 20. https://doi.org/10.1037/0033-2909.99.1.20

Foa, E. B., Molnar, C., & Cashman, L. (1995). Change in rape narratives during exposure therapy for posttraumatic stress disorder. *Journal of Traumatic Stress, 8*, 675–690.

Foa, E. B., & Rauch, S. (2004). Cognitive changes during prolonged exposure versus prolonged exposure plus cognitive restructuring in female assault survivors with posttraumatic stress disorder. *Journal of Consulting and Clinical Psychology, 72*, 879–884.

Foa, E. B., & Riggs, D. S. (1993). Posttraumatic stress disorder in rape victims. In J. Oldham, M. B. Riba, & A. Tasman (Eds.), *American psychiatric press review of psychiatry* (Vol. 12, pp. 273–303). Washington, DC: American Psychiatric Press.

Foa, E. B., & Rothbaum, B. O. (2001). *Treating the trauma of rape: Cognitive-behavioral therapy for PTSD*. New York, NY: Guilford Press.

Foa, E. B., Rothbaum, B. O., Riggs, D. S., & Murdock, T. B. (1991). Treatment of posttraumatic stress disorder in rape victims: A comparison between cognitive-behavioral procedures and counseling. *Journal of Consulting and Clinical Psychology, 59*, 715–723.

Foa, E. B., Zoellner, L. A., & Feeny, N. C. (2006). An evaluation of three brief programs for facilitating recovery after assault. *Journal of Traumatic Stress, 19*, 29–43. https://doi.org/10.1002/jts.20096

Frazier, P., Conlon, A., & Glaser, T. (2001). Positive and negative life changes following sexual assault. *Journal of Consulting and Clinical Psychology, 69*, 1048–1055. https://doi.org/10.1002/jts.20096

Gilboa-Schechtman, E., & Foa, E. B. (2001). Patterns of recovery from trauma: The use of intraindividual analysis. *Journal of Abnormal Psychology, 110*, 392–400. https://doi.org/10.1037/0021-843X.110.3.392

Gingerich, W. J., & Peterson, L. T. (2013). Effectiveness of solution focused-brief therapy: A systematic qualitative review of controlled outcome studies. *Research on Social Work Practice, 23*, 266–283. https://doi.org/10.1177/1049731512470859

Girardin, B. (2017). More steps to take after sexual assault. *Contemporary OB/GYN, 62*, 15–17.

Goodman, L. A., Rosenberg, S. D., Mueser, K. T., & Drake, R. E. (1997). Physical and sexual assault history in women with serious mental illness: Prevalence, correlates, treatment, and future research directions. *Schizophrenia Bulletin, 23*, 685–696. https://doi.org/10.1093/schbul/23.4.685

Harris, M., & Fallot, R. D. (2001). Trauma-informed inpatient services. *New Directions for Mental Health Services, 2001*, 33–46. https://doi.org/10.1002/yd.23320018905

Harris, M., & Landis, C. L. (2016). *Sexual abuse in the lives of women diagnosed with serious mental illness*. New York, NY: Routledge.

Hofmann, S. G., Asnaani, A., Vonk, I. J. J., Sawyer, A. T., & Fang, A. (2012). The efficacy of cognitive behav-

ioral therapy: A review of meta-analyses. *Cognitive Therapy and Research, 36*, 427–440. https://doi.org/10.1007/s10608-012-9476-1
Hovelson, S., Scheiman, L., & Pearlman, M. (2016). After a sexual assault: What to do: Ob/gyns have a responsibility to screen patients for sexual assault and to provide a safe and nonjudgmental environment. *Contemporary OB/GYN, 61*, 17.
International Association of Forensic Nurses. (2017). *Sexual assault nurse examiners*. Retrieved from http://www.forensicnurses.org/?page=aboutsane
Iverson, K. M., King, M. W., Cunningham, K. C., & Resick, P. A. (2015). Rape survivors' trauma-related beliefs before and after cognitive processing therapy: Associations with PTSD and depression symptoms. *Behaviour Research and Therapy, 66*, 49–55. https://doi.org/10.1016/j.brat.2015.01.002
Iveson, C. (2002). Solution-focused brief therapy. *Advances in Psychiatric Treatment, 8*(2), 149–156.
Jaycox, L. H., Zoellner, L., & Foa, E. B. (2002). Cognitive–behavior therapy for PTSD in rape survivors. *Journal of Clinical Psychology, 58*, 891–906. https://doi.org/10.1002/jclp.10065
Keefe, J. R., Wiltsey Stirman, S., Cohen, Z. D., DeRubeis, R. J., Smith, B. N., & Resick, P. A. (2018). In rape trauma PTSD, patient characteristics indicate which trauma-focused treatment they are most likely to complete. *Depression and Anxiety, 35*, 330–338. https://doi.org/10.1002/da.22731
Kim, J. S. (2008). Examining the effectiveness of solution-focused brief therapy: A meta-analysis. *Research on Social Work Practice, 18*, 107–116. https://doi.org/10.1177/1049731507307807
Koss, M., Woodruff, W., & Koss, P. (1991). Criminal victimization among primary care medical patients: Prevalence, incidence and physician usage. *Behavioral Sciences & the Law, 9*, 89–96.
Koss, M. P., & Harvey, M. R. (1987). *The rape victim: Clinical and community approaches to treatment*. Lexington, MA: Stephen Greene Press.
Landes, S. J., Garovoy, N. D., & Burkman, K. M. (2013). Treating complex trauma among veterans: Three stage-based treatment models. *Journal of Clinical Psychology, 69*, 523–533. https://doi.org/10.1002/jclp.21988
Lau, M., & Kristensen, E. (2010). Sexual revictimization in a clinical sample of women reporting childhood sexual abuse. *Nordic Journal of Psychiatry, 64*, 4–10. https://doi.org/10.3109/08039480903191205
Leiner, A. S., Kearns, M. C., Jackson, J. L., Astin, M. C., & Rothbaum, B. O. (2012). Avoidant coping and treatment outcome in rape-related posttraumatic stress disorder. *Journal of Consulting and Clinical Psychology, 80*, 317–321. https://doi.org/10.1037/a0026814
Linden, J. A. (2011). Care of the adult patient after sexual assault. *New England Journal of Medicine, 365*, 834–841. https://doi.org/10.1056/NEJMcp1102869
Linden, J. A., Oldeg, P., Mehta, S. D., McCabe, K. K., & LaBelle, C. (2005). HIV postexposure prophylaxis in sexual assault: Current practice and patient adherence to treatment recommendations in a large urban teaching hospital. *Academic Emergency Medicine, 12*, 640–646. https://doi.org/10.1197/j.aem.2005.01.015
Lindsay, J. K. (1996). Eye movement desensitization and reprocessing (EMDR) in the treatment of rape survivors. *Dissertation Abstracts International: Section B: The Sciences and Engineering, 56*(2-B), 1113.
Linehan, M. M. (1993). *Cognitive-behavioral treatment of borderline personality disorder*. New York, NY: The Guilford Press.
Lisak, D., Gardinier, L., Nicksa, S. C., & Cote, A. M. (2010). False allegations of sexual assault: An analysis of ten years of reported cases. *Violence Against Women, 16*, 1218–1334. https://doi.org/10.1177/1077801210387747
Luce, H., Schrager, S., & Gilchrist, V. (2010). Sexual assault of women. *American Family Physician, 81*, 489–495.
Markowitz, L. E., Dunne, E. F., Saraiya, M., Chesson, H. W., Curtis, C. R., Gee, J., … Unger, E. R. (2014). Human papillomavirus vaccination: Recommendations of the advisory committee on immunization practices (ACIP). *Morbidity and Mortality Weekly Report. Recommendations and Reports, 63*, 1–30.
Mason, F., & Lodrick, Z. (2013). Psychological consequences of sexual assault. *Best Practice & Research. Clinical Obstetrics & Gynaecology, 27*, 27–37. https://doi.org/10.1016/j.bpobgyn.2012.08.015
McGregor, M. J., Le, G., Marion, S. A., & Wiebe, E. (1999). Examination for sexual assault: Is the documentation of physical injury associated with the laying of charges? A retrospective cohort study. *Canadian Medical Association Journal, 160*, 1565–1569.
McHugh, R. K., Hearon, B. A., & Otto, M. W. (2010). Cognitive-behavioral therapy for substance use disorders. *The Psychiatric Clinics of North America, 33*, 511–525. https://doi.org/10.1016/j.psc.2010.04.012
Meichenbaum, D. (2007). Stress inoculation training: A preventative and treatment approach. In P. M. Lehrer, R. L. Woolfolk, & W. E. Sime (Eds.), *Principles and practice of stress management* (pp. 497–516). New York, NY: Guilford Press.
Melia, K., & Wagner, A. W. (2000). The application of dialectical behavior therapy to the treatment of post-traumatic stress disorder. *National Center for Post-Traumatic Stress Disorder Clinical Quarterly, 9*, 6–12.
Miller, W. R., Williams, A. M., & Bernstein, M. H. (1982). The effects of rape on marital and sexual adjustment. *American Journal of Family Therapy, 10*, 51–58. https://doi.org/10.1080/01926188208250436
Mueser, K. T., Rosenberg, S. D., Goodman, L. A., & Trumbetta, S. L. (2002). Trauma, PTSD, and the course of severe mental illness: An interactive model. *Schizophrenia Research, 53*, 123–143. https://doi.org/10.1016/S0920-9964(01)00173-6
Mulla, S. (2014). *The violence of care: Rape victims, forensic nurses, and sexual assault intervention*. New York, NY: NYU Press.
Nishith, P., Nixon, R. D., & Resick, P. A. (2005). Resolution of trauma-related guilt following treatment of PTSD in female rape victims: A result of cognitive processing therapy targeting comorbid depression?

Journal of Affective Disorders, 86, 259–265. https://doi.org/10.1016/j.jad.2005.02.013

Nishith, P., Resick, P. A., & Griffin, M. G. (2002). Pattern of change in prolonged exposure and cognitive-processing therapy for female rape victims with posttraumatic stress disorder. *Journal of Consulting and Clinical Psychology, 70*, 880–886. https://doi.org/10.1037/0022-006X.70.4.880

O'Hanlon, B. (1999). *Do one thing different: And other uncommonly sensible solutions to Life's persistent problems*. New York, NY: William Morrow & Company.

Olatunji, B. O., Deacon, B. J., & Abramowitz, J. S. (2009). The cruelest cure? Ethical issues in the implementation of exposure-based treatments. *Cognitive and Behavioral Practice, 16*, 172–180. https://doi.org/10.1016/j.cbpra.2008.07.003

Orchowski, L. M., & Gidycz, C. A. (2015). Psychological consequences associated with positive and negative responses to disclosure of sexual assault among college women: A prospective study. *Violence Against Women, 21*(7), 803–823. https://doi.org/10.1177/1077801215584068

Paul, L. A., Gray, M. J., Elhai, J. D., & Davis, J. L. (2009). Perceptions of peer rape myth acceptance and disclosure in a sample of college sexual assault survivors. *Psychological Trauma Theory Research Practice and Policy, 1*, 231–241. https://doi.org/10.1037/a0016989

Peterson, A. L., Foa, E. B., & Riggs, D. S. (2011). Prolonged exposure therapy. In B. A. Moore & W. E. Penk (Eds.), *Treating PTSD in military personnel: A clinical handbook* (pp. 42–58). New York, NY: Guilford Press.

Posmontier, B., Dovydaitis, T., & Lipman, K. (2010). Sexual violence: Psychiatric healing with eye movement reprocessing and desensitization. *Health Care for Women International, 31*, 755–768. https://doi.org/10.1080/07399331003725523

Regehr, C., Alaggia, R., Dennis, J., Pitts, A., & Saini, M. (2013). Interventions to reduce distress in adult victims of rape and sexual violence: A systematic review. *Research on Social Work Practice, 23*, 257–265. https://doi.org/10.1177/1049731512474103

Resick, P. A., Jordan, C. G., Girelli, S. A., Hutter, C. K., & Marhoefer-Dvorak, S. (1988). A comparative outcome study of behavioral group therapy for sexual assault victims. *Behavior Therapy, 19*, 385–401. https://doi.org/10.1016/S0005-7894(88)80011-X

Resick, P. A., Nishith, P., Weaver, T. L., Astin, M. C., & Feuer, C. A. (2002). A comparison of cognitive-processing therapy with prolonged exposure and a waiting condition for the treatment of chronic posttraumatic stress disorder in female rape victims. *Journal of Consulting and Clinical Psychology, 70*, 867–879. https://doi.org/10.1037/0022-006X.70.4.867

Resick, P. A., & Schnicke, M. (1993). *Cognitive processing therapy for rape victims: A treatment manual*. Thousand Oaks, CA: Sage Publications Inc.

Resick, P. A., Williams, L. F., Suvak, M. K., Monson, C. M., & Gradus, J. L. (2012). Long-term outcomes of cognitive–behavioral treatments for posttraumatic stress disorder among female rape survivors. *Journal of Consulting and Clinical Psychology, 80*, 201–210. https://doi.org/10.1037/a0026602

Resnick, H., Acierno, R., Waldrop, A. E., King, L., King, D., Danielson, C., … Kilpatrick, D. (2007). Randomized controlled evaluation of an early intervention to prevent post-rape psychopathology. *Behaviour Research and Therapy, 45*, 2432–2447. https://doi.org/10.1016/j.brat.2007.05.002

Resnick, H. S., Acierno, R., Amstadter, A. B., Self-Brown, S., & Kilpatrick, D. G. (2007). An acute post-sexual assault intervention to prevent drug abuse: Updated findings. *Addictive Behaviors, 32*, 2032–2045. https://doi.org/10.1016/j.addbeh.2007.01.001

Riviello, R. J., & Rozzi, H. V. (2013). *Evaluation and management of the sexually assaulted or sexually abused patient*. Dallas, TX: The American College of Emergency Physicians.

Rizvi, S. L., Vogt, D. S., & Resick, P. A. (2009). Cognitive and affective predictors of treatment outcome in cognitive processing therapy and prolonged exposure for posttraumatic stress disorder. *Behaviour Research and Therapy, 47*, 737–743. https://doi.org/10.1016/j.brat.2009.06.003

Rothbaum, B. O. (1997). A controlled study of eye movement desensitization and reprocessing in the treatment of posttraumatic stress disordered sexual assault victims. *Bulletin of the Menninger Clinic, 61*, 317–334.

Rothbaum, B. O., Astin, M. C., & Marsteller, F. (2005). Prolonged exposure versus eye movement desensitization and reprocessing (EMDR) for PTSD rape victims. *Journal of Traumatic Stress, 18*, 607–616. https://doi.org/10.1002/jts.20069

Rothbaum, B. O., Meadows, E. A., Resick, P., & Foy, D. W. (2000). Cognitive-behavioral therapy. In E. B. Foa, T. M. Keane, & M. J. Friedman (Eds.), *Effective treatments for PTSD: Practice guidelines from the International Society for Traumatic Stress Studies* (pp. 320–325). New York, NY: Guilford Press.

Scannell, M., MacDonald, A. E., Berger, A., & Boyer, N. (2018). The priority of administering HIV post-exposure prophylaxis in cases of sexual assault in an emergency department. *Journal of Emergency Nursing, 44*, 117–122. https://doi.org/10.1016/j.jen.2017.10.014

Shapiro, F., & Solomon, R. M. (1995). *Eye movement desensitization and reprocessing*. Somerset, NJ: John Wiley & Sons.

Shin, K. M., Chung, Y. K., Shin, Y. J., Kim, M., Kim, N. H., Kim, K. A., … Chang, H. Y. (2017). Post-traumatic cognition mediates the relationship between a history of sexual abuse and the post-traumatic stress symptoms in sexual assault victims. *Journal of Korean Medical Science, 32*, 1680–1686. https://doi.org/10.3346/jkms.2017.32.10.1680

Sigurvinsdottir, R., & Ullman, S. E. (2016). Sexual orientation, race, and trauma as predictors of sexual assault recovery. *Journal of Family Violence, 31*(7), 913–921. https://doi.org/10.1007/s10896-015-9793-8

Sobel, A. A., Resick, P. A., & Rabalais, A. E. (2009). The effect of cognitive processing therapy on cognitions: Impact statement coding. *Journal of Traumatic Stress, 22*, 205–211. https://doi.org/10.1002/jts.20408

Sommers, M. S. (2007). Defining patterns of genital injury from sexual assault: A review. *Trauma, Violence & Abuse, 8*, 270. https://doi.org/10.1177/1524838007303194

Substance Abuse and Mental Health Services Administration. (2014). *SAMHSA's Concept of Trauma and Guidance for a Trauma-Informed Approach.*. HHS Publication No. (SMA) 14–4884. Rockville, MD: Substance Abuse and Mental Health Services Administration.

Sugar, N. F., Fine, D. N., & Eckert, L. O. (2004). Physical injury after sexual assault: Findings of a large case series. *American Journal of Obstetrics and Gynecology, 190*, 71–76. https://doi.org/10.1016/S0002-9378(03)00912-8

Tambling, R. B. (2012). Solution-oriented therapy for survivors of sexual assault and their partners. *Contemporary Family Therapy, 34*, 391–401. https://doi.org/10.1007/s10591-012-9200-z

Tedeshi, R. G., & Calhoun, L. G. (2004). Posttraumatic growth: Conceptual foundation and empirical evidence. *Psychological Inquiry, 15*, 1–18. https://doi.org/10.1207/s15327965pli1501_01

Thompson, K. M., Crosby, R. D., Wonderlich, S. A., Mitchell, J. E., Redlin, J., Demuth, G., … Haseltine, B. (2003). Psychopathology and sexual trauma in childhood and adulthood. *Journal of Traumatic Stress, 16*, 35–38.

Ullman, S. E., & Brecklin, L. R. (2003). Sexual assault history and health related outcomes in a national sample of women. *Psychology of Women Quarterly, 27*, 46–57.

US Department of Justice Office of Violence Against Women. (2013). *A National Protocol for Sexual Assault Medical Forensic Examinations (NCJ 228119)*. Washington DC: U.S. Government Printing Office.

Van Deinse, T. B., Macy, R. J., Cuddeback, G. S., & Allman, A. J. (2018). Intimate partner violence and sexual assault among women with serious mental illness: A review of prevalence and risk factors. *Journal of Social Work*, 146801731876642. https://doi.org/10.1177/1468017318766425

Veronen, L. J., & Kilpatrick, D. G. (1982, November). *Stress inoculation training for victims of rape: Efficacy and differential findings*. Paper presented at the Sixteenth Annual Convention of the Association for the Advancement of Behavior Therapy, Los Angeles, CA.

Veronen, L. J., & Kilpatrick, D. G. (1983). Stress management for rape victims. In D. Meichenbaum & M. Jaremko (Eds.), *Stress reduction and prevention* (pp. 341–374). Boston, MA: Springer.

Vickerman, K. A., & Margolin, G. (2009). Rape treatment outcome research: Empirical findings and state of the literature. *Clinical Psychology Review, 29*(5), 431–448. https://doi.org/10.1016/j.cpr.2009.04.004

Wachen, J. S., Jimenez, S. S., Resick, K., & Patricia, A. (2014). Long-term functional outcomes of women receiving cognitive processing therapy and prolonged exposure. *Psychological Trauma Theory Research Practice and Policy, 6*, S58–S65. https://doi.org/10.1037/a0035741

Wagner, A. W., & Linehan, M. M. (2006). Applications of dialectical behavior therapy to post-traumatic stress disorder and related problems. In V. M. Follette & J. I. Ruzek (Eds.), *Cognitive-behavioral therapies for trauma* (2nd ed., pp. 117–145). New York: Guilford Press.

Walsh, K., Danielson, C. K., McCauley, J. L., Saunders, B. E., Kilpatrick, D. G., & Resnick, H. S. (2012). National prevalence of posttraumatic stress disorder among sexually revictimized adolescent, college, and adult household-residing women. *Archives of General Psychiatry, 69*, 935–942. https://doi.org/10.1001/archgenpsychiatry.2012.132

Walsh, K., Gilmore, A. G., Frazier, P., Ledray, L., Acierno, R., Ruggiero, K. J., … Resnick, H. S. (2017). A randomized clinical trial examining the effect of video-based prevention of alcohol and marijuana use among recent sexual assault victims. *Alcoholism: Clinical and Experimental Research, 41*, 2163–2172. https://doi.org/10.1111/acer.13505

Westwell, C. A. (1998). Cognitive processing therapy in the treatment of marital rape. *Psychotherapy in Private Practice, 17*, 63–77. https://doi.org/10.1300/J294v17n02_05

Wilson, L. C., & Jones, R. T. (2010). Therapists as trauma survivors: A case study detailing cognitive processing therapy for rape victims with a psychology graduate student. *Clinical Case Studies, 9*, 442–456. https://doi.org/10.1177/1534650110386106

Workowski, K. A., & Berman, S. (2010). Sexually transmitted diseases treatment guidelines. Centers for Disease Control and Prevention.

World Health Organization. (2003). *Guidelines for medico-legal care for victims of sexual violence*. Geneva: World Health Organization.

Zinzow, H. M., Resnick, H. S., Barr, S. C., Danielson, C. K., & Kilpatrick, D. G. (2012). Receipt of post-rape medical care in a national sample of female victims. *American Journal of Preventive Medicine, 43*, 183–187. https://doi.org/10.1016/j.amepre.2012.02.025

The Effectiveness of Psychoeducation and Brief Treatments in the Aftermath of Sexual Assault

30

Catalina Vechiu and Martha Zimmermann

For a significant proportion of US adult women, exposure to sexual assault victimization continues to be a pervasive reality. Since Koss, Gidycz, and Wisniewski's (1987) landmark study of rape prevalence among college women found that approximately 15% of respondents reported at least one experience that met the legal definition of rape, national prevalence rates indicate that sexual assault has remained a significant social problem that disproportionately affects women. More recent estimates indicate that roughly 20% of US adult women and 1.7% of men report being raped during their lifetime and an estimated 1.6% of women report being raped in the previous 12 months (Breiding et al., 2014). Rape is associated with both acute and long-term adverse psychological consequences. Immediate and long-term psychological responses include post-traumatic stress disorder (PTSD), depression, and other anxiety problems (Kessler, Sonnega, Bromet, Hughes, & Nelson, 1995). Sexual assault victimization is further associated with higher rates of revictimization, interpersonal difficulties, and social stigma. Survivors of sexual assault are also at an increased risk of abusing alcohol and drugs, even among those who did not abuse substances prior to the assault (Kilpatrick, Acierno, Resnick, Saunders, & Best, 1997a).

As such, there is an impetus to develop brief and evidence-based interventions that target the unique constellation of challenges faced by sexual assault victims. Several decades of research have yielded numerous trauma-focused psychological treatments aimed at ameliorating the most commonly experienced trauma-related sequelae with varying degrees of success (e.g., Foa, 2011). However, traditional modalities of service delivery are often characterized by high rates of attrition (Hembree et al., 2003). Furthermore, survivors of sexual assault are not likely to return for follow-up mental health services (Price, Davidson, Ruggiero, Acierno, & Resnick, 2014). Thus, it may be more prudent and efficacious to consider alternative intervention efforts, such as the provision of psychoeducation. Psychoeducation, or the delivery of information related to the nature and course of psychological responses to trauma and how to respond adaptively in the face of these reactions, in particular may represent a feasible, cost-effective method of preventing adverse psychological consequences of sexual assault and increasing effective help-seeking in this population. Research examining the provision of stand-alone psychoeducational interventions for sexual assault victimization is limited. This may be due in part to the inclusion of psychoeducation as a key component of the most widely utilized interventions for trauma-related disorders (i.e., prolonged exposure, trauma-focused cognitive

C. Vechiu (✉) · M. Zimmermann
University of Nevada, Reno, Reno, NV, USA

W. T. O'Donohue and P. A. Schewe (eds.), *Handbook of Sexual Assault and Sexual Assault Prevention*,
https://doi.org/10.1007/978-3-030-23645-8_30

behavioral therapy). While research is limited, it has been suggested that psychoeducation may not be indicated as a first-line treatment for individuals experiencing higher levels of distress and instead, they should be immediately referred for higher intensity intervention (Wessely et al., 2008). For these reasons, the aim of this chapter is to examine the available support for brief treatments and psychoeducational interventions in the aftermath of trauma and discuss limitations and future directions for research.

Prevalence and Adverse Mental Health Outcomes

Prevalence of Sexual Assault

Epidemiological studies yield high rates of sexual assault victimization among women, indicating that they are more likely to experience interpersonal assaults, such as sexual abuse in childhood or adulthood and rape in comparison to men (i.e., Breslau, Davis, Andreski, Peterson, & Schultz, 1997; Kessler et al., 1995). These findings suggest that exposure to traumatic events varies dramatically based on gender. Although men exhibit a higher propensity toward overall exposure to traumatic events (e.g., combat-related trauma, work-related injury), women are at a disproportionately higher risk for exposure to certain traumatic events (Breslau et al., 1997). For example, data from the National Intimate Partner and Sexual Violence Survey found that an estimated 43.9% of women and 23.4% of men reported experiencing other forms of sexual violence during their lifetimes, including unwanted sexual contact, noncontact unwanted sexual experiences, sexual coercion, and being made to penetrate (Breiding, Chen, & Black, 2014). This finding is consistent with previous national surveys that found the overall prevalence rate for sexual assault victimization to be 29.7%, with 15.8% of men reporting a history of sexual assault in comparison with 42.4% of women (Kilpatrick et al., 2013). Among specific age groups, 37.4% of women aged 18–24 reported experiencing a first-time rape (Centers for Disease Control [CDC], 2011). Of those who have been raped, 42.2% reported being raped before the age of 18 (CDC, 2011). Research further shows that eight of ten victims of rape knew the person who sexually assaulted them (Miller, Cohen, & Wiersema, 1996), and one in ten women report being sexually assaulted by an intimate partner, including attempted forced penetration, alcohol/drug-facilitated completed penetration, and completed forced penetration (Breiding, Chen, & Black, 2014).

In addition to the significant psychosocial costs to the victim, sexual assault victimization is associated with substantial public expenditure. For instance, in 2010, rape was associated with the highest US cost ($127 billion) in comparison with assault ($93 billion), murder ($71 billion), and drunk driving ($62 billion) (Delisi et al., 2010). Recent estimates indicate that the population economic burden of rape was $3.1 trillion in 2014 (Peterson, DeGue, Florence, & Lokey, 2017). The estimated lifetime cost of rape per victim is $122,461, including medical costs, lost work productivity, criminal justice activities, and other costs (i.e., victim property loss or damage), but excluding intangible costs, such as pain and suffering (Peterson et al., 2017). Despite the high costs of sexual victimization, 63% of sexual assaults are not reported to the police (Rennison, 2002). These data suggest that sexual assault occurs at alarming rates and is associated with a significant economic burden.

Psychosocial Consequences of Sexual Assault

There is considerable variability in emotional reactions following sexual assault victimization among individuals that may include subclinical symptoms of distress, resilience, or prolonged or clinically significant distress. The extant literature on outcomes following sexual assault victimization suggests that rape is associated with increased rates of psychopathology, particularly PTSD. Prevalence rates of both lifetime and current PTSD diagnosis are significantly higher for individuals who experience sexual assault, rape, and physical assault in comparison with individuals who experience a non-crime event (i.e., natural disaster). For instance, data from the National Comorbidity Study (NCS) indicate that the event with the highest conditional risk, that is the probability of having PTSD given exposure to a qualifying stressor, was rape among both women (46%) and men (65%) (Kessler et al., 1995). Among women, sexual violence accounted for almost half of the cases of PTSD (Kessler et al., 1995). PTSD is also comorbid with other disorders particularly depression and anxiety and is associated with chronic distress. Furthermore, individuals with PTSD are six times more likely to have a suicide attempt (Sareen et al., 2005). Many individuals with PTSD exhibit co-occurring symptoms of major depressive disorder (MDD), with epidemiological studies estimating that between 30 and 50% of individuals with PTSD meet diagnostic criteria for MDD (Kessler et al., 1995). Furthermore, research indicates that 46.4% of individuals with PTSD also met criteria for a substance use disorder (SUD) (Pietrzak, Goldstein, Southwick, & Grant, 2011), and individuals with PTSD are two to four times more likely to meet criteria for a SUD than individuals without PTSD (Kessler, Chiu, Demler, Merikangas, & Walters, 2005). In fact, PTSD and problem drinking are commonly co-occurring disorders following adult sexual assault (Walsh et al., 2014). Waldrop and Cohen (2014) found that interpersonal traumas (i.e., physical or sexual assault) and serious accidents were independently associated with self-reported alcohol and drug problems and/or smoking in comparison to other types of traumas, such as disasters. Some studies have found that drinking is often utilized as a maladaptive coping strategy to alleviate symptoms of PTSD but may in turn exacerbate symptoms and increases the risk for retraumatization (Najdowski & Ullman, 2009; Volpicelli, Balaraman, Hahn, Wallace, & Bux, 1999).

Several factors have been examined to explain the relationship between sexual assault victimization and psychological outcomes. Commonly explored variables include pre-, peri-, and posttraumatic variables, such as exposure to previous trauma, severity of assault, personality factors such as extraversion, openness to experience, and optimism (Tedeschi & Calhoun, 2004), and victim demographics, particularly low socioeconomic status, substance and alcohol abuse, presence of a psychiatric disease, and engaging in risky sexual behavior in adolescence (Bramsen, Lasgaard, Koss, Elklit, & Banner, 2012; Creighton & Jones, 2012; Wacker, Macy, Barger, & Parish, 2009). Although there is strong empirical evidence for the association between these characteristics and development of PTSD, MDD, and SUDs, other determinants of distress, such as coping skills, social support, and recovery environment (i.e., family functioning) may be important to explore and incorporate into brief psychoeducational interventions and early intervention. Pretrauma factors such as coping skills might be utilized to identify women who are at risk of developing PTSD and thus as the target audience for psychoeducational interventions. It is evident that trauma exposure is associated with short-term and long-term adverse mental health consequences, such as posttraumatic stress disorder, major depressive disorder, and substance use disorders. Extant data indicate that although PTSD is the most common trauma-related response, it is highly comorbid with MDD and SUDs. Paradoxically, individuals with PTSD do not receive adequate mental health treatment.

Psychoeducational Interventions in the Aftermath of Sexual Assault

There is an impetus to develop interventions that are brief, evidence-based, and target the unique constellation of symptoms and barriers experienced by sexual assault victims. The provision of psychoeducation may be a cost-effective prevention strategy for sexual assault victims. Psychoeducation is defined as the delivery of knowledge or information about the course of posttrauma psychological symptoms and appropriate responses to these symptoms with the "intention to ameliorate or mitigate the effects of exposure to extreme situations" (Wessely, et al., 2008, p. 287). The goal of psychoeducation in the context of trauma is to provide a "cognitive framework," which addresses maladaptive responses to trauma, such as negative and distorted cognitions that can function to maintain symptoms of PTSD (Phoenix, 2007, p. 123).

This includes responding to symptoms of hyperarousal as normal reactions rather than as pathological and uncontrollable responses. Psychoeducation should thus function to provide information that normalizes responses to trauma, teaches adaptive coping skills, and identifies when further intervention is warranted (Phoenix, 2007). Provision of psychoeducation can take the form of provider delivered (individual or group), reading material (e.g., articles brochures), bibliotherapy, internet, or videos (Whitworth, 2016). Psychoeducation is typically integrated into treatments such as cognitive behavior therapy (CBT) and prolonged exposure (PE), although the number of sessions specifically focused on psychoeducation varies from treatment to treatment. In the context of evidence-based treatment protocols, psychoeducation consists of identification of common reactions to trauma and adjustment difficulties, the normalization of experiences, and the identification of symptoms, coping skills, questions and barriers to treatment (Ghafoori, Fisher, Korestelova, & Hong, 2016).

The aim of providing psychoeducation at the onset of therapy is to increase knowledge and improve perceived need and attitudes toward treatment (Mendenhall, Fristad, & Early, 2009). Psychoeducation may constitute the first step of a "stepped-care" model of treatment. A stepped-care delivery system organizes treatment options in a hierarchy of intensity that is correlated with cost (Draper & O'Donohue, 2011). The default start position is the first step in the stepped care model, which should be an evidence-based treatment of low intensity (i.e., psychoeducation). Low-intensity treatments require less time from a professional than a conventional treatment and are more cost-effective. This model emphasizes the rationalization of mental healthcare systems by utilizing varying intensities (e.g., length and modality) of treatment. Stepped-care models utilize a first-line intervention (psychoeducation) and crucially include a monitoring component whereby nonresponders are "stepped-up," to higher levels of care (Bower & Gilbody, 2005). Given the brief and easily disseminable format (e.g., video, bibliotherapy), psychoeducation has the potential to serve as a first-line intervention for victims of sexual assault.

Psychoeducation as an intervention is advantageous for several reasons: (1) psychoeducation normalizes the aftermath of trauma by giving survivors information about what symptoms they may experience and that these symptoms are normal and expected; (2) psychoeducation may assist in help-seeking by providing information about evidence-based treatment options and sources of help; (3) psychoeducation may provide corrective information that modified a victim's perception of the event by dispelling myths and misconceptions; (4) psychoeducation is empowering by encouraging individuals to engage in self-help and designating the individual as the primary agent of change and (5) psychoeducation is inexpensive and easily disseminated as it is often delivered via brochure or leaflet (Wessely et al., 2008).

Efficacy of Early Interventions Utilizing Psychoeducation Only

Few studies consisting only of psychoeducation have been evaluated for efficacy in reducing distress following sexual assault. Resnick, Acierno, Holmes, Kilpatrick, and Jager (1999) first developed a 17-min psychoeducational video including information about forensic examinations, symptoms of psychological distress that may result from a sexual assault, and modeling of coping. In a preliminary study, 13 survivors of sexual assault viewed a brief video intervention and compared to participants (N = 33) enrolled in usual care in a hospital setting. Participants in the video intervention group reported lower distress (as measured by postexam Subjective Unit of Discomfort Scale (SUDS)) following a medical examination. Participants in the intervention condition also reported reduced anxiety when preexam distress was controlled for (Resnick et al.,

1999). The efficacy of the psychoeducational video was extended in the area of substance use and abuse with a larger sample of sexual assault survivors. This is particularly important as there is significant evidence in the literature that individuals with a history of trauma may engage in substance abuse as a means of coping with distress following the traumatic event (Kilpatrick, Acierno, Resnick, Saunders, & Best, 1997b; Stewart, 1996). The video appeared effective in reducing marijuana abuse at a 6-week follow-up assessment. Trends were also found in reducing quantity of alcohol and marijuana use after 6 weeks (Acierno, Resnick, Flood, & Holmes, 2003). In a subsequent investigation, survivors of sexual assault ($N = 140$) were randomized to receive the video intervention or receive usual care (Resnick et al., 2007). Participants were assessed after 6 weeks and again 6 months following the assault. At posttreatment, participants in the intervention condition demonstrated lower PTSD and depression symptom severity, although this effect was only found for women with a history of victimization. Depression severity was also lower at 6 months among this group.

Updated findings with a larger sample indicated a similar result with a dismantling study design (Resnick, Acierno, Amstadter, Self-Brown, & Kilpatrick, 2007). Participants were 268 victims of sexual assault assigned to one of several conditions. These included (1) a non-video usual care condition, (2) the full 17-min video intervention (as described by Resnick et al., 1999), (3) 7 min 40 s video containing only medical exam preparation and (4) 10-min video containing only the psychoeducation component related to common reactions following sexual assault and coping strategies to manage these reactions. Video conditions were not analyzed separately however, limiting the ability to determine differential effects of each component. Participants in any video condition reported reduced marijuana use frequency, but no association was found for abuse of alcohol or other drugs (Resnick, Acierno, Amstadter, et al., 2007).

Miller, Cranston, Davis, Newman, and Resnick (2015) examined the efficacy of a 9-min video intervention focusing on psychoeducation about trauma and sexual assault combined with instructions on coping strategies. The video also included a rationale for in-vivo exposure to cues related to the trauma. Survivors of sexual assault ($N = 164$) were randomly assigned to the psychoeducation condition or to usual care. Usual care consisted of meeting with a rape crisis counselor. The video intervention was provided by a forensic nurse following a sexual assault nurse examiner (SANE) examination within 3 days of the assault. Participants in both the psychoeducation condition and usual care demonstrated reductions in state anxiety at 2 weeks and 2 months follow-up regardless of prior exposure to sexual assault. Participants in the psychoeducation condition reported lower state anxiety both 2 weeks and 2 months follow-up than their counterparts in usual care. PTSD symptoms were reduced for survivors without a prior history of sexual assault (Miller et al., 2015). The effect of sexual assault history as a moderator was in contrast to the findings of Resnick and colleagues (Resnick, Acierno, Waldrop, et al., 2007), suggesting that more work is needed to understand the moderating effect of history on the effectiveness of psychoeducation in reducing distress.

It is noteworthy that these studies examined a format of psychoeducation that was brief, inexpensive, feasible, and targeted a population that has been found to be at high risk for developing initial symptoms of PTSD and maintenance of symptoms over time (Rothbaum, Foa, Riggs, Murdock, & Walsh, 1992). This is particularly important as rape victims who report the assault to authorities typically undergo a forensic rape exam within 72 h of the assault, which may function to serve as trauma reminders and increase distress (Kilpatrick, Cougle, & Resnick, 2008). Critically, sexual assault survivors are not likely to return for treatment following an initial medical examination (Price et al., 2014). Thus, initial medical examination may be a brief window during which the community may be able to intervene and provide preventative care and brief psychoeducation during this encounter may prove to be a viable option for intervention.

Efficacy of Early Interventions Containing Psychoeducation in the Aftermath of Trauma

There is little research to support the efficacy of stand-alone psychoeducation in the aftermath of trauma. It has been suggested that psychoeducation has been presumed to be effective just as education is considered clearly "good," that researchers have not deemed it worthy of investigation (Wessely et al., 2008). Studies investigating the specific effects of psychoeducation for trauma-exposed adults range in the length of treatment (i.e., some studies examine the effects of a single session, others of 16 sessions), trauma event type examined (i.e., some studies exclusively study combat veterans, others include all trauma types), and components of psychoeducation examined (i.e., some studies add interpersonal dialogue, CBT techniques while others do not provide a discussion of the core components (Ghafoori et al., 2016). For instance, Lubin, Loris, Burt, and Johnson (1998) tested the effectiveness of a 16-week trauma-focused psychoeducational group for multiply traumatized women, 83% of whom reported being sexually assaulted. The group was divided into three phases that explored the impact of trauma on: (1) the individual's sense of self, (2) interpersonal relationships, and (3) meaning-making despite the experience of trauma (Lubin et al., 1998). Each group was 90 min in duration and each session began with psychoeducation, followed by an interactive discussion, concluded with a wrap-up with an educational focus and included homework in between sessions. The authors reported that at termination, 38% of participants demonstrated clinically meaningful reductions in PTSD, with most participants showing significant reductions in PTSD symptoms (Lubin et al., 1998). Participants also demonstrated significant reductions in depressive symptoms. All improvements were maintained at 6-month follow-up (Lubin et al., 1998). It is important to note that the authors stated that they incorporated components from cognitive behavioral and direct exposure approaches. It is then unclear to what extent the psychoeducation portion of the group contributed to symptom reduction. The authors reported that the psychoeducational component of each session was approximately 15 min in duration, but details regarding this component were not provided. Additionally, although efficacious, the group did not specifically target victims of sexual assault.

Because research is limited with respect to testing the efficacy of psychoeducation alone for reducing psychological distress for victims of sexual assault, the extant literature on brief intervention with a psychoeducation component will be discussed. Some research has been conducted on early interventions designed to prevent and reduce psychological distress following trauma. This review may provide some insight into core aspects of psychoeducation that have proven to be effective within the context of brief interventions. However, definitive conclusions cannot be drawn given that psychoeducation is provided in conjunction with active treatment ingredients. Brief interventions have included some components of psychoeducation (e.g., common reactions to trauma) and not others (e.g., information regarding healthy coping). The inclusion of psychoeducation within psychotherapeutic interventions is nearly ubiquitous, rendering it difficult to parse the potentially differential effects of psychoeducation alone and the psychotherapeutic intervention (Wessely et al., 2008).

Kilpatrick and Veronen (1984) assigned 49 survivors of sexual assault to either a brief behavioral intervention, repeated assessment, or follow-up assessment. The brief intervention involved 4–6 h of interview about the event, relaxation training, common reactions to trauma, and a discussion of guilt and blame and coping skills such as assertiveness training. Participants in all groups demonstrated self-reported declines in symptoms after a 3-month follow-up assessment, suggesting that this intervention was not effective in reducing distress, as the intervention group did not report any benefit above the assessment or control groups. Similar results were found in a study conducted by Frank et al. (1988). Eighty-four treatment seeking survivors of sexual assault were assigned to receive systematic desensitization or cognitive behavioral therapy.

All participants appeared to demonstrate a decline in symptoms at the 3- to 4-month follow-up and no differences were found between conditions. Results should be interpreted with caution, as conditions were not randomly assigned.

Foa, Hearst-Ikeda, and Perry (1995) examined the effects of a Brief Prevention (BP) program consisting of four CBT sessions compared to repeated assessment control with 20 female survivors of sexual assault who met PTSD diagnostic criteria. The intervention included imaginal exposure and in vivo exposure, which is not psychoeducation to trauma-related cues. At the posttreatment assessment, the treatment group reported reductions in PTSD symptom severity, but these differences were not maintained at the 5-month follow-up. Participants in the treatment group did report lower depression symptom severity at follow-up. This BP protocol was extended to a five-session intervention that demonstrated some efficacy with non-sexual-assault victims of trauma (e.g., motor vehicle accident). BP appeared to reduce PTSD symptom severity, anxiety, and depression symptoms at posttreatment and 6-month follow-up, although sample sizes were small (Bryant, Harvey, Dang, Sackville, & Basten, 1998; Bryant, Sackville, Dang, Moulds, & Guthrie, 1999).

Foa, Zoellner, and Feeny (2006) also utilized a brief intervention among 90 survivors of sexual and non-sexual trauma meeting criteria for PTSD. Time since assault ranged from 2 to 46 days. Participants either received brief CBT, supportive counseling, or a matched-time repeated assessment. The intervention consisted of four weekly 2-h sessions of CBT procedures that included psychoeducation—specifically education about normal reactions to the assault in addition to imaginal exposure, in vivo exposure, and cognitive restructuring. At posttreatment, participants in the intervention condition experienced a greater reduction in PTSD symptom severity than the supportive counseling condition. The intervention condition also resulted in greater end-state functioning than the supportive counseling group. These differences were found again at 3 months but were not maintained at a 6-month follow-up assessment. The intervention did not appear to be superior in reducing symptoms to the repeated assessment condition (Foa et al., 2006). The authors suggest that limitations of the study design may have obscured effects of the intervention. Homework compliance was strongly associated with better outcomes in the intervention condition, a finding indicating that further investigation is warranted. The authors posit that when comparing the intervention to rates of natural recovery, early intervention may accelerate recovery but not improve it. Taken together, evidence appears to be mixed but promising regarding the utility of brief psychoeducational interventions. Brief interventions containing psychoeducation constitute a significant portion of the evidence for the use of psychoeducation following sexual assault and are thus reviewed here (for a review of psychoeducation for the prevention of distress following exposure to potentially traumatic events, see Krupnick & Green, 2008; Wessely et al., 2008; Whitworth, 2016).

Key Components of Psychoeducation & Best Practices

The risk of early intervention being at best unnecessary and at worst, iatrogenic, means that empirical support must be considered before psychoeducation is integrated into clinical practice. Despite limited evidence for the use of psychoeducation with sexual assault victims, its use warrants further examination. Perhaps most critically, key components of effective psychoeducation must be identified. "Normalizing" reactions to trauma appears to be relevant to all psychoeducation interventions. Phoenix (2007) suggests several key elements that should be thought of as essential components of psychoeducation to accomplish this goal. These elements include:

1. *Defining trauma and discussing prevalence of experiencing traumatic events*: This education should function to challenge beliefs that the individual is to blame or flawed because he or she was victimized. It can also include an assessment of mental health literacy, which

refers to the knowledge and beliefs about mental disorders which aid their recognition, management, or prevention (Jorm et al., 1997).

2. *Dispelling common myths about trauma*: This component may be particularly relevant to sexual assault survivors, who may have been exposed to myths that traumatic events and resulting PTSD reactions only occur among military populations. It may also be important to suggest that reactions to trauma may persist and that persistence of these reactions is not caused by weakness of the individual but other factors such as the contextual factors related to the trauma and available support systems. For sexual assault victims, dispelling rape myths (i.e., token resistance) should be particularly incorporated into this component (Shafer, Ortiz, Thompson, & Hyemmer, 2018).
3. *The impact of trauma on physical health*: Educating the survivor about the impact of trauma on physiological arousal may reduce the individual's self-blame and normalize these responses. This content may include information about the autonomic nervous system (See Phoenix, 2007 for a description of how these processes may be described) and strategies for managing physiological distress. Effective coping techniques can include breathing retraining and mindfulness exercises.
4. *Common reactions to trauma*: Describing common reactions to trauma may assist the survivor in identifying adaptive coping strategies. Reactions should be described as able to be changed over time in order to reduce cognitions common to trauma that the survivor is "broken," (Phoenix, 2007). This should include an "expectancy of resilience," (Wessely et al., 2008) so as not to "prescribe" symptoms by educating the survivor about them.
5. *Coping skills should include both adaptive and maladaptive* (Davis, Resnick, & Swopes, 2011): Miller et al. (2015) utilized Lewinsohn and Graf's (1973) reinforcement density theory to suggest increasing positive activities to address depressive symptoms and reduce drug use as a coping strategy. Addressing maladaptive coping strategies is particularly important given elevated risk for substance use in this population (Kilpatrick, 2000).

These features of psychoeducation are consistent with a cognitive-behavioral theoretical framework (e.g., challenging distorted cognitions and teaching coping strategies). Empirical studies, however, tend not to describe in detail the extent to which each of these components was included in the intervention studied. As such, it is difficult given the present state of the literature to determine empirically which of these features is essential for the efficacy of psychoeducation.

Key Gaps in Existing Literature

Research examining the impact of psychoeducation in the aftermath of trauma is characterized by significant weaknesses. First, psychoeducation is often confounded with psychological debriefing, or critical incident stress debriefing (CISD; Krupnick & Green, 2008). There is no question that psychological debriefing includes a great deal of psychoeducation. The aim of debriefing however is to reduce initial distress and prevent subsequent psychopathology by providing information *and* eliciting victims' first reactions, behaviors, and sensory impressions (Krupnick & Green, 2008). In contrast, the aim of psychoeducation is solely to provide information and correct misconceptions. The continued use of CISD often contributes to the misconception that psychoeducation exacerbates symptoms of PTSD and is ineffective. The confusion is in part due to the brief nature of CISD and timing of delivery directly following exposure to a traumatic event (Van Emmerik, Kamphuis, Hulsbosch, & Emmelkamp, 2002). Use of this intervention is widespread, despite several professional guidelines indicating that psychological interventions should not be provided within the first month of trauma exposure and the use CISD specifically has been discouraged. However, variants of CISD are still utilized as early interventions (within 1 week following a traumatic event) particularly following mass disasters or exposure to traumatic events on a large scale.

Systematic reviews and meta-analyses conducted to examine the efficacy of CISD have yielded little empirical support that would recommend its use (Van Emmerik et al., 2002; Rose et al., 2002; Devilly, Gist, & Cotton, 2006). Van Emmerik et al. (2002) identified seven studies utilizing CISD within 1 month of trauma exposure with non-sexual assault traumas and determined that symptom reduction did not result from CISD. Further, CISD was not more effective than no intervention or non-CISD interventions. This type of debriefing may actually result in greater distress. The authors suggest that the delivery of CISD may disrupt natural resilience trajectories and return to normal functioning by taking the place of other sources of support such as family and friends. It is also suggested that CISD may pathologize normal reactions to trauma by suggesting to the victim that intervention is warranted and necessary. Given the extant data, CISD should not be confused with trauma-informed psychoeducation and further not be utilized with sexual assault victims following victimization.

Second, there is concern that providing information about PTSD will cause people to develop symptoms of PTSD. While this seems reasonable, there is little empirical support that information leads to symptom reporting or development. Psychoeducation is designed to decrease the expectation of distress, particularly because most individuals exposed to trauma do not develop PTSD. Third, existing psychoeducational interventions target symptoms reduction. There is little empirical evidence to indicate that psychoeducation alone, without prolonged exposure, is sufficient in decreasing symptoms of PTSD. Several other limitations have been identified and are briefly reviewed in this section.

Timing of Intervention

Little evidence exists to support a determination of when psychoeducation should be provided. A systematic review indicated that the timing of the intervention does not appear to be associated with PTSD symptomology. Provider contact in this review, however, was widely varied and did not evaluate psychoeducation specifically (Dworkin & Schumacher, 2016). One early intervention study examined differences between early and late treatment seekers and found no differences in the effectiveness of treatment between groups (Frank et al., 1988). The timing of standalone psychoeducation has yet to be examined and warrants future examination.

This issue of timing is critical as individuals have more contact with responders during the first month following a sexual assault (Ahrens, Stansell, & Jennings, 2010). Peritraumatic distress is associated with the development of PTSD (Resnick, Acierno, Amstadter, et al., 2007). This association suggests that early intervention following a sexual assault may be a critical period in which to intervene. Further, early intervention may be more feasible as survivors are likely to seek healthcare services immediately following the assault (Miller et al., 2015). However, it is unclear the extent to which this timing provides clinical benefit over and above other time points. It has been suggested that psychoeducation could be delivered prior to exposure of the potentially traumatic event (Wessely et al., 2008) but this approach has yet to be empirically evaluated.

Method of Delivery (i.e., Printed Material, Website, Provider)

While many community interventions (e.g., hotlines, SANE examiners) do not have evidence for their efficacy in the reduction of PTSD or psychological distress following trauma, it is likely that these providers may be key in provision of psychoeducation (Dworkin & Schumacher, 2016). Theoretically, psychoeducation may be delivered in a variety of formats (Wessely et al., 2008), and early contact with community providers may be a critical window in which intervention is feasible (Miller et al., 2015). Existing evidence suggests that video (Resnick, Acierno, Waldrop, et al., 2007) and individual psychotherapy contexts (Foa et al., 2006) may be effective. All studies evaluating stand-alone psychoeducation that demonstrated effects utilized a video format (Acierno et al., 2003; Miller et al., 2015; Resnick, Acierno, Waldrop, et al., 2007; Resnick et al., 1999). Videos are often used in medical contexts for psychoeducational purposes, although long-term effects do not appear to be consistent (Krouse, 2001). Thus, future work should examine whether or not this format is optimal.

Length of Intervention (i.e., Single Session, 12 Sessions)

It remains unclear what the optimal dose of psychoeducation should be. Interventions evaluated were brief—consisting of four or five sessions (e.g., Bryant et al., 1998; Foa et al., 2006). All studies examining stand-alone psychoeducation utilized a video that ranged from 7 to 17 min (Acierno et al., 2003; Miller et al., 2015; Resnick, Acierno, Waldrop, et al., 2007; Resnick et al., 1999). That these studies were able to demonstrate an impact suggest that a relatively small dose of psychoeducation may enough to yield results. Future studies should evaluate the optimal length of intervention.

Indications for Use

Who is most likely to benefit from psychoeducation? Trauma history may be a critical moderator in need of future examination. Studies have yielded mixed findings regarding the effectiveness of psychoeducation for sexual assault based on past history of prior assault (Miller et al., 2015; Resnick, Acierno, Waldrop, et al., 2007). In one study, a history of sexual assault rendered psychoeducation effective (Resnick, Acierno, Waldrop, et al., 2007) and in another, the opposite was found (Miller et al., 2015). It may be that individuals at high risk should be selected as candidates for intervention (Wessely et al., 2008), but it is also possible that past sexual assault may have led to other maladaptive coping (e.g., substance use; Kilpatrick et al., 1997a) that may limit the utility of a brief intervention. Other moderators, such as mental health literacy, should be examined to determine for whom psychoeducation is effective and in what format. For example, Phoenix (2007) provides bibliotherapy suggestions but these may only be available to more educated consumers. It has also been suggested that studies have not examined prior knowledge about trauma, and the impact of this individual difference on the effectiveness of psychoeducation (Whitworth, 2016). For example, it may be that individuals who have prior knowledge about trauma, sexual assault, and its consequences may not benefit from psychoeducation.

Evaluation of Other Outcomes

Studies have begun to evaluate the effect of psychoeducation on PTSD symptoms, depression and anxiety (Resnick, Acierno, Waldrop, et al., 2007; Resnick et al., 1999) and alcohol and drug use (Acierno et al., 2003; Resnick, Acierno, Waldrop, et al., 2007). It may be that the expansion of investigation of other outcomes may be warranted. It is possible that psychoeducation may have other functions (e.g., reduce stigma, increase mental health literacy) that are presumed but have not been evaluated. Studies with individuals exposed to other trauma types also suggest that psychoeducation is effective in increasing help seeking (Gould et al., 2007). As such, the potential for psychoeducation to improve outcomes related to trauma should be examined in future studies.

Conclusion

Psychoeducation is increasingly used following exposure to trauma as a means of ameliorating or mitigating the effects of trauma exposure. Despite its ubiquity, there is a paucity of evidence regarding the effectiveness of psychoeducation in preventing or reducing symptoms of PTSD. Preliminary evidence suggests that a brief psychoeducational video intervention prior to a medical exam may be effective in reducing psychological distress including state anxiety, PTSD symptoms (Miller et al., 2015), anxiety related to the medical examination (Resnick et al., 1999), and marijuana abuse (Acierno et al., 2003; Resnick, Acierno, Amstadter, et al., 2007). While it is clear that well-controlled randomized trials are needed to establish the efficacy of psychoeducation, preliminary evidence suggests that psychoeducation should be further evaluated for use given its considerable advantages in cost-effectiveness, feasibility, and flexible nature. Psychoeducation has the unique advantage of being easily disseminated in the contexts in which survivors of sexual assault are likely to be present, and existing evidence establishes that a brief video (less than 17 min) may be sufficient to produce some positive effects.

While widely regarded as standard care, psychoeducation is in clear need of empirical support to optimize effectiveness and justify the use of stand-alone psychoeducational interventions. Future research should focus on identifying key components of psychoeducation. While "normalization" of symptoms appears to be common to most forms of psychoeducation, dismantling studies should examine whether this component is necessary to produce change. Mediation analyses should also be conducted to determine active ingredients. For example, does use of adaptive coping skills learned in psychoeducation account for meaningful changes in anxiety and posttraumatic stress symptoms? Optimization of intervention materials should also be determined. These conditions include the timing of psychoeducation, method of delivery, and length of intervention. Moderators should be investigated in order to determine for whom psychoeducation is appropriate. Finally, other outcomes should be explored, such as future help-seeking and reduction in shame and stigma related to psychoeducation provision.

References

Acierno, R., Resnick, H. S., Flood, A., & Holmes, M. (2003). An acute post-rape intervention to prevent substance use and abuse. *Addictive Behaviors, 28*(9), 1701–1715.

Ahrens, C. E., Stansell, J., & Jennings, A. (2010). To tell or not to tell: The impact of disclosure on sexual assault survivors' recovery. *Violence and Survivors, 25*(5), 631–648.

Bower, P., & Gilbody, S. (2005). Stepped care in psychological therapies: Access, effectiveness and efficiency: Narrative literature review. *The British Journal of Psychiatry, 186*(1), 11–17.

Bramsen, R. H., Lasgaard, M., Koss, M. P., Elklit, A., & Banner, J. (2012). Adolescent sexual victimization: A prospective study on risk factors for first time sexual assault. *European Child & Adolescent Psychiatry, 21*(9), 521–526.

Breiding, M. J., Chen J., & Black, M. C. (2014). Intimate partner violence in the United States — 2010. The Centers for Disease Control and Prevention, National Center for Injury Prevention and Control. Retrieved from http://www.cdc.gov/violenceprevention/pdf/cdc_nisvs_ipv_report_2013_v17_single_a.pdf

Breiding, M. J., Smith, S. G., Basile, K. G., Walters, M. L., Chen, J., & Merrick, M. T. (2014). Prevalence and characteristics of sexual violence, stalking, and intimate partner violence victimization: National Intimate Partner and Sexual Violence Survey, United States, 2011. *Surveillance Summaries, 63*(SS08), 1–18.

Breslau, N., Davis, G. C., Andreski, P., Peterson, E. L., & Schultz, L. R. (1997). Sex differences in posttraumatic stress disorder. *Archives of General Psychiatry, 54*, 1044–1048.

Bryant, R. A., Harvey, A. G., Dang, S. T., Sackville, T., & Basten, C. (1998). Treatment of acute stress disorder: A comparison of cognitive-behavioral therapy and supportive counseling. *Journal of Consulting and Clinical Psychology, 66*(5), 862.

Bryant, R. A., Sackville, T., Dang, S. T., Moulds, M., & Guthrie, R. (1999). Treating acute stress disorder: An evaluation of cognitive behavior therapy and supportive counseling techniques. *American Journal of Psychiatry, 156*(11), 1780–1786.

Centers for Disease Control. (2011). *National Intimate Partner and Sexual Violence Survey, 2010*. Atlanta, GA: National Center for Injury Prevention and Control. Centers for Disease Control and Prevention. Retrieved from http://www.cdc.gov.unr.idm.oclc.org/violenceprevention/pdf/nisvs_report2010-a.pdf

Creighton, C. D., & Jones, A. C. (2012). Psychological profiles of adult sexual assault victims. *Journal of Forensic and Legal Medicine, 19*, 35–39.

Davis, J. L., Resnick, H. S., & Swopes, R. M. (2011). Psychoeducation to reduce distress and promote adaptive coping among adult women following sexual assault. Surviving sexual violence: A guide to recovery and empowerment, (pp. 256–275).

Delisi, M., Kosloski, A., Sween, M., Hachmeister, E., Moore, M., & Drury, A. (2010). Murder by numbers: Monetary costs imposed by a sample of homicide offenders. *The Journal of Forensic Psychiatry & Psychology, 21*, 501–513. https://doi.org/10.1080/14789940903564388

Devilly, G. J., Gist, R., & Cotton, P. (2006). Ready! Fire! Aim! The status of psychological debriefing and therapeutic interventions: In the work place and after disasters. *Review of General Psychology, 10*(4), 318.

Draper, C., & O'Donohue, W. T. (2011). *Stepped care and e-health: Practical applications to behavioral disorders*. New York: Springer.

Dworkin, E. R., & Schumacher, J. A. (2016). Preventing posttraumatic stress related to sexual assault through early intervention: A systematic review. *Trauma, Violence & Abuse, 19*, 459. https://doi.org/10.1177/1524838016669518

Foa, E. B. (2011). Prolonged exposure therapy: Past, present, and future. *Depression and Anxiety, 28*(12), 1043–1047.

Foa, E. B., Hearst-Ikeda, D., & Perry, K. J. (1995). Evaluation of a brief cognitive-behavioral program for the prevention of chronic PTSD in recent assault survivors. *Journal of Consulting and Clinical Psychology, 63*(6), 948.

Foa, E. B., Zoellner, L. A., & Feeny, N. C. (2006). An evaluation of three brief programs for facilitating recovery after assault. *Journal of Traumatic Stress, 19*(1), 29–43.

Frank, E., Anderson, B., Stewart, B. D., Dancu, C., Hughes, C., & West, D. (1988). Efficacy of cognitive behavior therapy and systematic desensitization in the treatment of rape trauma. *Behavior Therapy, 19*(3), 403–420.

Ghafoori, B., Fisher, D. G., Korestelova, O., & Hong, M. (2016). A randomized, controlled pilot study of a single-session psychoeducation treatment for urban, culturally-diverse, trauma-exposed adults. *The Journal of Nervous and Mental Disease, 204*(6), 421–430. https://doi.org/10.1097/NMD.0000000000000512

Gould, M., Greenberg, N. & Hetherton, J. (2007). Stigma and the military: Evaluation of a PTSD psychoeducational program. Journal of Traumatic Stress, 20, 505–515.

Hembree, E. A., Foa, E. B., Dorfan, N. M., Street, G. P., Kowalski, J., & Tu, X. (2003). Do patients drop out prematurely from exposure therapy for PTSD? *Journal of Traumatic Stress, 16*(6), 555–562.

Jorm, A. F., Korten, A. E., Jacomb, P. A., Christensen, H., Rodgers, B., & Pollitt, P. (1997). Mental health literacy: A survey of the public's ability to recognise mental disorders and their beliefs about the effectiveness of treatment. Medical Journal of Australia, 166, 182–186.

Kessler, R. C., Chiu, W. T., Demler, O., Merikangas, K. R., & Walters, E. E. (2005). Prevalence, severity, and comorbidity of 12-month DSM-IV disorders in the National Comorbidity Survey Replication. *Archives of General Psychiatry, 62*(6), 617–627.

Kessler, R. C., Sonnega, A., Bromet, E., Hughes, M., & Nelson, C. B. (1995). Posttraumatic stress disorder in the National Comorbidity Survey. *Archives of General Psychiatry, 52*, 1048–1060. https://doi.org/10.1001/archpsyc.1995.03950240066012

Kilpatrick, D. G. (2000). Rape and sexual assault. National Violence Against Women Prevention Research Center, Medical University of South Carolina.

Kilpatrick, D. G., Acierno, R., Resnick, H. S., Saunders, B. E., & Best, C. L. (1997a). A 2-year longitudinal analysis of the relationships between violent assault and substance use in women. *Journal of Consulting and Clinical Psychology, 65*(5), 834.

Kilpatrick, D. G., Acierno, R., Resnick, H. S., Saunders, B. E., & Best, C. L. (1997b). The relationship between assault and alcohol, marijuana, and hard drug use in women. *Journal of Consulting and Clinical Psychology, 65*(5), 834–847.

Kilpatrick, D. G., Cougle, J. R., & Resnick, H. R. (2008). Reports of the death of psychoeducation as a preventative treatment for posttraumatic psychological distress are exaggerated. *Psychiatry, 71*(4), 322–328.

Kilpatrick, D. G., Resnick, H. S., Milanak, M. E., Miller, M. W., Keyes, K. M., & Friedman, M. J. (2013). National estimates of exposure to traumatic events and PTSD prevalence using DSM-IV and DSM-5 criteria. *Journal of Traumatic Stress, 26*, 537–547. https://doi.org/10.1002/jts.21848

Koss, M. P., Gidycz, C. A., & Wisniewski, N. (1987). The scope of rape: Incidence and prevalence of sexual aggression and victimization in a national sample of higher education students. *Journal of Consulting and Clinical Psychology, 55*, 162–170.

Krupnick, J. L., & Green, B. L. (2008). Psychoeducation to prevent PTSD: A paucity of evidence. *Psychiatry: Interpersonal and Biological Processes, 71*(4), 329–331.

Kilpatrick, D. G., and Veronen, L. J. (1984).Treatment of Fear and Anxiety in Victims of Rape (Final Report, Grant No. R01 MH29602), National Institute of Mental Health, Rockville, MD.

Krouse, H.J. (2001). Video modelling to educate patients. Journal of Advanced Nursing, 33, 748–757.

Lewinsohn, P. M., & Graf, M. (1973). Pleasant activities and depression. *Journal of Consulting and Clinical Psychology, 41*, 261–268.

Lubin, H., Loris, M., Burt, J., & Johnson, D. R. (1998). Efficacy of psychoeducational group therapy in reducing symptoms of posttraumatic stress disorder among multiply traumatized women. *American Journal of Psychiatry, 155*(9), 1172–1177.

Mendenhall, A. N., Fristad, M. A., & Early, T. J. (2009). Factors influencing service utilization and mood symptom severity in children with mood disorders: Effects of multifamily psychoeducation groups (MFPGs). *Journal of Consulting and Clinical Psychology, 77*, 463–473.

Miller, K. E., Cranston, C. C., Davis, J. L., Newman, E., & Resnick, H. (2015). Psychological outcomes after a sexual assault video intervention: A randomized trial. *Journal of Forensic Nursing, 11*, 129–136.

Miller, T. R., Cohen, M. A., & Wiersema, B. (1996). Victim costs and consequences: A new look (NCJ 155282). The U.S. Department of Justice, Office of Justice Programs, National Institute of Justice. Retrieved from https://www.ncjrs.gov/pdffiles/victcost.pdf

Najdowski, C. J., & Ullman, S. E. (2009). Prospective effects of sexual victimization on PTSD and problem drinking. *Addictive Behaviors, 34*, 965–968.

Peterson, C., DeGue, S., Florence, C., & Lokey, C. N. (2017). Lifetime economic burden of rape among U.S. adults. *American Journal of Preventive Medicine, 52*(6), 691–701. https://doi.org/10.1016/j.amepre.2016.11.014

Phoenix, B. J. (2007). Psychoeducation for survivors of trauma. *Perspectives in Psychiatric Care, 43*(3), 123–131.

Pietrzak, R. H., Goldstein, R. B., Southwick, S. M., & Grant, B. F. (2011). Prevalence and Axis I comorbidity of full and partial posttraumatic stress disorder in the United States: Results from wave 2 of the National Epidemiologic Survey on alcohol and related conditions. *Journal of Anxiety Disorders, 25*, 456–465. https://doi.org/10.1016/j.janxdis.2010.11.010

Price, M., Davidson, T. M., Ruggiero, K. J., Acierno, R., & Resnick, H. S. (2014). Predictors of using mental health services after sexual assault. *Journal of Traumatic Stress, 27*(3), 331–337.

Rennison, C. A. (2002). Rape and sexual assault: Reporting to police and medical attention, 1992–2000 [NCJ 194530]. The U.S. Department of Justice, Office of Justice Programs, Bureau of Justice Statistics. Retrieved from http://bjs.ojp.usdoj.gov/content/pub/pdf/rsarp00.pdf

Resnick, H., Acierno, R., Holmes, M., Kilpatrick, D. G., & Jager, N. (1999). Prevention of post-rape psychopathology: Preliminary findings of a controlled acute rape treatment study. *Journal of Anxiety Disorders, 13*(4), 359–370.

Resnick, H., Acierno, R., Waldrop, A. E., King, L., King, D., Danielson, C., … Kilpatrick, D. (2007). Randomized controlled evaluation of an early intervention to prevent post-rape psychopathology. *Behaviour Research and Therapy, 45*(10), 2432–2447.

Resnick, H. S., Acierno, R., Amstadter, A. B., Self-Brown, S., & Kilpatrick, D. G. (2007). An acute post-sexual assault intervention to prevent drug abuse: Updated findings. *Addictive Behaviors, 32*(10), 2032–2045.

Rothbaum, B. O., Foa, E. B., Riggs, D. S., Murdock, T., & Walsh, W. (1992). A prospective evaluation of post-traumatic stress disorder in rape victims. *Journal of Traumatic Stress, 5*, 455–475.

Rose, S., Bisson, J., Churchill, R., & Wessely, S. (2002). Psychological debriefing for preventing post traumatic stress disorder (PTSD). The Cochrane Databses of Systematic Reviews, 2.

Sareen, J., Cox, B. J., Afifi, T. O., de Graaf, R., Asmundson, G. J. G., ten Have, M., & Stein, M. B. (2005). Anxiety disorders and risk for suicidal ideation and suicide attempts. *Archives of General Psychiatry, 62*, 1249–1257.

Shafer, A., Ortiz, R. R., Thompson, B., & Hyemmer, J. (2018). The role of hypermasculinity, token resistance, rape myth, and assertive sexual consent communication among college men. *Journal of Adolescent Men, 62*(S3), S44–S50. https://doi.org/10.1016/j.jadohealth.2017.10.015

Stewart, S. H. (1996). Alcohol abuse in individuals exposed to trauma: A critical review. *Psychological Bulletin, 120*, 83–112.

Tedeschi, R.G. & Calhoun, L.G. (2004). Posttraumatic growth: Conceptual foundations and empirical evidence. *Psychological Inquiry, 15*, 1–18. https://doi.org/10.1207/s15327965pli1501_01.

Van Emmerik, A. A., Kamphuis, J. H., Hulsbosch, A. M., & Emmelkamp, P. M. (2002). Single session debriefing after psychological trauma: A meta-analysis. *The Lancet, 360*(9335), 766–771.

Volpicelli, J., Balaraman, G., Hahn, J., Wallace, H., & Bux, D. (1999). The role of uncontrollable trauma in the development of PTSD and alcohol addiction. *Alcohol Research and Health, 123*, 256–262.

Wacker, J., Macy, R., Barger, E., & Parish, S. (2009). Sexual assault prevention for women with intellectual disabilities: A critical review of the evidence. *Journal of Intellectual and Developmental Disability, 47*(4), 249–262. https://doi.org/10.1352/1934-9556-47.4.249

Waldrop, A. E., & Cohen, B. E. (2014). Trauma exposure predicts alcohol, nicotine, and drug problems beyond the contribution of PTSD and depression in patients with cardiovascular disease: Data from the Heart and Soul Study. *The American Journal on Addictions, 23*, 53–61. https://doi.org/10.1111/j.1521-0391.2013.12053.x

Walsh, K., Resnick, H., Danielson, C., McCauley, J., Saunders, B., & Kilpatrick, D. (2014). Patterns of drug and alcohol use associated with lifetime sexual revictimization and current posttraumatic stress disorder among three national samples of adolescent, college, and household-residing women. *Addictive Behaviors, 39*, 64–689.

Whitworth, J. D. (2016). The role of psychoeducation in trauma recovery: Recommendations for content and delivery. *Journal of Evidence-Informed Social Work, 13*(5), 442–451.

Wessely, S., Bryant, R.A., Greenberg, N., Earnshaw, M., Sharpley, J., & Hughes, J.H. (2008). Does psychoeducation help prevent post traumatic stress? Psychiatry, 71(4), 287–302.

The Good Lives Model and the Rehabilitation of Individuals Convicted of Sexual Offending

31

Roxanne Heffernan and Tony Ward

Introduction

The treatment of sexual offending has seen a number of developments across the last four decades, from a reliance on clinical intuition and behavioral therapies aimed at reconditioning, to the adoption of Relapse Prevention (RP) in the 1980s, and the discovery of recidivism correlates and development of risk measures in the 1990s (Marshall & Marshall, 2017). This shift saw the emergence of rehabilitation theories and principles based upon evidence concerning "what works" to reduce recidivism generally (Andrews & Bonta, 2010). Alongside this substantial work, theorists have developed and refined specific theories aimed at explaining sexual offending and empirically related phenomena (e.g., cognitive distortions, Ward & Keenan, 1999; self-regulation, Ward & Hudson, 2000). More recently, researchers have argued for the inclusion of personal strengths and values in correctional treatment, and a conceptualization of (sexual) offending as maladaptive goal-directed behavior. The *Good Lives Model* (GLM) was developed by Tony Ward (2002a, 2002b) as an augmentation to risk-management approaches, but has also been viewed as an alternative rehabilitation framework (Ward & Maruna, 2007; Ziv, 2018). This chapter will focus on the GLM, its core assumptions and implications, the empirical evidence supporting its use, and its relationship to practice—including its relationship with the Risk-Need-Responsivity model (RNR; Andrews & Bonta, 2010; Bonta & Andrews, 2017). We will conclude by highlighting areas for future development which will provide, in our opinion, a promising way forward for the treatment of individuals who have committed sexual offenses.

Rehabilitation theories contain (1) general principles, aims, and values, (2) causal assumptions about offending and related concepts, and (3) more concrete principles or tools to guide practice (Ward, Melser, & Yates, 2007). For example, the core RNR principles are practice guidelines derived from the *General Personality and Cognitive Social Learning* perspective of human beings, which values empirical evidence concerning variation in offending outcomes, and aims to decrease or manage risk of recidivism (Andrews & Bonta, 2010; Bonta & Andrews, 2017). This view is committed to respect for the complexity of human behavior and acknowledges that interactions between variables (rather than any variable on its own) are the causes of variation, and more recently has emphasized the critical role of personal

R. Heffernan
Victoria University of Wellington,
Wellington, New Zealand

T. Ward (✉)
School of Psychology, University of Ghent and
Victoria University of Wellington,
Wellington, New Zealand
e-mail: Tony.Ward@vuw.ac.nz

W. T. O'Donohue and P. A. Schewe (eds.), *Handbook of Sexual Assault and Sexual Assault Prevention*,
https://doi.org/10.1007/978-3-030-23645-8_31

autonomy in behavioral control (Bonta & Andrews, 2017). The probable causes of offending according to proponents of this model are a subset of dynamic risk factors known as the *central eight* (criminogenic needs), all of which influence the perceived costs and benefits associated with any particular behavior and thus the decision to engage in crime. In addition, the opposite of these risk factors have been labeled as "strengths," and interventions aim to cause shifts in these factors (i.e., from risk to strength) to reduce the likelihood of further offending (Andrews & Bonta, 2010; Bonta & Andrews, 2017). The central eight are: antisocial associates, antisocial attitudes, antisocial personality pattern, history of antisocial behavior (static factor), education and employment, leisure activities, relationships and family, and substance abuse (Bonta & Andrews, 2017). In short, treatment is most effective if it is proportionate to risk, prioritizes targeting criminogenic needs over non-criminogenic needs (i.e., those with a weaker statistical association with reoffending), and is responsive both to the evidence concerning which methods of intervention are most effective, and the particular needs of individuals (e.g., learning style, motivation). This is a simplified account of what is a large and enduring body of work, nevertheless, the RNR model is oriented towards objective and evidence-based prediction and intervention in order to reduce reoffending. Importantly, the authors of the model welcome sources of criticism and challenges which may advance the theory, as long as they demonstrate a respect for evidence.

The GLM was originally developed as a strength-based augmentation to enhance rather than replace the RNR. The underlying view of persons is as goal-directed agents with a range of priorities and capacities, who interact with their environments to pursue personally meaningful outcomes. According to the GLM, the aim of correctional treatment should be to reduce the likelihood of further offending via the promotion of a personally meaningful *Good Life*. These two priorities are not mutually exclusive, as offending is conceptualized as the result of problems in an individual's implicit *Good Life Plan*. A good life contains valued outcomes, termed *Primary Human Goods*, which are of varying importance to individuals, but should all be present to some degree. The GLM goods are: excellence in work, excellence in play, creativity, knowledge, relatedness, community, pleasure, life, inner peace, spirituality, and excellence in agency (Purvis, 2010). The means by which these are attained are termed *Secondary Human Goods*, and these can be more or less healthy, adaptive, and prosocial. For example, one person may achieve inner peace by practicing meditation, while another may use illegal substances. Use of secondary goods depends on internal capacities as well as environmental resources and opportunities. Problems with internal and external resources are considered to be causes or contributors to sexual offending (i.e., criminogenic needs), and as such should be the focus of intervention. The GLM acknowledges the importance of targeting criminogenic needs, but does so through the building of internal and external resources, rather than simply risk reduction.

According to Ward and colleagues (Ward, 2002a, 2002b; Ward & Fisher, 2005) there are four types of problems evident in the good life plans (priorities and means) of individuals who commit offenses. These are problems with: capacity, means, conflict, and scope, and they often interact or coexist. Briefly, when the *capacities* or resources (both internal and external) required for goods attainment are lacking, an individual may turn to antisocial behaviors such as offending (i.e., problematic or harmful *means*). *Conflict* occurs when these problematic behaviors and their consequences interfere with the attainment of other goods. For example, poor coping abilities (capacity) may lead to drug abuse (means) aimed at attaining inner peace, which may then impact negatively upon relationships (conflict). Lack of *scope* occurs when individuals prioritize certain goods at the expense of others, and not all are present within a person's life. For example, sexual offending could be aimed at seeking pleasure, but its consequences (e.g., prison, damage to reputation, remorse) create obstacles to attaining other goods such as excellence in work and inner peace. In addition, researchers have described two empirically established routes to offending, direct and indirect (Purvis, Ward, & Willis, 2011). The *direct route* is evident where capacities and resources are lacking, and an offense is a means to meet a need (e.g., intimacy or pleasure seeking). The *indirect route* involves conflict or problems with scope, whereby offending occurs as a ripple effect from other problematic means (e.g., substance use reducing control and inhibition).

GLM interventions center upon a personally meaningful good life plan, containing all primary goods to varying degrees (determined by the individual), and the secondary goods (goals and strategies) required to attain these without harming others. This can be linked with risk reduction by identification of the goods sought via offending (either directly or indirectly) in the past, and the barriers or problems (i.e., criminogenic needs) evident within the strategies used to attain these goods. For example, where sexual offending is used as a means to achieve relatedness or pleasure because of problems differentiating between appropriate partners (i.e., children are preferred as sexual partners because individuals feel emotionally safer with them). A new good life plan could incorporate relatedness and pleasure via the goal of seeking an intimate relationship with an age-appropriate consenting partner. Strategies may include attending social activities, creating an online dating profile, engaging in conversation, physical intimacy, vulnerable disclosure, conflict resolution, and so on. Individuals vary in their ability to engage in these normative practices; the capacities required for healthy intimacy are learned and shaped via social interaction. Treatment can target risk factors such as *emotional congruence with children* through the development or strengthening of internal and external capacities and resources. For example, developing healthy beliefs about the self, others, and relationships (e.g., "others are trustworthy", "I am safe"), communication and negotiation skills, emotion-management, perspective-taking, and so on. In addition, the availability of external resources (e.g., opportunity, finances, freedom) can support or obstruct goods attainment, and should also be included in a good life plan. To summarize, treatment should identify the most heavily weighted goods and those sought via offending, use these to construct a comprehensive good life plan, and then develop or strengthen the internal and external resources required to live a good life without reoffending. The GLM proposes a dual focus on promoting goods and overcoming barriers (i.e., criminogenic needs), it does this in collaboration with the individual to build upon strengths and focus on meaningful personal goals, rather than only avoiding reoffending.

The developers of the GLM have provided guidelines and tools to help practitioners integrate these principles into practice (e.g., Purvis et al., 2011; Willis, Yates, Gannon, & Ward, 2013). Its use extends to assessment and case conceptualization, case management, development of program content, and the therapeutic relationship. The GLM is currently used to guide practice internationally including in New Zealand, Australia, the United Kingdom, Belgium, France, Germany, Ireland, Norway, Hong Kong, the United States, Canada, and Singapore. In terms of its conceptualization, it is often seen as an "add on" to risk focused interventions, rather than being used in its intended role to guide the entirety of treatment. For example, when evaluating the operationalization of the GLM in North American programs Willis, Ward, and Levenson (2014) found that the GLM was typically evident within program delivery (i.e., positive therapist characteristics) and as an additional component to treatment focused on risk reduction (e.g., self-management plans at program completion). They conclude that "enhancing program consistency with the GLM requires using it as a comprehensive theoretical framework to guide interventions throughout the entirety of a program" (Willis et al., 2014, p. 77). Therefore, while the GLM is currently incorporated within treatment internationally, there are concerns about the appropriateness of its implementation, and inconsistencies are evident. The success of programs adopting this approach is still to be determined; this research is made more difficult by a number of features of treatment programs and their evaluation, which will now be discussed.

GLM Evidence Base

To engage with individuals who have committed sexual offenses in an ethically defensible way it is important that treatment programs are based on evidence concerning the sorts of interventions that are most effective in reducing reoffending. The Criminal Justice System exists to promote community safety via the effective management, rehabilitation, and reintegration of individuals who have harmed others. According to the RNR model, the best way to do this is to match intensity of treatment to risk level, target criminogenic needs, and to be responsive to individual needs and barriers to treatment (Bonta & Andrews, 2017). Indeed, adherence to these three principles has demonstrated relative success in reducing recidivism rates (Dowden & Andrews, 2000; Hanson, Bourgon, Helmus, & Hodgson, 2009), and so long as this continues they should be used to guide practice. However, we argue that this is a rather narrow view of the available knowledge, and we take a broader view of what constitutes evidence and success. The reasons for our focus are twofold; (1) recidivism is a difficult to measure and decontextualized outcome variable (Jung & Gulayets, 2011), and (2) the evidence concerning criminal behavior ought to be drawn from multiple disciplines, and should inform explanations of individual functioning rather than relying upon lists of correlates. Knowledge is cumulative, rather than one definitive study proving that treatment is effective or ineffective, our understanding of its effects will grow through the accumulation of many smaller studies using various methods (Collaborative Outcome Data Committee [CODC], 2007).

Recidivism Outcome Studies: Limitations

The effect of sexual offending treatment is currently moderately positive, although there is significant variation across studies—both in their findings and the quality of their methodology (Grady & Pettus-Davis, 2017; Lösel, 2017). Lösel and Schmucker (2017) highlight a number of weaknesses including combining different offense types, the range of treatment modalities used, small sample sizes, attrition, length of follow-up, and poorly controlled studies. While there are rigorous scientific methods that can overcome some of these issues and limit biases, there are often problems with implementing these in the real world. For example, it has been suggested that Randomized Controlled Trials (RCTs), considered the "gold standard" in experimental psychology, are inappropriate for use in sexual offending treatment outcome studies (Marshall & Marshall, 2007). This claim rests upon their low ecological validity (i.e., they do not approximate the real world), difficulties implementing these in clinical settings, and ethical concerns with random allocation (i.e., withholding treatment is dangerous). Thus, research is usually quasi-experimental in nature, comparing those who have already been allocated to treatment and those who have not.

In addition, "general statements about the effect or failure of sex offender treatment are inappropriate" (Lösel, 2017, p. 9). Interventions are complex and one should not assume that the relationship between treatment and (reductions in) recidivism is one of causality. It is important to acknowledge the composite and eclectic nature of treatment (Kim, Benekos, & Merlo, 2015), and consider the suggestion that evidence is most useful if it is able to differentiate aspects of treatment which moderate change (Lösel, 2017). Moderators suggested by Lösel (2017) include the programs' theoretical foundation, program integrity, and social context. Other influences include therapist characteristics and therapeutic alliance, participant characteristics (e.g., motivation, intelligence), setting (i.e., prison or community), involvement of support networks (personal and professional), and so on. Given that it is challenging (if not impossible) to control for the range of influences upon participants throughout a program and beyond (Grady & Pettus-Davis, 2017), it is difficult to say from the available research what (if anything) about treatment *causes* individuals to refrain from reoffending.

Recidivism is an undesirable outcome, an indication of failure—intervention has not "worked" when it precedes a re-offense. Its "success" is determined by the proportion of participants who *do not* reoffend, or in reality, those who are not detected (Lösel, 2017). Recidivism is difficult to accurately measure, with official records giving a conservative estimate (i.e., about a third of self-reported crime; Bonta & Andrews, 2017). There is variability in how recidivism is measured, defined, and reported (Grady & Pettus-Davis, 2017), for example, official records and/or self-report, rearrests and incarceration, and general, violent, and/or sexual recidivism. In addition, the dichotomous measure tells us nothing about the context, severity, frequency, or cause of the re-offense/s. The prevalence of reoffending is clearly relevant to the success or failure of interventions, however, important information about the range of behaviors (and causes) of interest to researchers and program developers is missing from most studies. In other words, recidivism outcome studies provide an effect size indicating the direction and magnitude of the relationship between two complex variables (i.e., treatment and recidivism), but cannot tell us about the causes or conditions of change.

We will now outline the relevant empirical research. Because the GLM is not a *treatment theory*, but rather a *rehabilitation model*, evidence supporting its use must come from evaluations of programs consistent with GLM values and assumptions, and their impact upon a range of practice-related outcomes. In addition, we propose that "success" involves more than reduced recidivism and include knowledge which falls outside treatment programs' efficacy in reducing recidivism.

The Empirical Research

The empirical research concerning GLM-consistent correctional treatment programs is limited, particularly in comparison to the abundance of papers advocating for and outlining its potential use in treating various populations. For example, it has been suggested as appropriate for youth (Fortune, 2017; Wylie & Griffin, 2013; Wainright & Nee, 2014), elderly (Di Lorito, Vollm & Dening, 2018), females (Van Damme, Hoeve, Vermeiren, Vanderplasschen, & Colins, 2016), mentally disordered (Barnao, Ward, & Casey, 2015, 2016; Gannon, King, Miles, Lockerbie, & Willis, 2011), intellectually disabled (Aust, 2010), and non-Western (Chu, Koh, Zeng, & Teoh, 2015; Leaming & Willis, 2016) offending populations. Furthermore, it has been extended beyond use in treatment for sexual offenses and proposed as useful for violent offending (Whitehead, Ward, & Collie, 2007), domestic violence (Langlands, Ward, & Gilchrist, 2009), general offending (Loney & Harkins, 2018), substance abuse (Thakker & Ward, 2010), and residential burglary (Taylor, 2017).

Much of the empirical research thus far has focused on case studies or relatively small sample sizes, although there have been several larger comparisons between GLM adaptations and traditional relapse prevention (i.e., risk avoidant) programs. Studies investigating the use of the GLM tend to focus on qualitative evidence such as perceptions of treatment, engagement and motivation, and other psychological and behavioral outcomes, rather than reduced recidivism. This makes sense given its dual focus on reducing reoffending *and* building good lives; targeting offense-related needs is already established as best practice, and so what the GLM adds is a more engaging focus on individual goals and strengths. Information concerning this added value is best accessed via first person accounts of the experience of treatment and personally meaningful outcomes or changes following treatment, rather than records of recidivism.

Approach Goals

Approach goals are central to the GLM, and are characterized by their orientation *towards* a desired outcome. For example, an approach goal would be to develop the skills and capacities necessary for a healthy and age-appropriate relationship, whereas an avoidant goal would be to abstain from viewing child exploitation material online. The desired outcome in both cases is a future free from sexual offending, however the approach goal emphasizes what is to be gained rather than just removing a means or source of goods without replacing it (what has been referred to as a "pin cushion" approach—Ward, Mann, & Gannon, 2007). While more motivating and engaging, approach goals also have a higher likelihood of being achieved and of their positive effects lasting longer than avoidance goals (Marshall & Serran, 2004). Simons, McCullar, and Tyler (2008) compared a sexual offending program focused on approach goals (n = 96) with an avoidant relapse prevention program (n = 100). Participants allocated to the GLM (approach) condition were much more likely to complete the program and were perceived as more motivated by their therapists. While both conditions produced improvement on psychometric measures relating to areas of need, participants in the GLM condition demonstrated significantly better improvement on coping skills and problem-solving scores, and were also more likely to have a social support system in place after treatment.

Similarly, Mann, Webster, Schofield, and Marshall (2004) compared an avoidant-goal intervention to an adapted approach-goal intervention, with individuals convicted of sexual offenses (n = 47) randomly allocated to each condition. They found that the approach-goal condition produced better engagement (i.e., task completion and disclosure), and therapists perceived more genuine motivation to live an offense-free lifestyle for participants in this condition, compared with the traditional approach. One disadvantage perceived by the therapists was the relative complexity of delivering the approach-goal intervention, and the potential that participants would lack an adequate understanding of their individual risk factors. However, use of the Relapse Prevention Questionnaire (a tool designed to measure awareness and understanding of risk factors and strategies to manage them—Beckett, Fisher, Mann, & Thornton, 1997) indicated that *both* groups had significantly improved, with no significant difference between groups. Nevertheless, it is important that interventions include a focus upon needs linked with offending, and include strategies to address risk alongside other positive outcomes. The delicate weaving of these dual aims requires adequate training of practitioners, so they are able to be flexible and responsive to individuals.

Prudential Values and Primary Human Goods

Values are an important consideration for forensic practice for a number of reasons, most of which will not be discussed here (see Ward & Heffernan, 2017). In terms of rehabilitation, it is important to consider the way that values (of different sorts) inform the goals of treatment. For example, the primary aim of the Criminal Justice System is to reduce harm through managing, reducing, or eliminating the causes of offending. However, the outcomes sought by participants (i.e., prudential values) are likely to be broader, and include aspects of life which make desistance a worthwhile process and reoffending undesirable. For example, while programs concentrate on needs such as impulsivity, deviance, and antisocial cognition, participants may be better motivated by the possibility of satisfying relationships, pleasure, and happiness. Practitioners should be concerned with both social and ethical values (i.e., harm reduction), and prudential values (i.e., well-being or flourishing)—these are not mutually exclusive. As the following studies suggest, the GLM concept of primary human goods is able to capture the role of prudential values in offending, and thus provide a way to link these two concerns.

A number of studies support the relevance of goods attainment, both in explaining past behavior (i.e., offending) and in guiding future behavior. For example, Barnett and Wood (2008) investigated the priority that untreated individuals imprisoned for sexual offending (n = 42) had placed upon the three goods thought to be most strongly associated with sexual offending (agency, relatedness, and inner peace; Ward & Mann, 2004) at the time of their offense. These individuals experienced problems with *prioritizing* inner peace (61.9% rated as high priority), relative to agency (71.4%) and relatedness (78.6%). They also found evidence to support the problems with scope, capacity, means, and conflict theorized to exist within the good life plans of individuals who engage in offending. For example, 47.6% had an "unbalanced" good lives conception, and 42.8% scored below average for problem-solving abilities. Participants' accounts of their attempts to achieve these goods contained problems with operationalizing their good life, difficulty for all participants in achieving one or more of these goods prior to or during offending, and for some participants offending was seen as a means (secondary good).

Further studies have supported the importance of primary human goods for individuals convicted of sexual offenses (e.g., Yates, Kingston, Simons, & Tyler, 2009), and others have investigated their importance and influence for other offending groups. For example, Chu et al. (2015) retrospectively identified the goods endorsed by youth who had engaged in sexual offending (n = 168) in Singapore. They found that pleasure (91.1%), relatedness (35.7%), and inner peace (17.3%) were most highly prioritized. Although retrospective (i.e., based on case notes), these findings suggest that pleasure may be more relevant for youth sexual offending, which makes sense considering the prevalence of pleasure seeking in adolescence. In addition, the use of sexually harmful behavior to meet needs of belonging (i.e., relatedness) and emotional health (i.e., inner peace) were reportedly common offense-related needs for youth engaged in sexual offending treatment in England (Wylie & Griffin, 2013). Investigating female youth (n = 95) in Belgium, Van Damme et al. (2016) examined the link between *quality of life* (QoL; physical, social, psychological, and environmental), future mental health, and offending. Although they did not find support for a direct negative pathway from QoL to offending, they found support for an indirect negative pathway via mental health problems to offending. This suggests that poor QoL increases risk of poor mental health, which in turn increases risk of offending for this population.

Loney and Harkins (2018) recently examined the utility of the GLM in explaining offending in the general population (students; n = 340), via a self-report questionnaire measuring life priorities and offending. Their study supported the importance of the GLM goods, and self-reported offending was linked with the absence of effective strategies or use of maladaptive strategies to meet needs. Interestingly, *life*, *knowledge*, and *happiness* were prioritized in this population, and *agency*, *inner peace*, and *happiness* were most highly sought via maladaptive means. In terms of offense types, they found links between *agency*, *inner peace*, and violence, and *inner peace*, *happiness*, and drug offenses. Similarly, Taylor (2017) found that various goods were relevant for a sample convicted of residential burglaries (n = 30) in the United Kingdom. For example, some individuals talked about the "buzz" (i.e., pleasure) from offending, whereas others spoke about being good at it (i.e., excellence in work). Overall, this study supported the importance of GLM goods, and suggested that the model is appropriate for use with this population. These findings highlight the possibility that particular goods are highly prioritized universally, while others may be more relevant for certain groups. Goods prioritization varies by individual, but it may also vary across culture, age, gender, and in its relevance for different behaviors (i.e., offending) and contexts (i.e., treatment, reintegration).

In applying the GLM to the process of reintegration, Harris, Pednault, and Willis (2017) interviewed males who had been convicted of sexual offending but who were deemed to be desisting (n = 42) in the United States. Their participants valued many of the GLM goods, but their means to achieve them were restricted considerably by their correctional status.

Specifically, *interpersonal relationships* and *life/survival* were identified as important for this sample, closely followed by *knowledge*. Barriers to achieving these highly valued goods included loss of relationships due to offending and the consequences of disclosing past behavior to new associates or potential partners, and difficulty obtaining employment and accommodation following a conviction for a sexual offense. Similarly, Willis and Ward (2011) found that released individuals previously convicted of sexual offenses (n = 16) endorsed the majority of the GLM goods as highly important. In addition, they found that attainment of these goods was associated with earlier positive experiences of re-entry. This suggests that successful re-entry experiences (e.g., accommodation, employment, social support) can facilitate or restrict goods attainment. These findings are important for the design and implementation of policies and initiatives that support rather than obstruct prosocial goods attainment after release, but are also worth considering in treatment.

Investigating the use of primary goods in treatment, Marshall, Marshall, Serran, and O'Brien (2011) evaluated a sexual offending program (n = 535) in Canada. This strength-based program contains a number of GLM concepts, including six areas of primary human good, alongside other targets relating to risk, self-esteem and motivation. Independent researchers found recidivism rates below expected (based on previous meta-analyses) and predicted prior to treatment. For instance, at 8.4 years follow-up, they found 5.6% sexual recidivism, and 8.4% violent recidivism, compared with expected (predicted via the STATIC-99 and Rapid Risk Assessment for Sexual Offence Recidivism) rates of 23.8% and 34.8%, respectively. It is worth noting that the program used a modified version of the GLM goods, introduced in the final phase, not guiding the whole intervention as intended. Nevertheless, Marshall et al. (2011) observed that "when programs target problems that are obstacles to treatment, and then focus on changing known criminogenic features by taking a positive, respectful, and process-oriented approach, the re-offense rates of the sexual offenders treated in this way are likely to be significantly reduced" (p. 92).

Overall, these findings provide support for the importance of primary human goods generally, and also the ways in which certain goods may be more relevant for different populations and offenses. They also suggest that the prioritization of goods and problems in their attainment may be linked (directly or indirectly) with offending, and offer preliminary support for the idea that their attainment may support desistance from offending.

Collaboration and Therapist Qualities

The GLM is able to facilitate a holistic and individualized approach to treatment because it is based upon a view of human beings as motivated towards *personally meaningful* outcomes, and universally desired goods. Primary human goods, while being empirically and theoretically grounded (Laws & Ward, 2011), are viewed as being both multiply realizable by a range of goals and strategies, and of varied importance for individuals. This avoids assumptions concerning what a good life looks like; the list of goods is provided as a guide to expand the scope of individuals' good lives plans, rather than to restrict or direct individuals towards meaningless outcomes. For example, attaining *knowledge* does not require individuals to gain a formal education, but rather that they identify the sorts of knowledge they value or which would support their other valued outcomes (e.g., vocational, self-knowledge). This flexible approach is responsive to individual differences and sensitive to persons' conceptions of a good life. The GLM is able to overcome the limitations of a "one size fits all" approach, based on lists of problems observed in "offenders" at the aggregate level. It is a collaborative approach (Yates & Ward, 2008), which means that it is able to prioritize participant agency and autonomy in the processes of treatment and treatment planning.

This collaborative relationship is often referred to as the *therapeutic alliance*, and accounts for as much as 30% of treatment-induced changes, compared with only 15% for specific techniques (Norcross, 2002). Therapist characteristics which influence this alliance include professional and interpersonal skills, but also their goals and expectations of treatment (Ross, Polaschek, & Ward, 2008), and it has been suggested that therapist variability is the most important factor in determining the alliance quality (Del Re, Flückiger, Horvath, Symonds, & Wampold, 2012). Marshall et al. (2002) reported that therapist attributes such as empathy and warmth, and a style that is both rewarding and directive enhanced therapeutic outcomes in sex offending programs. These are reflected within Bonta and Andrews' (2017) *Relationship Principle* and *Structuring Principle,* which state that "interpersonal influence is greatest in situations characterized by open, warm, enthusiastic, and non-blaming communication, and by collaboration, mutual respect, liking, and interest" and that practitioners use "effective authority practices, prosocial modeling, differential approval and disapproval, problem-solving, skill building, advocacy, the structuring aspects of motivational interviewing, and cognitive restructuring" (p. 238). In addition, *specific responsivity* requires sensitivity to individual priorities, strengths, and motivations, addressing low motivation (i.e., building on strengths, reducing barriers, addressing "matters of personal interest"), and attention to evidence concerning special populations (Bonta & Andrews, 2017).

While contained within the Risk-Need-Responsivity (RNR) model, on application specific responsivity is often secondary to a focus on risk factors (Polaschek, 2012). This is a limitation of the RNR model's translation into treatment contexts, and likely has a significant impact upon the therapeutic relationship. For example, Watson, Thomas, and Daffern (2017) found that 55.6% of their sample (sexual offending treatment participants, n = 75) experienced a rupture to the therapeutic alliance, caused largely by disagreement on treatment goals and tasks. This indicates that perceived discrepancies between the goals and priorities of treatment participants and providers can have a negative impact upon the therapeutic alliance, and consequently reduce effectiveness. Thus, it is important to carefully select and offer ongoing support to clinicians, respond to low treatment-readiness, and repair ruptures (Kozar & Day, 2012). The importance of interpersonal factors in therapy is currently acknowledged, and we argue that the GLM provides a practice framework which can guide therapeutic interactions that are experienced as respectful, warm, nonjudgmental, and engaging. Indeed, in treatment for youth who have engaged in sexual offending the GLM "appears to impact positively on the therapeutic alliance, promote self-efficacy and optimism and increase the client's capacity to succeed and address issues of risk" (Wylie & Griffin, 2013, p. 354).

Retaining and Engaging Participants

It has been argued that promoting complete engagement in the process of change is the answer to reducing sexual recidivism (Marshall et al., 2011). The prevalence of treatment dropout and higher rates of reoffending by non-completers (McMurran & Theodosi, 2007) suggest missed opportunities to engage with potential participants. For example, a meta-analysis including 17 cognitive-behavioral treatment outcome studies reported that 23.55% of participants allocated to treatment (n = 10,159) did not complete for various reasons, including voluntary exit, rule breaking, and administrative actions (McMurran & Theodosi, 2007). Of particular concern are the financial and social costs of attrition, and the fact that those who drop out tend to be those with higher levels of risk and need (Olver, Stockdale, & Wormith, 2011). While the content and focus of treatment determine the targets of change, it is impossible for treatment to work if individuals fail to engage and participate, or if they leave well before completion. Engagement is often measured via compliance with program requirements (e.g., attendance, homework completion, disclosure), however, meaningful engagement encompasses more than these behaviors; it depends on internal factors like motivation and commitment to change (Holdsworth, Bowen, Brown, & Howat, 2014). In addition, a number of external factors influence engagement, and it is important for researchers and practitioners to understand why some individuals choose to leave treatment, and how better to meet the needs of these often high-risk high-need individuals.

Sturgess, Woodhams, and Tonkin (2016) found that participants' who did not complete correctional treatment perceived it as ineffective, unnecessary, repetitive, boring, intrusive, stressful, challenging, patronizing, and incompatible with their personally meaningful goals. Barnao et al. (2015) found that forensic service users' perceptions of rehabilitation revolved around seven internal and external themes. For example, self-evaluations centered upon their psychological disorders (internal), and treatment lacked person-centeredness and featured relationships of varied quality (external). In response, Barnao et al. (2016) used a brief GLM program in an attempt at improving these perceptions, and findings suggested variation across themes and between participants ($n = 5$). Overall, two participants displayed "definite change," two "subtle change," and one "no change or negative change," following the GLM program. Potential sources of variation included level of exposure to the GLM (i.e., frequency and duration of sessions), readiness to change, and practitioners' adherence to and experience with the model. For instance, the two participants' with "definite change" received more treatment from an experienced clinical psychologist, and had expressed a desire and intention to change. These findings suggest that risk oriented treatment programs fail to engage a number of participants because they are perceived negatively, and that GLM concepts (when used effectively) can produce shifts in participants' perceptions of treatment.

In another investigation of this potential, Harkins, Flak, Beech, and Woodhams (2012) evaluated a "better lives" (BL) module ($n = 76$) as a replacement to relapse prevention (RP; $n = 701$) within a sexual offending program in England. The BL module followed a core module (i.e., targeting risk factors) and was developed according to a GLM perspective. While there was no difference between RP and BL in terms of changes during treatment or attrition, participants and therapists favored the GLM approach due to its emphasis on positive aspects of the future. This suggests that the BL module performed *as well as* the RP model in terms of treatment change, and that it was preferred. Therapists perceived that the BL module did not have enough emphasis upon risk, but interestingly this did not result in less positive change during treatment (i.e., it performed equally to RP). The omission of risk was rectified in an updated BL module, and Barnett, Manderville-Norden, and Rakestrow (2014) reported that participants in the GLM condition were more likely to attain a "treated profile" on a battery of psychometric tests. Similarly, Ware and Bright (2008) reported preliminary findings after GLM changes to a sexual offending program; attrition rates had reduced, clients had more autonomy, and therapists reported feeling more positive and effective in their work following these simple changes.

Gannon et al. (2011) conducted a small descriptive study, evaluating group-based application of the GLM with men diagnosed with a psychological disorder and convicted of sexual offenses ($n = 5$) in England. All five men engaged successfully and completed treatment, with one returning voluntarily after discharge. The authors noted that the inclusion of and focus upon goals and sources of motivation was crucial in promoting engagement. All participants understood the importance of goods and their prosocial attainment; however, some (i.e., those with lower intelligence or indirect routes to offending) struggled to link these with risk and appreciate the importance of addressing criminogenic needs. In addition, all participants reported experiencing benefits from the program, and the researchers noted that the GLM approach obviously appealed. Additional benefits included increased scores on the Relapse Prevention Questionnaire (Beckett et al., 1997), self-reported improvements in emotion tolerance, and decreased impersonal sexual fantasies, cognitive distortions, and emotional loneliness.

Lindsay, Ward, Morgan, and Wilson (2007) designed a GLM-based intervention for two men with histories of sexual offending.

Importantly, criminogenic needs were included alongside resources required for a future *Good Lives Pathway*. While both men were initially reluctant, they engaged in and successfully completed treatment. Positive outcomes included: volunteering for further treatment, completing homework, internalizing knowledge (i.e., risk management and anger control), constructing a future life plan incorporating goods and risk, reported wellbeing and life satisfaction, and control of alcohol use and debt. In addition, neither man had reoffended at a five-year follow-up. In a similar study, Whitehead et al. (2007) integrated the GLM into the community-based assessment, treatment planning, and monitoring of one high-risk male convicted of violent offending in New Zealand. This extended the GLM to violent offending and indigenous populations (Māori). While he had previously received the "best interventions available" (p. 586) and acquired the relevant knowledge to avoid reoffending, these experiences had not facilitated meaningful change in his life (i.e., continued drug use and gang involvement). During and after the GLM intervention, researchers observed expressions of guilt (not evident before), reduced drug use, a new prosocial peer group, prosocial goods attainment (i.e., University and leisure activities), and an identity based upon prosocial achievements rather than gang involvement. At the time of writing, the participant had abstained from violent offending for 14 months, which was not expected prior to the GLM intervention. In this case it seems that standard criminogenic interventions were unable to facilitate meaningful engagement with the change process, whereas the integration of GLM concepts was. While these case studies cannot provide sufficient evidence for reductions in recidivism, they suggest that the inclusion of personally meaningful targets in treatment can facilitate successful engagement with men who may otherwise refuse, and can also produce personally meaningful change.

Another factor influencing engagement and participation is the extent to which an individual is able to choose whether or not to complete a program. Volunteerism is thought to be related to treatment success, however, there are questions about whether or not any correctional intervention is truly voluntary given the context and the consequences of refusal (Parhar, Wormith, Derkzen, & Beauregard, 2008). One study looked at the extent to which forensic treatment programs were voluntary, coerced, or mandated, and the effect of this on recidivism (Parhar et al., 2008). The authors found that interventions that relied upon coercion or were mandated were less effective than those which were closer to being voluntary. In addition, it has been found that the positive effects of treatment are likely to last longer when an individual has intrinsic motivation, and that this can be eroded by coercion (Parhar et al., 2008; Ryan & Deci, 2000). Current practice often relies upon extrinsic sources of motivation such as sentence compliance and early parole (Parhar et al., 2008). A better approach may be to design treatment collaboratively around personally meaningful goals, and thereby foster intrinsic motivation to engage. Indeed, Andrews and Bonta (2010) suggest that participants who lack motivation may be engaged via an improved understanding of the way that interventions can benefit them personally. The GLM is able to do this through its focus on the attainment of valued goods.

Desistance and Protective Factors

Desistance is typically defined as the ongoing process from active offending to decreases in, and eventually cessation of, offending. The research into desistance from sexual offending is relatively sparse and tends to focus on the role of employment and relationships, and construction of a new non-offending identity centered upon valued activities and outcomes, and motivated by self-efficacy and hope (McAlinden, Farmer, & Maruna, 2017). Research suggests that desistance from sexual offending requires the development of a coherent explanation, or "self-narrative" which accounts for why the individual committed the sexual offense (Maruna, 2011), allowing the individual to make sense of their past and explain why it will not happen again. Agency and autonomy are crucial in taking control of the future, and building the resources necessary to meet needs (i.e., relationships, employment, skills)—what are often referred to in the literature as "protective factors" (PF). There has been much recent interest and debate about the status of PF as the opposite of risk or something different, and the mechanisms by which they exert their positive effects during desistance (Fortune & Ward, 2017). The term PF is often used alongside the terms "promotive factors" and "strengths," and they are generally defined as characteristics of the individual and their environment which are associated with decreases in recidivism. Empirical work by de Vogel, de Vries Robbé, de Ruiter, and Bouman (2011) identified a number of forensic PF falling into three domains: *internal* (e.g., self-control), *external* (e.g., intimate relationship), and *motivational* (e.g., life goals), and work continues to develop a PF assessment tool specific to sexual offending.

While we currently have some idea of the factors which can support desistance, we lack a coherent understanding of how they function to reduce risk (Ward, 2017), this is where the GLM can help. The concept of primary human goods can enhance our understanding of how PF or desistance "events" such as employment and relationships can reduce risk, and why they may vary in their function across individuals and situations. For example, being employed could be thought of as a secondary (instrumental) good which meets a range of needs, including (but not limited to) excellence in work and a sense of achievement, agency, creativity, relatedness, life (i.e., financial resources required for living), and inner peace (i.e., freedom from stress)—all of which contribute to a meaningful sense of self. Employment (or unemployment) that does not meet (or perhaps obstructs) these goods is less likely to support desistance, and may lead to the use of other secondary goods (e.g., substance abuse, theft, dishonesty). The concepts of internal and external resources required for a good life are useful in understanding the process of desistance, and "the agentic willingness to change on the part of individuals … needs to be accompanied by credible social opportunities for change and a range of external situational supports to help sex offenders achieve meaningful lives" (McAlinden et al., 2017, p. 278). The concept of a *good life plan* and its use in treatment can be linked with *possible futures* discussed in the desistance literature. For example, it is an important condition for change that individuals are able to see a personally meaningful and attainable future, and that they are able to construct a new identity—"the self is continually being projected into the future" (Farrall, 2005, p. 369).

Desistance requires both motivation and means to live a different, non-offending life, and while an exclusive focus on risk factors may temporarily provide some of the means (e.g., PF such as sobriety, problem-solving and coping skills), it cannot provide the motivation to maintain this lifestyle. In addition, it may be that the factors that are linked with offending are not necessarily the same factors that support desistance (McNeill, 2012); this is reflected in the differences between research into the correlates (and potential causes) of re/offending, and research into the process of desistance. The methods required to study desistance are similar to those used to investigate the GLM, for example, case studies, observation, interviews, and self-reported experiences (Farrall, 2005), and they uncover subjective processes such as: turning points or hooks for change, openness to change, maturation, life transitions, social bonds, knifing off, cognitive transformation, self-reflection and insight, and a new personally meaningful identity (Farrall, 2005; McNeill, 2012). Farrall (2005) makes the point that "without a willingness at least to consider in-depth the experiences of individuals who have successfully negotiated the transitions from "offender", it is unlikely that efforts to encourage desistance (e.g., the What Works movement) will produce the sorts of results so desperately needed" (p. 383). We argue that the focus of desistance research on agential processes such as the construction of a new prosocial identity, and the search for meaningful outcomes (e.g., mastery or success, interpersonal connection, and a purpose) is much better aligned with the GLM concepts than it is with risk reduction.

Ethical Practice

The Risk-Need-Responsivity (RNR) model assumes that effective intervention occurs via change in criminogenic factors through collaborative, compassionate, and dignified human service (Polaschek, 2012). However, in practice responsivity to the individual and their unique needs is often overlooked in favor of risk reduction and community safety. Indeed, it has been pointed out that needs unrelated to criminal activity are not the responsibility of Corrections (Bonta & Andrews, 2017; Polaschek, 2012). The targeting of predominantly risk-related features is recommended by the *need principle,* and needs which are not empirically linked with reoffending are largely seen as a responsivity issue—they may be targeted if they are barriers to treatment.

There are several treatment practices which may impinge upon participants' rights and dignity, including the language used in programs, the coercion or mandating of treatment, and the strong focus upon index offenses in assessment, treatment planning, and the content/delivery of sessions. Ethical treatment requires (at a minimum) viewing participants as human beings primarily, with their correctional status being a secondary property of the person, based upon their past actions—not necessarily representing an enduring character flaw (i.e., antisocial personality pattern, psychopathy). While this is likely the perspective of most therapeutic practitioners, its expression can be undermined by custodial processes and norms. One simple step towards more ethical treatment is using individuals' names or "participant" in conversations and program materials (rather than "offender" or "prisoner") and avoiding use of negative terms such as "antisocial," "offense-related," and "problem thinking" when referring to participants' characteristics and values (Willis, 2018; Willis et al., 2013). We argue that the GLM and its underlying view of humans as directed towards universal goods supports this nonjudgmental orientation, and that it encourages the use of language that is more respectful and motivating.

The effects of coercion and mandated treatment on motivation, engagement, and goal attainment were briefly discussed above. However, there are additional ethical issues with forcing or enticing participants to complete programs. While treatment is often presented as voluntary, there can be serious consequences associated with refusal, including being denied parole and being labeled as "unmotivated" or "non-compliant" with sentence conditions (Parhar et al., 2008). However, as the sections above suggest, there are a number of routes to desistance and it is not clear that individuals should be convinced that participation in the programs available is the only way to change. In other words, an individual can be motivated to change and live a non-offending future without being inclined to participate in criminogenic programs (Mann, Webster, Wakeling, & Keylock, 2013). We argue that it is unethical to require someone to engage in treatment that does not fit with their personal theory of change, and that the GLM, with its flexible and motivating orientation, is better able to fit with individuals' priorities than a program based upon externally imposed goals.

In addition, individuals who deny their crime are often excluded from treatment or encouraged to first disclose their sexual offense and agree with official charges and summaries of the facts, often creating tension and resistance. However, denial is not empirically linked with recidivism, and it has been suggested that attempts to reconcile participants' experiences with external accounts in treatment is "unnecessary and possibly iatrogenic" (Farmer, McAlinden, & Maruna, 2016, p. 23). A GLM approach can work with denial, due to its broad scope, collaborative aims, and orientation towards human goods in the form of approach goals (Dealey, 2018). It can account for denial as a secondary good aimed at various primary goods, for example inner peace, relatedness, agency, or spirituality. When practitioners view denial as instrumental in meeting persons' needs (rather than as manipulative or malicious), they can respond to it in a more effective way—working with the person rather than pushing them away. In addition, the GLM is compatible with culturally responsive practice and indigenous models (see

Leaming & Willis, 2016), and able to inform alternative avenues for ethical intervention such as Restorative Justice approaches (Walgrave, Ward & Zinsstag, 2019). There are numerous ethical concerns when providing treatment within a context concerned with punishment and justice. We suggest that the GLM can overcome many of these due to its view of persons, its flexibility, and its dual focus on risk and human needs.

Summary: The Evidence

This section outlined empirical studies providing support for the GLM in guiding treatment. Although mainly descriptive, they clarify the ways that the GLM can add to treatment with individuals who have engaged in sexual (and violent) offending. The most significant benefits include a focus on personally meaningful outcomes and approach goals which are attractive to the individual, and the engagement and commitment to change that follow this positive focus. In addition, due to their descriptive nature, these studies provide information about the potential pit falls when implementing GLM treatment. For example, it is important that participants understand the links between good lives and risk reduction, and that practitioners are adequately trained to use the GLM in case formulation. These requirements go hand in hand, and depend on a sound understanding of the nature of human beings as goal-directed and possessing a range of capacities and resources which support prosocial and healthy goods attainment.

It is important to note here that these suggestions do not require practitioners to abandon the RNR principles in favor of a strength-based GLM approach. Rather practitioners can use both models and integrate their best aspects into treatment—in fact the three major principles of risk, need and responsivity are woven into the model. The goals of the Criminal Justice System (i.e., reduced risk of recidivism/harm) and the individuals who exist within it (i.e., attainment of personally meaningful goods) are not mutually exclusive. If programs provide or assist individuals with the motivation, confidence, and resources to meet their needs without causing harm, they will maintain an offense-free good life in the long term. We suggest that the current dominant approach to risk reduction is failing, and it is time to adjust this in light of the broader evidence concerning correctional interventions and human nature in general.

Finally, given that the GLM prescribes adherence to RNR principles, it should be *at least equal* in its effectiveness, with the added benefit of being more motivating, and with the potential to produce long-lasting change. The findings discussed throughout this section offer preliminary support for its comparable effectiveness and added benefits. Arguably, if a GLM approach to treatment appeals to practitioners and participants, results in individualized and collaborative treatment planning, and can reduce some of the inherently negative aspects of treatment (e.g., avoidant goals, use of terms such as "antisocial" and "offender"), then it is an ethically important addition to correctional treatment. The question then is how the field can integrate these models in order to take advantage of a wider evidence base, and to inform treatment that can reduce recidivism and engage individuals in enduring and personally meaningful change.

Integrating The Good Lives Model

This section will briefly outline the GLM's relationship with the RNR model in practice. There are a number of excellent existing publications which outline the practical application of the GLM (e.g., Willis et al., 2013; Yates, Prescott, & Ward, 2010), and we will simply summarize what the GLM *adds* to each phase of intervention. It is important to note that the targeting of criminogenic needs remains a major goal of intervention, but this is communicated differently and explicitly combined with attention to personally meaningful outcomes. We suggest that these positive changes will result in interventions experienced as more motivating, respectful, and successful.

Table 31.1 draws upon suggestions for the integration of the GLM and the RNR model provided by Willis et al. (2013). This is a summary of key additions the GLM provides, and should not be considered a full description of a GLM-consistent intervention as these are available elsewhere (see Purvis et al., 2011; Ward, Mann, & Gannon, 2007). In terms of the *risk principle* and the GLM, risk assessment remains important, but the scope of its application is somewhat narrower. It is used for prediction, to inform the intensity of treatment, and to identify dynamic features implicated in offending—not to directly inform treatment. By this we mean that the terms and constructs used in prediction cannot guide treatment *on their own*—they are targets once reformulated as approach goals to support goods attainment. Dynamic risk factors are composite constructs and if they are to be effectively utilized in treatment require "stripping down" into their causal, contextual, and mental state facets—in effect, remodeled (see Ward, 2016; Heffernan, ward, Vandevelde & Van Damme, 2019). Integrating the GLM with the *need principle* involves the reconceptualization of dynamic risk factors as problems in the

Table 31.1 The additional value of the good lives model

Phase	RNR components	GLM additions
Communication of aims and orientation	Reduced risk/reoffending Criminogenic Need (CN)	Good Life: A range of Primary Human Goods (PHG) Good Life Plan (GLP), internal/external resources Collaboration and autonomy Positive language (verbal and written)
Assessment	Risk level determines dosage Targets = CN evident within offending Responsivity considerations	Open questions, reflective listening, validation of PHG, questionnaires PHG implicated in offending PHG prioritized, changes over time Flaws in past/current GLP Resources required for GLP Strengths Approach goals Holistic
Planning	CN, moving these towards strengths Addressing responsivity issues and barriers to engagement	Good Life Plan, Primary Human Goods, SHG Approach goals, sub-goals/steps Holistic—includes non-criminogenic needs, although these may not be explicitly addressed Draw links between SHG and offending Utilize existing strengths Collaborative, individualized, and ongoing
Program content	Modules based on CN, e.g.: Cognition and emotion Relationships Substance use Self-regulation and problem solving Sexual functioning Release planning	Structured guide, not rigid Description of GLM Developing GLP Modules based on capacities required for GLP (including CN) Positive language in sessions and materials Building upon strengths and resources to overcome barriers (CN)
Program delivery	Cognitive Behavioral Therapy (CBT) Responsive—e.g. motivational interviewing Relationship and structuring principles Program integrity	CBT techniques "wrapped around" goods and priorities Positive language Flexible/responsive to the individual Respectful and upholds dignity GLM used within treatment, and also surrounding environments Physical environment communicates equality and respect

attainment of goods. For example, where a traditional relapse prevention program might work on victim empathy in order to challenge cognitive distortions, a GLM approach would focus on gaining the knowledge/skills necessary (one of which may be empathy) for a satisfying adult relationship, and the goods this provides (e.g., pleasure and relatedness). Finally, in linking with *responsivity*, the GLM provides concepts (i.e., primary and secondary goods) for use alongside empirically supported techniques such as CBT and motivational interviewing. Individuals need reasons to want to change, not just the capacities to do so. The RNR model is concerned with providing resources, but links these with reducing risk (i.e., avoiding prison), rather than living the *good life*.

Areas for Development

The question of what constitutes effective treatment for persons convicted of sexual offenses remains open, and the evidence that will contribute to our knowledge ought to come from a range of sources and various methods of inquiry. While the existing research concerning the use of the GLM in treatment is promising, it is by no means conclusive, and there are problems with its use. For example, many GLM adaptations to programs do not use the model in the intended way; it should be used to guide the entire intervention (see Table 31.1 above) rather than added on to traditional approaches. It is important that future applications and evaluations of the GLM integrate it as intended, following the numerous guides provided by proponents of the model. Another limitation of some of the adapted programs reviewed here is the apparent absence of links between good lives and risk reduction. Although it doesn't seem that this negatively impacted upon outcomes, not all studies investigated subsequent risk management and recidivism. It is important to make these links clear to participants, and that staff are adequately trained in case formulation which incorporates offense-related needs as well as good lives goals. In addition, studies should evaluate various aspects of treatment addressing a range of outcomes of interest using multiple methods.

In considering the GLM's core concepts and assumptions, future research should continue to investigate the relative importance placed on primary human goods and their role in individuals' explanations of their offending. In addition, the field of correctional intervention may learn from evidence and conceptual issues in other areas, and theoretical developments within our own field. There is currently debate and concern surrounding the concepts of dynamic risk factors and protective factors, and the assumption that they explain the causes of offending (see Fortune & Ward, 2017; Ward, 2016, 2017). In order to properly link dynamic risk factors with individual goal-directed behavior, we need a better understanding of what they are and how they are causally linked. Theoretical developments and refinement of these concepts may facilitate the formation of more useful treatment targets, and treatment that is able to tap into the individual causes of and influences upon human agency. The application of these advancements should be evaluated in order to provide empirical support for theories and to justify their use in treatment.

In terms of the future integration of the GLM and the core RNR principles, responsivity is "the least developed of the three. It is theoretically unsophisticated: a catch-all category" (Polaschek, 2012, p. 8). It is important that future research prioritize the development of this principle, as it describes the way that treatment should be delivered, and how important issues such as low motivation or cultural barriers are addressed. A better understanding of potential participants can help practitioners overcome problems such as high rates of drop out, poor engagement, and ethical issues such as coercion. For example, more studies should look at why participants refuse treatment, and what their expectations of correctional interventions are (see Mann et al., 2013), and then use these findings to inform the communication of interventions' aims and orientation. In addition, while criminogenic targets *can be* framed positively (Polaschek, 2012), they are still an externally imposed list of treatment goals that are not explicitly linked with outcomes other than avoiding reoffending and associated consequences (i.e., future prison sentences). It would be useful to look at the impact of language and orientation of goals on expectations of treatment, subsequent engagement, and other meaningful outcomes.

Conclusions

It is clear that "there is much that is unknown about what is effective in reducing sexual and violent recidivism, and it is possible that the content included in the program model used is not effectively targeting the appropriate issues or risk areas" (Grady & Pettus-Davis, 2017, p. 259). The modest and heterogeneous effects of current sexual offending treatment programs suggest that progress is necessary, and the advancement of rehabilitation has arguably been overlooked in favor of enhanced risk prediction. Research aiming to advance the rehabilitation of those who have sexually offended cannot rely solely upon lists of correlates and statistical relationships, the variables involved are simply too complex. While the RNR model has undergone substantial improvements over the years and is based on an impressive body of empirical research, it is not the final word when it comes to what works to reduce sexual recidivism (Polaschek, 2012). It is based upon evidence gathered thus far, but this should encourage further innovation rather than acceptance of small effect sizes. Especially considering the consequences of treatment failure, and the likelihood of already disillusioned individuals giving up on the possibility of change.

The GLM offers a valuable addition to treatment which, in line with core RNR principles, is proportionate to risk level, targets variables which have demonstrated a relationship with offending, and is responsive to both the research concerning "what works" and the needs of individuals. This addition largely concerns what is considered to be related to offending (and the methods by which we have established this relationship), and being responsive to the needs of individuals. The research which has so far supported the use of the GLM in treatment has relied on different sources of evidence than the RNR, privileging the experiences of individuals within treatment and a range of outcomes alongside recidivism. By integrating the results of both bodies of research we can better understand what is happening in treatment and how best to increase the likelihood that individuals will meaningfully engage with the process of change. It will be important moving forward to use a range of research methods in order to discover the most effective ways to integrate the two models, rather than prioritizing one over the other. Just as the dual aims of GLM interventions are not mutually exclusive, practitioners need not commit to either the RNR *or* the GLM; they can instead integrate the two. We believe the result of careful and considered integration will be a treatment approach grounded in (holistic) evidence concerning aspects of the person and their environment which are relevant to offending, and which is engaging, motivating, and responsive to the individuals it seeks to rehabilitate.

References

Andrews, D. A., & Bonta, J. (2010). *The psychology of criminal conduct* (5th ed.). New Providence, NJ: LexisNexis.

Aust, S. (2010). Is the good lives model of offender treatment relevant to sex offenders with a learning disability? *Journal of Learning Disabilities and Offending Behaviour, 1*(3), 33–39.

Barnao, M., Ward, T., & Casey, S. (2015). Looking beyond the illness: Forensic service users' perceptions of rehabilitation. *Journal of Interpersonal Violence, 30*, 1025–1045.

Barnao, M., Ward, T., & Casey, S. (2016). Taking the good life to the institution: Forensic service users' perceptions of the Good Lives Model. *International Journal of Offender Therapy and Comparative Criminology, 60*, 766–786.

Barnett, G., & Wood, J. L. (2008). Agency, relatedness, inner peace, and problem solving in sexual offending: How sexual offenders prioritize and operationalize their good lives conceptions. *Sexual Abuse, 20*(4), 444–465.

Barnett, G. D., Manderville-Norden, R., & Rakestrow, J. (2014). The Good Lives Model or relapse prevention: What works better in facilitating change? *Sexual Abuse, 26*(1), 3–33.

Beckett, R. C., Fisher, D., Mann, R., & Thornton, D. (1997). The relapse prevention questionnaire and interview. *Therapists guide for maintaining change: Relapse prevention manual for adult male perpetrators of child sexual abuse*, pp. 445–473.

Bonta, J., & Andrews, D. A. (2017). *The psychology of criminal conduct* (6th ed.). New York, NY: Routledge.

Chu, C. M., Koh, L. L., Zeng, G., & Teoh, J. (2015). Youth who sexual offended: Primary human goods and offense pathways. *Sexual Abuse: A Journal of Research and Treatment, 27*, 151–172. https://doi.org/10.1177/1079063213499188

Committee, C. O. D. (2007). *Sex offender treatment outcome research: Guidelines for evaluation (CODC Guidelines), Part 1: Introduction and overview (Corrections User Report No 2007–002)*. Ottawa, ON: Public Safety Canada.

de Vogel, V., de Vries Robbé, M., de Ruiter, C., & Bouman, Y. H. (2011). Assessing protective factors in forensic psychiatric practice: Introducing the SAPROF. *International Journal of Forensic Mental Health, 10*(3), 171–177.

Dealey, J. (2018). Moving beyond the risk paradigm: Using the good lives model with offenders in denial of sexual offending. *European Journal of Probation, 10*(1), 28–43. https://doi.org/10.1177/2066220318755530

Del Re, A. C., Flückiger, C., Horvath, A. O., Symonds, D., & Wampold, B. E. (2012). Therapist effects in the therapeutic alliance–outcome relationship: A restricted-maximum likelihood meta-analysis. *Clinical Psychology Review, 32*(7), 642–649.

Di Lorito, C., Völlm, B., & Dening, T. (2018). Psychiatric disorders among older prisoners: A systematic review and comparison study against older people in the community. *Aging & Mental Health, 22*(1), 1–10.

Dowden, C., & Andrews, D. A. (2000). Effective correctional treatment and violent reoffending: A meta-analysis. *Canadian Journal of Criminology, 42*, 449.

Farmer, M., McAlinden, A.-M., & Maruna, S. (2016). Sex offending and situational motivation: Findings from a qualitative analysis of desistance from sexual offending. *International Journal of Offender Therapy and Comparative Criminology, 60*(15), 1756–1775. https://doi.org/10.1177/0306624X16668175

Farrall, S. (2005). On the existential aspects of desistance from crime. *Symbolic Interaction, 28*(3), 367–386.

Fortune, C. A. (2017). The good lives model: A strength-based approach for youth offenders. *Aggression and Violent Behavior*.

Fortune, C.-A., & Ward, T. (2017). Problems in protective factor research and practice. *Aggression and Violent Behavior, 32*, 1–3. https://doi.org/10.1016/j.avb.2016.12.008

Gannon, T., King, T., Miles, H., Lockerbie, L., & Willis, G. M. (2011). Good lives sexual offender treatment for mentally disordered offenders. *British Journal of Forensic Practice, 13*(3), 153–168. https://doi.org/10.1108/14636641111157805

Grady, M. D., Edwards, D., Jr., & Pettus-Davis, C. (2017). A longitudinal outcome evaluation of a prison-based sex offender treatment program. *Sexual Abuse, 29*(3), 239–266.

Hanson, R. K., Bourgon, G., Helmus, L., & Hodgson, S. (2009). The principles of effective correctional treatment also apply to sexual offenders: A meta-analysis. *Criminal Justice and Behavior, 36*(9), 865–891.

Harkins, L., Flak, V. E., Beech, A. R., & Woodhams, J. (2012). Evaluation of a community-based sex offender treatment program using a good lives model approach. *Sexual Abuse, 24*(6), 519–543.

Harris, D. A., Pedneault, A., & Willis, G. (2017). The pursuit of primary human goods in men desisting from sexual offending. *Sexual Abuse*, 1–23. https://doi.org/10.1177/1079063217729155

Heffernan, R., Ward, T., Vandevelde, S., & Van Damme, L. (2019). Dynamic risk factors and constructing explanations of offending: The risk-causality method. *Aggression and Violent Behavior, 44*, 47-56.

Holdsworth, E., Bowen, E., Brown, S., & Howat, D. (2014). Client engagement in psychotherapeutic treatment and associations with client characteristics, therapist characteristics, and treatment factors. *Clinical Psychology Review, 34*(5), 428–450.

Jung, S., & Gulayets, M. (2011). Using clinical variables to evaluate treatment effectiveness in programmes for sexual offenders. *Journal of Sexual Aggression, 17*(2), 166–180. https://doi.org/10.1080/13552601003802238

Kim, B., Benekos, P. J., & Merlo, A. V. (2015). Sex offender recidivism revisited: Review of recent meta-analyses on the effects of sex offender treatment. *Trauma, Violence, & Abuse, 17*(1), 105–117. https://doi.org/10.1177/1524838014566719

Kozar, C. J., & Day, A. (2012). The therapeutic alliance in offending behavior programs: A necessary and sufficient condition for change? *Aggression and Violent Behavior, 17*(5), 482–487.

Langlands, R. L., Ward, T., & Gilchrist, E. (2009). Applying the good lives model to male perpetrators of domestic violence. *Behaviour Change, 26*(2), 113–129.

Laws, D. R., & Ward, T. (2011). *Desistance from sex offending: Alternatives to throwing away the keys*. New York, NY: Guilford Press.

Leaming, N., & Willis, G. M. (2016). The good lives model: New avenues for Māori rehabilitation? *Sexual Abuse in Australia and New Zealand, 7*, 59–69.

Lindsay, W. R., Ward, T., Morgan, T., & Wilson, I. (2007). Self-regulation of sex offending, future pathways and the good lives model: Applications and problems. *Journal of Sexual Aggression, 13*(1), 37–50.

Loney, D. M., & Harkins, L. (2018). Examining the good lives model and antisocial behavior. *Psychology, Crime & Law, 24*(1), 38–51.

Lösel, F. (2017). Evidence comes by replication, but needs differentiation: The reproducibility issue in science and its relevance for criminology. *Journal of*

Experimental Criminology. https://doi.org/10.1007/s11292-017-9297-z

Lösel, F., & Schmucker, M. (2017). In T. Sanders (Ed.),. *The Oxford handbook on sex offences and sex offenders Treatment of sexual offenders: Concepts and empirical evaluations* (pp. 392–414). New York: Oxford University Press.

Mann, R. E., Webster, S. D., Schofield, C., & Marshall, W. L. (2004). Approach versus avoidance goals in relapse prevention with sexual offenders. *Sexual Abuse: A Journal of Research and Treatment, 16*(1), 65–75.

Mann, R. E., Webster, S. D., Wakeling, H. C., & Keylock, H. (2013). Why do sexual offenders refuse treatment? *Journal of Sexual Aggression, 19*(2), 191–206.

Marshall, W. L., & Marshall, L. E. (2007). The utility of the random controlled trial for evaluating sexual offender treatment: The gold standard or an inappropriate strategy? *Sexual Abuse: A Journal of Research and Treatment, 19*(2), 175–191.

Marshall, W. L., & Marshall, L. E. (2017). The treatment of adult male sexual offenders. In D. P. Boer (Ed.), *Theories, assessment, and treatment of sexual offending* (pp. 1227–1243). Chichester, England: Wiley Blackwell.

Marshall, W. L., Marshall, L. E., Serran, G. A., & O'Brien, M. D. (2011). *Rehabilitating sexual offenders: A strength-based approach*. Washington, DC: American Psychological Association.

Marshall, W. L., Serran, G., Moulden, H., Mulloy, R., Fernandez, Y. M., Mann, R., & Thornton, D. (2002). Therapist features in sexual offender treatment: Their reliable identification and influence on behaviour change. *Clinical Psychology & Psychotherapy, 9*, 395–405. https://doi.org/10.1002/cpp.335

Marshall, W. L., & Serran, G. A. (2004). The role of the therapist in offender treatment. *Psychology, Crime & Law, 10*(3), 309–320.

Maruna, S. (2011). Reentry as a rite of passage. *Punishment & Society, 13*(1), 3–28.

McAlinden, A. M., Farmer, M., & Maruna, S. (2017). Desistance from sexual offending: Do the mainstream theories apply? *Criminology & Criminal Justice, 17*(3), 266–283.

McMurran, M., & Theodosi, E. (2007). Is treatment non-completion associated with increased reconviction over no treatment? *Psychology, Crime & Law, 13*(4), 333–343.

McNeill, F. (2012). Four forms of 'offender'rehabilitation: Towards an interdisciplinary perspective. *Legal and Criminological Psychology, 17*(1), 18–36.

Norcross, J. C. (Ed.). (2002). *Psychotherapy relationships that work: Therapist contributions and responsiveness to patients*. New York, NY: Oxford University Press.

Olver, M. E., Stockdale, K. C., & Wormith, J. S. (2011). A meta-analysis of predictors of offender treatment attrition and its relationship to recidivism. *Journal of Consulting and Clinical Psychology, 79*(1), 6–21. https://doi.org/10.1037/a0022200

Parhar, K. K., Wormith, J. S., Derkzen, D. M., & Beauregard, A. M. (2008). Offender coercion in treatment: A meta-analysis of effectiveness. *Criminal Justice and Behavior, 35*(9), 1109–1135.

Polaschek, D. L. (2012). An appraisal of the risk–need–responsivity (RNR) model of offender rehabilitation and its application in correctional treatment. *Legal and Criminological Psychology, 17*(1), 1–17.

Purvis, M. (2010). *Seeking a good life: Human goods and sexual offending*. (Published PhD Manuscript). Germany: Lambert Academic Press.

Purvis, M., Ward, T., & Willis, G. (2011). The good lives model in practice: Offence pathways and case management. *European Journal of Probation, 3*(2), 4–28.

Ross, E. C., Polaschek, D. L., & Ward, T. (2008). The therapeutic alliance: A theoretical revision for offender rehabilitation. *Aggression and Violent Behavior, 13*(6), 462–480.

Ryan, R. M., & Deci, E. L. (2000). The darker and brighter sides of human existence: Basic psychological needs as a unifying concept. *Psychological Inquiry, 11*, 319–338.

Simons, D. A., McCullar, B., & Tyler, C. (2008, October). *The utility of the self-regulation model to re-integration planning*. Paper presented at the 27th Annual Association for the Treatment of Sexual Abusers Research and Treatment Conference.

Sturgess, D., Woodhams, J., & Tonkin, M. (2016). Treatment engagement from the perspective of the offender: Reasons for noncompletion and completion of treatment—A systematic review. *International Journal of Offender Therapy and Comparative Criminology, 60*(16), 1873–1896.

Taylor, E. (2017). 'I should have been a security consultant': The good lives model and residential burglars. *European Journal of Criminology, 14*(4), 434–450.

Thakker, J., & Ward, T. (2010). The good lives model and the treatment of substance abusers. *Behaviour Change, 27*(3), 154–175.

Van Damme, L., Hoeve, M., Vermeiren, R., Vanderplasschen, W., & Colins, O. F. (2016). Quality of life in relation to future mental health problems and offending: Testing the good lives model among detained girls. *Law and Human Behavior, 40*, 285–294.

Wainwright, L., & Nee, C. (2014). The good lives model—New directions for preventative practice with children. *Psychology, Crime & Law, 20*(2), 166–182.

Walgrave, L., Ward, T., & Zinsstag, E. (in press). When restorative justice meets the good lives model: Contributing to a criminology of trust. In E. Dieu & S. Corneille (Eds.), *The good lives model*. Routledge.

Ward, T. (2002a). Good lives and the rehabilitation of sexual offenders: Promises and problems. *Aggression and Violent Behavior, 7*, 513–528.

Ward, T. (2002b). The management of risk and the design of good lives. *Australian Psychologist, 37*, 172–179.

Ward, T. (2013). Addressing the dual relationship problem in forensic and correctional practice. *Aggression and Violent Behavior, 18*(1), 92–100.

Ward, T. (2016). Dynamic risk factors: Scientific kinds or predictive constructs. *Psychology, Crime & Law, 22*(1–2), 2–16.

Ward, T. (2017). Prediction and agency: The role of protective factors in correctional rehabilitation and desistance. *Aggression and Violent Behavior, 32*, 19–28.

Walgrave, L., Ward, T., & Zinsstag, E. (2019). When restorative justice meets the Good Lives Model: Contributing to a criminology of trust. *European Journal of Criminology*. https://doi.org/10.1177/1477370819854174

Ward, T., & Fisher, D. D. (2005). New ideas in the treatment of sexual offenders. In W. L. Marshall, Y. Fernandez, L. Marshall, & G. A. Serran (Eds.), *Sexual offender treatment: Issues and controversies* (pp. 143–148). Chichester: Wiley.

Ward, T., & Heffernan, R. (2017). The role of values in forensic and correctional rehabilitation. *Aggression and Violent Behavior, 37*, 42–51. https://doi.org/10.1016/j.avb.2017.09.002

Ward, T., & Hudson, S. M. (2000). A self-regulation model of relapse prevention). In R. Laws, S. M. Hudson, & T. Ward (Eds.), *Remaking relapse prevention with sex offenders: A sourcebook* (pp. 79–101). Thousand Oaks, CA: Sage Publications, Inc.

Ward, T., & Keenan, T. (1999). Child molesters' implicit theories. *Journal of Interpersonal Violence, 14*(8), 821–838.

Ward, T., & Mann, R. (2004). Good lives and the rehabilitation of offenders: A positive approach to sex offender treatment. *Positive Psychology in Practice*, 598–616.

Ward, T., Mann, R. E., & Gannon, T. A. (2007). The good lives model of offender rehabilitation: Clinical implications. *Aggression and Violent Behavior, 12*(1), 87–107.

Ward, T., & Maruna, S. (2007). *Rehabilitation: Beyond the risk paradigm*. London: Routledge.

Ward, T., Melser, J., & Yates, P. M. (2007). Reconstructing the risk–need–responsivity model: A theoretical elaboration and evaluation. *Aggression and Violent Behavior, 12*(2), 208–228.

Ware, J., & Bright, D. A. (2008). Evolution of a treatment programme for sex offenders: Changes to the NSW Custody-Based Intensive Treatment (CUBIT). *Psychiatry, Psychology and Law, 15*, 340–349.

Watson, R., Thomas, S., & Daffern, M. (2017). The impact of interpersonal style on ruptures and repairs in the therapeutic alliance between offenders and therapists in sex offender treatment. *Sexual Abuse, 29*(7), 709–728.

Whitehead, P. R., Ward, T., & Collie, R. M. (2007). Time for a change: Applying the good lives model of rehabilitation to a high-risk violent offender. *International Journal of Offender Therapy and Comparative Criminology, 51*, 578–598.

Willis, G. M. (2018). Why call someone by what we don't want them to be? The ethics of labeling in forensic/correctional psychology. *Psychology, Crime & Law*, 1–17.

Willis, G. M., & Ward, T. (2011). Striving for a good life: The good lives model applied to released child molesters. *Journal of Sexual Aggression, 17*, 290–303. https://doi.org/10.1080/13552600.2010.505349

Willis, G. M., Ward, T., & Levenson, J. S. (2014). The good lives model (GLM): An evaluation of GLM operationalization in North American treatment programs. *Sexual Abuse, 26*(1), 58–81.

Willis, G. M., Yates, P. M., Gannon, T. A., & Ward, T. (2013). How to integrate the good lives model into treatment programs for sexual offending: An introduction and overview. *Sexual Abuse, 25*(2), 123–142.

Wylie, L. A., & Griffin, H. L. (2013). G-map's application of the good lives model to adolescent males who sexually harm: A case study. *Journal of Sexual Aggression, 19*(3), 345–356.

Yates, P., & Ward, T. (2008). Good lives, self-regulation, and risk management: An integrated model of sexual offender assessment and treatment. *Sexual Abuse in Australia and New Zealand, 1*(1), 2–19.

Yates P. M., Kingston D. A., Simons D. A., Tyler C. (2009, October). *The good lives model of rehabilitation applied to treatment: Assessment and relationship to treatment progress and compliance.* Paper presented at the 28th Annual Convention of the Association for the Treatment of Sexual Abusers (ATSA), Dallas, TX.

Yates, P. M., Prescott, D. S., & Ward, T. (2010). *Applying the good lives and self-regulation models to sex offender treatment: A practical guide for clinicians.* Brandon, VT: Safer Society Press.

Ziv, R. (2018). *The future of correctional rehabilitation: Moving beyond the RNR model and good lives model debate*. New York, NY: Routledge.

Part VI

Sexual Assault and the Law

Understanding False Allegations of Sexual Assault

32

William T. O'Donohue

Sexual assault is a significant social problem, as commonly cited estimates suggest that approximately one in four individual and one in nine individuals report at least one incident of sexual assault sometime in their lives (e.g., Smith et al., 2017). However, these self-report estimates likely contain error, as it is impossible for these to accurately capture either the rates of underreporting or over-reporting. In addition, the large variance in definitions of sexual assault across legal jurisdictions and studies as well as a lack of sexual violence literacy held by the public (e.g., Koss, Gidycz, & Wisniewski, 1987) can add further error to these rates. For example, in Koss's (Koss et al., 1987) classic study, many fewer women responded affirmatively to questions of whether they were raped, than whether they ever had a sexual experience that they did not consent to. Importantly, there has been little effort to understand the rate of false allegations as inflating any of these sexual assault estimates due to the inability for researchers to conduct thorough investigations of the validity of their subjects' self-report. Instead the epidemiological data are usually constructed as if all self-reported allegations are true allegations, as well as all denials are accurate denials. This chapter will review the various limitations to understand these rates of sexual assault and propose ways to address these, as well as review literature regarding the purported rate of false allegations. In addition, this chapter will examine several issues related to false allegations of sexual assault: (1) Why does the rate of false allegations matter?; (2) What is meant by the construct, "false allegation of sexual assault?"; (3) What is known about pathways to false allegations?; (4) What does the empirical literature show regarding these rates?; and (5) How can future research regarding false allegations be improved?

The authors would like to thank Professors Ana Bridges and Lorraine Benuto for their assistance on portions of this chapter.

W. T. O'Donohue (✉)
University of Nevada, Reno, NV, USA

Why Do Rates of False Allegations Matter?

A basic question is why do the rates of false allegations matter? Of course, one can simply wish to discover descriptive information for its own sake—for example, an entomologist could attempt to discover the average width of the leg of a particular spider species for no other reason than he or she finds this information to be of interest. However, it does not appear that this situation is the case regarding rates of false allegations of sexual assault. It appears that this rate (or more precisely, rates—see below) is desired to be known as this information would have two major functions: (1) to demonstrate whether or

W. T. O'Donohue and P. A. Schewe (eds.), *Handbook of Sexual Assault and Sexual Assault Prevention*,
https://doi.org/10.1007/978-3-030-23645-8_32

not the rate of false allegations is sufficiently high to suggest that false allegations are an important social problem and (2) for its usefulness in determining the truth or falsity of a claim in a particular case of sexual assault.

The rate of false allegations has an obvious subtractive role in reported rape rates, that is, if the reported rape rate is 25% and the rate of false accusations contained in this is 10% then the true rape incident would be 22.5%. Of course, in general, the higher the frequency of the problem, the more important the problem is. For example, 30% of individuals contracting a deadly virus is more concerning than 15% of individuals contracting the virus. However, given the seriousness of rape it is not clear if there is a rate where sexual assault would suddenly become an unimportant problem. What if rape occurred in only 1% of the population, would then sexual assault become unimportant? What if 0.5%? It would seem that given the seriousness of this violation, its impact on victims and the effect it has on perceptions of safety and justice that sexual assault would still be regarded as an important social problem over a wide range of possible rape incidences.

Does this same logic hold true about the importance of false allegations? If false allegations occurred only 1% of the time, would this be a significant social issue? What if 10% of allegations were purposefully fabricated (and not just unfounded or a legitimate misperception of events)? Would this rise to the level of a significant social issue? Currently, false allegations are either considered rare enough to be insignificant or at most an uncomfortable anomaly. In the current social and political climate where all allegations of sexual assault are expected to be immediately believed, more carefully exploring the data around false allegations may be vitally important.

It might be instructive to briefly examine the more fundamental question of how useful these rates of false allegations, even if known, would actually be in clarifying whether or not rape occurred in some case under investigation. Let us examine five cases:

Case 1: If the rate of false allegations of sexual assault is zero then any allegation of sexual assault should be regarded as true. This seems to be a view that has increasing popularity at least among certain segments in the culture, for example, some activists. One sees slogans like "Believe survivors" that seem to imply that all allegations are true and therefore must be believed. This slogan and its cognates though are obviously question begging—that is, if someone is indeed a victim of a crime then by definition the underlying allegation that renders this person a victim is true. However, there is no study reviewed below that indicates that the rate of false allegations is zero.

It also should be noted that this a very extraordinary claim involving the view that it simply is empirically impossible that a person could ever lie or be mistaken about whether they have been sexually assaulted. There is an old saying that extraordinary claims require extraordinary evidence. Impossibility claims require either a logical contradiction (it is impossible to have round squares) or to be inconsistent with a universal scientific law (it is impossible for force not to equal mass x acceleration). However, no such logical contradiction or physical laws are relevant here. It is both logically possible and empirically possible for a person to make a false claim of sexual assault. Also, of course, we know that humans can be and are inaccurate about all sorts of claims. Besides misperceptions of intentions or events, false allegations can be purposeful as in divorce cases, child custody, extortion, retribution, alibi, etc. Thus, although this view of zero false allegations has been advanced and has been increasingly popular (e.g., it was expressed in the Kavanaugh Supreme Court hearings), it simply is mistaken. One must note that this view can be quite harmful—it is not a mere intellectual mistake—people can be seriously harmed and lives can be ruined. However, holding the factually erroneous view that all sexual assault allegations are true is today considered morally valid, while challenging this view can have significant consequences—not believing all claims of sexual assault can be seen by some as a serious moral failing.

Case 2: If all allegations of sexual assault are false, then any allegation of sexual abuse allegations is false. This is the converse of Case 1.

It, again, is an extraordinary claim requiring extraordinary evidence. Inflating the rate of false allegations of sexual abuse in the past due perhaps to significant sexism has certainly caused many legitimate claims of sexual assault to be disbelieved with many serious consequences—for example, trauma exacerbated, and rapists free to commit other acts of rape. However, similar considerations for Case 1 apply here; there is obviously empirical evidence that true claims are made; and there is no logical or empirical law to the effect that all sexual assault claims must necessarily be false. Again, one must note that this view can be quite harmful—it is not a mere intellectual mistake—people can be seriously harmed and lives can be ruined. Finally, unlike case 1, holding this factually erroneous view is rather universally seen as a moral failing.

Case 3: Some sort of inchoate base rate prediction might be attempted, that is, if the false allegation rate regarding sexual assault is 5% then this particular allegation is 95% likely to be true. The first problem is that results of studies are not converging on some clear population parameter for the rate of false allegations. The rates reported (see below) vary considerably and depend, as stated before, on sampling characteristics, definitions of sexual assault, rater reliability, and perhaps even researcher bias. With such variance in reported rates, reasoning from some single rate of false allegations of sexual assault is problematic. Perhaps with improved research this population parameter can be better approximated with confidence intervals to provide some information about variance in this estimate. However, given that the majority of studies show that most allegations of sexual assault are true, it does seem reasonable to say, *ceteris paribus*, that the allegation under question has a greater likelihood of being true than in being false.

In addition, if one assumes that only 50% of those who are sexually assaulted report the assault (see O'Donohue, Chap. 35, this volume) and assumes a 10% chance of an individual being raped and a 5% chance of a false allegation, then one can say that the rate of claims of rape are quite different in the group of people who have been raped versus those who have not been raped. In this example, the rate of claiming rape in people who were actually raped is 50% (by hypothesis), while the rate of claiming rape in people who have NOT been raped is only 0.26% (5/1895) (Table 32.1).

Table 32.1 Contingency table

	Rape	Not raped
Claim rape	95	5
Don't claim rape	95	1895
	190	1900

Finally, this picture is complicated by what is known as the "broken leg problem" in actuarial prediction (Meehl, 2013). That is, suppose that every Tuesday evening Anna plays basketball, therefore one would predict that on future Tuesdays there is essential a 1.0 probability that Anna will play basketball. But suppose Anna broke her leg this week—this relevant fact then obviates the prediction—Anna now has a 0% chance of playing basketball next week. Thus, predictions from base rates also need to be conditioned by a knowledge of factors that obviate or modify the accuracy of these predictions and as a field we have incomplete knowledge of these. For example, let us suppose that the rate of false allegations of sexual assault is 5%, then this would mean that if a person claims that President Obama sexually assaulted him or her that this is 95% likely to be true. But suppose we also know that this person is actively schizophrenic and has made a number of false allegations against Obama—this obviously would need to be properly considered in the probability estimate. This is related to the next case that will be considered.

Case 4: If one knows pathways for false allegations and this person has one or more of these pathways then the allegation is likely to be false. Again, there is the problem of reasoning from a sample statistic (both regarding the accuracy of the pathway as a legitimate pathway to a false allegation as well as the strength of this relationship) to the individual case. Thus, it is possible that despite the pathway the allegation is still true as none of the pathways to a false allegation is perfect, that is, the existence of the pathway precludes that a true allegation can occur. For example, say a diagnosis of x is associated with a pathway to a false allegation. It can still be the case that the person who suffers from x is actually assaulted. Finally, there can be measurement error associated with the claim that the individual actually has one of the pathways.

Case 5: If one knows pathways to false allegations and this person does not have any of these pathways then the allegation is true. This assumes that the known or theorized pathways are exhaustive—that is, that researchers have accurately identified all routes to false allegations. Of course, this is not the case—and no one makes this claim that the science is "complete." The actual case is that the science is just in its beginnings. In addition, there can be measurement error in ruling out a pathway and this would be compounded across individual pathways. Thus, either because some pathway was inappropriately ruled out or because there may be a pathway not identified by current research this information, although relevant, is not conclusive.

In sum, it would be useful for individuals using information about pathways to false allegations of sexual assault to be clearer on which one of the cases enumerated that they are attempting to utilize, their actual quantitative reasoning, as well as limitations of this.

What Is a False Allegation?

An important issue that needs to be resolved when attempting to determine the rate of false allegations of sexual assault is what constitutes a false allegation of sexual assault. O'Donohue, Cummings, and Willis (2018) argued that in some existing child sexual assault literature a false allegation has been interpreted to include allegations that are simply "unfounded" due to insufficient evidence to make a definitive substantiation, as well as those allegations where recantation occurs (as if in all recantations the original claim and not the recantation itself is false); as well as those that are only partly true (e.g., exaggerating the extent of the contact or the total number of incidents). In another words, allegations can be complex sets of claims and some of these individual statements can be true while others are false. Another definitional possibility is the issue of false negatives—sexual assaults that occurred but are denied or simply not reported (i.e., involve a false denial). Among the false positives (claims of sexual assault where no sexual assault occurred) are those that are intentional (e.g., lying), unintentional (e.g., misunderstanding of an innocent act or unintentional touching), allegations due to false memories, or allegations made due to suggestion. However, no study has examined the differences in rates of each of these sub-types.

Goodyear-Smith (2016) pointed out additional difficulties. This author acknowledges that sexual abuse and false accusations of abuse both occur, and both can do considerable harm. In addition, this author argued that an allegation of sexual assault may be true, partly true, or false. "Partly true" includes an embellished or distorted recollection, or a misinterpretation that the action of another involved sexual intent. A false allegation may be made knowingly and deliberately, or it may be the result of a belief that something happened that never took place. True and untrue allegations may be hard to distinguish: typically, there is no physical means of verifying or disproving an allegation. Sometimes, there is corroborative evidence that an event either did or did not occur. But most sexual abuse has happened in secret: there are no witnesses and, frequently, we cannot know for sure whether something happened or not. Further difficulties in uncovering the truth occur when allegations refer to events claimed to have occurred decades in the past.

The International Association of Chiefs of Police (IACP, 2015) proposed guidelines for investigating sexual assault allegations and argued that a false allegation can only be labeled as such when there is evidence to suggest that no crime was attempted or committed. Of course, there is a lot of judgments involved in ascertaining that "no evidence" exists. At a minimum one would have to interpret the victims' claims that they were assaulted as "no evidence." Logic suggests that the absence of evidence is not the same as evidence of falseness. These authors also argued for the distinction between a false allegation and an unsubstantiated one, with the latter being labeled as those which, after an investigation, do not have sufficient evidence to prove or disprove that an assault occurred—again a complex judgment. How does one define the dividing line between sufficient and insufficient? What if a woman claims a man grabbed her breast when no witnesses were present and the male denies this? There would be no medical evidence, no witness statements—how would one define "sufficient evidence in this kind of "he said she said" situation? This also begs important questions such as what is the standard of proof (e.g., beyond a reasonable doubt, clear and convincing, or preponderance of the evidence as well as complex variables such as the quality of evidence gathering). Currently in campus Title IX investigations of sexual assault, the standard of proof, per the "Dear Colleague" letter, has been set as preponderance of the evidence which is colloquially interpreted as "50-50 plus a feather." In "she said, he said" cases with no additional evidence, the mere presence of an accusation can be seen by some as serving as the feather.

Pathways to False Allegations

False allegations can occur at different stages in the investigatory process (e.g., report to friends, parents, Title IX), be made by reporters other than the purported alleged victims, and of particular relevance to this chapter, be made for various tangible or psychological motivations. Studies exploring the rate of false allegations sometimes explore the various pathways to filing a false allegation. DeZutter, Horselenberg, and van Koppen (2018) explored eight different motives for false allegations of sexual assault as originally outlined by Kanin (1994). These motives included material gain, producing an alibi, revenge, gaining sympathy, gaining attention, mental health diagnoses, relabeling and regret. Using a sample of 57 false allegations investigated by the Dutch National Police, the researchers explored the frequency at which these eight motives for filing a false report were endorsed by individuals who made false allegations of sexual assault. The false allegation cases were predominately motivated by the accuser's potential emotional gain (e.g., sympathy from loved ones) or as a means of diverting attention from some other behavior often associated with wrongdoing (e.g., infidelity, skipping school). Interestingly, 20% of the alleged victims could not provide a reason for filing their false allegation, indicating there could be some unlisted or more nebulous pathway to making a false allegation.

Campbell (1992) theorized that some false allegations can initially originate as rumors but eventually acquire the appearance of verified facts. Consequently, this author suggested that the dynamics of rumor formation and rumor transmission, combined with constructivist theory, can provide an explanatory model accounting for the origins and apparent credibility of these rumors/false allegations of sexual assault. The development of false allegations in this model includes elevated anxiety, rumor formation, reduction in ambiguity, credibility expansion, validating networks, and invalidating information. Ultimately, according to this view false allegations of sexual abuse influence and are influenced by the systemic context in which they occur. Thus, parents and children can report false allegations without consciously fabricating these. This etiological theory of false allegations indicates key psychological and psychosocial pathways for false allegations including the roles of anxiety and social processes that can be present in some cases.

In another examination of potential pathways to false allegations, Engle and O'Donohue (2012) proposed eleven pathways: lying, failure to recognize implied/behavioral consent, false memories, intoxication, antisocial personality disorder, borderline personality disorder, histrionic personality disorder, delirium, psychotic disorders, dissociation, and intellectual disability. Further, O'Donohue, Cirlugea, Bennett, and Benuto (2015) proposed seven pathways to false allegations of child sexual abuse, two of which may also be applicable to adolescent sexual assault. Specifically, adolescents alleging sexual assault may be susceptible to suggestive influences (e.g., by the forensic interviewer in the interview or by parents or close friends prior to the interview) and their report may be influenced if they have a stake in the outcome (e.g., findings may influence a custody decision or may distract from other wrongdoing). Given these various potential pathways for reporting a false allegation of sexual assault, a comprehensive review examining the rates of false allegations for each of these pathways is warranted, though little exists. Specifically, it is important to understand which pathway(s) to false allegations are most relevant to consider when determining whether an alleged sexual assault is substantiated or deemed false or unsubstantiated, as it may have implications on the rate of false allegations found.

Rates of False Allegations

Despite a lack of consensus regarding what constitutes a false allegation, researchers have attempted to understand the rate of false allegations of sexual assault that are made in naturalistic settings. A literature search was conducted in the EBSCOHost and PsycInfo databases with the following search terms: "sexual assault," "sexual harassment," "sexual abuse," "rape" and "false allegation," "false accusation," "recantation," "false rate," "report," "false claim." Papers were excluded if they involved content only on child sexual abuse or did not provide an estimated rate of false allegations, as the purpose of this review was to examine rates in the adult (18+) population. All materials reviewed were book chapters or peer-reviewed scholarly journals, and the reference section of each publication was reviewed to identify additional potential publications to include in the current review.

One of the earliest attempts to explore the rate of false allegations was conducted by Kanin (1994). Although the main aim of the study was to explore the pathways to false allegations (see below), Kanin provided some preliminary evidence for the frequency of these complaints. In a sample of 109 sexual assault allegations reported to a police agency in a small metropolitan area in the Midwest within a 9-year period of 1978–1987, 45 cases were determined to be false, yielding a false allegation rate of 41%. However, this study was conducted several decades ago and thus may not be representative of the current rate of false allegations. Further, the cases were deemed false *only* when the accuser admitted the sexual assault did not occur after making the allegation. As stated by the researchers, these recantations do not definitively indicate that the initial allegation was false since the recantation itself could be false perhaps as a result of some other concern (e.g., not wanting to testify in court; being threatened by the perpetrator), though with such a high recantation rate it is plausible to interpret that there is at least some significant rate of false allegations revealed in this study. Conversely, some of the allegations might have been false despite the absence of a recantation.

Gross (2009) reported that the United States Air Force Special Studies Division examined the 1218 reports of rape that were made between 1980 and 1984 on Air Force bases throughout the world. Of those, 460 were found to be "proven" allegations either because the "overwhelming preponderance of the evidence" strongly supported the allegation or because there was a conviction in the case. Another 212 (17.4%) of the total reports were found to be "disproved" as the alleged victim convincingly admitted the complaint was a "hoax" at some point during the initial investigation. The researchers then investigated the 546 (44.8%) remaining or "unresolved" rape allegations including having the accusers submit to a polygraph. Twenty-seven percent (27%) of these complainants admitted they had fabricated their accusation just before taking the polygraph or immediately after they failed the test. (It should be noted that whenever there was any doubt, the unresolved case was reclassified as a "proven" rape.) Combining this 27% with the initial 212 "disproved" cases, it was determined that approximately 45% of the total rape allegations were false.

Theilade and Thomsen (1986) conducted a study of sexual assault cases and found that 1 in 56 reports (1.5%) was false. Theilade and Thomsen (1986) defined a false case as "without any doubt… false" (p. 17; as cited by Hunt & Bull, 2012). However, it is unclear what evidence was used to demonstrate falsity "without any doubt," therefore the rate found should be interpreted with caution. Stewart (1981) conducted a review of 18 allegations of sexual assault reported to the precinct. Of those, 16 (88.9%) were deemed false, with 14 (87.5%) of those deemed false due to the alleged victim's retraction of the allegation. However, this was a small sample size, thus the reported rate may not be a good indicator of the actual population rate. Additionally, as mentioned previously recantations do not necessarily prove that the alleged assault was false, and the judgment did not have to be supported by additional evidence of falsity.

Greenfeld (1997) conducted a review of the Bureau of Justice Statistics report from the United States Department of Justice, that encompasses sexual assault cases reported to 16,000 different local and state agencies in 1995. All cases were labeled as "founded" and "unfounded," though it is unclear how each label was operationalized. Nonetheless, this study found that 8% of the total cases were unfounded. However, the review does include child sexual abuse cases that were unfounded, which, as discussed previously, does not necessarily indicate falsity but rather a lack of evidence to clearly demonstrate the veracity of the allegation.

Romney (2006) conducted a review of literature to examine the rates of false allegation worldwide. The review found a wide variability in studies based in England and Scotland, with the lowest rate found being 1.5% (Theilade & Thomsen, 1986) and the highest rate being 88.9% (Stewart, 1981). Of the studies based in the United States, there was less variability, with the lowest rate being 8% (Greenfeld, 1997) and the highest rate being 41% (Kanin, 1994). Romney (2006) also noted that the high discrepancy in false allegation rates reported by various researchers causes difficulty in gaining a thorough understanding to help guide decision-making in sexual assault cases.

In a recent meta-analysis, Ferguson and Malouff (2016) attempted to quantify the rate of false allegations of sexual assault. Using seven studies of confirmed false reports, the researchers found a range of 2.1% to 10.3% of false allegations with an overall rate of 5.2% (Ferguson & Malouf, 2016). However, this meta-analysis included some studies with reports of child sexual abuse, one study included was unpublished and thus not a product of peer review, and this large variance in rates was influenced by the year and country studied. Additionally, the interrater reliability was only reported in 2 of the 5 studies, thus there may be error and biases in the judgements regarding truth or falseness of the allegation. Future studies should also explore the rate of false allegations at each stage of the forensic process (e.g., reported to someone other than law enforcement, reported and investigated by police, district attorney's decision to proceed with prosecution, cases tried, and appellate decisions), as the studies reviewed do not sub-divide analyses based on this. Without this, the field will not have a sufficiently clear understanding of the frequency of false allegations.

Kelly (2010) reported two studies of false allegations of sexual assault in Europe. The first study examined data from the St. Mary's Sexual Assault Referral Centre tracking database between 2000 and 2002 (Kelly, Lovett, & Regan, 2005), which gathers detailed data of sexual assault cases referred to six different multidisciplinary, victims' services sites in the United Kingdom. Each case had data regarding: details of the assault, victim, perpetrator(s), forensic examination, and the proceedings/outcomes of the case. Of the 3527 cases seen at the centers, 2643 were reported to law enforcement agencies, and 299 (11.3%) of the cases investigated were judged "no crime" due to being either a false allegation (n = 216) or a lack of evidence of assault (n = 83), with the remaining cases either judged as true or unknown. Police statements describing why the case was labeled as being false were available for 120 of the cases and included 53 admissions of falsity with reasons such as revenge towards an ex-partner and covering up sexual relations with someone other than their partner, though these purported pathways of were not investigated or confirmed by the researchers. The remaining cases were deemed false due to other reasons, including inconsistencies in the initial statement given and witness statements which did not support the accuser's account. Further, it was found that false allegations occurred most often in cases involving individuals who were 16–25 years old, unemployed, disabled, and/or had mental health concerns. False allegations were also more likely to occur when the victim-perpetrator did not have a prior relationship and when the victim had previously made a prior allegation to police. Altogether, the findings suggested a false reporting rate of 8.2%. However, this rate includes retractions (n = 28; 1%), which, again, does not necessarily prove the allegation is indeed false, and the cases were deemed false based on one law enforcement official's judgment, thus both the reliability and validity of these judgments is unknown. Further, as the authors point out, the cases judged as false include those in which victim characteristics (e.g., prior allegation, perceived embellishment of victim report) were used to judge the veracity of their claim. Excluding those cases, the remaining false allegation rate is only 3% and only includes those cases in which the alleged victim admitted the allegation was false or there was some evidence to support the falsity of the claim.

Kelly (2010) reported a second study of attrition of sexual assault cases in Europe using similar methods as Kelly et al. (2005). In a sample of 100 consecutive cases in nine counties in Europe beginning in April 2004, the study found a false allegation rate ranging between 1% and 9% per country, which includes both cases that were unfounded and deemed "no crime" (Lovett & Kelly, 2009). However, the cases considered false did not include those with no evidence to support the allegation or those that had retractions. This is problematic because at least some of the cases with these properties may be false, thus the reported rate may be underestimated. Additionally, the cases included were only single perpetrator incidents, thus this study excluded an unknown number of additional cases that may have been falsely filed.

In a recent study of false allegations reported to university campus police within a 10-year period, Lisak, Gardinier, Nicksa, and Cote (2010) aimed to examine the generalization of the previously determined false allegation rate to the university setting. Case summaries were reviewed and false allegations were coded based on a literature review of procedures police departments use to classify sexual assault cases, personal discussions about report classification procedures with senior members of the police department, and the IACP's (International Association of Chiefs of Police) definition of false reports. One hundred and thirty-six cases of sexual assault during this period were categorized as one of the following: a false report, a case that did not proceed forensically, or a case that proceeded and insufficient information to assign a category. A false report was defined as a case that was thoroughly investigated (e.g., multiple interviews of the alleged perpetrator, victim and witnesses, forensic evidence gathered and considered) and a preponderance of evidence gathered suggested the assault had not occurred. Individual cases were coded by two independent raters, with an interrater agreement rate of 94.9%. Results indicated that there was a false report rate of 5.9% (n = 8), while 44.9% (n = 61) of the total cases did not proceed forensically, 35.3% (n = 48) proceeded, and 13.9% (n = 19) did not have sufficient information to be coded. The rationale for the eight allegations deemed false varied, with three including admissions of falsity/fabrication by the complainant, three with evidence suggesting fabrication though no admission was made, one with a partial admission of fabrication combined with evidence of fabrication, and one with a recantation and evidence that the initial report was false. The researchers concluded that false allegations reported to university police have a similar rate of false reporting as those cases reported to community police and examined in previous studies. However, it should be noted that these findings do not provide much insight regarding the pathways associated with false reports. Nonetheless, the methodology used in this study has the fewest limitations of the literature reviewed in this chapter and yet yielded similar false allegations rates to previous studies. However, a significant percentage—nearly 14% were not coded in this study and 45% did not proceed forensically. If any substantial subsample of these were actually false then the rate of false allegations would be significantly higher. Taking these unknown cases out of the equation results in a false allegation rate of 14/3% (8/56).

Summary of the Literature on Rates of False Allegations of Sexual Assault

This section reviewed the extant literature regarding false allegations of sexual assault. Combined, the literature suggests a need to develop an agreed upon operationalization of the construct "false allegation." Further, the majority of studies agreed that most allegations of sexual assault are in fact true, as only 3 studies (Gross, 2009; Kanin, 1994; Stewart, 1981) reported over 40% of claims to be false, while the remaining studies reviewed had an estimated false allegation rate range of 1.5% (Theilade & Thomsen, 1986) to 10.9% (Harris & Grace, 1999). Therefore, it can be presumed that false allegations do occur at some non-negligible rate, but there is a need to better decipher between those allegations that are true or false, as well as a willingness for researchers (and investigators) to label an allegation as unknown if the preponderance of evidence is too equivocal. It is also important to note that the studies reviewed each had significant methodological limitations, including small and unrepresentative samples, variable criteria to operationalize the construct of false allegation; equivocal use of "false allegation" and "unfounded allegation," unknown interrater reliabilities, and a lack of acknowledgement that these rates vary based upon the stage of investigation the sample was drawn from. Further, the majority of studies reviewed were published multiple decades ago, thus the rate of false allegations may have changed since the researchers' data collection timeframe.

False Allegations of Sexual Assault: Construct Validation

First, we recommend that increased sophistication and transparently be used to report the key classifications. We suggest that all three rates be reported: rates of true allegations, rates of false allegations, and rates of undecided cases. These should sum to 100%. One reason this is important is rates of false allegations can be altered by increased rates of undecided allegations—for example, the more undecided cases the lower the rates of identified false allegations. Reporting all three rates provides more transparency and clarity.

Second, we recommend that a confidence interval or indications of error terms be simultaneously reported with these rates. It would seem that there would be a fallacy of imprecision to suggest a precise rate, for example, 8.9%. In general, there are many recommendations for the use of confidence intervals and the use of these also provides some indication of the error term and this can decrease the likelihood that these figures will be misused.

Finally, we recommend that the question of "What are the rates of false allegations of sexual assault?" be viewed as simplistic. We suggest that it would be more accurate to use a paraphrase of Gordon Paul's (1969) "ultimate question" which was originally developed to combat another overly simplified and insufficiently nuanced question regarding psychotherapy, that is, "Is psychotherapy effective?" A more properly nuanced question regarding false allegations would be along the lines of "**What are the rates of false allegations (and true and undetermined cases), judged by what evidentiary standard (e.g., preponderance of evidence, clear and convincing, beyond reasonable doubt), by what operational definitions of false (e.g., recantations, medical evidence), in what population, with what other relevant characteristics (e.g., mental health diagnoses, past history of lying) with what sampling limitations (e.g., nonrandom convenience sample), made against whom (ex-lover, stranger, current partner), during what time period (e.g., 1960–1965), in what stage of the forensic process (e.g., court trial), with what interrater-reliability, with what possible researcher bias or general error rate?** This is obviously a complex question but the underlying phenomenon appears to be this complex. Certainly, if some parameter contained in this question above is shown empirically to be irrelevant to rates then it can and should be eliminated. However, we would argue that this question forces both researchers and consumers of this information to acknowledge the nuances and complexities involved with this question and combats misleading and simplistic answers like 8.9%.

Given these limitations, scholars and particularly expert witnesses should exercise caution in making claims about the veracity versus the falsity of allegations made, especially if stating a specific false allegation rate to support their claims. Socrates was one of the first to think deeply about issues such as truth and justice and he famously came to the conclusion that if he is wise it is because he knows that he does not know. We need to keep in mind Socrates' wisdom in this domain. Everyone interested in justice desires that all sexual assault victims to be believed; and all who have been falsely accused of sexual assault to be exonerated. Recently, our society has experienced a steady diet of possibly politically infused sexual abuse allegations (e.g., the Duke Lacrosse case as well as possibly the Kavanaugh Supreme Court nomination hearings) as well as individuals rendering public judgments about the alleged victim's credibility on faulty reasoning. It is interesting to note that one still can go a long way in uncovering someone's political orientation simply by asking them about the credibility of the sexual harassment accusations of Anita Hill against Justice Thomas, the rape accusations of Juanita Broderick against President Clinton, or the rape accusations of Christine Blasey-Ford against Judge Kavanaugh.

Improving Forensic Decision-Making in Sexual Assault Allegations

How can we best make more accurate decisions regarding "he said; she said" accusations of sexual assault? First, we need to realize that there are no markers of truth or falsity. A marker would be a property that every true allegation contains and no false accusations contains. Thus, all reasoning using a supposed marker, for example, "She did x and x never happens in actual rape so her report is false" are fallacious—there is no characteristic x or characteristics x1 to xn that have this power to infallibly parse true from false accusations. But can we reason probabilistically—perhaps we know some properties that individually or taken together would validly allow a correct decision that the allegation is more likely true than false—or the converse? Unfortunately, due to the limited science relating to sexual assault we don't know what these key properties would be or their probabilities. The following are examples of common properties that are used to try to make judgements about rape accusations, where only *intuition*, but too few data exist to support these claims:

Delay in disclosing to authorities: Some rapes are reported immediately, but research studies show that sizeable percentages of rape victims (often 40% or higher; see O'Donohue, Chap. 35, this volume) delay reporting for months or years. A person leveling a false accusation can either include or not include a delay in their accusation. So, unfortunately, any reasoning along the lines of "She failed to report immediately so the accusation is likely to be false" has no data to support this claim.

Disclosing to another person (such as a friend). Some rape victims do this; some don't (and again a false accusation could contain or not contain this characteristic). No data currently exists to confirm or deny whether false accusers are less likely to disclose to a close friend.

Obvious psychological symptoms. Many, but not all, victims suffer from post-traumatic stress disorder (PTSD) and other mental disorders (Foa, Cahill, Smelser & Bates, 2001). However, others, especially in less severe forms of sexual assault (e.g., one brief incident of groping), may not experience any symptoms. In addition, symptoms can be feigned or observed symptoms can be due to other causes (the observed depression may be due to an unrelated life event such as a relationship breakup). Also, individuals vary in their astuteness in seeing symptoms and victims vary in their ability to hide symptoms. Thus, reasoning along the lines of "She was fine" or "She was distressed" weeks or months after an alleged assault and therefore the allegation is more or less likely to be true/false also is not valid. Some distress immediately following an assault is probably likely in the case of a sexual assault. False accusers are often shown in videos or text messages following an alleged assault expressing positive emotions towards the sexual encounter or the person involved in the incident (See Mattress Girl).

Wouldn't forget details. Most rape victims remember key details of their rape (who, what, when, where) but can forget other details, especially after the passage of time or if there were many incidents (see memory chapter this volume). Finding that a person has forgotten or remembered a certain detail is not a valid way to discern whether the allegation is true or not. While it may be that false accusers may more likely to use selective memory or lack of memory to bolster their claim of sexual assault, no data is currently available that supports or disconfirms this.

No further contact with their perpetrator. Many victims do try to avoid their perpetrator, but some cannot (a close relative) and research into date rape has surprisingly found that a large percentage of women alleging date rape have further contact with their rapist (Koss et al., 1987). Of course, the definition of date rape has been expanded to include so many behaviors that many of the behaviors that researchers label as sexual assault are considered benign or inconsequential by those who we would label "victims." While it may be that victims of sexual assault are more likely to avoid their rapist than false accusers, no data are currently available that supports or disconfirms this claim.

Fighting back. Again, research shows that for a variety of factors (fear that fighting back could get them killed; being frozen in fear at the initial trauma of the attack), some victims do and some victims don't fight back. So, failure to resist should not be taken as an indication that an allegation was false. However, in the absence of significant threat or violence, a victim should indicate that he or she gave some indication to the perpetrator that their behavior was unwanted. While it may be that victims of sexual assault are more likely to fight back than false accusers, no data are currently available that supports or disconfirms this claim.

Never denying the assault. Some rape victims feel shame or even feel that they will be blamed for the rape and can be placed in situations where they will deny that they were raped. The circumstances surrounding a denial or a recantation should certainly be investigated for possible threats or coercion, or simply an unwillingness to disclose to a particular person or in a particular situation.

One vs. multiple independent complainants. In the recent case of the movie producer Harvey Weinstein, dozens of women have independently claimed that he has committed some form of sexual abuse. How likely would this happen if the allegations are false? This is a much sounder form of reasoning but still it has significant limitations: it does not mean that *each and every* allegation is true (a particular allegation can be caused by jumping on the bandwagon for some personal gain); and second, it would be fallacious to reason that a single complainant means the allegation is false—serial rapists all have their first victim.

Consistency in core details. My colleagues and I have conducted some research that shows that 97% of young children can consistently recount their sexual abuse (O'Donohue et al., 2013). However, inconsistencies can be caused by the victim not being comfortable in answering questions in some situations; or didn't understand some nuance in the question.

The Nobel Laureate Daniel (Kahneman & Tversky, 2000) has found that we as humans dislike uncertainty and use cognitive heuristics (shortcuts) to attempt to bring clarity to situations that are in fact unclear. Some of these heuristics are motivated reasoning—for example, because we wish to see our children as special we can "reason" in ways so that we can conclude that indeed they are so. We would be well advised to remember Socrates and be on guard regarding our motivations, especially political ones, and the problems in the quality of our reasoning regarding sexual assault.

There is also an important question of what ought to be done regarding individuals who knowingly make false allegations of sexual assault. Important distinctions need to be made here—making an inadvertent false allegation would seem to necessitate fewer consequences than knowingly making one. Making a false accusation as a result of a mental disorder might necessitate mandating mental health treatment (although it is unclear if in its current state mental health treatment could prevent someone from making additional false allegations). Perhaps effective psychotropic medication can decrease paranoid ideation in a person suffering from schizophrenia but there is no evidence that psychotherapy can reduce the likelihood of someone making a false accusation of sexual assault due to a Personality Disorder. There has been little scholarly discussion of the type of consequences (jail, fines, restitution, expulsion from school, etc.), or the magnitude of these in the literature. Perhaps it can be the case that these, if widely publicized, could have a preventative function and decrease the rate of false accusations. One would also need to be careful that these consequences do not have the effect of further inhibiting true allegations to be reported. However, if a person were punished for falsely reporting that their car is stolen (i.e., insurance fraud) and this punishment was widely publicized, would that result in others being less likely to report to the police if their car were stolen?

Conclusions

As sexual assault researchers and advocates, our focus on preventing sexual violence and achieving justice for individuals who are sexually assaulted continues to be of paramount importance. Our justice system has not yet progressed to the point where every individual who makes a rape accusation gets a proper police investigation or a fair hearing. However, seeking justice for victims of sexual assault should make us more concerned, not less, with justice for individuals who have been falsely accused. Promoting justice for all requires finding ways to support victims of sexual violence without equating accusation with guilt, and recognizing that the wrongly accused are real victims too. We must not assume that the only positive outcome of a sexual assault allegation is a conviction. Laws and campus policies that are rooted in the assumption that wrongful accusations are inconsequentially rare need to be resisted and reformed. Just like all other crimes, individuals accused of sex crimes should also be presumed innocent until proven guilty. While the general consensus on false allegations has been that 2–9% of allegations are false, a more careful examination of the research suggests that 2–41% may be false. Certainly, much more research is necessary.

References

Campbell, T. W. (1992). False allegations of sexual abuse and their apparent credibility. *American Journal of Forensic Psychology, 10*(4), 21–35.

Dezutter, A. Horselenberg, R. & van Koopen, P. (2018). Motivations for filing a false allegation of rape. Archives of sexual behavior, 47, 457–464.

DeZutter, A. Z., & Horselenberg, R. (2018). Motives for filing a false allegation of rape. *Archives of Sexual Behavior, 47*, 457–464.

Engle, J., & O'Donohue, W. (2012). Pathways to false allegations of sexual assault. *Journal of Forensic Psychology Practice, 12*, 97–123.

Foa E. B, Cahill S. P, Smelser N. L, Bates P. B. (2001). Psychological therapies: Emotional processing. International encyclopedia of the social and behavioral sciences; Oxford: Elsevier.

Ferguson, C. E., & Malouf, J. M. (2016). Assessing police classifications of sexual assault reports: A meta-analysis of false reporting rates. *Archives of Sexual Behavior, 45*, 1185–1193.

Goodyear-Smith, F. (2016). In R. Burnett (Ed.),. *Wrongful allegations of sexual and child abuse Why and how false allegations of abuse occur: An overview* (pp. 304–333). New York, NY: Oxford University Press.

Greenfeld, L. A. (1997). *Sex offenses and offenders: An analysis of data on rape and sexual assault.* Washington, DC: US Department of Justice, Office of Justice Programs.

Gross, B. (2009). False rape allegations: An assault on justice. *Forensic Examiner, 18*(1), 66.

Harris, J., & Grace, S. (1999). *A question of evidence? Investigating and prosecuting rape in the 1990s.* London: Home Office.

Hunt, L., & Bull, R. (2012). Differentiating genuine and false rape allegations: A model to aid rape investigations. *Psychiatry, Psychology and Law, 19*, 682–691.

International Association of Chiefs of Police. (2015). *Sexual Assault Response Policy and Training Content Guidelines*. Alexandria, VA: International Association of Chiefs of Police.

Kahneman, D., & Tversky, A. (Eds.). (2000). *Choices, values and frames*. New York: Cambridge University Press and the Russell Sage Foundation.

Kanin, E. J. (1994). False rape allegations. *Archives of Sexual Behavior, 23*, 81–92.

Kelly, L. (2010). The (in)credible words of women: False allegations in European rape research. *Violence Against Women, 16*, 1345–1355.

Kelly, L., Lovett, J., & Regan, L. (2005). *A gap or a chasm. Attrition in reported rape cases*. London: Home Office.

Koss, M. P., Gidycz, C. A., & Wisniewski, N. (1987). The scope of rape: incidence and prevalence of sexual aggression and victimization in a national sample of higher education students. *Journal of Consulting and Clinical Psychology, 55*(2), 162–170.

Lisak, D., Gardinier, L., Nicksa, S. C., & Cote, A. M. (2010). False allegations of sexual assault: An analysis of ten years of reported cases. *Violence Against Women, 16*, 1318–1334.

Lovett, J., & Kelly, L. (2009). *Different systems, similar outcomes? Tracking attrition in reported rape cases across Europe*. London, UK: Child and Women Abuse Studies Unit London Metropolitan University.

Meehl, P. E. (2013). *Clinical versus statistical prediction*. New York: Echo Point.

O'Donohue, W., Cummings, C., & Willis, B. (2018). The frequency of false allegations of child sexual abuse: A critical review. *Journal of Child Sexual Abuse, 27*(5), 459–475.

O'Donohue, W. T., Cirlugea, O., Bennett, N., & Benuto, L. (2015). Psychological and investigative pathways to untrue allegations of child sexual abuse. In W. O'Donohue & M. Fanetti (Eds.), *Forensic interview with children who may have been sexually abused*. New York: Springer.

Romney, P. N. (2006). False allegations of rape. *The Cambridge Law Journal, 65*, 128–158.

Smith, S. G., Chen, J., Basile, K. C., Gilbert, L. K., Merrick, M. T., Patel, N., ... Jain, A. (2017). *The National Intimate Partner and Sexual Violence Survey (NISVS): 2010–2012 State Report*. Atlanta, GA: National Center for Injury Prevention and Control Centers for Disease Control and Prevention.

Stewart, C. H. (1981). A retrospective survey of alleged sexual assault cases. *Police Surgeon, 28*, 32–35.

Theilade, P., & Thomsen, J. L. (1986). False allegations of rape. *Police Surgeon, 30*, 17–22.

Rape and the Jury

33

Peter O. Rerick, Tyler N. Livingston, and Deborah Davis

As we write this chapter, the nomination of Brett Kavanaugh to the United States Supreme Court is being exhaustively debated in public and private exchanges: much of the debate centering on the question of his alleged sexual assault of Christine Blasey Ford decades in the past. Ford's case has raised many issues common to allegations of rape litigated every day across America. Why did the victim fail to report for so long, and what does that reflect about her credibility? How do we assess memories for events where one or both parties were drinking, and perhaps to the point of blackout for one or both? What about memories for events so long in the past? How does intoxication affect responsibility for either party? What difference does it make for memory, or for responsibility, if the parties knew one another or were strangers? How does the context in which the accusation arose matter? How do we judge credibility when the evidence is "he said" versus "she said?" To what extent does it matter if others make similar allegations against the accused? Does character evidence (good or bad) matter—including testimony of women over a number of years of exemplary behavior? These issues and many other characteristics of the case evidence affect judgments of who is telling the truth.

And, there is the issue of who is going to believe whom and why. Judgments of Kavanaugh versus Ford tended to split along political lines. But what of jurors in everyday cases? Which jurors generally tend to vote for prosecution versus defense? How do specific items of evidence affect jurors, and for which jurors do they exert the strongest effects? What makes a good case for the prosecution and what are the elements of a good defense?

These are the issues we address in this chapter. We first address some unique features of allegations of rape versus other crimes. We then turn to the main topic of the chapter: What determines perceptions of alleged perpetrators and victims and determinations of rape?

Rape Is Unique Among Criminal Cases

Perhaps the most unique feature of rape cases is the extent to which alleged victims are essentially "on trial," arguably as much as alleged perpetrators. As we document throughout this chapter, victim blaming for rape tends to be pervasive, and much greater than for other crimes (e.g., Bieneck & Krahe, 2011). This victim blaming happens in part because a defendant can be acquitted if the jury can be convinced that the alleged victim actually consented (see Wood, Rikkonen, & Davis, this volume) to the sexual

P. O. Rerick (✉) · T. N. Livingston · D. Davis
University of Nevada, Reno, NV, USA
e-mail: prerick@nevada.unr.edu

W. T. O'Donohue and P. A. Schewe (eds.), *Handbook of Sexual Assault and Sexual Assault Prevention*,
https://doi.org/10.1007/978-3-030-23645-8_33

encounter: or, under many statues, if the alleged perpetrator had a "reasonable belief" that the alleged victim consented (i.e., the "mistake of fact" defense).

Even if observers believe the victim was raped, they can also be less motivated to find defendants guilty or to punish them harshly if the victim can be painted as unlikeable, disreputable, or unworthy of justice. Such defenses are a rarity for other types of crimes. A victim would never have to prove she did not consent to having her property stolen or her house burned to the ground. Thus, rape is one of the few crimes where the prosecution will benefit by trying to make the defendant appear as though she somehow invited, was responsible for, deserved, and/or was not harmed by the crime. These forms of victim blaming lead to a phenomenon known as "secondary victimization" (e.g., Williams, 1984), whereby victims of rape suffer ill treatment by professionals involved in their cases, sometimes the media, and others in the victim's social or professional networks. The victim's life is scrutinized for anything that might indicate he/she is to blame or not to be believed; he/she might actually be disbelieved or suffer criticism and rejection as the result of the allegation or even the fact of the victimization (see Reddington & Kreisel, 2017, for review). All of these reactions could be seen in the scrutiny and criticism of Dr. Blasey-Ford resulting from her claim against Judge Kavanaugh.

Given the fact and success of efforts to discredit alleged rape victims, researchers have extensively documented the difficulties in prosecuting cases of rape: ranging from initial evaluations by first responders, law enforcement, and medical personnel through attorney reactions and jury verdicts (see reviews in this volume; Allison & Wrightsman, 1993; Reddington & Kreisel, 2017; Ward, 1995). Though there are many reasons for such difficulties, prominent among them are tendencies to disbelieve and blame victims, and to believe or excuse perpetrators. Accordingly, a large body of research has examined both situational and personal determinants of these rape perceptions (see reviews by Allison & Wrightsman, 1993; Anderson, Cooper, & Okamura, 1997; Van der Bruggen & Grubb, 2014; Ward, 1995; Whatley, 1996). Broadly, these include (1) type of rape (stranger, acquaintance, spousal, etc.), (2) victim characteristics and behaviors, (3) perpetrator characteristics and behaviors, and (4) individual differences among perceivers.

Before we turn to discussion of this research, it is worth noting that alleged perpetrators can also be inappropriately presumed guilty, and treated unfairly as their cases proceed through the legal system. Though existing work on perceptions of rape allegations does address circumstances in which perpetrators are more or less likely to be blamed, researchers have tended to approach the problem from the perspective that alleged victims are inappropriately blamed and perpetrators inappropriately excused. As becomes apparent as we review the jury research below, there has thus far been little attention to characteristics or behaviors of either party that might lead to inappropriate blame and perceived guilt of the alleged perpetrator.

Effects of Type of Rape

Stranger Versus Acquaintance

A significant portion of research on rape distinguishes between rape by a stranger and rape by an acquaintance. Stranger rape is generally conceptualized as rape by someone the victim has never previously encountered, whereas acquaintance rape can range from someone the victim recently met to a long-time partner or spouse (Persson, Dhingra, & Grogan, 2018). Although people might think of rape as a crime usually committed by a stranger, acquaintance rape is more prevalent than stranger rape (Rainn, 2016); and yet it is reported at much lower rates than stranger rape (Fisher, Cullen, & Turner, 2000).

Attributions regarding rape and its victims seem to indicate that some observers do not perceive acquaintance rape as "real rape" (Estrich, 1987). In general, people place more blame on victims allegedly raped by acquaintances versus by strangers (e.g., Abrams, Viki, Masser, &

Bohner, 2003; Viki, Abrams, & Masser, 2004; see Van der Bruggen & Grubb, 2014, for review) and in turn attribute less blame to, and recommend shorter sentences for, perpetrators of acquaintance rape versus stranger rape (Frese, Moya, & Medias, 2004; McCormick, Maric, Seto, & Barbaree, 1998). The closer the relationship between a victim and perpetrator, the more blame the victim receives (see Van der Bruggen & Grubb, 2014, for review). Moreover, observers tend to minimize the harmful effects of acquaintance rape on the victim (e.g., Kirkwood & Cecil, 2001; Monson, Langhinrichsen-Rohling, & Binderup, 2000; Simonson & Subich, 1999).

Some have argued that gendered sexual scripts might explain the relationship between familiarity and blame in the context of rape. Generally speaking, these scripts dictate that men are the initiators of sexual acts, whereas women are sexual "gatekeepers" responsible for both their own and their partner's behavior (e.g., Jozkowski & Peterson, 2013). For someone who believes in these scripts, a woman is not responsible for the sexual behavior of a stranger, so she receives less blame for being raped by a stranger. However, because she is responsible for the sexual behavior of her friend, boyfriend, or husband, she is more blameworthy for being raped by a man in any of these roles.

These reactions to acquaintance rape are more likely among observers high in various gender and rape-relevant attitudes. For example, ambivalent sexism (Glick & Fiske, 1996) and gendered sexual scripts both seem to contribute to this familiarity-blame relationship. Ambivalent sexism is further categorized into two different but related categories: hostile sexism and benevolent sexism (with correlations between categories ranging from 0.4 to 0.5; Glick & Fiske, 2011). Hostile sexism refers to inherently negative views of women, such as that women are more dishonest and incompetent than men; whereas the latter encompasses seemingly beneficent but ultimately negative attitudes about women, such as that women should be protected because they are weaker and more vulnerable than men. People who endorse benevolent or hostile sexist attitudes tend to more often blame women for their own victimization when the rape was committed by an acquaintance rather than a stranger, especially if they view her as having violated traditional female gender roles (Abrams et al., 2003; Grubb & Turner, 2012; Viki & Abrams, 2002). This is also true for those high in Rape Myth Acceptance (Krahe, Temkin, & Bieneck, 2007; Frese et al., 2004; see section below on Juror Characteristics).

The Issue of Spousal Rape

Spousal rape has relatively recently become a topic of jury research. Historically, a "marital exemption" existed within the United States and other countries such that a woman had no right to say no to her husband because they were married (a concept known as "irrevocable consent"). Some jurisdictions defined rape as "sexual intercourse with a female, not his wife, by force and against her will" (Finkelhor & Yllö, 1987, p. 1). It wasn't until 1978 that the first man was prosecuted in Oregon for raping his wife while they were still living together; and marital rape did not become criminalized in all 50 states until 1993. Since then, however, exemptions have existed for marital rape in some states, including, for example, that marital rape is not criminal if the victim is sleeping or mentally or physically incapacitated (unless the perpetrator uses excessive force; for review, see Allison & Wrightsman, 1993; Bergen, 2016; Carline & Easteal, 2017; Reddington & Kreisel, 2017; Russell, 1990; Van der Bruggen & Grubb, 2014; Yllö & Torres, 2016).

As the above reviews indicate, though marital rape has been increasingly recognized by law, and research has burgeoned regarding the frequency, nature, and consequences of marital rape, a large body of research has shown that marital rape is taken less seriously than either stranger or acquaintance rape. Research participants judge marital rape as less traumatic or damaging to the victim, less consequential, as a lesser violation of victim rights, or less serious than other forms of rape (Bergen, 2016). Further reflecting the apparent perceptions of the relative triviality of marital rape, research has indicated that victims of marital rape tend to be blamed more (and their assailants less), including while the marriage is dissolving (Ewoldt, Monson, & Langhinrichsen-Rohling, 2000); and that alleged perpetrators are less likely to be found guilty of rape (Kirkwood & Cecil, 2001). Some research participants even fail to recognize marriage as a context in which rape can occur (e.g., Sullivan & Mosher, 1990). Even victims of marital rape tend to blame themselves (Russell, 1990).

A number of researchers have expressed frustration that historical views of women as the property of their husbands have not fully dissipated in our culture (and worldwide), and marital rape continues to be viewed as either a lesser form of rape, or as no rape at all by many (for review, see Bergen, 2016; Yllö & Torres, 2016). However, it should be noted that jury and public sentiment research on this topic is mostly 15–20 years old or more. More research is need to determine the extent to which marital rape still tends to be discounted, as well as the circumstances in which it is perceived as more or less serious.

Victim and Perpetrator Behaviors that Affect Perceptions of Rape Allegations

Pre-Rape Behaviors

With the exception of alcohol, most research on pre-rape behaviors has concerned those of the victim (almost exclusively female victims; for review see Allison & Wrightsman, 1993). What the victim does prior to the rape itself can be viewed as indicating her willingness to have sex (negating the fact of rape), as leading the perpetrator on (justifying the rape and excusing the perpetrator), as indicating the low worthiness or value of the victim (minimizing perceived consequences of the rape for the victim), or as increasing dislike of the victim (and increasing motivation for the preceding reactions; see Reddington & Kreisel, 2017, for review). Researchers have identified a number of pre-rape victim behaviors that promote one or more of these consequences.

Some behaviors occur independent of contact between the parties. These behaviors include the alleged victim's sexual history, promiscuity, involvement in sex professions such as prostitution or pornography, chronic drug or alcohol use, previously living in unconventional circumstances with a man (e.g., sharing an apartment), and so on. They nevertheless affect rape perceptions for both stranger and acquaintance rape, though more so for the latter (for reviews, see Allison & Wrightsman, 1993; Reddington & Kreisel, 2017).

Within the date rape context, a number of behaviors that *might* signal sexual availability (e.g., going to the perpetrator's residence), that might be viewed as obligating the woman to have sex (e.g., the man paying for expensive dates) or as provocative (e.g., wearing sexy clothing; flirtatious behaviors), those seemingly reflecting liking of the man, or as leading toward intercourse (e.g., sexual foreplay) have been associated with more positive judgments of the perpetrator and less positive judgments of the victim. Some of these behaviors also affect judgments of stranger rape (Viki et al., 2004). As with all behaviors and characteristics of perpetrators and defendants, many pre-rape victim behaviors affect the likelihood that their cases will be perceived as credible by law enforcement and prosecutors, worthy of prosecution (or likely to succeed if prosecuted), and therefore the likelihood they will reach trial (for review, see Allison & Wrightsman, 1993; Reddington & Kreisel, 2017).

Victim attire

Victim choice of attire is among the most frequently studied pre-rape behaviors, perhaps in part because it has been shown to affect judgments of both stranger and date rape. Reflecting cultural beliefs among both genders suggesting that dress reflects sexual willingness (see Wood et al., this volume, for review), or rape myths suggesting that women who dress sexily are "asking for it," (e.g., Burt, 1980), people who committed rape have often cited their victims' appearance and clothing as justification for their sexual aggression (see Feild, 1978; Scully & Marolla, 1984), and jury research has revealed similar rape justifying reactions. That is, particularly for male observers (who generally more strongly endorse rape myths; see Suarez & Gadalla, 2010), victims who dress in revealing or suggestive clothing are held more responsible (and the perpetrators less responsible) for their rapes (see Lennon, Adomaitis, Koo, & Johnson, 2017, for review). The victim's attire can also exert greater effects than her attractiveness, character, or acquaintance with the perpetrator (e.g., Whatley, 1996). More provocative attire has even promoted victim blame in the situation of marital rape (Whatley, 2005).

Alcohol and drugs

Among the most extensive research literatures on jury perceptions of rape is that concerning the role of intoxication (primarily alcohol). Given that alcohol use by one or both parties is pervasively involved in disputed sexual encounters (for review, see Abbey, Zawacki, Buck, Clinton, & McAuslan, 2004; Testa, 2002), it is important to understand how alcohol use by either party might affect perceptions of the alleged victim and the accused perpetrator.

Notably, many current rape statues and campus regulations specify that sufficient intoxication renders a person unable to consent to sex (see Wood et al., this volume, for review of state and federal statues). But, as we show below, effects of alcohol or other intoxication on rape perceptions seem to be incompatible with those the law suggests.

Alcohol is linked to actual and perceived sexual intentions in ways that suggest intoxicated persons are likely to be more sexually aroused and willing (Davis & Loftus, 2004). Alcohol expectancy studies have generally shown that alcohol is expected to increase sexual arousal and enjoyment and is used for that purpose, and there is evidence that intoxicated persons are viewed as more sexually willing. Substantial research indicates that perceivers, particularly males, tend to believe that alcohol use results in increased likelihood of sexual consent, promoting the idea that (in direct contradiction to many rape statutes) alcohol use is misperceived as consent itself (Abbey, 2011; Abbey & Harnish, 1995; Davis & Loftus, 2004; Johnson, Ju, & Wu, 2016; Schuller & Wall, 1998; see also Wood et al., this volume, for evidence that alcohol use is linked to perceived consent).

Research has more commonly addressed victim, rather than perpetrator, intoxication. A large body of studies demonstrates increased blame of intoxicated victims of both genders, and less punitive evaluations of the perpetrator: and, moreover, even if not intoxicated at the time of the alleged rape, a history of chronic drug or alcohol use leads to disbelief and blaming of the victim (for review, see Allison & Wrightsman, 1993; Brown, Horton, & Guillory, 2018; Davis & Loftus, 2004; Grubb & Turner, 2012). Reactions of professionals leading up to and including prosecution of rape cases are more negative for intoxicated alleged victims. Victims' claims are perceived as less credible by police, medical personnel, and prosecutors, and therefore their cases are less likely to be tried (see reviews by Allison & Wrightsman, 1993; Sleath & Bull, 2017; Ward, 1995). As these reviews indicate, a number of other factors moderate effects of alcohol use, such as who buys the drinks, which party or parties are drinking and their relative degree of intoxication, where the victim became intoxicated, and others. Perpetrators receive more blame the greater the relative intoxication of the victim, for example.

The Role of Resistance

Legal definitions of rape common in earlier years specified that a woman must have resisted for the sexual act to be rape (Anderson, 1998). Though such requirements are no longer included in rape statues for most of the United States, cultural definitions of rape and common rape scripts include victim resistance, as shown by a body of research indicating that victim resistance exerts strong effects on rape perceptions (see Allison & Wrightsman, 1993; Van der Bruggen & Grubb, 2014 for reviews).

Victims who do not resist are blamed more than those who do, and this difference is greater for male victims, who presumably should be better able to physically resist their attackers (Ong & Ward, 1999). Either verbal or physical resistance increases victim credibility and decreases victim culpability compared to no resistance (Angelone, Mitchell, & Grossi, 2015; McCaul, Veltum, Boyechko, & Crawford, 1990; Ong & Ward, 1999; Warner & Hewitt, 1993). In general, victims receive more favorable judgments when they resist more (Branscombe & Weir, 1992), perhaps because resistance helps convey a clear lack of consent. The effect of resistance is stronger among male than female observers, however (Angelone et al., 2015). Likely reflecting both homophobic attitudes and the presumed greater ability of males to defend themselves, homosexual victims who fail to defend themselves are blamed most and resistant heterosexual males are blamed least by male observers (see Van der Bruggen & Grubb, 2014, for review).

Timing of Resistance

Not only do sexual scripts dictate that a woman resist sex, she also is expected to resist early in the sexual encounter (Nyúl, Kende, Engyel, & Szabó, 2018; Weis & Borges, 1973). This idea might partially stem from beliefs about "leading a man on." Both males and females have endorsed beliefs that if a woman leads a man on, she forfeits her right to say no to further sexual advances (Quinn, Sanchez-Hucles, Coates, & Gillen, 1991). Reflecting these beliefs, several studies have shown that victim blame is greater, perpetrator blame is less, and the incident is less likely to be considered rape when victims resist later in an encounter rather than earlier (e.g., Kopper, 1996; Shotland & Goodstein, 1983; Yescavage, 1999). These effects were additionally supported by recent data from a large sample of U.K. police officers (Hine & Murphy, 2017).

Type of resistance

Although physical and verbal resistance strategies appear to be utilized about equally often (at least in a sample composed mainly of stranger rape victims), physical resistance is the more effective resistance strategy (Ullman & Knight, 1995), which might be one reason it is sometimes taken more seriously than verbal resistance. However, some research has found that verbal resistance alone resulted in more perpetrator blame than verbal and physical resistance together, (Black & Gold, 2008), although this finding seems to be uncommon. As most studies have shown the reverse, this finding needs replication.

Sexual scripts partially explain the way people perceive a victim's resistance to rape. First, cultural scripts for "real rape" include that the victim resists (see Nyúl et al., 2018). Additionally, a belief in a sexual script known as "token resistance to sex" affects reactions to verbal versus physical resistance. The token resistance script dictates that women are expected to provide "token resistance" to a man's sexual advances by saying no (again acting as a gatekeeper) when her true intention is to eventually have sex (Muehlenhard & Hollabaugh, 1988). Thus, verbal resistance might be seen as "token" rather than real; whereas physical resistance is taken more seriously. Accordingly, belief in the token resistance script has been linked to lower perceptions of rape when the victim uses verbal resistance only, compared to both verbal and physical resistance (Black & McCloskey, 2013; Osman, 2003).

Those who believe in token resistance also appear to require more evidence of resistance to recognize a woman's refusal. For example, a sample of men who believed in token resistance indicated that a woman needs to refuse sex an average of 2.6 times before they believed that she truly did not want to have sex (Mills & Granoff, 1992). Unfortunately, belief in women's token resistance stands out as particularly difficult to combat, as several studies show that a substantial portion of women, and in some cases a majority, indicate that they have engaged or do engage in token resistance when their true intentions are to have sex (Muehlenhard & Hollabaugh, 1988; Sprecher, Hatfield, Cortese, Potapova, & Levitskaya, 1994).

Perpetrator Use of Force

Past definitions of rape commonly specified perpetrator force as an element of the crime. For example, the FBI defined rape as "the carnal knowledge of a female forcibly and against her will" (Federal Bureau of Investigations, 2012). They and others have since changed their definitions to focus on the issue of consent (see Wood et al., this volume, for review of state and federal statutes). Nevertheless, force continues to be a prominent aspect of lay definitions of rape, and is central to the "real rape" cultural script (Nyúl et al., 2018). Although an uncommon topic of research, some evidence indicates that when a perpetrator uses force, he receives more blame and victim blame is reduced compared to when he uses no force (e.g., Brown et al., 2018; Mitchell, Angelone, Kohlberger, & Hirschman, 2009; Proite, Dannells, & Benton, 1993; Russell, Oswald, & Kraus, 2011).

Victim and Perpetrator Characteristics

Victim Gender and Sexual Orientation

Studies of effects of victim gender have been relatively sparse, yielding contradictory results. It has been assumed that males might be blamed more for their rapes than females because they are assumed to have greater ability to offer physical resistance. Yet, females might be blamed more based on character (e.g., Davies & Rogers, 2006). Much evidence supports these assumptions regarding male victims. For example, male victims of alleged stranger rape are blamed more, particularly when they failed to actively resist (sometimes mostly by male observers; e.g., Ayala, Kotary, & Hetz, 2018; Davies, Pollard, & Archer, 2001; Davies, Rogers, & Whitelegg, 2009; Davies, Smith, & Rogers, 2009; Fisher & Pina, 2013; Gerber, Cronin, & Steigman, 2004; Rye, Greatrix, & Enright, 2006; White & Kurpius, 2002) or when the perpetrator is a woman (Bourke, 2007). Like female victims, male victims are subject to secondary victimization by law enforcement and others, and their claims are disbelieved and go unprosecuted: but more so than for female victims (for review, see Fisher & Pina, 2013; Javaid, 2018; Lowe & Rogers, 2017).

Despite much evidence for more negative reactions to male victims and their claims, other research has shown greater blame of female victims, and more research is needed to understand the conditions that affect gender differences in blame (see Van der Bruggen & Grubb, 2014, for review).

Intertwined with victim gender, the sexual orientation of victims is an important determinant of rape perceptions. Male homosexual victims of same-sex attacks have been studied more than heterosexual male victims of either male or female perpetrators (Davies et al., 2001; Davies, Pollard, & Archer, 2006). Male homosexual victims are blamed more for both acquaintance and stranger rape, and perceptions of the impact of the rape are minimized (Davies, Rogers, & Whitelegg, 2009). Homophobia is associated with greater blame of both homosexual and heterosexual victims and with rape minimization for homosexual victims (Davies, Smith, & Rogers, 2009). Additionally, heterosexual males, in part because of their greater homophobia, blame homosexual victims more than females or homosexual males (see Van der Bruggen & Grubb, 2014, for review). As an additional reflection of lack of sympathy or concern for male victims, Katz (2015) found that men presented with a hypothetical party situation where a male perpetrator was leading a highly intoxicated victim (varying the gender of the victim) into a bedroom recommended greater inaction when the victim was male, in part because they felt less responsibility to help a male than a female. Less is known about reactions to lesbian victims, or to transgender or cross-dressing victims (see Van der Bruggen & Grubb, 2014, for review).

Perpetrator Gender and Sexual Orientation

Much less is known about reactions to female (vs. male) perpetrators. However, consistent with a meta-analysis showing greater leniency for females across crime types (Mazzella & Feingold, 1994), research has generally indicated greater leniency toward female perpetrators of sexual assault. Female perpetrators elicit less moral outrage, receive less blame, and receive more favorable perceptions, especially when the victim is male (but see Gerber et al., 2004, for an exception), and sometimes only by male observers (Ayala et al., 2018; Davies et al., 2006; Mackelprang & Becker, 2017; McCracken & Stevenson, 2017; Osman, 2011; Russell et al., 2011). Jurors might be more likely to perceive male victims as having invited the assault when the perpetrator was male compared to female (Smith, Pine, & Hawley, 1988), perhaps because male rape myths also seem to have larger effects when the perpetrator is female and the victim is male (Struckman-Johnson & Struckman-Johnson, 1992). Research has not specifically examined the effects of perpetrator sexual orientation, as that information can presumably be obtained from the sex of the victim.

Less research has focused on female perpetrators with female victims, primarily because the majority of research manipulating perpetrator gender uses only male victims. Some research has shown that male perpetrators are blamed more regardless of victim gender (e.g., Ayala et al., 2018). Other research notes that when women victimize other women, they are blamed more (Gerber et al., 2004) and receive less empathy (Osman, 2011) than when they victimize men (Gerber et al., 2004). Overall, male perpetrators generally receive more blame than female perpetrators, regardless of victim gender (Süssenbach, Eyssel, Rees, & Bohner, 2017).

The Role of Race

Meta-analyses of experimental data (Mitchell, Haw, Pfeifer, & Meissner, 2005; Sweeney & Haney, 1992) and secondary analyses of decades of real-world legal data (see Cochran et al., 2017) demonstrate a consistently significant effect of race on legal judgments. Black defendants are more likely to receive a guilty verdict and a longer sentence compared to their White counterparts across case types, including rape (Cochran et al., 2017). Victim race is just as important—and sometimes more important—as a predictor of juror perceptions than defendant race. Perpetrators of crimes against Black (vs. White) victims generally receive less harsh punishment (see Bornstein & Greene, 2017, for review).

For rape cases researchers have investigated main effects and interactions regarding perpetrator and victim race, and moderators of these effects (such as the relationship between the parties and others; see Maeder, Yamamoto, & Saliba, 2015, for review). Generally, researchers have expected that Black (vs. White) perpetrators and victims would receive more blame, particularly for interracial stranger rapes. But effects of race have been more complicated. Overall, race has not always exerted the expected effects, but when race has affected blame of either party, Blacks tended to receive more blame (see Maeder et al., 2015; van der Bruggen & Grubb, 2014). Nevertheless, research has often found moderators of this effect such as the nature of the perpetrator-victim relationship (Willis, 1992): and often inconsistent effects of the moderators (see Lynch, Golding, Jewell, Lippert, & Wasarhaley, 2018).

For example, the type of relationship between the defendant and the victim (e.g., strangers vs. prior dating partners) can interact with race to influence juror judgments: For stranger rape, rape myths suggesting that Black men lust after White women have been assumed to promote greater blame of Black (vs. White) men who rape White women, and less blame of their victims. But for acquaintance rape, a White victim might receive more blame when accusing a Black romantic partner, versus a White partner or a stranger, because she is seen as low class or morally deficient (Willis, 1992). Further, jurors assigned more blame to Black victims of rape perpetrated by a dating partner versus a stranger, but this difference between relationship types was nonsignificant for White victims, regardless of the perpetrator's race (e.g., Willis, 1992; cf. Lynch et al., 2018, for null effects of relationship type generally). Yet other studies have suggested that defendants in mixed-race rapes were treated more harshly, regardless of jurors' own race. Juror bias against victims of interracial rape might be due to unfavorable attitudes toward interracial relationships.

Other moderators of effects of race have not concerned the combination of victim and perpetrator race. For example, when both race and respectability of the victim were manipulated, observers reacted more favorably to Black victims compared to White victims, but the reverse was true for less respectable victims (Dupuis & Clay, 2013). As another example, an attractive White woman sexually assaulted by a White man is perceived as more responsible for her assault than is an attractive White woman sexually assaulted by a Black man, consistent with the rape myth that rape is sexually motivated when Black men lust after White women (Maeder et al., 2015). Indeed, physical attractiveness was the most influential variable in a meta-analysis of victim and defendant characteristics that affect jurors' perceptions, such that attractive defendants received the most lenient sentences (Mazzella & Feingold, 1994).

Researchers have also observed a race × gender interaction, where Black males had more negative attitudes toward rape victims than did White males, White females, and Black females (White males did not differ significantly from White or Black females; Nagel, Matsuo, McIntyre, & Morrison, 2005). However, participant race was associated with socioeconomic status (SES) in this study, which could explain the findings.

In sum, though many moderators of race effects have been observed, none have been sufficiently replicated to establish their reliability. Much more research is needed to fully understand effects of victim and defendant race on rape perceptions: including effects for additional races, and interactions with juror race.

Effects of Physical Attractiveness

The effects of physical attractiveness on interpersonal perception are reliable and wide-ranging across all demographic categories, all social or professional contexts, and many domains of interpersonal judgment (for review, see Rhode, 2010; Todorov, 2017) including legal judgments (see Davis, 1991, for review). Under most circumstances, attractive persons are perceived more positively, and enjoy better social, professional and legal outcomes. Not surprisingly, effects of attractiveness extend to the parties to rape allegations.

Victim Attractiveness

One might expect that attractive victims of sexual assault would receive more sympathy and be blamed less than unattractive victims. Some have argued, for example, that such reactions might be based on the implicit assumption that a man would not rape an unattractive woman without provocation because unattractive women are undesirable (Vrij & Firmin, 2001). A number of studies have indeed shown that attractive victims receive less blame and their assailants receive harsher sentences (Erian, Lin, Patel, Neal, & Geiselman, 1998; Ferguson, Duthie, & Graf, 1987; Ferrão, Gonçalves, Ginger, & Parreira, 2015; Gerdes, Dammann, & Heilig, 1988).

Nevertheless, some research suggests that jurors assign more blame to attractive victims of sex crimes (e.g., Clarke & Lawson, 2009). Attractive victims are sometimes perceived as more provocative (e.g., Jacobson & Popovich, 1983), perhaps because mock jurors view the appearance of attractive victims as being partially to blame for their victimization (Coates & Wade, 2004). Male participants also perceive attractive women as more interested in sex than unattractive women and consequently are less likely to consider an interaction as sexual assault when the victim is attractive (Perilloux, Easton, & Buss, 2012; Yndo & Zawacki, 2017), which might explain one study that found only males attributed lower responsibility to a defendant when the victim was attractive versus unattractive (i.e., Maeder et al., 2015).

Juror gender and attractiveness

Juror gender seems to be a particularly important moderator of the effects of victim attractiveness (Vrij & Firmin, 2001), typically such that male (vs. female) jurors are more certain of defendant guilt when the victim is attractive (Deitz, Litman, & Bentley, 1984; cf. Maeder et al., 2015, for the opposite pattern). This difference could be due to ceiling effects on guilt measures among female jurors in sexual assault cases. Women are often more empathic to sexual assault victims compared to men (see section on juror gender below), rendering women less likely to blame a victim regardless of the victim's level of attractiveness (Maeder et al., 2015; Vrij & Firmin, 2001). Alternatively, men's judgments might be more susceptible to influence from victim characteristics because men are less sure of defendant guilt from the onset (and generally less punitive than women in sexual assault cases; see subsequent section on juror gender).

Perpetrator Attractiveness

Research has been somewhat inconsistent regarding perpetrator attractiveness. Some studies have indicated that attractive alleged perpetrators are judged less harshly, particularly among observers high in Rape Myth Acceptance. Presumably, this effect occurs both because they are liked more, and because they are perceived as having no need to rape (e.g., Vrij & Firmin, 2001). Other research has indicated that attractiveness leads to less punitiveness for female, but not male, offenders: particularly among male observers (e.g., Mackelprang & Becker, 2017). Thus, it is premature to draw conclusions about the effects of perpetrator attractiveness

Although much research has investigated effects of physical attractiveness on rape perceptions (e.g., Westfall, Millar, & Lovitt, 2018), few studies have examined the effects of other victim and perpetrator physical characteristics such as body weight, tattoos, and piercings. These variables have significantly affected mock jurors' perceptions in crimes unrelated to rape in the direction that observers perceive defendants who appear unconventional (vs. conventional) more negatively (e.g., Brown, McKimmie, & Zarkadi, 2018; Funk & Todorov, 2013; Schvey, Puhl, Levandoski, & Brownell, 2013).

Social Status and Reputation

Victim and perpetrator social status also matters. Women who are more respectable (typically manipulated by varying marital status, virginity, manner of dress, or occupied positions of high social status) tend to receive less blame than women who are not deemed respectable: and their perpetrators tend to receive harsher punishments (Alexander, 1980; Cohn, Dupuis, & Brown, 2009; Kanekar & Kolsawalla, 1977, 1980; Omata, 2013; Whatley, 1996). Similar reactions occur among police officers, who are less likely to believe reports from victims who are sex workers (Page, 2010) and more often perceive cases involving sex workers as false (Venema, 2016).

SES *differential* also matters. When participants perceived the victim to be of lower SES than her attacker, they tended to minimize the responsibility of the rapist and blame the victim (see Black & Gold, 2008). However, the perception that the victim was higher SES than her attacker was not predictive of blame for either party.

High SES might serve as an indicator of responsibility or overall virtue (for review of just world theory, see Westfall et al., 2018). In one study supportive of this hypothesis, participants attributed more blame to a respectable rape victim than a nonrespectable victim, which the researchers suggested resulted from participants' greater need to blame the victim's actions because it was more difficult to blame her character (Jones & Aronson, 1973). However, this result appears to be unique and has failed to replicate in at least two attempts (Kahn, 1977; Kerr & Kurtz, 1977).

Perpetrator Social Status

As with alleged victims, the social status of alleged perpetrators matters. Perpetrators with higher SES are less likely to be convicted, are seen as less blameworthy, and are assigned shorter sentences than those of lower SES (for meta-analysis, see Devine & Caughlin, 2014). Field studies of perpetrator status and trial outcomes have supported mock jury research on this subject. Low status men are more commonly blamed (Mazzella & Feingold, 1994) and convicted of rape (Vaughan, 2001) than are higher status men. These results fit into the more general body of research suggesting that low status men tend to receive more blame for the same crime (such as assault; Gleason & Harris, 1975) than high status men.

Recently, philosophy professor Kate Manne coined the concept of "himpathy," which has since appeared in popular discourse. The term denotes "the inappropriate and disproportionate sympathy powerful men often enjoy in cases of sexual assault, intimate partner violence, homicide, and other misogynistic behavior" (Manne, 2018; Scene on Radio Podcasts: Men, Part 7). Supporting this concept, two studies indicated that observers perceive celebrities accused of rape more positively than they view non-celebrities accused of the same crime (Knight, Giuliano, & Sanchez-Ross, 2001), and that perceptions of the celebrity's degree of life and career success were positively associated with favorable perceptions of the accused (Nyúl et al., 2018). Even coercive sexual advances are judged as more acceptable when the perpetrator is of high (vs. low) SES (Black & Gold, 2003).

Victim Symptoms, Rape Trauma Syndrome, and Expert Testimony

Rape trauma syndrome is a group of symptoms or behaviors allegedly experienced by victims of rape in response to the trauma of rape (Burgess & Holmstrom, 1974; Tannura, 2014). Testimony about rape trauma syndrome is common when the defendant admits that intercourse occurred, but claims it was consensual. In this common scenario, the prosecution may call an expert on rape trauma syndrome to testify as to how rape commonly affects victims, and sometimes that the specific alleged victim's behavior and emotional state are consistent with that of rape victims (Frazier & Borgida, 1988). This use of rape trauma testimony is controversial, in that the message is that if a victim shows these symptoms, she was raped: even though there are many other causes for the same symptoms.

Rape trauma testimony is also offered to explain why victims might behave in ways that seem to indicate she is not credible. For example, the expert might explain such things as why a victim delayed reporting, is not as emotional as expected, why she showed unexpectedly positive reactions to the perpetrator at some points, or why she has gaps and inconsistencies in memory: things that might otherwise lead jurors to view the rape claim with skepticism. In fact, such behaviors suppress prosecution of perpetrators as well as affect jury reactions. Law enforcement and prosecutors might view a case as "unfounded" or unwinnable, based on victim failures or inconsistencies in memory, delay in reporting, failure to appear sufficiently upset, and others (see Reddington & Kreisel, 2017, for review). Thus, rape trauma information can prevent investigators, prosecutors and juries from viewing victim claims as invalid.

On the other hand, the scientific validity of rape trauma syndrome is not unequivocally accepted within the scientific community: and some have argued that the methodology originally used by Burgess and Holmstrom (1974) was not adequate enough to create a new kind of trauma diagnosis (Frazier & Borgida, 1992). Others have opposed the diagnosis on the basis that the empirical evidence for rape trauma syndrome is questionable. And, many have suggested that testimony about rape trauma syndrome should not be admissible in court (e.g., O'Donohue, Carlson, Benuto, & Bennett, 2014). This view is based on two primary objections: (1) the existence of symptoms consistent with rape trauma is not proof of rape, as many other causes of such symptoms are possible: and the implication that the victim's symptoms prove rape is prejudicial to the defendant, and (2) the testimony implies that virtually any victim reactions are consistent with rape (and there are none that should be taken as evidence against rape). In other words, if the victim reports immediately or later, whether she remembers clearly from the start and consistently or fails to remember at first and is inconsistent in her reports, she has still been raped. Others have argued in favor of rape trauma testimony, raising the issue of whether the tendency to blame victims and to misunderstand their reactions to rape may outweigh any prejudice to the defendant posed by expert testimony (see Cossins, 2013, for review).

Nonetheless, experts do testify about rape trauma syndrome, raising the question of how such testimony affects jury reactions. Unfortunately, there have been few relevant studies. Brekke and Borgida (1988) tested the effects of expert testimony specific to rape trauma syndrome, and found that jurors exposed to expert testimony were more likely to view the defendant as guilty, and recommended longer sentences than jurors who were exposed to standard expert testimony on rape. Testimony was also more effective when it was presented early in the trial, rather than later. The authors also noted that expert testimony made no difference in the recall of case facts, and that the expert was not always positively evaluated. Frazier and Borgida (1992) note that expert testimony takes several forms that may exert different effects, so more research specific to rape trauma testimony is necessary.

Effects of Juror Characteristics

Rape Myth Acceptance

Rape myth acceptance (RMA) is perhaps the most commonly studied construct related to rape trials, and has been purported to be the most powerful predictor of perceptions of rape (Basow & Minieri, 2011). RMA has been studied with a variety of instruments (e.g., Burt, 1980; Hust et al., 2013; King & Hanrahan, 2015), and scales to measure it continue to undergo development due to changes in societal perception of rape (e.g., McMahon & Farmer, 2011). Rape myths are widely held attitudes and beliefs that serve to justify sexual aggression by males against females (Lonsway & Fitzgerald, 1994; see also Burt, 1980), and recent research on rape is rarely conducted without inclusion of measures of RMA or related constructs. Rape myths vary by culture, but people who endorse rape myths consistently report greater victim blame for the rape, express disbelief toward claims of rape, assert that only "certain types" of women are raped, absolve the perpetrator of responsibility, and minimize the negative impact of rape on victims (for review, see Grubb & Turner, 2012; Van der Bruggen & Grubb, 2014). Findings also generally indicate men tend to endorse rape myths more than do women (e.g., Russell & Hand, 2017; see Suarez & Gadalla, 2010, for a meta-analysis), although some research has suggested that RMA is better predicted by sexually dysfunctional beliefs in both men and women rather than femininity and masculinity (Barnett, Hale, & Sligar, 2017). Religiosity and conservatism also are positively related to RMA (Barnett, Sligar, & Wang, 2016). Others have suggested that effects of RMA might be in part due to those high in RMA more often attending to information about the victim rather than the defendant (Süssenbach et al., 2017), which leads to increase victim blame, even when the information is irrelevant (Eyssel & Bohner, 2011).

Other Related Gender Attitudes

In addition to RMA, other gender related attitudes have been associated with perpetrator supportive perceptions of rape allegations. These constructs include traditional sex role stereotypes (e.g., Shotland & Goodstein, 1983; Simonson & Subich, 1999; Whatley, 2005; Whatley & Riggio, 1993; Willis, 1992); just world beliefs (e.g., Whatley & Riggio, 1993), though evidence for how this matters is mixed (for review, see Van der Bruggen & Grubb, 2014; Sleath & Bull, 2017); attitudes toward rape victim scale (Ward, 1988); negative attitudes toward women (Whatley, 1994); and benevolent sexism (e.g., Durán, Moya, Megías, & Viki, 2010; Viki et al., 2004). Both RMA and these additional attitudes occur in women and men, and some argue that they matter more than biological sex for perceptions of rape (e.g., Angelone, Mitchell, & Lucente, 2012). These various scales are highly intercorrelated and in many cases overlapping in content. The original RMA scale, for example, contained subscales tapping constructs assessed individually in other scales: such as traditional gender role stereotyping.

Finally, it is important to note that these measures sometimes include scale items asking the same question the experimental research design is testing. For example, the study may vary alcohol use, preliminary sexual behaviors such as necking, dress, and other variables expected to affect rape perceptions. And the measures often have directly relevant items: for example, "in the majority of rapes, the victim is promiscuous or has a bad reputation," "any healthy woman can successfully resist a rapist if she really wants to," "if a girl engaged in necking or petting and she lets things get out of hand, it is her own fault if her partner forces sex on her" (Burt, 1980). It is no wonder, then, that these personality assessments predict judgments of the same things they measure.

Male Rape Myths

Rape myth measurement for decades referred only to myths regarding females. However, several conceptual treatments and measures of male rape myths have been introduced into the literature (e.g., Graham, 2006; Kassing, Beesley, & Frey, 2005; Sleath & Bull, 2017), and these measures are associated with more negative reactions to male victims and their claims (see Fisher & Pina, 2013, for review).

Juror Gender

Not surprisingly, evidence suggests that in most situations females tend to have more prosecution friendly rape perceptions than males (see Van der Bruggen & Grubb, 2014, for review). Researchers have suggested that this gender difference is, in part, the result of greater rape myth acceptance (e.g., Russell & Hand, 2017, see Suarez & Gadalla, 2010, for a meta-analysis) and/or more conservative gender role attitudes (see Angelone et al., 2015; Hammond, Berry, & Rodriguez, 2011) among males; or greater empathy by males for male defendants. Regarding the latter, however, females have manifested more prosecution friendly rape judgments for defendants of both genders, whether homosexual or heterosexual: and for stranger, date and marital rape (Van der Bruggen & Grubb, 2014).

Despite this overall gender difference, some research has indicated that females can sometimes render harsher victim blaming rape judgments, particularly for female victims (e.g., Batchelder, Koski, & Byxbe, 2004). Some have offered just world explanations for women's reluctance to blame the perpetrator, suggesting that because women find rape more threatening than do men, women are more likely to blame the victim for the crime. If they can perceive the victim as different from themselves and those differences as responsible for the rape, the threat of rape to themselves is lessened (e.g., Shaver, 1985). However, this perspective has been contradicted by at least one empirical test showing that women with a high (vs. low) belief in a just world had more positive perceptions of a rape victim (Kleinke & Meyer, 1990).

Other studies suggest that women's hostility toward one another might also contribute their tendency to disbelieve alleged rape victims (see Allison & Wrightsman, 1993; Cowan, 2000; Cowan, Neighbors, DeLaMoreaux, & Behnke, 1998; Reddington & Kreisel, 2017). Hostility toward women is also related to acceptance of interpersonal violence (Cowan et al., 1998), which is a component of the Burt (1980) rape myth scale, and therefore likely to promote victim blaming. Cowan (2000) also found significant positive relationships between women's hostility toward other women, beliefs that rape is caused by victim precipitation, and other victim blaming beliefs.

As with most juror characteristics, gender exerts greater effects when evidence is weak, and exerts little to no effects when evidence is strong (e.g., Rumsey & Rumsey, 1977). Similarly, males (vs. females) were more likely to blame a respectable female victim, but no gender effect was found for victims who were not respectable (Luginbuhl & Mullin, 1981).

The Importance of Similarity to the Victim

The defensive attribution hypothesis (Shaver, 1970) suggests that victim blame will be less when the victim and observer are similar and/or when identification with the victim is greater. Van der Bruggen and Grubb (2014) reviewed evidence that (1) females blame rape victims who are similar to them less, (2) similarity predicts blame of both adult and child victims, and (3) the greater tendency for males to blame victims is in part because of their lesser identification with female victims.

Conclusions

At this point there is a relatively vast literature on determinants of perceptions related to rape. In general terms, this research supports the notion that judgments conform to scripts regarding "real rape:" in that cases are more likely to be perceived as rape, and result in more perpetrator and less victim blame, if the perpetrator is a male stranger, the victim is female, the perpetrator uses physical force, the victim attempts to resist, and the victim reports the rape quickly and cooperates with police (see Nyúl et al., 2018).

Although research has identified these and other regularities in determinants of rape perceptions, six important caveats are in order. First, our review was of necessity incomplete. Space did not permit us to explore the many nuances, contingencies, inconsistencies, and methodological issues of the studies addressing each topic. This is true of other major reviews of literature on jury perceptions of rape (e.g., Van der Bruggen & Grubb, 2014). This puts readers at risk of developing oversimplified views of given sets of findings.

Second, multiple dependent measures are common in rape perceptions research, including blame of each party and guilt judgments, among others. It is often the case that results for the various measures do not correspond. Predictions are often supported for some measures and not others, and in ways that are not replicated across studies. This makes it difficult to confidently identify replicable patterns of effects in some areas of rape perceptions research.

Third, many studies suffer from methodological flaws, yet are cited in support of their main hypotheses by subsequent researchers without report or discussion of those flaws (see Lindren, Parkhill, George, & Hendershot, 2008; van der Bruggen & Grubb, 2014, for discussions of such problems). Though this is true for other areas of research as well, we nevertheless caution readers of rape perceptions literature to go to original sources where possible to gain a better understanding of overall effects of the many variables studied in this domain.

Fourth, much of the foundational research done on the topic of rape was performed decades ago, and is in need of modern replication. Indeed, few things have changed as rapidly in recent times as our understanding and socialization surrounding gender, and very recently, sexual assault, underscoring increased need to ensure that foundational findings still hold true today.

Fifth, most research in this domain is conducted with samples of university students. Sample limitations are always an issue for who would wish to apply results in trial of rape cases. But it is arguably a greater issue recently, as campuses have provided sexual assault training classes and other rape-related education, and publish explicit policies covering issues such as those shown in this review to affect jury verdicts. When research concerns basic cognitive processes and behavioral principles, it is less likely that one will get fundamental differences between samples. But when the research domain concerns attitudes that are shaped by culture, including the micro culture of college campuses, such differences become more likely. It remains for future research to examine sample effects more closely to determine if there are significant differences in the way college students versus community members perceive rape cases. Research could also profitably address the issue of whether sexual assault training programs affect student rape perceptions in mock jury research such as that reviewed herein. This may be a vain hope, however, as indicated by the previously reviewed failures of training programs to affect police judgments of rape.

What about the issue of innocent alleged perpetrators?

A sixth and final caveat is in order, regarding the failure of existing jury research on rape perceptions to address the circumstances leading to inappropriate perpetrator blame. In the age of "#metoo", there may be a tendency to presume a man guilty of rape allegations, particularly when he possesses characteristics consistent with stereotypes of rape perpetrators: such as athletes (particularly Black athletes), for example. As for that matter, research is lacking concerning such stereotypes. What categories of males do we presume guilty and why? Other than degree of force used, how do the male's behaviors matter? What is our cultural script for false allegations of rape, and how does failure to fit that script affect perceived perpetrator blame and guilt? Though many such questions may seem to have been addressed in the existing literature (because some factors raise and others lower perpetrator blame), they have not been the focus of the research, and the research questions have been largely presented in the context of discussions of inappropriate victim blaming. This focus, of course, restricts what research questions are asked. Even if one adopts the view that errors are more likely to be made toward inappropriate disbelief of true victims, there are, nevertheless, wrongfully convicted innocent alleged perpetrators: and greater understanding of these errors is needed.

References

Abbey, A. (2011). Alcohol's role in sexual violence perpetration: Theoretical explanations, existing evidence and future directions. *Drug and Alcohol Review, 30*, 481–489. https://doi.org/10.1111/j.1465-3362.2011.00296.x

Abbey, A., & Harnish, R. J. (1995). Perception of sexual intent: The role of gender, alcohol consumption, and rape supportive attitudes. *Sex Roles, 32*, 297–313.

Abbey, A., Zawacki, T., Buck, P. O., Clinton, A. M., & McAuslan, P. (2004). Sexual assault and alcohol consumption: What do we know about their relationship and what types of research are still needed? *Aggression and Violent Behavior, 9*, 271–303. https://doi.org/10.1016/S1359-1789(03)00011-9

Abrams, D., Viki, T., Masser, B., & Bohner, G. (2003). Perceptions of stranger and acquaintance rape: The role of benevolent and hostile sexism in victim blame and rape proclivity. *Journal of Personality and Social Psychology, 84*, 111–125. https://doi.org/10.1037/0022-3514.84.1.111

Alexander, C. (1980). The responsible victim: Nurses' perceptions of victims of rape. *Journal of Health and Social Behaviour, 21*, 22–23. https://doi.org/10.2307/2136691

Allison, J. A., & Wrightsman, L. S. (1993). *Rape: The misunderstood crime*. New York, NY: Sage.

Anderson, K. B., Cooper, H., & Okamura, L. (1997). Individual differences and attitudes toward rape: A meta-analytic review. *Personality and Social Psychology Bulletin, 23*, 295–315. https://doi.org/10.1177/0146167297233008

Anderson, M. J. (1998). Reviving resistance in rape law. *University of Illinois Law Review, 1998*, 953–1012.

Angelone, D. J., Mitchell, D., & Grossi, L. (2015). Men's perceptions of an acquaintance rape: The role of relationship length, victim resistance, and gender role attitudes. *Journal of Interpersonal Violence, 30*, 2278–2303. https://doi.org/10.1177/0886260514552448

Angelone, D. J., Mitchell, D., & Lucente, L. (2012). Predicting perceptions of date rape: An examination of perpetrator motivation, relationship length, and gender role beliefs. *Journal of Interpersonal Violence, 27*, 2582–2602. https://doi.org/10.1177/0886260512436385

Ayala, E. E., Kotary, B., & Hetz, M. (2018). Blame attributions of victims and perpetrators: Effects of victim gender, perpetrator gender, and relationship. *Journal of Interpersonal Violence, 33*, 94–116. https://doi.org/10.1177/0886260515599160

Barnett, M. D., Hale, T. M., & Sligar, K. B. (2017). Masculinity, femininity, sexual dysfunctional beliefs, and rape myth acceptance among heterosexual college men and women. *Sexuality & Culture, 21*, 741–753. https://doi.org/10.1007/s12119-017-9420-3

Barnett, M. D., Sligar, K. B., & Wang, C. D. (2016). Religious affiliation, religiosity, gender, and rape myth acceptance: Feminist theory and rape culture. *Journal of Interpersonal Violence, 33*, 1219–1235. https://doi.org/10.1177/0886260516665110

Basow, S. A., & Minieri, A. (2011). "You owe me": Effects of date cost, who pays, participant gender, and rape myth beliefs on perceptions of rape. *Journal of Interpersonal Violence, 26*, 479–497. https://doi.org/10.1177/0886260510363421

Batchelder, J. S., Koski, D. D., & Byxbe, F. R. (2004). Women's hostility toward women in rape trials: Testing the intra-female gender hostility thesis. *American Journal of Criminal Justice, 28*, 181–200. https://doi.org/10.1007/BF02885871

Bergen, R. K. (2016). An overview of marital rape research in the United States: Limitations and implications for cross-cultural research. In K. Yllö & G. Torres (Eds.), *Marital rape: Consent, marriage, and social change in global context*. New York, NY: Oxford University Press.

Bieneck, S., & Krahe, B. (2011). Blaming the victim and exonerating the perpetrator in cases of rape and robbery: Is there a double standard? *Journal of Interpersonal Violence, 26*, 1785–1797. https://doi.org/10.1177/0886260510372945

Black, K. A., & Gold, D. J. (2003). Men's and women's reactions to hypothetical sexual advances: The role of initiator socioeconomic status and level of coercion. *Sex Roles, 49*, 173–178.

Black, K. A., & Gold, D. J. (2008). Gender differences and socioeconomic status biases in judgments about blame in date rape scenarios. *Violence and Victims, 23*, 115–128. https://doi.org/10.1891/0886-6708.23.1.115

Black, K. A., & McCloskey, K. A. (2013). Predicting date rape perceptions: The effects of gender, gender role attitudes, and victim resistance. *Violence Against Women, 19*, 949–967. https://doi.org/10.1177/1077801213499244

Bornstein, B. H., & Greene, E. (2017). Jurors in criminal cases can fairly punish wrongdoers. In *The jury under fire: Myth, controversy, and reform*. New York, NY: Oxford University Press.

Bourke, J. (2007). *Rape: A history from 1860 to the present*. London: Virago Press.

Branscombe, N. R., & Weir, J. A. (1992). Resistance as stereotype-inconsistency: Consequences for judgments of rape victims. *Journal of Social and Clinical Psychology, 11*, 80–102. https://doi.org/10.1521/jscp.1992.11.1.80

Brekke, N., & Borgida, E. (1988). Expert psychological testimony in rape trials: A social-cognitive analysis. *Journal of Personality and Social Psychology, 55*, 372–386.

Brown, A. L., Horton, J., & Guillory, A. (2018). The impact of victim alcohol consumption and perpetrator use of force on perceptions in an acquaintance rape vignette. *Violence and Victims, 33*, 40–52. https://doi.org/10.1891/0886-6708.33.1.40

Brown, K. A., McKimmie, B. M., & Zarkadi, T. (2018). The defendant with the prison tattoo: The effect of tattoos on mock jurors' perceptions. *Psychiatry, Psychology and Law, 25*, 386–403. https://doi.org/10.1080/13218719.2017.1412240

Burgess, A. W., & Holmstrom, L. L. (1974). Rape trauma syndrome. *American Journal of Psychiatry, 131*, 981–986. https://doi.org/10.1176/ajp.131.9.981

Burt, M. (1980). Cultural myths and supports for rape. *Journal of Personality and Social Psychology, 38*, 217–230. https://doi.org/10.1037/0022-3514.38.2.217

Carline, A., & Easteal, P. (2017). The court's response to intimate partner sexual violence perpetrators). In L. McOrmond-Plummer, J. Y. Levy-Peck, & P. Easteal (Eds.), *Perpetrators of intimate partner sexual violence: A multidisciplinary approach to prevention, recognition, and intervention* (pp. 143–152). New York, NY: Routledge.

Clarke, A. K., & Lawson, K. L. (2009). Women's judgments of a sexual assault scenario: The role of prejudicial attitudes and victim weight. *Violence and Victims, 24*, 248–264. https://doi.org/10.1891/0886-6708.24.2.248

Coates, L., & Wade, A. (2004). Telling it like it isn't: Obscuring perpetrator responsibility for violent crime. *Discourse & Society, 15*, 499–526. https://doi.org/10.1177/0957926504045031

Cochran, J. K., Marier, C. J., Jennings, W. G., Smith, M. D., Bjerregaard, B., & Fogel, S. J. (2017). Rape, race, and capital punishment: An enduring cultural legacy of lethal vengeance? *Race and Justice*, 1–18. https://doi.org/10.1177/2153368717702700

Cohn, E. S., Dupuis, E. C., & Brown, T. M. (2009). In the eye of the beholder: Do behavior and character affect victim and perpetrator responsibility for acquaintance rape? *Journal of Applied Social Psychology, 39*, 1513–1535. https://doi.org/10.1111/j.1559-1816.2009.00493.x

Cossins, A. (2013). Expert witness evidence in sexual assault trials: questions, answers and law reform in Australia and England. *International Journal of Evidence and Proof, 17*, 74–113. https://doi.org/10.1350/ijep.2013.17.1.419

Cowan, G. (2000). Women's hostility toward women and rape and sexual harassment myths. *Violence Against Women, 6*, 238–246. https://doi.org/10.1177/10778010022181822

Cowan, G., Neighbors, C., DeLaMoreaux, J., & Behnke, C. (1998). Women's hostility toward women. *Psychology of Women Quarterly, 22*, 267–284. https://doi.org/10.1111/j.1471-6402.1998.tb00154.x

Davies, M., Pollard, P., & Archer, J. (2001). The influence of victim gender and sexual orientation on judgments of the victim in a depicted stranger rape. *Violence and Victims, 16*, 607–619.

Davies, M., Pollard, P., & Archer, J. (2006). Effects of perpetrator gender and victim sexuality on blame toward male victims of sexual assault. *The Journal of Social Psychology, 146*, 275–291. https://doi.org/10.3200/SOCP.146.3.275-291

Davies, M., & Rogers, P. (2006). Perceptions of male victims in depicted sexual assault: A review of the literature. *Aggression and Violent Behavior, 11*, 357–367. https://doi.org/10.1016/j.avb.2006.01.002

Davies, M., Rogers, P., & Whitelegg, L. (2009). Effects of victim gender, victim sexual orientation, victim response and respondent gender on judgments of blame in a hypothetical adolescent rape. *Legal and Criminological Psychology, 14*, 331–338. https://doi.org/10.1348/978185408X386030

Davies, M., Smith, R., & Rogers, P. (2009). Police perceptions of rape as a function of victim gender and sexuality. *The Police Journal: Theory, Practice, and Principles, 82*, 4–12. https://doi.org/10.1350/pojo.2009.82.1.466

Davis, D. (1991). Facing justice and judging faces: What do they have in common? In D. Davis (Ed.), *From the Mind's eye* (Vol. 1, pp. 1–4).

Davis, D., & Loftus, E. F. (2004). What's good for the goose cooks the gander: Inconsistencies between the law and psychology of voluntary intoxication and sexual assault. In W. T. O'Donohue & E. Levensky (Eds.), *Handbook of forensic psychology: Resources for mental health and legal professionals* (pp. 997–1032). Boston, MA: Boston Academic Press.

Deitz, S. R., Litman, M., & Bentley, B. J. (1984). Attributions of responsibility for rape: The influence of observer empathy, victim resistance, and victim attractiveness. *Sex Roles, 10*, 261–280.

Devine, D. J., & Caughlin, D. E. (2014). Do they matter? A meta-analytic investigation of individual characteristics and guilt judgments. *Psychology, Public Policy, and Law, 20*, 109–134. https://doi.org/10.1037/law0000006

Dupuis, E. C., & Clay, J. A. (2013). The role of race and respectability in attributions of responsibility for acquaintance rape. *Violence and Victims, 28*, 1085–1096. https://doi.org/10.1891/0886-6708.VV-D-12-00013

Durán, M., Moya, M., Megías, J. L., & Viki, G. T. (2010). Social perception of rape victims in dating and married relationships: The role of perpetrator's benevolent sexism. *Sex Roles, 62*, 505–519. https://doi.org/10.1007/s11199-009-9676-7

Erian, M., Lin, C., Patel, N., Neal, A., & Geiselman, R. E. (1998). Juror verdicts as a function of victim and defendant attractiveness in sexual assault cases. *American Journal of Forensic Psychology, 16*, 25–40.

Estrich, S. (1987). *Real rape*. Camridge, MA: Harvard University Press.

Ewoldt, C. A., Monson, C. M., & Langhinrichsen-Rohling, J. (2000). Attributions about rape in a continuum of dissolving marital relationships. *Journal of Interpersonal Violence, 15*, 1175–1182. https://doi.org/10.1177/088626000015011004

Eyssel, F., & Bohner, G. (2011). Schema effects of rape myth acceptance on judgments of guilt and blame in rape cases: The role of perceived entitlement to judge. *Journal of Interpersonal Violence, 26*, 1579–1605. https://doi.org/10.1177/0886260510370593

Federal Bureau of Investigation. (2012). *UCR program changes definition of rape*. Retrieved from http://www.fbi.gov/about-us/cjis/cjis-link/march-2012/ucr-program-changesdefinition-of-rape.

Feild, H. S. (1978). Attitudes toward rape: A comparative analysis of police, rapists, crisis counselors, and citizens. *Journal of Personality and Social Psychology, 36*, 156–179. https://doi.org/10.1037/0022-3514.36.2.156

Ferguson, P. A., Duthie, D. A., & Graf, R. G. (1987). Attribution of responsibility to rapist and victim: The influence of victim's attractiveness and rape-related information. *Journal of Interpersonal Violence, 2*, 243–250. https://doi.org/10.1177/088626087002003001

Ferrão, M. C., Gonçalves, G., Ginger, J. C., & Parreira, T. (2015). Of rape and other demons: The impact of the victim's eye size and observer's gender on the attributions of responsibility. *Psychological Topics, 25*, 157–180.

Finkelhor, D., & Yllö, K. (1987). *License to rape: Sexual abuse of wives*. New York, NY: The Free Press.

Fisher, B., Cullen, F., & Turner, M. (2000). *The sexual victimization of college women*. Washington, DC: U.S. Department of Justice, National Institute of Justice and Bureau of Justice Statistics.

Fisher, N. L., & Pina, A. (2013). An overview of the literature on female-perpetrated adult male sexual victimization. *Aggression and Violent Behavior, 18*, 54–61. https://doi.org/10.1016/j.avb.2012.10.001

Frazier, P., & Borgida, E. (1988). Juror common understanding and the admissibility of rape trauma syndrome evidence in court. *Law and Human Behavior, 12*, 101–122.

Frazier, P. A., & Borgida, E. (1992). Rape trauma syndrome: A review of case law and psychological research. *Law and Human Behavior, 16*, 293–311.

Frese, B., Moya, M., & Medias, J. (2004). Social perception of rape: How Rape Myth Acceptance modulates the influence of situational factors. *Journal of Interpersonal Violence, 19*, 143–161. https://doi.org/10.1177/0886260503260245

Funk, F., & Todorov, A. (2013). Criminal stereotypes in the courtroom: Facial tattoos affect guilt and punishment differently. *Psychology, Public Policy, and Law, 19*, 466–478. https://doi.org/10.1037/a0034736

Gerber, G. L., Cronin, J. M., & Steigman, H. (2004). Attributions of blame in sexual assault to perpetrators and victims of both genders. *Journal of Applied Social Psychology, 34*, 2149–2165. https://doi.org/10.1111/j.1559-1816.2004.tb02694.x

Gerdes, E. P., Dammann, E. J., & Heilig, K. E. (1988). Perceptions of rape victims and assailants: Effects of physical attractiveness, acquaintance, and subject gender. *Sex Roles, 19*, 141–153.

Gleason, J. M., & Harris, V. A. (1975). Race, socioeconomic status, and perceived similarity as determinants of judgments by simulated jurors. *Social Behavior and Personality, 3*, 175–180. https://doi.org/10.2224/sbp.1975.3.2.175

Glick, P., & Fiske, S. (1996). The ambivalent sexism inventory: Differentiating hostile and benevolent sexism. *Journal of Personality and*

Social Psychology, 70, 491–512. https://doi.org/10.1037/0022-3514.70.3.491

Glick, P., & Fiske, S. (2011). Ambivalent sexism revisited. *Psychology of Women Quarterly, 35*, 530–535. https://doi.org/10.1177/0361684311414832

Graham, R. (2006). Male rape and the careful construction of the male victim. *Social & Legal Studies, 15*, 187–208. https://doi.org/10.1177/0964663906063571

Grubb, A., & Turner, E. (2012). Attribution of blame in rape cases: A review of the impact of rape myth acceptance, gender role conformity and substance use on victim blaming. *Aggression and Violent Behavior, 17*, 443–452. https://doi.org/10.1016/j.avb.2012.06.002

Hammond, E. M., Berry, M. A., & Rodriguez, D. N. (2011). The influence of rape myth acceptance, sexual attitudes, and belief in a just world on attributions of responsibility in a date rape scenario. *Legal and Criminological Psychology, 16*, 242–252.

Hine, B., & Murphy, A. (2017). The impact of victim-perpetrator relationship, reputation and initial point of resistance on officers' responsibility and authenticity ratings toward hypothetical rape cases. *Journal of Criminal Justice, 49*, 1–13. https://doi.org/10.1016/j.jcrimjus.2017.01.001

Hust, S. J., Lei, M., Ren, C., Chang, H., McNab, A. L., Marett, E. G., & Willoughby, J. F. (2013). The effects of sports media exposure on college students' rape myth beliefs and intentions to intervene in a sexual assault. *Mass Communication and Society, 16*, 762–786.

Jacobson, M. B., & Popovich, P. M. (1983). Victim attractiveness and perceptions of responsibility in an ambiguous rape case. *Psychology of Women Quarterly, 8*, 100–104. https://doi.org/10.1111/j.1471-6402.1983.tb00621.x

Javaid, A. (2018). Male rape, masculinities, and sexualities. *International Journal of Law, Crime and Justice, 52*, 199–210. https://doi.org/10.1016/j.ijlcj.2017.12.003

Johnson, K. K., Ju, H. W., & Wu, J. (2016). Young adults' inferences surrounding an alleged sexual assault: Alcohol consumption, gender, dress, and appearance schematicity. *Clothing and Textiles Research Journal, 34*, 127–142. https://doi.org/10.1177/0887302X15624550

Jones, C., & Aronson, E. (1973). Attribution of fault to a rape victim as a function of respectability of the victim. *Journal of Personality and Social Psychology, 26*, 415–419. https://doi.org/10.1037/h0034463

Jozkowski, K. N., & Peterson, Z. D. (2013). College students and sexual consent: Unique insights. *Journal of Sex Research, 50*, 517–523. https://doi.org/10.1080/00224499

Kahn, A. (1977). Attribution of fault to a rape victim as a function of respectability of the victim: A failure to replicate or extend. *Representative Research in Social Psychology, 8*, 98–107.

Kanekar, S., & Kolsawalla, M. B. (1977). Responsibility in relation to respectability. *The Journal of Social Psychology, 102*, 183–188. https://doi.org/10.1080/00224545.1977.9713263

Kanekar, S., & Kolsawalla, M. B. (1980). Responsibility of a rape victim in relation to her respectability, attractiveness, and provocativeness. *The Journal of Social Psychology, 112*, 153–154. https://doi.org/10.1080/00224545.1980.9924310

Kassing, L. R., Beesley, D., & Frey, L. L. (2005). Gender role conflict, homophobia, age, and education as predictors of male rape myth acceptance. *Journal of Mental Health Counseling, 27*, 311–328. https://doi.org/10.17744/mehc.27.4.9wfm24f52kqgav37

Katz, J. (2015). Effects of group status and victim sex on male bystanders' responses to a potential party rape. *Journal of Aggression, Maltreatment & Trauma, 24*, 588–602. https://doi.org/10.1080/10926771.2015.1029184

Kerr, N. L., & Kurtz, S. T. (1977). Effects of a victim's suffering and respectability on mock juror judgments: Further evidence on the just world theory. *Representative Research in Social Psychology, 8*, 42–56.

King, L. L., & Hanrahan, K. J. (2015). University student beliefs about sexual violence in prison: Rape myth acceptance, punitiveness, and empathy. *Journal of Sexual Aggression, 21*, 179–193. https://doi.org/10.1080/13552600.2013.820851

Kirkwood, M. K., & Cecil, D. K. (2001). Marital rape: A student assessment of rape laws and the marital exemption. *Violence Against Women, 7*, 1234–1253. https://doi.org/10.1177/10778012010070011003

Kleinke, C. L., & Meyer, C. (1990). Evaluation of rape victim by men and women with high and low belief in a just world. *Psychology of Women Quarterly, 14*, 343–353. https://doi.org/10.1111/j.1471-6402.1990.tb00024.x

Knight, J. L., Giuliano, T. A., & Sanchez-Ross, M. G. (2001). Famous or infamous? The influence of celebrity status and race on perceptions of responsibility for rape. *Basic and Applied Social Psychology, 23*, 183–190. https://doi.org/10.1207/S15324834BASP2303_4

Kopper, B. A. (1996). Gender, gender identity, rape myth acceptance, and time of initial resistance on the perception of acquaintance rape blame and avoidability. *Sex Roles, 34*, 81–93.

Krahe, B., Temkin, J., & Bieneck, S. (2007). Schema-driven information processing in judgements about rape. *Applied Cognitive Psychology, 21*, 601–619. https://doi.org/10.1002/(ISSN)1099-0720

Lennon, S. J., Adomaitis, A. D., Koo, J., & Johnson, K. K. (2017). Dress and sex: A review of empirical research involving human participants and published in refereed journals. *Fashion and Textiles, 4*, 1–21. https://doi.org/10.1186/s40691-017-0101-5

Lindren, K. P., Parkhill, M. R., George, W. H., & Hendershot, C. S. (2008). Gender differences in perceptions of sexual intent: A qualitative review and integration. *Psychology of Women Quarterly, 32*, 423–439. https://doi.org/10.1111/j.1471-6402.2008.00456.x

Lonsway, K. A., & Fitzgerald, L. F. (1994). Rape myths: In review. *Psychology of Women Quarterly, 18*, 133–164. https://doi.org/10.1111/j.1471-6402.1994.tb00448.x

Lowe, M., & Rogers, P. (2017). The scope of male rape: A selective review of research, policy and practice. *Aggression and Violent Behavior, 35*, 38–43. https://doi.org/10.1016/j.avb.2017.06.007

Luginbuhl, J., & Mullin, C. (1981). Rape and responsibility: How and how much is the victim blamed? *Sex Roles, 7*, 547–559.

Lynch, K. R., Golding, J. M., Jewell, J. A., Lippert, A., & Wasarhaley, N. E. (2018). "She is his girlfriend—I believe this is a different situation": Gender differences in perceptions of the legality of intimate partner rape. *Journal of Family Violence*, 1–18.

Mackelprang, E., & Becker, J. V. (2017). Beauty and the eye of the beholder: Gender and attractiveness affect judgments in teacher sex offense cases. *Sexual Abuse, 29*, 375–395. https://doi.org/10.1177/1079063215597646

Maeder, E. M., Yamamoto, S., & Saliba, P. (2015). The influence of defendant race and victim physical attractiveness on juror decision-making in a sexual assault trial. *Psychology, Crime, & Law, 21*, 62–79. https://doi.org/10.1080/1068316X.2014.915325

Manne, K. (2018, September). Brett Kavanaugh and America's "himpathy" reckoning. *The New York Times*. Retrieved from https://www.nytimes.com/2018/09/26/opinion/brett-kavanaugh-hearing-himpathy.html

Mazzella, R., & Feingold, A. (1994). The effects of physical attractiveness, race, socioeconomic status, and gender of defendants and victims on judgments of mock jurors: A meta-analysis. *Journal of Applied Social Psychology, 24*, 1315–1344. https://doi.org/10.1111/j.1559-1816.1994.tb01552.x

McCaul, K. D., Veltum, L. G., Boyechko, V., & Crawford, J. J. (1990). Understanding attributions of blame for rape: Sex, violence, and foreseeability. *Journal of Applied Social Science, 20*, 1–26. https://doi.org/10.1111/j.1559-1816.1990.tb00375.x

McCormick, J. S., Maric, A., Seto, M. C., & Barbaree, H. E. (1998). Relationship to victim predicts sentence length in sexual assault cases. *Journal of Interpersonal Violence, 13*, 413–420. https://doi.org/10.1177/088626098013003007

McCracken, E. W., & Stevenson, M. C. (2017). Rape perpetrator gender shapes liability judgments: Implications for disgust and moral outrage. *Translational Issues in Psychological Science, 3*, 153–166.

McMahon, S., & Farmer, G. L. (2011). An updated measure for assessing subtle rape myths. *Social Work Research, 35*, 71–81. https://doi.org/10.1093/swr/35.2.71

Mills, C. S., & Granoff, B. J. (1992). Date and acquaintance rape among a sample of college students. *Social Work, 37*, 504–509. https://doi.org/10.1093/sw/37.6.504

Mitchell, D., Angelone, D. E., Kohlberger, B., & Hirschman, R. (2009). Effects of offender motivation, victim gender, and participant gender on perceptions of rape victims and offenders. *Journal of Interpersonal Violence, 24*, 1564–1578. https://doi.org/10.1177/0886260508323662

Mitchell, T. L., Haw, R. M., Pfeifer, J. E., & Meissner, C. A. (2005). Racial bias in mock juror decision-making: A meta-analytic review of defendant treatment. *Law and Human Behavior, 29*, 621–637.

Monson, C. M., Langhinrichsen-Rohling, J., & Binderup, T. (2000). Does "no" really mean "no" after you say "yes": Attributions about date and marital rape. *Journal of Interpersonal Violence, 15*, 1156–1174. https://doi.org/10.1177/088626000015011003

Muehlenhard, C. L., & Hollabaugh, L. C. (1988). Do women sometimes say no when they mean yes? The prevalence and correlates of women's token resistance to sex. *Journal of Personality and Social Psychology, 54*, 872–879. https://doi.org/10.1037/0022-3514.54.5.872

Nagel, B., Matsuo, H., McIntyre, K. P., & Morrison, N. (2005). Attitudes towards victims of rape: Effects of gender, race, religion and social class. *Journal of Interpersonal Violence, 20*, 725–737. https://doi.org/10.1177/0886260505276072

Nyúl, B., Kende, A., Engyel, M., & Szabó, M. (2018). Perception of a perpetrator as a successful person predicts decreased moral judgement of a rape case and labelling it as rape. *Frontiers in Psychology, 9*, 1–12. https://doi.org/10.3389/fpsyg.2018.02555

O'Donohue, W., Carlson, G. C., Benuto, L. T., & Bennett, N. M. (2014). Examining the scientific validity of rape trauma syndrome. *Psychiatry, Psychology and Law, 21*, 858–876. https://doi.org/10.1080/13218719.2014.918067

Omata, K. (2013). Factors affecting bystanders' blame of a sex-crime victim and assessment of psychological damage: Reputation of victims and prejudice about women's desire for violent sex. *The Japanese Journal of Social Psychology, 29*(1), 1–10.

Ong, A. S. J., & Ward, C. A. (1999). The effects of sex and power schemas, attitudes toward women, and victim resistance on rape attributions. *Journal of Applied Social Psychology, 29*(2), 362–376. https://doi.org/10.1111/j.1559-1816.1999.tb01391.x

Osman, S. L. (2003). Predicting men's rape perceptions based on the belief that "no" really means "yes". *Journal of Applied Social Psychology, 33*, 683–692. https://doi.org/10.1111/j.1559-1816.2003.tb01919.x

Osman, S. L. (2011). Predicting rape empathy based on victim, perpetrator, and participant gender, and history of sexual aggression. *Sex Roles: A Journal of Research, 64*, 506–515.

Page, A. D. (2010). True colors: Police officers and rape myth acceptance. *Feminist Criminology, 5*, 315–334. https://doi.org/10.1177/1557085110384108

Perilloux, C., Easton, J. A., & Buss, D. M. (2012). The misperception of sexual interest. *Psychological Science, 23*, 146–151. https://doi.org/10.1177/0956797611424162

Persson, S., Dhingra, K., & Grogan, S. (2018). Attributions of victim blame in stranger and acquaintance rape: A quantitative study. *Journal of Clinical Nursing, 27*, 2640–2649. https://doi.org/10.1111/jocn.14351

Proite, R., Dannells, M., & Benton, S. L. (1993). Gender, sex-role stereotypes, and the attribution of responsibility for date and acquaintance rape. *Journal of College Student Development, 34*, 411–417.

Quinn, K., Sanchez-Hucles, J., Coates, G., & Gillen, B. (1991). Men's compliance with a woman's resistance to unwanted sexual advances. *Journal of Offender Rehabilitation, 17*, 13–31. https://doi.org/10.1300/J076v17n01_02

RAINN. (2016). *Statistics*. Retrieved from https://www.rainn.org/statistics

Reddington, F. P., & Kreisel, B. W. (2017). *Sexual assault: The victim, the perpetrator, and the criminal justice system*. Durham, NC: Carolina Academic Press.

Rhode, D. L. (2010). *The beauty bias: The injustice of appearance in life and law*. New York, NY: Oxford University Press.

Rumsey, M. G., & Rumsey, J. M. (1977). A case of rape: Sentencing judgments of males and females. *Psychological Reports, 41*, 459–465. https://doi.org/10.2466/pr0.1977.41.2.459

Russell, B. L., Oswald, D. L., & Kraus, S. W. (2011). Evaluations of sexual assault: Perceptions of guilt and legal elements for male and female aggressors using various coercive strategies. *Violence and Victims, 26*, 799–815.

Russell, D. E. H. (1990). *Rape in marriage*. Bloomington, IN: Indiana University Press. https://doi.org/10.1891/0886-6708.26.6.799

Russell, K. J., & Hand, C. J. (2017). Rape myth acceptance, victim blame attribution and just world beliefs: A rapid evidence assessment. *Aggression and Violent Behavior, 37*, 153–160. https://doi.org/10.1016/j.avb.2017.10.008

Rye, B. J., Greatrix, S. A., & Enright, C. S. (2006). The case of the guilty victim: The effects of gender of victim and gender of perpetrator on attributions of blame and responsibility. *Sex Roles, 54*(10), 639–649

Schuller, R. A., & Wall, A. M. (1998). The effects of defendant and complainant intoxication on mock jurors' judgments of sexual assault. *Psychology of Women Quarterly, 22*, 555–573. https://doi.org/10.1111/j.1471-6402.1998.tb00177.x

Schvey, N. A., Puhl, R. M., Levandoski, K. A., & Brownell, K. D. (2013). The influence of defendant's body weight on perceptions of guilt. *International Journal of Obesity, 37*, 1275–1281.

Scully, D., & Marolla, J. (1984). Convicted rapists' vocabulary of motive: Excuses and justifications. *Social Problems, 31*, 530–543. https://doi.org/10.2307/800239

Shaver, K. G. (1970). Defensive attribution: Effects of severity and relevance on the responsibility assigned for an accident. *Journal of Personality and Social Psychology, 14*, 101–113. https://doi.org/10.1037/h0028777

Shaver, K. G. (1985). *The attribution of blame*. New York, NY: Springer-Verlag.

Shotland, R. L., & Goodstein, L. (1983). Just because she doesn't want to doesn't mean it's rape: An experimentally based causal model of the perception of rape in a dating situation. *Social Psychology Quarterly, 46*, 220–232. https://doi.org/10.2307/3033793

Simonson, K., & Subich, L. M. (1999). Rape perceptions as a function of gender-role traditionality and victim-perpetrator association. *Sex Roles, 40*, 617–634.

Sleath, E., & Bull, R. (2017). Police perceptions of rape victims and the impact on case decision making: A systematic review. *Aggression and Violent Behavior, 34*, 102–112. https://doi.org/10.1016/j.avb.2017.02.003

Smith, R. E., Pine, C. J., & Hawley, M. E. (1988). Social cognitions about adult male victims of female sexual assault. *Journal of Sex Research, 24*, 101–112. https://doi.org/10.1080/00224498809551401

Sprecher, S., Hatfield, E., Cortese, A., Potapova, E., & Levitskaya, A. (1994). Token resistance to sexual intercourse and consent to unwanted sexual intercourse: College students' dating experiences in three countries. *Journal of Sex Research, 31*, 125–132. https://doi.org/10.1080/00224499409551739

Struckman-Johnson, C., & Struckman-Johnson, D. (1992). Acceptance of male rape myths among college men and women. *Sex Roles, 27*, 85–100.

Suarez, E., & Gadalla, T. M. (2010). Stop blaming the victim: A meta-analysis on rape myths. *Journal of Interpersonal Violence, 25*, 2010–2035. https://doi.org/10.1177/0886260509354503

Sullivan, J. P., & Mosher, D. L. (1990). Acceptance of guided imagery of marital rape as a function of macho personality. *Violence and Victims, 5*(4), 275–286. https://doi.org/10.1891/0886-6708.5.4.275

Süssenbach, P., Eyssel, F., Rees, J., & Bohner, G. (2017). Looking for blame: Rape myth acceptance and attention to victim and perpetrator. *Journal of Interpersonal Violence, 32*(15), 2323–2344. https://doi.org/10.1177/0886260515591975

Sweeney, L. T., & Haney, C. (1992). The influence of race on sentencing: A meta-analytic review of experimental studies. *Behavioral Sciences & the Law, 10*, 179–195. https://doi.org/10.1002/bsl.2370100204

Tannura, T. A. (2014). Rape trauma syndrome. *American Journal of Sexuality Education, 9*, 247–256. https://doi.org/10.1080/15546128.2014.883267

Testa, M. (2002). The impact of men's alcohol consumption on perpetration of sexual aggression. *Clinical Psychology Review, 22*, 1239–1263. https://doi.org/10.1016/S0272-7358(02)00204-0

Todorov, A. (2017). *Face value: The irresistible influence of first impressions*. Princeton, NJ: Princeton University Press.

Ullman, S. E., & Knight, R. A. (1995). Women's resistance strategies to different rapist types. *Criminal Justice and Behavior, 22*, 263–283.

Van der Bruggen, M., & Grubb, A. (2014). A review of the literature relating to rape victim blaming: An analysis of the impact of observer and victim characteristics on attribution of blame in rape cases. *Aggression and Violent Behavior, 19*, 523–531. https://doi.org/10.1016/j.avb.2014.07.008

Vaughan, A. E. (2001). The association between offender socioeconomic status and victim-offender relationship in rape offences. *Psychology, Evolution & Gender, 3*, 121–136. https://doi.org/10.1080/14616660110067357

Venema, R. M. (2016). Police officer schema of sexual assault reports: Real rape, ambiguous cases, and false reports. *Journal of Interpersonal Violence, 31*, 872–899. https://doi.org/10.1177/0886260514556765

Viki, G. T., & Abrams, D. (2002). But she was unfaithful: Benevolent sexism and reactions to rape victims who violate traditional gender role expectations. *Sex Roles, 47*, 289–293.

Viki, G. T., Abrams, D., & Masser, B. (2004). Evaluating stranger and acquaintance rape: The role of benevolent sexism in perpetrator blame and recommended sentence length. *Law and Human Behavior, 28*, 295–303. https://doi.org/10.1023/B:LAHU.0000029140.72880.69

Vrij, A., & Firmin, H. R. (2001). Beautiful thus innocent? The impact of defendants' and victims' physical attractiveness and participants' rape beliefs on impression formation in alleged rape cases. *International Review of Victimology, 8*, 245–255. https://doi.org/10.1177/026975800100800301

Ward, C. A. (1988). The attitudes toward rape victims scale: Construction, validation, and cross cultural applicability. *Psychology of Women Quarterly, 12*, 127–146. https://doi.org/10.1111/j.1471-6402.1988.tb00932.x

Ward, C. A. (1995). *Attitudes toward rape: Feminist and social psychological perspectives*. London, UK: Sage.

Warner, A., & Hewitt, J. (1993). Victim resistance and judgments of victim "consensuality" in rape. *Perceptual and Motor Skills, 76*, 952–954. https://doi.org/10.2466/pms.1993.76.3.952

Weis, K., & Borges, S. S. (1973). Victimology and rape: The case of the legitimate victim. *Issues Criminology, 8*, 71–116. Retrieved from https://heinonline.org/HOL/P?h=hein.journals/iscrim8&i=197

Westfall, R. S., Millar, M., & Lovitt, A. (2018). The influence of physical attractiveness on belief in a just world. *Psychological Reports*, 1–14. https://doi.org/10.1177/0033294118763172

Whatley, M. A. (1994). *Factors Affecting Attributions of Blame for Date Rape. Poster presented at the annual meeting of the Society for Southeastern Social Psychologists*. NC: Winston-Salem.

Whatley, M. A. (1996). Victim characteristics influencing attributions of responsibility to rape victims: A meta-analysis. *Aggression and Violent Behavior, 1*, 81–95. https://doi.org/10.1016/1359-1789(95)00011-9

Whatley, M. A. (2005). The effect of participant sex, victim dress, and traditional attitudes on causal judgments for marital rape victims. *Journal of Family Violence, 20*, 191–200. https://doi.org/10.1007/s10896-005-3655-8

Whatley, M. A., & Riggio, R. E. (1993). Gender differences in attributions of blame for male rape victims. *Journal of Interpersonal Violence, 8*, 502–511. https://doi.org/10.1177/088626093008004005

White, B. H., & Kurpius, S. E. R. (2002). Effects of victim sex and sexual orientation on perceptions of rape. *Sex Roles, 46*, 191–200. https://doi.org/10.1177/0886260514549466

Williams, J. E. (1984). Secondary victimization: Confronting public attitudes about rape. *Victimization: An International Journal, 9*, 66–81.

Willis, C. E. (1992). The effect of sex role stereotype, victim and defendant race, and prior relationship on rape culpability attributions. *Sex Roles, 26*, 213–226.

Yescavage, K. (1999). Teaching women a lesson: Sexually aggressive and sexually nonaggressive men's perceptions of acquaintance and date rape. *Violence Against Women, 5*, 796–812. https://doi.org/10.1177/10778019922181482

Yllö, K., & Torres, M. G. (2016). *Marital rape: Consent, marriage, and social change in global context*. New York, NY: Oxford University Press.

Yndo, M. C., & Zawacki, T. (2017). Factors influencing labeling nonconsensual sex as sexual assault. *Journal of Interpersonal Violence*, 1–25. https://doi.org/10.1177/088620517699948

Policing Sexual Assault: Lessons Learned in Los Angeles

34

Katharine Tellis and Cassia Spohn

In this chapter, we analyze police and prosecutorial decision making in sexual assault cases because our research in Los Angeles revealed that decisions made by police and prosecutors cannot be examined in isolation from one another (Spohn & Tellis, 2012, 2014, 2018). Examining only cases that are formally cleared by arrest or focusing only on charging decisions that follow the arrest of a suspect may be ignoring important aspects of police and prosecutorial decision making and may lead to misleading conclusions about the factors that influence arrest and charging decisions. It is important to disentangle these overlapping decisions and, in so doing, illuminate the ways that law enforcement policies and practices contribute to high rates of sexual assault case attrition.

Prior Research on Prosecuting Sexual Assault

There is very limited research on police decision making in sexual assault cases and much of the research that does exist is dated. Researchers have examined the decision to unfound the charges (Alderden & Ullman, 2012; Kerstetter, 1990; LaFree, 1989; Spohn, White, & Tellis, 2014), the decision to make an arrest (Alderden & Ullman, 2012; Bachman, 1998; Bouffard, 2000; Du Mont & Myhr, 2000; Horney & Spohn, 1996; LaFree, 1981), and the decision to present the case to the prosecutor for charge evaluation (Alderden & Ullman, 2012; Spohn & Tellis, 2014). These studies reveal that police decision making is influenced by a combination of legal and extra-legal factors. An early study (LaFree, 1981), for example, found that the decision to arrest was affected by the victim's ability to identify the suspect, the victim's willingness to prosecute, whether the victim engaged in any type of misconduct at the time of the incident, the promptness of the victim's report, whether the victim was assaulted by an acquaintance rather than a stranger, and the suspect's use of a weapon. On the other hand, the arrest decision was not affected by the victim's race, whether the victim resisted, the location of the incident, whether there was a witness who could corroborate the victim's allegations, or whether the victim was injured. These findings led LaFree (1981) to conclude that the emphasis on the role played by the victim's background characteristics was "greatly overstated" and that "legally relevant variables were paramount" (p. 592). However, more recent research calls this conclusion into question. Bouffard (2000) found that arrest was more likely if the victim and suspect had a prior relationship, the victim agreed to undergo a sexual assault exam,

K. Tellis (✉)
California State University at Los Angeles, Los Angeles, CA, USA
e-mail: ktellis@calstatela.edu

C. Spohn
Arizona State University, Phoenix, AZ, USA

W. T. O'Donohue and P. A. Schewe (eds.), *Handbook of Sexual Assault and Sexual Assault Prevention*, https://doi.org/10.1007/978-3-030-23645-8_34

and the credibility/seriousness score of the crime was higher. Alderden and Ullman (2012) similarly found that police decision making was determined primarily by extra-legal factors—the victim's preference for how the case should be handled, discrepancies in victim statements, and victim resistance—while Schuller and Stewart (2000) found that police officers' responses to sexual assault vignettes were affected by the intoxication and credibility of the complainant.

The findings regarding prosecutors' charging decisions in sexual assault cases are very similar. This research, which is much more extensive than the research on police decision making, reveals that although these decisions are strongly influenced by legally relevant factors such as the seriousness of the crime, the offender's prior criminal record, and the strength of the evidence in the case (Alderden & Ullman, 2012; Frazier & Haney, 1996; Kingsnorth, MacIntosh, & Wentworth, 1999; Spohn & Holleran, 2001; Tellis & Spohn, 2008), victim characteristics also play a role. Studies have documented the influence of the victim's age, occupation, and education (McCahill, Meyer, & Fischman, 1979), "risk-taking" behavior such as hitchhiking, drinking, or using drugs (Alderden & Ullman, 2012; LaFree, 1981; McCahill et al., 1979; Spohn & Holleran, 2001; Tellis & Spohn, 2008), and the character or reputation of the victim (Alderden & Ullman, 2012; Feldman-Summers & Lindner, 1976; Field & Bienen, 1980; Martin & Powell, 1994; McCahill et al., 1979; Reskin & Visher, 1986; Spohn, Beichner, & Davis-Frenzel, 2001).

Research also has demonstrated that the relationship between the victim and the accused has a significant effect on charging decisions in sexual assault cases. Consistent with Black's (1976) relational distance theory, these studies conclude that reports of sexual assaults by strangers are less likely than reports of sexual assaults by acquaintances or intimate partners to be rejected by the prosecutor (Alderden & Ullman, 2012; Spohn et al., 2001; Tellis & Spohn, 2008); sexual assaults involving strangers also are more likely to result in police and prosecutor agreement on the severity of charges to be filed (Holleran, Beichner, & Spohn, 2010). Other studies find that different predictors affect charging decisions in stranger and acquaintance cases (Kingsnorth et al., 1999; Spohn & Holleran, 2001). Spohn and Holleran (2001), for example, found that characteristics of the victim affected charging decisions only in cases involving non-strangers and that the suspect's use of a gun or knife affected charging only in cases involving strangers.

Two studies used qualitative data to explore in more detail the reasons why prosecutors reject charges in sexual assault cases (Frohmann, 1991; Spohn et al., 2001; see also, Frohmann, 1997). The notion that decisions in rape cases are affected by the "typifications of rape held by processing agents" (LaFree, 1989: 241) plays a central role in the research conducted by Frohmann (1991, 1997), who used data gathered during observations of the case screening process and interviews with prosecutors to analyze explanations of and justifications for case rejection. Frohmann (1991) asserted that prosecutors' concerns about convictability led them to question the credibility of the rape victim and the veracity of her story. She found that prosecutors used inconsistencies in the victim's story, incongruities between the victim's account and prosecutors' beliefs about "typical" rapes, and assertions about ulterior motives on the part of the victim to justify case rejection. Spohn and her colleagues (Spohn et al., 2001) used data on sexual assaults cleared by arrest in Miami to replicate and extend Frohmann's (1991) research. Their examination of prosecutors' written justifications for rejecting charges in these cases led them to conclude that the prosecutor's assessment of the likelihood of conviction was based on factors other than typifications of rape and rape victims. In a substantial number of their cases, the decision to reject charges could be traced to the victim's failure to appear for a pre-file interview, the victim's refusal to cooperate in the prosecution of the case, or the victim's admission that the charges were fabricated. As they noted, in these types of cases "the odds of conviction were low (or nonexistent), not because the prosecutor believed that the facts in the case contradicted potential jurors' assumptions about rape and rape victims, but because the unavailability of a victim who was willing to testify made it impossible to proceed with the case" (Spohn et al., 2001: 228).

In summary, prior research on police and prosecutorial decisions in sexual assault cases suggests that these decisions are affected by a combination of legal and extra-legal factors. As they evaluate cases and assess the likelihood of prosecution and conviction, police and prosecutors consider, not only the seriousness of the offense and the strength of evidence against the defendant but also the characteristics, behavior, and reputation of the victim, the relationship between the victim and the suspect, and the willingness of the victim to cooperate in the investigation of the case.

Theoretical Perspectives on Police and Prosecutor Decision Making

Research on police and prosecutor decision making is somewhat atheoretical. Black (1976, 1980, 1989) contended that police decision making is predictable from the sociological theory of law, which holds that the quantity of law applied in any particular situation depends on factors such as the social status of those involved, the relational distance between the parties, and the degree of informal social control to which the parties are subjected. In discussing the investigation of crimes by detectives, Black (1980) argued the amount of time and energy that will be devoted to a case will depend, not only on the seriousness of the crime but also on the social status, background, reputation, and credibility of the victim and suspect. Although this perspective has not been applied to decisions made by prosecutors, it clearly is relevant. Prosecutors, like police, will devote more resources to cases that have a strong likelihood of a successful outcome.

Another theoretical perspective applicable to decision making in sexual assault cases is the focal concerns perspective (Steffensmeier, Ulmer, & Kramer, 1997). Although this perspective was developed to explain judges' sentencing decisions, it has been applied to prosecutors' charging decisions (see, for example, Spohn et al., 2001) and, as we explain below, is also relevant to police decision making. According to this perspective, judges' sentencing decisions are guided by three focal concerns: their assessment of the blameworthiness of the offender; their desire to protect the community by incapacitating dangerous offenders or deterring potential offenders; and their concerns about the practical consequences, or social costs, of sentencing decisions. The first focal concern—offender blameworthiness—reflects judges' assessments of the seriousness of the crime, the offender's prior criminal record, and the offender's motivation and role in the offense. By contrast, the second focal concern—protecting the community—rests on judges' perceptions of the dangerousness and threat posed by the offender and the offender's likelihood of recidivism. Judges' concerns about the practical consequences or social costs of sentencing decisions reflect their perceptions regarding the offender's ability "to do time" and the costs of incarcerating offenders with medical conditions, mental health problems, or dependent children, as well as their concerns about maintaining relationships with other members of the courtroom workgroup and protecting the reputation of the court.

We suggest that the focal concerns that guide police and prosecutor decision making in sexual assault cases are similar, but not identical, to those that guide judges' sentencing decisions. Like judges, police officers and prosecuting attorneys consider the seriousness of the crime, the degree of injury to the victim, and the blameworthiness and dangerousness of the offender. They also are concerned about the practical consequences or social costs of their decisions, but their concerns focus more on the likelihood of conviction than the costs of incarceration. Although, technically, police decisions to unfound the report or arrest the suspect do not rest on an assessment of convictability, as a practical matter the police do take this into consideration. They view the decision to arrest as the first step in the process of securing a conviction in the case; as a result, they are reluctant to make arrests that are unlikely to lead to the filing of charges against the suspect.

We suggest that this concern with convictability creates what Frohmann (1997) refers to as a "downstream orientation" to decision makers who will handle the case at subsequent stages of the process (pg. 535). Whereas Frohmann (1997), whose work focused on charging decisions in sexual assault cases, argued that prosecutors consider how the judge, jury, and defense attorney will react to the case, we contend that the downstream orientation of detectives investigating sexual assault cases is to the prosecutors who make filing decisions. That is, detectives attempt to predict how prosecutors will assess and respond to the case. Because prosecutors' assessments of cases are based on a standard of convictability that encourages them "to accept only 'strong' or 'winnable' cases for prosecution" (Frohmann, 1991, p. 215), this means that detectives' decisions similarly will reflect their assessment of the likelihood of conviction should an arrest be made. In sexual assault cases, in which the victim's testimony is crucial, these assessments rest squarely on an evaluation of the victim's credibility. As a result, if the victim's allegations are inconsistent or do not comport with detectives' beliefs about the typical sexual assault or if the detective believes that the victim has ulterior motives for reporting the crime or will not cooperate as the case moves forward, the likelihood of arrest will decrease.

Both the sociological theory of law and the focal concerns perspective suggest that the "social structure" (Black, 1989) of the case influences how the case will be handled. As stated by Black (1989), "the handling of a case always reflects the social characteristics of those involved in it" (pg. 21) Similarly, the focal concerns perspective holds that the limited information available about the case, especially at early stages in the process, means that decision makers will "rely on attributional decision making processes that invoke societal stereotypes" (Johnson & Betsinger, 2009, p. 1055). In the context of police and prosecutor decision making generally and decisions to arrest and charge specifically, these perspectives suggest not only that the social status of the complainant and suspect will be influential, but that stereotypes of "real rapes" (Estrich, 1987) and "genuine victims" (LaFree, 1989) will also play a role. Thus, decisions to arrest and to charge the suspect will be based on a combination of factors related to crime seriousness and victim credibility. These perspectives suggest that arrest and prosecution will be more likely if the crime is serious, the victim and suspect are strangers, the victim was injured, the victim's allegations are consistent with detectives' "typifications of rape scenarios" (Frohmann, 1991, p. 217), and the victim is viewed as credible and without ulterior motives for making allegations against the suspect.

Policy and Practice in the Investigation and Prosecution of Sexual Assault in Los Angeles

Spohn and Tellis' (2012) research revealed that reports of sexual assault are handled differently by the Los Angeles Police Department (LAPD) and the Los Angeles County Sheriff's Department (LASD). Crimes reported to the LAPD are initially handled by a uniformed patrol officer in one of the LAPD's 21 divisions. The responding officer will prepare the initial report of the crime based on the statements of the victim and witnesses (if any); included will be a description of the suspect and, if known, identifying information about the suspect. If the crime was reported promptly, the responding officer also will collect evidence from the scene of the crime and from the victim and, if she agrees, transport the victim to a rape treatment center or other medical facility for a forensic medical exam. The case is then investigated by one of the detectives in that division who handles sex crimes.

At the time of data collection, the LASD had a bifurcated approach to the investigation of sexual assault based on the age of the victim (Spohn & Tellis, 2012). Crimes involving victims 18 years old or older were handled in much the same way as are all sexual assaults reported to the LAPD; the initial report is taken by a sheriff's deputy in the jurisdiction where the crime occurred and the case is then assigned to a detective from the station house in that jurisdiction. Crimes involving victims under the age of 18 were referred to the Special Victims Bureau; detectives assigned to this unit take the report from the victim and investigate the crime.

For both agencies the follow-up investigation is handled by the detective assigned to the case, who will pursue leads, interview the victim and any witnesses, and attempt to identify, locate, and interview the suspect. If the detective believes the complaint is false or baseless, s/he can unfound the report. If there is an identified suspect and probable cause to make an arrest, the detective can clear the case by arrest or, under specified circumstances, by exceptional means. If a suspect has not been identified or there is not probable cause to make an arrest, the case can be kept open or, in the vernacular of the LAPD, "IC'd" (investigation continuing).

Los Angeles County District Attorney's Office

Spohn and Tellis' (2012) study also included the Los Angeles County District Attorney's (LADA) office. Since 2001, the LADA has had a specialized sex crimes unit, the Victim Impact Program (VIP), that vertically prosecutes sexual assault. Each of the 11 branches of the District Attorney's Office utilizes a VIP team approach, with an experienced attorney designated as the VIP Deputy-in Charge (DIC). The VIP DIC works closely with the DDAs assigned to the VIP team to ensure that sexual assault cases are appropriately prepared and prosecuted. All DDAs assigned to a VIP team receive enhanced, ongoing training focusing on legal issues, potential defenses, and trial tactics.

Although all of the prosecutors interviewed during our study affirmed that the Victim Impact Program is philosophically committed to the notion of vertical prosecution, many noted the case screening process varied by branch and the VIP Deputy-in-Charge. In some branches case screening and filing decisions are handled by the DIC, in others there is a designated case screener, and in still others all members of the VIP team participate in case screening and make filing decisions. In branches where "everyone screens cases," if the DDA screening the case decides to file charges, s/he is assigned to prosecute the case. As one respondent noted, "After filing, we own the case so we take the filing decision very seriously." Another respondent expressed a more cynical attitude, noting that "If you file the dog, you walk the dog." In some branches, the VIP DIC screens cases initially and decides whether the case should be rejected; cases that are not rejected outright are assigned to a member of the VIP team, who will conduct the pre-filing interview with the victim and decide whether charges should be filed and, if so, what the charges should be. In other branches, the VIP DIC conducts the interview with the victim and makes the filing decision; cases that are filed are assigned to a member of the VIP team for prosecution.

It is important to note the Los Angeles County District Attorney's Office screens cases using a trial sufficiency standard (Jacoby, 1980). That is, the DDA will file charges only if there is sufficient evidence to prove the case beyond a reasonable doubt at a jury trial. Moreover, the policy in sexual assault cases is charges will not be filed without some type of corroboration of the victim's testimony—DNA evidence that establishes the identity of the perpetrator, injuries to the victim, witnesses who can corroborate the victim's testimony, or physical or medical evidence that is consistent with the victim's account of the incident. Although there are some exceptions, a pre-filing interview designed to assess the victim's credibility and willingness to cooperate in the prosecution of the case also is required. Many interviewees emphasized that rejection is likely if the incident is a "she said/he said" situation in which the victim is claiming she was forced to engage in sexual relations but the suspect contends the sexual acts were consensual and there is no corroboration of the victim's allegations. In fact, when asked directly whether there are any types of "she said/he said" cases that would be filed without corroboration of the victim's allegations, most admitted that there were not.

The Process of Case Clearance

According to the Uniform Crime Reporting Handbook (Federal Bureau of Investigation, 2004), law enforcement agencies can clear offenses either by arrest or by exceptional means. The handbook states that "an offense is cleared by arrest, or solved for crime reporting purposes, when at least one person is (1) arrested, (2) charged with the commission of the offense, and (3) turned over to the court for prosecution (whether following arrest, court summons, or police notice)" (p. 79). Regarding exceptional clearances, the handbook notes that there may be occasions where law enforcement has conducted an investigation, exhausted all leads, and identified a suspect but is nonetheless unable to clear an offense by arrest. In this situation, the agency can clear the offense by exceptional means, provided that each of the following questions can be answered in the affirmative (p. 80–81):

- Has the investigation definitely established the **identity** of the offender?
- Is the **exact location of the offender known** so that the subject could be taken into custody now?
- Is there **enough information** to support an arrest, charge,[2] and turning over to the court for prosecution?
- Is there some reason **outside law enforcement control** that **precludes arresting**, charging, and prosecuting the offender?

To illustrate the types of cases that might be cleared by exceptional means, the handbook provides a list of examples, many of which involve the death of the offender or an offender who is unable to be arrested because s/he is being prosecuted in another jurisdiction for a different crime or because extradition has been denied. One of the examples provided is when the "victim refuses to cooperate in the prosecution," but there is an added proviso, which states that this alone does not justify an exceptional clearance and that the answer must also be yes to the first three questions outlined above (Federal Bureau of Investigation, 2004, p. 81).

Analysis of case outcomes and interviews with detectives and district attorneys revealed that both the LAPD and the LASD have complicated rules for clearing cases, misinterpret UCR guidelines regarding the two types of case clearances (cleared by arrest and cleared by exceptional means), and overuse (misuse) the exceptional clearance. If the detective investigating the crime has identified a suspect and has probable cause to arrest the suspect, the detective will either arrest the individual and present the case to an DDA from the Victim Impact Program (VIP) of the Los Angeles County District Attorney's Office for a filing decision, or delay making an arrest and present the case to an DDA for a pre-arrest charge evaluation.

The DDA reviewing the case following the arrest of the suspect can either accept the case for prosecution, send the case back to the investigating officer for further investigation (although this is complicated by the fact that charges must be filed within 48 hours of the suspect's arrest), send the case to the city attorney for prosecution as a misdemeanor, or decline the case for prosecution. Because LAPD policy states that cases can be cleared by arrest only if the district attorney files charges, if charges are declined, the LAPD detective changes the case clearance category from cleared by arrest to cleared by exceptional means. The LASD does not have a similar policy, but, depending on the preferences of the detective's supervisor and/or the detectives own interpretation of UCR policies on exceptional clearances, a LASD detective may also recategorize the case from cleared by arrest to cleared by exceptional means if the district attorney declines to file charges against the suspect. Because the UCR Handbook clearly states that cases can be cleared by exceptional means only if there is something beyond the control of law enforcement that prevents them from making an arrest, this is a misuse of the exceptional clearance. Cases in which a suspect is arrested should be cleared by arrest, regardless of whether charges are filed by the district attorney.

Similar procedures are followed if the case is evaluated by the district attorney prior to the arrest of the suspect. If the evidence in the case meets the district attorney's standard for filing, the suspect will be arrested and the case will be cleared by arrest. If the case is sent back for further investigation or if the evidence is deemed insufficient to justify charging, the investigating officer will either continue the investigation and, once additional evidence is obtained, resubmit the case for a second review by the district attorney, or—and this is what more typically happens—end the investigation and clear the case by exceptional means. This, too, may be a misuse of the exceptional clearance. If the detective has probable cause to make an arrest but the victim tells the district attorney that s/he does not want the suspect arrested or is unwilling to cooperate in the prosecution of the case, the case can be cleared by exceptional means (provided that the identity and location of the suspect are known). Although one might argue that the suspect should be arrested if there is probable cause to make an arrest, the victim's unwillingness to cooperate is something that is beyond the control of law enforcement. On the other hand, the case should not be cleared by exceptional means if the district attorney declines to file charges because the evidence in the cases does not meet the filing standard of proof beyond a reasonable doubt. If there is probable cause to arrest the suspect and the victim is cooperative, the suspect should be arrested and the case cleared by arrest, as there is nothing beyond the control of law enforcement that *prevents* them from making an arrest. Alternatively, the detective could continue the investigation and, once additional evidence is obtained, resubmit the case to the district attorney.

Methodological Overview of the Los Angeles Study

Detailed information regarding the study's methodology are reported elsewhere (Spohn & Tellis, 2012, 2014), but the basis of findings discussed here come from case files involving female victims over the age of 12 reported in 2008. Because our focus is on arrest and charging decisions, and because arrest (and charging) is not possible unless there is an identified suspect, this analysis includes all rape and attempted rapes in which the police knew the identify and location of the suspect. Of the 650 cases in the original sample, 530 (81.5%) were cases with an identified suspect. Because there were very few victims who were not white, Black, or Hispanic, we also eliminated cases ($N = 31$) involving victims who were Asian American or other races. This resulted in a data file with 491 cases; 171 were cases reported to the LAPD and 320 were cases reported to the LASD.

Dependent and Independent Variables

Our dependent variables were measures of decisions made by police and prosecutors. We began with the decision to arrest, conceptualized in two ways. The first is a dichotomous measure of whether the case was *cleared by arrest* and the second is a dichotomous indicator of whether the *suspect was arrested*. As explained above, both the LAPD and, to a lesser extent, the LASD change the case clearance category from cleared by arrest to cleared by exceptional means in cases in which they make an arrest but the district attorney does not file felony charges. Focusing only on cases that were cleared by arrest, in other words, means that not all cases that resulted in the arrest of a suspect are "counted" as arrests. Our third dependent variable was a dichotomous indicator of whether the investigating detective presented the case to a DDA for pre-arrest charge evaluation. We also conceptualized the charging decision in two ways.[5] The first, which is the conceptualization used by prior research, examined charging outcomes only for cases that resulted in the arrest of a suspect ($N = 210$); the second, which we argue more accurately captures the decisions that prosecutors make, examined charging decisions in all cases that were presented to the district attorney for a charge evaluation, regardless of whether the suspect was arrested or not ($N = 357$). We used binary logistic regression analysis to analyze each of our dichotomous dependent variables.

Our independent variables include victim characteristics, indicators of crime seriousness, and measures of the strength of evidence in the case. The victim characteristics include the victim's age, race/ethnicity, relationship with the suspect, whether the victim engaged in any "risk-taking behavior" at the time of the incident, and whether the case file indicated that the victim had characteristics that would make police and prosecutors question her credibility. The "risk-taking" variable, which reflects legally *irrelevant* stereotypes about real rapes and genuine victims, was a composite variable because of the infrequency of any of these behaviors at the time of the incident. Of the cases in which the most serious charge was rape or attempted rape, 35.1% ($N = 125$) involved some type of risk-taking behavior, typically walking alone late at night or drinking alcohol.

The character/reputation variable was also a composite of several factors that might lead officials to question the victim's credibility, such as whether there was information in the case file indicating the victim had a pattern of substance abuse, had a "disreputable" job (e.g., stripper, exotic dancer), was a prostitute, or had a criminal record. There were 49 cases (13.8%) with one or more of these were present.[6] The final two victim characteristics measured whether the victim had mental health issues, or a noted motive to lie about being sexually assaulted.[8]

Our model also included a number of indicators of case seriousness, including whether the most serious charge was rape, whether the suspect used a weapon, whether the suspect physically as well as sexually assaulted the victim, and whether the victim suffered some type of collateral injury.[8] Finally, we measured whether the victim verbally or physically resisted the suspect.[9]

In terms of evidentiary factors, we measured the strength of evidence in the case, including whether the victim made a prompt report, number of witnesses, whether the victim was willing to cooperate,[10] whether evidence was collected from the victim or the scene of the incident, and whether the case was reported to LAPD or LASD.

Findings

Case Outcomes

The outcomes of the sexual assault cases reported to the LAPD and the LASD in 2008 are shown in Tables 34.1 and 34.2. The data presented in Table 34.1 indicate that, for both agencies, about one third of all rape and attempted rape cases with identified suspects were cases in which the final case clearance type was cleared by arrest. The rate was somewhat higher for the LASD (37.8%) than for the LAPD (25.1%). The percentage of cases in which a suspect was arrested (regardless of how the case was cleared) was 46.8% overall; it was 40.4% for the LAPD and 50.3% for the LASD. Considering both law enforcement agencies, there were 357 cases in which the district attorney made a charging decision. As shown in Table 34.2, 147 cases (41.2%) were presented to an DDA before the suspect was arrested and 210 cases (58.8%) were presented after the suspect was arrested. Of the cases presented before arrest, the DDA filed charges in only 9 (6.1%) cases. By contrast, charges were filed in 106 (50.5%) of the cases presented to the DDA following the arrest of the suspect.

The data presented in Table 34.2 also demonstrate that cases presented to the district attorney prior to the suspect's arrest and subsequently rejected by the prosecutor who reviewed the case were, with only three exceptions, cleared by exceptional means. By contrast, cases rejected following the arrest of the suspect were either cleared by arrest (43.3%) or cleared by exceptional means (56.7%). Use of the exceptional clearance is problematic for both types of cases.

Turning first to cases cleared by exceptional means without the arrest of the suspect, all were cases in which the suspect's identity was known, but we do not know whether the location of the suspect was known or whether the police had probable cause to make an arrest. Even assuming that criteria two and three were met, there is still a question of whether there was something beyond the control of law enforcement that prevented them from making an arrest. In 51 of the 133 cases (38.3%), the victim indicated she did not

Table 34.1 Indicators of arrest: rape and attempted rape cases with an identified suspect, 2008

	All cases ($N = 491$)		LAPD cases ($N = 171$)		LASD cases ($N = 320$)	
	N	%	*N*	%	*N*	%
Case formally cleared by arrest	164	33.4	43	25.1	121	37.8
Suspect was arrested	230	46.8	69	40.4	161	50.3
Suspect was arrested or case presented to DA prior to arrest but rejected by DA	364	74.1	121	70.8	243	75.9

Table 34.2 Outcomes of cases presented to the Los Angeles district attorney for charge evaluation before and after arrest of suspect, 2008

	Suspect arrested ($N = 210$)		Suspect not arrested ($N = 147$)	
	N	%	*N*	%
LDDA filed charges				
Yes	106	50.5	9	6.1
No	104	49.5	138	93.9
Case clearance—cases rejected by LDDA				
Cleared by arrest	45	43.3	0	0.0
Cleared by exceptional means	59	56.7	135	97.8
Unfounded	0	0.0	3	2.2

want the suspect arrested and/or was unwilling to cooperate in the investigation and prosecution of the suspect, but the victims in the remaining cases (82/133 or 61.7%) were willing to cooperate. Assuming in these latter cases the police had probable cause to make an arrest, they should not have been cleared by exceptional means given the victim was willing to cooperate and there was nothing beyond the control of law enforcement that prevented them from making an arrest.

The 59 cases cleared by exceptional means following the arrest of the suspect—34 of which were investigated by the LASD and 25 of which were investigated by the LAPD—clearly should not have been cleared exceptionally. Because these cases resulted in the arrest of the suspect, by definition there was nothing beyond the control of the law enforcement agency that prevented the suspect's arrest. These cases should have been cleared by arrest.

As these data indicate, 28.7% of the rape and attempted rape cases in which the police made an arrest were not cleared by arrest; rather, they were cleared by exceptional means when the district attorney refused to file felony charges. Moreover, a substantial proportion of rape and attempted rape cases were presented to the district attorney prior to the suspect's arrest, and the outcomes of these cases were very different than the outcomes of cases presented following the suspect's arrest. This suggests the decision to arrest is not adequately measured by examining only cases that were cleared by arrest and that the charging decision is not effectively measured by examining only cases that were evaluated following the arrest of the suspect.

Predictors of Police Decision Making

The results of our analysis of the two arrest variables and of the detective's decision to present the case to the district attorney for charge evaluation prior to the arrest of the suspect are presented in Table 34.3. The *decision to arrest the suspect* was not affected by any of the victim characteristics; instead, this decision was affected by all of the indictors of crime seriousness except the type of resistance offered by the victim and by all four measures of the strength of evidence in the case. Arrest was more likely if the crime was more serious, as measured by whether the suspect physically, as well as sexually, assaulted the victim, whether the suspect used a weapon, and whether the victim suffered some type of collateral injury; by contrast, arrest was less likely if the crime involved rape rather than attempted rape. The police were more likely to arrest the suspect if the victim reported the crime within one hour, the victim was willing to cooperate in the investigation, and there was physical evidence from the victim or the crime scene; the likelihood of arrest also increased as the number of witnesses increased.

In contrast to these results, which suggest arrest decisions are based on legally relevant factors, the results of the analysis of cases that were *officially cleared by arrest* indicate that this outcome was affected by a combination of indicators of crime seriousness and evidentiary strength and victim characteristics. The case was less likely to be cleared by arrest if the case file contained information that raised questions about the victim's reputation or character, the victim had a motive to lie, or the case involved rape rather than attempted rape. Consistent with the results for the arrest decision, the case was more likely to be cleared by arrest if the suspect used a weapon, the victim suffered collateral injuries, the victim reported the crime within one hour, and the victim was willing to cooperate in the investigation of the crime. Neither outcome, on the other hand, was affected by the victim's age, race/ethnicity, or relationship with the suspect; by whether the victim engaged in any risky behavior at the time of the incident or had a mental illness or mental health issues, or by the type of resistance offered by the victim.

We also analyzed whether the detective investigating the crime presented the case/case file to the district attorney for a pre-arrest charge evaluation. The frequency with which sexual assault cases are presented to the district attorney for charge evaluation prior to the suspect's arrest, coupled with the fact that the outcomes of cases evaluated prior to and following the arrest of the suspect differ significantly, suggests that it is important to identify the factors that predict whether cases will be evaluated before or after arrest. As shown in the third column of Table 34.3, only one victim characteristic—whether the victim engaged in any risky behavior at the time of the alleged assault—influenced whether the case would be presented to the district attorney for a pre-arrest charge evaluation. Cases involving victims who engaged in risk-taking behavior were 1.9 times more likely to be presented to the district attorney prior to the arrest of the suspect. Surprisingly, given the comments of detectives, many of whom stated that cases involving non-strangers were much more likely to be subjected to pre-arrest charge evaluation, the relationship between the suspect and the victim did not affect the likelihood that the case would be presented to the district attorney prior to the arrest of the suspect.

The odds of a pre-arrest charge evaluation also were affected by two indicators of crime seriousness and four measures of evidentiary strength. Compared to cases in which the most serious charge was attempted rape, cases in which rape was the most serious charge were over six times more likely to be presented to the district attorney before the suspect could be arrested. The likelihood of a pre-arrest charge evaluation was significantly lower for cases in which the suspect used some type of weapon, the victim reported the crime within one hour, the victim was willing to cooperate in the investigation, there was some type of physical evidence, and there were one or more witnesses.

Predictors of Prosecutors' Charging Decisions

The results of our analysis of these variables, shown in Table 34.4, reveal that different factors affect the two outcomes. Beginning with the more traditional conceptualization of charging—charging decisions that follow the arrest of the suspect—only three variables affect this outcome: victim age (charging is four and a half times more likely if the victim is under the age of 18); whether the victim had a motive to lie; and whether the victim was willing to cooperate in the investigation and prosecution of the case. In fact, prosecutors were nearly 19 times more likely to file charges if the victim was cooperative and they were about 6 times more likely to accept the case for prosecution if the victim did not have a motive to lie. Although our broader indicator of charging is affected in the same way by these three variables, it also is affected by the victim's risk-taking behavior, whether the most serious charge

Table 34.3 Results of the logistic regression analyses of three indicators of arrest outcomes

	Suspect arrested			Case cleared by arrest			Case presented to the DA for charge evaluation prior to suspect's arrest		
	B	SE	Exp(*B*)	*B*	SE	Exp(*B*)	*B*	SE	Exp(*B*)
Victim Characteristics									
Victim is Less Than 18	0.16	0.27	1.17	0.43	0.29	1.54	0.01	0.01	1.01
Race/Ethnicity									
Black	−0.14	0.34	0.87	0.36	0.37	1.43	−0.22	0.40	0.80
Hispanic	−0.07	0.28	0.93	0.38	0.30	1.47	−0.21	0.32	0.81
Relationship with									
Suspect	0.39	0.32	1.48	0.53	0.35	1.71	0.10	0.42	1.11
Non-stranger	0.66	0.36	1.93	0.49	0.40	1.63	0.19	0.45	1.21
Intimate partner									
Risk-taking behavior	−0.21	0.26	0.81	−0.03	0.28	0.97	**0.63***	**0.32**	**1.88**
Questions about character/reputation	−0.11	0.33	0.89	**−1.00***	**0.43**	**0.37**	0.24	0.40	1.28
Mental Illness or mental health issues	−0.35	0.40	0.71	−0.80	0.49	0.45	0.72	0.45	2.05
Has a motive to lie	−0.32	0.33	0.73	**−1.16***	**0.41**	**0.31**	−0.14	0.41	0.87
Indicators of crime seriousness									
Most serious charge is rape	**−1.43***	**0.40**	**0.24**	**−1.09***	**0.38**	**0.34**	**1.83***	**0.57**	**6.27**
Suspect physically assaulted victim	**0.61***	**0.24**	**1.84**	0.21	0.26	1.23	−0.52	0.30	0.60
Suspect used a weapon	**0.92***	**0.36**	**2.50**	**1.06***	**0.37**	**2.88**	**−1.27***	**0.50**	**0.28**
Victim suffered collateral injury	**0.46***	**0.22**	**1.58**	**0.72***	**0.26**	**2.06**	−0.31	0.29	0.73
Type of resistance									
Verbal resistance	−0.46	0.37	0.64	−0.59	0.41	0.56	0.60	0.42	1.82
only	0.05	0.49	1.05	−0.05	0.53	0.95	−0.28	0.64	0.76
Physical resistance	0.24	0.30	1.26	0.40	0.32	1.49	−0.30	0.36	0.74
only Both verbal and physical resistance									
Strength of evidence									
Victim reported crime within one hour	**0.96***	**0.29**	**2.61**	**0.55***	**0.26**	**1.73**	**−1.54***	**0.41**	**0.21**
Number of witnesses	**0.36***	**0.08**	**1.30**	**0.24***	**0.08**	**1.27**	**−0.33***	**0.10**	**0.72**
Victim is willing to cooperate	**1.80***	**0.28**	**6.03**	**2.28***	**0.36**	**9.77**	**−1.74***	**0.35**	**0.18**
Physical evidence	**0.58***	**0.25**	**1.78**	0.26	0.27	1.30	**−0.91***	**0.31**	**0.40**
Agency is LAPD	−0.15	0.25	0.86	−0.17	0.27	0.84	−0.12	0.30	0.89
Constant	−1.79*	0.63	0.17	3.30*	0.72	0.14	0.50	0.92	1.65
Nagelkerke R^2	0.38			0.41			0.40		

*$P \leq 0.05$. Significant coefficients are in bold

was rape rather than attempted rape, whether the suspect used a weapon, and whether the victim reported the crime within one hour. Consistent with the results of the arrest decisions, charging was not affected by the victim's race/ethnicity or relationship with the suspect, whether the victim had a mental illness or mental health issues, or the type of resistance offered by the victim.

Table 34.4 Results of the logistic regression analyses of charging decisions

	Suspect arrested and DA filed charges ($N = 210$)			Case presented To DA (before or after arrest) and DA filed charges ($N = 357$)		
	B	SE	Exp(*B*)	*B*	SE	Exp(*B*)
Victim characteristics						
Victim is less than 18	**1.53***	**0.45**	**4.60**	**1.58***	**0.36**	**4.81**
Race/ethnicity						
Black	0.78	0.54	2.19	0.57	0.45	1.77
Hispanic	0.78	0.43	2.19	0.54	0.36	1.72
Relationship with suspect						
Non-stranger	−0.29	0.54	0.75	−0.29	0.44	0.75
Intimate partner	−0.20	0.58	0.82	−0.13	0.46	0.88
Risk-taking behavior	−0.56	0.40	0.57	**−0.60***	**0.24**	**0.45**
Questions about character/reputation	−0.17	0.58	0.84	−0.63	0.52	0.53
Mental illness or mental health issues	−1.38	0.85	0.25	−0.95	0.60	0.39
Has a motive to lie	**−1.81***	**0.65**	**0.16**	**−1.52***	**0.58**	**0.22**
Indicators of crime seriousness						
Most serious charge is rape	−0.48	0.50	0.62	**−1.00***	**0.45**	**0.037**
Suspect physically assaulted victim	−0.61	0.39	0.54	−0.34	0.32	0.71
Suspect used a weapon	0.86	0.50	2.37	**1.16***	**0.44**	**3.20**
Victim suffered collateral injury	0.30	0.38	1.34	0.40	0.31	1.49
Type of resistance						
Verbal resistance only	0.28	0.62	1.32	0.25	0.47	1.29
Physical resistance only	0.13	0.75	1.14	0.68	0.65	1.97
Both verbal and physical resistance	0.80	0.49	2.23	0.96*	0.40	2.60
Strength of evidence						
Victim reported crime within one hour	0.42	0.42	1.52	**0.80***	**0.36**	**2.23**
Number of witnesses	−0.03	0.10	0.97	0.06	0.10	1.07
Victim is willing to cooperate	**2.94***	**0.72**	**18.84**	**2.70***	**0.54**	**14.80**
Physical evidence	−0.03	0.39	0.97	0.21	0.32	1.23
Agency is LAPD	0.69	0.40	1.99	0.38	0.33	1.46
Constant	−3.35*	1.18	0.04	−3.72*	0.92	0.02
Nagelkerke R^2	0.40			0.43		

*$P \leq 0.05$. Significant coefficients are in bold

Policing Sexual Assault: Research and Policy Implications

Our analyses reveal that arresting and charging decisions are affected by legally relevant indicators of case seriousness and evidentiary strength and, depending upon the way outcomes are operationally defined, by legally irrelevant indicators of the victim's behavior at the time of the incident and her character, reputation, and motivation in reporting the crime to the police. These findings are consistent with the focal concerns perspective and, to a lesser extent, with Black's sociological theory of law. They suggest that the decisions of police and prosecutors, like those of judges, are affected by perceptions of crime seriousness and offender dangerousness and by assessments of the likelihood of conviction, which are themselves influenced not only by the strength of evidence in the case but also by stereotypes (Johnson & Betsinger, 2009) or typifications (Frohmann, 1991, 1997) of rape and rape victims. Our results thus provide further evidence of the utility of the focal concerns perspective and its applicability to decisions other than sentencing.

Our findings are not consistent with Black's (1989) assertions that the "handling of a case always reflects the social characteristics of those involved in it" (p. 21). The race/ethnicity of the victim did not affect any of the case outcomes and the age of the victim affected charging, but not arrest, decisions. In contrast to prior research (Frazier & Haney, 1996; Holleran et al., 2010; Tellis & Spohn, 2008), which found that sexual assaults involving strangers were treated more harshly than those involving acquaintances or intimate partners, we also found that the victim/suspect relationship did not affect any of the outcomes we examined. This is surprising, given Black's (1976) contention that case outcomes are affected by the "relational distance" between the victim and the suspect and given that all of the cases included in our study were cases with an identified suspect. The fact that the relationship between the victim and suspect did not affect case outcomes once other victim characteristics, indicators of case seriousness, and measures of evidentiary strength were taken into consideration suggests that it is not the victim/suspect relationship per se that influences arresting and charging decisions; rather, the characteristics of cases and the strength of the evidence vary depending on the type of relationship.

The findings of this study make a number of important methodological contributions.

Prior research on police and prosecutorial decision making has been criticized for failure to control adequately for crime seriousness and strength of evidence in the case, with critics arguing that models that lack these measures are misspecified. Because we had access to the case files, we were able to collect detailed data on physical evidence, witnesses, whether the victim was willing to cooperate, and whether the victim reported the crime promptly. We also were able to collect several indicators of crime seriousness—whether the suspect used a weapon or physically assaulted the victim and whether the victim suffered some type of collateral injury. The fact that we were able to control for these legally relevant factors may explain why some of the factors identified by prior research did not affect the arrest and charging decisions we examined.

We also demonstrate the importance of the ways in which arrest and charging decisions are conceptualized and operationalized. The concept of "cleared by arrest" plays a key role in research on police and prosecutorial decision making. Policing researchers often operationalize the decision to arrest based on whether the crime was cleared by the arrest of a suspect and researchers examining prosecutorial charging decisions typically examine data on cases that resulted in an arrest and were presented by law enforcement for a formal charging decision. These operational definitions are based on assumptions that *all cases* that result in the arrest of a suspect are cases that are cleared by arrest and that the *only cases* on which prosecutors make charging decisions are cases in which a suspect was arrested. As we have shown, these assumptions are not necessarily valid. At least in Los Angeles and for sexual assault, a substantial proportion of cases in which a suspect was arrested were not cleared by arrest. Moreover, a significant number of cases were evaluated—and rejected for prosecution—by the district attorney prior to the arrest of the suspect. Defining the decision to arrest as cases that were formally cleared by arrest and operationalizing the charging decision as cases that were evaluated following arrest is misleading, as doing so undercounts both types of decisions.

Further evidence of this surfaced in our multivariate analyses of arresting and charging decisions. *We found that the predictors of these outcomes varied depending on the way in which the outcome was defined.* For example, none of the victim characteristics affected whether the suspect was arrested by the police, but whether there were questions about the victim's character or reputation and whether the victim had a motive to lie about the incident predicted the likelihood that the crime would be cleared by arrest.

These differences reflect the fact that many of the cases that resulted in the arrest of the suspect, but did not result in the filing of charges by the prosecutor, are not defined as cases that are cleared by arrest (due to the fact that the detective changed the case clearance from cleared by arrest to cleared by exceptional means). The cleared by arrest variable, in other words, conflates decisions made by police and prosecutors. The fact that these victim characteristics affected whether the case was cleared by arrest but not whether the police made an arrest suggests that the police are willing to make arrests in potentially problematic cases but that prosecutors are not willing to file charges in these cases. Alternatively, it may be that questions about the victim's character, reputation, or motivation for filing the complaint do not surface—or do not raise red flags if they do—until the victim is interviewed by the district attorney.

We also found that different variables affected our two indicators of charging. When we used the traditional operational definition—the suspect was arrested and the district attorney evaluated the case for prosecution—we found that only three variables (the victim's age, whether the victim was willing to cooperate, and whether the victim had a motive to lie) affected the likelihood of charging. Our analysis of the charging variable that combined cases screened before and after the arrest of the suspect revealed that four additional variables—whether the victim engaged in risky behavior, whether the most serious charge was rape, whether the suspect used a weapon, and whether the victim reported the crime within one hour—had an effect. These results suggest that detectives present problematic cases in which there is an identified suspect and in which there may be probable cause to make an arrest to the district attorney for a charge evaluation before arresting the suspect and that these cases are rejected for prosecution. That this is, in fact, what is occurring was confirmed by our analysis of the detective's decision to present the case to the district attorney for a pre-arrest charge evaluation. Detectives were significantly more likely to bring the case to the district attorney before arresting the suspect if the victim engaged in risky behavior, did not report the crime promptly, and was unwilling to cooperate as the case moved forward; if the suspect did not use a weapon; if there was no physical evidence, and if there were no or few witnesses. In fact, we found that the various measures of the strength of evidence in the case had a positive effect on whether the suspect would be arrested and whether the case would be cleared by arrest, but a negative effect on whether the case would be presented to the district attorney for charge evaluation prior to the arrest of the suspect. Coupled with the fact that all but 9 of the 147 cases evaluated by the district attorney prior to the arrest of the suspect were rejected for prosecution, this suggests that pre-arrest charge evaluation is an important component of both police and prosecutorial decision making.

Several of our other findings merit comment. We found that only one variable—whether the victim was willing to cooperate in the investigation and prosecution of the case—affected all five of the outcomes we examined. In fact, victim cooperation had a substantial effect on each outcome. The police were six times more likely to arrest the suspect and were nearly 10 times more likely to clear the case by arrest if the victim was cooperative; they were significantly less likely to present the case to the district attorney for a pre-arrest charge evaluation if the victim was willing to cooperate. The effect of victim cooperation on charging decisions was even more pronounced; cases with a cooperative victim were almost 15 times more likely to result in the filing of charges before or after the suspect's arrest and were almost 19 times more likely to result in the filing of charges following the arrest of the suspect. These findings, although not surprising, point to the importance of the individual-level dynamic between victims and detectives and between victims and prosecutors.

Our results have important policy implications. We found that law enforcement officials in Los Angeles overuse (in fact, misuse) the exceptional clearance in two important situations: when an arrest does not lead to the filing of felony charges and when cases are rejected for prosecution during the pre-arrest charge evaluation. Regarding the first situation, cases that result in the arrest of a suspect should be cleared by arrest, as these cases do not meet the fourth requirement for clearing cases by exceptional means. Given that the suspect was arrested, there is by definition nothing beyond the control of law enforcement that prevents an arrest. Thus, cases in which a suspect is arrested should be cleared by arrest. The second situation in which cases may be cleared incorrectly by exceptional means is where probable cause to arrest the suspect exists but the detective chooses instead to present the case to the district attorney's office, where charges are rejected based on insufficient evidence. Like the first scenario, this situation is problematic in that it does not involve something beyond the control of the law enforcement that prevents the arrest of the suspect. There is probable cause to make an arrest but the case is cleared exceptionally because a prosecutor determined that the evidence is insufficient to prove the case beyond a reasonable doubt to a jury.

Whether a suspect is arrested should not be contingent on whether the prosecuting attorney believes that the evidence meets the standard of proof beyond a reasonable doubt and that the case therefore would result in a jury conviction. Doing so subjects the decision to arrest to a higher standard of proof than is required by law and effectively gives the prosecutor control over the decision to arrest. It also means that individuals who may have committed a serious crime are not held accountable for their behavior and denies justice to victims who made a difficult decision to report the crime and are willing to cooperate with the police and prosecutor as the case moves forward. Failure to make an arrest in spite of probable cause to do so is reminiscent of police inaction in response to domestic violence prior to the implementation of mandatory arrest policies. Although we are not suggesting that police departments should adopt mandatory arrest policies for sexual assault cases, they should make an arrest when there is sufficient evidence that a crime occurred and that the suspect is the person who committed the crime.

Clearly, there are cases where the police cannot—indeed should not—make an arrest. If probable cause to arrest does not exist or if the prosecutor rejects the case for further investigation as a result of a pre-arrest screening process, the case should be left open and investigated further. These cases *should not* be cleared by exceptional means, as they do not meet the UCR criterion that there must be "enough information to support an arrest, charge, and turning over to the court for prosecution." The case cannot be solved—that is, cleared—if probable cause to make an arrest does not exist. Cases in which the police know who and where the suspect is and in which probable cause exists to make an arrest, but the victim refuses to cooperate with the police can legitimately be cleared by exceptional means if the victim's lack of cooperation means that the police cannot make an arrest.

We believe that our study, which was conducted in one of the largest and most diverse cities in the United States, makes important theoretical and methodological contributions to our understanding of police and prosecutorial decision making. However, our approach is not without limitations, the most important of which stems from our reliance on the information contained in official case files. Although we were provided with redacted copies of all documents in the case files, the material contained in the files ultimately reflects the perceptions and biases of individual law enforcement officers, who describe the incident, recount the victim's allegations, and document the results of interviews with victims, witnesses, and suspects. Although we have no reason to believe that their accounts were slanted or written in such a way as to make the department "look good," there is obviously a possibility of "biased reporting," which we cannot measure or take into consideration.

Conclusion

The findings of our study illuminate the ways in which the decisions of police and prosecutors overlap and influence one another. Our findings also illustrate that, at least in the context of sexual assault, it is misleading to assume that data on cases cleared by arrest accurately reflect police arrest decisions and that data on cases that were evaluated for charging following the arrest of the suspect accurately capture prosecutors' charging decisions. More importantly, our findings illustrate that the conclusions we draw about the factors that influence sexual assault case outcomes depend to some extent on the conceptualization and operationalization of decisions to arrest and charge. Our research has attempted to disentangle these complicated relationships in one jurisdiction and with respect to one type of crime. Future research should focus on determining whether these overlapping decision rules are found in other jurisdictions and for other types of crimes.

Notes

1. To enhance our understanding of policies and practices that guided the handling of sexual assault cases and to enable us to more accurately interpret the quantitative data, we also conducted interviews with LAPD and LASD detectives who had experience investigating sexual assaults, and DDAs from the Victim Impact Program. During June and July of 2010, we interviewed 52 detectives from the LAPD, 24 detectives from the LASD, and 30 attorneys from the Los Angeles County District Attorney's Office. For a more detailed description of the policies and procedures in Los Angeles, see (AUTHOR'S CITE).
2. This refers to a police booking procedure; not a prosecutorial filing decision (FBI Section Chief R. Casey, Personal Communication, January 14, 2011).
3. The LAPD currently has 21 divisions in 4 bureaus, but in 2008 there were only 19.
4. Our goal was to select 6 cases from each case closure type from each of the 19 divisions that existed in 2008. This would have produced a sample of 456 cases. Because each division did not necessarily have 6 cases from each case closure type in 2008, the final sample included 401 cases. We created a weighted sample that divided the percentage of each stratum (that is, each case closure type for each division) in the population of cases by the percentage of each stratum in the sample. We use the unweighted data when we are focusing on a particular type of case closure (e.g., unfounded cases or cases that were cleared by exceptional means). We use the weighted data when discussing 2008 case outcomes and when providing descriptive statistics for these cases. 5.
5. We were unable to separately analyze cases that were presented to an DDA for a pre-arrest charge evaluation due to the fact that all of 9 of these 147 cases were rejected for prosecution.
6. This variable was coded 1 if the case file indicated that the victim was currently or had been in the past a patient at a mental health facility, that the victim was taking medication for a mental health problem, or if a family member or friend told the responding officer or the detective that the victim had a mental illness or mental health issues.
7. Information about whether the victim had a motive to lie was obtained either from the victim's statement, the interview of the victim by the investigating officer, or the statement of witnesses. Examples of the types of statements found in the case file regarding the victim's motive to lie are the following: "all informants interviewed said the victim fabricated the incident because her parents found out she was sexually active," "victim was angry with suspect because he would not give her crack cocaine," "the victim was angry that the suspect returned to his wife," "the victim is involved in a custody dispute with the suspect," "victim was angry with suspect because he broke off the affair with her," "victim did not want her mother to find out what she did," "victim was cheating on her husband with the suspect," "suspect (victim's boyfriend) was flirting with another woman at a party," "suspect has nude photos of victim and victim found out that suspect has another girlfriend," "the girls were afraid that they would get in trouble for coming home late."
8. This information was obtained from the report of the sexual assault examination, from the responding officer's description of the victim's physical condition, and/or from the victim's and/or witnesses' statements in the case file.

9. The type of resistance was obtained from the victim's statement. We originally coded six types of verbal resistance (cried, screamed, refused/protested/said stop, attempt to dissuade/fool, calls names/denigrates suspect, passive/saying nothing) and five types of physical resistance (fled/attempted to flee, resisted/struggled, fought (hit, scratched, bit), used a weapon to defend, passive/did nothing to resist). Because there could be multiple types of verbal and physical resistance, we coded verbal resistance 1 if the case file indicated that there was any type of verbal resistance; similarly, we coded physical resistance 1 if the case filed indicated that there was any type of physical resistance.
10. Whether the victim was willing to cooperate with the detective assigned to the case was determined from the case file. If the victim was uncooperative, it would be noted in the file by the investigating officer (IO). For example, the IO might have noted that he/she had attempted to contact the victim but the victim refused to talk to him/her (either via telephone or in person), that the victim stated that she did not want anything to happen to the suspect/that she did not want the suspect arrested, that the victim said (for a variety of reasons) that she did not want to take the case to court, that the victim stated that she was no longer interested in pursuing a criminal prosecution, or that the victim refused to participate in a pre-filing interview with the district attorney's office.

References

Alderden, M. A., & Ullman, S. E. (2012). Creating a more complete and current picture: Examining police and prosecutor decision making when processing sexual assault cases. *Violence Against Women, 18*, 525–551.

Bachman, R. (1998). Factors related to rape reporting and arrest: New evidence from the NCVS. *Criminal Justice and Behavior, 25*, 8–29.

Black, D. J. (1976). *The behavior of law*. New York: Academic Press.

Black, D. J. (1980). *Manners and customs of the police*. New York: Academic Press.

Black, D. J. (1989). *Sociological justice*. New York: Oxford University Press.

Bouffard, J. (2000). Predicting type of sexual assault case closure from victim, suspect, and case characteristics. *Journal of Criminal Justice, 28*, 527–542.

Du Mont, J., Miller, K.-L., & Myhr, T. L. (2003). The role of "real rape" and "real victim" stereotypes in the police reporting practices of sexually assaulted women. *Violence Against Women, 9*, 466–486.

Du Mont, J., & Myhr, T. L. (2000). So few convictions: The role of client-related characteristics in the legal processing of sexual assaults. *Violence Against Women, 6*, 1109–1136.

Estrich, S. (1987). *Real rape*. Cambridge, MA: Harvard University Press.

Federal Bureau of Investigation. (2004). *Uniform crime reporting handbook*. Washington, DC: U.S. Government.

Feldman-Summers, S., & Lindner, K. (1976). Perceptions of victims and defendants in criminal assault cases. *Criminal Justice and Behavior, 3*, 135–150.

Field, H., & Bienen, L. (1980). *Jurors and rape: A study in psychology and law*. Lexington, MA: Lexington Books.

Frazier, P. A., & Haney, B. (1996). Sexual assault cases in the legal system: Police, prosecutor and victim perspectives. *Law and Human Behavior, 20*, 607–628.

Frohmann, L. (1991). Discrediting victims' allegations of sexual assault: Prosecutorial accounts of case rejections. *Social Problems, 38*, 213–226.

Frohmann, L. (1997). Convictability and discordant locales: Reproducing race, class, and gender ideologies in prosecutorial decision-making. *Law & Society Review, 31*, 531–555.

Holleran, D., Beichner, D., & Spohn, C. (2010). Modeling the charging agreement between the police and prosecutors in sexual assault. *Crime and Delinquency, 56*, 385–413.

Horney, J., & Spohn, C. (1996). The influence of blame and believability factors on the processing of simple versus aggravated rape cases. *Criminology, 34*, 135–162.

Jacoby, J. E. (1980). *The American prosecutor: The search for identity*. Lexington, MA: Lexington Books.

Johnson, B. D., & Betsinger, S. (2009). Punishing the 'model minority': Asian-American criminal sentencing outcomes in federal district courts. *Criminology, 47*, 1045–1090.

Kerstetter, W. A. (1990). Gateway to justice: Police and prosecutorial response to sexual assaults against women. *Journal of Criminal Law and Criminology, 81*, 267–313.

Kingsnorth, R., MacIntosh, R. C., & Wentworth, J. (1999). Sexual assault: The role of prior relationship and victim characteristics in case processing. *Justice Quarterly, 16*, 275–302.

LaFree, G. (1981). Official reactions to social problems: Police decisions in sexual assault cases. *Social Problems, 28*, 582–594.

LaFree, G. (1989). *Rape and criminal justice: The social construction of sexual assault*. Belmont, CA: Wadsworth.

Martin, P. Y., & Powell, R. M. (1994). Accounting for the "second assault": Legal organizations' framing of rape victims. *Law and Social Inquiry, 19*, 853–890.

McCahill, T. W., Meyer, L. C., & Fischman, A. M. (1979). *The aftermath of rape*. Lexington, MA: Lexington Books.

Reskin, B., & Visher, C. (1986). The impacts of evidence and extralegal factors in jurors' decisions. *Law & Society Review, 20*, 423–438.

Schuller, R. A., & Stewart, A. (2000). Police responses to sexual assault complaints: The role of perpetrator/complainant intoxication. *Law and Human Behavior, 24*, 535–551.

Spohn, C., Beichner, D., & Davis-Frenzel, E. (2001). Prosecutorial explanations for sexual assault case rejection: Guarding the gateway to justice. *Social Problems, 48*, 206–235.

Spohn, C., & Holleran, D. (2001). Prosecuting sexual assault: Comparison charging decisions in sexual assault cases involving strangers, acquaintances, and intimate partners. *Justice Quarterly, 18*, 651–689.

Spohn, C., & Horney, J. (1992). *Rape law reform: A grassroots movement and its impact*. New York: Plenum Press.

Spohn, C., & Tellis, K. (2012). *Policing and Prosecuting Sexual Assault in Los Angeles City and County: A Collaborative Study in Partnership with the Los Angeles Police Department, the Los Angeles County Sheriff's Department, and the Los Angeles County District Attorney's Office. National Institute of Justice*. Award No. 2009-WG-BX-0009. Retrieved from https://www.ncjrs.gov/pdffiles1/nij/grants/237582.pdf

Spohn, C., & Tellis, K. (2014). *Policing and prosecuting sexual assault: Inside the criminal justice system*. Boulder, CO: Lynne Rienner Publishers.

Spohn, C., & Tellis, K. (2018). Sexual assault case outcomes: Disentangling the overlapping decisions of police and prosecutors. *Justice Quarterly*,. Published online February 19. https://doi.org/10.1080/07418825.2018.1429645

Spohn, C., White, C., & Tellis, K. (2014). Unfounding sexual assault: Examining the decision to unfound and identifying false reports. *Law & Society Review, 48*, 161–192.

Steffensmeier, D., Ulmer, J., & Kramer, J. (1997). The interaction of race, gender and age in criminal sentencing: The punishment cost of being young, black, and male. *Criminology, 36*, 763–798.

Taylor, J. (1987). Rape and women's credibility: Problems of recantations and false accusations echoed in the case of Cathleen Crowell Webb and Gary Dotson. *Harvard Women's Law Journal, 10*, 59–115.

Tellis, K., & Spohn, C. (2008). The sexual stratification hypothesis revisited: Testing assumptions about simple versus aggravate rape. *Journal of Criminal Justice, 36*, 252–261.

Tjaden, P., & Thoennes, N. (2006). *Extent, nature, and consequences of rape victimization: Findings from the national violence against women survey*. Washington, DC: US Department of Justice, National Institute of Justice.

35 Reporting Sexual Assault: Process and Barriers Victims Experience

William T. O'Donohue

Sexual assault is a prevalent problem, with 18.3% of women and 1.4% of men endorsing an experience of sexual victimization within a single year (Basile et al., 2011). However, research has suggested that less than half of victims disclose the assault during the first 3 days post-assault, and approximately 33% wait over a year to do so (Ahrens, Stansell, & Jennings, 2010). Further, there is also evidence that less than half of all sexual assault incidents are ever reported to law enforcement (Greenfield, 1997; Rennison & Rand, 2002; as cited Zinzow & Thompson, 2011). Various explanations have been advanced to account for these findings, including a lack of awareness of what sexual assault is (e.g., Littleton, Rhatigan, & Axsom, 2007) and fear of being blamed or disbelieved (e.g., Tjaden & Thoennes, 2000). In addition, it has been alleged that if sexual assault reporting is handled poorly, a "second traumatization" can occur for the victim (Brown, Hamilton & O'Neill, 2007). Given these findings, further examination of the literature on the reporting of sexual assault, including a review of barriers victims experience that influence their decision to report, is warranted. The purpose of this chapter is to examine the definitions of sexual assault, how victims report an incident, and what factors make the process of reporting difficult for victims.

W. T. O'Donohue (✉)
University of Nevada, Reno, NV, USA

What Is Sexual Assault?

Littleton et al. (2007) conducted a literature review of "unacknowledged rape" to address the large percentage of undisclosed sexual assault, arguing that non-reporting may be at least partially attributable to a lack of awareness on the victim's part that the experience was indeed a sexual assault. These researchers found that as few as 42% and as high as 73% of participants in the reviewed studies were considered "unacknowledged victims." In one particular study, it was found that 44% of women had, by the legal definition in California, been victims of sexual assault based upon a series of 38 questions assessing for sexual assault history, but only 22% participants responded yes to the question "at any time in your life, have you ever been the victim of a rape or attempted rape?" (Russell, 1982). Koss, Gidycz, and Wisniewski Koss, Gidycz, and Wisniewski (1987) found similar findings, as their results indicated there was a 100–150% greater rate of self-reported sexual victimization in their sample than data gathered in the National Crime Statistics, which may be due to wording used by Koss and colleagues (Koss et al., 1987). Specifically, the researchers asked questions that avoided using the term "rape" and instead asked specific questions assessing whether participants had ever engaged in sexual intercourse without consenting. Given

W. T. O'Donohue and P. A. Schewe (eds.), *Handbook of Sexual Assault and Sexual Assault Prevention*,
https://doi.org/10.1007/978-3-030-23645-8_35

these findings, it may be that people's definition of what constitutes a sexual assault differs from state laws and researchers, which makes it troubling to accurately explore the rates of these crimes and assist victims with the recovery process and adjudication of perpetrators.

The Process of Reporting Sexual Assault

Reporting Sexual Assault to Law Enforcement

For victims of sexual assault, one pathway to reporting the incident is to disclose the assault to law enforcement. This pathway has a number of advantages including possibly increasing the victim's immediate safety and possible prosecution of the perpetrator which can have advantages for the victim and perhaps prevent further victimization. However, victims more frequently report the assault to informal sources (e.g., friends/family; 40–100%; Sabina & Ho, 2014) than to law enforcement (0–40%). The experience of reporting sexual assault to police is highly variable, with some victims affirming higher mean positive experiences than the overall victim population and others affirming more negative experiences (e.g., secondhand trauma), as demonstrated by retrospective, quantitative studies about victims' attitudes towards police and the legal system (Frazier & Haney, 1996). For example, some victims reported feeling that the detectives they interacted with were "concerned", "respectful", and informative, whereas others felt the criminal justice system overall grants perpetrators more rights than victims. To assuage these potential concerns and gaps in overall satisfaction with reporting to police and then subsequent involvement with the criminal justice system, upon reporting the assault to the police, victims are typically provided the option to have a victim advocate assist them in their testimony and forensic medical examination. Research has demonstrated that utilization of victim advocates can help to increase victims' willingness to participate with law enforcement through an increase in victims' confidence (Patterson & Tringali, 2014), though this has not yet been tested with a sample of victims of sexual assault and Patterson and Tringali's (Patterson & Tringali, 2014) study relied on victim advocates' perceived benefits of their advocacy based upon their own field experience. Nonetheless, the victim is typically provided with an ally to help them navigate the criminal justice system, which may be especially helpful for victims who do not have family or friends providing support and might experience further harm or fear of doing so alone.

During the initial stage of the police investigatory process, victims typically provide a video- or audio-recorded statement usually obtained in a forensic interview, detailing the allegation and, if possible, details about the perpetrator (Heydon & Powell, 2018). However, due to victims' concerns with confidentiality, there is also often an option for a victim to hand-write their initial, confidential, anonymous statement for the purposes of obtaining some initial information that can later be utilized for an official report once the victim is more willing to testify and assist in the adjudication process (see Heydon & Powell, 2018 for a detailed review). If the victim requires medical assistance, the initial interview may be very brief, or even delayed until after their physical recovery. Often, victims will also be provided the option to have a medical examination to check for sexual transmitted infections (STIs), provide emergency contraception, check for and treat physical damage, as well as collect forensic evidence to be used in court (e.g., sperm, skin under nails; Campbell, Patterson, & Bybee, 2012). After these initial steps, as well as interviews with any witnesses and the alleged perpetrator, law enforcement can advance this information to a district attorney who then makes the decision of whether or not to prosecute (see Kreiger chapter in this volume), which is a multifaceted process (Alderden & Ullman, 2012). It is important to note, however, that it is up to the law enforcement discretion about how to conduct the forensic interview. Therefore, not all of these steps necessarily occur in all investigations, thus the validity or reliability of the interview process is unknown.

Reporting Sexual Assault on College Campuses

For students attending a government-funded university, a separate pathway for reporting sexual assault is guided by Title IX of the Education Amendments of 1972 that states: "No person in the United States shall, on the basis of sex, be excluded from participation in, be denied the benefits of, or be subjected to discrimination under any education program or activity receiving Federal financial assistance" (34 CFR 106.51(a)(1)). The amendment mandates public institutions to investigate allegations of sexual assault and sexual harassment involving enrolled students (Walker, 2010). The process of reporting sexual assault includes disclosing the assault to a Title IX officer, or mandated reporter on campus (e.g., professor, office staff), which then initiates an investigation by the Title IX office (Nisenson, 2015). This process of investigation is similar to that of law enforcement, but does not require an in-depth gathering of evidence (e.g., sexual assault response team medical examination kit) and does not carry any criminal implications. Instead, there is a reliance on the victim and alleged perpetrator to present their own statements and evidence at a hearing, with the option of having assistance of an advisor present. The Title IX office then makes a ruling about whether or not the alleged sexual conduct occurred and, if so, determines the necessary steps to end the sexual violence, reduce the hostile environment, and prevent it from occurring again. The Title IX office will then provide a formal written document to both parties, indicating the decision made, rationale for the decision, and sanctions imposed if any. Schools do have the ability to provide the option to students who wish to appeal the decision, but the process is up to each school's discretion. If there is a preponderance of evidence (i.e., it is more likely than not the respondent is or is not responsible), the Title IX office can instill sanctions, such as rearrange the victim's class schedule to avoid any encounters with their accuser and even expel the perpetrator, suspend the perpetrator, or put them on academic probation if the investigation suggests that the allegation is valid (Nisenson, 2015). Despite the option to pursue this process, victims may still be hesitant to report to the college, as there has been recent criticism of the investigatory process guided by the Title IX mandate, driven by lawmakers' struggle to derive and pass rules that balance providing protections for those accused while also attempting to make the process fair and likely to find the truth (Anderson, 2015).

Reporting Sexual Assault to Informal Sources

Due to stigma with being a victim of sexual assault (see below about barriers), victims may often disclose the assault to informal personal supports (i.e., friends, family, religious leaders) and rely on them to provide assistance and support following the assault, instead of law enforcement or other specialty-trained individuals, such as Title IX officers (Baker, Campbell, & Straatman, 2012). In a recent review of sexual assault disclosure by college students, Sabina and Ho (2014) found across 45 studies that 41–100% students reported at least one incidence of sexual assault to informal sources, including friends, family, and other confidants. Fisher, Daigle, Cullen, and Turner (2003) found that individuals who were sexually assaulted (i.e., nonconsenting sexual contact was made) were more likely to disclose to informal sources than those who were verbally harassed. Additionally, those sexual assaults that resulted in physical injury were more likely to be disclosed than those that did not include injury (Fisher et al., 2003). Further, women (85%) were more likely than men (67%) to disclose to an informal source (Banyard, Ward, Cohn, & Plante, 2007), and those who were unacknowledged victims (Littleton, Axsom, Breitkopf, & Berenson, 2006) and had higher rape myth acceptance (Paul, Gray, Elhai, & Davis, 2009) were less likely to disclose (Littleton et al., 2006). Last, previous sexual victimization (Orchowski & Gidycz, 2012), self-blame (Orchowski, Meyer, & Gidycz, 2009), level of acquaintance (Orchowski & Gidycz, 2012), and substance use prior to the assault (Fisher et al., 2003; Orchowski & Gidycz,

2012) were also negatively associated with likelihood of disclosing to an informal source.

With the high rate of informal disclosure, the responses victims experience have been demonstrated to impact adjustment post-assault, with negative reactions (e.g., pressuring the victim to end the relationship, joking about the incident, giving bad advice) having a greater association with post-traumatic stress symptoms, depressive symptoms, anxiety, poor self-esteem, and poor reassurance of worth (Orchowski et al., 2009; Sabina & Ho, 2014). Combined, the findings reviewed provide strong evidence of the routine usage of informal supports for victims of sexual assault.

Barriers to Reporting Sexual Assault

Though the study of sexual assault has spanned several decades, little research has been conducted regarding specific reasons victims of sexual assault either delay their disclosure of the incident(s) or even decide to never disclose the assault. Often, researchers and other professionals instead rely on barriers previously explored by researchers Tjaden and Thoennes (2000) to guide their understanding of the victim's thought process. Therefore, a greater exploration of these variables is warranted to help guide public education, victim resources, and other efforts targeted at reducing the distress victims face post-assault with deciding whether or not to report the crime. This section will review the few studies that have explored potential barriers to reporting sexual assault.

Zinzow and Thompson (2011) conducted a study examining the endorsement of various barriers to reporting sexual assault victimization, using a sample of 127 female sexual assault victims enrolled as undergraduates at a university. All participants had experienced the sexual assault within their freshman year of college, as measured using the Sexual Experiences Survey (Koss et al., 1987). The findings demonstrated that 85% ($n = 108$) of victims had not reported the assault to law enforcement. Using barriers identified in the National Violence Against Women Survey (Tjaden & Thoennes, 2000), the researchers asked participants to identify if any of the following 12 barriers contributed to their decision to not report: thinking they would not be believed, belief that the incident would be viewed as their fault, belief the police could not do anything, fear of the offender, belief that it was not serious enough to be a crime, shame/embarrassment, not wanting anyone to know, not wanting involvement in the legal system, not wanting the perpetrator to be arrested/deported/stressed, desire to handle it themselves, not wanting the relationship to end, or reporting the incident to some other person except law enforcement (e.g., friend, therapist). Of the barriers explored, the most frequently endorsed barriers were wanting to handle it themselves (70%), believing the incident was not serious enough to report (68%), not wanting anyone to know (45%), not wanting involvement with law enforcement (43%), and personal shame/embarrassment (42%). Further, the researchers found that 8 of the 12 barriers, which were endorsed by at least 20 people, loaded onto two factors. Items from the first factor ("shame/not wanting others involved") were significantly and positively associated with various predictor variables of reporting, including physical injury from the assault ($p = 0.05$), relative as the perpetrator ($p < 0.01$), and self-blame ($p < 0.001$). Items from the second factor ("acknowledgment/handled it myself") were significantly and negatively associated with the victim's relative being the perpetrator ($p < 0.05$). The authors concluded that addressing help-seeking outside of law enforcement and public education/acknowledgement of sexual assault as a crime are both important to reduce delayed disclosure of rape. Specifically, they called for increased public knowledge of resources available for victims of sexual assault, as well as decreased victim blaming, especially in both informal and formal support networks. However, simply calling for this is insufficient for actually achieving these goals.

Miller, Canales, Amacker, Backstrom, and Gidycz (2011) conducted a similar study of 144 female victims of sexual assault while attending a university, only one of whom had reported the incident to law enforcement. The researchers were particularly interested in investigating how stigma threat, including fear of blame, doubt and insensitive treatment by the public, law enforcement, and/or one's social support network, influenced victims' nondisclosure and later revictimization. Therefore, they gathered a sample of women with a history of sexual assault (as determined via the Sexual Experiences Survey) and had them complete an interview and questionnaires assessing barriers to reporting, peri- and post-traumatic characteristics, and sexual experiences, then conducted a follow-up assessment at the end of the academic quarter to assess sexual revictimization. Barriers to reporting were assessed using open-ended, qualitative data from the interview and responses were coded into four categories: event minimization, self-responsibility taking, fear of getting the perpetrator in trouble, and minimization of the perpetrator's behavior, as well as stigma threat. Of particular relevance to this chapter was the finding that each barrier category was endorsed by victims, with 48.2% endorsing event minimization reasoning (e.g., "it wasn't that big a deal"), 34.8% endorsing self-responsibility reasons (e.g., "I felt I made a bad decision"), 22% endorsing stigma threat (e.g., "figured people wouldn't believe me"), 13.5% endorsing fear of trouble for the perpetrator (e.g., "I didn't want to screw things up for him"), and 12.8% endorsing minimization of the perpetrator's behavior as a reason (e.g., "he didn't mean to do anything wrong"). Miller and colleagues' study (2011) also built on prior research (e.g., Gibson & Leitenberg, 2001; Mackey et al., 1992) demonstrating that stigma threat-motivated nondisclosure was associated with poorer well-being and poorer coping, but extended the literature by examining its association with sexual revictimization.

Sable, Danis, Mauzy, and Gallagher (2006) conducted a study of 215 male and female college students, exploring a list of commonly reported barriers to reporting sexual assault. Specifically, the researchers asked participants to rate their perceived importance of 13 barriers to reporting on a 5-point Likert scale, then calculated participants' mean score of importance for each by gender. The findings demonstrated that respondents rated "shame, guilt, embarrassment," "confidentiality concerns," and "fear of not being believed" as the main barriers they perceived would make female and male victims hesitant to report the assault, though these were significantly more frequently endorsed as being potential problems for male victims than female victims. Additionally, participants perceived "fear of retaliation" and "financial dependence on perpetrator/perpetrator interference in seeking help", "does not want family member or friend to be prosecuted", "lack of resources to obtain help", and "cultural or language barriers to obtaining help" as being more likely barriers for female victims than male victims. Combined, the findings suggested that there are multiple barriers acknowledged by people who may later be victimized. Sable et al. (2006) concluded that the rape reform movement, which started 30 years prior to the study, has not yet appropriately addressed the barriers to reporting sexual assault, demonstrating a need to address these shortcomings in the field.

Thompson, Sitterle, Clay, and Kingree (2007) conducted a study of 492 college females at an undergraduate institution, 141 of which were victims of sexual assault (i.e., completed rape, attempted rape, sexual coercion—"intercourse subsequent to verbal pressure or misuse of authority"—and unwanted sexual conduct), to examine predictors of non-reporting of sexual violence, as derived by the National Violence Against Women Survey (Tjaden & Thoennes, 2000). Of the 141 victims, only 2 (1.4%) had reported that assault to police. The researchers found that, of those who did not report their sexual assault to law enforcement, belief that the assault would be viewed as their own fault (27.6%), belief that the police could not do anything (21.6%), belief that the crime was not serious enough (79.9%), shame/embarrassment (39.6%), not wanting the perpetrator to get into trouble (32.1%), not wanting anyone to know (48.5%), and not wanting police to be involved (47.0%) were most commonly endorsed as being barriers to reporting. Additionally, when the assault occurred on campus and/or the incident was more severe, victims were less likely to report the incident. The researchers concluded that college women have a low reporting rate, which is consistent with prior literature, and confirmed the purported reasons for nondisclosure to law enforcement, as outlined by the National Violence Against Women Survey (Tjaden & Thoennes, 2000).

Sabina and Ho (2014) conducted a literature review of 45 studies, examining the extant literature regarding disclosure of sexual assault and dating violence to informal and formal sources and utilization of services (e.g., healthcare providers, crisis center), 15 of which directly assessed barriers to reporting sexual assault to any source or service provider (Amar, 2008; Finkelson & Oswalt, 1995; Fisher et al., 2003; Fisher, Cullen, & Turner, 1999; Guerette & Caron, 2007; Kilpatrick, Resnick, Ruggiero, Conoscenti, & McCauley, 2007; Krebs, Lindquist, Warner, Fisher, & Martin, 2007; Littleton et al., 2006; Nasta et al., 2005; Orchowski et al., 2009; Orchowski & Gidycz, 2012; Paul et al., 2009; Sable et al., 2006; Thompson et al., 2007; Walsh, Banyard, Moynihan, Ward, & Cohen, 2010). For the purposes of this chapter, the overall results of the review will be discussed (please see the full review for detailed descriptions). The researchers found that across all studies of barriers to reporting to law enforcement, the most common barrier identified was disbelief that the assault was serious enough to report (Fisher et al., 2003; Krebs et al., 2007; Thompson et al., 2007). Additionally, lack of understanding that the assault was a crime and that the perpetrator wanted to harm them, fear of a lack of evidence, not wanting people to know, not wanting to be involved with law enforcement, fear of retaliation from the perpetrator, and belief of personal fault (e.g., being intoxicated, not keeping oneself safe) were all found to be significant barriers (Finkelson & Oswalt, 1995; Fisher et al., 2003; Kilpatrick et al., 2007; Krebs et al., 2007; Thompson et al., 2007). Further, shame/embarrassment (Sable et al., 2006) and not wanting to be labeled as a "victim" (Karjane, Fisher, & Cullen, 2002), as well as financial dependence on the perpetrator, lack of resources, and fear of not being believed (Sable et al., 2006) were additional barriers reported across studies. One particular study (Krebs et al., 2007) investigated factors that would increase a victim's willingness to report a sexual assault to law enforcement, which demonstrated a need for public education that rape can involve acquaintances as perpetrators, additional counseling and advocacy resources, free health services to address the health problems associated with sexual assault (e.g., pregnancy counseling, STI testing), and policy reform to provide victims more confidentiality when reporting.

In regard to barriers to reporting to service providers (i.e., medical doctors, religious officials, lawyers, psychiatrists/psychologists, social workers), shame and embarrassment (Guerette & Caron, 2007; Nasta et al., 2005; Walsh et al., 2010), as well as desire/belief of it being a private matter, belief that the sexual interaction was not serious enough, fear of lack of privacy/confidentiality, fear of the perpetrator, not wanting to deal with the assault any further, and denial of the assault (Guerette & Caron, 2007; Nasta et al., 2005; Walsh et al., 2010) were all negatively associated with likelihood of seeking these supports/services. Last, lack of knowledge of the services (e.g., campus rape crisis center, campus counseling center) available was a large predictor of service usage (Banyard et al., 2007). Given the findings, Sabina and Ho (2014) concluded that victims very often report sexual assault to informal sources (e.g., friends and family), but rarely to formal sources (e.g., law enforcement) and service providers, which demonstrates a need for additional exploration of the issue and increased availability of resources to be provided for victims.

Littleton et al. (2007) conducted a literature review to explore various predictors of being an unacknowledged rape victim (i.e., individual who has experienced unwanted sexual contact as reported on a survey, but do not label that experience as being sexual assault) and found that these individuals were more likely to be assaulted by a romantic partner and have prior consensual intimate experiences with the perpetrator. Additionally, they found that the incidents had less physical force involved, the victims were less resistant (e.g., physical restraint was not used) and more incapacitated (e.g., use of drugs/alcohol), and the incident usually resulted in less physical injury. They also found a general lack of understanding about sexual assault and its definition, and the fewer people in participants' social support network that have experienced a sexual assault, the higher likelihood that the participant will not disclose the assault. Last, Littleton et al. (2007) argued that rape script theory explains the difference between unacknowledged versus acknowledged rape, with unacknowledged victims having more disjunction in their experience of rape and their own person schema or "script" of rape. For example, those who are unacknowledged victims often presume that rape "script" solely involves an attack with severe physical force and sexual violence perpetrated by a stranger, whereas acknowledged victims include nonviolent, acquaintance rape within their rape "script." Rape script theory purports that the larger the mismatch in one's personal rape script and their experience of sexual assault, the less likely they are to consider the incident a sexual assault, which, in turn, results in reduced likelihood of reporting the crime. Given the findings, the researchers call for the examination of unacknowledged rape, as the research reviewed supports some unique experiences in comparison to those of acknowledged rape victim.

The studies reviewed provide insight into the commonly reported barriers to sexual assault; however, there are limitations in the studies reviewed. First, studies used a variety of definitions and questions to assess sexual assault. Many of the women whom researchers labelled as 'victims' would not self-identify as such. Furthermore, most studies (Thompson et al., 2007; Zinzow & Thompson, 2011) provided participants with a list of barriers, as outlined in the National Violence Against Women Survey (Tjaden & Thoennes, 2000) and did not allow for open-ended prompts. Therefore, there may be additional barriers victims face that are not otherwise identified in the extant literature. Additionally, the majority of samples used were college students (Miller et al., 2011; Sable et al., 2006; Thompson et al., 2007; Zinzow & Thompson, 2011), freshman (Sable et al., 2006; Zinzow & Thompson, 2011), mainly Caucasian (Miller et al., 2011; Sable et al., 2006; Thompson et al., 2007; Zinzow & Thompson, 2011), females (Miller et al., 2011; Thompson et al., 2007; Zinzow & Thompson, 2011), and none were large representative samples, thus the findings may not generalize to the general population. Additionally, Miller et al. (2011) only included sexual assaults that included oral, vaginal, or anal penetration, thus their findings may not translate to other forms of sexual violence (e.g., sexual harassment, fondling). Further, Sable et al. (2006) did not inquire whether participants had ever experienced a sexual assault, so it is unclear whether their findings would translate to actual victims who have not disclosed the assault experience. Last, Zinzow and Thompson (2011) did not assess for previous trauma history, and research demonstrates there is an increase in risk of victimization after an individual experiences a single sexual assault incident (Messman-Moore & McConnell, 2018). Despite these limitations, the research provides a preliminary understanding of the problems victims anticipate facing if they report and can help guide future efforts towards understanding potential barriers to reporting. One such effort is in the process of being conducted (O'Donohue, Chap. 35, this volume) and includes the testing of a barrier screen to be used routinely in investigations of sexual assault. This screen includes commonly reported barriers (see Appendix 1), with the option of listing any additional ones and provides pathways for addressing each (e.g., psychoeducation about sexual assault and common responses, referral to a victim advocate for information about the prosecutorial process; see Appendix 2).

The Effects of Delayed Disclosure

As previously stated, a large percentage of sexual assaults are not reported immediately post-assault (Ahrens et al., 2010), and there are multiple effects of the delay for the victim and the general public. One often cited effect of delayed disclosure is the considerable rate of recidivism of sexual assault. Hanson and Morton-Bourgon (2005) stated that there was a 13.7% rate of recidivism (i.e., re-offending upon release) of sexual assault, specifically across studies of sexual and nonsexual recidivism by child and adult sexual offenders. However, this rate is likely an underestimate and does not capture those sexual assaults where the perpetrator is never arrested. Immediate disclosure of the sexual assault may, theoretically, decrease the likelihood of serial perpetration, at least during the period that the offender is imprisoned. Therefore, addressing the problem of delayed disclosure is imperative for public health and safety.

Though victims often delay disclosure to avoid negative consequences (see above), lack of disclosure often still results in negative effects in the individual. In their study, Littleton et al. (2007) examined aftereffects associated with lack of self-acknowledgment of the assault and found equivocal findings in terms of whether the distress was higher than that in victims who did report their assault. Nonetheless, unacknowledged victims were highly likely to have more emotional turmoil, engage in riskier behavior (e.g., use alcohol), and suffer from post-traumatic stress disorder. Additionally, unacknowledged victims were likely to blame themselves for the assault (e.g., at fault for miscommunication, use of drugs/alcohol prior to the incident) and were likely to be revictimized later in life. Given these findings, there is a clear need to address these barriers to improve victim well-being and potentially provide some degree of personal comfort post-assault, as well as increase rates of perpetrators being held accountable for the crimes they commit.

Absence of Forensic Interview Protocol with Known and Acceptable Psychometrics.

Currently, investigation is hampered by the absence in the literature of a forensic protocol to use with adults that has known and good psychometric properties such as sensitivity, specificity, interrater reliability, social validity, and cultural appropriateness. Victims ought to expect to experience high-quality forensic tools but unfortunately there are no data to suggest that victims can expect this. Surprisingly, there has been much more effort to develop and test forensic interview protocols with child victims than with adult victims (see for example, O'Donohue & Fanetti, 2015).

Semi-structured protocols need to be developed and then tested on a number of dimensions (see O'Donohue, Chap. 35, this volume) for one such protocol. Protocols are necessary because psychometric investigations can only be conducted on a relatively fixed measurement process. However, given the large number of variables that can create variance in the reporting (age of victim, level of intoxication, number of perpetrators, mental health status of victim, etc.), the protocol can only be semi-structured as it needs to allow for latitude and flexibility to cover this variability.

For example, the following might serve as a basis for the major questions in such a semi-structured forensic interview protocol (O'Donohue, Chap. 35, this volume):

Victim-Centered Sexual Assault Forensic Interview Protocol

Preparation For the Interview

(a) **Determine whether interviewer matching is needed:** Ask the victim if she or he has a preference of the demographics of the interviewer, including gender or race/ethnicity. Emphasize that while matching may be desired, it may not always be possible. If matching is not possible, as determined by adequate attempts at accommodating, the interview may proceed, but let the interviewee know prior to the interview.

(b) **Assess the level of intoxication/ability:** (Is this problematic that interview cannot occur later?)

(c) **Assess the level of trauma:** If the victim has acute psychological or medical concerns, refer them to the appropriate professional. Psychological concerns may be determined by whether they are unable to speak coherently (e.g., in shock), if she or he is crying profusely, or express suicidal/homicidal ideation. Medical concerns may be determined by whether they have any open wounds or express large amounts of pain anywhere that are distracting or just need immediate medical attention.

(d) **Assess whether there are cognitive disabilities:** Use smaller words and shorter sentences in the interview. Cognitive disabilities may be determined by whether the victim speaks very slowly, appears confused, cannot speak in coherent sentences, or has a known history of developmental disabilities, etc.

(e) **Assess whether a language interpreter is required:** This can be determined by asking what their primary language is (i.e., what language they use at home, work, etc.) as well as assessing the victim's preferences. Request the appropriate interpreter, as needed. If there is a language barrier and one is not immediately available, reschedule the interview for when there will be one. Family members are not recommended as interpreters.

(f) **Ensure recording equipment is obscured and the room is comfortable, free from distractions, and does not have extreme temperatures. Gain victim's consent to have interview recorded.**

(g) **Ensure adequate amounts of water and Kleenex are available.**

Interview Steps

Introductions/Rapport Building

Hello, my name is (enter your name here) *and I am a(n)* (enter your profession). *I am here today to obtain your detailed statement of what occurred. I will ask questions but in a minute I will ask you first to give me a descriptive narrative of everything you remember from beginning to end. I know this can be an intimidating task. This is difficult and I realize that. I will try to make it as less difficult for you as I can. We will do this together. By the end of today, I will be able work with you to build a plan of what can happen next, although this is largely up to you, if you decide to move forward. I am here to help you decide what next steps are best for you and to support you in your decision. I may also be able to provide you with appropriate resources that you might find of help and we will identify those later. If you need breaks at any point, please let me know. Do you have any questions or concerns at this point?* Here you will want to provide reassurance if she or he is visibly upset. EXPLAIN VIDEOTAPING OR ONE WAY MIRROR.

Guidelines for the Interview

I know this is an unusual and difficult experience for you. If at any time you have any questions or concerns, please let me know. Also, if you want a break at any time just let me know. It is best if you can first tell me everything from beginning to end. I want you to tell me the truth and not to guess or exaggerate. It is very important you tell me, as they say in court, "the whole truth and nothing but the truth." Eventually, I will prompt for more details if you can remember these. I do not want to encourage you to guess and saying you are not sure is perfectly okay. If you do not understand one of my questions, please just let me know. Just say something like, "I don't understand that question". Also I want you to correct me if I am wrong or misunderstand what you say at any point. So if I try to summarize what I think I heard and say, so it was 8am but what you said was 8pm—just correct me. Also it is okay if you become emotional during parts of the process—most people do, so it is perfectly normal. I need to hear about difficult things as it is part of my job. I am going to record this so it can be referred to at a later time. Most importantly, I want you to know that you are in charge and you will make decisions about the next steps you want, if any.

Free Narrative

I want you to understand what I mean by a free narrative—essentially it means that you tell everything that happened from beginning to end without me saying much—I don't want to interrupt you. Later I will ask you some follow-up questions.

Here you will provide an example of a **free narrative** so the interviewee has a sense of what you're expecting in this section. *Last year on March 6th, 2016 it was my birthday. I woke up, but I'm not sure what time exactly. I brushed my* *teeth and took a shower. I drove to work in my Honda Civic and got there at 8:30 am as usual at 111 South Creek Street. My coworkers, Janet and Malcolm greeted me and gave me a chocolate cake with chocolate icing to celebrate my birthday. I left work at 5:30 pm and went to a bar down the street, though I cannot recall the name of it. I had a glass of wine with Malcolm, Janet, and Janet's husband, Michael. I then drove home where I had a glass of prosecco, steak, and potatoes. I went to sleep around 10:30 pm. This is an example of what a free narrative would look like. It is important to incorporate who, what, where, when, why, and how. Do you understand?* Answer questions as needed.

Okay, now I would like for you to start from the beginning—whatever beginning may make sense for you—maybe when you first met this person, and go through step by step as many details as you can remember until the end. In as much detail, tell me what happened from beginning to end. If there are multiple incidents, ask for them to tell you about the first incident and have them provide narratives for each event chronologically. After the end of each event, ask what happened next until the last event.

This is a chance for the interviewee to provide their own narrative with minimal prompts. The only prompts used should be: *Is there anything else you remember?* You will want to inquire about if they can remember vivid details (i.e., the five senses: sight, smell, touch, sound, and taste). This could include asking for example: *Do you remember anything else you heard?*

When they are finished, summarize what they have told you. *Let me see if I have this straight. Correct me at any point if I am wrong or left something out.* Here you will provide the summary.

Follow-up with Specific Questions

Thanks. You did a great job. I do have some follow-up questions. I want to go over specific details. Here you will go over gaps in the interview or anything that is not clear. You will want to ensure you have gathered all the elements of the possible crime.

You might want to start with the beginning—the first thing they said that was unclear or insufficiently detailed and then go through one by one until the end.

A good way to query is "So I remember when you said x—can you tell me a bit more about x if you remember?" or "You said y—I wasn't clear where y happened, can you tell me that if you can?"

By the end of this step, you will want to be clear on:

1. The jurisdiction, date, and time of the crime(s), the person(s) involved, and what forms of assault have been committed (i.e., vaginal penetration, oral sex, etc.)
2. Whether lack of consent was demonstrated and how. Possible specific follow-up questions to ask include:
   (a) How was it clear that you did not give consent?
   (b) How did you express that you were not consenting?
   (c) Was consent or lack thereof demonstrated by your emotions? Facial expressions? Body motions? Verbal dissent?
   (d) If they state that they pushed the perpetrator: How did you push them? Can you show me?
   (e) If they disclose consenting to certain sexual acts, but not others: What acts did you give consent to and how did you express this?
   (f) If there are multiple perpetrators involved: Who did you give consent to and for what act? Who did you not give consent to and for what act?
   (g) If the perpetrator is unknown: Describe what he or she looked like. What color and length of hair did they have? Can you remember their eye color? Did they have any distinguishing marks or tattoos, etc.?
3. Whether there were any witnesses. *Did anybody witness any part of what happened?* If yes: *What did they see? Could you provide me with their identity and contact info? Did anyone witness what happened before, or immediately after?*
4. Whether medical evaluation is needed. If there was physical contact in the assault and

medical examination has not yet occurred: *We want to make sure you are okay. We would like to provide you access to have a rape kit done with a medical provider. With this we can collect evidence, as well as check for any physical trauma or STDs.*

5. The amount of drugs or alcohol use, if any. Assure the victim that there typically is no need to worry about legal charges if they are underage or there was a usage of illegal substances. You will want to inquire about:
   (a) *Exactly what substances, how much, when, where, witnesses.*
   (b) *Do you think you might have been slipped a rape drug?*
   (c) Tolerance: *If you have ever used drugs or alcohol prior to the incident, how much would you typically have? How much would it typically take to become intoxicated?*
   (d) Body weight/height: *To further understand the standard influence of drugs or alcohol on someone similar to the same build as you, could you provide us with your body weight and height?*
   (e) Indicators of intoxication: *Were you visibly intoxicated?* If they do not understand the question, you may elaborate by asking: *Was there any slurring of words, stumbling while walking, or other signs of intoxication?*
   (f) The level of intoxication. Here you are trying to distinguish between whether they were tipsy or drunk to the point where consent was impossible to give. *On a level of 1 to 10 (with 1 being sober and 10 being passed out drunk/high), how intoxicated would you say that you were at the time of the assault?*
6. **Aftermath**
   What did you do following the assault(s)? Here you want to get an idea of how the interviewee responded to the events. For example, for medical examination purposes, you will want to know did they shower. You will want to know who they disclosed to or who witnessed their behavior immediately after the assault—you will want to get contact information for these individuals. Additionally, you want to know what negative consequences they may be able to identify as a result of these experiences.
   (a) First you should look for signs of anxiety, PTSD, suicide/homicide. *Sometimes people who have been victims of experiences such as yours report having physiological or psychological responses as a result of the assault(s), such as fear, sadness, or other emotions. Have you experienced any of these responses? If so, tell me about each of them:*
   (b) Provide the Modified Mini Screen (see Appendix 3) tool to assess for any mental health issues present. Refer to a specialist if "yes" is circled on any items.
   (c) You should create a safety plan as needed.

If the victim suggests in their narrative that there is any fear of retaliation from the perpetrator (both physical or verbal/emotional) ask *would you like me to help you to file a restraining order or gaining police protection?*. If yes, then provide them with information about how to do so at the end of the interview. If no, proceed to the next step.

If the victim suggests in their narrative that they are having financial issues as a result of the assault (i.e., damages to home, car, etc.), provide them with information about how to access victims of crime funds, shelters, or any other resources if available.

If the victim suggests in their narrative that they will need to seek somewhere else to live to avoid contact with the perpetrator, give them referrals to local options for temporary housing.

Referral to a therapist.

Explore Plausible Alternative Hypotheses

If you have any belief that one of the following alternative hypotheses may apply, say *I have to ask, because people accused of this may claim this, and I need to know what your response would be.*

1. The interviewee is mentally ill and it could be a false allegation.
   (a) *Are you under mental health treatment?*
   - If they say yes: *What is your diagnosis?*
   - If they say no: move to the next section.

2. Attention seeking.
3. Vindictiveness.
4. Misconstrued of consent.
5. False memories.
   (b) *Have you talked to anyone else about this?*
   - If they say yes:
   - If they say no: move to the next section.
6. Lying.

Assessing Potential Barriers to Further Steps

You did a good job. I want to remind you that you are in control of what happens next. Here is my contact information. Feel free to contact me if you remember anything else and want to provide more information or if you have any questions. I will contact you ___ (provide with a realistic amount of time, such as once weekly). *Here is what we can do next.* In this section, you will begin by discussing the next steps in the process (i.e., talking to a medical examiner, interviewing witnesses, doing a line-up with possible perpetrators, testifying in court). The purpose is to provide **forensic literacy** for the victim about the entire process of prosecution. Next, you will present various barriers they may identify.

How do you feel about doing these steps? If you move forward with pressing charges, what are your thoughts about pressing charges? Of testifying?

Note whether any issues with the next steps are included on the barriers sheet.

Now can I help you with any barriers that you may encounter. Provide the victim with a list of barriers (see Appendix 1). Allow them time to review the list and when they are finished, identify which ways to counteract those barriers applies to the individual. Write down on a pad of paper their "support plan," which will include the identified ways to counteract all barriers they identify with, so they can remember what to do after the interview.

Closing

You have done a good job today. Here, you will summarize the interview. Be sure to include details of the crime, details about the perpetrator, witnesses, consent, identified barriers and ways to counteract, and the next steps in the process. Ask if the interviewee has any questions and answer as necessary. Provide connections with your local victim's advocates. Inform them that different team members may contact them in the future and thank them for coming in.

Research Agenda regarding Forensic Interview Protocols

It must be emphasized that this is a proposed protocol that is in development. It would be useful to further study this protocol as well as others. There is some preliminary information regarding its content validity (as rated by various experts) as well as its social validity in that both male and female undergraduates rated it as inoffensive and generally as positive (O'Donohue, Chap. 35, this volume). These data were heartening, especially as this protocol contained questions about alternative hypotheses to actual sexual assault—but both males and females generally rated this feature positively. However, more research needs to be conducted. First, social validity ratings of actual sexual assault victims need to be conducted and modifications made to improve this. Second, its sensitivity (ability to detect actual abuse) and its specificity (ability to detect nonabuse) need to be determined. Information on its legal adequacy also needs to be collected (e.g., does it supply all the information desired by prosecutors). Information about whether it adequately identifies and effectively addresses these barriers also needs to be collected. Research into whether this can be taught to actual forensic interviewers and their fidelity to the protocol also needs to be done. Finally, the cultural appropriateness and any cultural accommodations need to be researched. However, it is important to emphasize that a forensic protocol with adults that has been investigated in this way currently does not exist.

Finally, more research is needed to devise and evaluate programs to combat both non-reporting and not proceeding with prosecution of perpetrators. Part of this would need to deal with a wide variety of barriers and also devising steps to address these barriers. In Appendices A and B, we have provided an example of this.

Conclusions

Sexual assault is a prevalent problem that affects victims, their families, and society as a whole. However, victims are faced with several problems, including a lack of awareness of what sexual assault is, what resources are available for them (e.g., victim advocates), and the process of how to report. These problems, combined with the other previously reviewed barriers to reporting, explain the large number of unreported sexual assaults. Given the literature reviewed, there is a need to increase public awareness and anticipate/counteract the barriers and problems victims have been found to face both immediately after the incident and in the long term. This may include providing victims with a barriers screen once they report and intervening in those that victims endorse, as well as incorporate educational efforts into colleges, high schools, and community forums about the resources available to victims. Without these efforts, the number of unreported sexual assaults will continue to grow, resulting in negative psychological and emotional outcomes for victims, as well as a large number of perpetrators who are never reprimanded.

Appendix 1: Barriers Screen

Sexual Assault Reporting/ Prosecution Barriers Screen

Below is a list of commonly reported barriers to reporting sexual assault and/or proceeding with prosecuting a sexual assault case. Please carefully read each item in the list. Indicate which, if any, you are currently experiencing or anticipate may be a possible future barrier for you assisting with the reporting and/or prosecution of your sexual assault case. By "reporting" we mean telling a legal professional, such as a police officer, attorney, or human resource professional, about the problem. By proceeding with legal action, we mean being willing to be interviewed and being willing to testify in court if needed. Please answer honestly and think about anything that will stop you from going all the way through the reporting/legal process.

1. I am afraid of how I will be treated by members of the criminal justice system.
   True False Not Sure
2. I am afraid how my coworkers or supervisors will treat me.
   True False Not Sure
3. I believe the situation is a private matter and do not want it to become public.
   True False Not Sure
4. I do not believe there is enough evidence for the case to be successfullyprosecuted.
   True False Not Sure
5. The police/law enforcement has been unsatisfactory during my contacts with them (i.e., from when I first contacted them to now).
   True False Not Sure.
6. I have not been provided with enough information about the prosecution process, or have not been given up-to-date information about my case, or have not been referred to support resources, and this makes me inclined to stop.
   True False Not Sure
7. The police or prosecutor's office has not handled my case to my satisfaction.
   True False Not Sure.
8. I have been encouraged by police or prosecutors to drop the charges or been told by them that my case is not winnable.
   True False Not Sure
9. I am scared, fearful or anxious, or traumatized.
   True False Not Sure.
10. I am depressed or feeling down, helpless, or hopeless.
    True False Not Sure.
11. I believe that the criminal justice system is unfair; perpetrators have more rights than victims; or victim's rights aren't protected.
    True False Not Sure.
12. I am scared of the actual trial process, testifying in court, or seeing the perpetrator in court.
    True False Not Sure.

13. I reunited with the perpetrator following the assault and do not want to make them go to court.
    True False Not Sure
14. I have felt pressure from my family to not continue with the prosecution.
    True False Not Sure.
15. I am still afraid of being revictimized, threatened, or hurt by the perpetrator.
    True False Not Sure.
16. I am scared that the judge, jury, prosecutors, or police will not believe me because I am a member of a minority group.
    True False Not Sure
17. I am afraid that police involvement will result in me being deported.
    True False Not Sure.
18. Society's attitudes about rape are negative and there is a negative stigma associated with sexual assault, so I am afraid of being embarrassed or judged.
    True False Not Sure
19. I am scared of being blamed by others for being sexually assaulted.
    True False Not Sure.
20. I do not believe the crime was serious enough to prosecute.
    True False Not Sure.
21. I feel embarrassed or ashamed.
    True False Not Sure.
22. I don't have a good enough support network to help me through the reporting process.
    True False Not Sure.
23. I used alcohol or other drugs during the assault, so I am afraid of how that will influence the outcome of the case.
    True False Not Sure.
24. I don't want to tell people about the assault because people may think I'm gay/lesbian/or bisexual.
    True False Not Sure
25. I don't want to tell people about my sexual life or interests.
    True False Not Sure
26. Please list any other barriers you are currently experiencing or believe you may in the future:

Appendix 2: Barriers Screen Resources

Resources for Combatting Sexual Assault Reporting/Prosecution Barriers

Below is a list of resources to refer sexual assault victims to following the "explore plausible alternative hypotheses" step of the interview protocol. Please refer to the victim's completed barrier screen. For each item that they responded "true" to, find the corresponding referral source(s) for that item (e.g., if they responded "true" to "fear of lack of evidence," refer them to a victim's advocate and provide education about the various forms of evidence that may be used). Continue down the list until you have provided the victim with all resources that may be useful. You will want to be sure these resources are available in your local area, prior to suggesting the victim seek these resources

Reasons for attrition	Ways to counteract the barriers
Fear of how they will be treated by members of the criminal justice system (secondary victimization)	1. Referral to victim's advocate, training of justice system members (prevention) 2. Psychoeducation 3. Provide stress coping assistance 4. Further meetings with prosecution
Perceptions of the situation as "private" and not wanting it to become public	1. Cognitive restructuring; 2. Assertiveness training regarding: rights; social phobia interventions; acceptance of negative

Reasons for attrition	Ways to counteract the barriers
Fear of lack of evidence	1. Referral to victim's advocate 2. Provide education about the various forms of evidence that may be used (i.e., rape kit, text messages)
Police were perceived as less effective at 6 to 12 months post-rape than at two weeks post-rape	1. Referral to victim's advocate 2. Increase contact with law enforcement (e.g., check-in with victim more)
Not provided with enough information about the process (i.e., not given up-to-date info or referred to support organizations)	1. Provide a general outline of the timeline of cases, communicate weekly with victim about the progress of the case 2. Referral to victim's advocates 3. Provide videos of the process
Cases not handled adequately by prosecutor's office	1. Referral to victim's advocate 2. Provide connection with the prosecutor
Encouragement by police or prosecutors to drop the charges (lack of "winnability")	1. Victim's advocate 2. Assertion skills 3. Social support
Fear, anxiety, depression	1. Normalization 2. Provide psychoeducational tools 3. Referral to a psychologist,
Belief that rapists have more rights than victims/ victim rights aren't protected/unfair system	1. Referral to victim's advocate 2. Meetings with law enforcement/DA 3. Cognitive reprocessing
Fear of actual trial process (i.e., testifying in court, seeing the assailant)	1. Referral to victim's advocate to help guide/advocate for the victim through the process and prepare them for each step
Reunited with the accuser/not wanting to make them go to court	1. Revictimization information 2. Values clarification work
Pressure from family	1. Provide family with educational tools about the court process, responses to rape (i.e., PTSD), and family therapy 2. Refer the family to a family therapist
Fear of further victimization by accuser	1. Offer help with filing a restraining order (i.e., provide information with how to do it)
Fear of not being believed because they are a minority	1. Ethnicity matching with police officer who will lead the process
Immigrant status (fear that police involvement will result in deportation)	1. Referral to legal aid/lawyer
Societal attitudes about rape/embarrassment and stigma associated with the crime	1. Provide information about the prevalence of the crime; psychoeducation 2. Cognitive restructuring
Fear of being blamed by others	1. Cognitive restructuring
Felt that crime was not "serious enough"	1. Provide information about the various types of sexual crimes
Use of alcohol or drugs during the assault	1. Psychoeducation 2. Referral to alcohol and drug counseling, if needed

Appendix 3: Modified Mini Screen

Section A—Please Circle "yes" or "no" for Each Question.

1. Have you been consistently depressed or down, most of the day, nearly every day, for the past two weeks? Yes No.
2. In the past two weeks, have you been less interested in most things or less able to enjoy the things you used to enjoy most of the time? Yes No.
3. Have you felt sad, low, or depressed most of the time for the last two years? Yes No.
4. In the past month, did you think that you would be better off dead or wish you were dead? Yes No.
5. Have you ever had a period of time when you were feeling up, hyper, or so full of energy or

full of yourself that you got into trouble, or that other people thought you were not your usual self? (Do not consider times when you were intoxicated on drugs or alcohol? Yes No.

6. Have you ever been so irritable, grouchy, or annoyed for several days that you had arguments, had verbal or physical fights, or shouted at people outside your family? Have you or others noticed that you have been more irritable or overreacted, compared to other people, even when you thought you were right to act this way? Yes No.

Section B – Please Circle "yes" or "no" for Each Question.

7. Have you had one or more occasions when you felt intensely anxious, frightened, uncomfortable, or uneasy, even when most people would not feel that way? Did these intense feelings get to be their worst within ten minutes? (If the answer to both questions is "yes," circle "yes"; otherwise circle "no.") Yes No.
8. Do you feel anxious or uneasy in places or situations where you might have the panic-like symptoms we just spoke about? Or do you feel anxious or uneasy in situations where help might not be available or escape might be difficult? Examples: ● being in a crowd, ● standing in a line, ● being alone away from home or alone at home, ● crossing a bridge, ● traveling in a bus, train, or car? Yes No.
9. Have you worried excessively or been anxious about several things over the past six months? (If you answer "no" to this question, answer "no" to Question 10 and proceed to Question 11.) … Yes No.
10. Are these worries present most days? Yes No.
11. In the past month, were you afraid or embarrassed when others were watching you or when you were the focus of attention? Were you afraid of being humiliated? Examples: ● speaking in public, ● eating in public or with others, ● writing while someone watches, ● being in social situations. Yes No.
12. In the past month, have you been bothered by thoughts, impulses, or images that you couldn't get rid of that were unwanted, distasteful, inappropriate, intrusive, or distressing? Examples: ● being afraid that you would act on some impulse that would be really shocking, ● worrying a lot about being dirty, contaminated, or having germs, ● worrying a lot about contaminating others, or that you would harm someone even though you didn't want to, ● having fears or superstitions that you would be responsible for things going wrong, ● being obsessed with sexual thoughts, images, or impulses, ● hoarding or collecting lots of things, ● having religious obsessions Yes No.
13. In the past month, did you do something repeatedly without being able to resist doing it? Examples: ● washing or cleaning excessively, ● counting or checking things over and over, ● repeating, collecting, or arranging things, ● other superstitious rituals. Yes No.
14. Have you ever experienced, witnessed, or had to deal with an extremely traumatic event that included actual or threatened death or serious injury to you or someone else? Examples: ● serious accidents, ● sexual or physical assault, ● terrorist attack, ● being held hostage, ● kidnapping, ● fire, ● discovering a body, ● sudden death of someone close to you, ● war, ● natural disaster. Yes No.
15. Have you reexperienced the awful event in a distressing way in the past month? Examples: ● dreams, ● intense recollections, ● flashbacks, ● physical reactions.

Section C – Please Circle "yes" or "no" for Each Question.

16. Have you ever believed that people were spying on you, or that someone was plotting against you, or trying to hurt you? Yes No.
17. Have you ever believed that someone was reading your mind or could hear your thoughts, or that you could actually read someone's mind or hear what another person was thinking? Yes No
18. Have you ever believed that someone or some force outside of yourself put thoughts in your mind that were not your own, or made you act in a way that was not your usual self? Or, have you ever felt that you were possessed? Yes No.

19. Have you ever believed that you were being sent special messages through the TV, radio, or newspaper? Did you believe that someone you did not personally know was particularly interested in you? Yes No.
20. Have your relatives or friends ever considered any of your beliefs strange or unusual? Yes No.
21. Have you ever heard things other people couldn't hear, such as voices? Yes No.
22. Have you ever had visions when you were awake or have you ever seen things other people couldn't see?

References

Ahrens, C. E., Stansell, J., & Jennings, A. (2010). To tell or not to tell: The impact of disclosure on sexual assault survivors' recovery. *Violence and Victims, 25*, 631.

Alderden, M. A., & Ullman, S. E. (2012). Creating a more complete and current picture: Examining police and prosecutor decision-making when processing sexual assault cases. *Violence Against Women, 18*, 525–551.

Amar, A. F. (2008). African-American college women's perceptions of resources and barriers when reporting forced sex. *Journal of National Black Nurses Association, 19*, 35–41.

Anderson, M. J. (2015). Campus sexual assault adjudication and resistance to reform. *Yale Law Journal, 125*, 1940–2005.

Baker, L. L., Campbell, M., & Straatman, A. L. (2012). *Overcoming barriers and enhancing supportive responses: The research on sexual violence against women*. London, ON: Centre for Research and Education on Violence Against Women and Children Learning Network.

Banyard, V. L., Ward, S., Cohn, E. S., & Plante, E. G. (2007). Unwanted sexual contact on campus: A comparison of women's and men's experiences. *Violence and Victims, 22*, 52–70. https://doi.org/10.1891/088667007780482865

Basile, K. C., Black, M. C., Breiding, M. J., Chen, J., Merrick, M. T., Smith, S. G., … Walters, M. L. (2011). *National Intimate Partner and Sexual Violence Survey: 2010 summary report*. Washington, DC: U.S. Department of Defense.

Brown, J. M., Hamilton, C., & O'Neill, D. (2007). Characteristics associated with rape attrition and the role played by scepticism or legal rationality by investigators and prosecutors. *Psychology, Crime & Law, 13*, 355–370.

Campbell, R., Patterson, D., & Bybee, D. (2012). Prosecution of adult sexual assault cases: A longitudinal analysis of the impact of a sexual assault nurse examiner program. *Violence Against Women, 18*, 223–244. https://doi.org/10.1177/1077801212440158

Finkelson, L., & Oswalt, R. (1995). College date rape: Incidence and reporting. *Psychological Reports, 77*, 526.

Fisher, B. S., Cullen, F. T., & Turner, M. G. (1999). *Extent & nature of the sexual victimization of college women: A national-level analysis* (Document No. 179977). Retrieved from https://www.ncjrs.gov/pdffiles1/nij/grants/179977.pdf.

Fisher, B. S., Daigle, L. E., Cullen, F. T., & Turner, M. G. (2003). Reporting sexual victimization to the police and others: Results from a national-level study of college women. *Criminal Justice and Behavior, 30*, 6–38. https://doi.org/10.1177/0093854802239161

Frazier, P. A., & Haney, B. (1996). Sexual assault cases in the legal system: Police, prosecutor, and victim perspectives. *Law and Human Behavior, 20*, 607–628.

Gibson, L. E., & Leitenberg, H. (2001). The impact of child sexual abuse and stigma on methods of coping with sexual assault among undergraduate women. *Child Abuse & Neglect, 25*, 1343–1361.

Greenfield, L. A. (1997). *Sex offenses and offenders: An analysis of data on rape and sexual assault*. Washington, DC: U.S. Department of Justice.

Guerette, S. M., & Caron, S. L. (2007). Assessing the impact of acquaintance rape: Interviews with women who are victims/ survivors of sexual assault while in college. *Journal of College Student Psychotherapy, 22*, 31–50. https://doi.org/10.1300/J035v22n02_04

Hanson, R. K., & Morton-Bourgon, K. E. (2005). The characteristics of persistent sexual offenders: A meta-analysis of recidivism studies. *Journal of Consulting and Clinical Psychology, 73*(6), 1154.

Heydon, G., & Powell, A. (2018). Written-response interview protocols: An innovative approach to confidential reporting and victim interviewing in sexual assault investigations. *Policing and Society, 28*, 631–646.

Karjane, H. M., Fisher, B. S., & Cullen, F. T. (2002). *Campus sexual assault: How American institutions of higher education respond* (Document No. 196676). Retrieved from https://www.ncjrs.gov/pdffiles1/nij/grants/196676.pdf.

Kilpatrick, D. G., Resnick, H. S., Ruggiero, K. J., Conoscenti, L. M., & McCauley, J. (2007). *Drug-facilitated, incapacitated, and forcible rape: A national study* (Document No. 219181). Retrieved from https://www.ncjrs.gov/pdffiles1/nij/grants/219181.pdf.

Koss, M. P., Gidycz, C. A., & Wisniewski, N. (1987). The scope of rape: incidence and prevalence of sexual aggression and victimization in a national sample of higher education students. *Journal of Consulting and Clinical Psychology, 55*, 162.

Krebs, C. P., Lindquist, C. H., Warner, T. D., Fisher, B. S., & Martin, S. L. (2007). *The campus sexual assault (CSA) study* (Document No. 221153). Retrieved from https://www.ncjrs.gov/pdffiles1/nij/grants/221153.pdf.

Littleton, H. L., Axsom, D., Breitkopf, C. R., & Berenson, A. (2006). Rape acknowledgment and postassault experiences: How acknowledgment status relates to disclosure, coping, worldview, and reactions received from others. *Violence and Victims, 21*, 761–778. https://doi.org/10.1891/vv-v21i6a006

Littleton, H. L., Rhatigan, D. L., & Axsom, D. (2007). Unacknowledged rape: How much do we know about the hidden rape victim? *Journal of Aggression, Maltreatment & Trauma, 14*, 57–74.

Mackey, T., Sereika, S. M., Weissfeld, L. A., Hacker, S. S., Zender, J. F., & Heard, S. L. (1992). Factors associated with long-term depressive symptoms of sexual assault victims. *Archives of Psychiatric Nursing, 6*, 10–25.

Messman-Moore, T. L., & McConnell, A. A. (2018). Intervention for sexual revictimization among college women. In L. M. Orchowski & C. A. Gidycz (Eds.), *Sexual assault risk reduction and resistance: Theory research and practice* (pp. 309–330). London, UK: Elsevier.

Miller, A. K., Canales, E. J., Amacker, A. M., Backstrom, T. L., & Gidycz, C. A. (2011). Stigma-threat motivated nondisclosure of sexual assault and sexual revictimization: A prospective analysis. *Psychology of Women Quarterly, 35*, 119–128.

Nasta, A., Shah, B., Brahmanandam, S., Richman, K., Wittels, K., Allsworth, J., & Boardman, L. (2005). Sexual victimization: Incidence, knowledge and resource use among a population of college women. *Journal of Pediatric and Adolescent Gynecology, 18*, 91–96. https://doi.org/10.1016/j.jpag.2005.01.002

Nisenson, A. (2015). Constitutional due process and title IX investigation and appeal procedures at colleges and universities. *Penn State Law Review, 120*, 963.

O'Donohue, W. T. & Fanetti, M. (2015). *Forensic interviews regarding child sexual abuse*. Hoboken, NJ: Springer.

Orchowski, L. M., & Gidycz, C. A. (2012). To whom do college women confide following sexual assault? A prospective study of predictors of sexual assault disclosure and social reactions. *Violence Against Women, 18*, 264–288. https://doi.org/10.1177/1077801212442917

Orchowski, L. M., Meyer, D. H., & Gidycz, C. A. (2009). College women's likelihood to report unwanted sexual experiences to campus agencies: Trends and correlates. *Journal of Aggression, Maltreatment & Trauma, 18*, 839–858. https://doi.org/10.1080/10926770903291779

Patterson, D., & Tringali, B. (2014). Understanding how advocates can affect sexual assault victim engagement in the criminal justice process. *Journal of Interpersonal Violence, 30*, 1987–1997.

Paul, L. A., Gray, M. J., Elhai, J. D., & Davis, J. L. (2009). Perceptions of peer rape myth acceptance and disclosure in a sample of college sexual assault survivors. *Psychological Trauma: Theory, Research, Practice, and Policy, 1*, 231–241. https://doi.org/10.1037/a0016989

Rennison, C. M., & Rand, M. R. (2002). *Criminal victimization*. Washington, DC: U.S. Department of Justice.

Russell, D. E. H. (1982). The prevalence and incidence of forcible rape and attempted rape of females. *Victimology: An International Journal, 7*, 81–93.

Sabina, C., & Ho, L. Y. (2014). Campus and college victim responses to sexual assault and dating violence: Disclosure, service utilization, and service provision. *Trauma, Violence, & Abuse, 15*, 201–226.

Sable, M. R., Danis, F., Mauzy, D. L., & Gallagher, S. K. (2006). Barriers to reporting sexual assault for women and men: Perspectives of college students. *Journal of American College Health, 55*, 157–162.

Thompson, M., Sitterle, D., Clay, G., & Kingree, J. (2007). Reasons for not reporting victimizations to the police: Do they vary for physical and sexual incidents? *Journal of American College Health, 55*, 277–282. https://doi.org/10.3200/JACH.55.5.277-282

Title IX of the Education Amendments of 1972, 20 U.S.C. A§ 1681 ET. SEQ.

Tjaden, P., & Thoennes, N. (2000). *Full report of the prevalence, incidence, and consequences of violence against women (NCJ 183781)*. Washington, DC: National Institute of Justice, Office of Justice Programs.

Walker, G. S. (2010). Evolution and limits of title IX doctrine on peer sexual assault. *Harvard Civil Rights-Civil Liberties Law Review, 45*, 95.

Walsh, W. A., Banyard, V. L., Moynihan, M. M., Ward, S., & Cohen, E. S. (2010). Disclosure and service use on a college campus after an unwanted sexual experience. *Journal of Trauma & Dissociation, 11*, 134–151. https://doi.org/10.1080/15299730903502912

Zinzow, H. M., & Thompson, M. (2011). Barriers to reporting sexual victimization: Prevalence and correlates among undergraduate women. *Journal of Aggression, Maltreatment & Trauma, 20*, 711–725.

The Forensic Sexual Assault Medical Legal Examination: The SANE Exam

36

Cari Caruso RN SANE-A

The SANE

The Sexual Assault Nurse Examiner (SANE) is an experienced Registered Nurse who has expanded their knowledge and skills, that come naturally for the time-honored nurse, and transitioned those proficiencies into the specialty of forensic nursing. The Sexual Assault Nurse Examiner will conduct comprehensive, compassionate, and exemplary forensic sexual assault medical legal examinations on reported victims and suspects of sexual assault events. It is an examination that requires distinct professional boundaries, nursing judgment, critical thinking, and the objectivity necessary for an independent, nonbiased forensic examination.

The "N" in "SANE" is for "Nurse." The first consideration, for the SANE, is the patient's health and well-being. The forensic nurse is always an advocate for the patients' health and well-being but not necessarily an advocate for the circumstances. That way, the nurse examiner will remain objective throughout the process, from the forensic examination to the courtroom, should the case should go to trial.

"SANE" is the designation for a Registered Nurse who has completed the 40-hour-plus didactic education, the 40-hour-plus preceptorship, and a clinical internship until competency has been achieved, to conduct an exemplary forensic medical legal examination, independently, and can be available for the "on-call" schedule. The "SANE" acronym can go *under* the nurse's name, indicating a Certificate of Completion.

The designations of SANE-A and SANE-P acronyms can go *beside* the nurse examiner's name; it is an earned credential of Board Certification. This is attained by sitting for a formal examination and passing, therefore earning the credential of SANE-A for adult/adolescent examiners and, with additional education, SANE-P for the credential in pediatric examiners. The age ranges overlap for the pediatric and adolescent examinations. The Board Certification examinations are given twice a year and require a fee. Board Certification is awarded to those nurse examiners who pass the examination. This chapter focuses primarily on the adult/adolescent examination.

The education, standards, and performance of the SANE, and others who conduct forensic examinations, are the same, regardless of degrees or positions held. The quality of the forensic medical legal examination should be complete, objective, and competent regardless of the designation held by the nurse examiner.

SANE programs strive to have someone on-call 24/7 unless otherwise arranged due to staffing or distance issues. The time frame for an

C. Caruso RN SANE-A (✉)
Forensic Nurse Professionals, Simi Valley, CA, USA

W. T. O'Donohue and P. A. Schewe (eds.), *Handbook of Sexual Assault and Sexual Assault Prevention*,
https://doi.org/10.1007/978-3-030-23645-8_36

acute forensic examination is up to 5 days to 7 days. The program will structure the call schedule according to policy.

The sexual assault nurse examiner position will most likely be a part-time position, which requires a full-time knowledge base. It is well worth it and rewarding for the registered nurse who is objective and detail oriented.

It is a capital mistake to theorize before you have all the evidence.
It biases the judgment.—Arthur Conan Doyle

Our Patients

The terms used by the SANE should reflect objective, understandable language and incorporate the words of the patient in quotation marks. As nurses, the interaction will be with patients. Persons are brought to the SANE, characterized as "victims" (v) by law enforcement. To the SANE, "reported victims" may present alone or with law enforcement (LE). "Reported victim," or, "Patient," is the terminology preferred by many practitioners, over "Survivor." "Survivor," is a term that may not reflect the objective language that is suitable for scientific medical professionals, at this place in time. The patient may become a survivor, at some point, but at the time of the examination, they are a patient reporting a crime of sexual assault or a patient being accused of a sexual offense.

The term, "suspect" (s), "accused," or "patient," is more appropriate than "perpetrator," or "assailant," for those suspected of committing a crime, because those persons have not been convicted of any crime; they have merely been accused, at this time.

The face of the sexual assault patient encompasses a wide variety of individuals. Most people imagine victims as they are portrayed on TV or in movies; the stereotypical encounter with a stranger. The fact is that the stranger assault is the rarest kind. Most reported sexual assaults are by someone the patient knows or has briefly encountered. Most cases are related to long- or short-term acquaintances and domestic events. Interpersonal and domestic violence are among the most dangerous and violent calls that law enforcement (LE) ever responds to.

For statistical purposes, the relationship between those involved in sexual assault events can be useful for classification purposes. Classifications may be:

- Stranger
- Nonstranger/Acquaintance
- Brief Encounter
- Interpersonal/Domestic Violence

The most recent category, by Dr. Sue Lindsay PhD, MSW, is the "brief encounter" (Archambault, 2001). This is when those involved have only known each other for a short time, usually under 24 h. That could mean that the persons had met and interacted but did know each other well and then, an untoward event occurred between them.

Many patients are ordinary people who lead seemingly safe, unassuming lives, interrupted by a random event. Particularly among the vulnerable are children, the elderly, the disabled, and the mentally challenged. The LGBTQ (Lesbian-Gay-Bisexual-Transgender-Queer) community are also subjected to violence and sexual assault. "According to the Centers for Disease Control and Prevention (CDC), lesbian, gay and bisexual people experience sexual violence at similar or higher rates than heterosexuals." The CDC's National Intimate Partner and Sexual Violence Survey found for LGBT people:

- 44% of lesbians and 61% of bisexual women experience rape, physical violence, or stalking by an intimate partner, compared to 35% of heterosexual women
- 26% of gay men and 37% of bisexual men experience rape, physical violence, or stalking by an intimate partner, compared to 29% of heterosexual men
- 46% of bisexual women have been raped, compared to 17% of heterosexual women and 13% of lesbians
- 22% of bisexual women have been raped by an intimate partner, compared to 9% of het-

erosexual women

- 40% of gay men and 47% of bisexual men have experienced sexual violence other than rape, compared to 21% of heterosexual men

Within the LGBTQ community, transgender people and bisexual women face the most alarming rates of sexual violence. Among both of these populations, sexual violence begins early, often during childhood.

- The 2015 U.S. Transgender Survey found that 47% of transgender people are sexually assaulted at some point in their lifetime.
- Among people of color, American Indian (65%), multiracial (59%), Middle Eastern (58%), and Black (53%) respondents of the 2015 U.S. Transgender Survey were most likely to have been sexually assaulted in their lifetime
- Nearly half (48%) of bisexual women who are rape survivors experienced their first rape between ages 11 and 17 (Human Rights Campaign, 2015) (Placeholder3) https://www.hrc.org/resources/sexual-assault-and-the-lgbt-community; National Center for Lesbian Rights, April 30, 2014 http://www.nclrights.org/sexual-assault-in-the-lgbt-community (National Center for Lesbian Rights, 2014)

Many patients are at higher risk due to age and lifestyle. Victims and suspects come from all walks of life, all socioeconomic levels, all educational levels, all cultures, all languages, all beliefs, all vocations, and don't necessarily fit the stereotypes. It is very important to be Culturally Competent (Lynch & Duval, 2011a). Patients may have engaged in behaviors that make them at higher risk for untoward actions, such as those who have mental health issues, either diagnosed or undiagnosed, runaways, homeless people, sex workers, those who use drugs and alcohol (ETOH), and those who fail to accurately assess their own safety.

It is vital that the SANE be knowledgeable about interacting with patients who have varied social, cultural, language, legal, and identity differences.

It is important to acknowledge that there are those who make reports of sexual assault which are not authentic. The fact that false reports do occur, regardless of frequency, should be an adequate reminder, to the forensic examiner, to remain objective and aware that all patients are not candid and forthcoming. It is not the role of the forensic nurse examiner to believe or to not believe the patient; the examiner's role is to document the patient's account of the event. Some patients may have motive or be otherwise troubled with issues that may have precipitated the report of sexual assault. The SANE may not be aware of the authenticity of the patient's report but regardless, exploring issues the patient may have and making appropriate referrals may be of great value to this patient. Sometimes, a report of sexual assault can be a gesture for attention or to cover up some type of transgression; sometimes, it is intentional that may or may not reveal itself, at a later time. Regardless, any false report of sexual assault is damaging for victims, accusers, and the falsely accused, and perpetuates skepticism among law enforcement and the community. No patient will be judged, or the objectivity of the examiner will be lost. All patients will be treated with the same compassion and professionalism.

Role of the Forensic Nurse Examiner

The sexual assault nurse examiner is the *link between nursing and the law* (Link Between Nursing and the Law, Lynch-Duval, 2005). The forensic nurse examiner will obtain a detailed event medical and history from the reported victim and gather vital evidence that will be analyzed by other forensic experts. The examination includes a carefully detailed account of the reported event, by the patient. There will be diagrams and photodocumentation of the any related findings observed on the patient, as well as appropriate specimen collection and collection locations, medication administration, and aftercare instructions (ACI). It is not the role of the SANE to come to any conclusions or pass judgment on whether anyone is being forthcoming or not; guilty or not guilty. That would cause the SANE to lose objectivity; being objective is the main point of being the neutral healthcare professional. The SANE, as an expert, does not give opinions or testimony to try to "help the case," for the prosecution; for whom the SANE will likely be called to trial, if that SANE has conducted the examination. SANEs who are appearing at the request of prosecution or consulting for defense, should not exaggerate, overstate, or appear biased toward one side or the other. However, the SANE's ethical opinion and testimony, regarding the forensic examination findings, may benefit one side of the aisle or the other, in the end. Many SANEs are defense consultants. They will be reviewing the forensic sexual assault examination and documentation for accuracy, quality, and completeness. The records can also be used for Peer Review, Chart Review, Quality Improvement, education, and annual competency evaluations. A SANE is an objective gatherer of reported information and potential scientific evidence; not a representative of the reporting patient or a victim advocate. The forensic exam is a neutral scientific process. The forensic nurse will be among other experts, who will be reviewing their aspect of the case.

The Sexual Assault Examiner must be objective, impartial, and neutral. Of course, in a court of law, there is no "innocent"; there is only "guilty" or "not guilty."

The Intake

EMTALA MSE

Reported victims present to the forensic setting in a variety of ways. Many are accompanied by law enforcement (LE) after a report of sexual assault has been made.

That is the best scenario because law enforcement knows where their SANE Centers are located.

Some patients enter via a hospital emergency department, alone or are accompanied by a partner, friend, or parent. If that particular facility does not have a SANE to do the examination, the patient should have a brief Medical Screening Examination (MSE) and be discharged. Then that patient can go to the SANE facility for the forensic Medical Legal Examination.

The urgent medical needs of the patient always take priority over the sexual assault evidentiary examination.

Very few (fewer than 2–3%) sexual assault patients need emergency medical care. This was specifically addressed by the Emergency Medical Treatment and Labor Act (EMTALA, 1986). EMTALA mandates that every patient who enters an Emergency Department receives a Medical Screening Examination (MSE). There are exceptions to EMTALA (Constantino, Crane, & Young, 2012). Most modern programs have set up protocols to bypass the Emergency Department (ED) completely. Many institutional programs have designated spaces which are, ideally, separate and away from the ED. Some have related programs but housed in separate facilities on or off campus, and there are those nurses in private forensic practice who offer a number of services to LE and the community.

EMTALA states, "When services are requested for a nonmedical condition or evidence of a crime has occurred and the patient is considered walking-well (E.G. sexual abuse/assault, blood alcohol) the facility is not obligated to conduct a MSE under EMTALA. However, if the individual, brought in by law enforcement may have sustained injury a MSE may be required to determine if the patient needs further medical treatment." Local policy will apply.

It is not uncommon for victims of Domestic and Interpersonal Violence to experience more physical body injury than other types of relationships. Interpersonal Violence evaluations, victim or crisis advocates (not the same as "patient advocates"; which is the role of the RN), offerings for counseling, and the provision of other services, are often included within the resources of forensic nursing programs and affiliates.

It is imperative that the SANE be attentive to the possibility of human trafficking. It is a special segment of awareness that should not be overlooked. The SANE will be familiar with indicators that their patient could be a victim of trafficking.

Patient Confidentiality

HIPAA

Patient personal information is protected by laws regarding who may access such personal information. The Health Information Portability and Accountability Act (HIPAA: Health Information Portability and Accountability Act, 1996; 2003 F.R. 82462) created privacy regulations for personal health information. Under this privacy regulation, "Covered Entities," who release medical information to unauthorized recipients, face heavy fines, whether intentional or unintentional. "Covered entities include healthcare plans, healthcare clearinghouses, and healthcare providers. Law enforcement officers are not considered to be covered entities under HIPAA. Although, HIPAA does impact how law enforcement can access healthcare information, police officers do not have to follow any HIPAA privacy regulations once they have obtained the personal health information of a patient" (Lynch-Duval, 2011; Chasson, 2011).

There are exceptions to HIPAA that relate to both reported victims and suspects of criminal events. Law enforcement may obtain some personal health information without the patient's consent for specific, purposes. Those specific purposes might include identifying and locating a suspect, a material witness, or a missing person. Some jurisdictions would include a welfare check. Some health information requires the authority of a court order or a warrant. All vital medical and psychiatric information, including DNA, dental records, and body fluids and their analysis, can be released and obtained with subpoena through the justice system.

Consent for the SANE Forensic Examination

The SANE should proceed through the examination with confidence and direction with the compassion and understanding of how personal and intimate the circumstances can be. If the patient chooses, one or more significant others should be allowed to remain with her/him, during this initial period. There will be times when the patient should only be with the investigating professionals, without any others present. Having other persons present during the interview can cause the patient to be inhibited when it comes to talking about their sexual history and the history of the event.

It is imperative that the patient give consent for all proceedings. Implied consent does not apply. This is not an emergency procedure; it is completely voluntary.

It is necessary for the SANE to be familiar with prevailing jurisdictional laws and policies concerning the ability of the reported victim to give consent for her/his own examination. In California, a person, 12 years old and older, can consent to her/his own forensic examination and should sign her/his own consents. **The age one may consent to control one's own reproductive health, including a sexual assault examination, is not necessarily the same as the Age of Consent. It is not the same for every state.**

If an adult or adolescent patient is able to understand what she/he is consenting to, then the exam may commence. The SANE will encounter patients who have been drinking, have taken drugs, or are otherwise impaired. The criteria for conducting an exam is when the patient can show desire to have the exam, can understand what will be included in the exam, understand the consents for the exam, and verbalize understanding to the SANE. This is not the same as "being under the influence," as with the intent to drive a car, so waiting for a toxicology screening for blood alcohol content (BAC) is not assistive, as far as consent is concerned. The SANE will explain all the aspects of the examination and assess and screen the patient for the patient's ability to understand what the examination involves and that the patient has the right to have the forensic examination or refuse or decline the exam or any parts of the examination.

If the SANE has assessed the patient as being unable to consent for the forensic examination, the patient should be allowed to rest for a period of time or come back when the patient is able to consent.

The time frame for an acute examination is up to 7 days so the patient should not be pressured to have the examination if not fully able to consent. The patient, having taken a shower, does not preclude that patient from having an examination and evidence collection.

It is the right of adolescent and adult patients to have, to decline, or delay the forensic examination. The patient should be informed that the more time that passes since the event, it decreases the possibility for the availability of biological evidence.

"However, the informed consent process includes making patients aware of the impact of declining a procedure, as it may negatively affect the quality of care and the usefulness of evidence collection" (U.S. Department of Justice, 2013). It may also have a negative impact on a criminal investigation because evidence that was not collected may have been useful. It is not the concern of the SANE to show partiality for either side of the aisle. Evidence may be of assistance to either party and should be introduced in an objective manner without overstating or editorializing. If the SANE appears biased the objectivity is lost. The SANE provides information and education; not conclusions. Consents will be required for the examination itself, which should include photography, the use of deidentified information for statistics, education, data collection, epidemiological studies, with whom the information will be shared. Also, consent for the administration of prophylaxis medications to prevent STI (Sexually Transmitted Infections) and emergency contraception (EC) to prevent pregnancy, screening for HIV, and any other procedure that might be assessed by the SANE or required by protocol.

A HIPAA authorization should also be included to inform the patient that her/his information is subject to disclosure, to law enforcement, the judicial system, and that a subpoena may be issued for records and photographs (U.S. Department of Justice, 2013).

History

The history of the event will be the words of the patient. It is best not to ask questions from a list but to allow the patient to tell her or his account of the event(s) in his/her own words, with little interruption except to clarify points and keep the patient focused. The attention should be on the patient; not a computer or a list of questions. It is not he nurse examiner's role to believe or not believe the history; the role is to assess the patient, physically, document what the patient states, using quotation marks, diagram, and photograph any physical findings, and to collect physical evidence.

There is a difference between the history that is taken by the SANE and a Forensic Interview. One does not necessarily replace the other although Forensic Interviews are recommended, if not mandated, for children/prepubescent patients. The SANE gathers information that will be specialized and contain different information than the interviews conducted by other forensic partners, who are not medical professionals. The medical history and the history of the event, taken prior to performing a forensic medical legal examination, is an integral part of the forensic examination and will be taken by the SANE. A forensic interview is typically conducted by a nonmedical person such as trained law enforcement officer, investigative social worker, or MDIT (Multi-Disciplinary Interview Team) (California Medical Protocol for Examination of Sexual Assault and Child Sexual Abuse Victims, with updates 3-9-2018, p. 23).

The SANE history taking should include details such as types of contact, time frames, physical locations, body contact locations, types of anogenital contact, number of times acts were reported to have occurred, positions employed, descriptions of surroundings, conditions and circumstances, and other pertinent information. Sometimes the SANE must keep the patient focused to stay on track. The SANE is the objective, medical professional, who collects information, potential evidence, and assesses the patient (SANE-SART Development and Operational Guide, Ledray, 1999).

The examiner's role is that of medical scientist administering medical care and assessment while collecting and preserving various kinds of evidence. These activities may require that the examiner testify to her/his observations, in court proceedings. The examiner must be viewed as impartial and objective. This should not take away from professional, sensitive care. The examiner must define her/himself as a neutral, compassionate practitioner while maintaining her/his role as a scientific medical professional. Bias, exaggeration, and overstatement will be evident if the case should go to trial. The forensic nurse examiner is always the "patient advocate" but, in California, for example, it is legislated that a "crisis advocate" must be called to accompany any reported victims to any interviews, examinations, or court proceedings (California Codes: Title 17 Penal Code Section 679.04 (California. Office of Criminal Justice Planning, 1987)).

The Forensic Examination

The forensic medical legal examination includes the thorough "head-to-toe" patient assessment by the SANE. The patient must be stable and free of any urgent medical issues. The forensic examination is not an urgent or lifesaving process. Should there be any emergent medical issues, clearly, those will take priority over the forensic examination.

For the rare patient who presents as a serious trauma victim, the patient's medical condition is always the first concern over the voluntary sexual assault exam. Trauma protocols can be initiated under the rule of "implied consent" but the sexual assault exam is not a priority and is not covered by implied consent. In these cases, the evidence collection is deferred until the patient is stabilized and able to give consent, or other approved legal protocols that have been put into place. Since it is most desirable that physical evidence be collected as soon as possible after a reported sexual assault, there is currently a window of opportunity, for biological evidence collection, for an **acute examination**, of about 120–168 h (5–7 days), for biological evidence collection. Clothing, vegetation, and other physical evidence can be held, in some cases, until consent can be obtained. California was among the first to institute State protocol and procedures with documentation forms for sexual assault events, for pediatric, adolescent, and adult reported victim exams, and a suspect examination (CA Penal Code Section 13823.5) (California Medical Protocol for Examination of Sexual Assault and Child Sexual Abuse Victims, with updates, 3-9-2018) (California Codes Title 17, 1986).

A **nonacute examination** would be one that is done after the time frame for the collection of viable biological evidence has passed. The same examination as the acute examination would take place, as far as interview, physical examination, and photography. Only the collection of samples would be omitted. Possibly STI testing would be done, depending on the timing and circumstances.

Forms can always use improving as the exam techniques improve and the progression of scientific methods advance. It is always best practice to make the examination observations and documentation as objective and nonbiased as possible. If the forensic exam can be said to be "consistent with the history," it could equally be consistent with something other than the history.

The forensic examination will include routine medical information, such as vital signs, complaints, illnesses, conditions, surgeries, allergies, psychological diagnoses, medications, and various other questions, depending upon the patient's age, development, and gender. The first day of the last menstrual period [FDLMP] or just [LMP], for women and girls, along with Gravida [pregnancies] Para [live births], Ab [abortions], M [miscarriages].

There is always the possibility that the forensic patient has engaged in recent consensual sexual activity. There will be no way to differentiate one finding from another. Forensic report forms ask about the last consensual intercourse (LCI) within 5–7 days. If the response is positive, there could be multiple samples of DNA present. It may be necessary for the patient's consensual partner to have an exemplar submitted as known DNA. If all persons agree that they were present and had had sexual contact, DNA would not be as significant in this case. The issue would be consent, which is necessary to note, since there could be more than one sexual contact or consensual partner, that could have resulted in anogenital findings, which would be indistinguishable from any current report of sexual assault.

The same way that DNA of the suspect can be found on the patient's body; the patient's DNA could be found on the suspect's body. The forensic nurse examiner should ask if the suspect (s) has been detained and if there might also be a suspect exam to be conducted. There is absolutely no reason that the suspect examination could not be done at the same facility and by the same SANE as the reported victim (RV) examination. If the facility maintains the same cleaning routine between patients, there should be the same routine applied for the next patient regardless if it is a suspect or reported victim. The nurse examiner will not ask the suspect any details of the event for which he/she is being examined. This could interfere with law enforcement business.

Sometimes, there are medical findings, hygiene issues, and skin conditions that can mimic and be mistaken for injury. The SANE will ask about anything that *may interfere* with the interpretation of the *current* examination findings.

Anatomy and Physical Development

The stages of physical growth and development affect the anogenital structures. Hormonal changes take place as the sexual anatomy matures. The anatomical structures that the forensic nurse must be familiar with, may be more detailed than the standard knowledge. The evolution and stages of the female hymen, from birth to death, may not be common knowledge to all; even some medical professionals.

"Anatomical position" is the patient's right and the patient's left, rather than the examiner, looking at the patient or a photograph in mirror image.

The location of anogenital findings are identified by using the face of the clock (Fig. 36.1).

Introitus also called the Vaginal Orifice: The introitus is empty space; it is air, or an opening to pass through into the vagina. There can be no injuries to the introitus because there is no actual structure there. The nearest actual structure is the hymen. When documenting findings, the SANE will list the physical structures being identified.

Hymen: It is not an indicator of virginity (Medical Response to Adult Sexual Assault-A Resource for Clinicians and Related Professionals, Ledray, Burgess, Giardino, p. 22, STM 2011). The hymen is the nearest physical structure to the Vaginal Introitus. It is a mucous membrane that is thick and elastic at birth due to estrogen from the mother. It loses the maternal estrogen and develops into a thin, translucent tissue that may tear easily. With puberty, the hormonal influence of estrogen causes the hymen to become thick and fluffy and elastic. There is no such thing as a "virgin exam" or a "virgin check." Minor superficial injury can be a natural by-product of consensual sexual contact as well as in nonconsensual contact. Whether or not the patient is reported to be a virgin is inconsequential. Injury can occur at about the same rate for both groups and there is no guarantee or method to predict when injuries may occur in sexual contact. Studies conducted regarding consensual sexual findings render the ability to tell what might be consensual and what might be nonconsensual, not possible from the physical examination. The studies from the past were less sophisticated and show mixed results from the more objective and recent studies. The statistical results of the studies reveal that the percentage of injuries are not so far apart that it could be determined what might be consensual

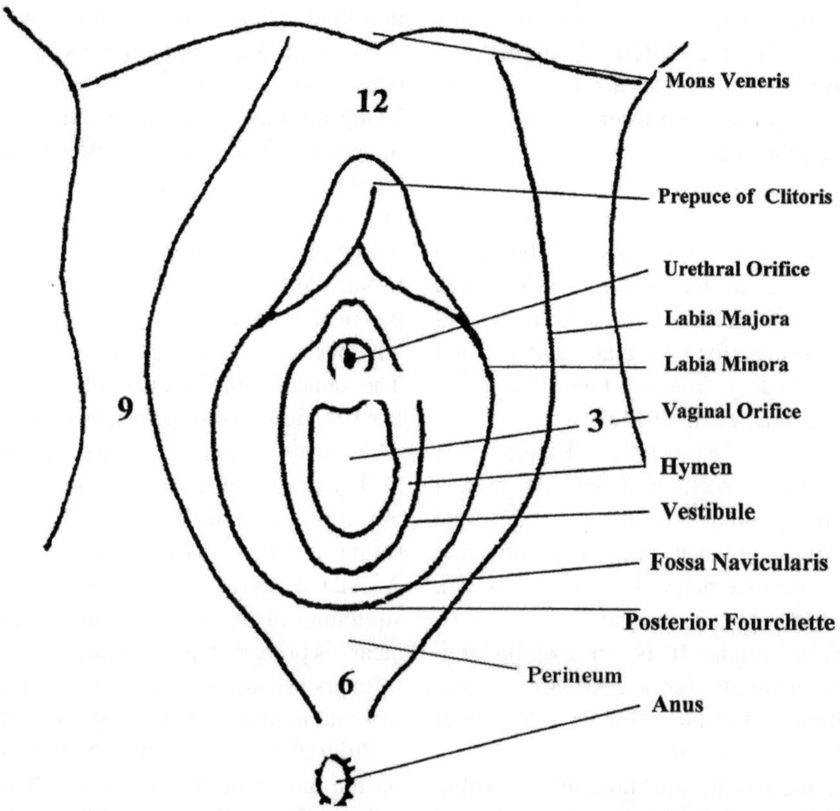

Fig. 36.1 This is the female vulva, also called the external genitalia, the perineum, and the anus. The vagina is not visible in this diagram

or nonconsensual or what patients may have been virginal. Jones et al. compared anogenital injury for adolescents reporting acute sexual assault with those following consensual sexual contact. Although data may not be completely reliable since the veracity of the history may not be known and some discrepancy exists regarding the types of findings that were defined as injury, both groups had a high rate of anogenital injury. The consensual group had 73% injuries and the nonconsensual group was at 85%. Sommer et al. concluded in their 2005 study that they could not differentiate injuries that occur as the result of consent versus nonconsent based on visual inspection, use of Toluidine Blue Dye, or the use of a colposcope (Kaplan, Adams, Starling, Giardino, 2011, Medical Response to Child Sexual Abuse, Chapter 11, SMT Learning, p. 226).

Vestibule: The "valley" or crevice between labium.

Fossa Naviculari s (FN): This is a slightly depressed area between the hymen and the Posterior Fourchette. *Posterior Fourchette (PF)*: It is where the labia minora join posteriorly and is just anterior to the Fossa Navicularis. This area is nonelastic and often a common site of injury. When viewed without traction or separation, it is web-like, similar to the tissue between your index finger and the thumb. When viewed with traction and separation, it flattens out and appears to be a part of the Fossa Navicularis.

Commissure: A site of union for the posterior fourchette. This term is used primarily for children whose commissure has not developed well enough to call it the Posterior Fourchette.

Perineum/Perineal Body: This is commonly referred to as the area between the Posterior Fourchette and the anus.

Anus: The anal area which is external to the rectum. The Dentate/Pectinate line defines the change of tissue types from anus and the Pectin Transitional Zone to the rectum of Stratified Epithelium (Medical Response to Adult Sexual Assault-A Resource for Clinicians and Related Professionals, Ledray, Burgess, Giardino, p. 45, STM 2011) (Ledray et al., 2011a).

"Internal" and "External": "External" is used to describe structures from the hymen forward and "internal" is used to describe structures from the hymen, back. The vulva and its structures are external, although, it is within the labium. The vagina is internal.

Pelvic examination: It is an examination, usually done annually for a PAP Smear, that includes a bimanual examination. It is NOT part of the forensic examination.

There are findings that are "normal" or "within normal limits" (WNL) and there are Normal Variants. The nurse examiner should be able to identify normal variants and common conditions such as venous pooling or venous congestion, which is the collection of venous blood, due to gravity, which can be mistaken for bruising by the unknowing examiner. If the area is pressed on, the blood will dissipate; if it does not dissipate, it could be a bruise.

The most common anogenital injury findings are superficial abrasions and tears. The mechanism of injury for abrasion is two skin surfaces rubbing together. The mechanism of injury for a tear is the stretching of the tissue, beyond its capacity, causing it to split or tear. These are common findings for sexual contact; it cannot be determined whether that contact was consensual or nonconsensual.

When two skin surfaces rub against each other, that contact can cause friction and abrasion. This is the action of persons having sexual intercourse. Sometimes, the external genital tissue is stretched, which is the mechanism of injury in sexual contact and can cause tears. Redness is nonspecific. Superficial injuries can occur in both consensual and nonconsensual sexual contact. Using the face of the clock for reference, when the participants are in "missionary position," for example, injury findings from penetration, are most commonly observed between the 4 and 8 o'clock position. There is no conclusive method to substantiate anogenital force. The degree of physical genital injury does not determine whether the acts have been consensual or not. The same findings can be observed when there has been reported nonconsensual intercourse and when there has been consensual intercourse.

The penis does not generally "strike" the genitals, as might be inferred in "blunt force trauma," so that is not usually the cause of injury findings. As stated above, the mechanism of injury is stretching of the tissue causing a tear. The term "tear" is preferred, to "laceration," by many practitioners because of the mechanism of injury and to avoid giving an overstated impression.

Injuries to the male may be varied, depending on the nature of the situation. Most frequently, the examiner will observe redness, abrasions, and tears to the anus. Foreign objects or other devices may be used on the penis and anus, either to constrict or bind or for insertion into the urinary meatus or anus. In these cases, ligature marks, redness and edema, bruising and/or tears may be present. It still cannot be concluded whether findings are from consensual or nonconsensual anogenital contact.

The suspect (s) examination is similar to the other forensic examinations but the suspect will not be asked about the reported event.

There can be injury or no injury when there is a report of sexual assault. There can be injury or no injury in consensual intercourse. There is no definitive way to tell them apart. The degree of the injury is not dependent upon whether an assault took place. There should be no expectation of injuries or the ability to substantiate anogenital force. The presence or absence of anogenital injury does not necessarily confirm or negate the possibility of sexual abuse or assault. Often, our patients will report that they cooperated to keep from getting hurt. Cooperation is not indicative of consent.

Even when injuries appear to be present, they may be due to consensual or nonconsensual contact. Some findings can be due to hygiene issues, such as tissue friability (breakdown), wiping back to front, infections and inflammations, or skin conditions such as rashes, excoriation, and dermatitis, which can mimic injuries. Naturally occurring findings, such as venous congestion, when blood, inside the veins, pools, due to gravity, in a dependent area of the body, the anus, in this example, causing it to have a blue hue and confusing it with bruising. Some conditions can mimic injuries.Some findings or lack of findings will depend on the timing of the examination. The patient's health and ability to heal will also be a factor to consider, along with the character and severity of the original injury, should there have been one.

When evaluating a patient in a nonacute examination, the conscientious examiner knows that it would only be speculation to attempt to "age" a possible nonacute finding unless the original, acute injury was observed and documented, at a specific location, and then followed-up through the healing process, to the nonacute phase, where a general time frame could be established. Findings can be naturally occurring, within normal limits (WNL), related to maturity and development, medical and skin conditions, hygiene, and can otherwise be misidentified and should always be included in differential diagnosis.

The forensic Examiner cannot substantiate anogenital force.

Of course, there is different criteria for prepubertal child exams because there is no consent for small children.

The adult and adolescent patient may choose to have a forensic examination but not participate in the investigation or the justice system and are not ready to make a decision about what they want to do. Rather than discourage any report at all, the patient may have the forensic medical legal examination with evidence collection and prophylaxis provided and have that exam held, for a limited amount of time, designated by the program, with limitations and notifications clearly defined. Then the patient will have time to decide what action to take and if action is taken the investigation will proceed. If not, the evidence kit will be destroyed.

It may not be known, at the time of the exam, what may or may not be valuable to the investigation.

All health care providers should be aware of the reporting requirements in the jurisdiction in which they work. In jurisdictions in which mandatory reporting by health care personnel is required, patients should be informed of the legal obligations of health care personnel, what triggers a mandatory report, that a report is being made, and the contents required to be contained in the report. Patients should understand that even if health care personnel make a mandatory report, they are not obligated to talk with law enforcement officials. Some jurisdictions mandate reporting for some or all violent crimes, requiring health care workers to notify law enforcement in cases involving a gunshot or knife wound, strangulation/choking, or other serious bodily injury. They vary, however, in whether they require acts of sexual violence without serious physical injuries to be reported. In addition, under VAWA 2005 as a condition of STOP Formula Grant funding, states must also certify that law enforcement officers, prosecutors, and other government officials do not ask or require victims of sex offenses to submit to polygraph exams or other truth telling devices as a condition for proceeding with the investigation or prosecution of the offense (VAWA, 2005).

In response to VAWA 2005, many jurisdictions have implemented alternatives to standard reporting procedures. Many SANE programs have joined with law enforcement and implemented alternatives to traditional reporting procedures, such as anonymous or blind reporting. These procedures are used when patients do not want to immediately report, do not want to cooperate with LE, or are undecided about reporting with their own name and contact information (but are willing to report anonymously) (U.S. Department of Justice, 2013).

Biohazards Associated with the Forensic Examination

There are few risks of biohazard contamination in the sexual assault forensic exam. There is a minimal amount of blood and body fluids, handled by the SANE and the nature of the examination makes the risk of exposure practically nil. Most exam rooms are not even required to have a red biohazard bag and all materials can be safely discarded in the general trash.

The evidence sets of swabs, collected for DNA analysis, must be protected from contacting one another and transferring DNA from one set of swabs to another. The samples, themselves will maintain their DNA, even if dropped on the ground, as evidenced from samples that are collected from less than pristine crime scene surfaces and locations. Fundamental to the Blood Borne Pathogen standard is the concept of "Standard Precautions." Once called "Universal Precautions," this concept is the primary mechanism for infection control. It requires medical personnel to treat all human blood, body fluids, or other potentially infectious materials as if it were contaminated with organisms such as hepatitis B (HBV), hepatitis C (HCV) and human immunodeficiency virus (HIV). Protective measures should be taken to avoid direct contact with these potentially infectious materials by using barrier protection, disposable, gloves without powder and changing them often, cover gown and mask, when appropriate.

All surfaces and nondisposable equipment should be wiped down with a solution of bleach diluted 1:10 or commercial 10% bleach preparation. The surfaces must be in contact for 10 min for proper disinfection and destruction of DNA.

The Forensic Exam Process

Generally, a patient, presenting for a forensic examination, should be in stable condition.

There are samples that will be routinely be collected. The patient history can guide any additional or unusual collections, when warranted.

When a patient states that, at the time of the event, she/he had experienced a loss of memory, for example, due to intoxication, or a loss of consciousness, due to a blow to the head, the SANE should use her/his experience and judgment to collect samples from every imaginable point of contact.

The goal is to conduct a proficient, objective, and meaningful examination for the patient and one that is appreciated by the justice system.

Elements of the Sexual Assault Examination

1. Initial Contact
2. Intake and Consents
3. Medical Assessment & Medical History
4. The History of the Event
5. Exam, Documentation, Photography, and Evidence Collection Procedures
6. Evidence Labeling, Drying, and Packaging
7. Sexually Transmitted Infections, Pregnancy Risk, other screenings: Prophylaxis, information, and resources
8. Discharge and Follow-up
9. Trial appearance as a neutral, objective witness who will educate the court and the jury.

There is no charge to the patient for the forensic examination.

In most circumstances the SANE will be "built in" to the prosecution's case, as an expert witness, and will likely be called by the prosecutor if the forensic medical legal examination becomes a significant element to be introduced. Unless other arrangements have been made, the district attorney's office does not compensate the SANE for the appearance at trial. However, the program for which the SANE works should have a system of compensating the SANE when a court appearance is warranted.

Of course, since the SANE would not say anything different should the SANE be called by prosecution or defense, the SANE could be called as a witness for either prosecution or defense.

SANEs who act as consultants and expert witnesses for defense should establish a fee schedule for review of the forensic medical legal examination documentation and photographs, along with other documents the SANE would likely review, pertinent to the case, such as transcripts, DNA and toxicology reports, CVs of opposition witnesses, law enforcement reports, and applicable medical records. SANE experts will likely charge by the hour for records review and have a daily rate and various rates for work product, travel, and expenses. A retainer and a time limit on the allotted hours for review, may be applicable.

> **We must remember that it is the 'Criminal Justice System,' not the, 'Victim Justice System.'** (*MADD* May 17, 2017 *DRUGGED DRIVING*) (Drunk Driver, 2017)

Most sexual assault adolescent and adult forensic examinations are conducted on females. The report forms are mainly focused on the female patient, but males are also subject to sexual assault and report forms should be created and modified to accommodate reports of acute and nonacute examinations of males, females, adult, adolescent, patients who do not want to cooperate with LE, at the time, pediatric patients, LGBTQ patients, and elderly patients. In some locations, consents should be made in more than one language

Most importantly, the SANE should think through the forensic examination using the patient history, critical thinking, nursing judgment, and applying evidence-based practice. "Evidence based practice (EBP) is the conscientious use of current best evidence in making decisions about patient care (Sackett, Straus, Richardson, Rosenberg, & Haynes, 2000)." (Improving healthcare quality, patient outcomes, and costs with evidence-based practice, Bernadette Mazurek Melnyk, p. 2, 10/23/2016) (Ledray, Burgess, & Giardino, 2011b).

The information gathering dialogue between the SANE and the patient takes about 45 min to an hour; a little longer if translation is needed or other barriers are encountered. The physical examination, with evidence collection, can take another 45 min to an hour. For the patient, the examination is about 2 h. For the SANE, it could be an average of about 4 h or more depending upon the complexity of the situation and the efficiency of the examiner.

Collections

A reference sample or exemplar. This is the known sample from the patient. Today, the most common form of DNA collection is with Buccal Swabs, which is a rubbing of the inside of the cheeks of the oral cavity, with a set of swabs to collect cells (not saliva) for an exemplar sample of the patient's own DNA.

The collection time has been expanded from 72 h to 5 to 7 days, since the early 2000s. Amazingly, the time frame was only recently updated in the California Protocol (2018). There are several methods that are passing trends and soon disappear as being unnecessary, outdated, or causing potential injury to the patient [dental tape flossing, using toothpicks or manicure sticks to scrape under fingernails] Neither of those things are currently approved.

Nasal swabs became popular, for a short while, as the exemplar or reference sample, but are not endorsed. A set of Buccal swabs is the current recommended method for the exemplar over liquid blood or blood cards (CCFMTC, 03-09-2018) (Sackett et al., 2000).

Control swabs and plucked head or pubic hair have not been necessary since the late 1990s when the advanced techniques for DNA analysis had evolved and a hair follicle root was no longer needed. Through the years, the techniques for collections and analysis have changed but they are slow to move ahead in policies, procedures, and protocols, leaving the older information "on the books." The use of antiquated collection methods and the citing of old literature, some of which has been invalidated, does not reflect well on the examiner, who is expected to keep up with current literature and Standards of Care.

Many changes that have been made, over time, and long-ago adopted, by the astute SANE who maintains contact with peers and affiliates and keeps current through professional organizations specifically the IAFN (International Association of Forensic Nurses), The Academy of Forensic Nurses, conferences and other educational venues and with the current literature. Some of the updated methods, annotated for the California State Protocol, March 2018) (Sackett et al., 2000):

- Eliminate all control swabs
- Eliminate routine head and pubic hair collections for reference or evidence unless a substance is suspected to be in the hair
- Eliminate oral and genital aspirate, wet mount exam, and all dry mount slides
- Collection for oral sample is expanded from 12 to 24 h [not the same and the exemplar]
- NO oral dental tape flossing
- Urine Toxicology expanded to 5 days
- Blood Toxicology/ETOH expanded to 24 h
- Alternate Light Source (ALS at least 450 nm, for use with orange goggles) has always been superior and recommended over the indiscriminate Wood's Lamp. Neither of those tools are specific for body fluids.
- Do not cut fingernails, use manicure sticks (orange sticks) or toothpicks [or anything else that may scrape or disrupt the tissue]. Use sets of moistened cotton-tipped swabs; preferably micro-tipped swabs.
- When there is an incomplete history or no history provided, collect sets of swabs from all imaginable points of contact:
  - Both sides of the neck
  - Both breasts
  - Perioral area
  - External genitalia (Vulva)
  - Vaginal swabs (4) and cervix (2) when appropriate for age]
  - Perianal and anal area
  - Rectal swabs if anoscopy is warranted [case-by-case basis]

The swabs will be identified, labeled, and placed in a swab dryer for an hour. It is the most efficient method, made specifically to dry forensic samples (Kinderprint, Martinez, CA). While the swabs are drying, the SANE will be going through the samples, sorting and labeling them, diagraming the location of collection, and filling out the forensic report form using the notes the SANE will have taken or recorded during the interview, so full attention could be given to the patient. After all the handling and packaging of the evidence, the exam room and all nondisposable equipment will be wiped down with a 10% bleach solution. The room should be ready for the next SANE and patient.

Law enforcement will sign Chain of Custody to receive the evidence, at the conclusion of the examination. Other arrangements can be made as long as Chain of Custody is maintained.

Taking Samples

Swab samples are collected by holding two swabs together, as a unit, lightly moistened with sterile or distilled water, and moved or rolled together, over the area of interest. This method is used for samples collected on dry areas. To collect from moist areas, distilled water is not needed. Some samples, like bite marks, can be collected using the double swab method where the set of moist swabs are followed by a set of dry swabs and labeled accordingly. Swabs are collected in twos, fours, or at least even numbers so there may be equal sample for the prosecution and defense to have tested independently.

The swabs must be dry for extended storage. The classic forensic swab dryer is ideal for this purpose, especially in areas of higher humidity where moisture may encourage mold growth. After drying, the swabs should be labeled, placed in designated boxes or envelopes, properly labeled with patient ID, contents, location of collection, and date.

If slides are used, a small, dime size sample should go onto the center of the slide.

The SANE will document all specimens collected and from where they were collected, on the forensic medical legal report form.

A urine sample (a few drops) will be used for a pregnancy test and the rest of the sample (the amount to be determined by the crime lab) can be used for toxicology, when appropriate.

Blood drawn to test for drugs, prescription medications, and for blood alcohol content (BAC), must be timely; those samples will also go to the crime lab for analysis.

The urine pregnancy test will not go to the crime lab and will not determine pregnancy from the existent event but will rule out current pregnancy, ensuring that it will be safe to provide the prophylaxis medications for STIs and pregnancy. If the patient has allergies to the proposed standard medications, alternative regimens can be ordered and consultation can be sought.

Generally, any testing for STIs, for the adolescent and adult patient, would be done at the two-week follow-up appointment since prophylaxis will be provided at the acute examination. However, any samples that are taken for medical purposes will go to the hospital lab. STI testing may be done for nonacute examinations. No forensic samples are collected, routinely, in nonacute examinations.

Underwear (panties) should be collected for evidence in an acute examination. If the patient has changed or washed the panties they should still be collected because semen can be detected, sometimes, even after an article of clothing has been laundered (Kafarowski, Lyon, & Sloan, 1996; Lynch & Duval, 2011b). Clothing can be photographed and may contain evidence of tears, rips, or debris. The patient may refuse to release articles of clothing for evidence, which is her/his privilege, as it is her/his option to refuse any parts of the examination.

Clothing is packaged separately in paper bags and sealed with evidence tape with the SANE's initials and the date, overlapping the tape edges. Body findings and anogenital findings may not be related and should be evaluated separately. One may have nothing to do with the other.

Sets of neck swabs, breast swabs, and external anogenital swabs are among the standard collections.

Other collections should be guided by history: suction marks, fingernail swabs, the abdomen, sites of piercings, and other areas of possible touch DNA or body fluids.

Accurate documentation and clear photography of visible injury, dirt, and debris on the body, could be assistive in the investigation. For the patient with an unknown history due to intoxication or other reasons, all imaginable points of contact should be swabbed. "Unknown history" refers to a patient who may have been too intoxicated with drugs or alcohol to know exactly what occurred at the time of the event. They may wake up later with a foggy memory and think that something may have happened. These patients can sometimes be unsure what, if anything untoward occurred. Regardless, the examination is conducted the same objective manner and it will be unknown if consent was given.

External genital or vulvar swabs will be taken separately from vaginal samples. Vaginal samples are taken with four swabs, held together as a unit which do not need moistening with distilled water. Two cervical swabs within the time parameters, will not need to be moistened. Each program will have their own policies, procedures, and protocols, that will be created to meet the needs of their community.

Nursing judgment and critical thinking, along with evidence-based practice, will guide the SANE throughout the exam. Some things are routine collections and some things could have been missed except for the astute forensic nurse examiner, who assesses the patient and the history provided in order to convert the intake information into individualized significant collections. The investigation is early; at this point, it is not known what might become significant, at a later time.

The forensic documentation and narrative should be complete with as much detail as possible but not so voluminous that it becomes burdensome to read by law enforcement, attorneys, jurors, reviewers, and other involved entities. The next people who are going to read the sexual assault forensic examination report and narrative will be law enforcement, not medical people. The anatomical structures have specific names and the correct terminology should be used. However, some terms can be used that are familiar to nonmedical persons. After all, the purpose of an expert witness, in the courtroom, is to educate the court and the jury so they can come to a fair and equitable decision. For example, "erythema" is a medical word for "redness," and "bruise" could be used instead of "ecchymosis." When the SANE knows who will be addressed, it is best to use the most understandable terms that to which the listener is accustomed.

Medical Photography

Medical photography is essential to the forensic process. It can be accomplished with a good quality digital camera. SANE programs should have a colposcope with a mounted camera or some other set-up for anogenital medical photography, and a handheld camera and even with use of a monopod. There are now a variety of methods for photographic and imaging software that are alternative to the colposcope with camera. Some are more portable but whatever the methods the program chooses, the photos should be clear, with good lighting, and enlarge well without losing quality. There is really no excuse for poor photography or for limiting the number of photographs. As many photos should be taken to demonstrate the observed finding.

The purpose of medical photography is to produce a fair and accurate representation of what was observed during the forensic SANE examination. These photographs will be reviewed for any potential value for use in legal proceedings. The examining SANE will be the expert called by prosecution. The SANE records and photographs will likely be reviewed by an expert working with defense.

The value of medical photography is to record and communicate that which cannot be communicated with the written word alone, since time will have passed since the reported event was acute. It is the responsibility of the SANE to take enough photographs to demonstrate the documented findings.

The controversy of using digital photography in the courts is long past. It was once thought, that with the ability to alter photos, the evidence was unreliable. There are many ways to authenticate the photos but first and foremost, it is the integrity of the photographer that brings ethical practice to the use of digital technology.

There are filters and software programs that can be used to amplify minor and superficial findings and can make them exaggerated and intensified in appearance. For example, a small area of redness can appear much worse and could be misleading if it is not made clear that it is being viewed with the use of a filter. It is not the same as photoshop, where you can actually change what is in the photo.

A head shot of the patient should be taken for patient identification. Body photos need not be taken if there are no injuries with one exception. If a patient has reported that an injury occurred to a body part, for example, being stabbed in the shoulder, and no evidence of injury is present on the shoulder, it would be prudent to take a few photos to show there is no injury on the shoulder.

Genital and anal photos should be taken with every SANE exam whether there are findings or not. This demonstrates that the examiner did a thorough examination and inspected all the anogenital structures. The anus should be always be inspected whether or not a report of anal penetration had been made.

Informed consent must be obtained for photography. It could be built into your consent for examination or a separate consent. The consent can ask for permission to use the photos for educational purposes, used in the investigation, and if the patient is a minor but has the ability to sign for her/his own examination, it would be necessary to ask consent from the patient before the SANE can share the information with the patient's mother, for example. That would be a violation of HIPAA so a separate release, should be signed and acknowledged by the patient.

The forensic report forms and the evidence collected will already have been collected by law enforcement with the chain of custody maintained. A copy of the forensic report should accompany the evidence in the sexual assault evidence kit (SAEK). Photographs can be held with the forensic records, in the secure SANE office, separate from medical records, until such a time that a trial is pending. Then a copy of the photos can be released, along with the entire file, to the subpoenaing body; usually the District Attorney's Office. Defense will obtain the documentation through discovery through the District Attorney's Office.

Forensic History and Evidence Collection

Information

- Date and time of arrival
- Date and time of event
- Patient name, age, date of birth, contact information, ethnicity, language spoken (translator name and position, if utilized)
- Vital statistics
- Location of the event: geographical area and physical location
- Acts reported
- What hygiene activities have been done since the reported event. Patients should be encouraged to have a forensic examination whether or not they have washed.
- Last menstrual period (LMP) (first day of last menstrual period: FDLMP)
- Pregnancy history: Pregnancies, Live Births, abortions, miscarriages (Para, Gravida, AB, Mis)
- Any other procedures, surgeries, unrelated injuries, or findings that WOULD AFFECT THE INTERPRETATION of the current exam findings
- Preexisting conditions
- Last consensual sexual contact within 5–7 days
- Alcohol (ETOH) or drug (prescription or street drugs) use
- Loss of memory
- Any of the reported acts consensual
- Pertinent physical surroundings
- Name of alleged suspect, age, gender, ethnicity, relationship (known, brief, unknown, interpersonal/domestic violence)
- Weapon
- Threats
- Physical assault
- Physical restraints (Ropes, duct tape, zip ties, handcuffs, other **physical** items of restraint; NOT a person).
- Strangulation
- Injuries inflicted on suspect by reported victim
- The history should indicate the number of times something occurred and whether any of the reported acts were completed, attempted, or the patient was unsure.
- If more than one suspect is reported to have been involved, they should be identified with a number (s-1), or by name.

The location of collections should be documented on body diagrams (Table 36.1).

Speculum examinations are done on female patients who have entered puberty as tolerated (case-by-case basis) and older. Speculum exams are not done on prepubertal females. Speculum exams will only be done on pubertal females when judged by the SANE to be accomplished without undue discomfort or injury to the patient.

In an extreme situation where the location of the reported sexual assault is unknown or the patient presents with debris of unknown origin on the clothing or body, have the patient stand and undress on two sheets of exam table paper. The patient will remove items of clothing, if it was the same clothing worn at the time, and each item will be placed in its own

Table 36.1 Possible forensic collections

History	Location	Collection
Kissing	Mouth, lips, neck, breasts	Circumoral, perioral, lip swabs, oral, if within 12 h of the reported event Neck swabs right, neck swabs left Breast swabs including nipples
Oral contact: fellatio, cunnilingus	Oral cavity, lips	Oral samples up to 24 h
Genital penetration, genital contact, attempted, unsure	Vulva, vagina	Genital swabs (2), vaginal swabs (4), cervical swabs (2).
Digital genital penetration	Vulva, vagina	Swabs, as above
Anal/rectal: digital, penetration, contact, attempted, unsure	No report of contact Anal penetration	Anal swabs (2) Rectal swabs (2)
Ejaculation	Location	Set of swabs
Condom use	Yes [ ] No [ ]	Collected
Foreign object	Yes [ ] No [ ]	Collected
Other		
Other		

paper bag, labeled and sealed. This process is not useful if the location is known or it is somewhere where the environment is not in question. Retain the top sheet of paper, where the debris has fallen, and bindle it and place in a paper bag. Label with patient's personal data and forensic evidence label and initial. Discard bottom sheet of paper. This process is not usually necessary.

Adjuncts to the Forensic Examination

The Colposcope

The colposcope is an instrument with low power magnification but a high-power light for visual inspection, using a system that can go from 4 to 35 X (or greater) magnification potential. It does not touch the patient or go inside of the patient. Once used only by gynecologic practitioners to visualize areas of cervical and vulvar tissue, using filters and screening methods, to aid in the diagnosis of vulvar and cervical pathology. The use of the colposcope with camera has been employed by the SANE, for forensic pediatric, adolescent, adult, male and female examinations for at least 25 years. When describing the SANE's use of the colposcope, in court, for example, it is not described as "colposcopy" by the forensic nurse. This is to differentiate it from the "diagnostic colposcopy" in women's health, as described above, rather than for forensic purposes. The SANE uses of the colposcope for its magnification purposes.

Regardless of whether a colposcope is used, a separate digital camera should be used for body photos, soiled or torn clothing, and other items that may become significant.

Alternate Light Source

Wood's Lamp

Some programs may still be using the Wood's Lamp, also called the "black light" or the "UV (ultraviolet) light." In a dark room, shining the ultraviolet light on an area of interest about 4–12 in. away, the examiner will look at the skin to see if there is any absorption, also called "fluorescence." The exam is painless and there are no adverse side effects.

The skin does not normally illuminate under the ultraviolet light. Fingernail beds, teeth, scars and the white of the eyes will. Things that will "fluoresce" are jewelry, soaps, make-up, creams, lotions, drinks, sodas, foods, acne, dust, lint, fibers, scars, fungal and bacterial infections, and many, many more substances, including the possibility of body fluids containing DNA, such as semen, sperm, amylase, and epithelial cells.

False negatives and false positives can be produced. There may be illumination of an area that has no sample and there may be no illumination where a valuable sample may be present. That is why the "results" of the UV lights are unreliable for any specific findings. The range of the Wood's Lamp ultraviolet light is about 360 nm and not very discriminating (Lynch & Duval, 2011a, 2011b).

The SANE will not know what substance, if any, is being collected.

Alternate Light Source

An alternate light source (ALS) is also an ultraviolet device but it is much more discriminating. It cuts down on the fine debris of lint, fibers, and dust that are commonly found on clothing that the Wood's Lamp does not. ALS are available in, small, handheld versions, up to the most powerful types used by crime labs. Orange goggles must be worn using this wavelength range. Other wavelength ranges may be visualized with various colors of goggles, to visualize absorption or "fluorescence," in a darkened room.

A forensic light source (ALS) is made up of a lamp containing the ultraviolet, visible, and infrared components of light at 400–475 nm or greater, where the Wood's Lamp is 360 nm.

Toluidine Blue Dye

Toluidine Blue Dye is a 1% aqueous solution of thiazine metachromatic nuclear stain, with an affinity for acidic tissue components. It is applied to determine the presence of nucleated squamous cells. Surface cells are nonnucleated cells and will not stain. Nucleated cells that are exposed will stain a dark blue, purplish color. The dye will adhere to any disruption of the tissue where nucleated cells are exposed, whether it is from an acute injury, hygiene issue, medical, or skin condition. Many observations are mistaken for injury.

The dye is applied with two cotton swabs to the genital and anal areas. It is not used to "find injury"; it is used to highlight findings observed by the SANE. It is NOT applied to mucous membranes (hymen) or internally. After the dye is applied and allowed to settle, the dye is removed. To remove the excess dye, it is decolorized with a 1% acetic acid (vinegar and water) solution spray, or some prefer a water-based lubricant. 4 × 4 gauze squares are used to gently pat the excess dye away. Baby wipes have also been successfully employed for this use.

Photos should be taken before application of the dye, after application of the dye, when the dye is present, and after the decolorization process. Some residue dye may be left on the skin, in folds, or textured skin surfaces. A skilled and experienced SANE will be able to recognize whether the tissue has been disturbed or not.

Accurate interpretation of the post-dye findings takes competence to avoid misinterpretation. Sometimes, the dye remains in tissue folds and adheres to tissue when there is no injury (residual dye). If the dye gets on mucous membrane, such as the hymen, it should not be "interpreted" at all.

Light blue, diffuse, and "weak uptake," should be interpreted as negative. Only dark purple/blue uptake will be considered positive. "Artifacts" may exist (Lynch & Duval, 2011b).

Anoscopy

Every patient should have an anal/perianal inspection, whether or not anal contact was reported. If, for no other reason, to make a record that the area was observed. In addition to separation and traction, of the anal folds, a photograph or two should be taken to document that you examined the anal area. If anal penetration is reported, external and internal swabs are collected. An anoscopy may be conducted, on a case-by-case basis, to examine the internal, mucosal surfaces of the anus and rectum.

It is not necessary to conduct anoscopy for every report of anal/penile penetration but, if there is active bleeding in which the SANE cannot visualize the source, an anoscopy may be in order. It also makes it easier to obtain the internal swabs, if desired.

The process is minimally uncomfortable, for the patient.

Baseline Status and Prophylaxis

The patient will be offered prophylaxis to prevent sexually transmitted infections (STI) (Gonorrhea, Chlamydia, and possibly Trichomonas, depending on local protocols) and screened for HIV post exposure (CDC Guidelines, 2015).

Female patients will be offered prophylaxis for pregnancy, when appropriate.

Aftercare instructions will be provided, and a 2-week follow-up examination should be recommended, with the patient's provider, for STI and pregnancy testing for the efficacy of the prophylaxis.

All female victims of childbearing age should be offered prophylaxis for pregnancy. Even the most conservative institutions, who do not favor birth control, make allowances in cases of sexual assault. Emergency contraception is **not an abortifacient** and should be taken as soon as possible after an event of unprotected sexual intercourse. Levonorgestrel (Plan B One Step) is one such emergency contraceptive which is one tablet (1.50 mg), or the newest emergency contraceptive, ELLA (AFAXYS Pharma, Charleston, SC), which is a progesterone agonist/antagonist called ulipristal which can be taken up to 5 days or 120 h after an unprotected sexual encounter.

Additional information on sexually transmitted infections/diseases and recommendations can be obtained from the Centers for Disease Control and Prevention, refer to Sexually transmitted diseases treatment guidelines, click on http://www.cdc.gov/STD/

Secure the Evidence

Each item collected by the SANE must be identified by patient number, name, or both, with date and time of collection, item description, from where it was collected, by whom, and the collector's initials.

Once evidence collection has commenced, the evidence should not be left out of the control of the examiner until chain of custody is signed, with the transfer of the evidence to LE or other secure arrangements are made with the program.

The Suspect Examination

The accused is a suspect until, he/she is designated as the defendant. He/she should not be referred to as a perpetrator or "perp" until he/she is proven to be so. He/she will be referred to as a defendant in a court trial. This suspect is a patient and should be treated with the same professionalism and respect as any patient, regardless of what he/she is accused. If we remember that anyone; our brothers, husbands, sons and fathers, could be accused of sexual assault, we will have a better grasp of keeping our objectivity.

There is absolutely no reason that the SANE should not collect evidence from both reported victims and suspects; even at the same facility and with the same examiner. The exam room is cleaned with the same regime between patients, regardless of whether the next patient will be a reported victim or a suspect.

Suspects will generally be brought to the facility in handcuffs with one or two law enforcement officers. The examiner will never be left alone with the suspect and LE will never leave the suspect alone. In California, it is not necessary to get the suspect's consent for the evidentiary exam, if the suspect is in custody. Check your local laws and State laws regarding a suspect in custody.

The suspect exam begins with the SANE introducing her/himself to the patient and the explanation that we are objective evidence collectors and have no bias toward the patient. A brief medical history is obtained, vital statistics (ht. wt., color hair and eyes), vital signs and information as to whether the patient is right or left handed and whether he is circumcised or has had a vasectomy.

The routine areas for specimen collection are the reference sample, fingernail/hand swabs, sets of swabs of penile shaft and glans (two swabs), and scrotum (two swabs). Other evidence should be considered as is appropriate. Although, pubic hair plucking has long been (or should be) eliminated for the reported victim, it is still occasionally done on the suspect (required by old school crime labs, like "control swabs").

The examiner should be thinking through every exam, whether the patient is a reported (v) or (s). The only difference between the exam for a reported (v) and a (s) is that only a health history will be taken; an interview about the circumstances of the event, is NOT done. Only law enforcement should talk to the suspect about the alleged accusations. The forensic nurse conducts and interview; not an interrogation. There could be severe legal repercussions, Miranda Rights, for one, should the forensic examiner be involved in this aspect of the investigation. Law enforcement interrogations must be conducted in a controlled environment and, in many jurisdictions, must be recorded.

Should the in-custody patient have the need for medical care or require routine medications, LE should be advised, in writing, and signed and dated, as acknowledged, on the advisement of the SANE's recommendations that the patient may need further care or treatment. The suspect exam takes much less time, than the reported (v) exam because no interview is conducted other than the patient's health and hygiene history.http://www.ccfmtc.org/pdf/calema_forms/SA%20Suspect%202-950.pdf http://www.cmtc.tv/forensic.asp

Forensic Examination Interpretation

The Forensic SANE will be responsible for recognizing, accurately identifying, and objectively documenting examination findings. The examiner will be utilizing contemporary scientific methods, and continually keeping pace with the most current literature. The anogenital photographs, taken during the examination, should depict the findings described by the examiner in the documentation and on the accompanying diagrams. The photographs should be clear, a fair, and an accurate representation of what the SANE exam reveals. The SANE who has had experience seeing patients with a variety of anogenital manifestations, knows what is within normal limits (WNL), what is a normal variant, what might be findings related to hygiene, what might be genetic, a medical or skin condition, and what might be related to a recent injury.

Patients do not look exactly alike, anatomically. There will be findings related to growth and development in the child, adolescent, and adult patient. There could be residual findings from naturally occurring findings such as hymenal remnants or labial adhesions. There may be misinterpretation of such findings as venous congestion and Linea Vestibularis (https://law.duke.edu/sites/default/files/ccjpr/cb_adams_classification_2015_update.pdf).

There might be no findings, upon physical examination, though genital penetration has been reported. It is possible that there was skin to skin contact but perceived penetration when none actually occurred. In the patient who has no physical anogenital injuries, the examiner still cannot say, positively, that there was no penetration; it may not be known if there was any actual penetration. Some persons might have expectations that there would be injury if there had been genital or anal penetration, especially in the child. It is not an unreasonable expectation but there are several factors that should be considered. There are certain sexual acts that have a low expectation of injury, as in most digital penetration and oral contact to the male and female patient, although bruises can sometimes be seen if there has been suction activity reported, to the genitalia.

Another point that will undoubtedly enter in to the options of differential assessment, is that the contact never occurred.

Misinformation regarding the presence or absence of injury might come from those who believe that there would be no injuries with consensual sexual contact. Anogenital abrasions and tears are equally common findings in consensual and nonconsensual sexual contact. In fact, vulvar tears and abrasions can be natural by-products from sexual contact, by the fact that two skin surfaces are rubbing against each other.

SANE examinations can and should be exemplary and objective. Some SANE exams can contain faulty information and show the bias of the examiner in the documentation and the manner of testimony in court. Sometimes anatomical findings can be misidentified, misinterpreted, overstated, and editorialized. It is possible that a knowledge deficit is the reason. It is hopeful that this is the case, rather than being intentionally misleading. Some examiners may believe that their role is to "help" the prosecution and defeat the defense, but like the crime lab, the SANE is a neutral, scientific entity, and is not subject to hyperbole. In court, the SANE role is to educate the court and jury with unbiased information.

Some exam findings will be designated as "normal" without physical findings and cannot confirm nor negate sexual contact or abuse. That doesn't mean nothing happened; it means that there is no evidence of anything that may have happened. Of course, the timing from the reported event, to the time of the exam will be a factor in whether the exam will be acute or nonacute.

Some examinations will be "nonspecific," meaning that the anogenital findings may be caused from sexual abuse/assault or other mechanisms. "Redness" would be an example of a nonspecific finding. It does not signify anything exclusive to sexual contact.

If the interpretation by the examiner is that there was "sexual abuse/assault by history," that means that the gatherer of information was merely told that something had happened, usually without physical evidence. Still, sexual abuse cannot be dismissed whether or not there are findings.

Keep in mind that people who frequent or live in the same household can leave one another's DNA throughout the residence.

Some summaries use verbiage such as "the exam is consistent with the history," whether or not there are findings. Anything that could be consistent with the history could also be consistent with something other than the history. "Consistent with …," only means "could be." Anything could be consistent with the history. It might be best practice not to make those types of statements. It is not the role of the SANE to come to any opinions or conclusions, that are the providence of the jury; rather the role is to provide education to assist the jury forming their decision (Federal Rules of Evidence, Rule 702, 704, 2018 version) (Lynch & Duval, (2005, 2011), Forensic Nursing Science, p. 555, 2011).

Some sexual assault cases carry with them a minimum of body injury charges. Body injuries should be evaluated separately from anogenital findings. Body findings may not be directly related to a sexual act. For example, a bruise on the patient's arm is not a sexual finding. Body injuries may have been sustained hours or days prior to or at a time after the actual sexual contact. Patients who are most likely to sustain body injuries are those related to violent interpersonal relationships. Some patients avoid body injuries by cooperating. Cooperation does not imply consent.

The forensic examiner cannot substantiate anogenital force.

Editorial statements made by the SANE that conclude that sexual assault did or did not occur are improper and for the trier of fact, alone (Federal Rules of Evidence 704). It is permissible for the SANE to say a particular finding may be indicative of sexual contact or common findings for sexual penetration but cannot come to the ultimate conclusion that there was or was not consent or a sexual assault; or that someone is guilty or not guilty. Best practice would be to accurately describe the physical findings observed to the patient without embellishment.

Case example: patient presents with a large (est. 3–4 cm × 2 cm) bruise to the external genitalia on the anterior Labia Majora. The history is that the patient fell in the bathtub while intoxicated. The location of the finding is not in a penetrable location and is typical, if not textbook, of a straddle injury. However, the examiner still cannot declare that there was no sexual contact; only that the finding is not indicative or characteristic of sexual contact. In this case, the finding would be "consistent with" or significant for a straddle injury;' a finding that is nonsexual in nature. The misidentification of this finding and errors of this type can have devastating consequences.

Case example: An adult/adolescent patient is examined and observed to have the finding of an acute hymenal tear and an abrasion to the Fossa Navicularis. These findings are observed in consensual and nonconsensual sexual contact. The examination reveals a hymenal transection. This finding may be indicative of a penetration injury; possibly sexual contact if that is the history, but it will not be known, from the physical examination, whether the transection was the result of nonconsensual or consensual contact.

Some cases involve patients who have had recent sexual contact, with someone other than the accused. Although, "rape shield" laws may be in place, in trial, there are exceptions that apply to the forensic examination (Federal Rules of Evidence 412). While findings in the examination may be related to either "partner" they will complicate the ability to assess the current findings.

One More Thing...

If a case should go to trial, it will be assigned to a prosecutor from the District Attorney's office. The SANE will be a very important resource for educating the prosecutor regarding the SANE medical legal examination. The SANE might even suggest some questions for the prosecutor to ask her/him since this is the SANE's area of expertise. It is the SANE's role to maintain objectivity and to educate the court; the attorneys, the judge, and the jury. The SANE should not have anything different to say whether called by prosecution or defense.

Some sexual assault/abuse forms may have items listed that can be construed as less than objective. For example, if the examiner is asked to list "assault-related findings." The examiner would not know if the findings were the result of the reported event or something else (consensual sexual contact, hygiene, medical/skin condition). The examiner does not come to a conclusion whether or not a sexual assault occurred. That is the providence of the jury.

Conclusion

Forensic nurses have taken the forefront and expanded their practice roles, using their extraordinary skills, to include overlapping specialties such as domestic and interpersonal violence, correctional nursing, child physical abuse, elder abuse and neglect, death investigation, human trafficking, public health, research, and the development of innovative roles to respond to issues affecting worldwide health, mass disasters, and violence prevention.

The science of nursing has emerged with the forensic sciences and the justice system to provide a distinctive discipline: forensic nursing science. This scientific discipline incorporates numerous applications to the major status of the registered nurse at all levels of practice, ranging from the basic or generalist role to advanced practice in forensic nursing (Lynch & Duval, 2011a, 2011b)

The Forensic Sexual Assault Medical Legal Examination: The SANE Examination Cari Caruso RN SANE-A.

References

Archambault (2001). Dr. Sue Lindsay, Brief Encounter.

California Codes Title 17 (1986). Penal Code Section 679.04A.

California Office of Criminal Justice Planning (1987, 2001). California Medical Protocol for Examination of Sexual Assault and Child Sexual Abuse Victims, with updates 3-9-2018.

CDC Guidelines (Centers for Disease Control). (2015). Guidelines for Sexually Transmitted Diseases. http://www.cdc.gov/std/.

Constantino, R. E., Crane, P. A., & Young, S. E. (2012). *Forensic nursing: Evidence-based principles and practice* (p. 126). Philadelphia, PA: FA Davis. (unit two).

Drunk Driver (2017). "Re: Drunk Driver: Sadly, far too often, there is no justice for victims. After all, as one victim said, it's called the "criminal" justice system, not the "victim" justice system. The complex and confusing justice system can be difficult and emotionally exhausting to navigate." By, DRUNK DRIVING https://www.madd.org/blog/seven-ways-the-justice-system-will-frustrate-you/.

EMTALA (1986).

HIPAA: Health Information Portability and Accountability Act (1996). 2003 F.R. 82462.

Human Rights Campaign (2015). https://www.hrc.org/resources/sexual-assault-and-the-lgbt-community.

International Association of Forensic Nurses, SANE-A and SANE-P (2002). *Designations and placement*.

Kafarowski, E., Lyon, A. M., & Sloan, M. M. (1996). The retention and transfer of spermatozoa in clothing by machine washing. *Journal of the Canadian Society of Forensic Science, 29*(1), 7–11.

Kaplan, R., Adams, J. A., Starling, S. P., Giardino, A. P. (2011). Medical Response to Child Sexual Abuse.

Ledray L. (1999). SANE-SART Development and Operational Guide (1999).

Ledray, L. E., Burgess, A. W., & Giardino, A. (2011a) STM 2011 Medical Response to Adult Sexual Assault: A Resource for Clinicians and Related Professionals.

Lynch & Duval (2005) Link Between Nursing and the Law, (2005). UC Riverside Extension, The Forensic Sexual Assault Examiner Course, Caruso C. (2005)

Lynch & Duval (2011). Forensic Nursing Science, 'Legal and Ethical Issues in Forensic Nursing Roles,' Susan Chasson (2011) (HIPAA 2003 F.R. 82462) Chapter 44, Legal and Ethical Issues in Forensic Nursing.

Lynch, V., & Barber Duval, J. (2011a). *Forensic Nursing Science, Global and Cultural Crimes, Global Expansion*. St. Louis, MO: Elsevier.

Lynch, V. A., & Barber Duval, J. (2011b). *Forensic Nursing Science* (2nd ed.). St. Louis, MO: Elsevier.

National Center for Lesbian Rights (2014, April 30). http://www.nclrights.org/sexual-assault-in-the-lgbt-community.

Office on Violence Against Women (OVW), United States Department of Justice (DOJ), Violence Against Women Act (VAWA) of 2005, Enacted by Congress, 42 U.S.C. and 3796gg-4(d) (n.d.). STOP violence against women grant federal program guidelines, p. 7.

Sackett, D., Straus, S., Richardson, W., Rosenberg, W., & Haynes, R. (2000). *The Academy of Medical-Surgical Nurses (AMSN) values evidence-based practice (EBP) as a way to affect best patient care*. Medical Response to Adult Sexual Assault.

U.S. Department of Justice. (2013). *A National Protocol for Sexual Assault Medical Forensic Examinations Adults/Adolescents* (2nd ed., p. 43). Washington, DC: DOJ.

Decision Making in Title IX Investigations: A Hypothesis Testing Approach to Overcome Cognitive Bias

37

William T. O'Donohue

Investigations into allegations of sexual assault and sexual harassment, including Title IX investigations, can be considered to be comprised of several phases. However, all phases are essentially about gathering relevant information (and defining what is "relevant") and then processing this information in some way to arrive at a final decision regarding the truth of the allegations. For example, an investigation may begin with some information about a pertinent issue, such as a formal complaint of sexual harassment or sexual assault and then gather information from the complainant, the respondent, as well as other witnesses judged relevant or materials judged relevant (e.g., a torn dress). This chapter will not examine the problems of victims not reporting actual assault or experiencing problems in following through with either the entire investigation or a police investigation or a criminal prosecution (see Cummings & O'Donohue, 2019; Richards, 2019). It has been well documented that many sexual assault or sexual harassment victims will not make a formal report due to being traumatized, fears of not being believed, concerns about retaliation, feelings of shame and embarrassment or even not wanting to hurt the perpetrator (see Cummings & O'Donohue, 2019). However, after an initial report of sexual misconduct is made, the next steps in the investigation can be informing the respondent and the collection of additional information, the processing of this information, and then using this information to arrive at some sort of ultimate judgment. All interested parties of course desire that this entire process be fair, comprehensive, and accurate.

Title IX investigations have been going on since 1972 when Title IX was initially passed into law. However, these investigations have been controversial as many have been subsequently overturned in courts of law (see Chap. 10 in this volume) often because the courts have determined that due process rights of the accused were violated. Moreover, officials associated with the most recent two Presidents have modified Title IX procedures—however in opposing ways. For example, during the Obama administration, the Department of Education Office for Civil Rights' 2011 'Dear Colleague Letter' suggested the investigator should tell the complainant that he or she is believed by the investigator; while under the Trump administration, Secretary of Education Betsy Devos has increased the due process rights

W. T. O'Donohue (✉)
University of Nevada,
Reno, NV, USA

W. T. O'Donohue and P. A. Schewe (eds.), *Handbook of Sexual Assault and Sexual Assault Prevention*,
https://doi.org/10.1007/978-3-030-23645-8_37

of the accused, for example, by allowing for cross-examination of the alleged victim. Although there are indications that many respondents believe that it is difficult to defend themselves against the charges they face in Title IX investigations, these concerns need to be balanced for the consideration that increasing those rights may expose victims to harsh questioning, increased stress, and possibly even renewed trauma, and feelings that they are not believed (Triplett, 2012). One set of scholars (Harper, Maskaly, Kirkner, & Lorenz, 2017) has pointed to the intersectionality of legal problems, methodological problems, and psychological problems associated with current Title IX investigations:

"In developing Title IX adjudication policies and procedures, IHEs (institutions of higher education) are left with the seemingly impossible task of balancing victims' rights under Title IX with respondents' constitutional due process rights. The result is unstandardized adjudication systems employing varying procedures that often fail to meet legal obligations to both parties. Title IX adjudication systems are bound by competing and conflicting student conduct policies, constitutional due process rights, Title IX, federal laws, case law, and contract law. The Constitution mandates the accused are provided with due process of law, while the OCR (Office for Civil Rights) requires that due process should not restrict or delay Title IX's protections for victims (Triplett, 2012). This latter requirement enhances victim safety and eliminates educational gender inequity, but also curbs due process protections for respondents, infringing on their ability to maintain innocence" (p. 305).

No doubt that these investigations are complex and difficult. But it is also important to point out that these have not been studied scientifically: to date there is no evidence of Title IX investigations' sensitivity (rate of false negatives) or specificity (rate of false positives). Thus, currently there is little evidence of the error rates of these Title IX investigations.

Most of the debate about how to effectively construct and conduct a Title IX investigation has been through a legal lens (see for example, Harper et al., 2017). Critics of the current practice of Title IX investigations have debated important legal issues involved with due process such as right to legal representation, standards of proof, subpoena powers, right to cross-examination, admissible evidence, and so on. This is reasonable as these legal issues have a great deal of bearing on defining a proper and just investigation. However, this chapter will examine the investigatory process from the lens of psychology, particularly common cognitive biases that can bias the investigator's decision making such as confirmation bias. Psychologists have constructed a large body of research showing that humans are prone to make errors in judgments—e.g., humans tend to seek out, recall more easily, favor, and overvalue evidence that conforms to prior beliefs—the so-called "*confirmation bias*". However, humans are also prone to a number of other cognitive biases which may interact with this confirmation bias: for example, humans use the *availability heuristic* to falsely conclude that airplane travel is more dangerous than car travel because air accidents are covered more extensively (i.e., are more available) in the media. The Princeton psychologist Daniel Kahneman (2011) won a Nobel prize for this work and has identified a few dozens of these heuristics (see Table 37.1 for those potentially most relevant to Title IX investigations). Some research has also indicated heuristic biases are stronger for emotionally charged issues and, certainly, sexual assault and the threats of punishment make Title IX investigations an emotionally charged process (Kahneman, 2011).

This chapter will suggest that Title IX investigations ought to be seen as a hypothesis testing process that needs to be done with some care so that common cognitive biases, particularly confirmation bias, do not distort the results. The investigator ought to collect and process information to test competing hypotheses regarding the allegation. This helps both focus on the investigation and, if done properly, make the investigation fairer and thorough, particularly as this process can help combat common heuristic errors. We will turn next to a discussion of the most frequent and perhaps pernicious heuristic error: confirmation bias.

Table 37.1 Other cognitive heuristics that may interact with confirmation bias

Anchoring effect: The order a human learns information biases their beliefs such that first things learned have more of an influence: does hearing the complainant first bias toward believing the complainant?
Availability heuristic: Human judgments are influenced by what springs more easily to mind. Are true allegations more easily recalled and therefore influence unduly investigatory judgments?
Group think: Do pervasive beliefs in some group unduly bias the investigation? For example, does the belief that "victims must be believed" influence investigatory judgments?
Backfire effect: When beliefs are challenged, this can cause you to believe them more strongly. Does the respondent's challenge of the complainant's claims cause the investigator to believe these more strongly?
Framing effect: Humans are influenced by context and delivery. Does an emotionally distraught narrative unduly influence the investigator's belief?
In-group bias. Humans unduly favor members of their own group. Does identification or non-identification with one of the key actors influence the investigator's judgment?
Halo effect: Humans are unduly influenced by attractiveness and their liking of someone. Does one of the participants create a positive halo that unduly affects judgments?
Attitude polarization: When a disagreement becomes more extreme, even though the different parties are exposed to the same evidence.

Confirmation Bias: Philosophical and Epistemological Background

Philosophers of science such as Sir Karl Popper (2005) and Carl Sagan (2011) have suggested science is essentially an antidote to confirmation bias. The seventeenth century philosopher Sir Francis Bacon once told a story about a church in which sailors, before their journeys, would pray for their safe return. When they did indeed return safely, they would hang in the church a picture of themselves in gratitude for the efficacy of their prayers. Some took all these paintings as indications that prayers do in fact work. However, Bacon (as quoted in Urbach, 1987) stated:

> And therefore it was a good answer that was made by one who when they showed him hanging in a temple a picture of those who had paid their vows as having escaped shipwreck, and would have him say whether he did not now acknowledge to the power of the gods,—"Aye," asked he again. "but where are they painted that were drowned after their vows?" (p. 88)

Thus, every good hypothesis should divide the set of all statements derivable from it into two subsets: one subset contains observation statements that are consistent with the hypothesis (e.g., after prayer, sailors return). This set is less interesting from an epistemological point of view. However, the complementary set that for every hypothesis should be nonempty, is the set of potential falsifiers (e.g., after prayer sailors fail to return). Hypothesis testing consists of efficiently and ardently attempting to see if one of these potential states of affairs actually happens. A successful hypothesis has what Popper (2005) called *verisimilitude*—literally "truth likeness" because the hypothesis has survived these attempts at falsification.

Popper pointed out that hypotheses can differ on the degree to which they are potentially falsifiable. Hypotheses that make point predictions (e.g., the average IQ of females is 106.4) are extremely falsifiable because their sets of falsifiers include as elements all points except the particular point predicted by the hypothesis in this instance. In general, the more precise the statement is, the more falsifiable the statement is. Popper also valued *severe* testing in which we attempt to deduce the most improbable consequences of the hypothesis and check on whether these happen. The general notion is that if one wants to falsify the claim that "Priests don't swear", it is better to observe them at a golf course or after jamming their toe than when they are in the pulpit or at a church social.

However, unfortunately, there is evidence from cognitive psychology that humans are not particularly good at attempting to falsify their hypotheses. It is worthwhile to examine how confirmation bias can affect hypothesis testing (see Poletiek, 2015 for an extended treatment). A classic series of experiments was based on Wason's (1960) rule discovery task or the "2-4-6 task". Wason asked subjects to discover the rule for the generation of a series of 3 numbers. Participants could test their hypotheses concerning the rule by providing 3 numbers and then the experimenter would tell them if these three numbers were in accordance with the real rule or not. The real rule was simply a sequence of three ascending numbers. The subjects' task was to generate the series of numbers until they discovered the real rule. Wason (1960) found that many participants formed the hypothesis that the real rule was a sequence of ascending even numbers and would generate series of three even numbers to "confirm" this hypothesis—for example, their response would be 12, 14, 16. The experimenter would tell them that their answer was correct (because these three numbers are ascending); however, the participants would interpret this as a "confirmation" of their hypothesis of the real rule being 3 ascending even numbers. Wason also categorized subjects' responses by confirming or falsifying attempts: e.g., the response "6-8-10" would be a confirming test of the rule ascending even numbers, while "7-9-11" would be a falsifying test. He then calculated the ratio of falsifying to confirming probes. Wason found that subjects who discovered the true rule had a higher ratio of falsifying tests to confirming tests (1.79) as compared to subjects who did not discover the real rule (.22). Wason concluded that "very few intelligent young adults spontaneously test their beliefs" (1960, p. 139).

Complications in Falsificatory Testing

This argument for the importance of attempting to gather potential falsificatory evidence to combat confirmation bias toward favored beliefs is complicated, however, by two factors: (1) the fact that even scientists who are supposed to be engaging in a process to prohibit confirmation bias can engage in what are known as Questionable Research Practices (QRP) that give the appearance of a scientific test without any or much of the substance—thus failing to actually combat confirmation bias; and (2) the so-called Quine-Duhem problem. Let's briefly examine these two problems as these are relevant to understanding how an investigator ought to conduct a Title IX investigation.

Questionable Research Practices and Confirmation Bias

Recently, there has been a crisis associated with replication failures in science and in psychology (see John, Loewenstein, & Prelec, 2012; as well as O'Donohue, Snipes, and Soto (2015) for a case of this in psychotherapy) as well as other scientific fields. Although this matter is complex, one of the key threads for this problem is that scientists are actually trying to confirm their favored beliefs instead of really trying to fairly test these. This again supports the general view that testing favored beliefs is hard for humans—even when that is exactly what they are supposed to be doing when conducing science. QRPs include key (mis)steps to favor beliefs including:

1. Reanalyzing data until confirmations are found.
2. Stopping data collection when a confirmation of favored belief is found.
3. If multiple observations are predicted from favored beliefs selectively reporting only the outcome variables that confirm the belief.
4. Using the "file drawer", i.e., simply not reporting failures to confirm.
5. Reporting an unexpected confirmatory finding as if it was predicted from the start.

The point is not to provide a detailed overview of QRPs and their role in science. The point simply is that even in science—the paradigm of rigorous hypothesis testing and what is designed to be the most thoroughgoing check against confirmation bias, some scientists still have found ways to consciously or unconsciously allow confirmation bias to protect favored beliefs. A key proposal to combat QRP is that scientists preregister their studies so that hypothesis and their mode of testing can antecedently and transparently be advanced. This safeguards against use of ad hoc strategies to "explain away" anomalous observations as well as decreases the bias use of confirmation bias by precommitting the investigator to a logic of research. This antecedent specification of the logic of testing will be explored further in the next section.

The Quine-Duhem Problem

The logic of falsifying hypothesis testing is based on the valid logical inference rule called *modus tollens*:

1. If Hypothesis, then Observation.
2. *Not Observation.*
3. Therefore, Not Hypothesis.

However, the logical problem is that it is never the hypothesis alone that is under test because the hypothesis alone does not entail the observation statement. There are a number of auxiliary hypotheses that are also necessary to the test, e.g., claims like, "The laboratory device is functioning properly", to "The sample is adequate and uncontaminated", to "My recording of the results are accurate and unbiased" and so on. In fact, Quine (e.g., Quine & Ullian, 1978) has convincingly argued that one's entire web of belief is directly or indirectly involved in the test. Thus, the actual logic of falsification hypothesis testing is more accurately depicted as:

1. Hypothesis and Auxiliary Hypothesis 1 and Auxiliary Hypothesis 2 … and Auxiliary Hypothesis n, therefore Observation.
2. *Not Observation.*
3. Therefore, Not Hypothesis or Auxiliary Hypothesis 1 or Auxiliary Hypothesis 2 … or Auxiliary Hypothesis n.

Logic alone no longer indicates what belief or beliefs are responsible for the prediction failure. The investigator is free to use judgment to allocate blame for the prediction failure. Quine and Ullian (1978) stated:

"Just about any hypothesis, after all, can be held unrefuted no matter what, by making enough adjustments in other beliefs- though sometimes doing so requires madness. We think loosely of a hypothesis as implying predictions when, strictly speaking, the implying is done by the hypothesis together with a supporting chorus of ill- distinguished background beliefs" (p. 48)

Quine and Ullian (1978) suggested that in revising beliefs in one's web of belief, five virtues of hypotheses should be kept in mind: (1) conservatism (roughly, coherence with other beliefs in the web); (2) modesty (the hypothesis entails less than alternative hypotheses); (3) simplicity (parsimony is to be favored); (4) generality (a wide scope is better); and (5) refutability (a falsifiable hypothesis is to be preferred). Here is an example of how ad hoc hypothesis could be used to "explain away" a prediction failure in a Title IX investigation and protect a favored hypothesis (i.e., the allegation is true). For example, if an investigator reasons along the following lines:

1. "This alleged sexual assault described in the allegation was so severe that if it is true, I would expect to observe the victim to show significant emotion when recounting it during the investigation".
2. *"The sexual assault claimant displayed no emotion when recounting the sexual assault"*.
3. Therefore, the sexual assault allegation is false.

However, this argument can be rejected because, due to the Quine-Duhem problem, the lack of emotion can also be taken not to be evidence that falsifies the allegation because, instead, the investigator can rely on one of more auxiliary hypotheses such as:

(a) Not all individuals who are severely sexually assaulted are emotional when recounting their abuse, and this individual is simply one who is not.

or

(b) The claimant was not comfortable with me during the investigatory interview and this decreased the likelihood that she would show emotion when recounting the abuse.

or

(c) Some significant time has passed and she has received support from key individuals, so now she can recount the abuse without intense emotion due to this passage of time and support.

or

(d) Although I did not see any intense emotion displayed, I did see attempts to control herself which resulted in no emotion being displayed.

Propositions a–d are examples of what are known as ad hoc *hypotheses*—beliefs from one's web of belief that are called on to "explain away" the failure to observe what is expected. These ad hoc hypotheses serve to protect the favored belief from falsification—e.g., to allow confirmation bias to work.

Therefore, a true test is an information gathering procedure which in principle can result in both confirming or disconfirming evidence. If the information gathering can result in only confirming evidence—it is not really a test at all—it is simply an exercise in confirmation bias. So let us take an example of a medical exam of a sexual assault victim: if the medical exam cannot, in principle, falsify the claim that the complainant was sexually assaulted, it can then in principle provide no confirmatory evidence that the complainant was sexually assaulted. For example, suppose the complainant states that, after a period of consenting sexual contact, he or she withdrew consent and yet the respondent persisted and thus engaged in non-consenting sexual contact. The respondent agrees that consensual sex took place, but states that the complainant never withdrew consent. Let's further suppose that a medical exam is conducted and the medical exam finds (to state it without jargon) both the respondent's DNA and physical evidence that sexual intercourse took place (by, for example, swelling or redness or irritation) and concludes: "the medical evidence is consistent with sexual abuse". However, the medical evidence could not even in principle rule out assault as this medical evidence is also entirely consistent with the consensual sex that the respondent claims happened. Therefore, in no way should it be counted as a "test" of the hypothesis that assault occurred.

What is necessary is that, antecedent to evidence gathering, the investigator needs to commit to something along these lines:

1. If values a–c are found, then this evidence will be judged to support the claim.
2. If values d–f are found, then this evidence will be judged to be inconsistent with the claim.
3. If values g–i are found, then this evidence will be judged to be neutral: it is neither supportive or inconsistent.

Let's explore this decision format with another example. Suppose the investigator gathers information about the complainant's behavior after the alleged assault. Suppose the decision rule that will be used is the following:

(a) If the complainant appears traumatized after the allegation, then this is consistent with sexual abuse claim.
(b) If the complainant does not appear traumatized, then this is also consistent with the abuse claim as some assault victims can cope with the abuse, or have delayed reactions.

Again, where is even the possibility of disconfirmatory evidence—and if there is none, how again is this part of the investigation actually a "test"—isn't the evidentiary outcome preordained?

One final example: suppose the investigator inquires whether the complainant disclosed the abuse relevantly co-temporaneous to the alleged abuse, but will reason along the following lines:

(a) If the complainant discloses to someone relatively soon after the assault, then this provides some confirmation that the assault took place.
(b) If the complainant does not tell anyone after the assault, then this also provides evidence that the assault took place because many individuals delay reporting because of barriers to reporting such as feeling shame or that they will not be believed and therefore tell no one.

Again, where is even the possibility of disconfirming evidence—all values of the inquiry are interpreted to provide confirmatory support for the sexual misconduct claim—i.e., the very definition of confirmation bias.

The view of the proper way to handle ad hoc hypothesis is to design the investigation *anteced-*

ently so that no ad hoc hypotheses will be used to "explain away" anomalous observations, so that there are values of the test that can both confirm or disconfirm hypotheses. That is, it is important that the investigator take utmost care to ensure that the auxiliary conditions associated with the Quine-Duhem problem do not come into play. In the next section, more details will be provided regarding how this can be done in Title IX investigations.

Overcoming Confirmation Bias in Title IX Investigations

Confirmation bias in Title IX investigations may be due partly to the robust human tendency to not properly test initial favored beliefs, but also to the well-intentioned aim to not harm victims in the adjudication procedure. It may also be a well-intentioned act to correct the historical wrongs done to rape victims of not believing them. In fact, part of the historical wrongdoing may have been due to confirmation bias operating against legitimate victims (e.g., seeing the way the woman dressed as confirming the belief that she was "asking for it").

Step 1: Forming two competing hypotheses. One step that can help combat confirmation bias is not exploring one hypothesis, but rather two competing hypotheses related to both confirming and disconfirming the allegation of sexual misconduct as this forces evidence to be gathered and judgments to be made on both sides of the issue. Thus, the investigator should first form two competing hypotheses (note that this recommendation is in some tension with the Dear Colleague Letter, which recommends that the complainant be told that she or he is believed). The two hypotheses are broadly:

(a) The complainant's allegations are true.
(b) The complainant's allegations are false.

Three notes here: (1) These are taken to be logically contradictory hypotheses and, therefore, one of these must be false; and it is the investigator's job to find out which one is indeed most likely false. It is beyond the scope of this chapter, but subjectivist approaches to truth in which contradictory propositions are considered as possibly true due to each participant's subjective "truth" are rejected here as irrationalist. (2) There can be a third alternative, i.e., that some of the complainant's allegations are true and some are false, but, for purposes of illustration, here this possibility will be ignored but still can be handled with the same principles. Considering a third hypothesis, however, is still consistent with unduly focusing on only one hypothesis. (3) These hypotheses can have different expressions, but would still be logically equivalent. For example, the second hypothesis could be reformulated as "The respondent's denials are true"—however, in general, this would be logically equivalent expressions of the same underlying proposition.

Step 2: Identifying a favored hypothesis: Does the investigator have a favored hypothesis?

This step requires some intellectual honesty on the part of the investigator. It would seem that in the Obama "Dear Colleague Letter", the investigator's favored hypothesis would be Hypothesis (a)—that the complainant's allegations are true. There can be other reasons for favoring this hypothesis: the low base rates of false allegations (see O'Donohue, Chap. 32, this volume); the compelling nature of the complainant's statements; the primacy of information from the complainant; and so on. The reason why this step is necessary is that the investigator also needs to realize that initial "buy in" to any hypothesis may allow confirmation bias to have a larger influence. The investigator needs, therefore, to try harder to falsify any favored hypothesis to combat confirmation bias.

Step 3: Antecedently state a data gathering and processing plan in which the investigator will gather information Ia through In, as well as antecedently specify that if the value of I is a–c, then this will be judged confirmatory of one hypothesis; if d–f neutral; and if g–j, then disconfirming one hypothesis, then gather this evidence. Note: values should always exist for both confirming and disconfirming the competing

hypotheses. No "test" can occur when only one kind of evidence can, in principle, be gathered.

This is an important but difficult step and really illustrates some of the key difficulties of investigating sexual assault claims. The difficulty may be stated this way: Given the state of the science of sexual assault, there are few falsifiers related to sexual assault claims. Those falsifiers that do exist may largely be related to pragmatic considerations and not part of the knowledge of science of sexual assault—e.g., alibis. An additional part of the problem with finding falsifiers may also be due to the use of the Quine-Duhem problem described above. That is, protecting the favored hypothesis by placing blame on some auxiliary hypothesis is one way that confirmation bias manifests itself. A prediction failure can simply be blamed on some auxiliary hypothesis. This is the reason that the interpretation of the evidentiary value of the information will be stated antecedently.

Let us consider some candidates for domains that the investigator might gather evidence on and the difficulties of antecedently committing to falsifying evidence. What evidence ought to be gathered to rule this in or out—how would this evidence need to be properly analyzed—how ought pieces of it be weighed to meet or not meet standard?

Dimension 1: Delay in disclosing to authorities. Many individuals delay in reporting to authorities, but some do not (see O'Donohue, Chap. 35, this volume for a review). In addition, "delay" is a relatively imprecise word: if 3 h pass is this a delay? 3 days? 3 weeks? 3 years? These seem to all involve a different order of magnitude, yet all could be properly considered a delay. Is the only event that is not a delay either a contemporaneous report or a report at the earliest possible moment, e.g., as soon as the claimant gained access to a phone? It would seem that, even though most victims delay, there is not a sufficient scientific regularity to specify values that would provide disconfirmatory or confirmatory evidence for the competing hypotheses. However, if an investigator is planning to examine delay in reporting, then he or she ought to antecedently precisely define the time period that counts as a delay and how this will be used to either confirm and disconfirm the competing hypotheses.

Dimension 2: Disclosing the sexual assault to another person (such as a friend). Some sexual misconduct victims do this; some do not (and again a false accusation could contain, or not contain, this characteristic). It would appear that there is not a sufficient scientific regularity that this dimension could provide evidence to rule in or rule out either competing hypothesis. However, again, if a Title IX investigator plans to gather evidence regarding this dimension, then he or she needs to state antecedently the values of this dimension that will confirm as well as the values that will disconfirm the competing hypotheses.

Dimension 3: Obvious psychological symptoms occurring at some time period after the sexual misconduct. Most sexual assault victims will be distressed and traumatized, but whether others correctly observe this is another matter (see Chap. 10 this volume). Moreover, not all sexual misconduct victims will display obvious psychological symptoms because they have the resources to cope and be resilient. Some have even offered the notion of post-traumatic growth (e.g., Calhoun & Tedeschi, 2014) and suggest that some victims will even be healthier after the assault. Therefore, again, any Title IX investigator planning to collect information regarding this dimension needs to antecedently state the values of this dimension that will count for and which ought to count against the competing hypotheses.

Dimension 4: The claimant recants. This dimension essentially shifts the question—from, is the abuse allegation true? to, is the recantation true? That is, individuals can recant a true allegation (e.g., due to pressures for others or due to an unwillingness to continue the stressful investigatory process) or individuals can recant a false allegation. There is some statistical evidence in child sexual abuse that children rarely recant a true allegation. Bradley and Wood (1996) found in an examination of over 240 cases in CPS records that only 3% of true allegations were recanted. The recantation rate of adult sexual misconduct victims is less clear. However, again, if this dimension is judged relevant by the investigator, they must antecedently specify what values count for or against the competing hypotheses.

Dimension 5: Presence of mental illness. Engle & O'Donohue (2012) have suggested that mental illnesses such as psychotic disorders and personality disorders are pathways to false allegations of sexual assault. However, individuals with these disorders can also be sexually assaulted. Therefore, the mere presence of a mental disorder is not decisive regarding the truth or falsity of the allegation. Again, if this dimension is to be part of the investigation, the investigator ought to antecedently state which values are to be considered confirmatory or discomfirmatory for the competing hypotheses.

Dimension 6: A history of lying (for either the complainant or respondent). It would seem to be a truism that all people lie, although some lie more than others and some lie about more important matters than others. An unusual history of lying (abnormally frequent or about important matters) could be relevant, although again not decisive: individuals who generally tell the truth can sexually assault and individuals who lie frequently can still be victims of sexual misconduct. Thus, again, the investigator needs to explicate antecedently how values of information relevant to this dimension will be used to confirm or disconfirm the competing hypotheses.

Dimension 7: Past false allegations of sexual assault or other false allegations. This would be a sub-case of the above. The presence of a history of false allegations is quite unusual, but again an individual who has such as history can still be a victim of actual sexual misconduct. Again, the investigator needs to antecedently specify how values of this variable will be used to evaluate the competing hypotheses.

Dimension 8: Past findings or convictions, especially for sexual misconduct. This is mainly relevant to the respondent. Certainly, having past findings or convictions of sexual misconduct is unusual and indicates that the person is capable of such wrongdoing. However, again, just because an individual committed these acts in the past does not entail that this person committed the acts under investigation. The investigator needs to antecedently specify the values of this dimension that will be judged to confirm or disconfirm the competing hypotheses.

Dimension 9: The respondent's memory of details of the assault. Most sexual misconduct victims remember key details of their rape (who, what, when, where), but can forget other more peripheral details, especially after the passage of time or if there were many incidents (see memory chapter this volume as well as McNally, 2003). If the investigator will use information about how key events are remembered, then again they need to antecedently specify the values that from this dimension will confirm or disconfirm the competing hypotheses.

Dimension 10: No further contact with their perpetrator. Many victims do try to avoid their perpetrator, but some cannot (e.g., the perpetrator is a close relative) and research into date rape has surprisingly found that a large percentage of date rape victims have further contact with their rapist, especially in so-called date rape (Koss, Gidycz, & Wisniewski, 1987). Thus, again, the investigator, if they will gather information from this dimension, ought to state antecedently what values confirm and what values disconfirm the competing hypotheses.

Dimension 11: Fighting back during the assault. Again, research shows that for a variety of factors (fear that fighting back could result in increased injury or even result in death), some victims do, and some victims don't, fight back against their perpetrator. Also, some victimization might be so quick that fighting back is not an option (a quick grope and then the perpetrator flees). Thus again, if the investigator is to gather information about this dimension, he or she needs to specify antecedently which values will confirm and which values will disconfirm the competing hypotheses.

Dimension 12: A single vs. multiple independent complainants regarding the same respondent. In the recent case of the movie producer Harvey Weinstein, dozens of women have apparently independently claimed that he has committed some form of sexual abuse. How likely would this happen if all the allegations are false? This is a much sounder form of reasoning, but still it has significant limitations: it does not mean that *each and every* allegation is true (a particular allegation can be caused by jumping on the bandwagon for some personal gain); and second, the converse is not true: i.e., it would be fallacious to reason that a single complainant means the allegation is false—serial rapists all necessarily must have a first victim. Thus, if the investigator plans to consider evidence regarding the number of victims, then he or she needs to antecedently state how values on this dimension will confirm and disconfirm the competing hypotheses.

Dimension 13: Affiliative behavior that seems inconsistent with the aftermath of sexual assault such as affectionate text messages. Koss et al. (1987) found that many women who reported unwanted sexual contact on dates continued to date the individual responsible for the unwanted contact. Thus, although many women will stop all contact, and avoidance is a diagnostic criterion of Post-Traumatic Stress Disorder which is a common diagnosis after sexual assault (see Chap. 10 in this volume), some women will have contact with their perpetrator. Thus, this criterion too fails to be a marker for abuse or for a false allegation. Thus, the investigator needs again to antecedently specify what values of the dimension will count as confirmatory or disconfirmatory for the competing hypotheses.

Dimension 14: History of aggressive or sexist behavior. What if the respondent has a history of problematic behavior that seems similar to sexual misconduct? What if the respondent, for example, has made sexist comments or if they were in fights or made threats against someone? Of course, prior misbehavior does not entail that the specific acts being alleged actually occurred. And it is possible that if the claimant had prior knowledge of this, then the claimant could come to believe that a false allegation would be more likely to be believed. Therefore, again, the investigator needs to make decisions about the values of this dimension that will count as supportive and disconfirming evidence.

Dimension 15: Presence of a stake or ulterior motive. What if the claimant has something to gain by the allegation—either revenge (e.g., for a failing grade or a relationship that ended), or attention, or monetary reward due to a lawsuit? Although these sorts of motivations can induce a false allegation, a true allegation can still be made in these contexts; so therefore again, the investigator needs to antecedently state how values on this dimension will be used for both disconfirming and confirming the competing hypotheses.

Dimension 16: Problematic behavior surrounding the sexual misconduct such as limiting autonomy. What if the claim also involves other problematic behavior such as isolating the claimant, or a temper outburst, or refusing to let her leave a car? Some of these behaviors themselves might constitute other crimes and may need to be reported to the proper authorities, but, again, just because someone committed one bad action doesn't mean they are necessarily guilty of another bad act. The investigator needs to make antecedent decisions about how to handle the values of these variables.

Dimension 17: Intoxication. Many sexual assaults involve substance use, particularly alcohol (see Chap. 10 this volume). This issue also relates to whether consent could be given and thus is relevant to the investigation. Again, the investigator needs to determine the level of intoxication and to indicate how this will be construed in supporting or disconfirming the competing hypotheses. Parts of this may be relatively straightforward: if legal intoxication limits are exceeded, then this would support the claim of sexual misconduct; and if legal intoxication limits are not exceeded, then this would not support the claim of sexual misconduct due to inability to give consent (sexual misconduct could still have occurred due to other reasons).

This is not to say that there are no other dimensions that might be relevant to at Title IX investigation. The above is an illustration of how some of the major dimensions need to be handled. Finally, there are two other steps to the investigation.

Step 4: Not allowing the use of ad hoc strategies to combat the Quine-Duhem problem to save favored hypotheses.

That is, switching from antecedent commitments of the evidentiary value of the information needs to be done rarely and only under extraordinary circumstances which need to be justified.

Step 5: Finally, explicating by listing the evidence for and against each of the hypotheses and making an argument regarding whether preponderance of evidence is met.

Each dimension investigated ought to have values that confirm and disconfirm the competing hypotheses and these ought to be explicated in the report. It is unclear how these will result in a quantified result—the so-called 50% and a feather. But arguments about the weight of each dimension, the number of supportive and disconfirming values, seem particularly relevant.

Conclusions

Title IX investigations are both important and difficult—a lot rides on these for the parties involved. They need to be conducted in a way that maximizes their accuracy as well as their transparency. Confirmation bias is a particularly troublesome source of error in human judgment and hypothesis testing. This chapter describes this heuristic error as well as provides a framework to attempt to combat it. Unfortunately, little research has been conducted on the accuracy of Title IX investigations. Hopefully in the future, this framework can be evaluated on both its accuracy and its consumer acceptability.

References

Bradley, A. R., & Wood, J. M. (1996). How do children tell? The disclosure process in child sexual abuse. *Child Abuse and Neglect, 20*, 881–891.

Calhoun, L. G., & Tedeschi, R. G. (2014). *Post-traumatic growth*. New York: Psychology Press.

Cummings, C. & O'Donohue, W. (2019). *A forensic interview protocol for adult sexual assault: Content validity and consumer acceptability*. Article submitted for publication.

Engle, J., & O'Donohue, W. (2012). Pathways to false allegations of sexual assault. *Journal of Forensic Psychology Practice, 12*(2), 97–123.

Harper, S., Maskaly, J., Kirkner, A., & Lorenz, K. (2017). Enhancing Title IX due process standards in campus sexual assault adjudication: Considering the roles of distributive, procedural, and restorative justice. *Journal of School Violence, 16*, 302–316.

John, L. K., Loewenstein, G., & Prelec, D. (2012). Measuring the prevalence of questionable research practices with incentives for truth telling. *Psychological Science, 23*(5), 524–532.

Kahneman, D. (2011). *Thinking, fast and slow*. New York: Farrar, Straus and Giroux.

Koss, M. P., Gidycz, C. A., & Wisniewski, N. (1987). The scope of rape: Incidence and prevalence of sexual aggression and victimization in a national sample of higher education students. *Journal of Consulting and Clinical Psychology, 55*(2), 162–170.

McNally, R. (2003). *Remembering trauma*. Cambridge, MA: Harvard University Press.

O'Donohue, W. T., Snipes, C., & Soto, C. (2015). A case study of the overselling of psychotherapy: ACT interventions for diabetes management. *Journal of Contemporary Psychology, 46*(1), 15–25.

Poletiek, F. H. (2015). *Hypothesis testing behavior*. New York: Routledge.

Popper, K. R. (2005). *The logic of scientific discovery*. New York: Routledge.

Quine, W. V. O., & Ullian, J. S. (1978). *The web of belief*. New York: McGraw Hill.

Richards, T. N. (2019). No evidence of "Weaponized Title IX" here: An empirical assessment of sexual misconduct reporting, case processing, and outcomes. *Law and Human Behavior, 43*(2), 180–192.

Sagan, C. (2011). *The demon haunted world: Science as a candle in the dark*. New York: Paw Print.

Triplett, M. R. (2012). Sexual assault on college campuses: Seeking the appropriate balance between due process and victim protection. *Duke Law Journal, 62*(2), 487–527.

Urbach, R. (1987). *Francis Bacon's philosophy of science*. London: Open Court.

Wason, P. C. (1960). On the failure to eliminate hypotheses in a conceptual task. *Quarterly Journal of Experimental Psychology, 12*, 129–140.

38 Can We Prevent Sexual Homicide? An Examination of Correlates of a Lethal Outcome in Sexual Assaults

Eric Beauregard and Kylie S. Reale

Cleveland—"A registered sex offender has been convicted of raping and killing a 14-year-old Ohio girl and could face the death penalty" (Calgary Sun, 2018). Such a headline illustrates one of the greatest fears in the field of sexual violence, namely that individuals who perpetrate sexual assaults will not only recidivate in sexual crimes but will also increase their level of violence to the point where they will eventually end up killing their victim. However, research shows that such fear is not rational. Only a minority of offenders convicted of a sexual crime recidivate (e.g., Hanson & Bussiere, 1998), and sexual homicide—the fact of killing a victim in a sexual context (Beauregard & Martineau, 2017)—represents only between 1% and 4% of all homicides internationally, and this trend has been decreasing over the past several years (James & Proulx, 2014). In Canada, Roberts and Grossman (1993) found that between 1974 and 1986, sexual homicides comprised 4% of all homicides. This proportion fell to 3% between 1985 and 1995 (Statistics Canada, 2013) and reached its lowest point at 2% between 1991 and 2001 (Kong, Johnson, Beattie, & Cardillo, 2003). A similar trend was observed in the United States where the proportion of homicide with a sexual component declined from 0.8% between 1976 and 2004 (Chan & Heide, 2008) to 0.7% between 1991 and 1995 (Meloy, 2000) and 0.2% in 2011 (U.S. Department of Justice, Federal Bureau of Investigation, Criminal Justice Information Services Divisions, 2012). Interestingly, a similar downward trend has been observed in the United Kingdom, where it was reported that in England and Wales between 1985 and 1994, 3.7% of homicides involved "sexual circumstances" (Francis & Soothill, 2000), whereas this number fell to 2.5% between 1995 and 2000 (Francis et al., 2004). A low base rate of sexual homicide has also been reported in other countries such as Australia (0.9%, Mouzos, 2003), Jamaica (5.0%, Lemard & Hemenway, 2006), and Finland (2.8%, Häkkänen-Nyholm, Repo-Tiihonen, Lindberg, Salenius, & Weizmann-Henelius, 2009). The only country for which data is available and that does not follow this trend appears to be South Africa. In 1999, 16% of female homicides were "suspected" of being rape-homicides (Abrahams et al., 2008), which was hypothesized to be related to their unusually high crime rate (Seedat, Van Niekerk, Jewkes, Suffla, & Ratele, 2009).

Despite their low-frequency occurrence, lethal outcomes in sexual crimes—or, more simply, sexual homicides—continue to attract a lot of attention from the media, the community, and the different actors of the criminal justice system. Media will often report on cases of sexual homicide due to the seriousness of the crime (see Wolfgang, Figlio, Tracy, & Singer, 1985), but

E. Beauregard (✉) · K. S. Reale
School of Criminology, Simon Fraser University, Burnaby, BC, Canada
e-mail: ebeaureg@sfu.ca

W. T. O'Donohue and P. A. Schewe (eds.), *Handbook of Sexual Assault and Sexual Assault Prevention*,
https://doi.org/10.1007/978-3-030-23645-8_38

also because these often involve unusual acts from the offender (e.g., dismemberment, insertion of foreign objects, mutilation of genitalia). Moreover, due in part to these gruesome acts but also to the apparent randomness of the victim selection, the community will rapidly develop fear that the perpetrator will strike again, becoming a serial killer. Finally, the different actors of the criminal justice system are concerned with cases of sexual homicide as few of them possess extensive experience handling and managing these cases (Beauregard & Martineau, 2017), while the decisions taken may carry important consequences for both the offender and the community that needs to be protected from these crimes.

Research on sexual homicide comes with an unavoidable paradox: despite being an unusual and relatively rare sexual crime, its consequences are too important to dismiss. At the same time, due to the fact that lethal outcomes in sexual crimes only represent less than 4% of all homicide, very few practitioners—whether clinicians or police investigators—have had contact with these offenders, leading to difficulties accumulating knowledge and experience with these types of crimes. This chapter attempts to partly remedy the situation by reviewing the different correlates associated with a lethal outcome in sexual assault cases.

Definition Problem

One of the first issues related to the study of sexual homicide is its definitional inconsistencies. Due in part to the absence of a legal definition (Roberts & Grossman, 1993), several authors have proposed different ways to define this specific form of sexual violence. At the broader level, Burgess, Hartman, Ressler, Douglas, and McCormack (1986) suggest that sexual homicides "result from one person killing another in the context of power, control, sexuality, and aggressive brutality" (p. 252). Similarly, others have simply proposed that sexual homicide should be defined as the intentional killing of a person where there is evidence of a sexual element to the murder (e.g., Beech, Fisher, & Ward, 2005; Douglas, Burgess, Burgess, & Ressler, 1992; Folino, 2000; Meloy, 2000; Myers, 2002; Porter, Woodworth, Earle, Drugge, & Boer, 2003). Some have also specified that sexual activity is not necessary for the murder to be sexual, as the act of killing itself may be sexually gratifying for the offender (Money, 1990; Schlesinger, 2004; Von Kraft-Ebing, 1886), whereas others have emphasized that certain acts performed by the perpetrator provide evidence of sexual homicide (e.g., mutilation, displacement of breasts, rectum, and/or genitals; Hazelwood & Douglas, 1980).

Another aspect implicitly related to the definition of sexual homicide is the motivation. According to Grubin (1994), it is crucial to distinguish between homicides that are sexually motivated and homicides associated with sexual activity. For instance, it is possible that offenders were not driven to kill their victim to satisfy sexual desires, but rather to eliminate a witness after a rape, to overcome victim resistance during a rape, or accidently killed the victim during a rape. Kerr, Beech, and Murphy (2013) argue that without a proper definition, this leaves considerable room for error as some cases might constitute false positives (e.g., staging a domestic homicide to appear as a sexual by removing the victim's clothing and exposing the genitals). These cases illustrate how some homicides may be associated with sexual activity without being necessary sexually motivated. This is problematic because it makes comparisons across studies difficult and creates inconsistencies in prevalence rates.

One problem with studying sexual homicide is that offenders' motivations and most of the definitions presented thus far rely on information known only to the offender and do not provide operationalized criteria that one may utilize in the classification process. For example, deviant sexual fantasies have been identified in research as a precipitating factor in sexual homicide; however, assessing deviant sexual fantasies relies entirely on the reliability and honesty of the offender. In order to remedy the situation, Ressler and Burgess (Ressler & Burgess, 1988) proposed a pragmatic definition of sexual homicide. According to such definition, to be considered sexual, a homicide has to present at least one of the following: (a) victim partially or completely undressed; (b) exposure of the sexual parts of the victim's body; (c) sexual positioning of the victim's body; (d) insertion of foreign objects into the victim's body cavities; (e) evidence of sexual intercourse; or (f) evidence of substitute sexual activity, interest, or sadistic fantasy. This definition is without a doubt the most widely used in the research on sexual homicide and encompasses the broadest range of factors.

Different Types of Sexual Homicides

The issues surrounding the definition of sexual homicide and how some could be sexually motivated while others not highlight the fact that sexual homicide constitutes a heterogeneous type of crime. When examining typological studies of sexual homicide, four main types are revealed, with each study describing between two and four types (see Beauregard, Proulx, & St-Yves, 2007 for an extensive review). However, the two types of sexual homicide that are consistently reported in the various studies are the angry and sadistic offender (Beauregard & Proulx, 2002).

The sadistic sexual homicide is often characterized by the offender having very elaborate and overwhelming fantasies, which are often used in the premeditation of the crime. These offenders use surveillance to select a specific victim who matches certain criteria. They often use alcohol before committing the crime and usually kill following a blow to their self-esteem or a situational stressor. Sadistic sexual murderers often use manipulation to approach an unknown victim and use a vehicle during the crime, and they often select an isolated crime scene, which is chosen in advance and one that is far from their home base. Their crime is characterized by the use of torture instruments or a so-called rape kit, tying up and gagging the victim, and the crime is also characterized by a prolonged and ritualized torture (e.g., mutilations to genitals). The sexual acts committed (i.e., fellatio, vaginal and anal penetration) may be recorded along with the murder, which is most often caused by strangulation. Sometimes, their homicides will include some unusual acts such as the insertion of objects into body cavities, dismemberment, and the retention of trophies or souvenirs belonging to the victim. They may also engage in behaviors during the crime commission process that indicate a conscious effort to avoid detection. For example, following the murder, offenders committing a sadistic sexual homicide may decide to move the victim's body, hiding it to delay or prevent recovery. These offenders may decide to move to a different city or change their job after the crime, while others may volunteer to help during the investigation. Some of these offenders may show some interest in the media coverage of the crime, but their behavior remains relatively normal following each crime. They usually show no remorse and even get some pleasure from describing the horror of their acts.

As to angry sexual murderers, the homicide is usually characterized by the absence of planning and a desire to kill, which often comes from some form of rage that is displaced toward the victim. The victim is usually selected opportunistically, often during the offenders' daily activities and from a location familiar to them. Before the crime, the offenders report suicidal ideations, depressive moods, and feelings of anger (Beauregard et al., 2007). The crime is characterized by the explosive and violent attack of a known victim who is usually older than the offender. The offender walks to the crime scene and is familiar with the location. There is a minimal use of restraints, but a weapon found at the crime scene may be used during the crime, even if death is usually caused by strangulation, just as in the sadistic sexual homicide. The homicide is often provoked by the victim's words or actions, resulting in humiliation and extreme violence (e.g., blows directed toward the victim's face, overkill). Sexual assault of the victim is possible (especially postmortem sexual acts), although no semen is found at the crime scene (Beauregard et al., 2007). After the murder, offenders committing an angry sexual homicide usually leave the victim's body on her back and in plain view at the crime scene. These offenders show no interest in media coverage of the crime, and they often report a feeling of relief after the murder (Beauregard et al., 2007).

As can be seen, although sadistic and angry sexual homicide may sometimes be difficult to distinguish due to the extreme violence of the acts and the cause of death by strangulation, the context, modus operandi, and behaviors following the crime are very different. As mentioned previously, another type of sexual homide has been identified in several studies; the offender whose primary intent is to sexually assault their victim and only kill the victim to eliminate witnesses. In these cases, the murder is merely instrumental. This type of offender is often described as seldom having long-term emotional relationships, and his victims are usually younger than 30 and unknown to him. The sexual assault is characterized by penetration of the victim and some sadistic elements. The murder may or may not be premeditated and is panicky or cold-blooded, depending on the murderer's criminal experience. Usually, the victim's wounds are restricted to a single site on the body, and the victim is found lying on her back. Often, the victim's corpse is found at the site at which first contact beween the murderer and the victim occurred (Beauregard et al., 2007).

More recently, another type of sexual homicide offender was identified: the forensically aware sexual homicide offender. Reale, Beauregard, and Martineau (2017a) found that some sexual homicide offenders are forensically aware, in that they will adapt their *modus operandi* or take precautions, before, during, or post-crime commission to decrease their chances of apprehension. The sadistic homicide offenders in this study were significantly more likely than non-sadistic sexual homicide offenders to engage in forensic awareness strategies such as destroying or removing evidence, taking precautions at the crime scene (e.g., disabling home alarms, wearing gloves or a mask), and dismembering the victim's body. Taking a different approach, Reale, Beauregard, and Martineau (2017b) used cluster analysis to separate sexual homicide offenders into distinct groups based on their crime scene behaviors. They identified three groups of sexual homicide offenders: (1) non-sadists; (2) mixed, engaged in sadistic offending behaviors but to a lesser frequency; and (3) severe sadists, engaged in the most sadistic behaviors. These three groups were then examined to determine whether forensic awareness would be associated with only the severe sadists or if it would be a feature of the mixed sadists as well. Findings indicated that when considering non-sadists, mixed, and severe sadists together, forensic awareness is still most associated with severe sadistic sexual homicide offenders.

Among the differences found in sexual murders of women, some studies have suggested that perpetrators of sexual homicide against children were different from those who targeted women. Firestone and colleagues (Firestone, Bradford, Greenberg, & Larose, 1998; Firestone, Bradford, Greenberg, Larose, & Curry, 1998; Firestone, Bradford, Greenberg, & Nunes, 2000) conducted three studies comparing sexual murderers of children to other groups of perpetrators of sexual crimes. Their findings showed that sexual murderers were rated significantly higher on the Psychopathy Checklist-Revised (PCL-R); had a greater incidence of psychosis, personality disorders (antisocial), paraphilias (sadism), and addictions; and showed more deviant phallometric responses to depictions of sexual assaults of children and adults. Moreover, findings revealed that sexual murderers were significantly more likely to have victimized strangers and to have been charged or convicted with past violent nonsexual and sexual offenses, when compared to a nonhomicidal group of sex offenders.

Following these studies, Beauregard, Stone, Proulx, and Michaud (2008) compared a group of 11 sexual murderers of children to a group of 66 sexual murderers of adults. Although their study did not find many differences between the groups of offenders, they did however identify differences in the pre-offense behavior and intent to commit the offense. For instance, sexual murderers of children were more likely to report having deviant sexual fantasies and to use pornography (deviant or not) prior to the crime and premediate their offense. Perhaps more interesting is the fact that sexual murderers of children were more likely to establish contact with the victim prior to the crime, to commit the crime during the day, to use strangulation to kill the victim, and to dismember and hide the victim's body, as compared to sexual murderers of adults. These behaviors are largely consistent with the literature of sadistic offending, which suggests a unique relationship between child sexual homicide offending and sadistic traits. Furthermore, in terms of pre-offense behavior, Beauregard et al. (2008) hypothesized that sexual murderers of children would spend time at home watching pornography—deviant or not—and then go to places that attract children (e.g., playgrounds, schools, and convenience stores) to establish prior contacts with victims (e.g., grooming). They are opportunistic and will wait for the absence of parents or guardians and then attract the child victim to an isolated location to commit the offense. According to Beauregard et al. (2008), most of the differences observed between sexual murderers of children and adults could also be explained through a routine activity perspective (Cohen & Felson, 1979).

Similarly, a study by Spehr, Hill, Habermann, Briken, and Berner (2010) compared a group of 35 sexual murderers who targeted children to a group of 100 sexual murderers who targeted adult victims. Findings revealed that sexual murderers of children were less likely to report alcohol abuse and drug dependency, as well as to present sexual dysfunctions or narcissistic personality disorders. There were no significant differences between the two groups on risk assessment scores, Psychopathy Checklist-Revised (PCL-R) scores, and rates of release and reconvictions. However, sexual murderers of children were more likely to have committed sexual abuse prior to the crime, although they were less likely to have committed rape or have caused bodily injury, than sexual murderers of adults. Unlike sexual murderers of adult victims, those who murdered children were more likely to have purposefully carried out the crime without any provocation from the victim (Spehr et al., 2010).

In a more recent study, Beauregard and Martineau (2015) compared a group of 79 sexual murderers of children to a group of 271 sexual murderers of adult women. Their findings also revealed a number of important differences between the two groups. For instance, sexual murderers of children were less likely to abuse drugs/alcohol and to leave the body in a residence, and the crimes were more like to be solved by the police, compared to cases against adult women. Further, the study showed that in cases of sexual homicide of children, the victims were more likely to be at home prior to the crime or outside on the street and living with an adult compared to sexual cases involving adult women. However, sexual murderers of children were more likely to beat the victim and kill using strangulation, compared to sexual murderers of adult women.

Once again, these findings illustrate the heterogeneity among perpetrators of sexual homicide. However, this heterogeneity has also been observed among serial and nonserial sexual murderers. Two important studies conducted by James and Proulx (2014, 2016) have highlighted several differences between the two groups. To summarize, the authors found that sexual preoccupations and sadism were key features of serial sexual murderers. Their modus operandi reflects sadistic sexual fantasies and organization which often results in these offenders planning their crimes to make them as congruent as possible with their fantasies. At the same time, these serial murderers are socially isolated, rejected, and humiliated and will often take refuge in compulsive masturbation. As to the nonserial sexual murderers, they are typically versatile criminals who are easily angered when their immediate needs are not met. They are also impulsive and extremely violent and use sexual homicide to diminish their internal tension. These sexual murderers often view themselves as the victim, and the sexual homicide serves as a way of exacting vengeance and an outlet for their anger. This is why their modus operandi is characterized by an explosion of anger.

Another study by Chan, Beauregard, and Myers (2015) also found several important differences between serial and nonserial sexual homicide offenders. In terms of crime characteristics, findings revealed that in comparison to nonserial sexual murderers, serial sexual murderers were more than twice as likely to choose victims based on physical features or personality characteristics and were more likely to target strangers. Serial sexual homicide offenders were also more likely to report having deviant sexual fantasies 48 hours prior to the crime, and a higher percentage of serial offenders also humiliated their victim, a behavioral indicator commonly associated with sadism. Interestingly, serial murderers were more than twice as likely than nonserial sexual murderers to have narcissistic personality features and to have comorbid personality disorders (e.g., obsessive-compulsive, schizoid, and narcissistic personality).

Comparing Sexual Homicide to Other Crimes

According to Felson and Messner (1996), there are two main perspectives to explain the lethal outcome in sexually violent crimes (see Beauregard & Mieczkowski, 2012). In the first perspective, homicide and other criminal violence are representative of the same type of behavior and involve the same processes, differing only in the outcome (Doerner & Speir, 1986; Harries, 1990). Consequently, based on such a perspective, one would expect no distinct patterns of behavior when examining sexual assaults that result in either physical injury or the death of the victim. The alternative perspective suggests that there are distinct factors that differentiate those who kill and those who do not. According to this perspective, some homicide offenders are motivated and have the intention to kill the victim, which differentiates them from sexual aggressors. Therefore, the lethal outcome is not incidental nor is it due to situational factors (Beauregard & Mieczkowski, 2012; Felson & Messner, 1996). This last perspective suggests that the sexual homicide offender is a unique type of offender. This perspective has been the focus of several recent studies. If we are going to predict sexual homicide, we need to be able to answer the following question: is the sexual homicide offender a unique type of offender?

To better understand sexual homicide offenders (SHOs) and their crimes, several studies have compared this group to a group of nonhomicidal sex offenders (NHSOs). The assumption underlying most of these studies is that by comparing these two groups, it is possible to identify factors that are related to a lethal outcome in a sexual crime. For instance, studies have shown that SHOs are more likely to target stranger victims who are older (Chene & Cusson, 2007; Firestone, Bradford, Greenberg, Larose, & Curry, 1998; Oliver, Beech, Fisher, & Beckett, 2007; not in Langevin, Ben-Aron, Wright, Marchese, & Handy, 1988). Contextually, SHOs more frequently live alone at the time of the crime (Grubin, 1994; not in Milsom, Beech, & Webster, 2003) and present a motive of anger or of both sex and anger (Chene & Cusson, 2007; Langevin et al., 1988). As to the criminal event, prior studies have shown that SHOs are more likely to use and/or abuse drugs and alcohol prior to crime (Chene & Cusson, 2007; Davis & Langevin, 2003), to use a weapon (Chene & Cusson, 2007; Firestone, Bradford, Greenberg, & Larose, 1998; Salfati & Taylor, 2006), and to engage in expressive violence (Firestone, Bradford, Greenberg, Larose, & Curry, 1998; Langevin et al., 1988; Salfati & Taylor, 2006). SHOs have also been shown to more frequently use strangulation (Langevin et al., 1988) as well as anal penetration and the insertion of an object in a body cavity (Salfati & Taylor, 2006).

Similar studies have investigated the "risk" of a lethal outcome in sexual crimes by considering the combination of factors instead of individual comparisons of one factor at a time. Mieczkowski and Beauregard (2010) used conjunctive analysis to look at the combination of victim, situation, and crime characteristics that are associated with a lethal outcome in cases of sexual assault. Their study findings revealed that the most lethal combination of factors involved actions taken by the offender during the crime, not victim or situational factors. More specifically, results indicated that a victim was almost 25 times more likely to be killed if the offender had brought a weapon, was intoxicated, and took more than 30 minutes to complete the offense but did not force the victim to commit sexual acts or commit any sexual intrusive acts on the victim. Although this may appear counterintuitive for the crime of sexual homicide—i.e., no sexual activity between the offender and the victim during a "sexual" homicide—it may be hypothesized that an inchoate sexual assault linked to a weapon in hand may be the worst possible combination of factors in the criminal situation leading to a lethal outcome.

Despite a modest effect of the situational factors on the lethality of the sexual assault, some victim characteristics were noteworthy. For instance, when a victim comes from a criminogenic environment (e.g., sex trade worker) and is less than 14 years old, his/her chances of survival are greater. Once again, it was hypothesized by Mieczkowski and Beauregard (2010) that coming from a criminogenic environment acted as a protective factor for potential victims, in the sense that they may be more effective at detecting early indicators of potentially dangerous behaviors or they may be better able to escape the circumstances at an earlier moment. This could be a result of having experienced socialization through other criminals. Alternatively, they may be more equipped to handle the circumstances once an assault has begun, which in turn leads them to act in ways more strategically likely to save their lives. Children, on the other hand, were hypothesized to be more likely to comply with sexual assaults, presenting less resistance, and thus may escape homicidal outcome as a result.

Using risk estimation as an alternative analytical strategy to look at the combination of factors leading to a lethal outcome in sexual assault cases, Beauregard and Mieczkowski (2012) found that several factors consistently contribute to the homicidal risk and appear distinctly separate from factors historically considered important. For example, a particularly dangerous situation is when the offender targets a stranger victim or is intoxicated during the crime. In fact, out of the ten most dangerous scenarios involving the event and context, targeting a stranger occurred seven times. Their study also highlighted potential factors that may serve to "protect" the victim. In addition to coming from a criminogenic environment, as identified in Mieczkowski and Beauregard (2010), the completion of a sexual act—either the victim completing a forced sexual act on the offender or the offender successfully initiating sexual contact with the victim—is associated with a greater chance of survival during a sexual assault. Beauregard and Mieczkowski (2012) hypothesized that in these cases the offender's primary motivation is sexual activity, which is not intrinsically related to violent behavior beyond the sexual activity itself. Moreover, the absence of a weapon appears to be important in increasing the victim's chance of survival during the sexual offense. This is likely because a weapon would make it easier for the offender to commit a homicide, but it also gives the offender an advantage if the victim resists.

Despite the fact that by comparing SHOs to NHSOs some factors appear to be related to a lethal outcome in sexual crimes, most of the existing studies have shown that overall, both groups of offenders present more similarities than differences (Langevin et al., 1988; Proulx, Beauregard, Cusson, & Nicole, 2007). However, it is important to point out that most of these previous studies did not use multivariate analyses in their design. Moreover, several of these studies suffered from small sample size. But more importantly, these studies have divided their sample into SHOs and NHSOs, leaving the NHSO group to include both violent and nonviolent perpetrators of sexual crimes. Such strategy may have introduced noise in the analyses, which resulted in finding more similarities than differences between the two groups of perpetrators.

In order to counteract these limitations, Beauregard and colleagues have conducted a series of studies comparing three groups of offenders who have committed sexual crimes: the nonhomicidal offender, the violent nonhomicidal offender, and the homicidal offender. Beauregard and Martineau (2017) have examined differences among these three groups of offenders on several offender characteristics. Among the factors investigated, they have looked specifically at the differences related to paraphilias and personality disorders. Results showed that perpetrators of sexual homicide significantly differ in terms of paraphilic behaviors. These offenders are significantly more likely to have engaged in paraphilic behavior both as a juvenile and as an adult. Although individuals who have perpetrated sexual homicides are significantly more likely to have engaged in a lifetime of paraphilic behavior, they are significantly less likely than the two other groups of sex offenders to be involved in the paraphilias involving nonconsenting adult and child partners (i.e., rape and pedophilia). Interestingly, it was the group of nonhomicidal offenders who were most likely to engage in pedophilia, whereas the violent nonhomicidal offenders were most likely to engage in rape.

In terms of personality disorders and constructs, several significant differences emerged between the three groups of offenders. Offenders who have committed a sexual homicide are significantly more likely than both groups to have diagnoses of schizoid and borderline personality disorders. The group of nonhomicidal offenders are more likely than the two other groups to present with avoidant personality, whereas both the nonhomicidal offenders and the violent nonhomicidal offenders were more likely than offenders who have committed a sexual homicide to present with avoidant personality, dependent personality, passive-aggressive personality, and immature personality. The violent nonhomicidal sex offenders were more likely than the two other groups to present with antisocial and impulsive personality disorders.

Although interesting, these findings were mainly exploratory and did not involve multivariate analyses. Beauregard and DeLisi (2018a, 2018b) further investigated the issue of personality in perpetrators of sexual homicide by comparing the same three groups, but this time using multivariate analyses and controlling for other factors that have been associated with the commission of sexual homicide. They determined that the personality profile of the perpetrators of sexual homicide is comprised primarily of schizoid and borderline personality disorders. These offenders were also significantly more likely to select a victim, use a weapon, and use drugs and alcohol before their offenses, but less likely to force their victim to engage in sexual acts or humiliate them. Beauregard and DeLisi (2018a, 2018b) argued that the comorbidity of schizoid, borderline, and antisocial personality disorder features presents unique personality dysfunction that facilitates the lethal sexual violence of SHOs relative to their nonhomicidal sexual offender counterparts.

In a different study, Beauregard, DeLisi, and Hewitt (2018) have examined differences among the three groups of offenders on their criminal career. Despite the fact that all three groups have extensive and serious offending records, some important distinctions were found. The nonhomicidal offenders had more convictions for rape/sexual abuse and other sexual offenses relating to exhibitionism as well as more specialization in their offending repertoires. Violent nonhomicidal offenders were more versatile in their offending patterns and had more assaults, homicides, kidnappings, and aggravated sexual assaults. Offenders who have committed sexual homicides were similarly versatile and had extensive histories of armed robbery, kidnapping, and homicide. Interestingly, the group that presented with the most prolific criminal career profile was the violent nonhomicidal offenders, characterized with the greatest number of prior convictions and the most varied criminal career. They were more likely to be versatile, as they committed a wide variety of crime, going from nonviolent nonsexual crimes to violent sexual crimes (see Lussier, 2005).

In another study, Beauregard and DeLisi (2018a, 2018b) compared the same three groups of offenders but this time on several developmental factors. Their analyses identified a number of developmental factors that are more likely to be found in offenders who have committed sexual homicide. The findings show that offenders who commit sexual homicide present a background characterized by abuse and a variety of problematic behaviors. For instance, of the 12 behavioral indicators examined in the study, 10 proved to be statistically different. Specifically, offenders who commit sexual homicides experience more problem behaviors such as chronic lying, angry temperament, running away, and recklessness. Moreover, they are more likely to report cruelty against animals, whereas the violent nonhomicidal offenders are more likely to report rebellious attitude and neuropsychological deficits compared to offenders committing sexual homicides. Such findings show that offenders committing sexual homicides learn specific sexual behaviors early in childhood that suggest a strong need for sexual gratification, and they also may not adequately address their sexual needs, which potentially contributes to the seriousness of their sexual offending. Beauregard and DeLisi (2018a, 2018b) hypothesized that this investment in solitary, illegal, or obsessive sexual behaviors is the result of their need to regain some control over their lives, as suggested by several of the theoretical models of sexual homicide.

Recently, Chopin and Beauregard (2018) have taken a similar approach to answer the same question but this time including a group of nonsexual homicidal offenders. Comparing a large sample of sexual homicide offenders, violent sexual abusers, and nonsexual homicidal offenders, they found that perpetrators of sexual homicide presented several differences that were consistent with the other two groups. These convergent differences suggested that offenders who perpetrated a sexual homicide were different not only from perpetrators of sexual crimes but also from individuals who had committed a nonsexual homicide. Even more interesting was the fact that these differences were not only identified as to the crime characteristics but on the offender characteristics as well.

Taken together, these findings suggest that perpetrators of sexual homicide present several differences with other perpetrators of sexual crimes as well as nonsexual homicides. The differences observed are not only related to the way the crime is committed but mainly consist of differences in personality and developmental characteristics. These differences have important implications for homicide investigations, corrections, and offender management and treatment. Finally, as Chopin and Beauregard (2018) have concluded, it appears that perpetrators of sexual homicide represent a unique type of offender that should be examined on its own.

Implications

If we are correct in assuming that the perpetrators of sexual homicides represent a unique type of offender, this may have several potential implications for the different actors of the criminal justice system and their practices. Looking at law enforcement first, although cases of sexual homicide are suggestive that the police should be looking for offenders who have previous sexual convictions, previous studies show that such a recommendation would be ill-advised. Most individuals who have committed sexual homicides do not have prior convictions for sexual crimes and have only a few prior convictions for violent crimes. Therefore, focusing exclusively on known sex offenders represents an ineffective strategy and constitutes a waste of valuable resources for the police.

However, this is not to say that the criminal career of perpetrators of sexual homicide cannot be useful to the criminal investigation. For example, Beauregard et al. (2018) have found that sexual murderers could be distinguished from violent and nonviolent nonhomicidal sex offenders by one particular offense: armed robberies. Before having committed their sexual homicide, many of these individuals committed other crimes—predominantly property crime—but it seems that a large proportion of them also committed armed robberies. Similar to the study by Soothill, Francis, Sanderson, and Ackerley (2000), some offenses are related to a higher risk of committing homicide. What these researchers found was that manslaughter, blackmail, and kidnapping increased the relative risk of homicide by 19, 5, and 4 times, respectively. Moreover, the offense of robbery—not necessarily armed robbery—doubled the risk of homicide. These findings are important for the police in charge of investigating these cases. Instead of exclusively focusing on known sex offenders, the findings suggest that sexual murderers may in fact have modest to no sexual criminal histories but are instead are more often characterized by property offenses, especially armed robberies. Such findings suggest that an offender's criminal history gains great investigative importance when one goes beyond simply examining the presence or absence of prior convictions for sexual crimes.

Arguably more important are the implications for corrections. The fact that sexual murderers represent a unique type of offender, different from both sex offenders and homicide offenders, has practical implication from the admission of the offender to his supervision if/when returned to the community. As suggested by Chopin and Beauregard (2018), individuals convicted of sexual homicide pose specific challenges for corrections, and this starts right at their admission. For instance, perpetrators of sexual homicide do not typically enter the correctional system with a label of "sex offender." Being considered as murderers first and foremost, these offenders will typically be incarcerated within the general population. However, in some cases, offenders who have been widely publicized in the media will face a different reality. Instead of seeing their homicidal act being the focus of correctional administrators and other inmates, it is the sexual nature of the act that will be predominant. As sex offenders do not typically benefit from the same status inside as other inmates, a decision will need to be made by correctional authorities as to whether the sexual murderer should be put in protective custody with sex offenders or if they can risk a placement in the general population. Such decision will have an impact not only for the security of the inmate but also for the security in the institution.

Knowing that the sexual murderer represents a unique type of offender also has implications for the treatment programming, inside as well as outside prison. The fact that the sexual murderer does not follow the same trajectory of a typical sex offender seems to suggest that the "one-size-fits-all" treatments for sex offenders would be ineffective. At the same time, we believe it would be a mistake to assume that these offenders do not require treatment adapted to their specific problems. As previous studies have shown, sexual murderers present several problems that are unique to them, some of which are of a sexual nature (e.g., sexual preoccupations). This suggests that correctional authorities should consider the adoption of more tailored or individualized treatment programs, instead of the more generic ones. This may be even more important for juvenile sexual murderers as they have a greater opportunity to be released back into the community.

Beyond the correctional functioning of sexual murderers, findings of previous studies may inform the assessment of these offenders as well as the decision-making involved in such cases. As mentioned previously, studies on the developmental factors of sexual murderers (Beauregard & DeLisi, 2018a, 2018b; Beauregard & Martineau, 2017; DeLisi & Beauregard, 2018) have shown that these offenders present specific problems during their childhood. In fact, the findings suggest that it is not enough to identify whether or not the offender has experienced victimization in childhood. Instead, they show the importance of detailing these experiences and to take into account the variety of these adverse childhood experiences. Therefore, it would be important for risk assessment tools to consider this crucial piece of information to not only predict the risk of recidivism but also to predict the risk of a lethal outcome in the case of a sexual recidivism. As to the contribution of the findings to decision-making by correctional officials, the findings suggest that it would be important to identify cases which present a myriad of adverse childhood experiences in order to offer them an intensive treatment intervention to "solve" some of these traumas before being released back to the community. Establishing intervention strategies that adequately address the resultant issues to attempt to prevent relapse—or worse a homicidal relapse—seems to be of the utmost importance to interfere with the cycle of violence.

Finally, it is important to consider that in some cases, sexual murderers will eventually be released back into the community and that supervision conditions will need to be put in place. What type of supervision will be required for this specific type of offender is something that remains unknown as no study has investigated this aspect of sexual homicide yet. However, this is still an important question. Myers, Chan, Vo, and Lazarou (2010) looked specifically at juvenile sexual murderers and found that of the 11 cases for which follow-up community recidivism data was available, 5 remained free of further convictions for an average of 8.9 years, whereas 6 offenders recidivated after only 4.4 years later on average. While three of the offenders who recidivated committed nonsexual offenses, the three other offenders survived an average of 5.3 years before committing additional sexual homicides (Myers et al., 2010). This suggests that despite sexual homicide being rare and uncommon, some of these offenders will eventually reintegrate society and will need to be monitored adequately if we want to avoid recidivism for the same type of crime. Further the public response to recidivism in a previously convicted sexual homicide offender would have drastic public policy implications and would likely result in moral panic. In order to promote public confidence in community corrections, more research on reintegration is essential. Moreover, protective factors are equally important to consider as early intervention efforts tailored to the unique needs of high-risk offenders could help to ensure the risk of escalation to homicide is reduced.

Conclusion

Ultimately, although researchers have shed light onto correlates of lethal outcomes in sexual homicide, there are still many unanswered questions. The extant literature has been limited by small sample sizes, incomplete comparison groups, and a lack of more complex statistical analyses. As a result, more research that uses larger samples and more complex models are needed and should not only compare perpetrators of sexual homicide with perpetrators of nonsexual homicide but also nonhomicidal sexual crimes. Further, cross-cultural comparisons of sexual homicide offenders would be beneficial to determine whether culture influences, victim selection, crime scene behaviors, and other aspects of the crime commission process.

Although future studies need to continue comparing differences between types of sexual and nonsexual and violent and nonviolent homicide offenders, more research is needed that examines a wider range of clinical features associated with these offenders as well. For instance, despite the interest and usefulness of police data, they are often limited in terms of the offender characteristics. Clinical data such as personality diagnostics (e.g., personality disorders, psychopathy, sadism) would be important to consider as well in the comparisons of these three types of offenders. Further, most studies are retrospective in nature, and the utility of longitudinal studies that include sexual homicide offenders is imperative to identifying pathways to sexual homicide.

Similarly, future studies should focus on the identification of the different pathways leading to sexual homicide paying specific focus to developmental risk factors. Despite the sexual murderer being a unique type of offender, there exists different types of sexual homicides (e.g., Beauregard & Proulx, 2002), and it is possible that different pathways have led these offenders to commit these different types of sexual homicides. To achieve this, it will be important to conduct qualitative interviews with individuals who have committed sexual homicide, from their childhood to the moment of their crime. Such information would also be valuable to investigate the decision-making involved in the killing of the victim during or following a sexual assault.

DeLisi and Wright (2014) have highlighted the fact that mainstream criminological research has by and large refused to scientifically investigate sexual homicide. The result of this large slight has been an almost quasi absence of sexual homicide research by mainstream criminologists. Future studies need to test some of the main concepts of criminological theories to explain sexual homicide (e.g., low self-control, strain, opportunity). In addition, instead of looking at sexual homicide as a distinct category of sexual violent crime, future studies need to look at the lethal outcome in sexual crimes as a continuum of violence.

Furthermore, as confusion still persists as to the definition of sexual homicide and what constitutes a real sexual homicide, future studies need to test different ways to compare cases of sexual homicide where the perpetrator clearly indicated his intent to kill the victim with cases where such intent was absent.

Chan and Frei (2013) also contend that female sexual homicide offenders have been largely ignored in the extant literature of sexual homicide. This is in part due to the rarity of these offenses; however this does not discredit the need for more research as studies that have examined female sexual homicide offenders have identified unique characteristics associated with these offenders.

Finally, we shall return to the question with which we began. Can we predict sexual homicide? Unfortunately, previous findings do not provide us with a definitive answer to this question. However, when considering the findings reviewed in this chapter, we can conclude that the sexual murderer is a unique type of offender, one that presents with specific characteristics. Although it is still too early to do, we believe that after replicating some of these findings and taking into account the interactions between some of the important factors related to a lethal outcome in sexual crimes, it will be possible to at least suggest "red flags" or risk factors associated with the commission of a sexual homicide.

References

Abrahams, N., Martin, L. J., Jewkes, R., Mathews, S., Vetten, L., & Lombard, C. (2008). The epidemiology and pathology of suspected rape homicide in South Africa. *Forensic Science International, 178*, 132–138.

Beauregard, E., & DeLisi, M. (2018a). Stepping stones to sexual murder: The role of developmental factors in the etiology of sexual homicide. *Journal of Criminal Psychology, 8*(3), 199–214.

Beauregard, E., & DeLisi, M. (2018b). Unraveling the personality profile of the sexual murderer. *Journal of Interpersonal Violence*.

Beauregard, E., DeLisi, M., & Hewitt, A. (2018). Sexual murderer: Sex offender, murderer, or both? *Sexual Abuse: A Journal of Research and Treatment, 30*(8), 932–950.

Beauregard, E., & Martineau, M. (2015). An application of CRAVED to the choice of victim in sexual homicide: A routine activity approach. *Crime Science, 4*, 24.

Beauregard, E., & Martineau, M. (2017). *The sexual murderer: Offender behaviour and implications for practice*. London: Routledge.

Beauregard, E., & Mieczkowski, T. (2012). Risk estimations of the conjunction of victim and crime event characteristics on the lethal outcome of sexual assaults. *Violence and Victims, 27*, 470–486.

Beauregard, E., & Proulx, J. (2002). Profiles in the offending process of nonserial sexual murderers. *International Journal of Offender Therapy and Comparative Criminology, 46*, 386–399.

Beauregard, E., Proulx, J., & St-Yves, M. (2007). Angry or sadistic: Two types of sexual murderers. In J. Proulx, E. Beauregard, M. Cusson, & A. Nicole (Eds.), *Sexual murder: A comparative analysis and new perspectives* (pp. 123–141). Winchester: Wiley.

Beauregard, E., Stone, M. R., Proulx, J., & Michaud, P. (2008). Sexual murderers of children: Developmental, pre-crime, crime, and post-crime factors. *International Journal of Offender Therapy and Comparative Criminology, 52*, 253–269.

Beech, A. R., Fisher, D., & Ward, T. (2005). Sexual murderers' implicit theories. *Journal of Interpersonal Violence, 20*, 1336–1389.

Burgess, A. W., Hartman, C. R., Ressler, R. K., Douglas, J. E., & McCormack, A. (1986). Sexual homicide: A motivational model. *Journal of Interpersonal Violence, 1*, 251–272.

Calgary Sun. (2018). Sex offender convicted in rape and murder of 14-year-old girl—Could face death penalty. Retrieved from http://calgarysun.com/news/crime/sex-offender-convicted-in-rape-and-murder-of-14-year-old-girl-could-face-death-penalty/wcm/7f67a179-bf30-4b4e-b2a5-c53875c23f9d.

Chan, H., Beauregard, E., & Myers, W. (2015). Single-victim and serial sexual homicide offenders: Differences in crime, paraphilias and personality traits. *Criminal Behaviour and Mental Health, 25*(1), 66–78.

Chan, H. C. O., & Heide, K. M. (2008). Weapons used by juveniles and adult offenders in sexual homicides: An empirical analysis of 29 years of US data. *Journal of Investigative Psychology and Offender Profiling, 5*, 189–208.

Chan, H. C. (Oliver), & Frei, A. (2013). Female sexual homicide offenders: An examination of an underresearched offender population. *Homicide Studies, 17*(1), 96–118. https://doi.org/10.1177/1088767912449625

Chene, S., & Cusson, M. (2007). Sexual murderers and sexual aggressors: Intention and situation. In J. Proulx, E. Beauregard, M. Cusson, & A. Nicole (Eds.), *Sexual murderers: A comparative analysis and new perspective* (pp. 71–97). Chichester: Wiley.

Chopin, J., & Beauregard, E. (2018). Is the sexual murderer a unique or hybrid type of offender? *Journal of Criminal Justice*.

Cohen, L., & Felson, M. (1979). Social change and crime rate trends: A routine activity approach. *American Sociological Reviews, 44*, 588–608.

Davis, F. A., & Langevin, R. (2003). A study of the psychosexual characteristics of sex killers: Can we identify them before it is too late? *International Journal of Offender Therapy and Comparative Criminology, 47*, 366–382.

DeLisi, M., & Beauregard, E. (2018). Adverse childhood experiences and criminal extremity: New evidence for sexual homicide. *Journal of Forensic Sciences, 63*(2), 484–489. https://doi.org/10.1111/1556-4029.13584

DeLisi, M., & Wright, J. (2014). Social control theory of sexual homicide offending. In G. Bruinsma & D. Weisburd (Eds.), *Encyclopedia of criminology and criminal justice* (pp. 4916–4922). New York: Springer.

Doerner, W. G., & Speir, J. C. (1986). Stitch and sew: The impact of medical resources upon criminally induced lethality. *Criminology, 24*, 319–330.

Douglas, J. E., Burgess, A. W., Burgess, A. C., & Ressler, R. (1992). *Crime classification manual*. Lexington, MA: Lexington Books.

Felson, R. B., & Messner, S. F. (1996). To kill or not to kill? Lethal outcomes in injurious attacks. *Criminology, 34*(4), 519–545. https://doi.org/10.1111/j.1745-9125.1996.tb01218.x

Firestone, P., Bradford, J. M., Greenberg, D. M., & Larose, M. R. (1998). Homicidal sex offenders: Psychological, phallometric, and diagnostic features. *Journal of the American Academy of Psychiatry and Law, 26*, 537–552.

Firestone, P., Bradford, J. M., Greenberg, D. M., Larose, M. R., & Curry, S. (1998). Homicidal and nonhomicidal child molesters: Psychological, phallometric, and criminal features. *Sexual Abuse: A Journal of Research and Treatment, 10*, 305–323.

Firestone, P., Bradford, J. M., Greenberg, D. M., & Nunes, K. L. (2000). Differentiation of homicidal child molesters, nonhomicidal child molesters, and nonoffenders by phallometry. *The American Journal of Psychiatry, 157*(11), 1847–1850. http://dx.doi.org/10.1176/appi.ajp.157.11.1847

Folino, J. O. (2000). Sexual homicides and their classification according to motivation: A report from Argentina. *International Journal of Offender Therapy and Comparative Criminology, 44*, 740–750.

Francis, B., Barry, J., Bowater, R., Miller, N., Soothill, K., & Ackerley, E. (2004). *Using homicide data to assist murder investigations. London: Home Office Online Report 26/04*. Retrieved from http://www.homeoffice.gov.uk/rds.

Francis, B., & Soothill, K. (2000). Does sex offending lead to homicide? *Journal of Forensic Psychiatry, 11*, 49–61.

Grubin, D. (1994). Sexual murder. *British Journal of Psychiatry, 165*, 624–629.

Häkkänen-Nyholm, H., Repo-Tiihonen, E., Lindberg, N., Salenius, S., & Weizmann-Henelius, G. (2009). Finnish sexual homicides: Offence and offender characteristics. *Forensic Science International, 188*, 125–130.

Hanson, R. K., & Bussiere, M. T. (1998). Predicting relapse: A meta-analysis of sexual offender recidivism studies. *Journal of Consulting and Clinical Psychology, 66*, 348–362.

Harries, K. D. (1990). *Serious violence: Patterns of homicide and assault in America*. Springfield, IL: Thomas Books.

Hazelwood, R. R., & Douglas, J. E. (1980). The lust murderer. *FBI Law Enforcement Bulletin, 49*, 18–22.

James, J., & Proulx, J. (2014). A psychological and developmental profile of sexual murderers: A systematic review. *Aggression and Violent Behavior, 19*, 592–607.

James, J., & Proulx, J. (2016). The modus operandi of serial and nonserial sexual murderers: A systematic review. *Aggression and Violent Behavior, 31*, 200–218.

Kerr, K. J., Beech, A. R., & Murphy, D. (2013). Sexual homicide: Definition, motivation and comparison with other forms of sexual offending. *Aggression and Violent Behavior, 18*, 1–10.

Kong, R., Johnson, H., Beattie, S., & Cardillo, A. (2003). *Sexual offences in Canada*. Canadian Centre for Justice Statistics.

Langevin, R., Ben-Aron, M. H., Wright, P., Marchese, V., & Handy, L. (1988). The sex killer. *Annals of Sex Research, 1*, 263–301.

Lemard, G., & Hemenway, D. (2006). Violence in Jamaica: An analysis of homicides 1998–2002. *Injury Prevention, 12*, 15–18.

Lussier, P. (2005). The criminal activity of sexual offenders in adulthood: Revisiting the specialization debate. *Sexual Abuse: A Journal of Research and Treatment, 17*, 269–292. https://doi.org/10.1177/107906320501700303

Meloy, J. R. (2000). The nature and dynamics of sexual homicide: An integrative review. *Aggression and Violent Behavior, 5*, 1–22.

Mieczkowski, T., & Beauregard, E. (2010). Lethal outcome in sexual assault events: A conjunctive analysis. *Justice Quarterly, 27*, 332–361.

Milsom, J., Beech, A. R., & Webster, S. D. (2003). Emotional loneliness in sexual murderers: A qualitative analysis. *Sexual Abuse: A Journal of Research and Treatment, 15*, 285–296.

Money, J. (1990). Forensic sexology: Paraphilic serial rape (biastophilia) and lust murder (erotophonophilia). *American Journal of Psychotherapy, 44*, 26–36.

Mouzos, J. (2003). Homicide in the course of other crime in Australia. In *Trends & issues in crime and justice No. 252*. Canberra: Australian Institute of Criminology.

Myers, W. C. (2002). *Juvenile sexual homicide*. San Diego, CA: Academic Press.

Myers, W. C., Chan, H. C., Vo, E., & Lazarou, E. (2010). Sexual sadism, psychopathy, and recidivism in juvenile sexual murderers. *Journal of Investigative Psychology and Offender Profiling, 7*(1), 49–58. https://doi.org/10.1002/jip.113

Oliver, C. J., Beech, A. R., Fisher, D., & Beckett, R. (2007). A comparison of rapists and sexual murderers on demographic and selected psychometric measures. *International Journal of Offender Therapy and Comparative Criminology, 51*, 298–312.

Porter, S., Woodworth, M., Earle, J., Drugge, J., & Boer, D. (2003). Characteristics of sexual homicides committed by psychopathic and non-psychopathic offenders. *Law and Human Behavior, 27*, 459–469.

Proulx, J., Beauregard, E., Cusson, M., & Nicole, A. (2007). *Sexual murderers: A comparative analysis and new perspectives*. Winchester: Wiley.

Reale, K., Beauregard, E., & Martineau, M. (2017a). Is investigative awareness a distinctive feature of sadism? *Journal of Interpersonal Violence*, 1–18.

Reale, K., Beauregard, E., & Martineau, M. (2017b). Classifying sexual homicide offenders: Using sadistic crime scene behaviours to identify distinct groups.

Journal of Criminal Psychology, 7, 120–133. https://doi.org/10.1108/CJP-11-2016-0042
Ressler, R. K., Burgess, A. W., & Douglas (1988). *Sexual homicide: Patterns and motives*. New York, NY: Lexington.
Roberts, J. V., & Grossman, M. G. (1993). Sexual homicide in Canada: A descriptive analysis. *Annals of Sex Research, 6*, 5–25.
Salfati, C. G., & Taylor, P. (2006). Differentiating sexual violence: A comparison of sexual homicide and rape. *Psychology, Crime and Law, 12*, 107–125.
Schlesinger, L. B. (2004). *Sexual murder: Catathymic and compulsive homicides*. Boca Raton, FL: CRC Press.
Seedat, M., Van Niekerk, A., Jewkes, R., Suffla, S., & Ratele, K. (2009). Violence and injuries in South Africa: Prioritising an agenda for prevention. *Lancet, 374*, 1011–1022.
Soothill, K., Francis, B., Sanderson, B., & Ackerley, E. (2000). Sex offenders: Specialists, generalists or both? *British Journal of Criminology, 40*, 56–67. http://www.jstor.org/stable/23638530
Spehr, A., Hill, A., Habermann, N., Briken, P., & Berner, W. (2010). Sexual murderers with child or adult victims: Are they different? *Sexual Abuse: A Journal of Research and Treatment, 22*, 290–314.
Statistics Canada. 2013. *Homicide Survey (Record No. 3315)*. Retrieved from http://www.statcan.gc.ca/dli-ild/data-donnees/ftp/hs-eh-eng.htm.
U.S. Department of Justice, Federal Bureau of Investigation, Criminal Justice Information Services Divisions. 2012. *Uniform Crime Reports: Crime in the United* States *2012*. Retrieved from http://www.fbi.gov/about-us/cjis/ucr/crime-in-the-u.s/2012/crime-in-the- u.s.-2012/offenses-known-to-law-enforcement/expandedhomicide/expanded_homicide_data_table_10_murder_circumstances_by_relationship_2012.xls.
Von Kraft-Ebing, R. (1886). *Psychopathia sexualis* (C. G. Chaddock, Trans.). Philadelphia: Butterworth-Heinemann.
Wolfgang, M., Figlio, R., Tracy, P., & Singer, I. (1985). *The National Survey of Crime Severity*. Washington, DC: U.S. Department of Justice, Bureau of Justice Statistics.

Part VII
Special Populations

Sexual Violence in LGBTQ Communities

39

Adam M. Messinger and Sarah Koon-Magnin

It is really daunting to talk about sexual abuse that happened when you were presenting as your birth gender after you have transitioned. I was not ready to talk about it for a long time after it had happened. However, when I was ready to disclose, I was presenting as a man and then I encountered two problems; one) I didn't want to remember when I was a girl and two) men are perceived as not having experienced sexual abuse so I wasn't sure how I would be received.

Rymer and Cartei (2015), p. 158

The scale of prevention efforts, survivor support services, and public awareness regarding sexual violence has increased dramatically over the past 40 years. The majority of sexual assaults and rapes are perpetrated by cisgender (i.e., non-transgender) men against women (e.g., see Black et al., 2011; Planty, Langton, Krebs, Berzofsky, & Smiley-McDonald, 2013). Perhaps understandably, most published research and societal interventions focus on sexual violence involving this pairing. Unfortunately, as a consequence of this nearly singular focus, scholarship and societal efforts to address sexual violence are severely lacking in their consideration of lesbian, gay, bisexual, transgender, and queer (LGBTQ)-identified individuals (Girshick, 2002; Menning & Holtzman, 2014). This is despite the fact that research repeatedly concludes that LGBTQ people are at an elevated risk of sexual violence victimization (Coulter et al., 2017; Katz-Wise & Hyde, 2012; Walters, Chen, & Breiding, 2013). It is the very invisibility of LGBTQ lives within the public discourse on sexual violence that makes this problem seemingly so intractable. As exemplified in the story above about a transgender victim's quandary of whether to disclose, LGBTQ survivors too often face a minefield of risks when seeking help: from service providers turning them away, to having their experiences and identities devalued, to being outed, or worse (Girshick, 2002; Messinger, 2017). In this chapter, we review the research literature on the experience of sexual violence within LGBTQ communities: its prevalence, risk factors, interpersonal contexts, and barriers to help-seeking. We conclude with recommendations for future research, policy, and service provision.

A. M. Messinger (✉)
Justice Studies Department and Women's & Gender Studies Program, Northeastern Illinois University, Chicago, IL, USA
e-mail: a-messinger@neiu.edu

S. Koon-Magnin
Department of Political Science and Criminal Justice, University of South Alabama, Mobile, AL, USA

Prevalence of LGBTQ Sexual Violence

Methodological Concerns

Prevalence estimates of LGBTQ sexual violence are necessarily influenced by methodological decisions in how to operationalize sexual violence. There is substantial variation in the way

W. T. O'Donohue and P. A. Schewe (eds.), *Handbook of Sexual Assault and Sexual Assault Prevention*,
https://doi.org/10.1007/978-3-030-23645-8_39

that people understand the words "rape" and "sexual assault" and what acts are involved in each (Schulze, Koon-Magnin, & Bryan, 2019). However, this is not surprising, given that there is also significant variation in the meaning of these terms across jurisdictions. Definitions of what constitutes a sexual offense, as well as the name and assigned severity of the offense, differ across jurisdictions and have changed significantly over time. For instance, through 2012, the federal definition of rape for the purposes of data collection in the United States was "Carnal knowledge of a woman forcibly and against her will" (Federal Bureau of Investigation, 2014). This narrow definition limits who can be recognized as a victim (a woman), or a perpetrator (a man), and what sexual acts constitute rape (penile-vaginal penetration). As a result, under this definition, many acts of sexual violence against an LGBTQ victim would not be legally recognized as "rape." The new and much more inclusive federal definition of rape—"Penetration, no matter how slight, of the vagina or anus with any body part or object, or oral penetration by a sex organ of another person, without the consent of the victim" (Federal Bureau of Investigation, 2014)—has important implications for all victims of rape, but it is particularly impactful for those in LGBTQ communities in two ways. First, the definition is now gender-neutral and recognizes that both men and women can be victims of rape and that both men and women can be perpetrators of rape. Second, the revised definition reflects a more accurate understanding of sexual violence by including various penetrative violations (oral, anal, or vaginal) and not requiring that a penis be the penetrating object.

An additional benefit of the updated definition is that the use of force is no longer a requirement in this definition. Rather, the focus is on a lack of consent. This difference is critical because a victim may be unable to provide consent to sex for a variety of reasons that would not require the offender employ physical force (e.g., the victim may be asleep, unconscious, or incapacitated by alcohol or other drugs). Recent research indicates that some individuals in traumatic situations like sexual assault experience a complete though temporary paralysis, a phenomenon termed "tonic immobility" (for an excellent discussion, see Campbell, 2012). Individuals who experience this "freeze" response are unable to fight back against an assailant, negating the need for force by the attacker (Bucher & Manasse, 2011). However, statutes that emphasize lack of consent rather than physical force still recognize these violations as rape because they are being completed against the will of the victim. Importantly, not all state statutes are as inclusive as the new federal definition, meaning that certain sexual acts that are more likely to affect sexual minority victims of sexual assault are not recognized as "rape" in all states. While such acts are usually still illegal and can be prosecuted as sexual offenses, in many states, they are given a label other than "rape" (e.g., "forcible sodomy" or "sexual battery"), which may make a victim feel marginalized in their experience.

Scholars of sexual violence tend to take a broader view of rape and sexual assault than many legal codes and may define sexual violence as any non-consensual sexual activity, including sexual touching or penetration without permission, through coercion, by force or threat of force, or with a victim who is unable to consent. Despite the absence of force in such cases, non-consensual sexual touching or penetration can still have extremely serious effects on victims (Tark & Kleck, 2014).

In addition to the question of whether to define sexual violence as non-consensual versus force-facilitated sexual activities, researchers also have to decide which sexual activities to assess: non-consensual, non-penetrative sexual contact and oral sex (often termed "sexual assault") or non-consensual sexual penetration of the vagina or anus by a penis, finger, or object (often termed "rape"). Even among the most highly regarded studies for measuring crime prevalence (e.g., Uniform Crime Reports, *National Crime Victimization Survey*, *National Violence Against Women Survey*, and *National Intimate Partner and Sexual Violence Survey*), there are differences in the ways that rape and sexual assault are defined and measured (Panel on Measuring Rape and Sexual Assault in Bureau of Justice Statistics Household Surveys 2014). Criminal justice researchers, mirroring many criminal statutes, often narrow this definition of sexual violence to include only sexual activity involving force or threat of force (Girshick, 2002; Messinger, 2017). Such force-based sexual violence survey measures risk excluding equally troubling cases of non-forced, non-consensual sexual activities. Despite the absence of force, unwanted and coerced sexual activity can be extremely harmful to the victim, as much psychological literature demonstrates. Moreover, studies of rape may overlook a substantial portion of LGBTQ sexual violence given that sexual penetration is not always as central to conceptions of sexual intercourse and rape in female same-gender relationships. Ultimately, decisions about how to measure sexual violence—whether as non-consensual or force-facilitated, as sexual contact or sexual penetration—will have a significant impact on LGBTQ sexual violence prevalence estimates. Specifically, studies that focus exclusively on the older definition of "rape" as penile-vaginal penetration will likely have lower prevalence estimates than those that include a more inclusive definition of sexual violence. With that in mind, as reviewed in the following section, research finds LGBTQ individuals to be at an elevated risk of sexual violence victimization, particularly bisexuals, cisgender women, and transgender and nonbinary individuals assigned female at birth.

Prevalence of Sexual Violence Victimization Among Sexual Minorities

Regarding sexual minorities (i.e., lesbian, gay, bisexual, queer, and other non-heterosexual-identified individuals), the *National Intimate Partner and Sexual Violence Survey* is a recent nationally representative study ($N = 16{,}507$, 97% heterosexual) that offers some of the most accurate estimates available of sexual violence prevalence among sexual minorities in the United States (Walters, Chen, & Breiding, 2013). Findings indicated that, relative to heterosexual women (17.4% victimization rate), lesbian women were at similar risk (13.1%) and bisexual women were at substantially higher risk (46.1%) of experiencing forced or substance-facilitated rape in their lifetimes (measured as oral, vaginal, or anal penetration or attempted penetration using a penis, fingers, or object, with either force or the use of substances). Rates for those experiencing coerced rape (penetration through the use of coercion but not force), sexual assault (measured as unwanted non-penetrative sexual contact), or non-contact unwanted sexual experiences (such as exposing sexual body parts or being made to participate in sexual movies or photos) were again similar for heterosexual (43.3%) and lesbian women (46.4%) and higher for bisexual women (74.9%). Because of low base rates of male sexual victimization within the sample, male estimates of rape could not be provided across sexual orientations. However, regarding coerced rape, sexual assault, and non-contact unwanted sexual experiences, gay men (40.2%) and bisexual men (47.4%) were at approximately double the risk of victimization as compared to heterosexual men (20.8%; Walters et al., 2013). Thus, with the exception of lesbian women being at a similar risk of forced and substance-facilitated rape as compared to heterosexual women, sexual minorities were generally at higher risk of sexual violence than heterosexuals. In the United Kingdom, an analysis of the 2007–2010 *British Crime Survey* was consistent with these findings in that bisexual men and women were at significantly higher risk of sexual assault victimization than heterosexual men and women (Mahoney, Davies, & Scurlock-Evans, 2014). The *2015 Asexual Community Census* ($N = 8663$ people on the asexual spectrum, including asexual, demisexual, or graysexual) found similarly alarming rates of lifetime sexual violence victimization among asexual individuals, 43.5% of whom reported rape or sexual assault (Bauer et al., 2017).

These findings are echoed by past research. For instance, a meta-analysis of 65 studies found that sexual minorities were significantly more likely to experience sexual violence than heterosexuals (Katz-Wise & Hyde, 2012), and a review of 25 population-based studies confirmed that sexual minority women experienced sexual violence in their lifetimes at greater rates than sexual minority men (Rothman, Exner, & Baughman, 2011).

An emerging area of research explores methods used by perpetrators. Coercion and pressure are often key tools in sexual violence, but research suggests that they may be used significantly more often with bisexual victims compared to victims of other sexual orientations (Menning & Holtzman, 2014). Relatedly, both gay and bisexual men often report that they participate in unwanted sexual activity out of a sense of guilt (i.e., feeling that they owed something to the assailant) or because they feel like they deserve to be treated badly—yet neither of these reasons for engaging in unwanted sex are typically expressed by heterosexual men (Menning & Holtzman, 2014). Research also indicates that sexual minorities are significantly more likely than heterosexuals to experience sexual assault while incapacitated due to substance use (Martin, Fisher, Warner, Krebs, & Lindquist, 2011; Richardson, Armstrong, Hines, & Palm Reed, 2015).

Prevalence of Sexual Violence Victimization Among Transgender Individuals

Regarding sexual violence among transgender individuals, the *US Transgender Survey* is the largest national study to date (*N* = 27,715 transgender people), albeit a study using a less representative and thus potentially less accurate non-probability sampling design (James et al., 2016). Findings revealed that 47% of respondents reported that they had experienced a sexual assault or rape within their lifetime (measured as "unwanted sexual contact, such as oral, genital, or anal contact, penetration, forced fondling, or rape"; James et al., 2016). Furthermore, the *US Transgender Survey* indicated that male-identified (i.e., transgender men) as well as nonbinary-identified transgender people assigned female at birth (51% and 58%, respectively) were more likely to experience sexual assault or rape within their lifetimes than female-identified (i.e., transgender women) as well as nonbinary-identified transgender people assigned male at birth (37% and 41%, respectively; James et al., 2016). Gender identity also played an important role in the *2015 Asexual Community Census*, in which trans (22.0%) and nonbinary (17.9%) respondents reported higher rates of sexual violence than women (12.6%) and men (8.9%).

These prevalence rates are similar to those found in a review of 11 studies on transgender samples (rates ranged between 14% and 66%; Stotzer, 2009). Limited research also suggests that transgender people are substantially more likely to experience sexual violence than cisgender people. For instance, according to analyses of the 2012–2014 *National College Health Assessment* (*N* = 71,421 undergraduate students from 120 schools, 99.75% cisgender), transgender people experienced sexual assault (measured as non-consensual sexual contact) or rape (measured as attempted or completed non-consensual oral, vaginal, or anal penetration) in the past year (20.9%) at rates 2–6 times greater than that of cisgender women (8.6%) and cisgender men (3.6%; Coulter et al., 2017).

Risk Factors for LGBTQ Sexual Violence

Cross-sectional studies—which gather data only once from a sample—inhibit the ability of scholars to establish the time order of risk factors and victimization (Messinger, 2017). In some instances, risk factors may be true outcomes, caused by the victimization itself (e.g., a victim begins abusing alcohol specifically to cope with past victimization). In other instances, risk factors may actually precede and contribute to the likelihood of victimization (e.g., an attacker intentionally targets a victim experiencing alcohol abuse issues because the victim is perceived to be less likely to resist). Still in other instances, the associations between victimization and risk factors may be purely coincidental (e.g., an attacker intentionally targets a victim engaging in sex work because such victims are perceived to be less likely to report victimization to police, and the victim's alcohol abuse preceded the sexual violence victimization because it was intended to be used to cope with the trauma associated with sex work; Messinger, 2017). Thus, given that research to date on LGBTQ sexual violence has largely been cross-sectional rather than longitudinal, it remains unclear whether identified risk factors are precipitating factors for or outcomes of LGBTQ sexual violence victimization—or perhaps both.

That said, according to research on predominantly heterosexual cisgender samples, victims of sexual assault or rape are likely to experience a variety of negative mental and physical health issues (see Campbell, Dworkin, & Cabral, 2009). The severity of outcomes may vary between individuals, but it is common for sexual violence survivors to suffer both acute, immediate problems and long-term consequences of the assault. The psychological sequelae of sexual violence are known to include post-traumatic stress disorder (PTSD), depression, anxiety, substance abuse, and suicidal thoughts and behaviors (Campbell et al., 2009). Negative health covariates of sexual violence victimization likely extend beyond heterosexual-cisgender survivors to LGBTQ survivors. Regardless of whether these are precipitating factors or outcomes for a particular victim, the unfortunate reality is that LGBTQ survivors often contend with debilitating mental health and medical issues that clearly warrant increased attention by scholars and service providers. This section reviews this still-emerging yet critically important body of research.

Risk Factors for Sexual Violence Victimization Among Sexual Minorities

Research on sexual minorities suggests that adult sexual violence victimization predicts sexual risk-taking (e.g., a greater number of sexual partners) and alcohol abuse (Hequembourg, Livingston, & Parks, 2013; Hequembourg, Parks, Collins, & Hughes, 2015). Among sexual violence survivors, research on undergraduates indicates that sexual minorities are more likely than heterosexual respondents to report that an injury resulted from the assault, which may indicate that their assaults involved more violence (Richardson et al., 2015).

Research remains inconclusive as to the exact role played by the acceptance of homophobic attitudes by sexual minorities (often termed "internalized homophobia"). Conflicting studies have found that internalized homophobia and sexual violence victimization do *not* covary in a sample of sexual minority men (Hequembourg et al., 2015), *do* covary in a sample of undergraduate sexual minority students (Murchison, Boyd, & Pachankis, 2017), and, specifically within intimate relationships, covary among sexual minorities in the United Kingdom and South Africa but not in Australia, Brazil, Canada, or the United States (Finneran, Chard, Sineath, Sullivan, & Stephenson, 2012). Further research is clearly needed to better understand the role of internalized homophobia in the lives of LGBTQ victims of sexual violence.

Finally, little research on the experience of sexual assault among sexual minorities has examined whether health-based risk factors tend to covary with one another. However, as one indication that risk factors may indeed cluster together, studies of sexual minority sexual violence survivors suggest that higher levels of internalized homophobia covary with more severe depression and PTSD symptoms (Gold, Dickstein, Marx, & Lexington, 2009; Gold, Marx & Lexington, 2007). In addition, in a study of lesbian women, heterosexual women, and gay men, Balsam, Lehavot, and Beadnell (2011) found that experiencing repeat sexual assault victimization was associated with an increase in multiple negative mental health consequences (e.g., suicidal thoughts, self-harm).

Risk Factors for Sexual Violence Victimization Among Transgender Individuals

In comparison to research on sexual minorities, research on sexual violence among transgender individuals has lagged considerably farther behind, including with regard to risk factors. For instance, unlike the comparatively robust literature emerging on the risk factor internalized homophobia, the literature is largely silent on whether the internalization of transphobic attitudes serves as a risk factor for sexual violence victimization among transgender individuals. That said, Testa et al. (2012) identified several important risk factors for sexual violence victimization among transgender individuals, including an increased risk of suicide attempts and substance abuse (Testa et al., 2012). In addition, hinting at the possibility that perpetrators target victims who are perceived to be less likely to resist or report victimization, the aforementioned *US Transgender Survey* concluded that rates of lifetime sexual violence are higher for transgender people who have a disability, are homeless, or have engaged in sex work (James et al., 2016). Findings such as these underscore the need for a nuanced understanding of sexual assault. The contexts in which individuals are situated impact the experience of sexual violence, as the next section demonstrates.

Interpersonal Contexts for LGBTQ Sexual Violence

Contrary to popular stereotypes in society of the unknown rapist who jumps out of bushes, victims usually know their attacker personally prior to the assault (e.g., Planty et al., 2013). According to the *National Intimate Partner and Sexual Violence Survey*, most victims of rape reported that the offender was an intimate partner (51.1%) or acquaintance (40.8%). In far fewer cases was the offender reported to be a stranger (13.8%) or family member (12.5%; Black et al., 2011). Likewise, research on sexual minorities (Tjaden, Thoennes, & Allison, 1999) and transgender individuals (James et al., 2016; Stotzer, 2009) finds that sexual violence against LGBTQ people is far more often perpetrated by someone the victim knows than by a stranger. With this in mind, four interpersonal contexts for LGBTQ sexual violence are briefly reviewed in this section: hate crime sexual violence, sexual violence among the incarcerated, childhood sexual violence, and sexual intimate partner violence.

Anti-LGBTQ Hate Crime Sexual Violence

At least two unique methodological issues hinder the study of anti-LGBTQ hate crime sexual violence. First, as Messinger (2017) notes, hate crimes—crimes motivated by a bias against the actual or perceived demographic identity of the victim—are often difficult to disentangle from other interpersonal crimes in research. This is due to the fact that anti-bias motivations can be held not only by strangers but also family members, intimate partners, peers, and other acquaintances (Messinger, 2017). Thus, in the absence of research more clearly delineating anti-LGBTQ sexual hate violence that is stranger-perpetrated versus acquaintance-perpetrated, it is unclear whether this crime is largely a subtype of or wholly distinct from LGBTQ child abuse, sibling abuse, intimate partner violence, and peer bullying.

In addition, complicating research further is that hate crimes have the potential to be motivated by a bias against multiple demographic identities intersecting in the same victim, and victims participating in studies may not always be aware of which bias was the primary motivator of their attacker. For instance, some research suggests that, among those who have experienced an anti-LGBTQ bias-motivated hate crime, LGBTQ people of color may be less likely than white LGBTQ people to perceive that their attacker was motivated by an anti-LGBTQ bias rather than an anti-racial minority bias (Meyer, 2008).

Importantly, because hate crime perpetrators are motivated by a bias against an entire demographic community rather than a single victim, hate crimes have the potential to generate high degrees of fear among targeted communities. Indeed, according to the *Trans Mental Health Survey* (N = 889 transgender individuals in Scotland), over 40% of transgender people self-reported knowing someone who had experienced anti-LGBTQ bias-motivated sexual violence, and 42% personally feared becoming a victim in the future (McNeil, Bailey, Ellis, Morton, & Regan, 2012). These fears may be founded, as research indicates that anti-LGBTQ bias-motivated sexual violence is startlingly common. One review of five studies in the literature found median prevalence rates of 14% for sexual minority men and 5% for sexual minority women (Rothman, Exner, & Baughman, 2011). Regarding transgender people, findings from the *Trans Mental Health Survey* indicate that 20% of transgender people have experienced anti-transgender bias-motivated sexual violence in their lifetimes (McNeil et al., 2012). While not nationally representative, the lifetime victimization rate identified by the *Trans Mental Health Survey* may be given more credence because the study's *past-year* victimization rate (4%; McNeil et al., 2012) is strikingly similar the past-year rate found in the much larger, national *US Transgender Survey* (approximately 2.6%, arrived at by extrapolating from the reported rates of past-year anti-transgender attacks and rates of past-year sexual violence; James et al., 2016).

Given disturbingly high rates lifetime rates, as well as high rates of those knowing a victim, it is disconcerting that hate crime laws often do not recognize anti-LGBTQ bias-motivated violence as a type of hate crime. While the *Matthew Shepard and James Byrd, Jr. Hate Crimes Prevention Act* criminalizes federal-level hate crimes in the United States motivated by an anti-LGBTQ bias, the majority of criminal hate crime prosecutions occur at the state level where federal law is less relevant (Human Rights Campaign, 2014). As of this writing, 20 US states still do not have hate crime laws covering anti-sexual minority bias (including Wyoming, where Matthew Shepard was murdered), and 32 states do not have hate crime laws covering anti-transgender bias (Human Rights Campaign, 2018).

Sexual Violence Among Incarcerated LGBTQ People

Sexual violence is an ongoing concern in corrections systems throughout the United States. According to *The National Former Prisoner Survey* (N = 18,526 former state prisoners under active supervision), during their most recent period of incarceration, gay (38.6%) and bisexual men were significantly more likely than heterosexual men to experience sexual assault or rape perpetrated by another inmate (38.6% of gay male inmates, 33.7% of bisexual male inmates, and 3.5% of heterosexual male inmates) and were significantly more likely to be sexually assaulted or raped by prison staff (11.8%, 17.5%, and 5.2%, respectively). Lesbian women were at similar risk and bisexual women were at significantly greater risk as compared to heterosexual women of being sexually assaulted or raped by another inmate (12.8% of lesbian inmates, 18.1% of bisexual female inmates, and 13.1% of heterosexual female inmates), and both lesbian and bisexual women were at significantly greater risk than heterosexual women of being sexually assaulted or raped by prison staff (8.0%, 7.5%, and 3.7%, respectively; Beck & Johnson, 2012).

By comparison, according to the *US Transgender Survey*, 17% of transgender people incarcerated in the past year had been sexually assaulted or raped by another inmate, and 11% had been sexually assaulted or raped by facility staff. To place these rates in context, relative to comparable past-year sexual violence victimization rates in the predominantly cisgender general incarcerated population, transgender people are over nine times more likely to experience sexual violence by another inmate and over five times more likely to experience sexual violence by facility staff (James et al., 2016). Moreover, of those transgender individuals who had been sexually assaulted or raped while incarcerated in the past year, approximately half had been victimized more than once in that same time period (James et al., 2016).

These high rates of sexual violence victimization among LGBTQ inmates must be understood in the broader context of discrimination in corrections systems. Research finds that LGBTQ people experience a wide variety of discrimination and assaults while incarcerated (Beck & Johnson, 2012; James et al., 2016). The 2012 update to the *Prison Rape Elimination Act* (PREA) was designed in part to improve many of the discriminatory conditions facing transgender inmates that may give rise to increased sexual violence risk. For instance, PREA requires the corrections system to place transgender inmates in wings corresponding with their gender identity rather than sex assigned at birth, prohibiting the use of isolation units (traditionally used as punishment) as a means of protection for transgender inmates, and permitting transgender inmates wishing to do so to shower separately. However, a major flaw in PREA is that its requirements are limited to corrections systems receiving federal funding. Because state corrections systems often receive the majority of their funding from state governments, it is financially possible for state corrections systems to forgo federal funding and the accompanying PREA regulations (American Civil Liberties Union, 2015).

Childhood Sexual Violence Against LGBTQ People

Estimates of the prevalence rates of LGBTQ childhood sexual violence are necessarily impacted by methodological decisions. For instance, a recent meta-analysis found that rates may be artificially depressed when researchers choose to limit the tactics assessed, require that participants identify the abuse as against their will (despite such a requirement not being included in most statutes of sexual violence against minors), narrow the assessed age range during which victimization can occur, and use telephone interview methods (rather than face-to-face interviews or questionnaires; Xu & Zheng, 2015).

With this in mind, across 25 population-based studies included in their review, Rothman and colleagues found that a median of 21% of sexual minority men and 28% of sexual minority women experienced sexual violence in childhood (Rothman, Exner, & Baughman, 2011). These rates are similar to a meta-analysis of 32 studies, which concluded that 28% of sexual minorities have experienced sexual violence perpetrated by a family member not including an intimate partner (Katz-Wise & Hyde, 2012). These rates are also nearly identical to the rate of childhood sexual violence victimization (27%) among men who have sex with men, as found in a meta-analysis of 12 studies (Lloyd & Operario, 2012). Two meta-analyses have also confirmed that sexual minorities were significantly more likely than heterosexuals to experience childhood sexual violence (Friedman et al., 2011; Katz-Wise & Hyde, 2012). Research suggests that sexual minority women were at an increased risk of childhood sexual violence victimization relative to sexual minority men (Rothman, Exner, & Baughman, 2011; Xu & Zheng, 2015).

Childhood sexual violence victimization among LGBTQ people is associated with a variety of negative health-related covariates. Research on men who have sex with men finds that childhood sexual violence victimization is positively associated with substance abuse, HIV-positive status, and sexual risk-taking behaviors (e.g., more frequent sexual partners, having sex under the influence of substances, and having recent unprotected sex; Lloyd & Operario, 2012). Whether physical force was present may also impact the likelihood of negative sequelae, as research indicates that the presence of force is significantly associated with a host of negative health covariates, including anxiety, depression, unsafe sex practices, and suicidality (Arreola, Neilands, & Diaz, 2009; Welles et al., 2009). In addition, individuals who experienced sexual violence as children are also at increased risk of sexual violence victimization as adults (Hequembourg et al., 2015).

Sexual Intimate Partner Violence Against LGBTQ People

Intimate partner violence (IPV)—psychological, physical, or sexual abuse in a romantic or sexual intimate relationship—has been found to be more prevalent in same-gender relationships (relative to different-gender relationships) as well as in relationships involving at least one LGBTQ-identified partner (Messinger, 2011, 2017; Walters et al., 2013). A recent comprehensive review of the LGBTQ IPV literature by Messinger (2017) found a broad range of rates of lifetime sexual IPV victimization for sexual minority women (4–33%) and men (1–29%; Messinger, 2017). The most accurate estimates currently available come from the nationally representative *National Intimate Partner and Sexual Violence Survey*, which found that 22% of bisexual women experience sexual IPV victimization in their lifetimes, as compared to just 9.1% of heterosexual women. Interestingly, prevalence rates were so low as to not be accurately estimated for lesbian women, bisexual men, gay men (likely due to the limited sample size of these groups), and heterosexual men (likely due to the low base rate of victimization of this group in the broader population; Walters et al., 2013). The finding that sexual minorities are more likely than heterosexuals to experience sexual IPV has been confirmed by several other probability-sampled studies (McLaughlin, Hatzenbuehler, Xuan, & Conron, 2012; Porter & Williams, 2011), as has the finding that sexual minority women are at an increased risk relative to sexual minority men (Blosnich & Bossarte, 2009; Messinger, 2011). Limited research suggests that sexual IPV can take on unique forms with sexual minority victims, such as when perpetrators justify raping or sexually assaulting bisexual victims by relying on false myths that bisexuals are hypersexual and thus must always want sex (Girshick, 2002).

Regarding transgender people, studies find lifetime sexual IPV victimization rates for transgender people range between 8% and 47% (Messinger, 2017). The *US Transgender Survey*, which offers arguably the most accurate data available, found that 19% of transgender people experience sexual IPV in their lifetimes (James et al., 2016). Compare such rates with those of the predominantly cisgender *National Intimate Partner and Sexual Violence Survey*, for which 9.4% of all female participants reported sexual IPV victimization in their lifetimes and for which rates were too low to calculate accurate estimates among all male participants (Black et al., 2011). One Australian study suggests that transgender men (14%) may be more likely than transgender women to experience sexual IPV victimization (8%; Pitts, Mitchell, Smith, & Patel, 2006). Scholars suggest that sexual IPV may exhibit unique tactics with transgender victims, such as when perpetrators intentionally sexually assault pieces of a transgender victim's body that had or have gendered meaning (such as genitals or breasts) or when perpetrators justify raping transgender victims by arguing that "real" women or men prefer rough sex (Goodmark, 2013; Messinger, 2017; Tesch & Bekerian, 2015). These types of pervasive beliefs about gender, sexual orientation, and sexual assault also have important implications for the availability of and likelihood of utilizing support services following a sexual assault.

Barriers to Help-Seeking

Research shows that most people disclose their sexual violence victimization to a friend or family member (Ullman & Filipas, 2001a), a finding that has been replicated in a sample of LGBTQ respondents (Koon-Magnin & Schulze, 2016). These disclosure experiences have important implications for the victim's eventual healing. If, upon disclosure, a victim is disbelieved, judged, or blamed for the assault, that victim is likely to experience more severe PTSD symptoms (Ullman & Filipas, 2001b). The risk of receiving such negative reactions is higher for victims who disclose their assaults to formal support networks (e.g., medical professionals, law enforcement) than those who disclose only to informal support networks (e.g., friends, family; Starzynski, Ullman, Filipas, & Townsend, 2005). Perhaps reflecting the fear of secondary victimization, the rates of reporting sexual violence in the United States to law enforcement are extremely low (e.g., Sinozich & Langton, 2014). In Richardson et al. (2015) study, none of the sexual minority respondents whose survey responses indicated that they had experienced sexual violence reported that they sought help from a formal on-campus support provider, as compared to nearly 11% of heterosexual respondents. Sexual minorities were also less likely than heterosexual respondents to report that they had sought help from formal sources off campus, but this difference was not significant. When asked why they did not seek help, sexual minority respondents were nearly three times more likely than heterosexual respondents to report that they thought they would be blamed for the assault, a statistically significant difference (Richardson et al., 2015).

In a study of mental health help-seeking among sexual violence survivors, lesbian and bisexual women were more likely than heterosexual women to seek help from mental health professionals (Starzynski, Ullman, Townsend, Long, & Long, 2007). The authors attributed this finding to a general trend among sexual minority women to seek mental health treatment at higher rates than heterosexuals. Though there are few studies addressing the post-assault experience for LGBTQ victims of sexual violence, existing works suggest that there are important considerations that must be addressed in order to adequately serve this population.

A key problem facing LGBTQ sexual violence survivors is that many existing programs and services have been designed from a cisnormative and heteronormative perspective. This in turn may generate mistrust and decreased help-seeking by LGBTQ sexual violence victims. For instance, in a primarily LGBQ-identified sample of college students, a substantial number of students were not aware of any services available to victims following a sexual assault (Schulze & Perkins, 2017). After disaggregating by sexual orientation, heterosexual respondents had the highest rates of awareness of both on-campus (76.5% of heterosexual respondents were aware of a resource, compared to 65.5% overall) and off-campus services (64.7% of heterosexual respondents were aware of a resource, compared to 51.8% overall).

A mixed method study that assessed existing responses to LGBTQ survivors of sexual violence points to three major themes that may contribute to low reporting and low rates of service use among LGBTQ communities (Todahl, Linville, Bustin, Wheeler, & Gau, 2009). First, participants reported feeling that LGBTQ communities were poorly understood or not accepted within the larger society. It is a difficult experience for any victim of sexual violence to disclose or report, but the experience would be even more intimidating if the victim felt that they may be judged for their sexual orientation or gender identity while in this vulnerable position. Second, respondents cited a lack of available resources that were LGBTQ-friendly. A survivor feeling secure to come forward with an assault is a necessary first step for help-seeking, but if they have nowhere to go or no one that they believe will help them, they are unlikely to receive help or support. Third, respondents emphasized the need for better training for first responders (e.g., law enforcement) who are likely to encounter victims following a sexual assault. If not trained in how to speak with LGBTQ victims in a respectful and sensitive way, the interactions between victims and practitioners can be unproductive and potentially harmful.

Lastly, a potentially valuable yet underexplored avenue for improving societal responses rests with LGBQ-specific rape myths. A theme throughout this handbook is the existence of victim blaming and the harm that it can cause, both to sexual violence victims personally and to society more broadly in the form of case attrition from the criminal justice system. The most widely used rape myths instruments (e.g., the Illinois Rape Myth Acceptance Scale; Payne, Lonsway, & Fitzgerald, 1999) focus on statements depicting female victims of male perpetrators, though there are a handful of other instruments that depict male victims of sexual violence (e.g., the Male Rape Survey; Struckman-Johnson & Struckman-Johnson, 1992). However, the sexual orientations of the individuals depicted in these scenarios are never specified and in most cases are implied to be heterosexual. The first instrument to take both gender identity and sexual orientation into account, the Identity-Inclusive Sexual Assault Myth Scale (IISAMS; Schulze, Koon-Magnin, & Bryan, 2019) will provide researchers with the ability to better understand how sexual assaults involving lesbian, gay, bisexual, transgender, and queer individuals are perceived. Such information will allow empirical evaluation of beliefs about sexual violence committed within or against members of LGBTQ communities. Only once the precise content of such myths is understood can programs be designed and implemented to address those beliefs. The pilot test of IISAMS indicated that respondents were significantly more likely to support myths depicting LGBTQ individuals than heterosexual victims (as depicted in the IRMAS). If these beliefs are prevalent throughout society, they serve to undermine the victimization experience of sexual minorities and gender minorities by trivializing the assault, placing blame on the victim, and removing culpability from the perpetrator. All of these outcomes are problematic in that they devalue, delegitimize, and deny justice to LGBTQ victims of sexual violence.

Conclusions

The studies outlined in this chapter demonstrate that the prevalence of sexual violence is higher for sexual minorities compared to heterosexuals. National samples, community samples, and meta-analyses all suggest a disproportionate risk of sexual violence among sexual minorities. This trend was consistent regardless of the operationalization of sexual violence (e.g., rape, sexual assault, coercive or unwanted sex). Research discussed in this chapter also indicates that transgender people are at a greater risk of sexual violence than both cisgender men and women.

A small but growing body of literature focused on sexual violence in LGBTQ communities suggests that the risk and contextual factors associated with sexual violence warrant further exploration. While there are important similarities with the experience of sexual violence in both the LGBTQ and heterosexual-cisgender communities (e.g., the perpetrator is usually known to the victim, drugs or alcohol are often used to facilitate the assault), there are also important differences that remain poorly understood (e.g., the role of anti-LGBTQ bias in motivation for the assault, the impact of internalized homophobia on victimization risk and post-assault healing). Additional research is needed to address these issues and others that may be unique to the experience of sexual violence in LGBTQ communities.

These foundational studies illustrate the need not only to identify differences between how sexual violence is experienced by LGBTQ and heterosexual-cisgender people but also among LGBTQ subgroups. A fuller understanding of these differences will require intentional oversampling of LGBTQ respondents in research samples, providing a more exhaustive list of choices and an open-ended response option for both sexual orientation and gender identity in survey research, and the use of more inclusive sexual violence instruments (e.g., IISAMS; Schulze, Koon-Magnin, & Bryan, 2019).

Future research should continue to explore how people define the terms "rape" and "sexual assault." Instruments like the Sexual Experiences Survey (Koss & Gidycz, 1985) circumvent this issue by describing specific sexual acts without attaching a label such as "rape." However, some surveys ask respondents to self-report whether they have ever been raped or sexually assaulted, and, because people define these words differently, the validity of such measurements is undermined. It may be that the terms "rape" and "sexual assault" hold different meanings for sexual minorities than they do for heterosexuals. If this is the case as research suggests (Schulze, Koon-Magnin, & Bryan, 2019), then additional work is needed to identify these differences and their implications for disclosure, reporting, and service provision.

A major issue that impacts sexual violence in the LGBTQ community is the way that such acts are legally defined. Jurisdictions that have not yet incorporated more inclusive statutes should do so. Failure to broaden these statutes likely has a disproportionate impact on the LGBTQ community, but all victims of sexual violence are better served by laws that reflect a more complete picture of sexual violence and its various forms.

Another problem faced by many sexual minority and transgender victims of sexual violence is the lack of available resources following an assault. The resources that do exist are typically designed to address the most common type of sexual assault: a penetrative act committed by a cisgender male perpetrator against a cisgender female victim. However, the emphasis on this type of sexual assault may result in the exclusion or marginalization of individuals who experience victimization that does not fit this paradigm (e.g., same-gender victims, transgender victims). The risk of secondary victimization following a negative disclosure experience and the harm that it causes the victim is too significant to disregard. To truly address the phenomenon of sexual violence, laws, policies, and programs must be responsive to and supportive of all victims. There is substantial work to be done by researchers and practitioners alike to ensure that all survivors of sexual violence receive the respect and justice that they deserve.

References

American Civil Liberties Union. (2015). *Prison Rape Elimination Act (PREA) toolkit: End the abuse: Protecting LGBTI prisoners from sexual assault.* Retrieved from https://www.aclu.org/sites/default/files/assets/012714-prea-combined.pdf.

Arreola, S. G., Neilands, T. B., & Diaz, R. (2009). Childhood sexual abuse and the sociocultural context of sexual risk among adult Latino gay and bisexual men. *American Journal of Public Health, 99*(S2), S432–S438.

Balsam, K. F., Lehavot, K., & Beadnell, B. (2011). Sexual revictimization and mental health: A comparison of lesbians, gay men, and heterosexual women. *Journal of Interpersonal Violence, 26*(9), 1798–1814.

Bauer, C., Miller, T., Ginoza, M., Chiang, A., Youngblom, K., Baba, A., … Ramaraj, V. (2017). *The 2015 Asexual Census Summary Report.* Retrieved from https://asexualcensus.files.wordpress.com/2017/10/2015_ace_census_summary_report.pdf.

Beck, A. J., & Johnson, C. (2012). *Sexual victimization reported by former state prisoners, 2008.* Office of Justice Programs, Bureau of Justice Statistics: U.S. Department of Justice.

Black, M. C., Basile, K. C., Breiding, M. J., Smith, S. G., Walters, M. L., Merrick, M. T., … Stevens, M. R. (2011). *The National Intimate Partner and Sexual Violence Survey (NISVS): 2010 Summary Report.* Atlanta, GA: National Center for Injury Prevention and Control, Centers for Disease Control and Prevention.

Blosnich, J. R., & Bossarte, R. M. (2009). Comparisons of intimate partner violence among partners in same-sex and opposite-sex relationships in the United States. *American Journal of Public Health, 99*(12), 2182–2184.

Bucher, J., & Manasse, M. (2011). When screams are not released: A study of communication and consent in acquaintance rape situations. *Women & Criminal Justice, 21*(2), 123–140.

Campbell, R. (2012). The neurobiology of sexual assault: Implications for first responders in law enforcement, prosecution, and victim advocacy. In *NIJ Research for the Real World Seminar.* Washington, DC: National Institute of Justice.

Campbell, R., Dworkin, E., & Cabral, G. (2009). An ecological model of the impact of sexual assault on women's mental health. *Trauma, Violence, & Abuse, 10*(3), 225–246.

Coulter, R. W., Mair, C., Miller, E., Blosnich, J. R., Matthews, D. D., & McCauley, H. L. (2017). Prevalence of past-year sexual assault victimization among undergraduate students: Exploring differences by and intersections of gender identity, sexual identity, and race/ethnicity. *Prevention Science, 18*(6), 726–736.

Federal Bureau of Investigation. (2014). *Uniform Crime Report: Crime in the United States, 2013, Rape Addendum.* U.S. Department of Justice.

Finneran, C., Chard, A., Sineath, C., Sullivan, P., & Stephenson, R. (2012). Intimate partner violence and social pressure among gay men in six countries. *Western Journal of Emergency Medicine, 13*(3), 260–271.

Friedman, M. S., Marshal, M. P., Guadamuz, T. E., Wei, C., Wong, C. F., Saewyc, E. M., & Stall, R. (2011). A meta-analysis of disparities in childhood sexual abuse, parental physical abuse, and peer victimization among sexual minority and sexual nonminority individuals. *American Journal of Public Health, 101*(8), 1481–1494.

Girshick, L. B. (2002). *Woman-to-woman sexual violence: Does she call it rape?* Lebanon, NH: University Press of New England.

Gold, S., Dickstein, D., Marx, B. P., & Lexington, J. M. (2009). Psychological outcomes of lesbian sexual assault survivors: An examination of the roles of internalized homophobia and experiential avoidance. *Psychology of Women Quarterly, 33*(1), 54–66.

Gold, S., Marx, B. P., & Lexington, J. M. (2007). Gay male sexual assault survivors: The relations among internalized homophobia, experiential avoidance, and psychological symptom severity. *Behaviour Research and Therapy, 45*(3), 549–562.

Goodmark, L. (2013). Transgender people, intimate partner abuse, and the legal system. *Harvard Civil Rights-Civil Liberties Law Review, 48*, 51–104.

Hequembourg, A. L., Livingston, J. A., & Parks, K. A. (2013). Sexual victimization and associated risks among lesbian and bisexual women. *Violence Against Women, 19*(5), 634–657.

Hequembourg, A. L., Parks, K. A., Collins, R. L., & Hughes, T. L. (2015). Sexual assault risks among gay and bisexual men. *The Journal of Sex Research, 52*(3), 282–295.

Human Rights Campaign. (2014). *A guide to state-level advocacy following enactment of the Matthew Shepard and James Byrd, Jr. Hate Crimes Prevention Act*. Retrieved from https://assets2.hrc.org/files/assets/resources/HRC-Hate-Crimes-Guide-2014.pdf?_ga=2.44892644.1580109581.1523843307-1373807809.1512938529.

Human Rights Campaign. (2018). *Hate crimes*. Retrieved from https://www.hrc.org/state-maps/hate-crimes/pdf.

James, S. E., Herman, J. L., Rankin, S., Keisling, M., Mottet, L., & Anafi, M. (2016). *The Report of the 2015 U.S. Transgender Survey*. Washington, DC: National Center for Transgender Equality.

Katz-Wise, S. L., & Hyde, J. S. (2012). Victimization experiences of lesbian, gay, and bisexual individuals: A meta-analysis. *Journal of Sex Research, 49*(2–3), 142–167.

Koon-Magnin, S., & Schulze, C. (2016). Providing and receiving sexual assault disclosures: Findings from a sexually diverse sample of young adults. *Journal of Interpersonal Violence, 34*(2), 416–441.

Koss, M., & Gidycz, C. (1985). Sexual Experiences Survey: Reliability and validity. *Journal of Consulting and Clinical Psychology, 53*(3), 422–423.

Lloyd, S., & Operario, D. (2012). HIV risk among men who have sex with men who have experienced childhood sexual abuse: systematic review and meta-analysis. *AIDS Education and Prevention, 24*(3), 228–241.

Mahoney, B., Davies, M., & Scurlock-Evans, L. (2014). Victimization among female and male sexual minority status groups: Evidence from the British Crime Survey 2007–2010. *Journal of Homosexuality, 61*(10), 1435–1461.

Martin, S., Fisher, B., Warner, T., Krebs, C., & Lindquist, C. (2011). Women's sexual orientations and their experiences of sexual assault before and during university. *Women's Health Issues, 21*(3), 199–205.

McLaughlin, K. A., Hatzenbuehler, M. L., Xuan, Z., & Conron, K. J. (2012). Disproportionate exposure to early-life adversity and sexual orientation disparities in psychiatric morbidity. *Child Abuse & Neglect, 36*(9), 645–655.

McNeil, J., Bailey, L., Ellis, S., Morton, J., & Regan, M. (2012). Trans mental health study 2012. Scottish Transgender Alliance.

Menning, C. L., & Holtzman, M. (2014). Processes and patterns in gay, lesbian, and bisexual sexual assault: A multimethodological assessment. *Journal of Interpersonal Violence, 29*(6), 1071–1093.

Messinger, A. M. (2011). Invisible victims: Same-sex IPV in the national violence against women survey. *Journal of Interpersonal Violence, 26*(11), 2228–2243.

Messinger, A. M. (2017). *LGBTQ intimate partner violence: Lessons for policy, practice, and research*. Oakland, CA: University of California Press.

Meyer, D. (2008). Interpreting and experiencing anti-queer violence: Race, class, and gender differences among LGBT hate crime victims. *Race, Gender & Class, 15*(3/4), 262–282.

Murchison, G. R., Boyd, M. A., & Pachankis, J. E. (2017). Minority stress and the risk of unwanted sexual experiences in LGBQ undergraduates. *Sex Roles, 77*(3–4), 221–238.

Panel on Measuring Rape and Sexual Assault in Bureau of Justice Statistics Household Surveys; Committee on National Statistics; Division on Behavioral and Social Sciences and Education; National Research Council (2014). *Estimating the incidence of rape and sexual assault*. Kruttschnitt, C., Kalsbeek, W. D., House, C. C., (Eds).Washington, DC: National Academies Press; Comparison of Rape and Sexual Assault Across Data Sources. Retrieved from https://www.ncbi.nlm.nih.gov/books/NBK202258/.

Payne, D. L., Lonsway, K. A., & Fitzgerald, L. F. (1999). Rape myth acceptance: Exploration of its structure and its measurement using the Illinois Rape Myth Acceptance Scale. *Journal of Research in Personality, 33*(1), 27–68.

Pitts, M., Mitchell, A., Smith, A., & Patel, S. (2006). *Private lives: A report on the health and wellbeing of GLBTI Australians*. Melbourne: Australian Research Centre in Sex, Health and Society, La Trobe University.

Planty, M., Langton, L., Krebs, C., Berzofsky, M., & Smiley-McDonald, H. (2013). *Female victims of sexual violence, 1994–2010*. Washington, DC: US Department of Justice, Office of Justice Programs, Bureau of Justice Statistics.

Porter, J., & Williams, L. M. (2011). Intimate violence among underrepresented groups on a college campus. *Journal of Interpersonal Violence, 26*(16), 3210–3224.

Richardson, H. B., Armstrong, J. L., Hines, D. A., & Palm Reed, K. M. (2015). Sexual violence and help-seeking among LGBQ and heterosexual college students. *Partner Abuse, 6*, 29–46.

Rothman, E. F., Exner, D., & Baughman, A. L. (2011). The prevalence of sexual assault against people who identify as gay, lesbian, or bisexual in the United States: A systematic review. *Trauma, Violence, & Abuse, 12*(2), 55–66.

Rymer, S., & Cartei, V. (2015). Supporting transgender survivors of sexual violence: learning from users' experiences. *Critical and Radical Social Work, 3*(1), 155–164.

Schulze, C., Koon-Magnin, S., & Bryan, V. (2019). Gender Identity, Sexual Orientation, and Sexual Assault: Challenging the Myths. Boulder, CO: Lynne Rienner Publishers, Inc.

Schulze, C., & Perkins, W. (2017). Awareness of sexual violence services among LGBQ-identified college students. *Journal of School Violence, 16*(2), 148–159.

Sinozich, S., & Langton, L. (2014). *Rape and sexual assault victimization among college-age females, 1995–2013*. Washington, DC: US Department of Justice, Office of Justice Programs, Bureau of Justice Statistics.

Starzynski, L. L., Ullman, S. E., Filipas, H. H., & Townsend, S. M. (2005). Correlates of women's sexual assault disclosure to informal and formal support sources. *Violence and Victims, 20*(4), 417.

Starzynski, L. L., Ullman, S. E., Townsend, S. M., Long, L. M., & Long, S. M. (2007). What factors predict women's disclosure of sexual assault to mental health professionals? *Journal of Community Psychology, 35*(5), 619–638.

Stotzer, R. L. (2009). Violence against transgender people: A review of United States data. *Aggression and Violent Behavior, 14*(3), 170–179.

Struckman-Johnson, C., & Struckman-Johnson, D. (1992). Acceptance of male rape myths among college men and women. *Sex Roles, 27*(3–4), 85–100.

Tark, J., & Kleck, G. (2014). Resisting rape: The effects of victim self-protection on rape completion and injury. *Violence Against Women, 20*(3), 270–292.

Tesch, B. P., & Bekerian, D. A. (2015). Hidden in the margins: A qualitative examination of what professionals in the domestic violence field know about transgender domestic violence. *Journal of Gay & Lesbian Social Services, 27*(4), 391–411.

Testa, R. J., Sciacca, L. M., Wang, F., Hendricks, M. L., Goldblum, P., Bradford, J., & Bongar, B. (2012). Effects of violence on transgender people. *Professional Psychology: Research and Practice, 43*(5), 452.

Tjaden, P., Thoennes, N., & Allison, C. J. (1999). Comparing violence over the life span in samples of same-sex and opposite-sex cohabitants. *Violence and victims,14*(4), 413.

Todahl, J. L., Linville, D., Bustin, A., Wheeler, J., & Gau, J. (2009). Sexual assault support services and community systems: Understanding critical issues and needs in the LGBTQ community. *Violence Against Women, 15*(8), 952–976.

Ullman, S. E., & Filipas, H. H. (2001a). Correlates of formal and informal support seeking in sexual assault victims. *Journal of Interpersonal Violence, 16*(10), 1028–1047.

Ullman, S. E., & Filipas, H. H. (2001b). Predictors of PTSD symptom severity and social reactions in sexual assault victims. *Journal of Traumatic Stress, 14*(2), 369–389.

Walters, M. L., Chen, J., & Breiding, M. J. (2013). *The National Intimate Partner and Sexual Violence Survey (NISVS): 2010 Findings on Victimization by Sexual Orientation*. Atlanta, GA: National Center for Injury Prevention and Control, Centers for Disease Control and Prevention.

Welles, S. L., Baker, A. C., Miner, M. H., Brennan, D. J., Jacoby, S., & Rosser, B. S. (2009). History of childhood sexual abuse and unsafe anal intercourse in a 6-city study of HIV-positive men who have sex with men. *American Journal of Public Health, 99*(6), 1079–1086.

Xu, Y., & Zheng, Y. (2015). Prevalence of childhood sexual abuse among lesbian, gay, and bisexual people: A meta-analysis. *Journal of Child Sexual Abuse, 24*(3), 315–331.

Sexual Victimization Among Sexual and Racial/Ethnic Minority Women: Bridging the Gap Between Research and Practice

40

Gabriela López, Elizabeth A. Yeater, Ryan S. Ross, and Kristen N. Vitek

Sexual victimization is a public health concern for all women in our society and particularly for sexual minority women (e.g., lesbian, bisexual). Approximately 4% of the US population identifies as lesbian, bisexual, or gay, which equates to about 9 million people (Priola, Lasio, De Simone, & Serri, 2014). Sexual minority women report rates of sexual victimization between 21% and 40%, rates that are higher than those reported by heterosexual women (e.g., Balsam, Lehavot, & Beadnell, 2011; Rothman, Exner, & Baughman, 2011). Although sexual minority women are more likely to be victimized relative to heterosexual women, the majority of research has examined heterosexual women's experiences of sexual victimization, leading to a significant gap in the literature regarding sexual minority women.

Although the literature is limited, research indicates additional discrepancies in rates of sexual victimization among lesbian and bisexual women (Heidt, Marx, & Gold, 2005; Hughes, McCabe, Wilsnack, West, & Boyd, 2010). For instance, Krahé and Berger (2013) found that women who had sex with both men and women had a victimization rate of 47.4%, as compared to 8.7% of women who had sex with only women. This finding is consistent with other studies that have found that bisexual women experience higher rates of sexual victimization than lesbian women (Hequembourg, Livingston, & Parks, 2013; Hughes, McCabe, Wilsnack, et al., 2010).

It is well documented that sexually victimized women are at increased risk of developing long-term negative psychological sequelae as a result of their sexual victimization (Campbell, Dworkin, & Cabral, 2009; Simmons & Granvold, 2005). This relationship appears particularly relevant for lesbian and bisexual women who report greater negative mental health consequences post-victimization relative to heterosexual women (Jorm, Korten, Rodgers, Jacomb, & Christensen, 2002), including higher rates of depression (Acierno et al., 2002), drug and alcohol use (Resnick et al., 2012), low self-esteem (Campbell et al., 2009), posttraumatic stress disorder (PTSD) (Littleton & Ullman, 2013; Roberts, Austin, Corliss, Vandermorris, & Koenen, 2010), and sexual dysfunction (Faravelli, Giugni, Salvatori, & Ricca, 2004).

In this chapter, we will review the current state of the literature regarding sexual minority women's experiences of sexual victimization, their post-victimization recoveries, and the major gaps in the literature regarding these experiences. We then will discuss theoretical frameworks that elucidate additional psychosocial stressors that sexual

G. López (✉) · E. A. Yeater · R. S. Ross · K. N. Vitek
Department of Psychology, University of New Mexico, Albuquerque, NM, USA
e-mail: glopez28@unm.edu

W. T. O'Donohue and P. A. Schewe (eds.), *Handbook of Sexual Assault and Sexual Assault Prevention*,
https://doi.org/10.1007/978-3-030-23645-8_40

minority and triple minority (e.g., both sexual and racial/ethnic minority) women may encounter during their victimization and post-victimization recovery experiences. While there is an abundance of interventions aimed to decrease the rates of sexual assault, interventions specifically tailored for sexual minority women who have been sexually victimized have yet to be developed. Thus, we will not review the literature on sexual assault interventions. Finally, we will discuss cultural and ethical considerations for working with sexual minority women and avenues for improving cultural humility (i.e., cultural competence) among clinicians who may work with this population.

Coping

Because of the negative and long-term sequelae associated with sexual victimization, research has sought to identify factors that may influence women's post-victimization recovery. Coping is a crucial factor that has been explored extensively in victimized heterosexual populations but remains an understudied factor among sexual minority women. Women can use various coping strategies after they have been victimized, and these strategies are important because they have been shown to affect women's post-victimization psychological health (Campbell et al., 2009). There are two general categories of coping: adaptive and maladaptive. Adaptive coping can be conceptualized as positive and helpful coping; examples include expressing emotions, reducing stress, and seeking social support and/or mental health services (Campbell et al., 2009; Ullman, 2010). On the other hand, maladaptive coping can be best conceptualized as "negative" coping and includes behaviors such as alcohol use and withdrawal from others (Campbell et al., 2009). Engaging in maladaptive coping, as opposed to utilizing more adaptive coping strategies, has been shown to hinder women's post-victimization recovery by exacerbating negative psychological symptoms (e.g., depression and anxiety) (Campbell et al., 2009; Ullman & Najdowski, 2011).

Not only can maladaptive coping hinder women's post-victimization recoveries; it is also associated with increased risk of being revictimized (Najdowski & Ullman, 2011; Ullman, 1996). For instance, Najdowski and Ullman (2011) found that individuals who had been sexually victimized and engaged in maladaptive coping were twice as likely to be revictimized, as compared to individuals who did not engage in maladaptive coping. Furthermore, maladaptive coping has been shown to be a significant predictor of psychological distress in sexually victimized women (Filipas & Ullman, 2006). Therefore, how a woman copes with her sexual victimization experience can lead to increased psychological symptoms, making coping an important factor to consider during post-victimization recovery (Ullman, 1996).

Seeking Social Support and Disclosure

Seeking positive social support, such as having supportive friends and/or family members to turn in times of need, can strengthen women's ability to adaptively cope, which can protect against the effects of trauma (Ullman, 2010). A specific example of how women may seek social support is by disclosing their sexual assault experience to others and having people validate that disclosure (Ullman, 1999); disclosure is an adaptive coping strategy that women can employ to assist them during their post-victimization recovery. However, negative social support (e.g., blaming the victim, taking away control from the victim) has various harmful effects to women recovering from a sexual assault (Relyea & Ullman, 2015). Women who receive more negative social support when they disclose are more likely to utilize maladaptive coping (i.e., less engagement in problem-focused coping), which can lead to increased symptoms of PTSD, depression, and anxiety (Orchowski, Untied, & Gidycz, 2013).

Indeed, Relyea and Ullman (2015) found support for an association between social support and coping, such that women who had others turn against them (e.g., victims were blamed, stigmatized, and/or infantilized) reported more maladaptive coping as compared to women who received unsupportive acknowledgment (e.g., trying to distract the victim regarding the sexual assault, trying to hurt the perpetrator) or positive supportive reactions (e.g., believing the victims, supporting their decisions). Women who disclosed and had others turn against them reported more maladaptive coping (e.g., social withdrawal, self-blame, decreased sexual assertiveness) compared to women who disclosed and received unsupportive acknowledgment or positive supportive reactions. On the other hand, women who disclosed and had others responded with unsupportive acknowledgement reported more maladaptive coping and also sought additional adaptive individual coping strategies (e.g., planning or reframing the assault in a positive way) compared to women who disclosed and had others turn against them. Receiving positive supportive reactions was associated with more adaptive social and individual coping strategies and less maladaptive coping. These findings demonstrate that although disclosure is an adaptive coping strategy for sexual assault victims, it can be detrimental to their post-victimization recovery if others respond negatively.

Sexual minority women also use disclosure as a strategy to attempt to cope positively with their traumatic experiences, but there are both differences and similarities in disclosure between lesbian and bisexual women (Long, Ullman, Long, Mason, & Starzynski, 2007). For example, bisexual women are more likely to disclose to a formal source, but they also tend to receive fewer positive reactions than lesbian or heterosexual women (Long et al., 2007). On the other hand, lesbian women, relative to bisexual women, are less likely to disclose their victimization experiences to anyone (Lehavot, Molina, & Simoni, 2012). In addition, both lesbian and bisexual women often perceive that they receive unequal medical treatment based on their sexual minority status. This perception may color their outlook of resources available to them, both personal and professional, and add an additional layer to the recovery process (Long et al., 2007). Bisexual women also express being dissatisfied by the support they receive from mental health professionals (Long et al., 2007). For example, bisexual women face unique challenges when seeking help as most of the services targeted for sexual minority women are generally focused on the needs of lesbian women (Balsam, 2003). This finding is alarming as bisexual women have been found to encounter more adverse life events, less support from family, more negative support from friends, and more financial difficulties than lesbian women (Jorm et al., 2002). These are important differences that may be harmful to a bisexual woman's ability to seek more individualized treatment or support (Jorm et al., 2002).

Resiliency

Resiliency is a phenomenon that may occur during women's post-victimization recoveries. To place resiliency into the context of sexual assault, it is important to first consider posttraumatic stress disorder (PTSD), a debilitating mental health disorder that can occur for people who experience a traumatic or stressful life event (e.g., sexual assault, physical assault, perceived death) (Masho & Ahmed, 2007). Only about 15–24% of individuals exposed to a traumatic event will develop PTSD (Simmons & Granvold, 2005). In other words, most women who experience sexual assault do not develop PTSD (Simmons & Granvold, 2005).

One hypothesis used to explain this is that women who do not develop PTSD may have been more resilient at that time in their life. Resiliency is a difficult construct to define, and there is no universally accepted definition for resiliency in the literature (Thompson, et al., 2016). Bonanno (2004) defines resiliency as the ability to maintain relatively stable and healthy levels of psychological and physical functioning after experiencing a traumatic event. He posits that resiliency is conceptually different from recovery, in which an individual's healthy levels of psychological and physical functioning are temporarily disrupted, causing threshold or subthreshold psychopathology (e.g., anxiety, depression, PTSD) for a period of time, with the individual gradually returning to pre-traumatic levels of psychological and physical functioning. Other researchers, such as Smith and Trimble (2016), have posited that although resiliency does entail the ability to bounce back or recover from stress, personal and social resources are important in facilitating recovery. That is, resiliency should be considered within a person's ability to access resources (e.g., access to health, mental health care, and social support).

Although resiliency can occur following a sexual victimization, some women do experience a disruption of psychological and physical functioning following sexual assault (Calhoun & Tedeschi, 2006). This disruption in functioning is best characterized as experiencing a change in cognitions (e.g., thinking that the world is unsafe) and emotions (e.g., having a difficult time regulating emotions) following the traumatic event (Calhoun & Tedeschi, 2006). Once the person is able to redefine their cognitions and emotion in an adaptive way (e.g., "I can handle difficult situations"), it is thought that people experience positive changes that results in posttraumatic growth. For example, experiencing any positive psychological change (e.g., personal strength—feeling more confident in one's ability to handle difficult emotional situations) that occurs as a result of the struggle with traumatic events (e.g., sexual assault, being the victim of a violent crime) is an example of posttraumatic growth (Tedeschi & Calhoun, 2004).

Posttraumatic growth has been explored among female sexual assault victims (Grubaugh & Resick, 2007; Ullman, 2004), but sexual identity was not assessed and/or reported as part of the study demographics; thus, this process remains understudied and unclear among sexual minority women. Frazier, Conlon, and Glaser (2001) examined levels of distress and posttraumatic growth among adult women who had been sexually victimized. Most of the women in the sample reported experiencing positive changes such as increased empathy, better relationships, and greater appreciation of life only 2 weeks after their sexual assault. Women who had reported more positive life changes 2 weeks and 12 months after their sexual victimization had lower levels of distress during the 12-month follow-up. This finding demonstrates that posttraumatic growth is beneficial for sexual assault victims in decreasing their levels of distress long term or helping them return to their original levels of psychological functioning.

Mental Health Disparities

Although not every woman who has been sexually victimized develops PTSD, there are certain psychosocial factors (e.g., abusive family members, abusive partners, child sexual abuse, overall levels of stress in women's environment) that make women particularly vulnerable to developing PTSD and other forms of psychopathology (Ullman, Peter-Hagene, & Relyea, 2014). Notably, research suggests that sexual minority women experience more negative psychosocial factors relative to heterosexual women (Jorm et al., 2002). These differences in psychosocial factors might contribute to the mental health disparities demonstrated between sexual minority and heterosexual women (Hughes, Szalacha, & McNair, 2010).

Notably, numerous research studies have provided compelling evidence of mental health disparities among nonvictimized lesbian, bisexual, and heterosexual women (Bostwick, Boyd, Hughes, & McCabe, 2010; Hughes, Szalacha, & McNair, 2010; Kuyper & Vanwesenbeeck, 2011; Meyer, 2003). Bisexual women report higher levels of perceived stress, depression symptoms, anxiety symptoms, self-harm, binge drinking, and use of illicit drugs than lesbian and heterosexual women (Hughes et al., 2010). Consistent with this finding, Duncan and Hatzenbuehler (2014) found that bisexual women were at higher risk for poorer health-related quality of life compared to lesbian women. Bisexual women were also twice as likely as lesbian women and four times as likely as heterosexual women to report suicidal ideation (Hughes, Szalacha, Johnson, et al., 2010; Hughes, Szalacha, & McNair, 2010).

Indeed, suicidal ideation is a pervasive problem in sexual minority populations and the third leading cause of death for youth between the ages of 15 and 24 in the USA (Grossman & D'Augelli, 2007). D'Augelli et al. (2005) found that about one-third of a community-based sample of 529 lesbian, gay, and bisexual (LGB) youth, ages 15–19, had attempted suicide. This rate is considerably higher than the 8.5% attempted suicide rate in a recent survey of high school students (Center for Disease Control and Prevention, 2004). Higher rates of psychopathology might place lesbian and bisexual women at a higher risk for developing additional negative psychological sequelae post-victimization, compared to heterosexual women (Eaton, 2014).

Research has also demonstrated mental health disparities between sexually victimized and non-victimized lesbian, bisexual, and heterosexual women. Heidt et al. (2005) found that lesbian and bisexual nonvictims reported significantly less depression, symptoms of PTSD, and general distress compared to lesbian and bisexual women who had experienced child sexual victimization only, adult sexual assault only, or sexual revictimization. Likewise, Jorm et al. (2002) found that bisexual women reported poorer mental health compared to heterosexual women on different measures of psychological distress (e.g., anxiety symptoms, depression symptoms, suicidality, alcohol misuse, negative affect, positive affect), with lesbian women falling in between the two with respect to distress. Thus, it appears that experiencing sexual victimization places sexual minority women at a higher likelihood for experiencing additional negative mental health symptoms.

Alcohol use. It is common for women to use alcohol as a form of maladaptive coping to manage the mental health problems experienced as a result of sexual victimization (Bryant-Davis, Chung, & Tillman, 2009; Carlson & Dalenberg, 2000; Filipas & Ullman, 2006; Littleton & Ullman, 2013; Messman-Moore, Ward, & Brown, 2009; Resnick et al., 2012; Ullman, 2003). Alcohol use is a particularly harmful coping mechanism, as studies show that women who consume more alcohol are less likely to seek additional help from sexual assault services (e.g., therapy) and less likely to report their assault to police (Cohn, Hagman, Moore, Mitchell, & Ehlke, 2014; Wolitzky-Taylor et al., 2011).

Alcohol use also plays an important role in women's sexual assault experiences. Women who report consuming alcohol prior to their sexual victimization experience report more self-blame, experience more stigma, receive fewer positive reactions when disclosing their victimization experience, and experience more violent assaults (e.g., greater number of injuries, greater use of force) (Bedard-Gilligan, Kaysen, Desai, & Lee, 2011; Koss, Figueredo, & Prince, 2002; Littleton, Axsom, & Grills-Taquechel, 2009) relative to women who do not report consuming alcohol prior to their sexual victimization experience.

López and Yeater (2018) examined the contextual features of sexual minority and heterosexual women's victimization experiences and found that there were no differences with respect to the frequency by which alcohol was involved in their assaults. However, they did find that sexual minority women were more likely to cope through substances (i.e., alcohol) relative to heterosexual women, with sexual minority women reporting more substance use than heterosexual women.

Notably, alcohol use and hazardous drinking are higher among victimized sexual minority women than victimized heterosexual women (Drabble, Trocki, Hughes, Korcha, & Lown, 2013). Hazardous drinking among sexual minority women also has been shown to be associated with a history of child and adult sexual victimization experiences (Han et al., 2013; Hughes, Johnson, & Wilsnack, 2001; Hughes, Szalacha, Johnson, et al., 2010). Bisexual women are also thought be at higher risk for victimization because they report higher rates of hazardous drinking than lesbian women (Hughes, Szalacha, & McNair, 2010). For example, Hequembourg et al. (2013) assessed child and adult sexual victimization history, risky drinking patterns (e.g., having more than four drinks at a time), and number of lifetime sexual partners among lesbian and bisexual women. They found that bisexual women, relative to lesbian women, reported significantly more severe victimization experiences both in childhood and adulthood, more heavy episodic drinking days, and more lifetime male sexual partners.

Child Sexual Abuse

Child sexual abuse (CSA) disproportionately burdens sexual minority women (Balsam, Molina, Beadnell, Simoni, & Walters, 2011; Hughes et al., 2001; Hughes, McCabe, Wilsnack, et al., 2010). Although the mechanisms responsible for this disparity among groups still remain unclear, studies have highlighted other types of abuse that could contribute to these increased rates such as childhood physical abuse (e.g., not having enough to eat, being physically punished) and emotional abuse (e.g., being told they are not loved, called names). Childhood physical and emotional abuse have been found to be strongly associated with a higher likelihood of being sexually victimized in childhood (Gold, Feinstein, Skidmore, & Marx, 2011). Lesbian and bisexual women have been found to have higher rates of childhood physical and emotional abuse compared to their heterosexual siblings (Balsam, Rothblum, & Beauchaine, 2005). Not only does a history of childhood abuse and physical abuse predispose sexual minority women to an increased likelihood of being sexually victimized in childhood; it also predisposes them to being sexually victimized again in adulthood, relative to women who do not report a history of childhood abuse and physical abuse (Heidt et al., 2005).

Sexual Revictimization. Sexual revictimization is commonly defined as experiencing sexual victimization during childhood and subsequent sexual revictimization in adulthood or as having two or more sexual victimization experiences after the age of 14. Although the mechanisms responsible for revictimization are not well understood, the literature demonstrates that once women have been victimized, their chances of being victimized again are significantly higher, relative to women who have never been victimized (Banyard, Williams, & Siegel, 2001; Gidycz, Coble, Latham, & Layman, 1993; Messman-Moore, Long, & Siegfried, 2000). As noted previously, women who are victimized during childhood are also more likely to be victimized in adulthood; in fact, they are four times more likely to be revictimized in adulthood (Gidycz et al., 1993).

Research has demonstrated that lesbian and bisexual women are more likely to be revictimized than heterosexual women (Martin, Fisher, Warner, Krebs, & Lindquist, 2011). That is, a history of CSA is strongly associated with a higher risk of future sexual assaults in adulthood among lesbian and bisexual women (Gilmore et al., 2014; Morris & Balsam, 2003). For instance, Heidt et al. (2005) assessed the severity of CSA and its associations with revictimization in a sample of lesbian and bisexual women. They found that lesbian and bisexual women who reported more severe CSA experiences were more likely to be revictimized than lesbian and bisexual women who reported less severe CSA experiences. Moreover, research suggests that rates of revictimization between lesbian and bisexual women are disparate, with bisexual women being at greater risk than lesbian women for being revictimized (Hequembourg et al., 2013). One explanation for this discrepancy in revictimization rates is that bisexual women are more likely to have male sexual partners in adulthood, which might explain their higher rates of revictimization as men are the primary perpetrators of sexual violence (Heidt et al., 2005).

Summary of Sexual Minority Women's Experiences of Sexual Victimization

While there is a growing body of literature investigating sexual minority women's experiences of sexual victimization, many questions remain unanswered with respect to this group of women (Balsam, 2003; Gold, Dickstein, Marx, & Lexington, 2009; Han et al., 2013). Researchers are often forced to collapse bisexual and lesbian women into one group due to difficulties recruiting this population, thereby obscuring important differences that likely exist between these groups of women (Balsam, 2003; Gold et al., 2009; Han et al., 2013). This practice is particularly problematic as research suggests that bisexual women, relative to lesbian women, report more maladaptive coping, mental health symptoms post-victimization, CSA, adult sexual victimization, and revictimization (Heidt et al., 2005; Hequembourg et al., 2013; Long et al., 2007; Martin et al., 2011). In other words, they appear to be a particularly high-risk group for experiencing both victimization and the negative psychological consequences of sexual violence; thus, in research studies, bisexual women should be studied separately from lesbian women. Although it is clear that bisexual women are a high-risk group, it remains unclear what factors might be placing bisexual women at risk of having higher rates of substance use, CSA, and revictimization. Longitudinal work with bisexual women might profitably examine potential causal factors responsible for their increased risk for adverse events. In the section that follows, we discuss additional theoretical explanations for these negative outcomes among victimized sexual minority women.

Theoretical Explanations for Increased Risk for Adverse Outcomes Among Sexually Victimized Sexual Minority Women

Minority stress, as defined by Meyer (2003), is "excess stress to which individuals from stigmatized social categories are exposed as a result of their social position, often a minority, position" (Meyer, 2003, p. 675). Meyer originally developed the theoretical framework of minority stress to explain the mental and health disparities unique to sexual minorities, but it is commonly used to explain the experience of other minority groups. The minority stress theory posits that lesbian and bisexual women are at greater risk for mental health problems because of the constant stress associated with living in a heterosexist society (Meyer, 2003). For example, sexual minority women may experience physical attacks, job discrimination, microaggressions (verbal or nonverbal negative messages due to their sexual identity), negative expectations, and difficulties with "coming out" to various people because of living in a heteronormative world (Meyer, 2003). The constant stress that arises from worrying about experiencing discrimination, or actual experienced discrimination, is thought to result in minority stress.

Minority Stress, Sexual Minority Women, and Sexual Victimization

Research has focused on examining factors that might explain physical health discrepancies among sexual minorities (Meyer, 2003). In one longitudinal study, Frost, Lehavot, and Meyer (2013) examined the effects of minority stress on the physical health of lesbian women, gay men, and bisexual men/women. Frost et al. (2013) found that health problems between baseline and follow-up were associated with having experienced prejudice events and more daily discrimination, as well as holding higher expectations of rejection. At the 1-year follow-up, sexual minorities who experienced a prejudice event were three times more likely to report a physical health problem than sexual minorities who did not experience a prejudice event.

In addition to physical health problems, men and women identifying as sexual minorities are at greater risk of interpersonal violence (Eaton, 2014). Research suggests that LGB adults and youth are more likely to experience violence related to their sexual identity (i.e., verbal abuse, verbal threats, physical threats, physical attacks, and sexual assault) compared to heterosexual adults and youth (D'Augelli & Grossman, 2001). In fact, a recent survey assessing experiences of violence in sexual minority youth found that 72% of participants reported having experienced verbal abuse, 11% had been victims of physical attacks, and 3% of the participants had experienced verbal and physical threats. Notably, participants reported they were targets of this violence because they identified as sexual minorities (Dragowski, Halkitis, Grossman, & D'Augelli, 2011).

These findings are particularly alarming because being the victim of violence increases the risk of negative mental health consequences. As noted, sexual minority women experience both sexual victimization and negative mental health issues at higher rates than heterosexual women (Balsam, et al., 2011; Bostwick, Boyd, Hughes, & McCabe, 2010). Given that nonvictimized sexual minority women report higher rates of negative mental health symptoms, being a victim of sexual assault might exacerbate preexisting psychopathology (Balsam, et al., 2011). Indeed, minority stress theory posits that sexual victimization experienced by sexual minority women might lead to more negative mental health consequences, as compared to sexually victimized heterosexual women, due to the additional psychosocial stressors that these women face as a result of their minority identity (Meyer, 2003).

Minority Stress and Other Psychosocial Stressors

Microaggressions. According to minority stress theory, sexual minority women are at heightened risk for experiencing microaggressions, which are thought to increase levels of stress. Microaggressions are usually brief demonstrations of implicit bias toward minority individuals, which can be social or environmental, verbal or nonverbal, as well as intentional or unintentional (Sue et al., 2007; Robinson & Rubin, 2016). Individuals who engage in microaggressions often are not aware that their interpersonal interactions are discriminatory. In fact, many individuals believe that microaggressions are innocent and harmless, and they may not understand the potential negative impact of these acts on recipients (Sue, Capodilupo, Nadal, & Torino, 2008). Regardless of individuals' intent or understanding of the impact of microaggressions, research has demonstrated that microaggressions are associated with more negative mental health consequences (e.g., depression, perceived stress, PTSD symptoms) among sexual and racial/ethnic minority groups (Balsam, et al., 2011; Robinson & Rubin, 2016).

Being the victim of sexual identity microaggressions also can exacerbate existing mental health problems for sexual minorities. Robinson and Rubin (2016) examined the association between sexual identity microaggressions and PTSD symptoms in a sample of lesbian, gay, bisexual, and heterosexual adults. They found that participants who experienced a higher number of microaggressions (i.e., being told that sexual identity was a choice, being sexualized for being gay, experiencing homophobia, and experiencing heterosexist language or terminology) were more likely to report a higher number of PTSD symptoms. Furthermore, sexual minorities reported a higher negative impact (e.g., self-reported intensity of the perceived impact) of microaggressions compared to heterosexual participants, and this discrepancy in negative impact was significantly associated with more trauma-related symptoms.

Coming out. "Coming out" is a process that occurs for sexual minorities because of the assumption of heterosexuality in our society (Coleman, 1982). The "coming out" process includes sexual minorities disclosing their sexual identity to others, which plays a key role in sexual identity development (Balsam, 2003). However, this process can be disrupted by sexual assault or violence that can either slow down or speed up the process, which has potential detrimental effects such as experiencing violence or negative mental health symptoms (Balsam, 2003). For example, "coming out" can be accelerated if a sexual minority woman experiences a sexual assault and disclosing her assault would force her to also "come out" to others (Balsam, 2003). Relatedly, the process of "coming out" and maintaining a positive concept of your self-identity may be disrupted if a sexual minority woman is targeted because of recent disclosure of her sexual identity. The "coming out" process is important for sexual minority women, and this process is made difficult by the heteronormative assumptions of the extant society (Balsam, 2003).

Overall, there is general disagreement in the literature as to whether "coming out" is a protective factor for sexual minorities or an additional psychosocial stressor. For instance, the identifiability/vulnerability hypothesis posits that disclosure of sexual identity, appearing more obviously gay or lesbian to others, and being more gender atypical increases the likelihood of victimization (Pilkington & D'Augelli, 1995). Pilkington and D'Augelli (1995) tested this hypothesis and found that when sexual minority youth disclosed their sexual identity at an earlier age, their "coming out" process did not serve as a protective factor, but rather increased their chances of being abused by others around them. They found that 22% ($n = 41$) of the sample of youth that self-identified as lesbian, bisexual, or gay and who had disclosed their sexual identity to others reported a consequent sexual assault, and 1 in 10 youth had been sexually assaulted on more than once occasion (Pilkington & D'Augelli, 1995). Approximately 40% (n = 78) of the youth experienced verbal attacks by immediate family members because of their sexual identity. Most of the youth expressed fear about being out at home, work, or school and interacting with professionals in their community such as police officers and doctors. Youth that had self-identified as lesbian or bisexual from a younger age or who disclosed their sexual identity earlier reported more victimization relative to youth who self-identified and disclosed their sexual identity at a later age. These findings provide support for the target identifiability/vulnerability hypothesis (Pilkington & D'Augelli, 1995).

Balsam (2003) discussed a more holistic approach to "coming out" for sexual minority women; she acknowledged that traumatic events such as sexual assault might hinder women's ability/desire to come out. However, she also argued that "coming out" after a sexual victimization experience might help women regain a sense of control that may facilitate their post-victimization recovery. Although Balsam's argument is based on a contextual approach and is intended to inform and educate clinicians working with lesbian and bisexual sexual assault survivors, her individualistic approach to the "coming out" process highlights that it is a unique process for each sexual minority woman and that disclosure of sexual identity can either serve as a protective or risk factor. In sum, it remains unclear what role the "coming out" process plays for sexual minority adult women who have experienced sexual victimization.

Internalized homophobia. Internalized homophobia is an additional psychosocial stressor that can have a negative impact on LGB identity and "coming out." Internalized homophobia is a psychological phenomenon in which people take on negative societal attitudes toward sexual identity minorities as part of their own self-concept (Herek, Gillis, & Cogan, 2009). Internalized homophobia is relevant to sexual minority women and sexual victimization because internalized homophobia is associated with increased guilt and shame and poorer physical and mental health for these women (Frost & Meyer, 2009; Greene & Britton, 2012; Herek et al., 2009; Ueno, 2010). Given that internalized homophobia exacerbates negative physical and mental health symptoms in nonvictimized sexual minority women, it may have even more deleterious effects on the physical and mental health of victimized sexual minority women who are also experiencing mental health difficulties (Robinson & Rubin, 2016).

Race/Ethnicity, Sexual Victimization, and Triple Minority Status

Minority stress theory can also be used as a framework to further understand racial and ethnic minority women's experiences of sexual victimization. Indeed, it appears that there are significant differences among racial and ethnic groups in victimization rates. American Indian/Alaska Native (AI/AN) women consistently have higher rates of victimization compared to non-Hispanic White, African American, Asian, and Hispanic women (Lehavot, Walters, & Simoni, 2010; Morris & Balsam, 2003). Hispanic women also have higher rates of sexual coercion relative to non-Hispanic White women (Basile et al., 2015). These discrepancies are not well understood; however, according to minority stress theory, racial/ethnic minority women would be more likely to have negative mental health outcomes relative to their Caucasian counterparts (Meyer, 2003).

It is also possible for women to hold more than one minority identity, such as being a sexual, racial/ethnic, and gender minority, which is called a *triple minority status*. Women who are both racial/ethnic and sexual minorities might be at greater risk of sexual victimization and increased negative consequences associated with sexual victimization due to the burden of experiencing homophobia, racism, and sexism. Indeed, triple minority women have been identified as a population that has the highest risk for sexual victimization compared to their non-Hispanic

White heterosexual counterparts (Gold et al., 2009). However, research indicates that triple minority women who are relatively young (i.e., 18–25) appear to be particularly resilient to experiencing the negative psychological sequelae of trauma exposure (Balsam et al., 2015).

Research on triple minority women and their experiences of sexual victimization is scarce. Balsam et al. (2015) examined the rates of sexual victimization in a racially/ethnically diverse sample of 1106 lesbian, bisexual, and heterosexual women. Balsam et al. (2015) found that although there were statistically significant differences across racial and ethnic groups for socioeconomic variables, degree of "outness" to family, CSA (child sexual abuse), and forcible rape, there were almost no differences between groups (e.g., non-Hispanic White, African American, Latina, Asian) with respect to mental health and substance use (i.e., smoking and marijuana). These findings are the opposite of what one would expect from minority stress theory and suggest instead that triple minority women might be resilient to the negative physical and mental health consequences that often are associated with a sexual victimization experience. The reasons for these findings are unclear; thus, future research should examine resiliency and protective factors among sexual minority women, particularly sexual minority women of color who have experienced sexual victimization.

Cultural Considerations when Working with Sexual Minority Women

It is important to conduct research that is culturally and ethically appropriate for sexual minority women in order to improve this populations' participation and retention in research studies. Similar considerations need to be taken when working with sexual minority women in mental health settings. One cultural consideration is a concept called *intersectionality*, which posits that sexual minority women hold memberships in other minority groups, such as race/ethnicity, gender, social class, cultural background, religion, and disabilities (Cole, 2009; Crenshaw, 1989). Combinations of several minority identities may lead to diverse clinical presentations (Sue & Sue, 2012). For instance, a bisexual Latina woman might report more somatic complaints than a bisexual non-Hispanic White woman when presenting for treatment. This discrepancy in clinical presentation might be due to Latina populations unknowingly somaticizing psychological complaints because it is more culturally appropriate (Sue & Sue, 2012). Indeed, it is a cultural and ethical necessity to use intersectionality theory to conceptualize sexual minority women who are seeking treatment for sexual assault (Zea & Nakamura, 2014).

Furthermore, research indicates that lesbian and bisexual women are not a homogenous group and perceive mental health differently (Daley, 2010). To assess these differences in perception, Das (2012) conducted in-person interviews with a sample of LGBTQ (e.g., lesbian, gay, bisexual, transgender, and queer) women and asked them to define the term mental health recovery, a term often used in mental health treatment centers. Das (2012) found three distinct responses across the sample group's definitions: (1) some women were unable to define it, (2) some women were sensitive to the medical field's drive to "fix" patients and its use to shame people for not progressing toward being mentally healthy, and (3) some women report that they needed extra time to recover from the stigma of being a minority before being able to address their mental health recovery. Overall, the study highlights the complexity of treating sexual minority women and the importance of using cultural and ethical sensitivity in regard to terminology they might use to describe mental health and recovery.

Given that clients who have diverse cultural identities are seeking treatments at higher rates than previously (Rutter et al., 2016), graduate programs should strongly encourage rigorous training in cultural competence (i.e., cultural humility) (Boroughs, Bedoya, O'Cleirigh, & Safren, 2015). The American Psychological Association (APA), an accreditation system for psychology graduate and internship programs, is cognizant of the complex presentation of sexual minority women and has published 21 guidelines for psychological practice with lesbian, gay, and bisexual (LGB) clients (APA, 2012). APA's guidelines are aspirational and not standards, which does not guarantee that clinical psychologists from APA-accredited training programs have achieved LGB client cultural competence. One potential strategy to help bridge the gap between guidelines and practice, and subsequently improve clinical competence with sexual minorities, might be to (1) introduce theoretical models of cultural competence to clinical psychologists during the beginning of their training [e.g., multicultural competence framework (Inman & Ladany, 2014)], (2) model behaviors that are judged as competent (i.e., use all-inclusive pronouns, not assume heterosexuality, etc.) by a supervisor, and (3) receive ongoing feedback on ways to improve culturally competent behavior. A discussion of the implementation of these theoretical models is beyond the scope of this paper but should be considered when discussing cultural and ethical considerations for working with sexual minority women in clinical and research settings.

Suggested Avenues for Future Research with Sexual Minority Women

Research on the prevalence of sexual assault among sexual minority women highlights the need for additional studies to examine risk factors for and consequences of sexual assault among this vulnerable population. By examining additional risk and protective factors for sexual victimization, it might be possible to identify variables that mediate and/or moderate the relationship between these risk factors and sexual assault experiences. However, in order to facilitate future research with sexual minority women, efforts need to be made to improve recruitment among this population. Currently, most methods of recruitment for studies on sexual minority women involve snowball sampling (i.e., asking enrolled study participants to recruit their friends or acquaintances into the study). This sampling method is convenient but ultimately limits the generalizability of the findings. For example, most studies that have used snowball sampling recruit women who are actively involved within the LGB community or have indicated on their social media web page (i.e., Facebook) that they are interested in women. Although this method can recruit a large number of women relatively efficiently, it does not offer the opportunity for women who are not out (i.e., who may not have indicated that they are interested in women through social media or who are not involved with the LGB community) to participate in this important research. This is a significant limitation of snowball sampling. However, random probability sampling is still not feasible for this population of women due to low base rates and stigma associated with having a sexual minority identity.

Longitudinal Research. Longitudinal research is needed to determine potential causation between identified risk factors and sexual assault victimization. Likewise, longitudinal research could also establish whether certain risk factors (i.e., alcohol use) are a cause or consequence of sexual victimization. Further, given the high occurrence of sexual assault and sexual revictimization in this population, measures of sexual assault that incorporate both severity and frequency may be able to provide more sensitive predictors of health consequences (Rhew, Stappenbeck, Bedard-Gilligan, Hughes, & Kaysen, 2017).

Qualitative Research. In addition to longitudinal study designs, research on sexual minority women would benefit from qualitative research. Qualitative methods have the capacity to explore the meaning, lived experiences, and complex relationships between factors that are often ignored in quantitative research designs. Qualitative research on the victimization experiences of sexual minority women would allow for the study of characteristics of the sexual assault not traditionally captured by quantitative measures, but also the victim's perspective and perceptions which may differ from those of the researchers (López & Yeater, 2018). These perceptions are particularly relevant when examining help-seeking behaviors and barriers to receiving both formal and informal social support. Additionally, qualitative data on sexual minority women's coping strategies could provide researchers with new insights regarding sexual minority women's protective factors against mental health symptoms. By providing open-ended in-person interview questions that could be answered in a qualitative fashion, participants presumably would have free reign to describe their victimization experiences and post-victimization recoveries in detail.

Help-Seeking Behaviors and Social Support. Seeking help and social support following sexual victimization may ameliorate some of the long-term consequences of sexual assault, with a majority of sexual minority women not disclosing their sexual assault experiences to any formal or informal sources (Sylaska & Edwards, 2014). In the context of sexual assault, low levels of social support have been found to be associated with more severe PTSD and depression symptoms for sexual minority women (Weiss, Garvert, & Cloitre, 2015). Furthermore, there may be a lack of resources perceived to be safe for sexual minority survivors of sexual assault (National Coalition of Anti-Violence Programs, 2012; as reported in Ollen, Ameral, Palm Reed, & Hines, 2017). When reporting anti-LGBT violence, sexual minority women may fear that authorities will mistreat them, they will not be believed, services will not be culturally sensitive, and disclosing their sexual identities will have negative consequences (Dworkin & Yi, 2003). These fears may be amplified (and for valid reasons) in our current sociopolitical climate. A qualitative study found that sexual minority students have concerns that others in their lives may generalize specific information about their sexual assault to the entire sexual minority community, and thus would be reluctant to disclose victimization to others (Ollen et al., 2017). Additionally, LGBTQ survivors of color may face additional barriers to seeking criminal or civil legal services for interpersonal violence due to fear of experiencing anti-LGBTQ, racist, and/or xenophobic violence by law enforcement (National Coalition of Anti-Violence Programs (NCAVP), 2016).

Coming Out. Many have suggested that the "coming out" process is an important step for sexual minority women. While early theoretical models of sexual identity development suggest this process unfolds in a linear manner, more recent work proposes that sexual identity development may follow various pathways (Rosario, Schrimshaw, & Hunter, 2008; Savin-Williams, 2001; Schneider, 2001). Although there is some research to suggest that there is variability in the development of sexual identity, it is still unclear as to which individual factors (e.g., sexual victimization) may impact the expression of these different patterns. Additionally, little is known about how sexual victimization experiences influence sexual identity integration over time (Rosario et al., 2008).

There appears to be disagreement among researchers as to whether the "coming out" process serves as a protective factor or as an additional source of stress for sexual minority women, with some suggesting that disclosing one's sexual identity may increase the likelihood of being victimized (e.g., Pilkington & D'Augelli, 1995) and others positing that "coming out" may promote healthy recovery post-victimization (e.g., Balsam, 2003). More research is needed to investigate the complex relationship between "coming out" and victimization experiences among sexual minority women. Robohm, Litzenberger, and Pearlman (2003) examined the relationships between childhood sexual abuse and the "coming out" process among lesbian and bisexual women. Results suggested that over half of women in the study did not report an association between CSA and feelings of their sexual identity or their "coming out" process, suggesting that there is still much we do not know about various protective factors that are associated with resiliency.

Internalized Homophobia. In addition to "coming out" considerations, special consideration should be taken for internalized homophobia in sexual minority clients. Internalized homophobia should be assessed through measures developed for sexual minority populations prior to treatment for the effects of sexual victimization because these patients are at greater risk for more negative mental health (i.e., anxiety and depression) that may interfere with treatment or need to be addressed in treatment. Understanding levels of internalized homophobia in lesbian and bisexual women might be useful to better effectively target their experience of negative psychological sequelae post-victimization and to individualize treatment.

Intersectionality Theory. To address sexual minority women's treatment barrier concerns, service providers should strive to be sensitive to the specific identities, and how these identities interconnect, for the particular individual they are providing services to. Intersectionality theory attempts to identify how various forms of social stratification (i.e., race/ethnicity, gender, sexual orientation, class, age, etc.) interlock to marginalize members of society (Crenshaw, 1989). Thus, sexual minority women may experience discrimination based on multiple facets of their identity, not only based on their sexual identity. Racial/ethnic minority women have been found to experience discrimination and marginalization based on the interplay of multiple social categories following sexual assault (Leung, 2017). Further attention is warranted around the intersectionality of culture, race/ethnicity, and sexual identity of sexual assault survivors.

To address potential multifaceted discrimination, service providers might include measures of cultural and racial/ethnic identity in order to adequately care for the needs of sexual assault survivors. By examining the survivor's cultural identity and how their identities may affect treatment, clinicians may be able to address some of the client's concerns of being understood by mental health professionals. Psychologists, social workers, and any other mental health providers working with minority individuals should consider a comprehensive framework for addressing multicultural competence such as the framework proposed by Inman and Ladany (2014). This framework conceptualizes multicultural competence as incorporating an understanding of how social contexts and larger ecosystems intersect with multiple identities to influence psychologist's knowledge, skills, and self-awareness.

In sum, acknowledging that women's experiences with sexual victimization might be different across race/ethnicities and sexual identities could aid researchers in further understanding various contexts in which diverse women experience sexual victimization. Using culturally appropriate approaches could also help foster a stronger relationship between minority women and investigators that, in turn, would increase participation and retention in research studies and ultimately improve services for sexual minority populations (Long et al., 2007).

References

Acierno, R., Brady, K., Gray, M., Kilpatrick, D. G., Resnick, H., & Best, C. L. (2002). Psychopathology following interpersonal violence: A comparison of risk factors in older and younger adults. *Journal of Clinical Geropsychology, 8*, 13–23.

American Psychological Association. (2012). *Guidelines for psychological practice with lesbian, gay, and bisexual clients*. Retrieved from http://www.apa.org/pi/lgbt/resources/guidelines.aspx.

Balsam, K. F. (2003). Traumatic victimization in the lives of lesbian and bisexual women. *Journal of Lesbian Studies, 7*(1), 1–14.

Balsam, K. F., Lehavot, K., & Beadnell, B. (2011). Sexual revictimization and mental health: A comparison of lesbians, gay men, and heterosexual women. *Journal of Interpersonal Violence, 26*(9), 1798–1814.

Balsam, K. F., Molina, Y., Beadnell, B., Simoni, J., & Walters, K. (2011). Measuring minority stress: The LGBT people of color microaggressions scale. *Cultural Diversity and Ethnic Minority Psychology, 17*(2), 163–174.

Balsam, K. F., Molina, Y., Blayney, J. A., Dillworth, T., Zimmerman, L., & Kaysen, D. (2015). Racial/ethnic differences in identity and mental health outcomes among young sexual minority women. *Cultural Diversity and Ethnic Minority Psychology, 21*(3), 380–390.

Balsam, K. F., Rothblum, E. D., & Beauchaine, T. P. (2005). Victimization over the life span: A comparison of lesbian, gay, bisexual, and heterosexual siblings. *Journal of Consulting and Clinical Psychology, 73*(3), 477–487.

Banyard, V. L., Williams, L. M., & Siegel, J. A. (2001). The long-term mental health consequences of child sexual abuse: An exploratory study of the impact of multiple traumas in a sample of women. *Journal of Traumatic Stress, 14*(4), 697–715.

Basile, K. C., Smith, S. G., Walters, M. L., Fowler, D. N., Hawk, K., & Hamburger, M. E. (2015). Sexual violence victimization and associations with health in a community sample of Hispanic women. *Journal of Ethnic & Cultural Diversity in Social Work, 24*(1), 1–17.

Bedard-Gilligan, M., Kaysen, D., Desai, S., & Lee, C. M. (2011). Alcohol-involved assault: Associations with posttrauma alcohol use, consequences, and expectancies. *Addictive Behaviors, 36*(11), 1076–1082.

Bonanno, G. A. (2004). Loss, trauma, and human resilience: Have we underestimated the human capacity to thrive after extremely aversive events? *American Psychologist, 59*, 20–28.

Boroughs, M. S., Bedoya, C. A., O'Cleirigh, C., & Safren, S. A. (2015). Toward defining, measuring, and evaluating LGBT cultural competence for psychologists. *Clinical Psychology: Science and Practice, 22*(2), 151–171.

Bostwick, W. B., Boyd, C. J., Hughes, T. L., & McCabe, S. E. (2010). Dimensions of sexual orientation and the prevalence of mood and anxiety disorders in the United States. *American Journal of Public Health, 100*(3), 468–475.

Bryant-Davis, T., Chung, H., & Tillman, S. (2009). From the margins to the center: Ethnic minority women and the mental health effects of sexual assault. *Trauma Violence Abuse, 10*(4), 330–357.

Calhoun, L. G., & Tedeschi, R. G. (2006). The foundations of posttraumatic growth: An expanded framework. In L. G. Calhoun (Ed.), *Handbook of posttraumatic growth: research & practice* (pp. 3–23). Mahwah, NJ: Lawrence Erlbaum Associates Publishers.

Campbell, R., Dworkin, E., & Cabral, G. (2009). An ecological model of the impact of sexual assault on women's mental health. *Trauma, Violence, & Abuse, 10*(3), 225–246.

Carlson, E. B., & Dalenberg, C. J. (2000). A conceptual framework for the impact of traumatic experiences. *Trauma, Violence, and Abuse, 1*(1), 4–28.

Center for Disease Control and Prevention. (2004). Surveillance summaries: Youth risk behavior surveillance. *MMWR, 53*(SS-2).

Cohn, A., Hagman, B. T., Moore, K., Mitchell, J., & Ehlke, S. (2014). Does negative affect mediate the relationship between daily PTSD symptoms and daily alcohol involvement in female rape victims? Evidence from 14 days of interactive voice response assessment. *Psychology of Addictive Behaviors, 28*(1), 114–126.

Cole, E. R. (2009). Intersectionality and research in psychology. *American Psychological Association, 64*(3), 170–180.

Coleman, E. (1982). Developmental stages of the coming out process. *Journal of Homosexuality, 7*(2–3), 31–43.

Crenshaw, K. (1989). Demarginalizing the intersection of race and sex: A black feminist critique of antidiscrimination doctrine, feminist theory and antiracist politics. *The University of Chicago Legal Forum, 1*(8), 139–167.

D'augelli, A. R., & Grossman, A. H. (2001). Disclosure of sexual orientation, victimization, and mental health among lesbian, gay, and bisexual older adults. *Journal of Interpersonal Violence, 16*(10), 1008–1027.

D'Augelli, A. R., Grossman, A. H., Salter, N. P., Vasey, J. J., Starks, M. T., & Sinclair, K. O. (2005). Predicting the suicide attempts of lesbian, gay, and bisexual youth. *Suicide and Life-threatening Behavior, 35*(6), 646–660.

Daley, A. E. (2010). Being recognized, accepted, and affirmed: Self disclosure of lesbian/queer sexuality within psychiatric and mental health service settings. *Social Work in Mental Health, 8*, 336–355.

Das, A. (2012). LGBTQ women and mental health "recovery". *Psychiatric Rehabilitation Journal, 35*(6), 474–475.

Drabble, L., Trocki, K. F., Hughes, T. L., Korcha, R. A., & Lown, A. E. (2013). Sexual orientation differences in relationship between victimization and hazardous drinking among women in the national alcohol survey. *Psychology of Addictive Behaviors, 27*(3), 639–648.

Dragowski, E. A., Halkitis, P. N., Grossman, A. H., & D'Augelli, A. R. (2011). Sexual orientation victimization and posttraumatic stress symptoms among lesbian, gay, and bisexual youth. *Journal of Gay & Lesbian Social Services, 23*(2), 226–249.

Duncan, D. T., & Hatzenbuehler, M. L. (2014). Lesbian, gay, bisexual, and transgender hate crimes and suicidality among a population-based sample of sexual-minority adolescents in Boston. *American Journal of Public Health, 104*(2), 272–278.

Dworkin, S. H., & Yi, H. (2003). LGBT identity, violence, and social justice: The psychological is political. *International Journal for the Advancement of Counselling, 25*(4), 269–279. https://doi.org/10.1023/B:ADCO.0000005526.87218.9f

Eaton, N. R. (2014). Transdiagnostic psychopathology factors and sexual minority mental health: Evidence of disparities and associations with minority stressors. *Psychology of Sexual Orientation and Gender Diversity, 1*(3), 244–254.

Faravelli, C., Giugni, A., Salvatori, S., & Ricca, V. (2004). Psychopathology after rape. *The American Journal of Psychiatry, 161*(8), 1483–1485.

Filipas, H. H., & Ullman, S. E. (2006). Child sexual abuse, coping responses, self-blame, posttraumatic stress disorder, and adult sexual revictimization. *Journal of Interpersonal Violence, 21*(5), 652–672.

Frazier, P. A., Conlon, A., & Glaser, T. (2001). Positive and negative life changes following sexual assault. *Journal of Consulting and Clinical Psychology, 69*(6), 1048–1055.

Frost, D. M., Lehavot, K., & Meyer, I. H. (2013). Minority stress and physical health among sexual minority individuals. *Journal of Behavioral Medicine, 38*(1), 1–8.

Frost, D. M., & Meyer, I. H. (2009). Internalized homophobia and relationship quality among lesbians, gay men, and bisexuals. *Journal of Counseling Psychology, 56*, 97–109.

Gidycz, C. A., Coble, C. N., Latham, L., & Layman, M. J. (1993). Sexual assault experience in adulthood and prior victimization experiences: A prospective analysis. *Psychology of Women Quarterly, 17*, 151–168.

Gilmore, A. K., Koo, K. H., Nguyen, H. V., Granato, H. F., Hughes, T. L., & Kaysen, D. (2014). Sexual assault, drinking norms, and drinking behavior among a national sample of lesbian and bisexual women. *Addictive Behaviors, 39*(3), 630–636.

Gold, S. D., Dickstein, B. D., Marx, B. P., & Lexington, J. M. (2009). Psychological outcomes among lesbian sexual assault survivors: An examination of the roles of internalized homophobia and experiential avoidance. *Psychology of Women Quarterly, 33*, 54–66.

Gold, S. D., Feinstein, B. A., Skidmore, W. C., & Marx, B. P. (2011). Childhood physical abuse, internalized homophobia, and experiential avoidance among lesbians and gay men. *Psychological Trauma: Theory, Research, Practice and Policy, 3*(2), 50–60.

Greene, D. C., & Britton, P. J. (2012). Stage of sexual minority identity formation: The impact of shame, internalized homophobia, ambivalence over emotional expression, and personal mastery. *Journal of Gay & Lesbian Mental Health, 16*(3), 188–214.

Grossman, A. H., & D'Augelli, A. R. (2007). Transgender youth and life-threatening behaviors. *Suicide and Life-threatening Behavior, 37*(5), 527–537.

Grubaugh, A. L., & Resick, P. A. (2007). Posttraumatic growth in treatment-seeking female assault victims. *Psychiatry Quarterly, 78*, 145–155.

Han, S. C., Gallagher, M. W., Franz, M. R., Chen, M. S., Cabral, F. M., & Marx, B. P. (2013). Childhood sexual abuse, alcohol use, and PTSD symptoms as predictors of adult sexual assault among lesbians and gay men. *Journal of Interpersonal Violence, 28*(12), 2505–2520.

Heidt, J. M., Marx, B. P., & Gold, S. D. (2005). Sexual revictimization among sexual minorities: a preliminary study. *Journal of Traumatic Stress, 18*(5), 533–540.

Hequembourg, A. L., Livingston, J. A., & Parks, K. A. (2013). Sexual victimization and associated risks among lesbian and bisexual women. *Violence Against Women, 19*(5), 634–657.

Herek, G. M., Gillis, J. R., & Cogan, J. C. (2009). Internalized stigma around sexual minority adults: Insights from a social psychological perspective. *Journal of Counseling Psychology, 56*(1), 32–43.

Hughes, T., McCabe, S. E., Wilsnack, S. C., West, B. T., & Boyd, C. J. (2010). Victimization and substance use disorders in a national sample of heterosexual and sexual minority women and men. *Addiction, 105*(12), 2130–2140.

Hughes, T., Szalacha, L. A., & McNair, R. (2010). Substance abuse and mental health disparities: comparisons across sexual identity groups in a national sample of young Australian women. *Social Science & Medicine, 71*(4), 824–831.

Hughes, T. L., Johnson, T., & Wilsnack, S. C. (2001). Sexual assault and alcohol abuse: a comparison of lesbians and heterosexual women. *Journal of Substance Abuse, 13*(4), 515–532.

Hughes, T. L., Szalacha, L. A., Johnson, T. P., Kinnison, K. E., Wilsnack, S. C., & Cho, Y. (2010). Sexual victimization and hazardous drinking among heterosexual and sexual minority women. *Addictive Behaviors, 35*(12), 1152–1156.

Inman, A. G., & Ladany, N. (2014). Multicultural competences in psychotherapy supervision. In F. T. L. Leong (Ed.), *APA handbook of multicultural psychology, Vol 2, applications and training* (pp. 643–658). Washington, DC: American Psychological Association.

Jorm, A. F., Korten, A. E., Rodgers, B., Jacomb, P. A., & Christensen, H. (2002). Sexual orientation and mental health: Results from a community survey of young and middle-aged adults. *The British Journal of Psychiatry, 180*(5), 423–427.

Koss, M. P., Figueredo, A. J., & Prince, R. J. (2002). Cognitive mediation of rape's mental, physical and social health impact: Tests of four models in cross-sectional data. *Journal of Consulting and Clinical Psychology, 70*(4), 926–941.

Krahé, B., & Berger, A. (2013). Men and women as perpetrators and victims of sexual aggression in heterosexual and same-sex encounters: A study of first-year college students in Germany. *Journal of Aggressive Behavior, 39*, 391–404.

Kuyper, L., & Vanwesenbeeck, I. (2011). Examining sexual health differences between lesbian, gay, bisexual, and heterosexual adults: The role of sociodemographics, sexual behavior characteristics, and minority stress. *Journal of Sex Research, 48*(2–3), 363–274.

Lehavot, K., Molina, Y., & Simoni, J. M. (2012). Childhood trauma, adult sexual assault, and adult gender expression among lesbian and bisexual women. *Sex Roles, 67*(5–6), 272–284.

Lehavot, K., Walters, K. L., & Simoni, J. M. (2010). Abuse, mastery, and health among lesbian, bisexual, and two-spirit American Indian and Alaska Native women. *Psychology of Violence, 1*(S), 53–67.

Leung, L. (2017). Intersectional challenges: Marginalization of ethnic minority sexual assault survivors in Hong Kong. *Journal of Women & Social Work, 32*(2), 217–229. https://doi.org/10.1177/0886109916678026

Littleton, H., Axsom, D., & Grills-Taquechel, A. G. (2009). Sexual assault victims' acknowledge status and revictimization risk. *Psychology of Women Quarterly, 33*(1), 34–42.

Littleton, H., & Ullman, S. E. (2013). PTSD symptomatology and hazardous drinking as risk factors for sexual assault revictimization: Examination in European American and African American women. *Journal of Traumatic Stress, 26*, 345–353.

Long, S. M., Ullman, S. E., Long, L. M., Mason, G. E., & Starzynski, L. L. (2007). Women's experiences of male-perpetrated sexual assault by sexual orientation. *Violence and Victims, 22*(6), 684–701.

López, G., & Yeater, E. A. (2018). Comparisons of sexual victimization experiences among sexual minority and heterosexual women. *Journal of Interpersonal Violence.* https://doi.org/10.1177/0886260518787202

Martin, S. L., Fisher, B. S., Warner, T. D., Krebs, C. P., & Lindquist, C. H. (2011). Women's sexual orientations and their experiences of sexual assault before and during university. *Women's Health Issues, 21*(3), 199–205.

Masho, S. W., & Ahmed, G. (2007). Age at sexual assault and posttraumatic stress disorder among women:

Prevalence, correlates, and implications for prevention. *Journal of Women's Health, 16*(2), 262–271.
Messman-Moore, T. L., Long, P. J., & Siegfried, N. J. (2000). The revictimization of child sexual abuse survivors: An examination of the adjustment of college women with child sexual abuse, adult sexual assault, and adult physical abuse. *Child Maltreatment, 5*(1), 18–27.
Messman-Moore, T. L., Ward, R. M., & Brown, A. L. (2009). Substance use and PTSD symptoms impact the likelihood of rape and revictimization in college women. *Journal of Interpersonal Violence, 24*, 499–521.
Meyer, I. H. (2003). Prejudice, social stress, and mental health in lesbian, gay, and bisexual populations: Conceptual issues and research evidence. *Psychological Bulletin, 129*(5), 674–697.
Morris, J. F., & Balsam, K. F. (2003). Lesbian and bisexual women's experiences of victimization: Mental health, revictimization, and sexual identity development. *Journal of Lesbian Studies, 7*(4), 67–85.
Najdowski, C. J., & Ullman, S. E. (2011). The effects of revictimization on coping and depression in female sexual assault victims. *Journal of Traumatic Stress, 24*(2), 218–221.
National Coalition of Anti-Violence Programs (NCAVP). (2016). *Lesbian, gay, bisexual, transgender, queer, and HIV-affected intimate partner violence in 2015*. New York, NY: Emily Waters.
National Coalition of Anti-Violence Programs. (2012). *Report of LGBT and HIV-affected intimate partner violence*. In Ollen, E. W., Ameral, V. E., Palm Reed, K., & Hines, D. A. (2017). Sexual minority college students' perceptions on dating violence and sexual assault. *Journal of Counseling Psychology, 64*(1), 112–119. Retrieved from http://avp.org/wp-content/uploads/2017/04/2011_NCAVP_IPV_Report.pdf
Ollen, E. W., Ameral, V. E., Palm Reed, K., & Hines, D. A. (2017). Sexual minority college students' perceptions on dating violence and sexual assault. *Journal of Counseling Psychology, 64*(1), 112–119. https://doi.org/10.1037/cou0000180
Orchowski, L. M., Untied, A. S., & Gidycz, C. A. (2013). Social reactions to disclosure of sexual victimization and adjustment among survivors of sexual assaults. *Journal of Interpersonal Violence, 28*(10), 2005–2023.
Pilkington, N. W., & D'Augelli, A. R. (1995). Victimization of lesbian, gay and bisexual youth in community settings. *Journal of Community Psychology, 23*, 34–56.
Priola, V., Lasio, D., De Simone, S., & Serri, F. (2014). The sound of silence. Lesbian, gay, bisexual and transgender discrimination in 'inclusive organizations'. *British Journal of Management*. https://doi.org/10.1111/1467-8551.12043
Relyea, M., & Ullman, S. E. (2015). Unsupported or turned against: Understanding how two types of negative social reactions to sexual assault relate to post-assault outcomes. *Psychology of Women Quarterly, 39*(1), 37–52.
Resnick, H. S., Walsh, K., McCauley, J. L., Schumacher, J. A., Kilpatrick, D. G., & Acierno, R. E. (2012). Assault related substance use as a predictor of substance use over time within a sample of recent victims of sexual assault. *Addictive Behaviors, 37*, 914–921.
Rhew, I. C., Stappenbeck, C. A., Bedard-Gilligan, M., Hughes, T., & Kaysen, D. (2017). Effects of sexual assault on alcohol use and consequences among young adult sexual minority women. *Journal of Consulting and Clinical Psychology, 85*, (5), 424–433. https://doi.org/10.1037/ccp0000202
Roberts, A. L., Austin, B., Corliss, H. L., Vandermorris, A. K., & Koenen, K. C. (2010). Pervasive trauma exposure among US sexual orientation minority adults and risk of posttraumatic stress disorder. *American Journal of Public Health, 100*(12), 2433–2441.
Robinson, J. L., & Rubin, L. J. (2016). Homonegative microaggressions and posttraumatic stress symptoms. *Journal of Gay and Lesbian Mental Health, 20*(1), 57–69.
Robohm, J. S., Litzenberger, B. W., & Pearlman, L. A. (2003). Sexual abuse in lesbian and bisexual young women: Associations with emotional/behavioral difficulties, feelings about sexuality, and the "coming out" process. *Journal of Lesbian Studies, 7*(4), 31–47.
Rosario, M., Schrimshaw, E. W., & Hunter, J. (2008). Predicting different patterns of sexual identity development over time among lesbian, gay, and bisexual youths: A cluster analytic approach. *American Journal of Community Psychology, 42*(3–4), 266–282.
Rothman, E. F., Exner, D., & Baughman, A. L. (2011). The prevalence of sexual assault against people who identify as gay, lesbian, or bisexual in the United States: A systematic review. *Trauma, Violence, & Abuse, 12*(2), 55–66.
Rutter, T. M., Flentje, A., Dilley, J. W., Barakat, S., Liu, N. H., Gross, M. S., Muñoz, R. F., & Leykin, Y. (2016). Sexual orientation and treatment-seeking for depression in a multilingual worldwide sample. *Journal of Affective Disorders, 206*, 87–93.
Simmons, C. A., & Granvold, D. K. (2005). A cognitive model to explain gender differences in rate of PTSD diagnosis. *Brief Treatment and Crisis Interventions, 5*(3), 290–299.
Smith, T. B., & Trimble, J. E. (2016). Mental health service utilization across race: A meta-analysis of surveys and archival studies. In T. B. Smith & J. E. Trimble (Eds.), *Foundations of multicultural psychology: Research to inform effective practice* (pp. 67–94). Washington: American Psychological Association. Retrieved from http://content.apa.org/books/14733-004
Sue, D. W., Capodilupo, C. M., Nadal, K. L., & Torino, G. C. (2008). Racial microaggressions and the power to define reality. *American Psychologist, 63*(4), 277–279.
Sue, D. W., Capodilupo, C. M., Torino, G. C., Bucceri, J. M., Holder, A. M. B., Nadal, K. L., & Esquilin, M. (2007). Racial microaggressions in everyday life: Implications for clinical practice. *American Psychologist, 62*(4), 271–286.

Sue, D. W., & Sue, D. (2012). *Counseling the culturally diverse: Theory and practice*. Hoboken, NJ: John Wiley & Sons.

Sylaska, K. M., & Edwards, K. M. (2014). Disclosure of intimate partner violence to informal social support network members: A review of the literature. *Trauma, Violence & Abuse, 15*, 3–21. https://doi.org/10.1177/1524838013496335

Savin-Williams, R. C. (2001). Chapter 2: Differential developmental trajectories. In *Mom, dad. I'm gay. How families negotiate coming out* (pp. 7–21). Washington, DC: American Psychological Association.

Schneider, M. S. (2001). Toward a reconceptualization of the coming-out process for adolescent females. In A. R. D'Augelli & C. J. Patterson (Eds.), *Lesbian, gay, and bisexual identities and youth: Psychological perspectives* (pp. 71–96). New York, NY: Oxford University Press.

Tedeschi, R. G., & Calhoun, L. G. (2004). A clinical approach to posttraumatic growth. In P. A. Linkey (Ed.), *Positive psychology in practice* (pp. 405–419). Hoboken, NJ: John Wiley & Sons.

Thompson, S. J., Ryan, T. N., Montgomery, K. L., Lippman, A. D. P., Bender, K., & Ferguson, K. (2016). Perceptions of resiliency and coping: Homeless young adults speak out. *Youth & Society, 48*(1), 58–76.

Ueno, K. (2010). Mental health differences between young adults with and without same-sex contact: A simultaneous examination of underlying mechanisms. *Journal of Health and Social Behavior, 51*(4), 391–407.

Ullman, S. E. (1996). Social reactions, coping strategies, and self-blame attributions in adjustment to sexual assault. *Psychology of Women Quarterly, 20*(4), 505–526.

Ullman, S. E. (1999). Social support and recovery from sexual assault: A review. *Aggression and Violent Behavior, 4*(3), 343–358.

Ullman, S. E. (2003). A critical review of field studies on the link of alcohol and adult sexual assault in women. *Aggression and Violent Behavior, 8*, 471–486.

Ullman, S. E. (2010). Social reactions and their effects on survivors. In *Talking about sexual assault: Society's response to survivors* (pp. 59–82). Washington, DC: American Psychological Association.

Ullman, S. E., Peter-Hagene, L. C., & Relyea, M. (2014). Coping, emotion regulation, and self-blame as mediators of sexual abuse and psychological symptoms in adult sexual assault. *Journal of Child Sexual Abuse, 23*(1), 74–93.

Ullman, S. E., & Najdowski, C. J. (2011). Prospective changes in attributions of self-blame and social reactions to women's disclosures of adult sexual assault. *Journal of Interpersonal Violence, 26*(10), 1934–1962.

Ullman, S. E. (2004). Sexual assault victimization and suicidal behavior in women: A review of the literature. *Aggression and Violent Behavior, 9*(4), 331–351.

Weiss, B. J., Garvert, D. W., & Cloitre, M. (2015). Ptsd and trauma-related difficulties in sexual minority women: The impact of perceived social support. *Journal of Traumatic Stress, 28*(6), 563–571. https://doi.org/10.1002/jts.22061

Wolitzky-Taylor, K. B., Resnick, H. S., McCauley, J. L., Amstadter, A. B., Kilpatrick, D. G., & Ruggiero, K. J. (2011). Is reporting of rape on the rise? A comparison of women with reported versus unreported rape experiences in the National Women's Study-Replication. *Journal of Interpersonal Violence, 26*(4), 807–832.

Zea, M. C., & Nakamura, N. (2014). Sexual orientation. In F. T. L. Leong (Ed.), *APA handbook of multicultural psychology, vol 1, theory and research* (pp. 395–410). Washington, DC: American Psychological Association.

41 Homelessness and Sexual Assault

Kimberly A. Tyler and James D. Wright

Homeless individuals, people who lack a permanent place to live, are difficult to count because their housing dynamics are very fluid. On a single night in January 2017, using the Department of Housing and Urban Development's point-in-time estimation procedures, it was found that over 553,000 people were experiencing homelessness in the United States (Henry, Watt, Rosenthal, Shivji, & Abt Associates, 2017). Approximately 39% of these individuals were women, and 70% were over the age of 24 (Henry et al., 2017). The National Network for Youth (2018) estimates that between 1.3 and 1.7 million youth have experienced at least one night of being homeless within a specific year. Some of the main reasons youth leave home include family conflict (Tyler & Cauce, 2002), child abuse (Bender, Brown, Thompson, Ferguson, & Langenderfer, 2015), and parental drug abuse (Tyler & Melander, 2015). Among adults, there are also numerous reasons for becoming homeless such as domestic violence, job loss, divorce, and physical and mental health problems (Lee, Tyler, & Wright, 2010). Experiencing homelessness is also a well-known risk factor for sexual assault (Jasinski, Wesely, Wright, & Mustaine, 2010).

Each year, millions of women and men experience sexual violence.[1] In the United States alone, it is estimated that 23 million women (19.1%) and 1.6 million men (1.5%) have been the victim of rape or an attempted rape at some point in their lives (Smith et al., 2017). Moreover, in the United States, approximately 1 in 3 women (36.3%) and nearly 1 in 6 men (17.1%) have experienced some form of contact sexual violence during their lifetime. Contact sexual violence refers to rape, being made to penetrate, sexual coercion, or unwanted sexual contact[2] (Smith et al., 2017, p. 17). Sexual violence is a serious public health issue that can have long-term effects including poor physical and mental health. Moreover, experiencing sexual violence early in one's life increases the risk for revictimization. Though both men and women experience sexual violence, women tend to experience higher rates and more serious outcomes compared to men (Kaukinen, 2014).

K. A. Tyler (✉)
Department of Sociology, University of Nebraska-Lincoln, Lincoln, NE, USA
e-mail: kim@ktresearch.net

J. D. Wright
Department of Sociology, University of Central Florida, Orlando, FL, USA

[1]The terms "sexual violence," "sexual assault," and "sexual victimization" are used interchangeably throughout this chapter.

[2]Unwanted sexual contact is defined as "unwanted sexual experiences involving touch but not sexual penetration, such as being kissed in a sexual way, or having sexual body parts fondled, groped, or grabbed" (Smith et al., 2017, p. 17).

W. T. O'Donohue and P. A. Schewe (eds.), *Handbook of Sexual Assault and Sexual Assault Prevention*,
https://doi.org/10.1007/978-3-030-23645-8_41

Although these prevalence rates for sexual violence among the general population are high, rates among homeless individuals often exceed general population numbers. Research comparing rates of sexual victimization based on where homeless women stay revealed that 27% of homeless women living in a shelter had been sexually assaulted as an adult compared to 36% of homeless women living on the streets (Nyamathi, Leake, & Gelberg, 2000). A study of adult homeless women found that 34% had been raped as adults (Hudson et al., 2010). Similarly, among homeless young people ages 18 to 24, research has found that 32% have been sexually assaulted since being on the street (Tyler & Beal, 2010).

In this chapter, we review research studies focused on *outcomes* of sexual violence among homeless adult women and men, youth and adolescents. Though most research on sexual victimization has examined risk factors (e.g., child sexual abuse, mental illness, substance abuse), fewer studies have looked at long-term outcomes. The studies that do exist on "outcomes" of sexual victimization have focused on substance abuse, poor mental health, HIV risk behaviors, and revictimization. Regarding study inclusion, all studies that focused on outcomes of sexual violence as their main concern are included in this review. Additionally, studies that are cross-sectional and include findings on associations between sexual victimization and one of the outcomes listed above are also included as directionality of these relationships cannot be assessed with cross-sectional data. Though most studies included only women, we incorporate findings for men if information was provided. Studies not included are those that combined different forms of violence (e.g., physical and sexual) into a single measure, and thus their individual effects could not be determined. Finally, the reader should keep in mind that though we focus on "outcomes" of sexual violence, these studies are generally cross-sectional; therefore, causal ordering is sometimes ambiguous.

Theoretical Explanations of Sexual Assault

Countless studies have found that the greatest risk factor for being a victim of sexual assault while homeless is having a history of child sexual abuse (e.g., Edalati, Krausz, & Schütz, 2016; Hudson et al., 2010; Tyler & Melander, 2015). What is it about early sexual abuse that continues to put women (and men) at risk for repeated sexual assault in later years? Understanding this link is important as repeated sexual assault has devastating consequences for all victims including substance abuse, poor mental health, and revictimization. Though few studies include theory to explain the link between early sexual abuse and later revictimization, there are at least four perspectives that have been utilized to explain this relationship among homeless and general population youth and young adults. The first explanation is Finkelhor and Browne's (1985) *traumatic sexualization model.* This model suggests that the trauma of being sexually abused shapes the child's sexuality in ways that are developmentally inappropriate (e.g., promiscuity, sexual aggression), and this negative self-concept and behavior make these adolescents vulnerable to exploitive males and others who may take advantage of them (Finkelhor & Browne, 1988). Similarly, those who have been abused may also learn maladaptive behaviors and have difficulty trusting others (Desai et al., 2002). Additionally, because children who have been sexually abused often experience numerous emotional problems, including heightened loneliness, anxiety, and depression (Turner, Finkelhor, & Ormrod, 2010; Tyler, 2002), these young people may be at increased risk for being taken advantage of socially including sexual victimization. Relatedly, it is possible that being sexually abused as a child increases the likelihood that these youths will become involved in high-risk behaviors such as substance use and HIV risk behaviors (e.g., having multiple sexual partners; Harris, Rice,

Rhoades, Winetrobe, & Wenzel, 2017), which increases the likelihood for revictimization (Simons & Whitbeck, 1991). In terms of gender, females are more likely to experience child sexual abuse and subsequent lowered self-esteem because of this abuse compared to males (Tyler, 2002). As such, having lower self-esteem may be another risk factor that makes young women more vulnerable to sexual revictimization once on the street (Harris et al., 2017; Widom, Czaja, & Dutton, 2008).

The risk amplification model (Whitbeck, Hoyt, & Yoder, 1999) argues that early negative experiences within the family of origin, such as child sexual or physical abuse, set in motion a negative chain of events that lead to youth running away from home at an earlier age and spending more time on the street, which increases their involvement in risky behaviors such as trading sex and delinquency, both of which increase young people's chances for being a victim of sexual (and physical) assault. Research examining child abuse and sexual victimization has found support for this model among samples of homeless youth and young adults (Tyler, Gervais, & Davidson, 2013; Tyler & Melander, 2015).

Social learning theory, a third explanation, holds that violence directed at others is learned from one's social environment through the process of observational learning (Bandura, 1977). Children exposed to violence in their family may later imitate the behavior they have observed, especially if they witness its positive outcomes. Gelles (1997) further argued that children who grow up in violent homes learn the techniques of being violent and the justifications for this behavior. Owens and Straus (1975) also hold that those exposed to interpersonal violence at a young age, either as victims or perpetrators, report greater approval of interpersonal violence as adults. Moreover, early exposure to family violence such as sexual abuse and witnessing family violence are related to the development of unique forms of aggression in later life (Bevan & Higgins, 2002; Straus, Douglas, & Medeiros, 2013).

A related model, *the background situational model,* suggests that those who are more accepting of aggression are more likely to engage in perpetration (McNaughton Reyes, Foshee, Niolon, Reidy, & Hall, 2016; Temple, Shorey, Tortolero, Wolfe, & Stuart, 2013). This acceptance is not restricted to exposure to violence within the home, but may also be a result of being a victim of interpersonal violence as a child (Owens & Straus, 1975). Exposure to familial violence may lead children to view aggression as a normative aspect of relationships and increase their tolerance for it and likelihood of using it to establish compliance (Foshee, Bauman, & Linder, 1999). Previous work supports this notion of intergenerational violence, or the creation of expectations or norms related to interpersonal relationships based on experiences in childhood (Straus & Gelles, 1990). Thus, childhood victims of violence not only learn how to be perpetrators, but they may also be vulnerable to becoming victims. There has been empirical support for these findings as a history of child sexual abuse has been linked to street sexual victimization among homeless youth (Hudson et al., 2010; Tyler & Melander, 2015).

Rates of Sexual Violence

Though rates of sexual assault among homeless populations vary somewhat, many studies put the prevalence rate at approximately one-third. For example, in their study of 202 homeless women staying in shelters or living on the street, 34% had been raped as adults and 31% had been sexually harassed as adults (Hudson et al., 2010). Similarly, Edalati et al. (2016) in their study of 500 homeless adults aged 19+ found that 29% experienced adult sexual victimization. Among homeless youth, Bender et al. (2015) found that 21% of their sample of 600 homeless youth (ages 18–24) had been sexually assaulted since being on the street. Among homeless adolescents, Tyler et al. found that 35% of these young people had been sexually victimized at least once since leaving home.

Moreover, gender comparisons revealed that 23% of adolescent females and 11% of adolescent males reported one or more experiences of sexual victimization while on the street (Tyler, Whitbeck, Hoyt, & Cauce, 2004).

Outcomes of Sexual Victimization

Prior research has found that various negative outcomes are associated with sexual victimization among several homeless populations. These outcomes have included substance use and abuse (e.g., Tyler et al., 2004; Wenzel, Leake, & Gelberg, 2000), poor health (e.g., D'Ercole & Struening, 1990; Rattelade, Farrell, Aubry, & Klodawsky, 2014), HIV risk behaviors (Harris et al., 2017; Melander & Tyler, 2010), and revictimization (e.g., Edalati et al., 2016; Hudson et al., 2010). The following section summarizes each of these outcomes among samples of homeless adults, youth, and adolescents.

Substance Use

Research has examined the link between sexual victimization and alcohol, marijuana, and illicit drug use, and meeting criteria for substance abuse disorder. One of the earlier studies (D'Ercole & Struening, 1990) examined correlates of victimization using a representative sample of 141 sheltered women in New York City. In-depth structured interviews were conducted with the women, the majority of whom were African American (67%) with a median age of 31. At the bivariate level, the authors found alcohol problems to be a significant correlate of both lifetime sexual assault and recent sexual harassment. At the multivariate level, however, only lifetime sexual assault remained a significant correlate of alcohol problems (D'Ercole & Struening, 1990).

Another study of adult homeless women, conducted by Wenzel and colleagues (2000), examined the association between rape and substance use or abuse among a probability sample of 974 adult homeless women in Los Angeles. The women completed a 45-minute structured interview and were sampled from shelters and meal programs. Approximately one-half (56%) of their sample was African American with ages ranging from 15 to 44 years. Their results revealed that women who experienced rape at least once had more lifetime alcohol abuse or dependence and more lifetime drug abuse or dependence than women who had not been raped. The results from logistic regression revealed that alcohol abuse or dependence was no longer significantly associated with rape when controlling for other factors. However, lifetime drug abuse or dependence and using illicit drugs in the past 30 days were more likely to be reported among women who had been raped compared to those who had not been raped (Wenzel et al., 2000).

Research with homeless youth and young adults also has found a positive link between sexual victimization and illicit drug use. Using a large sample of 966 homeless youth (71% male) aged 14–24 years, Harris et al. (2017) found that sexual victimization was positively associated with heroin use among males and positively associated with methamphetamine use among females. The authors note that youth who experienced sexual victimization use substances at higher rates and may use them to cope with the trauma related to the experience of victimization.

Research using a sample of 137 homeless female adolescents, ages 14–21 from the Midwestern United States, found that though alcohol use was not a significant correlate of sexual victimization, adolescent females who had more frequent marijuana use experienced higher rates of sexual victimization (Tyler et al., 2013). Though marijuana use was modeled in this study as the dependent variable, the study was cross-sectional; thus, marijuana may have led to sexual victimization, but the reverse is also plausible (Tyler et al., 2013).

A study based in Seattle examined correlates of sexual victimization among 372 homeless youth ages 13–21 years. The results of this study revealed that 35% of the sample had been sexually victimized. Male acquaintances were the main perpetrators of sexual violence against females (41%), whereas male strangers were the main sexual perpetrators for victimized males. In terms of outcomes, the authors found that sexual victimization was associated with the use of illicit drugs but only among females (Tyler et al., 2004).

Finally, a recent review of 23 studies by Heerde and Hemphill (2016) revealed that only four studies out of a possible 23 investigated the association between substance use and sexual victimization. Of these four studies, alcohol, marijuana, and stimulants were the most frequently reported substances. Overall, their review showed that substance use was associated with sexual victimization, but the authors note that the direction of these relationships remains ambiguous given the cross-sectional nature of the studies. Moreover, Heerde and Hemphill note that studies examining the link between substance use and sexual victimization are scarce indicating the need for more research in this area.

Mental and Physical Health

Research on mental and physical health issues as outcomes of sexual victimization has focused on depression, post-traumatic stress disorder (PTSD), self-mutilation, and general mental and physical health functioning. The first study, by D'Ercole and Struening (1990), conducted in-depth structured interviews with a representative sample of 141 homeless women staying in shelters in New York City. The majority of their sample was African American (67%), and the overall median age was 31 years. The authors measured depressive symptoms using the 20-item CES-D scale (Radloff, 1977), as well as a 7-item adapted scale to measure psychoticism over the past year. Though the authors used a combined scale of sexual and physical victimization, they also looked at recent sexual harassment. Results from correlational analysis revealed that both depressive and psychotic symptoms were positively associated with sexual victimization (D'Ercole & Struening, 1990).

A probability study of 974 adult homeless women examined the association between rape and physical and mental health using a 45-min structured interview (Wenzel et al., 2000). Just over half (56%) of their sample was African American, and 13% of women reported being raped in the previous year. Their results showed that women who were raped reported overall poorer general health, more gynecological symptoms, more serious physical health symptoms, and more likely to have had at least one physical health limitation. Moreover, women who had been raped reported more depression in the past year and more psychological distress in the past month compared to women who had not been raped. These results remained significant even when controlling for potential confounders at the multivariate level (e.g., age, education, ethnicity, recruitment site). Though cross-sectional, this study highlights the association between rape and numerous physical and mental health limitations (Wenzel et al., 2000).

The relationship between victimization and mental health functioning has also been examined among homeless youth and adults. Rattelade et al. (2014) conducted interviews with 325 homeless youth and adults; the average age was 39 for adults and 19 for youth. The authors used a mental health summary measure, which consisted of four subscales on vitality, social functioning, emotional role, and mental health. Twenty-eight percent of the total sample experienced child sexual abuse with females being significantly more likely to have had this experience than males. Taken together, however, rates of child sexual abuse did not differ between homeless adults and youth. Multiple victimization experiences also were reported by 39% of the sample. Their results showed that those who experienced child sexual abuse had lower mental health scores than those without this experience. Having a recent experience of victimization, however, was not associated with mental health functioning. The authors note that the lack of significant findings between adults and youth is surprising and conclude that perhaps it is not current age but rather age at time of victimization that matters for mental health. This cross-sectional study did not solely examine sexual victimization; thus, its relationship with mental health could not be determined in this study (Rattelade et al., 2014).

The following study focused on female veterans. Decker, Rosenheck, Tsai, Hoff, and Harpaz-Roitem (2013) interviewed 509 homeless female veterans including those with and without a history of military sexual assault. The majority of their sample (66%) were racial/ethnic minorities with a mean age of 43 years. Overall, the authors found that 41% of female veterans reported a history of military sexual assault. Those who reported having this experience were more likely to have lower self-esteem and greater past year victimization (though victimization combined physical and sexual items). Their results revealed that having experienced military sexual assault was associated with greater severity of PTSD and other psychiatric symptoms. Given that our search only yielded one study on female veterans that met our inclusion criteria, more research on this population is needed.

The final study examined the association between sexual victimization and self-injurious behavior (e.g., intentionally cutting oneself) using a 16-item scale of self-injury among a sample of 172 homeless young adults, ages 19–26. Results of this study revealed that those who experienced more sexual victimization while on the street were likely to report engaging in a greater number of self-injurious behaviors compared to those young adults with fewer experiences of sexual assault (Tyler, Melander, & Almazan, 2010). The authors found no significant differences in self-injurious behavior between males and females and attribute this to the similar levels of stress that homeless males and females likely experience due to meeting daily survival needs over and above those associated with gender.

HIV Risk Behaviors

Only four studies were found that looked at HIV risk behavior and its relationship with sexual victimization. Though definitions vary somewhat, HIV risk behavior may include having numerous sexual partners, unprotected sex, concurrent sex, and trading sex for specific items such as food or shelter (Harris et al., 2017; Melander & Tyler, 2010). Using a large sample of 966 homeless youth 14–24 years of age, Harris et al. found that for males, experiencing sexual victimization prior to being homeless was positively associated with numerous HIV risk behaviors including multiple partners, unprotected vaginal sex, unprotected anal sex, and exchanging sex for food, money, drugs, a place to stay, or any other commodity. They also found support for mediation effects: use of cocaine and crack served as mediators between sexual victimization and concurrent sex among males. For females, sexual victimization was positively associated with concurrent sex and unprotected vaginal sex. Harris et al. also found one mediating effect for females: PTSD mediated the relationship between sexual victimization and exchanging sex for specific items. Overall, the pathways from sexual victimization to HIV risk behavior differed significantly for males and females.

A second study by Melander and Tyler (2010) examined the relationship between sexual victimization and HIV risk behaviors among 172 homeless young adults, ages 19–26 years. Their results revealed that those who experienced more sexual victimization on the street were more likely to have engaged in more types of HIV risk behaviors, such as having a greater number of sexual partners, an earlier age at first voluntary sexual intercourse, and ever having traded sex or engaged in prostitution.

Based on a sample of 372 homeless youth (ages 13–21) in Seattle, Tyler et al. (2004) found that over one-third of their sample had been sexually victimized with the rate more than double among females (23%) compared to males (11%). In terms of HIV risk behavior, the authors examined the exchange of sex for specific items of necessity. Their results revealed that exchanging sex was a significant correlate of sexual victimization for both male and female adolescents.

A final study looking at HIV risk behavior was based on data from 150 homeless youth in the Midwest where Tyler and Schmitz (2018) examined the relationship between sexual victimization and the likelihood of these youth trading sex for specific items of necessity. Their results showed that for each additional type of sexual victimization homeless youth experienced while on the street, their odds of trading sex for food, money, drugs, and shelter increased by 106%, 66%, 125%, and 147%, respectively. Given the cross-sectional nature of this study, it is also possible that youth who lack basic necessities and resort to trading sex are also at high risk for being a victim of sexual assault.

Revictimization

Early life experiences including being a victim of child sexual abuse can pave the way to future victimization. Among general population studies, research finds that individuals with a history of childhood sexual abuse are at much greater risk of experiencing revictimization as an adult (Aosved, Long, & Voller, 2011; Elliott, Mok, & Briere, 2004). For example, Messman-Moore et al. found that approximately 30% of child sexual abuse victims experienced subsequent rape as an adolescent or adult (Messman-Moore, Walsh, & DiLillo, 2010). Moreover, according to Browne (1993), women who suffer repeat victimization may experience long-term negative outcomes such as "emotional numbing, extreme passivity, and helplessness" (1993, p. 375). Specifically, early victimization may decrease social support networks of those who have been victimized and thus increase their risk of becoming homeless at some future time point (Browne, 1993). Though child sexual abuse is a risk factor rather than outcome, below we review studies that examine the link between early sexual abuse and subsequent sexual revictimization given that research finds that the strongest and most consistent risk factor for sexual victimization in both general population studies and studies on homeless adolescents and adults is a history of child sexual abuse.

In terms of revictimization, the first study focused on adult homeless women. Hudson et al. (2010) examined the likelihood of sexual revictimization among 202 homeless women residing in shelters or living on the street in the Skid Row area of Los Angeles. Twenty-nine percent of these women have been raped and 31% have been sexually harassed as adults. Moreover, 22% reported being raped prior to the age of 18. Results from logistic regression analyses revealed that those women who reported rape as a child were 3.88 times more likely to have been sexually assaulted as an adult. Additionally, women who reported engaging in trading sex at any point in their lifetime, another form of sexual victimization (Tyler & Schmitz, 2018), were over three times more likely to have been sexually assaulted as an adult. This study reveals the strong link between early sexual trauma and risk for subsequent sexual assault in the lives of homeless adult women.

Additionally, four studies focused on samples of homeless young adults. Edalati et al. (2016) gathered data from 500 homeless young adults 19–25 years of age, 39% of whom were female. The authors sampled from three different cities in British Columbia, Canada. Their results revealed that 29% of young adults had experienced sexual victimization, which included "rape, forced sexual advances or non-consensual sexual acts" (2016, p. 2496). Additionally, Edalati et al. found that child sexual abuse was strongly associated with adult sexual victimization, controlling for other types of child abuse. No significant gender interactions were found in the effect of child maltreatment and adult victimization. Though there were no differences between men and women regarding adult victimization, this study found strong support for the link between early sexual abuse and subsequent sexual revictimization. Three remaining studies, all of which focused on homeless young adults 19–26 years of age, all found a positive association between child sexual abuse and experiencing a greater amount of sexual victimization while on the street regardless of control variables used (Melander & Tyler, 2010; Tyler et al., 2004; Tyler & Melander, 2015).

The following study combined youth and adults into a single sample. Though Rattelade et al.'s (2014) sample of 325 homeless youth and adults did not examine sexual victimization as an adult, they did find that 28% of their total sample experienced child sexual abuse, 64% reported being victimized, and 10% reported a recent victimization experience though the specific form of victimization could not be disentangled. Overall, 39% experienced multiple victimizations. Though the exact form of victimization is unknown, it is relevant that their results show a considerable risk for revictimization when exposed to child sexual abuse.

The remaining study, which focused only on female homeless adolescents (Tyler et al., 2013), found a positive correlation between a history of child sexual abuse and experiencing more sexual victimization while on the street.

Summary

Most studies on sexual victimization among homeless populations have focused on risk factors rather than outcomes. Of those studies that have examined outcomes of sexual assault, we included four main areas: substance use/abuse, mental and physical health, HIV risk behaviors, and sexual revictimization. Overall, the results from the studies included in this review are generally consistent in finding that those who experienced sexual abuse as a child are at greater risk for being revictimized and that sexual assault is associated with numerous negative health outcomes, regardless of respondent age (i.e., youth versus adult), geographic location (e.g., west coast versus the Midwest), and sample size (e.g., $n = 150$ versus $n = 500$). Though fewer studies examined sexual victimization among men, results from these studies show that men also have this experience, though their prevalence of sexual victimization is lower than the rate for women.

In considering the overall findings in this review, the reader should keep in mind that these studies are cross-sectional and even though sexual victimization was generally viewed as an independent variable in studies, it is feasible that sexual victimization was an *outcome* of one of the four areas examined (e.g., HIV risk behaviors). Cross-sectional studies cannot generally determine the direction of causation. Also, the results should be interpreted in the context of a particular study. That is, some studies included respondents from shelters (e.g., D'Ercole & Struening, 1990), whereas other studies included respondents from both shelter and the street (e.g., Tyler & Melander, 2015). Definitions of what constitutes child sexual abuse and street sexual victimization also varied. These issues as well as additional limitations are discussed below.

Limitations of Existing Research

Though there are limitations to the studies reviewed in this paper, it is important to keep in mind that homeless people are a difficult group to sample, to study, and to follow longitudinally (Wright, Allen, & Devine, 1995) given their nomadic lifestyle (Tyler & Whitbeck, 2004) and their multiple housing transitions (Tyler & Schmitz, 2013). Study limitations are organized into the following categories: samples, study design, measures, and theory.

Samples

Though three studies included only adult homeless women or female youth, most of the research included large enough numbers of males and females to allow for gender comparisons (see, e.g., the Harris et al., 2017 comparison of male and female homeless youth on HIV risk behaviors). Given that the majority of sexual abuse victims tend to be female, focusing only on young women is not necessarily a limitation. However, a group in which more research is needed includes that of lesbian, gay, bisexual, and transgender (LGBT) homeless youth and adults. Given that recent research has found that this group of homeless young people experience higher rates of child sexual abuse and more street sexual victimization compared to heterosexual homeless youth (Tyler & Schmitz, 2018), this is a subsample of the homeless population in need of further study. Although there has been more research on LGBT homeless youth in the past 10–15 years (e.g., Gattis, 2013; Rew, Whittaker, Taylor-Seehafer, & Smith, 2005; Tyler & Schmitz, 2018; Whitbeck, Chen, Hoyt, Tyler, &

Johnson, 2004), the samples generally are not large enough to examine lesbians or gays, for example, individually. Thus, most research has combined sexual minority youth (regardless of gender) into a single group.

Another potential concern regarding sampling is that although studies combine a wide range of age groups such as 13–24 years, some studies do not control for age in their analyses. For example, it is possible that some older youth have been on the street for longer periods of time and may have different experiences from those who are new to the street. Also, those who have been on the street for a longer time may also have more knowledge about obtaining resources such as shelter, social services, and other essentials. Thus, their risk for victimization may be lower compared to those with little street knowledge who might be younger. Though studies include a wide age range, this can be managed by controlling for age or testing for age interactions between different developmental age groups.

Study Design

The studies included in this review, as is typical with most of the research on homeless populations, are cross-sectional. Though these studies allow researchers to make claims about associations between variables such as that of sexual victimization and substance use, we cannot ascertain from these studies which event came first. That is, some homeless individuals may be using substances to cope with sexual victimization and other traumas (Kidd & Carroll, 2007), but it is also possible that using substances occurred prior to a victimization episode. Alternatively, it is also conceivable that sexual victimization and substance use occurred simultaneously. Moreover, cross-sectional studies that use retrospective reporting cannot determine *which* sexual victimization experience was associated with a specific drinking or drug use episode. As such, we can only conclude that sexual victimization is *associated* with a range of factors including substance use, poorer mental and physical health, HIV risk behavior, and revictimization among homeless youth and adults.

Measures

Another limitation is that different definitions were used to measure child sexual abuse and street sexual victimization; therefore, the prevalence rates vary. For example, some studies used detailed questions about sexual abuse (see, e.g., Hudson et al., 2010), while others left the definition up to the respondent (e.g., did you experience sexual abuse while you were a child?). This is problematic given that prior research comparing these two formats (i.e., detailed questions versus single item) has found that when the definition is left up to the respondent (i.e., single item), they are more likely to underreport child sexual abuse (Tyler & Melander, 2009). Specifically, Tyler and Melander (2009) found a discrepant reporting rate of 38% for noncontact sexual abuse and a 27% discrepant reporting rate for contact sexual abuse indicating that the way questions are asked influences prevalence rates. Another limitation is that some studies combined sexual, physical, and emotional abuse into a single measure of child abuse; therefore, the individual effects of child sexual abuse could not be examined. Relatedly, some of the studies examined here also combined both physical and sexual street victimizations into a single measure, so we were unable to examine the specific outcomes for these studies.

Theory

The final area of limitations surrounds the use of theory. Though we outlined four theories that have been previously used to examine the link between child abuse and revictimization among both homeless and general population samples, only one of these theories was utilized by the studies in this review. Moreover, several of the studies reviewed here did not include any theory. As a result, they are unable to explain their findings in a larger context making it more difficult for other researchers to build upon their work. The theories that were used in the current review included the risk amplification model, victimization theories (e.g., lifestyle exposure theory), and a social stress framework. These three theories were used to explain the link between early child abuse and subsequent sexual victimization. Given the lack of theory in the studies examined, this is an area for future research.

Future Research Priorities

There are several research priorities which we believe will improve research in this area and continue to move the field forward. First, more innovative methods are needed to improve data collection with homeless populations and to better understand their experiences. Given that homeless individuals are regularly on the move, using cell phones to collect data from them seems a worthy endeavor. Recent work tested the feasibility of using cell phones to collect daily data from homeless youth over a 30-day period (Tyler & Olson, 2018). Their results revealed that on average, homeless youth completed almost 19 days of texts, but 30% of youth had texting data on 28 or more days (out of 30). Moreover, youth answered an average of 8.49 texts per day (out of a possible 11), and 73% of youth reported that responding to texts was very easy or somewhat easy (Tyler & Olson, 2018). Work by Freedman and colleagues (2006) tested the feasibility of cell phones and automated telephone interviewing to collect daily data from 30 homeless crack cocaine-addicted adults in treatment; 80% of adults completed the full 2 weeks of data collection. These results reveal that using cell phones to collect real-time data from homeless populations is feasible. Moreover, this type of data collection can be used to address issues of time ordering regarding the link between street sexual victimization and substance use.

A second priority for future research is the use of multiple item scales (standardized if possible) so that prevalence rates can be compared across studies. Relatedly, studies should avoid combining different forms of victimization into a single measure as previous research finds that the association between child abuse and street victimization varies by type (i.e., child sexual abuse versus child physical abuse; Tyler & Melander, 2015).

Third, future studies need to incorporate theory so that they can justify the inclusion of study variables and offer context for how their findings fit into a larger picture. This will also help future researchers build upon their work in this area. Moreover, the use of theory will aid in providing a more holistic understanding of the life histories of homeless individuals as well as their present situation and future prospects.

Fourth, more research is needed on the topic of sexual victimization and both short- and long-term outcomes. Heerde and Hemphill (2016), for example, noted that studies examining the link between substance use and sexual victimization were scarce, recalling that their review of the literature only yielded four studies on this topic, making this an area ripe for future studies. Additionally, given that our search only yielded one study on homeless female veterans that met our inclusion criteria, and the high rates of sexual assault that many of these women experienced while in the military (Decker et al., 2013), this is another subgroup in which further research is warranted.

Finally, there are numerous other negative outcomes that have yet to be explored within a homeless population. Some of these outcomes are difficult to study (e.g., suicide), and others are challenging given the difficulties of longitudinally studying homeless populations (Wright et al., 1995). Despite this, fruitful areas for future research regarding outcomes of sexual violence include suicide ideation, loss of education (dropping out of school), loss of employment and income, reduced long-term life chances, difficulties in family formation, marital disruption and dissolution, gang involvement, adult criminality, and incarceration.

Implications and Future Policy

When we consider the policy implications of the research we have reviewed, two separate concerns come to mind: (1) how to reduce or eliminate sexual violence against homeless individuals in the first place and (2) how to mitigate the effects of sexual violence on long-term outcomes once the violence has occurred.

One approach to (1) would be to eliminate homelessness altogether. If there were no homeless people, no sexual violence could be perpetrated against them. This, unfortunately, is unrealistic. The current wave of homelessness began in the late 1970s and has been with us for a half-century. Very little evidence suggests that the problem is abating. Many forces in the political economy of capitalism create homelessness despite efforts to reduce or eliminate it, among them the recurring crisis in low-income or "affordable" housing, wage stagnation, and an inadequate social safety net. Homelessness will be with us for the long run.

How, then, might we reduce the violence (sexual or otherwise) committed against homeless individuals? This too is a difficult proposition since by definition, homeless people live in environments that make them vulnerable to predation. If we put homeless people in safe, stable, permanent housing, then they would no longer be homeless. The so-called Housing First model (Tsemberis, 2010) would do exactly that (Housing First defers providing services to homeless individuals until they are stably housed and has been the official federal homeless policy for about a decade), and as Housing First expands to more and more cities, we should begin to see some decline in the violence that (formerly) homeless people experience. But Housing First is no panacea, is costly, and is not nearly as successful as its proponents sometimes claim (Groton, 2013).

Homeless people experience violence at elevated rates because they are often perceived as valueless, contemptible human beings. Massey (2008) argues that people carry around cognitive schemas in their heads that sort others into categories (usually stereotypical categories) and that these schemas form the basis of social stratification (the unequal distribution of wealth, income, power, prestige, or other valued items). These schemas, Massey argues, are aligned across the two dimensions of competence and warmth. Persons and groups perceived as both warm and competent define our "esteemed in-group," the people to whom we feel attracted, people we respect. The warm but incompetent are the "pitied outgroup"—the disabled, the elderly, and the mentally challenged. Those neither warm nor competent are the "despised outgroup." "Being neither likable nor capable, people within these outgroups are socially despised, and the dominant emotion is disgust" (2008:13). In modern American (and most other) societies, the chronically homeless are a "despised outgroup" and therefore subject to all manner of dehumanization, including being subject to sexual victimization and degradation.

Stigma is inherent in the process of dehumanization, and homeless individuals are a heavily stigmatized group (Belcher & DeForge, 2012; Phelan, Link, Moore, & Stueve, 1997). Some people stigmatize the homeless because they are smelly and ill-kempt; others may stigmatize them because, as Ronald Reagan put it, "many are, well, we might say, homeless by choice." In this view, the miseries of homelessness are self-inflicted, and that makes them beneath contempt. The results of this contempt include the well-documented practice of bum-bashing (where homeless people are set upon, beaten, and otherwise violated just because they are homeless) and the patterns of sexual and physical abuse documented earlier. Here the apparent antidote is the recognition that homeless people are, first and foremost, people—each with his or her own history, talents, desires and aspirations—and this too seems unlikely in what seems to be an increasingly intolerant age. We are left, then, with policies to mitigate the effects of violence once it has occurred. Promising developments on this front include Safe Housing Partnerships, the body of interventions known as Housing First, so-called Trauma-Informed Shelters, and a policy known as Rapid Rehousing.

Safe Housing Partnerships are intended to prevent abused women from becoming homeless. Approximately three homeless women in four have experienced violence in their homes, and about one in four cites domestic violence as the cause of their current homeless episode (Jasinski et al., 2010). Thus, if we could prevent victimized women from becoming homeless, we would make a significant dent in the overall homeless problem. Safe Housing Partnerships attempt to achieve this goal with "flexible funding" and "intensive mobile advocacy." Flexible funding provides access to immediate funds that keep victimized women in their homes; advocacy provides the necessary support and direction. Many partnerships embrace some version of a housing resource center to help victims locate and obtain safe housing. Many are also linked to:

Rapid Rehousing programs attempt to get victims out of the shelters and back into safe, stable housing as rapidly as possible. Rapid rehousing is an acknowledgment that extended stays in domestic violence and homeless shelters, which many victims turn to for short-term safety and relief, are not therapeutic, and probably create as many problems as they solve (e.g., extended shelter stays promote dependency, interfere with job searches, and erode self-esteem; see Housing and Urban Development, 2013), although shelter operators often disagree with this assessment). These programs attempt to stabilize victims quickly and get them back into stable housing.

Unfortunately, both Safe Housing Partnerships and Rapid Rehousing are relatively recent policy innovations. Evaluation studies that would demonstrate their efficacy are at best embryonic. Both seem like "good ideas" but have yet to attain the status of "best practice."

Housing First is also a fairly recent policy initiative that recognizes that homeless people, including homeless trauma victims, need safe, stable housing more than they need shelter, counseling, or treatment for mental health and substance abuse disorders (Padgett, Gulcur, & Tsemberis, 2006; Stergiopoulos et al., 2015). Housing First recognizes that victims of violence often face discrimination in housing markets and acknowledges that safe, stable, and permanent housing is often the best defense against future violence, another proposition yet to be systematically investigated in the evaluation research literature.

Trauma-Informed Shelters recognize that most homeless women (and some homeless men) are seeking shelter mainly as relief from violent home situations and that the proper care of such people requires more than a hot meal and a place to sleep for a few nights. Most homeless people have clearly been exposed to trauma of various kinds, so trauma-informed care can be recommended as a paradigm for all homeless services. Alas, "there is no consensus on a definition that clearly explains the nature of [trauma-informed care]" (Hopper, Bassuk, & Olivet, 2010, p. 80). Key elements of a definition include awareness of the extent of trauma in homeless peoples' lives and an understanding of its effects, an emphasis on safety and on assisting victims to rebuild control, and a strengths-based vs. needs-based approach to intervention. And yet here as in most other places, "We do not know whether trauma-informed services are effective specifically within homeless services" (Hopper et al., 2010, p. 87). Much the same as rapid rehousing, safe housing partnerships, and Housing First, trauma-informed care seems like a "good idea," but firm evidence on its effectiveness as an intervention is lacking.

To conclude, it is obvious beyond all doubt that homeless individuals, particularly homeless women, suffer from sexual assault and violence at starkly elevated rates and that these experiences generate life-long and strongly negative outcomes. There are many good reasons to intervene in the ongoing homelessness crisis on both the private and public sides, and alleviating the short-term miseries and long-term outcomes of sexual assault and violence is surely one of them. But increasingly, a societal commitment to being rid of homelessness once and for all has become the dues we are asked to pay for our membership in the community of civilized nations.

References

Aosved, A. C., Long, P. J., & Voller, E. K. (2011). Sexual revictimization and adjustment in college men. *Psychology of Men & Masculinity, 12*, 285–296.

Bandura, A. (1977). *Social learning theory*. Englewood Cliffs, NJ: Prentice Hall.

Belcher, J. R., & DeForge, B. R. (2012). Social stigma and homelessness: The limits of social change. *Journal of Human Behavior in the Social Environment, 22*, 929–946.

Bender, K., Brown, S. M., Thompson, S. J., Ferguson, K. M., & Langenderfer, L. (2015). Multiple victimizations before and after leaving home associated with PTSD, depression, and substance use disorder among homeless youth. *Child Maltreatment, 20*, 115–124.

Bevan, E., & Higgins, D. J. (2002). Is domestic violence learned? The contribution of five forms of child maltreatment to men's violence and adjustment. *Journal of Family Violence, 17*, 223–245.

Browne, A. (1993). Family violence and homelessness: The relevance of trauma histories in the lives of homeless women. *American Journal of Orthopsychiatry, 63*, 370–384.

D'Ercole, A., & Struening, E. (1990). Victimization among homeless women: Implications for service delivery. *Journal of Community Psychology, 18*, 141–152.

Decker, S., Rosenheck, R., Tsai, J., Hoff, R., & Harpaz-Roitem, I. (2013). Military sexual assault and homeless women veterans: Clinical correlates and treatment preferences. *Women's Health Issues, 23*, e373–e380.

Desai, S., Arias I., Thompson, M.P., and Basile, K.C. (2002). Childhood victimization and subsequent adult revictimization assessed in a nationally representative sample of women and men. Violence & Victims, 17, 639–653

Edalati, H., Krausz, M., & Schütz, C. G. (2016). Childhood maltreatment and revictimization in a homeless population. *Journal of Interpersonal Violence, 31*, 2492–2512.

Elliott, D. M., Mok, D. S., & Briere, J. (2004). Adult sexual assault: Prevalence, symptomatology, and sex differences in the general population. *Journal of Traumatic Stress, 17*, 203–211.

Finkelhor, D., & Browne, A. (1985). The traumatic impact of child sexual abuse: A conceptualization. *American Journal of Orthopsychiatry, 55*, 530–541.

Finkelhor, D., & Browne, A. (1988). Child sexual abuse: A review and conceptualization. In G. T. Hotaling, D. Finkelhor, J. T. Kirkpatrick, & M. A. Straus (Eds.), *Family abuse and its consequences: New directions in research* (pp. 270–284). Newbury Park, CA: Sage.

Foshee, V. A., Bauman, K. E., & Linder, G. F. (1999). Family violence and the perpetration of adolescent dating violence: Examining social learning and social control processes. *Journal of Marriage and the Family, 61*, 331–342.

Gattis, M. N. (2013). An ecological systems comparison between homeless sexual minority youths and homeless heterosexual youths. *Journal of Social Service Research, 39*, 38–49.

Gelles, R. J. (1997). *Intimate violence in families* (3rd ed.). Thousand Oaks, CA: Sage Publications.

Groton, D. (2013). Are housing first programs effective? A research note. *Journal of Sociology and Social Welfare, 40*, 51–63.

Harris, T., Rice, E., Rhoades, H., Winetrobe, H., & Wenzel, S. (2017). Gender differences in the path from sexual victimization to HIV risk behavior among homeless youth. *Journal of Child Sexual Abuse, 26*(3), 334–351.

Heerde, J., & Hemphill, S. (2016). Sexual risk behaviors, sexual offenses, and sexual victimization among homeless youth: A systematic review of associations with substance use. *Trauma, Violence & Abuse, 17*, 468–489.

Henry, M., Watt, R., Rosenthal, L., Shivji, A., & Abt Associates. (2017). *Part 1: Point-in-time estimates of homelessness: The 2017 annual homeless assessment report (AHAR) to congress, December 2017*. Retrieved from https://www.hudexchange.info/resources/documents/2017-AHAR-Part-1.pdf.

Hopper, E. K., Bassuk, E. L., & Olivet, J. (2010). Shelter from the storm: Trauma-informed care in homelessness services settings. *The Open Health Services and Policy Journal, 3*, 80–100.

Housing and Urban Development. (2013). *Homeless Prevention and Rapid Rehousing Program (HPRP): Year 2 Summary*. Washington, DC: HUD. Retrieved from https://www.hudexchange.info/resources/documents/HPRP_Year2Summary.pdf.

Hudson, A., Wright, K., Bhattacharya, D., Sinha, K., Nyamathi, A., & Marfisee, M. (2010). Correlates of adult assault among homeless women. *Journal of Health Care for the Poor and Undeserved, 21*, 1250–1262.

Jasinski, J. L., Wesely, J. K., Wright, J. D., & Mustaine, E. E. (2010). *Hard lives, mean streets: Violence in the lives of homeless women*. Boston: Northeastern University Press.

Kaukinen, C. (2014). Dating violence among college students: The risk and protective factors. *Trauma, Violence & Abuse, 15*, 283–296.

Kidd, S. A., & Carroll, M. R. (2007). Coping and suicidality among homeless youth. *Journal of Adolescence, 30*, 283–296.

Lee, B. A., Tyler, K. A., & Wright, J. D. (2010). The new homeless revisited. *Annual Review of Sociology, 36*, 501–521.

Massey, D. (2008). *Categorically unequal: The American stratification system*. New York: Russell Sage Foundation.

McNaughton Reyes, H. L., Foshee, V. A., Niolon, P. H., Reidy, D. E., & Hall, J. E. (2016). Gender role attitudes and male adolescent dating violence perpetration: Normative beliefs as moderators. *Journal of Youth and Adolescence, 45*, 350–360.

Melander, L. A., & Tyler, K. A. (2010). The effect of early maltreatment, victimization, and partner violence on

HIV risk behavior among homeless young adults. *Journal of Adolescent Health, 47*, 575–581.
Messman-Moore, T. L., Walsh, K. L., & DiLillo, D. (2010). Emotion dysregulation and risky sexual behavior in revictimization. *Child Abuse & Neglect, 34*, 967–976.
National Network for Youth. (2018). *How many homeless youth are in America*? Retrieved from https://www.nn4youth.org/learn/how-many-homeless/.
Nyamathi, A., Leake, B., & Gelberg, L. (2000). Sheltered versus nonsheltered homeless women: Differences in health, behavior, victimization, and utilization of care. *Journal of General Internal Medicine, 15*, 565–572.
Owens, D. J., & Straus, M. A. (1975). The social structure of violence in childhood and approval of violence as an adult. *Aggressive Behavior, 1*, 193–211.
Padgett, D. K., Gulcur, L., & Tsemberis, S. (2006). Housing First services for people who are homeless with co-occurring serious mental illness and substance abuse. *Research on Social Work Practice, 16*, 74–83.
Phelan, J., Link, B. G., Moore, R. E., & Stueve, A. (1997). The stigma of homelessness. The impact of the label "homeless" on attitudes toward poor persons. *Social Psychology Quarterly, 60*, 323–337.
Radloff, L. S. (1977). The CES-D scale: A self-report depression scale for research in the general population. *Applied Psychological Measurement, 1*, 385–401.
Rattelade, S., Farrell, S., Aubry, T., & Klodawsky, F. (2014). The relationship between victimization and mental health functioning in homeless youth and adults. *Journal of Interpersonal Violence, 29*, 1606–1622.
Rew, L., Whittaker, T. A., Taylor-Seehafer, M. A., & Smith, L. R. (2005). Sexual health risks and protective resources in gay, lesbian, and bisexual, and heterosexual homeless youth. *Journal for Specialists in Pediatric Nursing, 10*, 11–19.
Simons, R. L., & Whitbeck, L. B. (1991). Sexual abuse as a precursor to prostitution and victimization among adolescent and adult homeless women. *Journal of Family Issues, 12*, 361–379.
Smith, S. G., Chen, J., Basile, K. C., Gilbert, L. K., Merrick, M. T., Patel, N., … Jain, A. (2017). *The National Intimate Partner and Sexual Violence Survey (NISVS): 2010–2012 State Report*. Atlanta, GA: National Center for Injury Prevention and Control, Centers for Disease Control and Prevention.
Stergiopoulos, V., Hwang, W. W., Gozdick, A., Nisenbaum, R., Latimer, E., Rabouin, D., … Goering, P. N. (2015). Effect of scattered-site housing using rent supplements and intensive case management on housing stability among homeless adults with mental illness: A randomized trial. *Journal of the American Medical Association, 313*, 905–915.
Straus, M., & Gelles, R. J. (1990). *Physical violence in American families*. New Brunswick, NJ: Transaction.
Straus, M. A., Douglas, E. M., & Medeiros, R. A. (2013). *The primordial violence: Spanking children, psychological development, violence, and crime*. New York: Routledge.
Temple, J. R., Shorey, R. C., Tortolero, S. R., Wolfe, D. A., & Stuart, G. L. (2013). Importance of gender and attitudes about violence in the relationship between exposure to interparental violence and the perpetration of teen dating violence. *Child Abuse & Neglect, 37*, 343–352.
Tsemberis, S. (2010). *Housing First: The pathways model to end homelessness for people with mental health and substance abuse disorders*. New York: Hazelden.
Turner, H. A., Finkelhor, D., & Ormrod, R. (2010). The effects of adolescent victimization on self-concept and depressive symptoms. *Child Maltreatment, 15*, 76–90.
Tyler, K., & Olson, K. (2018). Examining the feasibility of ecological momentary assessment using short message service surveying with homeless youth: Lessons learned. *Field Methods, 30*, 91–104.
Tyler, K., & Schmitz, R. (2013). Family histories and multiple transitions among homeless young adults: Pathways to homelessness. *Children and Youth Services Review, 35*, 1719–1726.
Tyler, K., & Schmitz, R. (2018). A comparison of risk factors for various forms of trauma in the lives of lesbian, gay, bisexual and heterosexual homeless youth. *Journal of Trauma & Dissociation, 19*, 431–443.
Tyler, K. A. (2002). Social and emotional outcomes of childhood sexual abuse: A review of recent research. *Aggression and Violent Behavior, 7*, 567–589.
Tyler, K. A., & Beal, M. R. (2010). The high-risk environment of homeless young adults: Consequences for physical and sexual victimization. *Violence and Victims, 25*, 101–115.
Tyler, K. A., & Cauce, A. M. (2002). Perpetrators of early physical and sexual abuse among homeless and runaway adolescents. *Child Abuse & Neglect, 26*, 1261–1274.
Tyler, K. A., Gervais, S. J., & Davidson, M. M. (2013). The relationship between victimization and substance use among homeless and runaway female adolescents. *Journal of Interpersonal Violence, 28*, 474–493.
Tyler, K. A., & Melander, L. A. (2009). Discrepancies in reporting of physical and sexual abuse among homeless youth. *Journal of Child Sexual Abuse, 18*, 513–531.
Tyler, K. A., & Melander, L. A. (2015). Child abuse, street victimization, and substance use among homeless young adults. *Youth & Society, 47*, 502–519.
Tyler, K. A., Melander, L. A., & Almazan, E. (2010). Self-injurious behavior among homeless young adults: A social stress analysis. *Social Science & Medicine, 70*, 269–276.
Tyler, K. A., & Whitbeck, L. B. (2004). Lost childhoods: Risk and resiliency among runaway and homeless adolescents. In P. Allen-Meares & M. W. Fraser (Eds.), *Intervention with children & adolescents: An interdisciplinary perspective* (pp. 378–397). Boston, MA, Pearson Education.
Tyler, K. A., Whitbeck, L. B., Hoyt, D. R., & Cauce, A. M. (2004). Risk factors for sexual victimization among male and female homeless and runaway youth. *Journal of Interpersonal Violence, 19*, 503–520.

Wenzel, S. L., Leake, B. D., & Gelberg, L. (2000). Health of homeless women with recent experienced of rape. *Journal of General Internal Medicine, 15*, 265–268.

Whitbeck, L. B., Chen, X., Hoyt, D. R., Tyler, K. A., & Johnson, K. D. (2004). Mental disorder, subsistence strategies, and victimization among gay, lesbian, and bisexual homeless and runaway adolescents. *The Journal of Sex Research, 41*, 329–342.

Whitbeck, L. B., Hoyt, D. R., & Yoder, K. A. (1999). A risk-amplification model of victimization and depressive symptoms among runaway and homeless adolescents. *American Journal of Community Psychology, 27*, 273–296.

Widom, C. S., Czaja, A. J., & Dutton, M. A. (2008). Childhood victimization and lifetime revictimization. *Child Abuse & Neglect, 32*, 785–796.

Wright, J. D., Allen, T. L., & Devine, J. A. (1995). Tracking non-traditional populations in longitudinal studies. *Evaluation and Program Planning, 18*, 267–277.

Military Sexual Assault

42

Michelle L. Bourgeois and Brian P. Marx

Background and History

Awareness of military sexual assault (MSA) and sexual trauma has increased significantly in the last several decades. These issues first came into the national spotlight in 1992, following the sexual harassment and/or assault of 87 female and seven male soldiers by Navy and Marine Corps officers at the 35th Annual Tailhook Association Symposium in Las Vegas, Nevada (Sughrue, 2013). This event highlighted the dangerous intersection of deeply entrenched components of military culture, including hypermasculinity, strict adherence to rank and authority structures (often male dominated), and alcohol use, which interacted to promote an environment of hostility and aggression towards women. An investigation by the Inspector General of the U.S. Department of Defense (DoD) directly led to policy revisions allowing women to serve in many combat assignments throughout the armed forces, a crucial move to establish gender equality and promote authority and respect for military women. In addition, the Sexual Assault Prevention and Response Office (SAPRO) was created in 2004 to improve sexual assault prevention, survivor support and advocacy, and reporting and accountability for sexual crimes. Still, major incidents of sexual assault continue to occur at alarming rates in the military and highlight the need to better understand, prevent, and treat MSA.

This chapter provides an overview of MSA, beginning with operational definitions of MSA and related phenomena (e.g., military sexual harassment, military sexual trauma); their measurement in active-duty service members, reservists, and veterans; as well as prevalence estimates. Next, we will examine the impact of MSA on survivors by focusing on the known psychological, physical, and psychosocial correlates. Finally, we will present current psychotherapeutic treatments for MSA and related psychological conditions and discuss prevention efforts.

Definition

Military sexual trauma broadly includes any sexual assault or harassment that occurs during military service, including during active-duty service, active-duty training, and inactive-duty training. Historically, definitions of military sexual trauma have been inconsistent across the research literature (Williamson, Holliday, Holder, North,

M. L. Bourgeois
VA Boston Healthcare System, Boston, MA, USA

B. P. Marx (✉)
VA Boston Healthcare System, Boston, MA, USA

National Center for PTSD, Boston, MA, USA

Boston University School of Medicine, Boston, MA, USA
e-mail: brian.marx@va.gov

W. T. O'Donohue and P. A. Schewe (eds.), *Handbook of Sexual Assault and Sexual Assault Prevention*,
https://doi.org/10.1007/978-3-030-23645-8_42

& Surís, 2017), with some studies including only certain forms of sexual assault and others including both assault and harassment under a broad sexual trauma category. Definitions of sexual assault and sexual trauma also differ across academic and legal disciplines. For example, research definitions of trauma and assault are generally more inclusive than legal definitions in order to capture the prevalence and wide-ranging effects of such behaviors. Notably, legal definitions of unwanted sexual acts have grown in both breadth and specificity over the last several years due to the influence of survivor advocacy groups (Ormerod & Steel, 2018). For example, some military definitions of sexual assault no longer require the use of physical force and instead acknowledge other important factors associated with non-consent, such as the use of substances that interfere with consciousness or behavioral control.

Military definitions of sexual assault are derived from the Uniformed Code of Military Justice (UCMJ; Manual for Courts-Martial, 2016), which outlines punitive articles related to sex-related offenses including rape, sexual assault, and aggravated or abusive sexual contact (e.g., Article 120: Rape and Sexual Assault Generally; Article 125: Forcible Sodomy; Article 80: Attempts). Rape is the most severely punishable offense and is defined as the penetration, no matter how slight, of the vulva, anus, or mouth with a body part or object through the use of physical force, threat of death, serious bodily harm, or kidnapping of any person, rendering a person unconscious, or administering a substance that impairs a person's ability to provide consent or control their conduct (Manual for Courts-Martial, 2016). In contrast, sexual assault refers to any of the above unwanted sexual acts that occur through inducing fear, using or threatening physical force that would not result in grievous bodily harm, misrepresenting one's rank or identity, quid pro quo promises of job benefits or threats of job loss, or committing sexual acts on people who are unaware of the act or unable to provide consent due to being asleep, impairment by substances, or a mental or physical disability (Manual for Courts-Martial, 2016). Attempts to commit any of these sexual offenses are also prosecutable. Aggravated or abusive sexual contact refers to touching or causing others to touch any body part above or below the clothes with the intent to arouse or gratify sexual desire. Based on these articles, the DoD SAPRO defines MSA as "intentional sexual contact characterized by the use of force, threats, intimidation, or abuse of authority or when the victim does not or cannot consent" (Department of Defense, 2015, p. 122).

Military sexual trauma is defined by the Veterans Health Administration (VHA) as "sexual harassment that is threatening in character or physical assault of a sexual nature that occurred while the victim was in the military, regardless of geographic location of the trauma, gender of victim, or the relationship to the perpetrator" (Department of Veterans Affairs, 2004, p. 1). Sexual harassment may take the form of any sexual behavior that is intentionally threatening or disturbing, such as unwanted sexual attention or advances; engaging in threatening verbal or physical behavior that is sexual in nature; creating a hostile work environment through the use of sexual comments, threats, or offensive remarks; or attempting to coerce others into engaging in sexual acts for professional purposes (Fitzgerald, Swan, & Magley, 1997). Although sexual harassment does not qualify as a Criterion A event in the diagnosis of post-traumatic stress disorder (PTSD), these acts often function as a precursor to sexual assault and are strongly related to PTSD symptoms (Street, Stafford, Mahan, & Hendricks, 2008).

Measurement

Since 2002, the DoD has administered the Workplace and Gender Relations survey to track sexual assault and harassment in active-duty (WGRA) and reserve (WGRR) service members. Within these surveys, sexual harassment and sexual assault have been measured using the Sexual Experiences Questionnaire (SEQ; Fitzgerald, Magley, Drasgow, & Waldo, 1999), a self-report measure with sound reliability and validity. In addition, the RAND Corporation has conducted independent evaluations of unwanted sexual contact in both active duty and reservists as part of the RAND Military Workplace Study (RMWS; Morral, Gore, & Schell, 2015). This survey provides data about sexual assault, sexual harassment, and gender discrimination. Given that the RMWS measure included more descriptive, UCMJ-consistent definitions of sexually abusive behavior and non-consent factors than the SEQ, it was added to the most recent version of the WGRA (Davis & Grifka 2017). The strength of these surveys is their ability to provide full population estimates through the use of best practice sampling and weighting procedures. However, these estimates are limited by their low response rates and the exclusion of individuals who have experienced MSA but left the military prior to survey administration.

In 2002, the VA implemented universal military sexual trauma (MST) screening and free treatment for MST and related conditions. As a result, veterans of Operation Enduring Freedom and Operation Iraqi Freedom (OEF/OIF) were the first generation of returning VA patients to receive comprehensive MST screening and treatment (Kimerling, Gima, Smith, Street, & Frayne, 2007), which allowed for the first national, population-based investigations of the prevalence and correlates of MST in veterans. Within the VA, screenings for MST often, but not always, occur in-person during medical appointments. Given the stigma related to experiencing sexual trauma and that veterans may not be seeking treatment specifically for conditions related to trauma exposure, positive screens for MST likely reflect a conservative estimate of true MST prevalence in this population (Kimerling et al., 2010).

One limitation of the VA's measurement of MST is that medical record documentation of MST does not provide information on the specific nature of the incident (sexual assault or sexual harassment). As a result, it is difficult to estimate the prevalence or differentiate the effects of each type of sexual aggression among veterans. Researchers have further suggested that several important factors of the sexual assault incidents be documented, such as the relationship between the perpetrator and survivor, the specific nature of the unwanted sexual behavior, methods used by the perpetrator, and the form of non-consent (Cook, Gidycz, Koss, & Murphy, 2011; Koss, White, & Kazdin, 2010). Further elucidating the nature and context of MST in these ways would likely aid in the development of more precisely targeted prevention efforts.

Prevalence

Prevalence estimates of MSA have been shown to vary based on the operationalization of sexual assault, sampling methods (e.g., anonymous surveys, legal reports of alleged or prosecuted crimes, in-person interviews), and type of study sample (e.g., active duty, veteran, treatment seeking versus nontreatment seeking) (Hoyt, Klosterman Rielage, & Williams, 2011; Surís & Lind, 2008; Turchik & Wilson, 2010). The timeframes of MSA studies also vary significantly, with some examining recalled incidents of MST within the past 6 months and others examining retrospective reports of MST in veterans separated from active service for decades. Moreover, assessment of MSA can be challenging due to reporting biases.

The 2016 WGRA (Davis et al., 2017) included 151,010 service members and revealed a 12-month sexual assault prevalence of 4.3% and 0.6% for cisgender women and men, respectively, and 4.5% for lesbian, gay, bisexual, or transgender (LGBT) personnel. In addition, 21.4% of women, 5.7% of men, and 22.8% of LGBT personnel reported experiencing sexual harassment. In contrast, the prevalences of sexual assault within reserve components are significantly lower, with 3.13% of women and 0.38% of men reporting MSA (Morral, Gore, & Schell, 2015). Notably, 69% of active-duty women and 85% of active-duty men who endorsed experiencing MSA never considered reporting it (Davis et al., 2017). These respondents cited reasons including shame and the desire to avoid thinking about the incident or to conceal it from others. Indeed, MSA tends to be underreported (Blais, Brignone, Fargo, Galbreath, & Gundlapalli, 2018) due, in part, to concerns about negative reactions from others, confidentiality, and stigma (Burns, Grindlay, Holt, Manski, & Grossman, 2014). This reluctance to report may be moderated by assessment modality, such that more private modes of survey response (e.g., computerized self-report measures) may encourage more complete reporting than those associated with less privacy (e.g., face-to-face interviews; Kataoka, Yaju, Eto, & Horiuchi, 2010).

According to recent WRGA data, roughly one-quarter of active-duty service members who endorsed MST reported taking steps to leave or separate from the military as a result of the incident. Given that this survey did not include individuals who had already left the military as a result of MSA, it is possible that reported prevalence of MSA among veterans may more accurately reflect the scope of the problem. One comprehensive review of MST in veterans seeking treatment at VA facilities concluded that the prevalence of MST (including both sexual harassment and sexual assault) lies between 20% and 43%, with women reporting a higher prevalence of MST than men (Surís & Lind, 2008). For example, a recent epidemiological study of 125,729 OEF/OIF veterans who received healthcare at VA facilities between 2001 and 2007 revealed that 15% of female and 0.7% of male veterans screened positive for MST (Kimerling et al., 2010). Taking into account the larger number of men serving in the military than women, however, the actual number of veterans endorsing MST within each gender is fairly equal (Kimerling et al., 2007).

Prevalence numbers observed exclusively among veterans seeking treatment at VA facilities stand in sharp contrast to recent findings from the 2009 to 2011 National Health Study for New Generation of U.S. Veterans, an anonymous, population-based survey of 60,000 OEF/OIF era veterans, which included veterans who have not sought healthcare at a VA facility (Barth et al., 2016). Of the 20,563 survey responders, 41% of female and 4% of male veterans reported experiencing MST. In addition, 10% of female and 0.5% of male veteran endorsed the MST item corresponding to experiences of sexual assault. These findings were corroborated in a more recent nationally representative sample of US veterans ($n = 1468$) collected between September and October 2013, in which 32.4% of female and 4.8% of male veterans reported experiencing MST (Klingensmith, Tsai, Mota, Southwick, & Pietrzak, 2014). Prevalence numbers observed in these samples may have been higher than VA-based samples due to anonymous nature and Internet administration of the surveys.

Studies of MSA among LGBT service members are only recently emerging, due to the military's repeal of bans related to the open service of gay, lesbian, and bisexual personnel ("Don't Ask, Don't Tell") in 2010 and transgender personnel in 2016. Prevalence estimates from the 2016 WGRA indicate greater endorsement of sexual harassment and sexual assault among LGBT personnel compared with cisgender and heterosexual personnel (Davis et al., 2017). Studies of MST among LGBT veterans reveal similarly high numbers of sexual harassment and sexual assault. For example, VA administrative data collected between 2000 and 2013 of 78 transgender men and 254 transgender women serving in Iraq and Afghanistan showed that 19.5% of transgender men and 13.5% of transgender women screened positive for MST (Lindsay et al., 2016). In an anonymous Internet survey of 445 LGBT veteran respondents, 8% endorsed experiencing MSA (Burks, 2011). Continued assessment of the occurrence and effects of sexual assault and sexual harassment in this vulnerable population is especially important as more personnel choose to openly serve as their true gender identity and/or sexual orientation.

Risk Factors

One of the most consistently observed risk factors for MST is gender. Specifically, the research literature on MST prevalence provides robust evidence that women report significantly greater amounts of sexual harassment, coercion, and assault than men across studies of active-duty, reserve, and veteran samples (Street, Gradus, Stafford, & Kelly, 2007). In addition, a developing literature on LGBT service members indicates that gender and sexual minority status confers greater risk for MST (Davis et al., 2017; Lindsay et al., 2016; Mattocks et al., 2013).

Other individual difference factors associated with heightened risk for MSA and MST include a history of childhood sexual abuse, enlisted rank, younger age, non-married status, lower education, and lower socioeconomic status (SES; Kimerling et al., 2007; Surís & Lind, 2008; Turchik & Wilson, 2010). Collectively, these studies highlight the increased vulnerability of service members belonging to groups with lower sociocultural power (e.g., gender and sexual minorities, younger, non-married, lower SES) and lower authority status within the military (i.e., enlisted rank, lower pay grade).

Situationally, alcohol and substance use by either the perpetrator or the victim is commonly associated with MSA, especially among women (Morral et al., 2015). However, alcohol and substance use do not appear to be related to instances of MSA that occur in the context of hazing and bullying, which are situations more commonly reported by men than women (Davis et al., 2017). Although deployment in the absence of combat exposure has been associated with *lower* risk for MST among male OEF/OIF veterans (Barth et al., 2016), combat exposure conferred greater risk of MST for both men and women in this sample (Adjusted Odds Ratios = 1.57/1.42, men/women). Lastly, branch of service appears to be differentially related to experiences of sexual harassment and assault in active-duty men and women (LeardMann et al., 2013; Morral et al., 2015). For example, Air Force male and female service members reported the lowest estimated occurrences of sexual harassment (men = 3.3%, women = 12.4%) and assault (men = 1%, women = 11.9%) in the past year, even after adjusting for demographic variables and certain military factors (e.g., months deployed, pay grade, years of service, relative proportion of men to women across jobs, units, and installations; Morral et al., 2015). Compared with Air Force members of the same gender, Marine Corps women and Navy men were the most likely to experience MSA in the past year (unadjusted relative risks = 2.71 [Marine Corps women] and 5.11 [Navy men]). Further analyses revealed that demographic variables (e.g., age, marital status, education level) accounted for nearly all the difference in relative risk for MSA among men and women in the Army, Navy, and Marines. Sexual response and prevention efforts would likely benefit from research examining possible individual difference factors or environmental characteristics (e.g., training, policy, aspects of work and living conditions) underlying the relatively low prevalence of MSA in the Air Force.

Regarding environmental risk factors, several unique aspects of military culture likely contribute to sexual harassment and violence. Specifically, military leadership continues to be heavily male dominated, and its culture has historically supported highly masculine norms and values, such as strength, competition, dominance, heterosexuality, and rigid sex and gender roles (Turchik & Wilson, 2010). In addition, military training includes components of deindividualization, violence desensitization, objectification of the enemy, and the frequent use of violent and sexualized language (Hunter, 2007). Combined with a hypermasculine environment, these unique components of military training likely contribute to problematic negative attitudes towards women, tolerance of harassment, and the promotion of sexual violence.

Perpetrators of Sexual Crimes

Little is known about the perpetrators of or risk factors for perpetrating sexual violence among military service members. One longitudinal study of sexual harassment and sexual assault of Navy women by male enlisted personnel revealed that prior history of male perpetration of sexual harassment conferred greater risk for sexual assault perpetration (OR = 4.66; Stander, Thomsen, Merrill, & Milner, 2018). Within the same sample, male perpetrators of attempted and completed rape reported engaging in multiple previous incidents of attempted and completed rape, using substances rather than physical force to incapacitate victims, and targeting known victims rather than strangers (McWhorter, Stander, Merrill, Thomsen, & Milner, 2009). There was no significant association between perpetration and demographic variables.

According to 2016 WGRA data gathered from sexual assault survivors, alleged perpetrators of military sexual harassment and assault overwhelmingly tended to be fellow male service members. In addition, these alleged perpetrators were more likely to be enlisted soldiers who were of a slightly higher rank than the survivor. One recent study modeled perpetration risk with machine learning methods using administrative data of reported sexual assault crimes from the Historical Administrative Data System (HADS) of the Army Study to Assess Risk and Resilience in Servicemembers (Army STARRS) (Rosellini et al., 2017). Results revealed that prior crime perpetration (sexual or violent) and the presence and treatment of mental or substance use disorders predicted sexual crime perpetration. Furthermore, mental and substance use disorders requiring inpatient treatment were only included in prediction models of nonfamily sexual assault perpetration, whereas prior perpetration of major physical violence or nonfamily sexual assault was only included in prediction models of sexual assault perpetration against family members. The findings of this study, however, were limited by the lack of available data related to pre-enlistment historical factors (e.g., crime perpetration prior to military service, child sexual abuse victimization) and crimes perpetrated by those who were never apprehended. Future research on MSA perpetration would be improved by including such historical data and extensively surveying all service members to elicit anonymous self-report of perpetration.

Taken together, the limited data on military sexual crime perpetration suggest a need for careful monitoring of service members for signs of threatening or sexually violent behavior. Prevention efforts may also be optimally targeted at men with any history of sexual or physical violence perpetration.

Impact of MSA

MSA and MST are strongly associated with psychiatric conditions, most commonly PTSD, major depressive disorder (MDD), personality, and alcohol or substance use disorders (Kimerling et al., 2007, 2010). A recent retrospective study of 595,525 OEF/OIF veterans seeking VA healthcare revealed that veterans with a history of MST are roughly twice as likely as those without MST to develop eating disorder diagnoses within 1 and 5 years of establishing VA care (Blais et al., 2017). In addition, MST increases risk for suicidal ideation, even after taking into account age, gender, combat exposure, depressive disorder, PTSD, negative affect, and prior suicide attempts (Monteith et al., 2016). Of note, the association between suicidal ideation and MST was stronger for male veterans than for female veterans. Furthermore, a growing body of evidence suggests that male and female veterans who screen positive for MST within VA settings are at increased risk for attempting and dying by suicide (Kimerling et al., 2007, 2016; Pavao et al., 2013). These findings highlight the importance of better understanding factors contributing to higher suicidal ideation risk in veterans, and especially men, who have experienced MST.

Despite the fact that many men have experienced MST during their time in the military, much of the research on the impact of MST has been conducted with female veterans. Multiple studies suggest that female veterans with a history of MST have been significantly more likely to receive PTSD, MDD, and alcohol use disorder diagnoses than female veterans with no MST history (Breland et al., 2018; Kimerling et al., 2007), as well as greater PTSD and MDD symptom severity (Street et al., 2008). One study of 673 OEF/OIF female Army or Marine veterans found that MSA uniquely predicted MDD diagnosis and symptom severity (but not PTSD diagnosis or severity) after controlling for deployment-related stressors (e.g., combat exposure, postbattle experiences), various demographic variables, and general harassment (Kearns et al., 2016).

Although there is robust evidence that MST increases the odds of developing PTSD for male and female veterans (Kimerling et al., 2010), far less is known about diagnostic comorbidity in veterans with MST and PTSD compared with veterans with PTSD and no history of MST. To date, the only study of PTSD comorbidity in veterans with and without MST revealed that the presence of MST was related to higher occurrence of comorbid mental health diagnoses as well as gender differences in patterns of comorbidity (Maguen et al., 2012). Specifically, female veterans with MST and PTSD were more likely to receive comorbid depression, anxiety, and eating disorder diagnoses, whereas male veterans with MST and PTSD were more likely to receive comorbid substance use disorder diagnoses. Increasing knowledge of the unique clinical presentations for veterans with MST-related PTSD will likely improve person-centered evaluation and treatment of veterans seeking trauma-focused mental healthcare.

Aside from related psychiatric problems, research has consistently linked MST to a wide range of physical problems, such as chronic pain, cardiovascular disease, gastrointestinal illness, respiratory conditions, genitourinary problems, sexually transmitted infections, liver disease, and obesity (Cichowski et al., 2017; Kimerling et al., 2010; Surís, Holliday, Weitlauf, North, & Veteran Safety Initiative Writing Collaborative, 2013; Surís & Lind, 2008; Turchik, Pavao, Nazarian, Iqbal, McLean, & Kimerling, 2012). Regarding impairment in quality of life, MST has been associated with increased difficulties adjusting to civilian life and unemployment in female veterans (Skinner et al., 2000), as well as increased risk of homelessness in both male and female veterans after adjusting for the effects of comorbid mental health and substance use disorders (Brignone et al., 2016). Lastly, MST has been associated with important and understudied intimacy problems (Tsai, Rosenheck, Decker, Desai, & Harpaz-Rotem, 2012), decreased sexual satisfaction, and sexual dysfunction among male and female veterans (Allard, Nunnink, Gregory, Klest, & Platt, 2011).

Given that the majority of research on the consequences of MSA and MST has been conducted with female veterans, further research on these issues among male survivors is needed to better understand their unique healthcare needs. Moreover, many of these studies are limited by their cross-sectional design and retrospective reporting of MST. Therefore, inferences about causality cannot be conclusively drawn. Researchers are beginning to employ prospective, longitudinal methods to study the effect of sexual assault and sexual harassment on military members' mental and physical health. One such prospective study of 226 female and 91 male Marine recruits revealed that incidents of sexual harassment within a 6-month timeframe were significantly related to PTSD symptoms and worse perceived physical health (Shipherd, Pineles, Gradus, & Resick, 2009). In this sample, MST showed a greater effect on both symptoms of PTSD and worse perceived physical health among men than among women. The authors hypothesize that the nature of MST, which goes against male gender expectations and proscribed masculine norms, may contribute to these differences. Collectively, these correlational studies of the psychological and physical health effects associated with military sexual harassment and assault highlight the importance of repeated, universal MST screening across all current and former military service members.

Treatment

VA and DoD recommend the use of individual psychotherapies that incorporate elements of cognitive, emotional, and/or behavioral processing of the trauma as the first-line treatment for PTSD (U.S. Department of Veterans Affairs & Department of Defense, 2017). This recommendation includes a wide variety of manualized psychotherapies that have demonstrated efficacy for reducing PTSD symptoms among male and female veterans with a variety of index traumas. In particular, cognitive processing therapy (CPT; Resick & Schnicke, 1992), prolonged exposure therapy (PE; Foa, Hembree & Cahill, 2005), and eye movement desensitization and reprocessing (EMDR; Shapiro, 1989) have garnered the strongest evidence for reducing PTSD among veterans (Foa, Keane, Friedman, & Cohen, 2009). CPT is a 12-session, primarily cognitive therapy that focuses on identifying and restructuring negative beliefs related to safety, power/control, trust, esteem, and intimacy as a result of trauma exposure. In contrast, the main component of PE and EMDR involves repeated sessions of exposure to the trauma memory through narrative recall (and in the case of PE, in vivo exposures assigned outside of session). During in-session exposures, the client is encouraged to imagine the trauma in vivid detail while observing any thoughts, emotions, and physical sensations that arise. Exposures are processed afterwards and are continued until a significant reduction in Subjective Units of Distress (SUDs) occurs within and across sessions. EMDR also includes the use of hand motions by the therapist to direct the client's eye movements from side to side, or other alternating bilateral stimulations (e.g., auditory, tactile), during the exposure. Of note, PTSD treatment using one of these recommended therapies can be initiated in the presence of comorbid psychological disorders (e.g., depression, substance use) as long as there are no immediate safety concerns (e.g., acute suicidality) and the client is able to abstain from using substances before, during, and shortly after sessions. Other recommended trauma-focused therapies include specific, trauma-focused cognitive-behavioral therapy protocols, brief eclectic psychotherapy (BEP), narrative exposure therapy (NET), and written exposure therapy (WET).

Despite the strong evidence of these approaches for treating PTSD in veterans (Watts et al., 2013), there is a paucity of literature examining how well these treatments work specifically for veterans with a history of MST. One randomized clinical trial compared PE with present-centered therapy (PCT, a supportive therapy control condition) for PTSD in female veterans ($n = 277$) and active-duty personnel ($n = 7$), 70% of whom had a history of MST (Schnurr et al., 2007). Results showed that both PE and PCT were associated with significant reductions in PTSD symptoms and self-reported depression and anxiety symptoms, as well as improvements in quality of life. However, veterans receiving PE showed superior reductions in self-reported PTSD symptoms during treatment and at 3- and 6-month follow-up. They were also more likely to no longer meet PTSD diagnostic criteria and achieve total remission than veterans in the PCT group (ORs = 1.80 and 2.43, respectively). Notably, treatment dropout was higher in PE (38%) than PCT (21%). Given the high rate of MST in this sample and that the majority of women across both conditions focused their treatment on sexual trauma, these results provide promising evidence for the efficacy of PE for MST-related PTSD.

In another randomized clinical trial, Surís and colleagues (2013) found that both CPT and PCT were effective in reducing PTSD and depression related to MST among male ($n = 13$) and female ($n = 73$) veterans. However, CPT demonstrated a larger posttreatment effect on PTSD symptoms than PCT. In addition, both CPT and PCT were associated with significant improvement in psychosocial, emotional, and physical functioning. CPT also demonstrated greater reductions in self-reported physical limitations than PCT (Holliday, Williams, Bird, Mullen, & Surís, 2015). Notably, neither intervention was associated with improvements in perceived mental health, pain, vitality, or overall life satisfaction, all of which represent important areas of recovery and wellness. In addition, 35% of veterans in the CPT group and 18% of veterans in the PCT group dropped out of treatment, which indicates the need for more tolerable and effective psychotherapies for MST.

One potential avenue for improving treatments for PTSD involves the use of technology-assisted exposures to promote fear habituation. There is some preliminary evidence that virtual reality exposure therapy (VRET) is tolerable and effective for the treatment of MST-related PTSD (Loucks et al., 2018). In VRET, the therapist provides psychoeducation about PTSD and the rationale for exposure therapy, works with the client to create an exposure hierarchy, and then tailors a virtual reality simulation to include perpetrator and environment characteristics that align with the client's trauma memory. The client then completes exposures using the virtual reality simulation, and reactions are processed afterwards. A recent open trial of VRET with 15 veterans with MST-related PTSD revealed marked reductions in clinician-rated and self-report PTSD and depression symptoms (PTSD: Cohen's $ds = 1.11–1.14$; depression symptoms: $d = 0.94$) following 6–12 sessions of VRET. At 3-month follow-up, the majority of participants no longer met diagnostic criteria for PTSD. However, similar to attrition rates reported in PE trials, 40% of this study's participants dropped out prior to treatment completion.

Despite the high efficacy of evidence-based treatments for PTSD, large dropout numbers and the significant amount of veterans who retain a PTSD diagnosis at posttreatment are concerns. Efforts to improve treatment retention could include the use of intensive outpatient programs, rather than the standard outpatient format of meeting once or twice per week for 60–90 min. Indeed, emerging research on intensive outpatient programs for PTSD related to combat trauma has revealed more favorable treatment retention rates (Beidel, Frueh, Neer, & Lejuez, 2017; Harvey et al., 2017). Future research is also needed to better understand which treatments work and for whom. The ability to identify client characteristics and features of clinical presentations (e.g., demographic variables, type of MST, symptomatology) that best respond to specific treatments would help clinicians optimize the delivery of interventions.

Prevention

The DoD (2015) has responded to the problem of MSA by creating several large-scale sexual assault prevention programs (SAPPs) across all military branches. Following evidence from public health sexual violence prevention efforts, these SAPPs aim to increase knowledge of sexual harassment, sexual assault, and gender diversity in order to change the behavior of potential perpetrators (DeGue et al., 2012). To increase accountability, annual prevalence figures of sexual assault and harassment within the Military Service Academies and all active-duty and reserve military branches (Air Force, Army, Coast Guard, Navy, Marine Corps) are generated. All service branches are further evaluated on their attention to the following five programmatic goals: sexual assault prevention, sexual assault victim assistance and advocacy, investigation, accountability, and assessment (Department of Defense, 2015).

Independent, objective evaluations of the efficacy of these SAPPs are lacking (Turchik & Wilson, 2010). Furthermore, the DoD primarily measures the success of SAPPs on whether rates of sexual harassment and assault decrease as a result of these programs. Continued high rates of MSA suggest a need for increased attention to the content and process of SAPPs. For example, one recent systematic review of four U.S. Air Force SAPPs revealed no specific guidance on the timing of SAPPs (e.g., early versus later in service career, during military campaigns), potentially inadequate dosing (i.e., one-session trainings), potential underuse of professionally trained educators, and a lack of robust outcome assessment measures (Gedney, Wood, Lundahl, & Butters, 2018). These authors suggested that SAPP development efforts would benefit from a systematic examination of the effect of isolated program improvements on outcomes, such as changes in bystander helping behaviors, reduction in risky behaviors (e.g., alcohol consumption), or shifts in the attitudes or behaviors of potential perpetrators.

MSA prevention may also benefit from focusing on individual difference factors. For example, recent evidence from machine learning analyses of ARMY STARRS administrative data suggests that targeting a subset of high-risk female military service members in prevention efforts could significantly reduce the prevalence of sexual crimes (Street et al., 2016). However, given the relative low proportion of women in the military, and even lower number of women at high risk for sexual assault, such narrowly targeted prevention efforts could be costly and difficult to implement. Nonetheless, additional theory-driven development and empirical evaluation of SAPPs tailored to specific subgroups within the military known to exhibit risk for MSA victimization or perpetration (e.g., gender identity and sexual orientation, enlisted status, marital status, occupational specialty, personality factors, prior victimization/perpetration, etc.) may improve prevention outcomes.

Conclusions

In summary, MSA continues to be experienced by large numbers of military service members despite the military's extensive MSA response and prevention efforts. This chapter has outlined a number of directions for future research on the nature, treatment, and prevention of MSA. First, researchers would benefit from using consistent definitions across studies and incorporating the use of anonymous, computer-administered surveys to more accurately estimate prevalence. Second, the majority of research on MSA has occurred using female veteran samples. Given that men who experience MSA are significantly less likely to report these crimes or seek treatment, more research on male survivors is needed. In addition, studies should further examine the mental, physical, and psychosocial effects of MSA in racial, ethnic, gender, and sexual minorities, especially as military membership and leadership continue to evolve and grow increasingly diverse. Third, further research should be conducted examining the efficacy and effectiveness of evidence-based treatments specifically for MST-related PTSD, with the goal of PTSD remission for all active-duty service members and veterans. Fourth, prevention research should seek to better understand and effectively target individual, situational, and environmental factors related to the perpetration of MSA. Finally, MSA prevention programs could be improved by employing rigorous, evidence-based methods for ongoing development, implementation, and evaluation.

References

Allard, C. B., Nunnink, S., Gregory, A. M., Klest, B., & Platt, M. (2011). Military sexual trauma research: A proposed agenda. *Journal of Trauma & Dissociation, 12*, 324–345. https://doi.org/10.1080/15299732.2011.542609

Barth, S. K., Kimerling, R. E., Pavao, J., McCutcheon, S. J., Batten, S. V., Dursa, E., … Schneiderman, A. I. (2016). Military sexual trauma among recent veterans. *American Journal of Preventative Medicine, 50*, 77–86. https://doi.org/10.1016/j.amepre.2015.06.012

Beidel, D. C., Frueh, B. C., Neer, S. M., & Lejuez, C. W. (2017). The efficacy of trauma management therapy: A controlled pilot investigation of a three-week intensive outpatient program for combat-related PTSD. *Journal of Anxiety Disorders, 50*, 23–32. https://doi.org/10.1016/j/janxdis.2017.05.001

Blais, R. K., Brignone, E., Fargo, J. D., Galbreath, N. W., & Gundlapalli, A. V. (2018). Assailant identity and self-reported nondisclosure of military sexual trauma in partnered women veterans. *Psychological Trauma, 10*, 470–474. https://doi.org/10.1037/tra0000320

Blais, R. K., Brignone, E., Maguen, S., Carter, M. E., Fargo, J. D., & Gundlapalli, A. V. (2017). Military sexual trauma is associated with post-deployment eating disorders among Afghanistan and Iraq veterans. *International Journal of Eating Disorders, 50*, 808–816. https://doi.org/10.1002/eat.22705

Breland, J. Y., Donalson, R., Li, Y., Hebenstreit, C. L., Goldstein, L. A., & Maguen, S. (2018). Military sexual trauma is associated with eating disorders, while combat exposure is not. *Psychological Trauma: Theory, Research, Practice, and Policy, 10*, 276–281. https://doi.org/10.1037/tra0000276

Brignone, E., Gundlapalli, A. V., Blais, R. K., Carter, M. E., Suo, Y., Samore, M. H., … Fargo, J. D. (2016). Differential risk for homelessness among US male and female veterans with a positive screen for military sexual trauma. *JAMA Psychiatry, 73*, 582–589. https://doi.org/10.1001/jamapsychiatry.2016.0101

Burks, D. J. (2011). Lesbian, gay, and bisexual victimization in the military: An unintended consequence of "Don't Ask, Don't Tell"? *American Psychologist, 66*, 604–613. https://doi.org/10.1037/a0024609

Burns, B., Grindlay, K., Holt, K., Manski, R., & Grossman, D. (2014). Military sexual trauma among U.S. servicewomen during deployment: A qualitative study. *American Journal of Public Health, 104*, 345–349. https://doi.org/10.2105/AJPH.2013.301576

Cichowski, S. B., Rogers, R. G., Clark, E. A., Murata, E., Murata, A., & Murata, G. (2017). Military sexual trauma in female veterans is associated with chronic pain conditions. *Military Medicine, 182*(9), e1895–e1899. https://doi.org/10.7205/MILMED-D-16-00393

Cook, S. L., Gidycs, C. A., Koss, M. P., & Murphy, M. (2011). Emerging issues in the measurement of rape victimization. *Violence Against Women, 17*, 201–218. https://doi.org/10.1177/1077801210397741

Davis, L., & Grifka, A. (2017). In K. Williams & M. Coffey (Eds.), *Workplace and gender relations survey of active duty members: Overview report*. Alexandria, VA: Office of People Analytics (OPA). Retrieved from http://www.sapr.mil/index.php/research

DeGue, S., Simon, T. R., Basile, K. C., Yee, S. L., Lang, K., & Spivak, H. (2012). Moving forward by looking back: Reflecting on a decade of CDC's work in sexual violence prevention, 2000–2010. *Journal of Women's Health, 21*, 1211–1218. https://doi.org/10.1089/jwh/2012.3973

Department of Defense. (2015). *Sexual Assault Prevention and Response (SAPR) program procedures (DoD Instructive 6495.02)*. Washington, DC: DoD.

Department of Veterans Affairs. (2004). *Military sexual trauma* (Independent study course). Retrieved from http://www1.va.gov/vhi/docs/MST_www.pdf.

Fitzgerald, L. F., Magley, V. J., Drasgow, F., & Waldo, C. R. (1999). Measuring sexual harassment in the military: The sexual experiences questionnaire (SEQ-DoD). *Military Psychology, 11*, 243–263.

Fitzgerald, L. F., Swan, S., & Magley, V. J. (1997). But was it really sexual harassment? Legal, behavioral, and psychological definitions of the workplace victimization of women. In W. O'Donohue (Ed.), *Sexual harassment: Theory, research and treatment* (pp. 5–28). Boston, MA: Allyn & Bacon.

Foa, E. B., Hembree, E. A., & Cahill, S. P. (2005). Randomized trial of prolonged exposure for posttraumatic stress disorder with and without cognitive restructuring: Outcome at academic and community clinics. *Journal of Consulting and Clinical Psychology, 73*(5), 953–964.

Foa, E. B., Keane, T. M., Friedman, M. J., & Cohen, J. A. (2009). *Effective treatments for PTSD: Practice guidelines from the International Society for Traumatic Stress Studies* (2nd ed.). New York: Guilford Press.

Gedney, C. R., Wood, D. S., Lundahl, B., & Butters, R. P. (2018). Sexual assault prevention efforts in the U.S. Air Force: A systematic review and content analysis. *Journal of Interpersonal Violence, 33*, 421–441. https://doi.org/10.1177/0886260515608801

Harvey, M. M., Rauch, S. A. M., Zalta, A. K., Sornborger, M. H., Pollarck, B. O., Rothbaum, B. O., … Simon, N. M. (2017). Intensive treatment models to address posttraumatic stress in post 9/11 warriors: The warrior care network. *FOCUS: The Journal of Lifelong Learning in Psychiatry, 15*, 378–383.

Holliday, R., Williams, R., Bird, J., Mullen, K., & Surís, A. (2015). The role of cognitive processing therapy in improving psychosocial functioning, health, and quality of life in veteran with military sexual trauma-related posttraumatic stress disorder. *Psychological Services, 12*, 428–434. https://doi.org/10.1037/ser0000058

Hoyt, T., Klosterman Rielage, J., & Williams, L. F. (2011). Military sexual trauma in men: A review of reported rates. *Journal of Trauma & Dissociation, 12*, 244–260. https://doi.org/10.1080/15299732.2011.542612

Hunter, M. (2007). *Honor betrayed: Sexual abuse in America's military*. Barricade Books Incorporated.

Kataoka, Y., Yaju, Y., Eto, H., & Horiuchi, S. (2010). Self-administered questionnaire versus interview as a screening method for intimate partner violence in the prenatal setting in Japan: A randomised controlled trial. *BMC Pregnancy and Childbirth, 10*, 1–7. https://doi.org/10.1186/1471-2393-10-84

Kearns, J. C., Gorman, K. R., Bovin, M. J., Green, J. D., Rosen, R. C., Keane, T. M., & Marx, B. P. (2016). The effect of military sexual assault, combat exposure, postbattle experiences, and general harassment on the development of PTSD and MDD in female OEF/OIF veterans. *Translational Issues in Psychological Science, 2*, 418–428. https://doi.org/10.1037/tps0000098

Kimerling, R., Gima, K., Smith, M. W., Street, A. E., & Frayne, S. (2007). The veterans health administration and military sexual trauma. *American Journal of Public Health, 97*, 2160–2166. https://doi.org/10.2105/AJPH.2006.092999

Kimerling, R., Makin-Byrd, K., Louzon, S., Ignacio, R. V., & McCarthy, J. F. (2016). Military sexual trauma and suicide mortality. *American Journal of Preventative Medicine, 50*, 684–691. https://doi.org/10.1016/j.amepre.2015.10.019

Kimerling, R., Street, A. E., Pavao, J., Smith, M. W., Cronkite, R. C., Holmes, T. H., & Frayne, S. M. (2010). Military-related sexual trauma among veterans health administration patients returning from Afghanistan and Iraq. *American Journal of Public Health, 100*, 1409–1412. https://doi.org/10.2105/AJPH.2009.171793

Klingensmith, K., Tsai, J., Mota, N., Southwick, S. M., & Pietrzak, R. H. (2014). Military sexual trauma in US veterans: Results from the national health and resilience in veterans study. *The Journal of Clinical Psychiatry, 75*, e1133–e1139. https://doi.org/10.4088/JCP.14m09244

Koss, M. P., White, J., & Kazdin, A. E. (2010). Violence against women and children: Perspectives and next steps. In M. P. Koss, J. W. White, & A. E. Kazdin (Eds.), *Violence against women and children* (*Navigating solutions*) (Vol. 2, pp. 261–305). Washington DC: American Psychological Association. https://doi.org/10.1037/12308-013

LeardMann, C. A., Pietrucha, A., Magruder, K. M., Smith, B., Murdoch, M., Jacobson, I. G., … the Millennium Cohort Study Team. (2013). Combat deployment is associated with sexual harassment or sexual assault in a large, female military cohort. *Women's Health Issues, 23*, 215–223. https://doi.org/10.1016/j.whi.2013.05.002

Lindsay, J. A., Keo-Meier, C., Hudson, S., Walder, A., Martin, L. A., & Kauth, M. R. (2016). Mental health of transgender veteran of the Iraq and Afghanistan conflicts who experienced military sexual trauma. *Journal of Traumatic Stress, 29*, 563–567. https://doi.org/10.1002/jts.22146

Loucks, L., Yasinski, C., Norrholm, S. D., Maples-Keller, J., Post, L., Zwiebach, L., … Rothbaum, B. O. (2018). You can do that?!: Feasibility of virtual reality exposure therapy in the treatment of PTSD due to military sexual trauma. *Journal of Anxiety Disorders*. https://doi.org/10.1016/j.janxdif.2018.06.004

Maguen, S., Cohen, B., Ren, L., Bosch, J., Kimerling, R., & Seal, K. (2012). Gender differences in military sexual trauma and mental health diagnoses among Iraq and Afghanistan veterans with posttraumatic stress disorder. *Women's Health Issues, 22*, e61–e66. https://doi.org/10.1016/j.whi.2011.07.010

Manual for Courts-Martial. (2016). *Manual for Courts-Martial, United States*. Retrieved from http://jsc.defense.gov/Portals/99/Documents/MCM2016.pdf?ver=2016-12-08-181411-957

Mattocks, K. M., Sadler, A., Yano, E. M., Krebs, E. E., Zephyrin, L., Brandt, C., ... Haskell, S. (2013) Sexual victimization, health status, and VA healthcare utilization among lesbian and bisexual OEF/OIF veterans. *Journal of General Internal Medicine, 28*(Suppl 2), S604-S608. https://doi.org/10.1007/s11606-013-2357-9.

McWhorter, S. K., Stranger, V. A., Merrill, L. L., Thomsen, C. J., & Milner, J. S. (2009). Reports of rape reperpetration by newly enlisted male Navy personnel. *Violence Victims, 24*, 204–218. https://doi.org/10.1891/0886-6708.24.2.204.13

Monteith, L. L., Bahraini, N. H., Matarazzo, B. B., Gerber, H. R., Soberay, K. A., & Forster, J. E. (2016). The influence of gender on suicidal ideation following military sexual trauma among veterans in the Veterans Health Administration. *Psychiatry Research, 244*, 257–265. https://doi.org/10.1016/j.psychres.2016.07.036

Morral, A. R., Gore, K. L., & Schell, T. L. (Eds.). (2015). *Sexual assault and sexual harassment in the U.S. military: Vol. 2. Estimates for Department of Defense service members from the 2014 RAND military workplace study*. Santa Monica, CA: RAND. Retrieved from https://www.rand.org/pubs/research_reports/RR870z2-1.html

Ormerod, A. J., & Steel, J. (2018). Sexual assault in the military. In C. B. Travis & J. W. White (Eds.), *APA Handbook of the Psychology of women: Perspectives on women's private and public lives* (pp. 195–213). Washington DC, US: American Psychological Association. https://doi.org/10.1037/0000060-011

Pavao, J., Turchik, J. A., Hyun, J. H., Karpenko, J., Saweikis, M., McCutcheon, S., & Kimmerling, R. (2013). Military sexual trauma among homeless veterans. *Journal of General Internal Medicine, 28*, 536–541. https://doi.org/10.1007/s11606-013-2341-4

Resick, P. A., & Schnicke, M. K. (1992). Cognitive processing therapy for sexual assault victims. *Journal of Consulting and Clinical Psychology, 60*, 748–756. https://doi.org/10.1037/0022-006X.60.5.748

Rosellini, A. J., Monahan, J., Street, A. E., Petukhova, M. V., Sampson, N. A., Benedek, D. M., … Kessler, R. C. (2017). Predicting sexual assault perpetration in the U.S. Army using administrative data. *American Journal of Preventative Medicine, 53*, 661–669. https://doi.org/10.1016/j.amepre.2017.06.022

Schnurr, P. P., Friedman, M. J., Engel, C. C., Foa, E. B., Shea, M. T., Chow, B. K., … Bernardy, N. (2007). Cognitive behavioral therapy for posttraumatic stress disorder in women: A randomized control trial. *Journal of the American Medical Association, 297*, 820–830. https://doi.org/10.1001/jama.297.8.820

Shapiro, F. (1989). Eye movement desensitization: A new treatment for post-traumatic stress disorder. *Journal of Behavior Therapy and Experimental Psychiatry, 20*, 211–217.

Shipherd, J. C., Pineles, S. L., Gradus, J. L., & Resick, P. A. (2009). Sexual harassment in the Marines, posttraumatic stress symptoms and perceived health: Evidence for sex differences. *Journal of Traumatic Stress, 22*, 3–10.

Skinner, K. M., Kressin, N., Frayne, S., Tripp, T. J., Hankin, C. S., Miller, D. R., & Sullivan, L. M. (2000). The prevalence of military sexual assault among female Veterans' Administration outpatients. *Journal of Interpersonal Violence, 15*, 291–310. https://doi.org/10.1177/088626000015003005

Stander, V., Thomsen, C., Merrill, L., & Milner, J. (2018). Longitudinal prediction of sexual harassment and assault by male enlisted Navy personnel. *Military Psychology, 30*, 229–239. https://doi.org/10.1037/mil0000171

Street, A. E., Rosellini, A. J., Ursano, R. J., Heeringa, S. G., Hill, E. D., Monahan, J., … Kessler, R. C. (2016). Developing a risk model to target high-risk preventive interventions for sexual assault victimization among female U.S. Army soldiers. *Clinical Psychological Science, 4*, 939–956. https://doi.org/10.1177/2167702616639532

Street, A. E., Gradus, J. L., Stafford, J., & Kelly, K. (2007). Gender differences in experiences of sexual harassment: Data from a male-dominated environment. *Journal of Consulting and Clinical Psychology, 75*(3), 464–474. https://doi.org/10.1037/0022-006X.75.3.464.

Street, A. E., Stafford, J., Mahan, C. M., & Hendricks, A. (2008). Sexual harassment and assault experienced by reservists during military service: Prevalence and health correlates. *Journal of Rehabilitation Research and Development, 45*, 409.

Sughrue, K. (2013). *The legacy of Tailhook*. Retrieved from https://www.retroreport.org/transcript/the-legacy-of-tailhook/

Surís, A., Holliday, R., Weitlauf, J. C., North, C. S., & Veteran Safety Initiative Writing Collaborative. (2013). Military sexual trauma in the context of veterans' life experiences. *Federal Practitioner, 30*, 16s–20s.

Surís, A., & Lind, L. (2008). Military sexual trauma: A review of prevalence and associated health consequences in veterans. *Trauma, Violence, and Abuse, 9*, 250–269. https://doi.org/10.1177/1524834419

Surís, A., Link-Malcolm, J., Chard, K., Ahn, C., & North, C. (2013). A randomized clinical trial of Cognitive Processing Therapy for veterans with PTSD related to military sexual trauma. *Journal of Traumatic Stress, 26*, 28–37. https://doi.org/10.1002/jts.21765

Tsai, J., Rosenheck, R. A., Decker, S. E., Desai, R. A., & Harpaz-Rotem, I. (2012). Trauma experience among homeless female veterans: Correlates and impact on housing, clinical, and psychosocial outcomes. *Journal of Traumatic Stress, 25*, 624–632. https://doi.org/10.1002/jts.21750

Turchick, J. A., Wilson, S. M. (2010). Sexual assault in the U.S. military: A review of the literature and recommendations for the future. *Aggression and Violent Behavior, 15*, 267–277.

Turchik, J. A., Pavao, J., Nazarian, D., Iqbal, S., McLean, C., & Kimerling, R. (2012). Sexually transmitted infections and sexual dysfunctions among newly returned veterans with and without military sexual trauma. *International Journal of Sexual Health, 24*, 45–49.

U.S. Department of Veterans Affairs & Department of Defense. (2017). *VA/DoD clinical practice guideline for the management of posttraumatic stress disorder and acute stress disorder.* Retrieved from https://www.healthquality.va.gov/guidelines/MH/ptsd/VADoDPTSDCPGFinal012418.pdf.

Watts, B. V., Schnurr, P. P., Mayo, L., Young-Xu, Y., Weeks, W. B., & Friedman, M. J. (2013). Meta-analysis of the efficacy of treatments for posttraumatic stress disorder. *Journal of Clinical Psychiatry, 74*, e541–e550. https://doi.org/10.4088/JCP/12r08225

Williamson, M. C., Holliday, R., Holder, N., North, C. S., & Surís, A. (2017). A reexamination of military sexual trauma and posttraumatic stress disorder. *Psychiatric Annals, 47*, 134–138. https://doi.org/10.3928/00485713-20170206-01

43 The Prison Rape Elimination Act: The Development of a Social Problem and Response to the Problem?

Roberto H. Potter and Richard Tewksbury

Being raped in a jail or prison has been a topic of comedy and literary genres for decades (Levan, Polzner, & Downing, 2011). Nonconsensual and consensual sex between inmates and correctional staff has been a staple of X-rated videos for nearly as long. For some of us, especially poorer African-American, Latino, and White males, the specter of being sexually assaulted in lockup was used by adults as a disincentive for us to engage in criminal behavior. And, regardless of the perspectives we will outline in this chapter, many in our society being sexually victimized by other prisoners is still viewed as almost a "just desert," or one of the "pains of imprisonment" (Sykes, 1958) to be suffered by inmates and prisoners. We might argue those themes and fantasies continue to be part of the cultural background in Western society.

In this chapter, we want to explore the development of "prison rape" from an almost acceptable pain of imprisonment to a social problem worthy of legislation from the Congress of the United States, the Prison Rape Elimination Act (PREA). Consistent with a social constructionist perspective (Blumer, 1971; Spector & Kitsuse, 1981), we will discuss briefly how something seemingly non-problematic to the broader society came to be defined as a felony offense in every state and the federal government requiring one of the few "government-unique standards" (Potter & Humiston, 2017), or "mandatory" standards, in the accreditation process utilized by the American Correctional Association (ACA) and the National Commission on Correctional Health Care (NCCHC).

We will then turn to the academic literature on sex and rape in correctional settings. A brief review of the empirical literature prior to the enactment of PREA will be offered, leading to a review of the nationally representative data on sexual assault in correctional facilities from the PREA surveys. Within these we will look at characteristics of the facilities with higher rates of sexual assault, as well as offenders and victims of these acts. Attention will be paid to the role of correctional staff in the sexual assault phenomenon. Responses to sexual assault in correctional facilities will be examined, and a canvas of the prevention efforts that are being taken will be provided.

Returning to our social problems perspective, we will examine how PREA has been implemented as a response to the putative problem. We will examine the development of what we might term the creation of a "PREA industrial complex" by multiple organizations and individuals to address this problem. Consistent with this perspective, we will examine perceptions of the effectiveness of PREA by groups who helped to

R. H. Potter
Department of Criminal Justice, University of Central Florida, Orlando, FL, USA

R. Tewksbury (✉)
Louisville, KY, USA

W. T. O'Donohue and P. A. Schewe (eds.), *Handbook of Sexual Assault and Sexual Assault Prevention*,
https://doi.org/10.1007/978-3-030-23645-8_43

bring the legislation into being. We believe we can offer a unique perspective on this issue given the involvement of both authors in the PREA development process.

The Development of a Social Problem—A Brief Primer

Sociologists generally distinguish between two primary ways of approaching social problems. One approach, which Hills (1980) labeled "absolutist," would argue that social problems are self-evident to those in a society. The other approach, labeled "relativist" by Hills, argues that social problems are created through a process of definition and action by social groups. This relativist perspective is consistent with the symbolic interactionist approach typified by Herbert Blumer (1971) and the "social constructionist" approach of Spector and Kitsuse (1981) and others. These writers and others developed the idea that there is a *process* in the *creation* of social problems. That is, a social problem does not spring into full view one morning in the newspaper, radio, or television. Rather, it comes to our attention through the activities of many people and organizations.

Let us outline the process. First, some individual or group must come to view a situation or behavior as causing them a "problem." This group (*claims makers*) must then set about convincing others that the situation or behavior is "really" a problem, a problem for everyone, not just them. Sometimes the group will enlist the help of celebrities to put their case to the media or governmental bodies in an effort to legitimate their claims. After all, if such an auspicious person can recognize the problem, surely everyone will. At this stage, if the group has been successful, some appropriate governmental body will recognize the problem and formulate plans to deal with the problem. The problem is legitimated and a solution to the problem is undertaken.

Blumer ended his analysis at that point; Spector and Kitsuse continued. Social problems were defined by Spector and Kitsuse (p. 146) as "the activities of groups making assertions of grievances and claims to organizations, agencies, and institutions about some putative conditions." They call these complainant groups "claims makers." It is important that the claims-making group gain some form of legitimacy. Again, this is where the role of celebrities and/or politicians becomes important. Once recognized as legitimate, some form of official (government) action is instigated, such as legislative hearings. Following such hearings, some form of reform proposal and/or outcome results to address the putative problem.

Spector and Kitsuse noted that often the original claims-making group may feel that the governmental body charged with solving the problem is not taking things seriously or just is not approaching the problem correctly. In short, they have got it all wrong. Often these groups find that once the governmental body has taken over the problem, the claims-making group members are no longer needed or allowed to work on the problem. They may find also that members of the claims-making group have been co-opted into the official government organization now charged with overseeing the solution to the problem. The claims-making groups then set about making their dissatisfaction with the way in which the governmental instrumentality is not handling the problem known to the wider community. The claims-making group will attempt to establish community-based organizations to tackle the alleged problem in the manner it really needs to be dealt with, from their perspective, at least.

More recently, McAdam and Scott (2005) have examined how these claims-making groups move from relatively disorganized collective behavior into institutionalized solutions via government and other organizational structures. To be very brief, by incorporating the work of Campbell (2005) into the analysis of social movements and social problems, we can begin to examine the organizational processes involved in the raising, recognition, and success or failure of claims-making activities. Potter and Humiston (2017) employ this combined framework to examine the role of rights movements to affect and/or be affected by the criminal justice system.

The constructionist approach to social/public problems emphasizes that social problems are *negotiated* in the public sphere in a manner which more often involves conflict among groups than societal consensus. The role of celebrities and the media in the public definition of the problem and awareness raising campaigns is key. The claims-making group must have the right people putting its case to the rest of the social world. There are many groups vying to have their problems recognized as legitimate and worthy of all our attention. Their plight must strike a resonant chord with enough of us to bring about attention to the matter. Or it must fit with some political party's agenda.

Prison rape (as an inclusive term) represents an interesting test of social problems theory. As noted in the introduction, there is a general sense in society that such victimization is either "part of the sentence," or a pain of imprisonment, or that its effects are minimal for those who are victimized. The manner in which the claims-making groups who championed the development of the Prison Rape Elimination Act and its subsequent implementation worked will be examined in the next section of the chapter. The "rights" organizations will play a key role in this analysis.

Academic Research on Sex and Rape in Confinement Prior to PREA[1]

One of the first areas to be explored is the scope of the problem according to claims makers and the nature of the victims. In general terms, having a victim with whom one can be sympathetic is a good starting point. Individuals in correctional facilities do not always fit this category. One of the starting points must be to typify the victim in a manner that elicits sympathy and/or action from the broader society. Our analysis begins with the published knowledge of victims of sexual assault in correctional settings prior to the passage of PREA.

Tucked away in the work of Alfred Kinsey (Kinsey, Pomeroy, & Martin, 1948) was a notation that many of Kinsey's interviewees were men imprisoned for same-sex behavior ("homosexuality"). In his interviews, Kinsey discovered that, when these men did engage in sex during confinement, it was often later in the term of confinement. They were careful to develop relationships that were as non-abusive as possible in their environment. After that, most studies of sex within confinement facilities turned to sexual assaults. The earliest known study of prison rape was conducted by Davis (1968) in the Philadelphia prison system (in other states, this would be a local jail facility). His research revealed that sexual assaults were relatively common, with one-in-twenty (4.7%) inmates who reported being sexually assaulted while in the Philadelphia prison system.

Potter and Tewksbury (2005) noted that there was, at that time, no systematic monitoring or surveillance system to measure sexual assaults in correctional facilities. Lacking systematic surveillance data, cross-sectional studies of prisoners' sexual behavior were examined to estimate the incidence and prevalence of sexual behavior in correctional settings. The relatively small amount of literature on the incidence of the sexual behavior of incarcerated populations (primarily men's prisons) had been reviewed by Tewksbury (1989), Saum et al. (1995), and Hensley, Struckman-Johnson, and Eigenberg (2000; see also Hensley, 2002). Saum et al. noted the need to differentiate between consensual and nonconsensual sex that takes place in prisons, a distinction that remained often overlooked in the research literature (Tewksbury & West, 2000). Even when that distinction is recognized, and there is some administrative opinion that there is no longer consensual sex under PREA, most studies are of nonconsensual sexual behavior, partly because of the potential effect sexual violence can have on the individuals victimized and on the climate of the correctional system.

Regardless of the context, most research between 1980 and the early 2000s reported low (i.e., 2–24% consensual; 0–27% coerced, broadly defined) sexual activity between inmates. Studies

[1] This section draws heavily on Potter, R.H. & Tewksbury, R. (2005). Sex and Prisoners: Criminal Justice Contributions to a Public Health Issue. *Journal of Correctional Health Care, 11*(2):171–190.

before 1980 reported high rates of "homosexual rape" in prisons (Fishman, 1934; Weiss & Friar, 1974; Lockwood, 1980; Smith & Batiuk, 1989; Struckman-Johnson & Struckman-Johnson, 2000). Looking abroad, health surveys conducted by the New South Wales (Australia) Correctional Health Service in 1997 and 2001 (Butler, 1997; Butler & Milner, 2003) asked state prisoners about their sexual activity before and during their incarceration. Fifteen percent (15%) of the women and 5% of the men reported consensual sex during their imprisonment in 1997; in 2001, 23% of the women and 3% of the men reported consensual sex while in prison. In the 1997 survey, 2% of the women and 2% of the men reported engaging in nonconsensual sex in prison; by 2001, 1% of the women and 0.4% of the men reported the experience of nonconsensual sex while imprisoned.

It was not only incarcerated men or correctional officers involved in coercive or assaultive sexual incidents; female inmates also have been shown to be sexually predatory. Such behaviors by incarcerated women were argued to be increasingly common (Alarid, 2000; Greer, 2000), but remain less frequent than by incarcerated men. In part this may be due to different attitudes regarding homosexuality; female inmates were reported to be more tolerant or even positive about consensual same-sex sexual behaviors than were male inmates (Hensley, 2000).

Complicating the study of prison rape is that inmates may fear retaliation if they report their victimization in surveys or to prison staff members. Concerns of reprisal for speaking out about sexual victimization are a rational fear given that inmates reported a higher rate of actual retaliation (33.3%) than the fear of retaliation (18.2%). Inmates who have spoken about their sexual assault are often placed in solitary confinement for their protection. At the same time, some victimized inmates have opted to accept their (sexual) relationship with their male attacker (Tewksbury & Mahoney, 2009).

The typical profile of a prison rape victim is a young, educated, heterosexual, White, male, with a history of sexual victimization (Beck et al., 2013; Carroll, 1977; Struckman-Johnson & Struckman-Johnson, 2000; Wooden & Parker, 1982). However, there is no stereotypical profile of a typical victim. Previous research indicated that slightly older men had a greater likelihood of being victimized sexually (Struckman-Johnson et al., 1996).

Using a "public health" or applied science approach, Potter and Tewksbury (2005) summarized the risk and protective factors for sexual victimization while incarcerated across these studies. The risk factors included physical weakness, youth, attractiveness, first-time offender and/or incarceration, no gang affiliation, appearing frightened, and being greedy (Chonco, 1989). In Canada, Cooley (1993) summarized risk factors as youth, in the early stages of their incarceration, and in higher security settings.

The role of being "white" as a risk factor has produced mixed results over the years. Racial conflicts are possibly heightened in prisons as a result of being in an arena that is mainly comprised of Blacks. Under that social circumstance, White inmates may be more likely to be targeted for sexual and physical harassment because they are outnumbered and, consequently, less powerful than the opposing group (Carroll, 1977). In most research before 2000, and some since then, a majority of sexual assaults were interracial with a Black male attacker and a White male victim, followed by Black-on-Black and then White-on-White (Davis, 1968; Hensley et al., 2003, 2005). Notably, prison rape literature for the past 25 years indicated that the perpetrator of prison sexual assault is most likely a Black individual while the victim is White (Hensley et al., 2005).

Outside of demographic characteristics, there are also social features that are influential predictors of inmates' susceptibility to sexual victimization. Gonsalves et al. (2012) surveyed staff perceptions of potential risk factors of inmate sexual victimization, and staff members reported that inmates who expressed concern (or fear) of sexual victimization were in fact at a higher risk of (sexual) assault. Even the type of offense committed by the inmate that resulted in their incarceration heightened their risk. For instance, one-third (34%) of inmates who were sexually victimized while imprisoned had committed sexual crimes (Struckman-Johnson et al., 1996), which was a finding consistent with later research. Social awkwardness was another risk factor for inmates as reported by staff persons, which is hard for some not to exhibit as they may have a mental disorder.

Sexual orientation has yielded mixed results as a predictor of an inmate's vulnerability to being sexually victimized. Past literature demonstrates the rate of sexual victimization was highest for homosexuals (41%) followed by heterosexuals (9%) and then bisexuals (2%) (Wooden and Parker, 1982). Since Wooden and Parker's (1982) study, other literature portrayed the relationship between vulnerability and sexual orientation differently. Specifically, homosexuals are not consistently the primary target for sexual victimization (Hensley et al., 2003, 2005; Struckman-Johnson et al., 1996).

There was a growing body of literature in disagreement with the claim that a significantly larger portion of homosexuals are targets of prison rape. Contrary to popular belief, Hensley et al. (2003) discovered that bisexuals (42%) and heterosexuals (42%) comprised a larger portion of being a target of sexual assault than homosexuals (16%). Further, Struckman-Johnson et al. (1996) reported a higher rate of heterosexuals (70%) and bisexuals (26%) being targeted sexually. In both these studies, homosexuals were the least likely group to be sexually victimized.

Struckman-Johnson and Struckman-Johnson (2000) also focused on institutional-level risk factors in Midwestern prisons. Sexual assault appeared more likely to occur in prisons of higher security levels. Struckman-Johnson et al. (1996) reported that 22% of male prisoners in maximum- and medium-security prisons and 16% of male inmates in minimum-security facilities experienced coerced sexual activity during confinement. Later research reported similar findings of inmates in maximum- (46%) and medium-security prisons (46%) who experienced greater rates of sexual victimization than those that resided in minimum-security prisons (8%) (Hensley et al., 2003).

Their institutional risk factors included institutions with large populations, racial conflict, dormitory housing, inadequate security, and large portions of inmates incarcerated for crimes against persons. The role of correctional staff in studies prior to PREA revealed that correctional officers, while not necessarily perpetrating sexual assaults, may be facilitating or encouraging sexual assaults by other inmates through their actions and attitudes and because of their difficulties in distinguishing between consensual and coercive sexual incidents (Dumond, 2000; Eigenberg, 1994, 2000; Nacci & Kane, 1984a, 1984b; Wooden & Parker, 1982). Many of the protective factors were what Tewksbury and West (2000) termed organizational factors. Essentially, these are social environmental factors that play a role in facilitating or hindering sexual behavior, including violence. Highly controlled interactions between inmates from different dormitories and cell blocks that limit the quality of information flow and discourage embellishment of rumors is one environmental protective factor.

In the public events conducted by the Prison Rape Elimination Commission, these individual-level factors were often evident in the victims who testified. They tended to be younger men and attractive women. In this manner, the typification (some might use the term stereotypes) of the victims was consistent with what we might construct as a "true" victim. In this manner, the claims-making groups attempted to make the victims of prison rape as sympathetic as possible to the broader public. However, we will argue later that this was not the primary focus of the claims-making groups. It is difficult to put "rights talk" into risk factors.

Offenders as a Risk Factor

Offenders constitute a type of risk factor, as well. The literature has shown that the typical aggressor is a strong, heterosexual, Black male (Carroll, 1977; Davis, 1968; Hensley et al., 2003, 2005; Struckman-Johnson & Struckman-Johnson, 2000; Wooden & Parker, 1982). To elaborate on the physical features associated with the offender, these individuals who were described as slightly more powerful and dangerous are also more likely to have been charged with violent felonies compared to the victims (Davis, 1968). Other similar traits associated with dangerousness are multiple incarcerations and prison experiences. Interestingly, staff persons' predictions of the likelihood of becoming a sexual offender in prison are highly accurate (Gonsalves et al., 2012).

Correctional staff, of all levels and types of jobs, are also known to offend against inmates sexually. It is not uncommon for the number of inmates victimized by staff to be very similar to the number of inmates victimized by other inmates (Beck et al., 2013; Struckman-Johnson et al., 1996; Struckman-Johnson & Struckman-Johnson, 2000; Tewksbury & Mahoney, 2009; Wolff & Shi, 2011), and in some cases, females, as with males, were more likely to be sexually victimized by another inmate than by staff (Wolff & Shi, 2011).

PREA as a Methodological Boon

As noted earlier, rates of sexual assault victimization in pre-PREA research ranged widely. A wide-ranged estimate of sexual victimization while incarcerated can be attributed to differences in the types of inmates surveyed, settings, data collection procedures, underreporting, definitions of sexual assault, and the validity of self-report statements.

To illustrate, Struckman-Johnson et al. (1996) surveyed 516 prisoners from four prison facilities in Nebraska and found that 22% of the male and 7% of the female prisoners surveyed reported sexual victimization. Later, Struckman-Johnson and Struckman-Johnson (2000) examined seven Midwestern prisons of varying security levels and uncovered that one-in-five (21%) prisoners surveyed reported an unwanted sexual experience. Three Oklahoma-based prisons yielded an average of 13.8% prisoners who had reported being sexually assaulted, with roughly 1-in-100 (1.1%) prisoners being raped (Hensley et al., 2003). Results from a Southern-based maximum-security prison reported 18.3% of the inmates who were targets of sexual threats with a higher rate of prisoners being raped (8.5%) (Hensley et al., 2005). Wolff and Shi (2011) surveyed inmates from 13 prisons in one state and dichotomized their inmates by gender and revealed that roughly 1-in-20 (4%) male inmates and a much higher 1-in-five (22%) female inmates reported wide-ranged sexual victimization. Additional recent research suggests that anywhere from 3.2% to 22% of inmates have been victimized while in prison (Beck et al., 2013; Hensley, Tewksbury, & Castle, 2003; Wolff & Shi, 2011).

One of the many outcomes of Prison Rape Elimination Act (PREA) was the standardization of a sophisticated process of collecting estimates of prison rape that would be known as the National Inmate Survey (NIS): "The Prison Rape Elimination Act of 2003 (PREA; P.L. 108-79) requires the Bureau of Justice Statistics (BJS) to carry out, for each calendar year, a comprehensive statistical review and analysis of the incidence and effects of prison rape. PREA further specifies that the review and analysis shall be based on a random sample, or other scientifically appropriate sample of not less than 10% of all prisons, and a representative sample of municipal prisons" (BJS, 2017). In 2014 the American Association for Public Opinion Research awarded the Bureau of Justice Statistics and contractors with the Policy Impact Award in recognition of the pioneering efforts to standardize collection of this very sensitive data (https://www.justice.gov/archives/opa/blog/bureau-justice-statistics-recognized-studies-prison-rape).

The survey is conducted by the Bureau of Justice Statistics (BJS) and contractors. From February 2011 to May 2012, 91,177 inmates from federal and state prisons and jails completed the survey. Four percent of state/federal prison inmates and a lower rate of jail inmates (3.2%) reported being sexually victimized by another inmate or staff person while they were incarcerated (Beck et al., 2013).

In addition to the inmate-level surveys, the "Survey of Sexual Victimization" (earlier "sexual violence"), since 2004, "collects data annually from administrative records on incidents of sexual victimization in adult and juvenile correctional facilities … The survey includes measures of five different types of sexual victimization and is administered to a sample of at least 10% of all correctional facilities covered under PREA. It gathers information on allegations and substantiated incidents that occur each calendar year" (BJS, 2017, p. 3). We might also note that surveys were also conducted for juvenile facilities (Heaton et al., 2016). There is also a "National Former Prisoner Survey" that seeks to obtain information from parolees about their sexual victimization experiences during their previous incarceration. No separate reports on these data are currently available. A full list of PREA-related publications is listed at the end of the PREA data collection activities documents.

By having a series of surveys that address the individual and facility levels of risk (and potentially protective) factors, it is hoped that a national-level picture of the scope of sexual victimization and perpetration can emerge. Once the baseline is set, it will be easier to determine whether PREA efforts are having an impact at the national level. As revealed in the surveys to date, the prevalence of sexual victimization in jails and prisons is lower than predicted by many. So far the results show that victimization among juveniles and of juveniles by staff is up to three times higher than for adult populations. Thus, reduction of the incidence and prevalence may be difficult, especially if there is some "floor effect" in these settings.

It should be noted that the PREA survey is intended to provide national-level data on the incidence of unwanted sexual contact in prisons and jails. We will address at least one study at state-level utilizing the same methodology below. Thus, the reader is discouraged from generalizing results of the national-level PREA study to their state prison system or local jail.

Offender Characteristics

Inmates victimized by staff persons exhibit similar features to those victimized by other inmates. Inmates who experienced greater rates of sexual victimization by staff were non-heterosexuals, had a history of sexual victimization, and spent more time at the facility (5 years or more). With that said, staff focused on younger inmates, who reported to not have been forced or pressured into their sexual victimization with staff (Beck et al., 2013). Gender has exhibited contradictory findings as a vulnerability to inmate-staff sexual misconduct. In one study, young females reported lower levels of sexual misconduct by staff when compared to young male inmates (Beck et al., 2013). In another study of one state system, a slightly higher rate for female inmates (8%) than male inmates (7%) reported a sexual victimization by staff persons (Wolf & Shi, 2011).

Why "Prison Rape" at This Time?

Consistent with our social constructionist approach, the question of why and how "prison rape" became a social problem at the end of the twentieth and beginning of the twenty-first centuries must be posed. As noted earlier, the phenomenon has been a part of our social narrative for many years. One of the first issues to be addressed is what "claims-making groups" mobilized to bring the putative problem to the attention of government officials. In the same vein, how did these claims-making groups put their case forward that this phenomenon is worthy of a major governmental expenditure? In the space remaining, we want to outline the basic case. It is our hope to fill in the gaps in later works.

As noted by Potter and Tewksbury (2005) and others (e.g., Jenness & Smyth, 2011), penological and academic interest in prison sex has existed since at least the late 1920s. The motivations for interest were varied. For example, our 2005 article was written from the perspective of the health-related issues that were being associated with unsafe sex in correctional settings. The penological interests most often cited had to do with the maintenance of "good order" within correctional facilities. Yet others were interested in the psychological impacts of these traumatic events on those who experienced them. The exportation of those traumas into the community after release from incarceration was another area of interest.

We would contend that, by themselves, these penological and academic interests were insufficient to get the attention of the United States Congress. Jenness and Smyth (2011) agreed, but took a slight different constructionist approach, from a view of PREA as a "newly politicized corrections problem" into "symbolic legislation" with "very little in the way of legally binding mandates for state action designed to address the problem" (p. 493). Their focus was on the "endogeneity of law" to examine the way in which the sector being regulated plays a "decisive role" in the development or lack of development of regulation. In this case, they focus on how certain claims-making groups influenced the development of the PREA standards, as opposed to the original authorizing legislation. We would argue that these are two separable issues, though clearly interrelated. First, and more of our focus, is how the genesis of the National Prison Rape Elimination Commission (NPREC) came into being through the passage of the Prison Rape Elimination Act of 2003 (43 U.S.C. 15,601 (12)). The focus of Jenness and Smyth (2011) appears to be aimed more at the development of the PREA standards, though their data are taken from the NPREC and earlier testimonies.

Like Jenness and Smyth (2011), we would agree that an unusual coalition of claims-making groups coalesced around this issue. Jenness and Smyth focused on three groups: "Prison Fellowship Ministries, Stop Prisoner Rape (SPR—now Just Detention International), and the correctional profession as represented by the National Institute of Corrections and the American Correctional Association." Three of these, Prison Fellowship, Just Detention International (JDI), and the American Correctional Association (ACA), are nongovernmental organizations (NGOs), while the National Institute of Corrections (NIC) is a federal agency organizationally attached to the Federal Bureau of Prisons.

We would argue that a broader view of who constituted the NPREC reveals more. The dominant political parties (Republicans and Democrats in Congress) were allowed to appoint three members each of NPREC members, with the chair (Judge Reggie Walton) and two others appointed by President Bush. The remaining committee members were as follows: Vice-Chair John A. Kaneb (attorney, businessman), James E. Aiken (attorney, expert witness on prison conditions), Jamie Fellner (attorney, Human Rights Watch), Pat Nolan (attorney, legislator, and former federal inmate—Prison Fellowship), Gus Puryear (attorney, former legal counsel for Corrections Corporation of America—now CoreCivic), Brenda V. Smith (civil rights attorney, professor), and Cindy Struckman-Johnson (psychology professor). The Commission, on the surface, appears to have a balance of interests more toward the inmate and civil rights perspective than the interests of the prison industrial complex.

The Commission itself was tasked with holding public hearings and given subpoena powers to compel witnesses. Hearings were held in major cities around the nation, where victims, family members, corrections professionals, and others testified. Within this process was the development of a set of draft standards to guide the development of federal-, state-, and local-level prisoner/inmate sexual assault programs and efforts. These draft standards were developed by volunteer groups appointed by the NPREC executive director. This is a good point at which to inform the reader that one author (Tewksbury) was a consultant to both the Bureau of Justice Statistics (BJS) and the NPREC on the data collection and standards development process. The other author (Potter) chaired the committee to develop the medical and behavioral health draft standards and was on the BJS workgroup. These experiences allow us to "fill in" some of the gaps missed by those who rely on the formal records and academic publications regarding the PREA process.

In answer to the question of why "prison rape" became an issue worthy of multiple years and millions of taxpayer dollars, we offer the hypothesis that the unique confluence of the prison experiences of former political elites and human rights attorneys spurred the development of the initial authorizing legislation and the PREA Commission (NPREC). We would add also that this represented a unique opportunity to extend the civil and human rights "project" with regard to prisons and jails that began with the riots at Attica in 1971. We believe a closer examination of the history or what Jenness and Smyth call the "genealogy of the politics of prison rape" will show this to be an exemplar of how elites construct social problems and impose putative solutions without the involvement of significant segments of the population. As we and Jenness and Smythdate have pointed out, there was probably not a groundswell of public opinion that "prison rape" was a significant social problem. When the testimonies of witnesses at the NPREC hearings are examined, one will see a balance of "celebrities" such as Senators Kennedy and Sessions, Representative Danny Davis, and others, along with victims, academics, and correctional and public health officials (Potter among them) from all levels of government, are included. We would also suggest a review of the academic literature of the time, to include law review articles to determine whether there was a positive deviation in the number of articles devoted to this topic immediately prior to and during the NPREC lifetime and compare those to publications since that time.

The Official Response

As noted earlier, Blumer (1971) stopped his analysis when the official government response occurred. For the prison rape problem, this would be the passage of the PREA in 2003 and the establishment of the PREA standards. In the Spector and Kitsuse (1981) model of social problem construction, the official response to the problem marks one "victory" point for the claims-making group. They argue it is almost inevitable that something about the proposed solution and/or its implementation will not be acceptable to the claims makers. This provides us with another area we believe is ripe for further exploration.

As outlined above, the initial process of developing the PREA standards was conducted by appointed volunteer groups from a range of perspectives. Potter (as an employee of the Centers for Disease Control and Prevention—CDC) chaired the health and behavioral health standards development group, with Robert Dumond as co-chair and primary lead on the behavioral health side. Like our group, others met at various conferences and by telephone conference and email communications to hammer out drafts. The committees were as balanced as the volunteers who comprised them. There were, to be sure, lively discussions and philosophical debates about whether standards were to be based on the realities of the correctional world or more aspirational. We hoped the proposed standards would be a mixture of both. Toward the end of the process, without notice from the NPREC Executive Director, we were joined by "interns" from a justice reform group who observed our processes. When the draft timeline expired, all committees submitted their drafts to the NPREC staff. What was promulgated by NPREC as the draft standards for public comment were not the drafts that went forward to the NPREC staff.

It is interesting that Jenness and Smyth (2011) employ the concept of "endogeneity" as an explanatory device for how the PREA standards were brought back, after the public comment period, to those more consistent with what the volunteer committees had produced. This is in contrast to what was submitted for public comment. Jenness and Smyth (2011, p. 497) write:

> The focus is on how an organizational field that lies relatively dormant during the incipient stages of lawmaking can nonetheless emerge to define the parameters of its own regulation—or lack thereof … . The development and installation of implementation structures and processes are effectively denied at the moment of formulation by the very organizations the implementation would otherwise target for control. The law as a form of administrative regulation is not 'co-opted' (in the classic formulation); rather, it is denied *in toto*." The result is the same, however: the social control *of* organizations is, in a very real sense, social control *by* organizations; in the case of prison reform, the correctional industry looms large in setting the parameters of the regulation of prisons (italics in original).

We believe that if Jenness and Smyth were to examine the process by which the draft standards came into being and how they were "co-opted" (in the traditional sense) by an organization not involved in the NPREC's open process, they might view the "symbolic" nature of their analysis somewhat differently. Depending upon which claims-making group one uses for one's lens on the PREA process and standards, the view of the process changes dramatically. We would note further that the denial of PREA as regulatory is overstated. As Thomas and Thomas (1928) put it years ago, if situations are defined as real, they are real in their consequences. We would remind the reader that there are substantive penalties to the states and NGOs that promulgate voluntary consensus standards (e.g., ACA and the National Commission on Correctional Health Care) should they not certify adoption of the PREA standards. For the states, this affects a variety of corrections-related funding programs at state and local levels. It was revised from earlier language that would have also affected victims' services funding. Never underestimate the coercive power of the federal purse.

The PREA standards were promulgated in 2012, and we would argue that not enough time has passed to allow all claims-making groups to determine whether their claims have been satisfied. We would argue this is true especially of the victims' groups. For others, we would argue that the eventual development of the PREA Resource Center and the processes of auditor certification have provided exactly the type of co-optation Jenness and Smyth deny. We would recommend an analysis of the scope of the "PREA industrial complex" that has developed since the promulgation of the standards and the development of the partnerships that underlie the Resource Center. We hypothesize that the manner in which the resources are distributed by the PREA Resource Center flow, and the assumption of continued funding into the future, will be primary determinants of whether or not the final phase of the Spector and Kitsuse (1981) model—a renewed call for action to address the original problem—will eventuate.

Conclusion

The Prison Rape Elimination Act of 2003 and its subsequent modification, standards, and application provide rich ground for a range of research efforts. Not the least among these is the question of most relevance to practitioners—do the standards produce the desired outcomes of reduced sexual assaults in correctional facilities? This is an evaluation question of interest to many in the academic world, as well. Equally interesting to academic researchers, we argue, is the reasons why prison rape and its analogs became and/or remains a social phenomenon worthy of the expenditure of substantial sums of public monies. We hope that our excursion through some (occasionally provocative to our friends) of the controversies associated with PREA will inspire other researchers to address more than simply the questions of efficacy.

References

Alarid, L. F. (2000). Sexual assault and coercion among incarcerated women prisoners: Excerpts from prison letters. *The Prison Journal, 80*(4), 391–406.

Beck, A. J., Berzofsky, M., Caspar, R., & Krebs, C. (2013). *Sexual Victimization Reported in Prisons and Jails by Inmates, 2011-2012*. Washington, D.C.: Bureau of Justice Statistics.

Blumer, H. (1971). Social problems as collective behavior. *Social Problems, 18*(3), 298–306.

Bureau of Justice Statistics. (2017). *Prison Rape Elimination Act of 2003: PREA Data Collection Activities, 2017*. Washington, DC: Bureau of Justice Statistics.

Butler, T. (1997). *Preliminary Findings from the Inmate Health Survey*. Sydney, NSW: New South Wales Corrections Health Service.

Butler, T., & Milner, L. (2003). *The 2001 New South Wales Inmate Health Survey*. Sydney, Australia: Corrections Health Service.

Campbell, J. (2005). Where Do We Stand? Common Mechanisms in Organizations and Social Movements Research. In: Davis, G. F., McAdam, D., Richard Scott, W., and Zald, M. N. (Eds.) Social Movements and Organization Theory. pp. 41–68. Cambridge, UK: Cambridge University Press.

Carroll, L. (1977). Humanitarian reform and biracial sexual assault in a maximum security prison. *Urban Life, 5*(4), 417–437.

Chonco, N. R. (1989). Sexual assaults among male inmates: A descriptive study. *The Prison Journal, 69*(1), 72–82.

Cooley, D. (1993). Criminal victimization in male federal prisons. *Canadian Journal of Criminology, 35*(4), 479–495.

Davis, A. J. (1968). *Report on Sexual Assaults in the Philadelphia Prison System and Sheriff's Vans*. Philadelphia: District Attorneys Office and Police Department.

Dumond, R. W. (2000). Inmate sexual assault: The plague that persists. *The Prison Journal, 80*(4), 407–414.

Eigenberg, H. M. (1994). *Male Rape: An Empirical Examination of Correctional Officers' Attitudes Toward Rape in Prison*. Sam Houston State University: Unpublished doctoral dissertation.

Eigenberg, H. M. (2000). Corrections officers and their perceptions of homosexuality, rape. *and prostitution in male prisons. The Prison Journal, 80*(4), 415–433.

Fishman, J. F. (1934). *Sex in Prison: Revealing Sex Conditions in American Prisons*. New York: National Library.

Gonsalves, V. M., Walsh, K., & Scalora, M. J. (2012) Staff perceptions of risk for rape perpetration and victimization. *Prison Journal 92*(2), 253–273.

Greer, K. R. (2000). The changing nature of interpersonal relationships in a women's prison. *The Prison Journal, 80*(4), 442–468.

Heaton, L., Cantor, D., Bruce, C., Ren, W., Hartge, J., & Beck, A. J. (2016). *Facility-level and individual-level correlates of sexual victimization in juvenile facilities* (p. 2012). Washington, DC: Bureau of Justice Statistics. https://www.bjs.gov/content/pub/pdf/flilcs-vjf12.pdf

Hensley, C. (2000). Attitudes toward homosexuality in a male and female prison: An exploratory study. *The Prison Journal, 80*(4), 434–441.

Hensley, C. (Ed.). (2002). *Sex in Prison: Pratice & Policy*. Boulder, CO: Lynne Reinner.

Hensley, C., Tewksbury, R., & Castle, T. (2003). Characteristics of prison sexual assault targets in male Oklahoma correctional facilities. *Journal of Interpersonal Violence, 18*(6), 595–607.

Hensley, C., Tewksbury, R., & Wright, J. (2005). The characteristics and motivations behind female prison sex. *Women and Criminal Justice.*

Hills, S. L. (1980). *Demystifying social deviance*. New York: McGraw-Hill Book Company.

Jenness, V., & Smyth, M. (2011). The passage and implementation of the Prison Rape Elimination Act: Legal endogeneity and the uncertain road from symbolic law and instrumental effects. *Stanford Law & Policy Review, 22*(2), 489–527.

Kinsey, A. C., Pomeroy, W. B., & Martin, C. E. (1948). *Sexual behavior in the human male*. Philadelphia: W.B. Saunders Company.

Levan, K., Polzner, K., & Downing, S. (2011). Media and prison sexual assault: How we got to the "don't drop the soap" culture. *International Journal of Criminology and Sociological Theory, 4*(2), 674–682.

Lockwood, D. (1980). *Prison Sexual Violence*. New York: Elsevier.

McAdam, D., & Richard Scott, W. (2005). Organizations and Movements. In: Davis, G. F., McAdam, D., Richard Scott, W., and Zald, M. N. (Eds.) Social Movements and Organization Theory. pp. 4–40. Cambridge, UK: Cambridge University Press.

Nacci, P. L., & Kane, T. R. (1984a). The incidence of sex and sexual aggression in federal prisons. *Federal Probation, 47*(4), 31–36.

Nacci, P. L., & Kane, T. R. (1984b). Sex and sexual aggression in federal prisons. *Federal Probation, 48*(1), 46–53.

Potter, R. H., & Humiston, G. S. (2017). *Criminal justice organizations: Structure, relationships, control, and planning*. St. Paul, MN: West Academic Publishing.

Potter, R. H., & Tewksbury, R. (2005). Sex and prisoners: Criminal justice contributions to a public health issue. *Journal of Correctional Health Care, 11*(2), 171–190.

Saum, C. A., Surratt, H. L., Inciardi, J. A., & Bennett, R. E. (1995). Sex in prison: Exploring the myths and realities. *The Prison Journal, 75*(4), 413–430.

Smith, N., & Batiuk, M. E. (1989). Sexual victimization and inmate social interaction. *The Prison Journal, 69*(2), 29–38.

Spector, M., & Kitsuse, J. I. (1981). *Constructing social problems*. Hawthorne, NY: Walter de Gruyter.

Struckman-Johnson, C., & Struckman-Johnson, D. (2000). Sexual coercion rates in seven midwestern prison facilities for men. *The Prison Journal, 80*(4), 379–390.

Struckman-Johnson, C., Struckman-Johnson, D., Rucker, L., Bumby, K., & Donaldson, S. (1996). Sexual coercion reported by men and women in prison. *The Journal of Sex Research, 33*(1), 67–76.

Sykes, G. (1958). *The Society of Captives*. Princeton: Princeton University Press.

Tewksbury, R. (1989). Fear of Sexual Assault in Prison Inmates. *The Prison Journal, 69*(1), 62–71.

Tewksbury, R., & West, A. (2000). Research on sex in prison during the late 1980s and early 1990s. *The Prison Journal, 80*(4), 368–378.

Tewksbury, R., & Mahoney, M. (2009). Sexual victimization and requests for assistance contained in inmates' letters to the National Prison Rape Elimination Commission. *Federal Probation, 73*(3), 56–61.

Thomas, W. I., & Thomas, D. S. (1928). *The child in America: Behavior problems and programs*. New York: Knopf.

Weiss, C., & Friar, D. J. (1974). *Terror in the Prisons: HomosexualRape and Why Society Condones It*. New York: Bobbs-Merrill.

Wolff, N., & Shi, J. (2011). Patterns of victimization and feelings of safety inside prison: The experience of male and female inmates. *Crime & Delinquency, 57*(1), 29–55.

Wooden, W. S., & Parker, J. (1982). *Men Behind Bars: Sexual Exploitation in Prison*. New York: Plenum Press.

Sexual Assault and Intercollegiate Athletes

44

Kristy L. McCray

Introduction

Prior to the women's movement of the 1960s and 1970s in the United States, sexual assault, rape, and other forms of violence against women were rarely discussed in public forums, let alone studied in academic settings. During the era of the women's rights movement, rape crisis centers and other support mechanisms for women were created nationwide, though little research into either victimization or perpetration was conducted during this time (Sable, Danis, Mauzy, & Gallagher, 2006). The 1980s began to see general research in the field of violence against women. After a multitude of high-profile athletes garnered media attention specifically for violent acts against women in the 1980s and 1990s (many of which are detailed in Benedict, 1997), researchers in fields ranging from sociology to psychology to higher education took notice and began conducting studies to assess the prevalence of student-athlete violence against women (i.e., Crosset, Ptacek, McDonald, & Benedict, 1996; Koss & Gaines, 1993).

Empirical results regarding the prevalence of student-athlete violence against women from the 1990s were mixed and, as such, were subject to criticisms from the field. Further, there is a definitive gap in the literature in the 2000s. In the last 15 years, only two new empirical studies sought to question whether male student-athletes are more likely to perpetrate sexual assault (Sawyer, Thompson, & Chicorelli, 2002; Young, Desmarais, Baldwin, & Chandler, 2017), and many studies have documented the generally positive effects of sexual assault prevention programming with student-athletes (Foubert & Perry, 2007; Jackson & Davis, 2000; McMahon & Farmer, 2009; Moynihan & Banyard, 2008; Moynihan, Banyard, Arnold, Eckstein, & Stapleton, 2010).

This chapter begins with an overview of rape culture, followed by an examination of hypermasculinity, particularly as it pertains to sexual assault and college athletics. Next, there is a brief overview of sexual assault at the university level, which is followed by information about sexual assault within intercollegiate athletics. This section includes an examination of perpetration by male student-athletes, criticisms and gaps in this research, and a brief overview of prevention education efforts. This chapter concludes with a look at how college athletic departments may be identified as rape-prone cultures.

Rape Culture

Prior to the 1980s, rape was assumed to be a consequence of male nature, in that men were "programmed for rape" (Sanday, 1981, p. 6). However,

K. L. McCray (✉)
Otterbein University, Westerville, OH, USA
e-mail: kmccray@otterbein.edu

W. T. O'Donohue and P. A. Schewe (eds.), *Handbook of Sexual Assault and Sexual Assault Prevention*,
https://doi.org/10.1007/978-3-030-23645-8_44

through her study of 156 tribal societies, Sanday (1981) posited that rape is not a biological need, but something that can be attributed a society's culture; thus, the term *rape culture* was born. Herman (1984) was the first to label America as a rape culture. In a society where the majority of the nation's leaders, both in the workplace and in elected government, are men, "the eroticization of male dominance means that whenever women are in a subordinate position to men, the likelihood for sexual assault is great" (p. 52). Herman concluded, "To end rape, people must be able to envision a relationship between the sexes that involves sharing, warmth, and equality, and to bring about a social system in which those values are fostered" (Herman, 1984, p. 52). The ideal of a rape-free environment was supported by Messner and Sabo (1994), who wrote:

> Compelling as the evidence is, we want to emphasize two points. First, *nothing inherent in men leads them to rape women.* Peggy Sanday, an anthropologist, and other researchers have found that there *are* rape-free societies in the world, and that they tend to be characterized by low levels of militarization, high levels of respect for women, high levels of participation by women in the economy and the political system, and high levels of male involvement in child care. (p. 34; emphasis original)

Thus, rape cultures are often characterized by high levels of tolerance for violence and strict sex segregation and gender roles, which foster lack of respect for women.

These characteristics of a rape culture are often cultivated and supported by rape myths. According to Burt (1980), these are "stereotypes and myths—defined as prejudicial, stereotyped, or false beliefs about rape, rape victims, and rapists—in creating a climate hostile to rape victims" (p. 217). Examples of rape myths are "look at how she was dressed—she was asking for it" or "he couldn't help himself—he's a guy just following his sexual urges; what do you expect?" Rape myths include stereotypes about both victims and perpetrators, but hold only the victim accountable for the sexual assault (Burt, 1980). Lonsway and Fitzgerald (1994) further contributed to the field's understanding of rape myths, noting they are "attitudes and beliefs that are generally false but are widely and persistently held, and that serve to deny and justify male sexual aggression against women" (p. 134).

Rape myths and stereotypes often uphold traditional views on sex, gender, and masculinity (i.e., women are to be pure and chaste, men are celebrated for sexual conquest). Burt's findings indicated that rape myth acceptance is "strongly connected to other deeply held and pervasive attitudes such as sex role stereotyping, distrust of the opposite sex (adversarial sexual beliefs), and acceptance of interpersonal violence" (p. 229). This last finding is particularly worrisome, as the acceptance of interpersonal violence was found to be the strongest predictor of rape myth support. In sum, rape myths and their acceptance contribute to a culture that is supportive of rape (i.e., a rape culture).

Thus, rape cultures are those that (1) "display a high level of tolerance for violence, male dominance, and sexual segregation" and (2) "lack the social constraints that discourage sexual aggression or contain social arrangements that encourage it" (Crosset, 1999, p. 245). In the realm of higher education, Sanday (1990) noted that many facets of American society, including intercollegiate athletics, are often considered to be rape cultures or display elements of rape culture. Curry (2002) exposed rape culture in college athletics through an examination of locker room talk. He found that locker room talk about women "promotes harmful attitudes and creates an environment supportive of sexual assault and rape" (p. 183). Further, Messner and Sabo (1994) connected locker room talk to peer support of violence:

> And when verbal sparring and bragging about sexual conquests led to actual behavior, peer group values encouraged these young men to treat females as objects of conquest. This sort of masculine peer group dynamic is at the heart of what feminists have called "the rape culture." (p. 50)

Peer support of violence is cited as the main reason for acting in a sexually aggressive way. According to Schwartz and DeKeseredy (1997), "We argue that North American is a 'rape-supportive culture,' where values and beliefs that support and encourage the sexual victimization of women are widely available to all men" (p. 52).

However, just because someone is supportive of rape myths does not necessarily mean that they will act upon those beliefs. Schwartz and DeKeseredy propose that perpetrators of sexual assault do so based on perceived peer support for violence against women (Schwartz & DeKeseredy, 1997).

Hypermasculinity

Rape cultures can be aggravated by hypermasculinity (Sanday, 1990). However, an examination of masculinity within the context of sport is necessary first. Crosset (1990) argued that in the Victorian era, "physical educators and ideologues of early modern sport professed inherent connections between sport, morality, and manliness" (p. 45). This early connection between sport, manliness, and masculinity has been supported throughout current sport manifestations. Messner and Sabo (1994) contended that to display masculinity in sport, men must be "competitive, successful, dominating, aggressive, stoical, goal-oriented, and physically strong," and therefore "many athletes accept this definition of masculinity and apply it in their relationships with women" (p. 38). However, they also argued that sport in itself does not make athletes more likely to sexually assault women. Drawing upon rape culture characteristics, they wrote, "*Nothing inherent in sports makes athletes especially likely to rape women. Rather, it is the way sports are organized to influence developing masculine identities and male peer groups that leads many male athletes to rape*" (p. 34; emphasis original).

In her work on male violence against women, Brackenridge (2002) argued that violence against women in sport (i.e., against female athletes themselves) is due to a crisis of masculinity facing men in sport. She described sex discrimination, sexual harassment, and sexual abuse as a continuum of violence against women that began in the 1970s and continued throughout the 1990s. Further, she acknowledged that "under-reporting is a common problem in research studies of rape, for obvious reasons of confidentiality and post-disclosure victimization" (p. 258), thus limiting her arguments to mostly those of sexual harassment, as there are little existing data on sexual assault victimization of female adult athletes.

While Brackenridge (2002) theorized that male athlete violence against women is due to a crisis of masculinity, others attributed it to the concept of hypermasculinity. As noted, rape cultures can be aggravated by hypermasculinity (Sanday, 1990). Corprew and Mitchell (2014) thoroughly explored hypermasculinity, noting that a more classical definition includes "an exaggerated adherence to traditional male gender role beliefs" which "encapsulates a belief by men that they should be tough, be independent, act as provider and protector, and be resistant to femininity" (p. 549). This was expanded to include "characteristics such as a supervaluation of competitive and aggressive activities" as well as "higher levels of status and self-reliance [that] are important to the hypermasculine male and that sensation-seeking, dominance over others, and interpersonal violence become necessary components of the hypermasculine male's perception of maleness" (p. 549).

Murnen and Kohlman (2007) defined hypermasculinity as values associated with all-male groups (e.g., fraternities, the military). Hypermasculinity is three-pronged in promoting (1) "the idea that violence is 'manly'"; (2) "that men are naturally aggressive and dominant over women;" and (3) "that the 'sexual conquest' of women is an important aspect of masculinity" (p. 146). As such, hypermasculinity has also been linked heavily with sport participation of men and violence against women. Brackenridge (2002) noted:

> This hyper masculine, heterosexual culture of sport, with its sexually intense initiation rituals, excessive use of alcohol and demeaning attitudes towards women, can remove inhibitions for sexual abuse and assault, both by males to females (singly or in groups) or by males to other males. (p. 262)

In a study on professional football players, Welch (1997) found that players in certain positions—namely, "scoring" positions, such as receivers or running backs—were more likely to commit violence against women. He said, "due to the degree that violence, aggression, domination, and physicality are rewarded in the context of the sport, it ought not be surprising that some football players enthusiastically embrace versions of hypermasculinity" off the field (p. 394). Welch's study appeared to be the only one attempting to measure the differences in hypermasculinity between specific positions. In addition, Corprew and Mitchell (2014) warned that studies attempting to measure masculinity were flawed as they exhibited mixed results; thus, it is inconclusive if hypermasculinity is a correlate or a cause of violent behaviors, particularly sexual assault. It is important to remember this in the next section about sexual assault on college campuses, which outlines information on both perpetrator and victim characteristics.

Sexual Assault on College Campuses

Victimization

It is often difficult to survey sexual assault due to the sensitive and confidential nature of the subject (Brackenridge, 2002; Crosset, 1999). However, the National Intimate Partner and Sexual Violence Survey (NISVS) released in 2010 is widely accepted by those within the rape crisis field as the most current and accurate picture of victimization of sexual assault in the United States (Black et al., 2011). The NISVS indicated that one in five women has experienced rape in their lifetime, with more than half reporting the perpetrator as their intimate partner and 40% reporting an acquaintance as perpetrator. Further, the study showed that almost 80% of female victims experienced a completed rape prior to the age of 25, making college one of the highest risk time periods in a young woman's life (Black et al., 2011). This supported the findings of the 2007 Campus Sexual Assault (CSA) Study released by the National Institute of Justice, which found that one in five undergraduate female students was the victim of attempted or completed sexual assault while in college.

As there are high numbers of women assaulted each year on college campuses, the National Institute of Justice compiled research on victimization statistics (Fisher, Cullen, & Turner, 2000). According to the report:

> Although exceptions exist, most sexual victimizations occur when college women are alone with a man they know, at night, and in the privacy of a residence. Most women attempt to take protective actions against their assailants but are then reluctant to report their victimization to the police (p. 34).

Additional risk factors for female sexual assault victimization included being single (i.e., unmarried), living on campus, prior victimization, and "frequently drinking enough to get drunk" (p. 23). The role of alcohol is clearly present in campus sexual assault, with research finding it consistently present in at least 50% of campus assaults (Abbey, Zawacki, Buck, Clinton, & McAuslan, 2001; Crowe & George, 1989; Crowell & Burgess, 1996; Littleton & Breitkopf, 2006; Logan, Cole, & Capillo, 2006; Pope & Shouldice, 2001; Ullman, Karabatsos, & Koss, 1999). In sum, campus sexual assault victimization often involved women who live on campus, are intoxicated, and know their perpetrator, which leads to the next section on campus perpetrators.

Perpetration

As noted, alcohol was present in more than half of campus sexual assaults, with both victims and perpetrators exhibiting intoxication. However, more important from the standpoint of perpetration is peer support. Schwartz and DeKeseredy (1997) noted that many cultures exhibit rape-supportive attitudes, but just because someone believes rape myths do not necessarily mean that he will engage in sexual assault. The authors noted that male peer support for sexual assault might lead men to commit the act. Peer support and the need for bystander intervention are discussed further in prevention efforts.

There is no typical "profile" of a campus perpetrator. However, Lisak and Miller's (2002) work "has been instrumental in highlighting the role of the 'undetected rapist,' a male who is an average person, who commits repeated assaults yet is not reported" (McMahon, 2011, p. 5). The "undetected rapist" was one who does not self-identify as a rapist, but when asked questions about sexual encounters, reported sexually violent behaviors.

For example, the perpetrators admitted to using physical violence, such as holding down a victim who is struggling, only after verbal and/or psychological coercion did not work (Lisak & Miller, 2002). Using physical violence as a last resort was also demonstrated by Carr and VanDeusen (2004), whose research found:

> Few men acknowledged using physical force to obtain sex, whereas more men acknowledged some form of sexual coercion. This included pressuring women and saying things they did not mean to obtain sex, using alcohol to obtain sex, and having sex with a woman even when she wanted to stop. (p. 286)

There is a strong link between alcohol, lack of force, and coercion by perpetrators of sexual assault. This is often upheld through peer support and rape-supportive attitudes in rape cultures on college campuses. The next section is a comprehensive review of sexual assault in college athletics, beginning with male student-athletes as perpetrators of sexual assault.

Sexual Assault in College Athletics

Male Student-Athletes' Violence Against Women

Until the 1990s, research in the field of student-athlete violence against women was nonexistent. Melnick (1992) was one of the first in the sport field to call upon colleagues to examine the relationship between intercollegiate athletic participation and sexual assault by male student-athletes. He proposed five potential reasons for the prevalence of student-athlete perpetration: (1) male bonding; (2) sport as a masculine proving ground; (3) combative sports (i.e., contact sports) and violence; (4) the athletic justice system (i.e., athletes believe that they are subject to more lenient rules by coaches); and (5) big-man-on-campus syndrome (i.e., athlete are so accustomed to "easy" sex that they are not used to hearing "no"). Based upon these presumptive reasons, Melnick also laid out the case for five reforms: (1) elimination of student-athlete specific residences; (2) elimination of sexist talk in the sporting environment; (3) tougher, swift punishment for perpetrators; (4) rape prevention education for student-athletes; and (5), the most radical, "reformation of the male sport experience" (p. 35), which one can see echoed in sport sociology literature (Coakley, 2015; Messner & Sabo, 1994). Coakley (2015) argued that hegemonic masculinity, the dominant form of manhood today, leads to a masculine power dynamic that many men, especially those in sports, are unwilling to give up. In contrast, Messner and Sabo (1994) wrote that many men are unhappy with the rigid strictures under which they must perform a stereotypical masculinity. The authors suggested a variety of reforms to be made, including more co-ed sports opportunities, ending excessive violence in sports, and the confrontation of sexist "locker room talk," among others. However, despite calls from Melnick and other scholars, no one is reforming the male sport experience in ways that are comprehensive and/or focus on masculinity, rather through nitpicking one element of a sport experience (i.e., alcohol abuse).

Perhaps in response to Melnick's (1992) call to action, the mid-1990s saw the development of research on violence against women perpetrated by male athletes, particularly intercollegiate student-athletes. Mostly quantitative in nature, empirical findings were mixed. What follows is a review of the literature detailing research indicating higher rates of student-athlete perpetrators of sexual assault, criticism of the field, and the positive impact of rape education prevention programming with student-athletes. It is important to note that in studies of sexual assault, other campus factors (e.g., fraternity affiliation, drug and/or alcohol use) were addressed; however, due to the focus of this study, only athletic participation is considered here.

One of the first studies, by Fritner and Rubinson (1993), provided early data on student-athlete perpetration of sexual assault. Their study focused on the correlation between fraternity affiliation, alcohol use, and student-athlete involvement with violence against women. The authors sampled 925 randomly selected women. Responses categorized women as experiencing one of four crimes: (1) sexual assault; (2) attempted sexual assault; (3) sexual abuse; and (4) battery, illegal restraint, and/or intimidation. Results indicated that 27.1% of women were victims of one of these crimes. Additionally, many women experienced more than one form of abuse. Victims identified their perpetrators, with student-athletes representing 22.6% of perpetrators of sexual assaults; 13.7% of perpetrators of attempted sexual assaults; 13.6% of perpetrators of sexual abuse incidences; and 11.09% of perpetrators of battery, illegal restraint, and/or intimidation incidences. During the time of the study, student-athletes represented less than 2% of the overall male student body. As such, Fritner and Rubinson (1993) indicated that student-athletes were "vastly overrepresented as offenders of these crimes" (p. 282) and noted that future research into this area should be undertaken. The need for further study is noted throughout the decade by other researchers.

As with much of the literature, Koss and Gaines (1993) explored the link between fraternity affiliation, athletic participation, and sexual assault. Taking an approach different than Fritner and Rubinson (1993), the authors surveyed 530 male students, including 140 student-athletes, of which 16% participated in revenue-producing sports (i.e., football and basketball). Scored on such attributes such as sexual nonaggression, uninvited sexual advances, unwanted sexual contact, sexual coercion, and attempted or completed rape, the authors found true the "prediction of sexual aggression by participation in organized athletics" (Koss & Gaines, 1993, p. 104). However, the authors did indicate that the association between being a student-athlete and sexual aggression was less than that of alcohol and/or nicotine use (i.e., alcohol and/or nicotine use is a higher predictor of sexual aggression than athletic participation).

While Koss and Gaines (1993) relied on students' self-reports, Crosset et al. (1996) examined the incidences of sexual assault reported to campus judicial affairs. In their study of ten judicial affairs offices during a three-year period, they found an overrepresentation of male student-athletes as perpetrators of sexual assault and battering (i.e., domestic violence). Though the intent was to study battering, not all schools in the dataset kept complete records, and thus, both sexual assault and battering were analyzed. In the ten participating schools, 35% of the reported perpetrators of sexual assault and battering were student-athletes, though they comprised only 3% of the student body. The authors did acknowledge the small sample (69 reports of sexual assault, 21 reports of battering) and cautioned that the reports only constitute a small number of actual assaults occurring on any campus at any given time, due to the stigma, fear, and negative stereotypes experienced by victims of reporting these crimes, which, by their nature, are intimate and taboo.

Though previous research found a link between athletic participation and sexually aggressive behavior and actions, Boeringer (1996, 1999) found a link between sport participation and sexually aggressive attitudes. After surveying 477 male undergraduates, of whom 16.2% were student-athletes, he found that student-athletes displayed a "greater rape proclivity" (Boeringer, 1996, p. 134). Further, student-athletes were more likely than their non-athlete counterparts to report *potential* use of coercion, alcohol and drugs, and force. Participants were asked to indicate their likelihood in engaging in acts such as coercion, force, etc., if there was no chance they would be caught. Due to the hypothetical nature of the survey, the dataset does not indicate that student-athletes were more likely to *actually* use coercion, drugs and alcohol, and/or force; thus, Boeringer (1996) was only able to measure attitudes or behavioral intentions. As such, he reported that while student-athletes were more likely to hypothetically engage in sexual force, they were not more likely than non-athletes to *hypothetically* engage in sexual aggression. He concluded by noting that this study did not allow for variances between different types of student-athletes, and he suggested longitudinal research in the future to determine whether or not student-athletes who enter the sports world are already predisposed to violence and aggression, or whether participation in sports may encourage this aggression.

Boeringer (1999) followed his 1996 study with additional information about the likelihood of student-athletes to support rape myths, which are "beliefs and situational definitions that excuse rape or define assaultive situations as something other than rape" (p. 82). For example, a rape myth is that a woman "asked for it" by wearing a short skirt or revealing clothes. Within a sample of undergraduate men (detailed in Boeringer, 1996), he found that student-athletes were significantly more likely to report agreement with 14 rape-supportive myths than non-athletes. Boeringer hypothesized that hypermasculine environments were responsible for student-athletes' endorsement of rape myth. Fifty-six percent of student-athletes responded positively to rape-supportive myths, whereas only 8% of non-athletes agreed with the same statements.

Despite student-athletes' self-reports and campus records indicating higher proclivity and incidences of sexual assault among student-athletes, other research indicated otherwise. Crosset, Benedict, and McDonald (1995) surveyed 20 campus police departments and found that student-athletes were not represented as perpetrators of sexual assault at higher rates than non-athletes. A significant limitation of this study is that more than 80% of all rapes go unreported to police, and thus, the campus police reports are not necessarily a representative sample (Crosset et al., 1995).

Criticisms and Gaps in the Literature

The bulk of research on student-athlete violence against women was conducted and published in the mid-1990s. During this time, Koss and Cleveland (1996) detailed the methodological and conceptual concerns with the studies that led to such mixed empirical results. The authors noted problems such as convenience sampling, as well as the need for larger and more representative samples. They also indicated that "qualitative richness has not been matched by quantitative rigor" (Koss & Cleveland, 1996, p. 181). Additionally, they addressed the nature of self-selection: Are more aggressive, rape-supportive men joining sports teams because they are naturally aggressive, or do sports make student-athletes more aggressive? Their findings from this time period do not address this concern. Lastly, they discussed a need to measure sport subcultures. Boeringer (1996) acknowledged this as a limitation, and Crosset (1999) focused on this in his critique.

Similar to Koss and Cleveland (1996), Crosset (1999) addressed the variance of sports and their individual cultures, and he noted that future research "should focus on why some positions, teams, sports, or programs are prone to committing specific types of violence against women" (p. 249). It does not appear that this research has been undertaken since Crosset's criticism in 1999. He also wrote that much of the research relied too broadly upon rape culture and called for both specificity in methods as well as theoretical constructs in future research. Lastly, Crosset indicated a need to focus on structural changes within intercollegiate athletics and higher education, instead of relying upon individual and punitive responses to incidences of sexual assault against women by student-athletes.

Despite the calls to re-evaluate the methods and conceptual frameworks and continue to study student-athlete sexual assault (Crosset, 1999; Koss & Cleveland, 1996), there is a significant time gap in the research, with only three publications addressing student-athlete violence against women during the last 15 years. One study sought new empirical data on whether male student-athletes are more likely than non-athletes to perpetrate sexual assault (Sawyer et al., 2002). While the authors did narrow their focus and sample a variety of student-athlete groups (e.g., team-based versus individual sports, class rank), they did so with a convenience sample, one of the issues noted by Koss and Cleveland (1996) as a limitation in this field of study. Sawyer et al. (2002) found higher rape myth acceptance in male student-athletes, first and second year male athletes, male athletes who play team-based sports, and female athletes at Division I schools. Though these results cannot be generalized, their findings do support the idea that student-athletes are not a homogeneous group and should be studied accordingly.

Next, Murnen and Kohlman (2007) conducted a meta-analytic review of both behaviors and attitudes that support sexual aggression. Through statistical analysis, they discovered a moderate effect between athletic participation and hypermasculinity, an attribute that positively contributes to rape culture (Sanday, 1990). Further, small but significant associations were found between athletic participation and sexual aggression and rape myth acceptance. Murnen and Kohlman (2007) recommended longitudinal studies with this student population, as well as distinct studies among student-athlete subcultures and teams.

Finally, the most recent study discovered that both intercollegiate athletes and recreational athletes exhibited similar rates of sexual coercion, notably higher rates than non-athletes (Young et al., 2017). Further, when compared to non-athletes, the male athletes reported higher rape myth acceptance and poor attitudes toward women, considered to be a risk factor for sexual assault (Gage, 2008; Kimble, Russo, Bergman, & Galindo, 2010).

In summary, findings indicated student-athletes disproportionately represented perpetrators of incidences of violence against women (Crosset et al., 1996; Fritner & Rubinson, 1993) and possessed rape-supportive attitudes and rape myth acceptance (Boeringer, 1996, 1999; Koss & Gaines, 1993; Murnen & Kohlman, 2007; Sawyer et al., 2002; Young et al., 2017). One study found that student-athletes were not overrepresented as perpetrators of sexual assaults in campus police reports (Crosset et al., 1995). It is important to remember the methodological criticisms of and differences in these studies. Few examined actual perpetration—and those that did used a variety of methodologies. Many of the studies focused on attitudes, not behaviors (e.g., rape myth acceptance, perceived sexual aggression). As a whole, this body of research suggests that college athletes may be more sexually violent, but one should be cautioned that these studies do not definitively prove that student-athletes rape at higher rate than non-athletes.

Sexual Assault Prevention Efforts

Regardless of the complicated findings in sexual assault perpetration by athletes, many universities understood the critical need to reduce sexual assault on campus and began implementing both awareness and prevention education programs on campuses. Though athletic participation is only one correlate of sexual assault, efforts have been made to document the effects of programming with student-athletes. Jackson and Davis (2000) outlined an athlete-specific rape prevention program, similar to what many universities provide to student-athletes. Unfortunately, while the abstract noted that "the program has been in place for 10 years and has demonstrated several uniquely positive results" (Jackson & Davis, 2000, p. 589), these results were not detailed in a methodologically sound way within the paper. Several other programs, however, have documented success with empathy-based prevention (Foubert & Perry, 2007) and bystander intervention (Katz, 1995; McMahon & Farmer, 2009; Moynihan & Banyard, 2008).

Though the above studies related to awareness and prevention programming were specific to student-athletes, studies throughout the literature noted the impact and success of general and/or campus-wide efforts not specific to student-athletes (Anderson & Whiston, 2005; Berkowitz, 2002; Berg, Lonsway, & Fitzgerald, 1999; Breitenbecher, 2000; Heppner, Neville, Smith, Kivlighan, & Gershuny, 1999; Rothman & Silverman, 2007; Thatcher, 2011). According to Breitenbecher, however, "most published investigations have reported favorable, short-term results on at least one outcome variable measured in the study" (p. 39), with the most consistent support for programs that reduce rape myth acceptance. These positive findings should be interpreted with some caution however, as "studies that result in nonsignificant findings are often less likely to be published" (Breitenbecher, 2000, p. 40).

Rape-Prone Environments and Athletic Cultures

What may contribute to male student-athlete violence against women? As previously noted, regardless of athletic status, higher rape myth acceptance and poor attitudes toward women may be a risk factor for perpetrating sexual assault (Gage, 2008; Kimble et al., 2010). The hypermasculine attributes that contribute to rape culture help foster environments in which sexual assault victims are blamed while the perpetrators are not held accountable for their actions. However, in light of the literature criticisms above, it is imperative to note that not all athletes, teams, and athletic departments are rape cultures. Instead, it is critical to consider what factors may help to identify "rape-prone subcultures" (Crosset, 2016; Sanday, 1990).

Crosset (2016) outlined the four main factors that contribute to a rape-prone culture in intercollegiate athletics: (1) peer support for violence against women; (2) normativity of interpersonal violence (i.e., off the field/court violence); (3) institutional support for male privilege; and (4) institutional practices that fail to hold athletes accountable for criminal behavior. He noted that while the presence of merely one of these factors is not ideal, it is not until all four are present that universities, athletic departments, and/or teams are in danger of creating a hostile environment for women on campus. Examples of these factors in high-profile and recent incidences may be found in the athletic departments at University of Montana, Michigan State University, Baylor University, and Florida State University (see Krakauer, 2015; Lavigne & Noren, 2018; Luther, 2016). Baylor's sexual assault scandal clearly exhibits these four attributes. First, the peer support for violence against women may be seen in multiple gang rapes, in which more than one football player was involved in a specific act of violence against women (Reagan, 2016). Second, many players displayed a history of off-the-field violence. Notable in the Baylor case is Sam Ukwuachu, a transfer student from Boise State, where he was dismissed from the institution for violence against women (Ellis, 2016). Many scholars have noted that, essentially, the person most likely to commit a sexual assault is the one who has done it before (see Murphy, 2017). Baylor coach Art Briles was aware of Ukwuachu's violence and dismissal from Boise State (Ellis, 2016), exhibiting the third rape-prone factor. The institutional support for football and football players was so strong, that even previous violence against women was ignored in the quest to field a strong football team. Further, reports indicated that Briles knew of other sexual assaults by his players, but did not report them to the police or the university's Title IX office (Reagan, 2016). Fourth, multiple reports indicated that coaches failed to hold football players accountable for their behavior (see Ellis, 2016; Reagan, 2016). For example, Ukwuachu was allowed to participate in some team activities even after his indictment, an example of what independent investigators described as "improper conduct that reinforced an overall perception that football was above the rules, and that there was no culture of accountability for misconduct" (Belkin & Futterman, 2016). Baylor's athletic department is but one case of a rape-prone culture.

In addition to Crosset's (2016) four factors for a rape-prone environment, there are three types of athletic department cultures that exist in college sports (McCray, Sutherland, & Pastore, 2018). This qualitative study, in which 15 former athletes from "big time" athletic institutions were interviewed, provided an overview of how athletic departments both prevent and respond to sexual assault. Based on participant narratives, the study characterized athletic department responses based on attitudes and behaviors as either proactive or reactive, culminating in three types of athletic department cultures. The Zero Tolerance Culture is one that actively prevents sexual assault through educational efforts, perpetration accountability, and victim support. The Checkbox Culture is one that appears to "check a box" by meeting any educational or reporting requirements as set by the university or through Title IX. The Rape Culture is one that reflects the traditional meaning of a rape culture in its support of perpetrators and lack of meaningful action to prevent sexual assault. However, the results were not generalizable and more research is needed in the field to further explore the intertwined nature of sexual assault and college athletics.

There is still much to be learned about sexual assault in the context of intercollegiate athletics. While much of the research in the 1990s indicated that male student-athletes were more likely than non-athletes to be perpetrators or hold sexually aggressive attitudes, there is little research in the last two decades. However, violence against women continues to happen, particularly visible at "big time" athletic departments around the country. More research on rape-prone environments and athletic cultures may be helpful in designing and implementing effective sexual violence prevention education programs for athletes.

References

Abbey, A., Zawacki, T., Buck, P. O., Clinton, A. M., & McAuslan, P. (2001). Alcohol and sexual assault. *Alcohol Research and Health, 25*(1), 43–51.

Anderson, L. A., & Whiston, S. C. (2005). Sexual assault education programs: A meta-analytic examination of their effectiveness. *Psychology of Women Quarterly, 29*(4), 374–388.

Belkin, D., & Futterman, M. (2016, May 26). Baylor plans to fire Art Briles, demotes Ken Starr over scandal. *Wall Street Journal*. Retrieved from https://www.wsj.com/articles/baylor-plans-to-fire-art-briles-demotes-ken-starr-over-scandal-1464284169

Benedict, J. (1997). *Public heroes, private felons: Athletes and crimes against women*. Boston, MA: Northeastern University Press.

Berg, D. R., Lonsway, K. A., & Fitzgerald, L. F. (1999). Rape prevention education for men: The effectiveness of empathy-induction techniques. *Journal of College Student Development, 40*(3), 219–234.

Berkowitz, A. (2002). Fostering men's responsibility for preventing sexual assault. In P. A. Schewe (Ed.), *Preventing intimate partner violence: Developmentally appropriate interventions across the lifespan* (pp. 163–196). Washington, DC: American Psychological Association.

Black, M. C., Basile, K. C., Breiding, M. J., Smith, S. G., Walters, M. L., Merrick, M. T., … Stevens, M. R. (2011). *The National Intimate Partner and sexual violence survey (NISVS): 2010 summary report*. Atlanta, GA: National Center for Injury Prevention and Control, Centers for Disease Control and Prevention.

Boeringer, S. B. (1996). Influences of fraternity membership, athletics, and male living arrangements on sexual aggression. *Violence Against Women, 2*(2), 134–147.

Boeringer, S. B. (1999). Associations of rape-supportive attitudes with fraternal and athletic participation. *Violence Against Women, 5*(1), 81–90.

Brackenridge, C. (2002). Men loving men hating women: The crisis of masculinity and violence to women in sport. In S. Scraton & A. Flintoff (Eds.), *Gender and sport: A reader* (pp. 255–268). New York: Routledge.

Breitenbecher, K. H. (2000). Sexual assault on college campuses: Is an ounce of prevention enough? *Applied & Preventive Psychology, 9*(1), 23–52.

Burt, M. R. (1980). Cultural myths and supports for rape. *Journal of Personality and Social Psychology, 38*(2), 217–230.

Carr, J. L., & VanDeusen, K. M. (2004). Risk factors for male sexual aggression on college campuses. *Journal of Family Violence, 19*(5), 279–289.

Coakley, J. (2015). *Sports in society: Issues and controversies*. New York: McGraw-Hill.

Corprew, C. S., & Mitchell, A. D. (2014). Keeping it frat: Exploring the interaction among fraternity membership, disinhibition, and hypermasculinity on sexually aggressive attitudes in college-aged males. *Journal of College Student Development, 55*(6), 548–562.

Crosset, T. (1990). Masculinity, sexuality, and the development of early modern sport. In M. A. Messner & D. F. Sabo (Eds.), Sport, men, and the gender order: Critical feminist perspectives (pp. 45–54). Champaign, IL: Human Kinetics Books.

Crosset, T. (1999). Male athletes' violence against women: A critical assessment of the athletic affiliation, violence against women debate. *Quest, 51*, 244–257.

Crosset, T. W. (2016). Athletes, sexual assault, and universities' failure to address rape-prone subcultures on campus. In S. C. Wooten & R. W. Mitchell (Eds.), *The crisis of campus sexual violence: Critical perspectives on prevention and response* (pp. 74–91). New York: Routledge.

Crosset, T. W., Benedict, J. R., & McDonald, M. A. (1995). Male student-athletes reported for sexual assault: A survey of campus police departments and judicial affairs offices. *Journal of Sport & Social Issues, 19*(2), 126–140.

Crosset, T. W., Ptacek, J., McDonald, M. A., & Benedict, J. R. (1996). Male student athletes and violence against women: A survey of campus judicial affairs offices. *Violence Against Women, 2*(2), 163–179.

Crowe, L., & George, W. (1989). Alcohol and human sexuality: review and integration. *Psychological Bulletin, 105*, 374–386.

Crowell, N., & Burgess, A. (1996). Understanding violence against women. Washington, DC: National Academy Press.

Curry, T. J. (2002). Fraternal bonding in the locker room: A profeminist analysis of talk about competition and women. In S. Scraton & A. Flintoff (Eds.), Gender and sport: A reader (169–187). London: Routledge.

Ellis, Z. (2016). A timeline of the Baylor sexual assault scandal. *Sports Illustrated*. Retrieved from https://www.si.com/college-football/2016/05/26/baylor-art-briles-sexual-assault-ken-starr

Fisher, B. S., Cullen, F. T., & Turner, M. G. (2000). *The sexual victimization of college women* (NCJRS Document No. 182369). Retrieved from https://www.ncjrs.gov/pdffiles1/nij/182369.pdf

Foubert, J. D., & Perry, B. C. (2007). Creating lasting attitude and behavior change in fraternity members and male student athletes. *Violence Against Women, 13*(1), 70–86.

Fritner, M. P., & Rubinson, L. (1993). Acquaintance rape: The influence of alcohol, fraternity membership, and sports team membership. *Journal of Sex Education and Therapy, 19*, 272–284.

Gage, E. (2008). Gender attitudes and sexual behaviors: Comparing center and marginal athletes and non-athletes in a collegiate setting. *Violence Against Women, 14*, 1014–1032.

Heppner, M. J., Neville, H. A., Smith, K., Kivlighan, D. M., & Gershuny, B. S. (1999). Examining immediate and long-term efficacy of rape prevention programming with racially diverse college men. *Journal of Counseling Psychology, 46*(1), 16–26.

Herman, D. F. (1984). The rape culture. In J. Freeman (Ed.), *Women: A feminist perspective*. Mayfield: Palo Alto, CA.

Jackson, T. L., & Davis, J. L. (2000). Prevention of sexual and physical assault toward women: A program for male athletes. *Journal of Community Psychology, 28*(6), 589–605.

Katz, J. (1995). Reconstructing masculinity in the locker room: The Mentors in Violence Prevention project. *Harvard Educational Review, 65*(2), 163–174.

Kimble, N., Russo, S., Bergman, B., & Galindo, V. (2010). Revealing an empirical understanding of aggression and violent behavior in athletics. *Aggression and Violent Behavior, 15*, 446–462.

Koss, M. P., & Cleveland, H. H. (1996). Athletic participation, fraternity membership, and date rape. *Violence Against Women, 2*(2), 180–190.

Koss, M. P., & Gaines, J. A. (1993). The prediction of sexual aggression by alcohol use, athletic participation, and fraternity affiliation. *Journal of Interpersonal Violence, 8*(1), 94–108.

Krakauer, J. (2015). *Missoula: Rape and the justice system in a college town*. New York, NY: Doubleday.

Lavigne, P., & Noren, N. (2018). *OTL: Michigan State secrets extend far beyond Larry Nassar case. ESPN*. Retrieved from http://www.espn.com/espn/story/_/id/22214566/pattern-denial-inaction-information-suppression-michigan-state-goes-larry-nassar-case-espn

Lisak, D., & Miller, P. M. (2002). Repeat rape and multiple offending among undetected rapists. *Violence and Victims, 17*(1), 73–84.

Littleton, H., & Breitkopf, C. (2006). Coping with the experience of rape. *Psychology of Women Quarterly, 30*, 106–116.

Logan, T., Cole, J., & Capillo, A. (2006). Program and sexual assault survivor characteristics for one SANE program. *Journal of Forensic Nursing, 2*, 66–74.

Lonsway, K. A., & Fitzgerald, L. F. (1994). Rape myths: In review. *Psychology of Women Quarterly, 18*, 133–164.

Luther, J. (2016). *Unsportsmanlike conduct: College football and the politics of rape*. New York, NY: Akashic Books.

McCray, K. L., Sutherland, S. L., & Pastore, D. L. (2018). Creating change in intercollegiate athletics: The sexual assault prevention paradigm for athletic departments. *Journal of Higher Education, Athletics, & Innovation, 1*(4), 25–53.

McMahon, S. (2011). *Changing perceptions of sexual violence over time*. Harrisburg, PA: VAWnet, a project of the National Resource Center on Domestic Violence. Retrieved http://www.vawnet.org/Assoc_Files_VAWnet/AR_ChangingPerceptions.pdf

McMahon, S., & Farmer, G. L. (2009). The bystander approach: Strengths-based sexual assault prevention with at-risk groups. *Journal of Human Behavior in the Social Environment, 19*, 1042–1065.

Melnick, M. (1992). Male athletes and sexual assault. *Journal of Physical Education, Recreation & Dance, 63*(5), 32–35.

Messner, M. A., & Sabo, D. F. (1994). *Sex, violence, & power in sports: Rethinking masculinity*. Freedom, CA: The Crossing Press.

Moynihan, M., Banyard, V., Arnold, J., Eckstein, R., & Stapleton, J. (2010). Engaging intercollegiate athletes in preventing and intervening in sexual and intimate partner violence. *Journal of American College Health, 59*(3), 197–204.

Moynihan, M. M., & Banyard, V. L. (2008). Community responsibility for preventing sexual violence: A pilot study with campus Greeks and intercollegiate athletes. *Journal of Prevention & Intervention in the Community, 36*(1/2), 23–39.

Murnen, S. K., & Kohlman, M. H. (2007). Athletic participation, fraternity membership, and sexual aggression among college men: A meta-analytic review. *Sex Roles, 57*, 145–157.

Murphy, H. (2017, October 30). What experts know about men who rape. *New York Times*. Retrieved from https://www.nytimes.com/2017/10/30/health/men-rape-sexual-assault.html

Pope, E., & Shouldice, M. (2001). Drugs and sexual assault: a review. *Trauma, Violence, & Abuse, 2*, 51–55.

Reagan, B. (2016, October 28). Baylor regents found sexual assaults by football players "horrifying". *Wall Street Journal*. Retrieved from https://www.wsj.com/articles/baylor-details-horrifying-alleged-sexual-assaults-by-football-players-1477681988

Rothman, E., & Silverman, J. (2007). The effect of a college sexual assault prevention program on first-year students' victimization rates. *Journal of American College Health, 55*(5), 283–290.

Sable, M. R., Danis, F., Mauzy, D. L., & Gallagher, S. K. (2006). Barriers to reporting sexual assault for women and men: Perspectives of college students. *Journal of American College Health, 55*(3), 157–162.

Sanday, P. R. (1981). The socio-cultural context of rape: A cross-cultural study. *Journal of Social Issues, 37*(4), 5–27.

Sanday, P. R. (1990). *Fraternity gang rape: Sex, brotherhood, and privilege on campus*. New York: New York University Press.

Sawyer, R. G., Thompson, E. E., & Chicorelli, A. (2002). Rape myth acceptance among intercollegiate student athletes: A preliminary examination. *American Journal of Health Studies, 18*(1), 19–25.

Schwartz, M. D., & DeKeseredy, W. S. (1997). *Sexual assault on the college campus: The role of male peer support*. Thousand Oaks, CA: Sage Publications.

Thatcher, W. G. (2011). Preliminary evaluation of "playing the game" sexual assault prevention theatre program. *International Electronic Journal of Health Education, 14*, 109–121.

Ullman, S. E., Karabatsos, G., & Koss, M. P. (1999). Alcohol and sexual assault in a national sample of college women. *Journal of Interpersonal Violence, 14*(6), 603–625.

Welch, M. (1997). Violence against women by professional football players: A gender analysis of hypermasculinity, positional status, narcissism, and entitlement. *Journal of Sport & Social Issues, 21*(4), 392–411.

Young, B. R., Desmarais, S. L., Baldwin, J. A., & Chandler, R. (2017). Sexual coercion practices among undergraduate male recreational athletes, intercollegiate athletes, and non-athletes. *Violence Against Women, 23*(7), 795–812.

Exhibitionism

45

Leah E. Kaylor and Elizabeth L. Jeglic

Historically, exhibitionism comes from the Latin word *exhibere* meaning "to show or to present" (Hanafy, Clervoy, & Brenot, 2016, p. e61). In 300 B.C., Theophrastus coined the term exhibitionist; however, it was not until 1824 that this behavior became illegal in England under the *Vagrancy Act* (Hanafy et al., 2016). In 1877, exhibitionism was specifically defined by French physician, Ernest-Charles Lasègue, as an individual revealing parts of his body, but going no further (Lasègue, 1877; Murphy & Page, 2008). Further acknowledgement of exhibitionism as a deviant sexual act resulted from the publication *Psychopathia Sexualis* by German psychiatrist Richard von Krafft-Ebing (Långström, 2010; von Krafft-Ebing, 1965).

Although exhibitionism dates back to 300 B.C., it was not included in the Diagnostic and Statistical Manual of Mental Disorders [DSM] until 1980 (American Psychiatric Association) (APA, 1980; Grant, 2005). Consequently, there is a dearth of literature on this specific type of sexual offense. The limited research on the topic may be reflective of the perception that exhibitionism is considered more of a nuisance behavior as opposed to a sexual crime (Långström, 2010; Morin & Levenson, 2008; Murphy & Page, 2008). This chapter comprehensively examines exhibitionism including how it is defined, gaps in the literature, best practices for working with those who engage in exhibitionistic behaviors, future research directions, and prevention measures.

L. E. Kaylor (✉)
Saint Louis University, St. Louis, MO, USA
e-mail: Leah.kaylor@slu.edu

E. L. Jeglic
John Jay College of Criminal Justice,
New York, NY, USA

Definition

Exhibitionism was first introduced into the DSM in its third edition in 1980 and was defined as "repetitive acts of exposing the genitals to an unsuspecting stranger for the purpose of achieving sexual excitement, with no attempt at further sexual activity with the stranger" (APA, 1980, p. 272). Since that time, the clinical definition of exhibitionistic disorder in the DSM has remained relatively unchanged (Långström, 2010). The latest edition, the DSM-5, now refers to this behavior as exhibitionistic disorder, which is one of eight conditions classified in the DSM-5 as a paraphilic disorder, referring to persistent and intense atypical sexual arousal which causes clinically significant distress or impairment (American Psychiatric Association, 2013; Hanafy et al., 2016).

According to the DSM-5, exhibitionistic disorder involves persistent and intense sexual arousal from exposing one's genitals to a nonconsenting person, typically a stranger, as manifested

W. T. O'Donohue and P. A. Schewe (eds.), *Handbook of Sexual Assault and Sexual Assault Prevention*,
https://doi.org/10.1007/978-3-030-23645-8_45

by fantasies, urges, or behaviors (APA, 2013). Over a period of at least 6 months, individuals with this disorder must have "acted on these sexual urges with a nonconsenting person, or the sexual urges or fantasies have caused clinically significant distress or impairment in social, occupational, or other important areas of functioning" (APA, 2013, p. 689). There are several subtypes of exhibitionistic disorder depending upon the age of the nonconsenting person. For example, exhibitionists may prefer to expose themselves to prepubescent children, adults, or both (APA, 2013).

Some individuals with exhibitionistic disorder may deny that they expose their genitals to others or they may deny that acting on these fantasies causes distress. Regardless of the denial component of this disorder, an individual can still be diagnosed with exhibitionistic disorder if they have exposed themselves repeatedly to nonconsenting persons (APA, 2013). Recurrent genital exposure is typically interpreted as three or more victims on separate occasions. If there are fewer than three victims, the diagnostic criteria can still be met if there were multiple occasions of exposure to the same victim (APA, 2013).

The International Classification of Diseases 10th revision [ICD-10] defines exhibitionism as "recurrent or persistent tendency to expose one's genitals, without desiring or attempting to obtain closer contact" (World Health Organization, 1992). This definition specifies that exposures may be limited to times of emotional distress and may disappear for long periods of time (Hanafy et al., 2016; WHO, 1992). This chapter relies on the DSM-5 definition of exhibitionistic disorder.

Legally, exposing one's genitals is considered to be a sexual offense. Sexual offenses can be divided into two categories: contact (hands-on) and noncontact (hands-off) offenses (MacPherson, 2003). During a contact offense, the perpetrator makes physical contact with a victim and encompasses acts such as forcible rape and other forms of sexual assault. Conversely, exhibitionism is considered a noncontact sexual offense as the perpetrator does not touch their victim during the commission of the offense (McNally & Fremouw, 2014).

Exhibitionism and Gender

Prevalence

The exact prevalence for exhibitionistic disorder is unknown; however, researchers have estimated that based upon exhibitionistic acts in the general population that the highest possible prevalence for this condition in males is 2–4% (APA, 2013). Even less is known about the prevalence for exhibitionistic disorder in females, yet it is assumed to be much lower than that of males (Murphy & Page, 2008). Interestingly, although we do not know the exact prevalence for this disorder, exhibitionistic behavior it not uncommon (Firestone, Kingston, Wexler, & Bradford, 2006; Rabinowitz-Greenberg, Firestone, Bradford, & Greenberg, 2002). Researchers believe exhibitionistic acts are the most commonly reported of all sex offenses, accounting for one-third (Rooth, 1973) to two-thirds of all reported sexual offenses (Abel, Becker, Cunningham-Rathner, Mittelman, & Rouleau, 1988; Firestone et al., 2006; Gebhard, Gagnon, Pomeroy, & Christenson, 1965; McNally & Fremouw, 2014). Estimating the incidence of exhibitionism is difficult as the majority of research has been drawn from clinical samples, which may only represent individuals with chronic and serious sexual offense histories or comorbid mental health disorders (Bader, Schoeneman-Morris, Scalora, & Casady, 2008; Murphy, 1997).

There appears to be gender differences in the prevalence of exhibitionism. A national survey completed on 4800 randomly selected Swedish individuals ranging from 18–60 years of age, revealed 4.3% of men and 2.1% of women admitted to acts of exhibitionism (Långström & Seto, 2006). Despite this data showing females do engage in exhibitionism, the vast majority of exhibitionists who are apprehended by authorities are male (Blair & Lanyon, 1981; Gebhard et al., 1965; McGrath, 1991; Swindell et al., 2011). Some researchers go as far as considering exhibitionism to be exclusively a male disorder (Rickles, 1955); however, most recognize the existence of female exhibitionists, but highlight that it is a rare phenomenon (Schneider, 1982;

Stekel, 1952). Although the bulk of available research describes male exhibitionists, Carnes (2001) found that females in treatment for sexual addiction reported higher levels of exhibitionistic behavior compared to their male counterparts. Yet, many of these women describe receiving few legal ramifications for their exhibitionistic behavior and were often rewarded in the form of sexual attention from others (Carnes, 2001; Hopkins, Green, Carnes, & Campling, 2016). Of note, this study revealed that although the proportion of females in treatment who reported exhibitionistic acts were higher than males, the total number of women in treatment was far less than the total number of men (Carnes, 2001).

In another study comparing men and women in treatment for problematic sexual behaviors, female exhibitionists scored above males on measures of prostitution, forcible sex, pimping, exploitation of authority figures, and engagement in illegal behaviors (Hopkins et al., 2016). While female exhibitionists reported engaging in illegal behaviors at a greater frequency, men are disproportionately arrested for sexual offenses (Hopkins et al., 2016). Explanations for the disproportion in arrest rates may be accounted for by different laws (e.g., it is not illegal to show breasts in certain jurisdictions), gender bias (i.e., men are considered to be more dangerous), or low reporting rates against women by men who welcome seductive behavior (Hopkins et al., 2016). Stekel (1952) describes exhibitionism as more socially acceptable in women via occupations that involve exotic dancing, strip tease, burlesque, and fashion (Schneider, 1982). Contrary to explanations of exhibitionism in men, the primary motivation for women is thought to be attention seeking rather than sexual gratification, which by definition would not meet criteria for exhibitionistic disorder (Hollender, Brown, & Roback, 1977; Schneider, 1982). Additional research needs to be done on females who expose themselves to understand their motivations to determine whether this behavior would meet criteria for exhibitionistic disorder or if this behavior is a form of attention seeking.

One of the challenges in estimating the prevalence of exhibitionistic disorder is significant underreporting (Långström & Seto, 2006). According to Grant (2005), many exhibitionists have exposed themselves on numerous occasions without arrest (Swindell et al., 2011). Researchers believe that acts of exhibitionism may occur up to 150 times more often that what is reflected in official police statistics (Abel et al., 1988; Bader et al., 2008). To further support this claim, a study conducted by Riordan (1999) revealed that 43% of individuals who had been subject to an exhibitionistic act did not report the crime to the police. Perpetrator self-reports may also underestimate the frequency of these behaviors as they may be motivated to underreport these acts in clinical or criminal justice settings (Abel et al., 1987; Bader et al., 2008; Bhugra, Popelyuk, & McMullen, 2010; Clark, Jeglic, Calkins, & Tatar, 2016). In spite of measurement challenges, the available research using official and perpetrator reports suggest that not only does exhibitionistic exposure take place frequently (Firestone et al., 2006; Rabinowitz-Greenberg et al., 2002), but also that each perpetrator has a large number of victims (Abel & Rouleau, 1990; Clark et al., 2016; Kafka & Hennen, 1999; Långström & Seto, 2006).

Due to the combination of a high number of victims per perpetrator and the low frequency of reporting, rates of exhibitionism may be more accurately calculated through the use of victim self-reports (Clark et al., 2016). In stark contrast to official police statistics, victim self-report studies estimate that lifetime victimization for exhibitionistic acts range from 33% to 52% (Clark et al., 2016; Cox, 1988; Rhoads & Borjes, 1981; Riordan, 1999). Exhibitionism studies have revealed that perpetrators primarily target young females with no relationship to the perpetrator (Clark et al., 2016; Riordan, 1999). One study found that 88.5% of female victims of exhibitionism were under the age of 21 at the time of the incident (Riordan, 1999). In addition to being young and female, many exhibitionists (68.1%) prefer exposing themselves to strangers (Cox, 1988; Freund, Watson, & Rienzo, 1988). Since incidences of exhibitionism are rarely reported to the authorities, it has been hypothesized that girls and young women are purposely targeted because they may believe that due to their age, they are more scared and timid, and thus less likely to yell/scream, or report the exposure (Clark et al., 2016). Underreporting exhibitionistic acts may result from younger victims not recognizing this behavior as a crime or having the ability to report to offense to the police (Bader et al., 2008; Clark et al., 2016).

Location

The location of exhibitionistic crimes varies based upon geographic locale of the study. For instance, police reports from a Midwestern police department revealed 25% of genital exposure occurred in parking lots, 21% occurred on a public street, and in 20.8% of the cases, the perpetrator exposed himself while inside a vehicle (Bader et al., 2008; Clark et al., 2016). Another study completed in a major U.S. city found that many instances of exhibitionism occur at public transportation stops (i.e., subway station) (53%) (Clark et al., 2016). Moreover, a study completed on 100 female nurses in the United Kingdom found that 39% of reported exhibitionistic acts occurred in parks or wooded areas (Clark et al., 2016; Gittleson, Eacott, & Mehta, 1978). Exhibitionism offenses may also take place in the victim's neighborhood or near their residence (Clark et al., 2016).

Development and Course

Adult males with exhibitionistic disorder often report that their interest in exposing their genitals to nonconsenting persons began during adolescence or early adulthood. There is no minimum age requirement for exhibitionistic disorder, thus it can be difficult to differentiate exhibitionistic behavior with age-appropriate sexual curiosity in adolescence (APA, 2013; Murphy & Page, 2008). Impulses to expose oneself typically begin in adolescence or young adulthood and are thought to decrease with age. Little information is available on the persistence and progression of this disorder over time (APA, 2013).

Etiology

Little is known about the development of exhibitionistic disorder (Swindell et al., 2011). This section will review popular etiology theories of exhibitionistic disorder including the behavioral theory, psychoanalytic theory, physiological approach, and the courtship disorder hypothesis.

Behavioral Theory

The most common etiological theory for the development of exhibitionistic disorder is the behavioral theory of classical conditioning. According to classical conditioning theory, a stimulus that would not usually initiate a response (in this case, the stimulus is exposing one's genitals to an unsuspecting person) is presented shortly before the unconditioned stimulus that will initiate the response (in exhibitionism, the stimulus is masturbation to achieve and maintain an erection with or without ejaculation) and this pattern of events is repeated often enough for the individual to associate these acts together (Hoffmann, Janssen, & Turner, 2004; Kantorowitz, 1978a, 1978b; Lalumi'ere & Quinsey, 1998; Plaud & Martini, 1999; Rachman, 1966; Rachman & Hodgson, 1968; Swindell et al., 2011). It is common for a perpetrator to masturbate during an exhibitionistic act, thus masturbating both before and after each exhibitionistic episode will result in classical conditioning to the exposure behavior (Firestone et al., 2006; Freund et al., 1988; Grant, 2005; Swindell et al., 2011).

Researchers who subscribe to the behavioral theory of conditioning believe that the first step towards developing exhibitionism occurs by random chance at an early age in which the individual exposes his or her genitals to someone and finds the experience to be pleasurable and sexually stimulating (Bandura, 1982; Kinsey, Pomeroy, Martin, & Gebhard, 1953; Kinsey, Reichert, Cauldwell, & Mozes, 1955). Since the individual found that experience to be pleasurable, the act will likely be repeated. The next step towards developing exhibitionistic disorder occurs when the individual begins to fantasize about exposing themselves, planning on how to engage in this behavior without being caught by the authorities, and masturbating to fantasies about exposing oneself (Langevin et al., 1979; Swindell et al., 2011). According to this theory, the urge to engage in exhibitionistic acts becomes more powerful and the frequency of exposing oneself increases (Grant, 2005).

Three categories of events were hypothesized to initiate exhibitionism and start the conditioning process: sharing a bathtub, appearing nude before family members, and children looking at one another's genitals during early sex play (Swindell et al., 2011). Moreover, the experience of a post-pubertal male seeing his mother naked was considered to be a form of modeling exhibitionism on the mother's part (Bandura, 1986). Such an experience is hypothesized to lead to sexual arousal in response to the mother's exhibitionism and serve as the foundation for incorrectly concluding that if he exposes himself to women, they will also become sexually aroused (Swindell et al., 2011).

When developing exhibitionistic disorder, exposing oneself is pleasurable; however, when exposing one's genitals follows an aversive feeling this behavior is used to self-soothe. Eventually, an aversive mood, feeling, or specific location (e.g., stress, boredom, sadness, feelings of inadequacy, interpersonal conflict, attractive person, and particular location) become the conditioned stimulus that evokes an urge to expose oneself (Grant, 2005; Grob, 1985; Swindell et al., 2011). A cycle in formed in which engaging in exhibitionism results in urges to expose oneself, thus acting on these urges serves as further conditioning (Grant, 2005). Therefore, a mood, feeling, urge, or location can all trigger the conditioned response of exhibitionistic behavior.

Psychoanalytic Theory

Historically, exhibitionism and other sexual deviations were first explained by psychoanalytic theory. This approach emphasizes interacting motives, intrapsychic forces, drives, conflicts, past behavior, and unconscious impulses in an effort to account for genital exposure (Blair & Lanyon, 1981). Psychoanalytic theory posits that exhibitionistic behavior in males is a defense against castration anxiety. By exposing oneself, the exhibitionist receives verification via the victim's response that his penis does exist (Blair & Lanyon, 1981; Enelow, 1969; Fenichel, 1964; Freud, 1905, 1914; Holtzman & Kulish, 2012; Rosen, 1964). Freud describes exhibitionism in women as defense against a narcissistic wound from castration by instead accentuating other parts of her body, particularly breasts, to display her attractiveness and draw attention away from her lack of penis (Blair & Lanyon, 1981; Freud, 1905, 1914; Holtzman & Kulish, 2012). Another factor thought to contribute to exhibitionistic behavior is a masochistic need to be caught and punished by the police (Blair & Lanyon, 1981; Enelow, 1969; Stekel, 1952).

Physiological Approach

Neuroscientists believe exhibitionistic behavior is a result of excessive neuronal discharges in the subcortical areas of the brain, particularly in the limbic system (Blair & Lanyon, 1981; Monroe, 1976). Excessive neuronal discharges are thought to account for impulsively acting upon deviant sexual urges (Monroe, 1976). Neuroscientists conceptualize sexual paraphilias to be on the obsessive-compulsive spectrum and encourage selective serotonin reuptake inhibitors (SSRIs) as the treatment of choice for this disorder (Abouesh & Clayton, 1999).

Courtship Disorder Hypothesis

Another explanation for the development of sexual paraphilias is the courtship disorder hypothesis, which postulates that exhibitionism is part of a larger progression of sexual behaviors that are socially abnormal yet are thought to function as the equivalent to normal dating patterns (Freund, 1990). Freund and Watson (1990) describe a typical sexual courtship beginning with visually selecting an appealing partner, followed by a nonphysical interaction, leading to physical touching, and culminating in sexual intercourse. According to this hypothesis, voyeurism can be conceptualized as a disturbance in the visual selection stage, exhibitionistic disorder can be understood as a disturbance in the second stage of nonphysical exchange, frottuerism and toucherism are disturbances in the touching phase, and rape as the nonconsensual final step (Clark et al., 2016; Freund, 1990; Freund & Watson, 1990; Hopkins et al., 2016). The courtship disorder hypothesis has been used to explain the highly comorbid nature of sexual paraphilias as well as the escalation to more severe sexual offending (McNally & Fremouw, 2014).

The primary goal of exhibitionism is to forcefully attract the attention of others (Carnes, Delmonico, & Griffin, 2007; Murphy & Page, 2006). There is debate as to whether exhibitionists experience sexual gratification without the wish for sexual contact (Hopkins et al., 2016; Murphy & Page, 2006). There are studies that provide support for the courtship disorder hypothesis, whereby exhibitionistic acts are an invitation for sexual contact (Freund et al., 1988; Hopkins et al., 2016; Lang, Langevin, Checkley, & Pugh, 1987). The overlap of various paraphilias may be better conceptualized from the courtship disorder hypothesis, where voyeurism, exhibitionism, frotteurism, toucherism, and rape are all progressive expressions of the same disorder (Freund & Watson, 1990).

Risk Factors and Comorbidity

Childhood emotional and sexual abuse as well as a preoccupation with sex/hypersexuality have been cited as risk factors for developing exhibitionistic disorder (APA, 2013). Acting on exhibitionistic impulses goes against both social norms as well as criminal law, thus a risk factor for engaging in exhibitionism may be a propensity for risk-taking (Långström & Seto, 2006; Quinsey, Skilling, Lalumière, & Craig, 2004). An inclination for risk-taking behavior may be explained by sex differences, drug and alcohol usage, and antisocial tendencies (Lalumère, Harris, Quinsey, & Rice, 2005; Långström & Seto, 2006; Seto & Barbaree, 1997; Quinsey, Skilling, & Lalumi'ere, & Craig, 2004).

Much of the information on known comorbidities is largely based on research on individuals who have been convicted for exposing themselves. Therefore, these comorbidities may not apply to everyone meeting criteria for exhibitionistic disorder. According to the DSM, exhibitionistic disorder is highly comorbid with anxiety, depression, substance use, bipolar disorder, attention-deficit/hyperactivity disorder, other sexual paraphilias, hypersexuality, and antisocial personality disorder (APA, 2013). Moreover, characteristics most often seen in individuals with exhibitionistic disorder are poor social skills and difficulty controlling their anger or hostility (Bader et al., 2008; Lee, Pattison, Jackson, & Ward, 2001; Raymond, Coleman, Ohlerking, Christenson, & Miner, 1999). A study by Bader et al. (2008) found that based on police reports from 106 exhibitionists: 37 were thought to have been abusing illegal drugs, 29 were suspected of abusing alcohol, 26 individuals showed symptoms of a mental disorder, and four perpetrators showed signs of developmental disabilities at the time they were arrested for exposing themselves.

Exhibitionism is highly comorbid with other sexual paraphilias (Bader et al., 2008; Kafka & Hennen, 1999; Price, Gutheil, Commons, Kafka, & Dodd-Kimmey, 2001). In a study of 241 individuals with exhibitionistic disorder, 32% also engaged in voyeurism and 30% also engaged in frotteurism (Bader et al., 2008; Freund, 1990). Another study of 142 exhibitionists found that 93% of the sample also engaged in pedophilia, rape, or voyeurism (Abel et al., 1988; Bader et al., 2008). Literature on exhibitionism suggests a high comorbidity with telephone scatologia, which entails calling unsuspecting individuals but does not involve physical touching for the perpetrator to become aroused. Scatologia is considered to be a verbal form of exhibitionism (Bader et al., 2008; Dalby, 1988; Price et al., 2001).

Recidivism and Escalation

Historically, exhibitionistic behavior was considered a nuisance and individuals exposing themselves were not considered to be sexually aggressive; however, empirical research has provided evidence that not only do exhibitionists recidivate at high rates but some also escalate to contact sexual offenses (Rabinowitz-Greenberg et al., 2002; Rooth, 1973). Measuring recidivism can be a challenge since many exhibitionists may not come into contact with authorities (Bader et al., 2008; Bartosh, Garby, Lewis, & Gray, 2003; Doren, 2002). Those exhibitionists who do come into contact with the criminal justice system or treatment programs typically have committed a contact offense (Bader et al., 2008; Sugarman, Dumughn, Saad, Hinder, & Bluglass, 1994). Despite the difficulty in measuring recidivism, there is evidence to support that exhibitionists recidivate at a very high rate—estimates range from 18.6% to 56.9% (Bader et al., 2008; Berlin et al., 1991; Gebhard et al., 1965; Swindell et al., 2011). Furthermore, exhibitionists who masturbated during exposure had more exhibitionism charges compared to those who did not masturbate during exposure (Bader et al., 2008). According to the American Psychiatric Association (2013), pedophilic sexual preference, antisocial history, alcohol misuse, and antisocial personality disorder may increase the risk of recidivism in individuals with exhibitionistic disorder.

Not only is exhibitionism highly comorbid with other sexual paraphilias, but also there is evidence to suggest that some exhibitionists may escalate to more serious sexual crimes. McNally and Fremouw (2014) found that approximately 25% of exhibitionists will recidivate with any type of sexual offense; whereas, 5–10% of exhibitionists will escalate to a subsequent contact offense during a five-year follow-up period. Exhibitionistic behavior has been associated with past, current, and future acts of pedophilia, attempted and completed rape, and sexual murder (Gebhard et al., 1965; McNally & Fremouw, 2014; Rooth, 1973). A study completed by Abel et al. (1988) found that 46% of exhibitionists also sexually assaulted children or engaged in an incestuous offense. Moreover, in a sample of 241 exhibitionists, 15% admitted to raping an adult (Bader et al., 2008; Freund, 1990).

Researchers have been working to identify risk factors that may contribute to the escalation from noncontact genital exposure to contact sexual offenses. Both hypersexuality and excessive libido have been posited as the underlying mechanism that lead to more serious contact offenses (Kafka, 2003a, 2003b; McNally & Fremouw, 2014; Morin & Levenson, 2008; Sugarman et al., 1994). Moreover, exhibitionists who masturbated during exposure, touched, or communicated with their victims were found to be more likely to escalate to sexually assaultive acts (Bader et al., 2008; Petri, 1969; Sugarman et al., 1994). Another predictor of escalation to contact offending is a preference toward exposing oneself to children (McNally & Fremouw, 2014; Mohr, Turner, & Ball, 1962). Bluglass (1980) has suggested that low intelligence as well as features of conduct or personality disorders pose a risk for escalation (McNally & Fremouw, 2014).

In an effort to better understand risk factors for exhibitionistic behavior, Sugarman et al. (1994) analyzed criminal records of 210 English males convicted of indecent exposure. The exhibitionists who went on to commit contact offenses were more likely to be intellectually impaired and have a family history of substance use. Moreover, escalated offenders were more likely to have a personality disorder, excessive libido (as measured by more than one orgasm per day), and a childhood diagnosis of conduct disorder (Sugarman et al., 1994). Contact offenders were also found to expose themselves at more than one location, corner, touch, and speak to victims, display an erect penis, and masturbate during exposure compared to exhibitionists who did not escalate to contact offenses (McNally & Fremouw, 2014; Sugarman et al., 1994).

There exists some data to suggest that exhibitionists also engage in other nonsexual criminal behaviors (Abel et al., 1988; Bader et al., 2008; Maletzky, 1997). It is estimated that between 17% and 30% of exhibitionists who are arrested for exposing themselves have a conviction history for committing other nonsexual crimes (Bader et al., 2008; Berah & Myers, 1983; Blair & Lanyon, 1981). An Australian study of 151 male exhibitionists found that 69% were also convicted for another offense other than exposing oneself, including violating parole, driving infractions, assault, and property crime (Bader et al., 2008; Berah & Myers, 1983). Furthermore, evidence from several studies suggest that exhibitionists who later committed contact sexual offenses were more likely to have prior criminal charges compared to noncontact recidivists (Firestone et al., 2006; McNally & Fremouw, 2014; Rabinowitz-Greenberg et al., 2002; Sugarman et al., 1994). These findings suggest that those who engage in exhibitionism may also be engaging other criminal acts (Hackett, 1971; Murphy, 1997; Rooth, 1971).

Assessment

Mental health professionals are often asked to assess recidivism risk. Determining whether an exhibitionist will escalate to a contact sexual offense can be a challenge, especially since research is lacking and available data have historically found mixed results (McNally & Fremouw, 2014; Rooth, 1973). There is no standardized risk assessment battery for those engaging in exhibitionistic behavior; however, a battery of tests including psychological, behavioral, self-report, and collateral information is recommended as best practice (Adams & Sturgis, 1977; Adams, Webster, & Carson, 1980; Barlow, 1977; Blair & Lanyon, 1981).

The cornerstone of an accurate assessment is understanding the behavior of interest (Bader et al., 2008). Important information for determining risk hinges upon the frequency, severity, and extent of deviant sexual behaviors. Especially when assessing exhibitionists, it is critical to obtain a comprehensive history of exposure, masturbation during exposure, libido levels, touching or communicating with victims during exposure (Bader et al., 2008; Petri, 1969; Sugarman et al., 1994). Since many exhibitionistic acts do not come to the attention of authorities, self-report is the primary method of data collection. However, given sexual offenders tend to underreport their offense history, accurate assessment can be challenging (Maletzky, 1997; McConaghy, 1993). Collateral information can be acquired from police reports, victim statements, and other sources of information (Bader et al., 2008). Other risk factors for escalation include substance use and abuse and thus gathering information on the offender's drug and alcohol usage is another an important component of the risk assessment (Bader et al., 2008). If the assessment is being completed for treatment purposes, information pertaining to cognitive distortions, denial of behavior, and instances of minimization should also be gathered in an effort to manage risk (Bader et al., 2008; Doren, 2002; Marshall, Anderson, & Fernandez, 1999).

Since there is not a specific psychological assessment battery given to exhibitionists, evaluators often pull assessment measures from tests completed with contact sex offenders. Due to the lack of exhibitionist-specific literature, it is recommended that similar assessment procedures completed on general sex offenders be followed until more research is conducted. A commonly used measure for discriminating between recidivists and nonrecidivists for criminal and violent crimes is the Psychopathy Checklist—Revised [PCL-R], which has been touted as a superior measure for predicting violent behavior (Fulero, 1995; Hare, Forth, & Strachan, 1992; Harris, Rice, & Quinsey, 1993; Rabinowitz-Greenberg et al., 2002; Serin, Malcolm, Khanna, & Barbaree, 1994). The PCL-R is a 20-item semi-structured interview, which takes into consideration the offender's personality traits and criminal history to assess for the presence of psychopathy (Venables, Hall, & Patrick, 2013). While it has been suggested that exhibitionists may engage in fewer antisocial behaviors compared to contact sex offenders, obtaining an accurate offense history is critical in determining risk for recidivism. Previous research has revealed that sexual recidivists had significantly more offenses in the sexual and criminal categories compared to nonrecidivists (Rabinowitz-Greenberg et al., 2002). Moreover, there is a growing body of literature suggesting those with elevated PCL-R scores are at a higher risk to recidivate, will reoffend sooner, and the next offense is more likely to be violent in nature compared to nonpsychopaths (Hare et al., 1992; Harris et al., 1993; Rabinowitz-Greenberg et al., 2002; Serin et al., 1994).

Phallometric assessment, also known as penile plethysmography, is an objective assessment measure used to identify deviant sexual interests in males. Phallometry measures changes in penile circumference in response to both nonsexual and sexual stimuli. Rabinowitz-Greenberg et al. (2002) used audiotaped vignettes depicting sexual activity varying the sex, age, and degree of consent, coercion, and violence on a group of exhibitionists. They found that penile plethysmography arousal to vignettes involving rape, especially those involving children were useful in determining a subgroup of exhibitionists who would escalate their behavior to more serious contact offenses (Rabinowitz-Greenberg et al., 2002). A Canadian study reviewed criminal records for 221 individuals with exhibitionistic disorder found that the contact recidivists scored significantly higher in psychopathy as well as on phallometric arousal to pedophilia and rape audio scenarios compared to noncontact recidivists (Rabinowitz-Greenberg et al., 2002). Overall, exhibitionists high in psychopathy as well as deviant sexual arousal patterns as measured by the phallometric assessment were more likely to escalate to contact offenses (McNally & Fremouw, 2014; Rabinowitz-Greenberg et al., 2002).

Another way exhibitionists have been examined for risk of reoffending and escalating their behavior is through the two-pronged typology of perpetrators (Rooth, 1971). Rooth described the first type of exhibitionists as inhibited through the exposure of a flaccid penis. According to Rooth, these individuals have low levels of comorbid psychopathology and little criminal history (Type I). The second type is described as sociopathic and sadistic through the exposure of an erect penis, these individuals typically have comorbid psychological and sexual disorders (Type II) (McNally & Fremouw, 2014; Rooth, 1971). Type II offenders, who characteristically expose an erect penis, were at higher risk for future contact offenses (Sugarman et al., 1994). Researchers are yet to determine how long an exhibitionist is at risk for future sexual offending after the initial exposure (McNally & Fremouw, 2014). Firestone et al. (2006) found exhibitionists who had been offense-free for 8 years were a very low risk of violent or sexual reoffending.

Electronic Manifestations

The classic image of an exhibitionist is a man in a trench coat who exposes his genitals to unsuspecting strangers. In actuality, exhibitionists may use many techniques to expose themselves such as cutting a hole in the crotch of their pants for men or strategically leaving a shirt unbuttoned for women (Carnes, 1991; Hopkins et al., 2016). The popularity of the Internet and invention of the webcam have given exhibitionists new avenues to engage in deviant sexual behavior similar to that of traditional exhibitionism (Hanafy et al., 2016; Kaylor, Jeglic, & Collins, 2016). When considering electronic manifestations of exhibitionism, we must consider whether the behavior is part of normal adolescent/young adult courtship behaviors, such as sexting, or if this behavior is more indicative of electronic exhibitionism (Kaylor et al., 2016). Retrospectively, individuals with exhibitionistic disorder report that the desire to expose themselves to others began in adolescence/early adulthood (APA, 2013; Murphy & Page, 2008; Kaylor et al., 2016). Moreover, the DSM-5 does not require a minimum age to meet criteria for exhibitionistic disorder; therefore it can become unclear at what point sexting with an unsuspecting person or nonconsenting individual changes from an attempt at flirting to a paraphilic act (APA, 2013; Kaylor et al., 2016; Lang et al., 1987).

When considering adolescent behavior, this population may be more likely to use technology to express their sexuality, since they are experiencing a period of identity development which is notable for increased interest and engagement in sexual exploration (Kaylor et al., 2016; Korenis & Billick, 2013; Sadhu, 2012). Moreover, adolescence is also marked by impulsivity and narcissism (i.e., excessive interest in oneself or one's physical appearance), thus it is hypothesized that individuals who expose themselves do so for sexual pleasure and erotic satisfaction from an audience rather than from sexual contact (Kaylor et al., 2016; Korenis & Billick, 2013; Lang et al., 1987; Sadhu, 2012).

Kaylor et al. (2016) completed a study on 959 participants ages 18–30 years, who were surveyed about traditional exhibitionistic behaviors as well as technological sexual behaviors, such as sending explicit pictures. Traditional exhibitionism was assessed as flashing one's nude or partially nude body parts (i.e., breasts, penis, or vagina) in a public place; whereas, digital exhibitionism was assessed as sending a sexually explicit image to a stranger or person known for less than 24 hours (Kaylor et al., 2016). Researchers found a significant proportion of participants reported engaging in both technological and traditional exhibitionistic-like behaviors (e.g., mooning), and they described their motivations for engaging in such behaviors were confidence, excitement, and arousal. While individuals with exhibitionistic disorder report similar motivations for their exposures, this study revealed that many participants' motivations aligned most closely with normal adolescent/young adult sexual exploration and courtship. Although some exhibitionist behavior amongst adolescents is considered harmless, this study revealed a small group of participants whose behavior went above and beyond that of normal teenage shenanigans, which may be indicative of a nascent paraphilia (Kaylor et al., 2016).

Due to the ever-evolving nature of technology, future research would benefit from gathering information on the motivations behind electronic exhibitionism. Researchers believe the anonymity and distance the Internet provides creates a protective barrier where individuals may feel more confident to expose themselves via the Internet. Moreover, technological exhibitionism may allow the sender to feel safer as the chance of rejection is lower compared to exposing oneself in person (Kaylor et al., 2016). Since the Internet and smartphones can provide exhibitionists with unlimited access to a large number of people to expose their genitals to websites and social media networking services are being misused, such as Snapchat and Chatroulette to expose oneself to unsuspecting victims (Hopkins et al., 2016; Kaylor et al., 2016). It is currently unclear how the use of technology to expose oneself will impact legislation, victims, and the diagnostic criteria for exhibitionistic disorder.

Treatment of Exhibitionistic Disorder

Much of the existing literature on treating exhibitionistic disorder relies heavily on case study subjects with the consensus that this paraphilia is often chronic and refractory to treatment (Blair & Lanyon, 1981; Grant, 2005; Swindell et al., 2011). Many exhibitionists may not come into contact with treatment programs, thus those who voluntarily seek treatment describe an inability to resist powerful urges to expose their genitals that intensify over time. Often times these urges are brought on by sadness, boredom, inadequacy, stress, interpersonal conflict, a specific location, or an attractive person (Grant, 2005; Swindell et al., 2011).

One form of treatment described for those with exhibitionistic disorder is aversion therapy. For instance, ammonia aversion treatment is a combination of aversive relief and punishment in which the exhibitionist carries a small bottle of smelling salts at all times. When the urge to expose oneself arises, the client inhales the ammonia mixture and clears their mind of any offense-related thoughts and replaces those thoughts with a prosocial image (e.g., enjoyable activities) (Marshall, 2006). Ammonia aversion treatment functions as a positive punishment in which the ammonia fumes create a pain-mediated response instead of an olfactory response, thus suppressing one's exhibitionistic urges (Barker, 2001). Over time, the association of the relief brought on by the ammonia and the prosocial thoughts are believed to reduce the urge to expose. This self-managing technique requires the client to diligently keep daily records of urges and continuously carry the ammonia mixture with them, if clients are inconsistent, the problematic behaviors are likely to return (Marshall, 2006).

Despite many studies describing the difficulties of treating exhibitionism, there has been some support for serotonergic antidepressant treatment. Terao and Nakamura (2000) described a case in which a low dose of trazadone was found to be effective in reducing the impulse to expose one's genitals in a client with exhibitionistic disorder. The client was administered 50 mg of trazadone daily for 1 year, then the dosage was decreased to 25 mg per day, and decreased further until it was discontinued at the two-year mark. During regular follow-up sessions, the client did not experience any urges or exposures. Although low dose trazadone has been suggested to be the best pharmacological treatment for exhibitionism, trazadone may lead to an overall decrease in sex drive, erectile dysfunction, and reduced libido, which may result in high rates of attrition (Terao & Nakamura, 2000).

Although medication can be helpful in controlling exhibition urges, medication alone will not impact the underlying psychological problem, thus the gold standard treatment is the combination of both psychotherapy and psychopharmacology (Chopin-Marcé, 2001). The success of psychotherapy depends on the client's motivation for seeking treatment and level of intelligence. Many treatment-seeking exhibitionists report that they do not know why they expose themselves and feel pushed by a force beyond their control that feels obsessive-compulsive in nature (Chopin-Marcé, 2001).

Imagery treatment, which examines deviant fantasies and encourages them to be replaced with appropriate ones, has been a well-established treatment for exhibitionists (Dandescu & Wolfe, 2003). Paraphilic fantasies are seen as a fundamental part of the etiology and maintenance of exhibitionistic behavior (O'Donohue, Letourneau, & Dowling, 1997). Research has found that after their first exposure, exhibitionistic offenders have a greater number of deviant masturbatory offenses compared to the number of fantasies prior to this first exposure. This information suggests a behavior/fantasy loop is created, where exposure triggers fantasies, which in turn leads to more exhibitionistic acts (Abel & Blanchard, 1974). Unfortunately, imagery instructions for exhibitionism are typically incomplete or missing from research reports, making replication difficult (Blair & Lanyon, 1981). Moreover, previous studies have reported conflicting data about the efficacy of this type of treatment (Dandescu & Wolfe, 2003; Marshall & Serran, 2000).

Similar to the behavior/fantasy loop described above, exhibitionism has been hypothesized to be triggered by dysphoric mood states in which the individual exposes oneself to self-soothe leading to a conditioned stimulus (Swindell et al., 2011). In order to break the cycle of dysphoric mood and exhibitionism, the individual needs to learn healthy ways to self-soothe that do not involve exposure or other addictive behaviors. In addition, any cognitive distortions or rationalizations involving exhibitionism need to be addressed (Swindell et al., 2011). Some mental health professionals also conceptualize exhibitionists as being stuck in an immature developmental phase, thus the importance of recognizing the suffering of their victims as people not as objects is highly emphasized (Chopin-Marcé, 2001).

Consequences

The earliest study on victims of exhibitionism reported that victims were not harmed from the exposure, but rather surprised and inconvenienced (Davis & Davis, 1976). More recent research has shown that victims of exhibitionism actually experience considerable distress (Clark et al., 2016; Cox, 1988; Krueger & Kaplan, 2000; Riordan, 1999). Contrary to the long-standing belief that exhibitionism is a nuisance offense, a study revealed that 18% of female victims of exhibitionism reported severe distress from the exposure (Cox, 1988). Moreover, another study found that 28% of female victims endorsed exhibitionism has impacted their social activities and movements, suggesting that exhibitionism has negative long-term consequences for victims (Clark et al., 2016; Riordan, 1999).

Although research has shown that victims of exhibitionism are significantly impacted by exposure, only a small percentage of individuals report the offense to the police. Clark et al. (2016) found that the majority of exhibitionism incidents were not reported to the police; in fact less than 10% of their sample endorsed reporting the offense to authorities. Consistent with research on contact sexual offenses, approximately two-thirds of victims of exhibitionism will disclose their experience to someone in their social network; however, the vast majority will not make an official police report (Clark et al., 2016; Golding, Siegel, Sorenson, Burnam, & Stein, 1989; Koss, Dinero, Seibel, & Cox, 1988; Ullman & Filiaps, 2001).

Prevention Measures

Exhibitionistic acts often occur in public places, thus addressing the problem at a situational level (e.g., posters on public transportation) may increase reporting rates, thereby decreasing the prevalence of the behavior. Such prevention methods are thought to decrease exhibitionistic acts, as well as increase victim disclosure and bystander mobilization (Clark et al., 2016). Moreover, situation crime prevention (SCP) methods such as increased police presence and better lighting have served to deter crime and may discourage exhibitionism (Clark et al., 2016; Farrington & Welsh, 2002; Painter, 1996; Sherman & Weisburd, 1995). By implementing SCP measures, subway crime in the Washington D.C. metro system saw a decrease in paraphilic offenses (Clark et al., 2016). Through the use of other crime prevention strategies, such as removing benches, eliminating public restrooms, and closing stairways during off-peak hours, the Washington D.C. metro was able to prevent offenders from lingering in places where exhibitionism was most likely to occur (La Vigne, 1997). Expanding such SCP efforts to other places where exhibitionism takes place such as parks and parking lots can potentially result in a decreased incidence of exhibitionistic acts (Clark et al., 2016).

Since the majority of exhibitionistic behaviors are not reported to the authorities, public education campaigns directed towards girls and young women may be an effective method to increase reporting rates of exhibitionism (Clark et al., 2016). Educational efforts aimed to identifying boundary violations and uncomfortable sexual situations may decrease guilt or self-blame experienced by victims, which in turn may alleviate negative long-term consequences of exposure (Finkelhor, 2009). Moreover, education on victim-blaming and training in empathic responding for criminal justice, medical, and mental health professionals may make victims feel more comfortable when speaking with individuals in positions of authority (Clark et al., 2016; Ullman & Filiaps, 2001). Through SCP and public education campaigns, the hope is to decrease exhibitionistic acts and increase reporting of such offenses.

Future Directions

Although exhibitionistic disorder has been identified as a crime for centuries, research on this disorder remains sparse. In order to get a better sense of the incidence, prevalence, and scope of this paraphilia large population-based studies are needed. One limitation of assessing exhibitionism remains the lack of standardized assessment tools to evaluate the risk for recidivism. While several methods for assessing exhibitionism exist, there are no gold standard assessment batteries for determining the risk for recidivism or escalation to contact offenses. Moreover, there exists many sexual paraphilias that not only share similar symptoms but are also highly comorbid. The lack of assessment tools for measuring this behavior speaks to the great need for a high level of specificity when evaluating for the presence of other sexual paraphilias. Furthermore, several methods for treating exhibitionism exist in the literature; however, many of these research studies rely on case studies or have little evidence to support the treatment of choice. The literature points to several methods for preventing the act of exhibitionism from occurring (e.g., increased police presence, better lighting), yet there is insufficient research on preventing an individual from developing exhibitionistic disorder. With the recent realization that exhibitionism is much more than a nuisance, we can hope that future research will fill the many gaps in what we know about diagnosing, assessing, and treating this paraphilic disorder.

References

Abel, G. G., Becker, J. V., Cunningham-Rathner, J., Mittelman, M., & Rouleau, J. (1988). Multiple paraphilic diagnoses among sex offenders. *Bulletin of the American Academy of Psychiatry and the Law, 16*(2), 153–168.

Abel, G. G., & Blanchard, E. (1974). The role of fantasy in the treatment of sexual deviation. *Archives of General Psychiatry, 30*(4), 467–475.

Abel, G. G., & Rouleau, J. L. (1990). The nature and extent of sexual assault. In W. L. Marshall, D. R. Laws, & H. E. Barbaree (Eds.), *Handbook of sexual assault: Issues, theories, and treatment of the offender* (pp. 9–21). New York, NY: Plenum Press.

Abouesh, A., & Clayton, A. (1999). Compulsive voyeurism and exhibitionism: A clinical response to paroxetine. *Archives of Sexual Behavior, 28*(1), 23–30.

Adams, H. E., & Sturgis, E. T. (1977). Status of behavioral reorientation techniques in the modification of homosexuality: A review. *Psychological Bulletin, 84*, 1171–1188.

Adams, H. E., Webster, J. S., & Carson, T. P. (1980). Appropriate behavioral assessment and modification of sexual deviation: A comment on "biosyntonic" therapy. *Journal of Consulting and Clinical Psychology, 48*, 106–108.

American Psychiatric Association. (1980). *Diagnostic and statistical manual of mental disorders* (3rd ed.). Washington, DC: Author.

American Psychiatric Association. (2013). *Diagnostic and statistical manual of mental disorders* (5th ed.). Arlington VA: American Psychiatric Publishing.

Abel, G. G., Becker, J. V., Mittelman, M., Cunningham-Rathner, J., Rouleau, J. L., & Murphy, W. D. (1987). Self-reported sex crimes of nonincarcerated paraphiliacs. Journal of interpersonal violence, 2(1), 3-25

Bader, S. M., Schoeneman-Morris, K. A., Scalora, M. J., & Casady, T. K. (2008). Exhibitionism: Findings from a Midwestern police contact sample. *International Journal of Offender Therapy and Comparative Criminology, 52*(3), 270–279.

Bandura, A. (1982). The psychology of chance encounters and life paths. *American Psychologist, 37*, 747–755.

Bandura, A. (1986). *Social foundations of thought and action, a social cognitive theory*. Englewood Cliffs, NJ: Prentice Hall.

Barker, L. M. (2001). *Learning and behavior: Biological, psychological, and sociocultural perspectives* (3rd ed.). Upper Saddle River, NJ: Prentice Hall.

Barlow, D. H. (1977). Assessment of sexual behavior. In R. A. Ciminero, K. S. Calhoun, & H. E. Adams (Eds.), *Handbook of behavioral assessment*. New York: Wiley.

Bartosh, D. L., Garby, T., Lewis, D., & Gray, S. (2003). Differences in predictive validity of actuarial risk assessments in relation to sex offender type. *International Journal of Offender Therapy and Comparative Criminology, 47*, 422–438.

Berlin, F. S., Hunt, W. P., Malin, H. M., Dyer, A., Lehne, G. K., & Dean, S. (1991). A five-year plus follow-up survey of criminal recidivism within a treated cohort of 406 pedophiles, 111 exhibitionists and 109 sexual aggressives: Issues and outcome. *American Journal of Forensic Psychiatry, 12*(3), 5–28.

Berah, E. F., & Myers, R. G. (1983). The offense records of a sample of convicted exhibitionists. *Bulletin of the Academy of Psychiatry and Law, 11*, 365–369.

Bhugra, D., Popelyuk, D., & McMullen, I. (2010). Paraphilias across cultures: Contexts and controversies. *Journal of Sex Research, 47*, 242–256.

Blair, C. D., & Lanyon, R. I. (1981). Exhibitionism: Etiology and treatment. *Psychological Bulletin, 89*(3), 439–463.

Bluglass, R. (1980). Indecent exposure in the West Midlands. Sex offenders in the criminal justice system, 171-180

Carnes, P. J. (1991). Don't call it love: Recovery from sexual additction. New Yrok, NY: Bantom Books.

Carnes, P. J. (2001). *Out of the shadows: Understanding sexual addiction*. Center City, MN: Hazelden.

Carnes, P. J., Delmonico, D. L., & Griffin, E. (2007). *In the shadows of the net: Breaking free of compulsive online sexual behavior*. Center City, MN: Hazelden.

Clark, S. K., Jeglic, E. L., Calkins, C., & Tatar, J. R. (2016). More than a nuisance: The prevalence and consequences of frotteurism and exhibitionism. *Sexual Abuse: Journal of Research and Treatment, 28*(1), 3–19.

Cox, D. J. (1988). Incidence and nature of male genital exposure behavior as reported by college women. *Journal of Sex Research, 24*(1), 227–234.

Chopin-Marcé, M. J. (2001). Exhibitionism and Psychotherapy: A Case Study. International Journal of Offender Therapy and Comparative Criminology, 45(5), 626–633

Dalby, J. T. (1988). Is telephone scatologia a variant of exhibitionism? *International Journal of Offender Therapy and Comparative Criminology, 32*, 45–49.

Dandescu, A., & Wolfe, R. (2003). Considerations on fantasy use by child molesters and exhibitionists. *Sexual Abuse: Journal of Research and Treatment, 15*(4), 297–305.

Davis, S. K., & Davis, P. W. (1976). Meanings and process in erotic offensiveness: An expose of exposees. *Journal of Contemporary Ethnography, 5*, 377–396.

Doren, D. M. (2002). *Evaluating sex offenders: A manual for civil commitments and beyond*. Thousand Oaks, CA: Sage.

Enelow, M. L. (1969). Public nuisance offenses: Exhibitionism, voyeurism and transvestism. In S. G. Kling (Ed.), *Sexual behavior and the law*. New York: Pocket Books.

Farrington, D. P., & Welsh, B. C. (2002). Improved street lighting and crime prevention. *Justice Quarterly, 19*, 313–342.

Fenichel, O. (1964). On acting. *Psychoanalytic Quarterly, 15*, 144–160.

Finkelhor, D. (2009). The prevention of childhood sexual abuse. *The Future of Children, 19*, 169–194.

Firestone, P., Kingston, D. A., Wexler, A., & Bradford, J. M. (2006). Long-term follow-up of exhibitionists: Psychological, phallometric, and offense characteristics. *Journal of the American Academy of Psychiatry and the Law, 34*(3), 349–359.

Freud, S. (1905). Three essays on sexuality. *SE, 7*, 130–243.

Freud, S. (1914). On narcissism: An introduction. *SE, 14*, 73–102.

Freund, K. (1990). Courtship disorders. In W. L. Marshall, D. R. Laws, & H. E. Barbaree (Eds.), *Handbook of sexual assault: Issues, theories, and treatment of the offender* (pp. 195–207). New York: Plenum.

Freund, K., & Watson, R. (1990). Mapping the boundaries of courtship disorder. *Journal of Sex Research, 27*, 589–606.

Freund, K., Watson, R., & Rienzo, D. (1988). The value of self-reports in the study of voyeurism and exhibitionism. *Sexual Abuse: A Journal of Research and Treatment, 1*, 244–262.

Fulero, S. M. (1995). Review of the hare psychopathy checklist-revised. In J. C. Conoley & J. C. Impara (Eds.), *The twelfth mental measurements yearbook* (pp. 453–454). Lincoln, NE: Buros Institute of Mental Measurements.

Gebhard, P. H., Gagnon, J. H., Pomeroy, W. B., & Christenson, C. V. (1965). *Sex offenders: An analysis of types*. London: Heinemann.

Gittleson, N. L., Eacott, S. E., & Mehta, B. M. (1978). Victims of indecent exposure. *British Journal of Psychiatry, 132*, 61–66.

Golding, J. M., Siegal, J. M., Sorenson, S. B., Burnam, M. A., & Stein, J. A. (1989). Social support sources following sexual assault. *Journal of Community Psychology, 17*, 92–107.

Grant, J. E. (2005). Clinical characteristics and psychiatric comorbidity in males with exhibitionism. *The Journal of Clinical Psychiatry, 66*(11), 1367–1371.

Grob, C. S. (1985). Female exhibitionism. *The Journal of Nervous and Mental Disease, 173*, 253–256.

Hackett, T. P. (1971). The psychotherapy of exhibitionism in a court clinic setting. *Seminars in Psychiatry, 3*, 297–306.

Hanafy, I., Clervoy, L., & Brenot, P. (2016). Exhibitionists, so much inhibition. *Sexologies: European Journal of Sexology and Sexual Health/Revue Européenne De Sexologie Et De Santé Sexuelle, 25*(4), e61–e63.

Hare, R. D., Forth, A. E., & Strachan, K. E. (1992). Psychopathy and crime across the life span. In R. D. Peters, R. J. McMahon, & V. L. Quinsey (Eds.), *Aggression and violence throughout the lifespan* (pp. 285–300). Newbury Park, CA: Sage.

Harris, G. T., Rice, M. E., & Quinsey, V. L. (1993). Violent recidivism of mentally disordered offenders: The development of a statistical prediction instrument. *Criminal Justice and Behavior, 20*(4), 315–335.

Hoffmann, H., Janssen, E., & Turner, S. L. (2004). Classical conditioning of sexual arousal in women and men: Effects of varying awareness and biological relevance of the conditioned stimulus. *Archives of Sexual Behavior, 33*, 43–53.

Hollender, M. H., Brown, W., & Roback, H. D. (1977). Genital exhibitionism in women. *American Journal of Psychiatry, 134*(4), 436–438.

Holtzman, D., & Kulish, N. (2012). Female exhibitionism: Identification, competition and camaraderie. *The International Journal of Psychoanalysis, 93*(2), 271–292.

Hopkins, T. A., Green, B. A., Carnes, P. J., & Campling, S. (2016). Varieties of intrusion: Exhibitionism and voyeurism. *Sexual Addiction & Compulsivity, 23*(1), 4–33.

Kafka, M. P. (2003a). Sex offending and sexual appetite: The clinical and theoretical relevance of hypersexual desire. *International Journal of Offender Therapy and Comparative Criminology, 47*(4), 439–451.

Kafka, M. P. (2003b). The monoamine hypothesis for the pathophysiology of paraphilic disorders: An update. *Annals of the New York Academy of Sciences, 989*(1), 86–94.

Kafka, M., & Hennen, J. (1999). The paraphilia-related disorders: An empirical investigation of nonparaphilic hypersexuality disorders in outpatient males. *Journal of Sex & Marital Therapy, 25*, 305–319.

Kantorowitz, D. A. (1978a). An investigation of preorgasmic reconditioning and post-orgasmic deconditioning. *Journal of Applied Behavior Analysis, 11*, 23–34.

Kantorowitz, D. A. (1978b). Personality and conditioning of tumescence and detumescence. *Behavior Research and Therapy, 16*, 117–123.

Kaylor, L., Jeglic, E. L., & Collins, C. (2016). Examining the impact of technology on exhibitionistic behavior. *Deviant Behavior, 37*(10), 1152–1162.

Kinsey, A. C., Pomeroy, W. B., Martin, C. E., & Gebhard, P. H. (1953). *Sexual behavior in the human female*. Philadelphia, PA: W. B. Saunders.

Kinsey, A. C., Reichert, P., Cauldwell, D. O., & Mozes, E. B. (1955). The causes of homosexuality: A symposium. *Sexology, 21*, 558–562.

Korenis, P., & Billick, S. (2013). Forensic implications: Adolescent sexting and cyberbullying. *Psychiatric Quarterly, 85*(1), 97–101.

Koss, M. P., Dinero, T. E., Seibel, C. A., & Cox, S. (1988). Stranger and acquaintance rape: Are there differences in the victim's experience? *Psychology of Women Quarterly, 12*, 1–24.

Krueger, R. B., & Kaplan, M. S. (2000). The nonviolent serial offender: Exhibitionism, frotteurism, and telephone scatologia. In L. B. Schlesinger (Ed.), *Serial offenders: Current thoughts, recent findings* (pp. 116–131). Washington, DC: CRC Press.

La Vigne, N. G. (1997). *Visibility and vigilance: Metro's situational approach to preventing subway crime (National Institute of Justice Research Brief)*. Washington, DC: U.S. Department of Justice, Office of Justice Programs, National Institute of Justice.

Lalumi'ere, M. L., Harris, G. H., Quinsey, V. L., & Rice, M. E. (2005). *The causes of rape: Understanding individual differences in male propensity for sexual aggression*. Washington, DC: American Psychological Association.

Lalumi'ere, M. L., & Quinsey, V. L. (1998). Pavlovian conditioning of sexual interests in human males. *Archives of Sexual Behavior, 27*, 241–252.

Lang, R. A., Langevin, R., Checkley, K. L., & Pugh, G. (1987). Genital exhibitionism: Courtship disorder or narcissism? *Canadian Journal of Behavioural Science, 19*(2), 216–232.

Langevin, R., Paitich, D., Ramsay, G., Anderson, C., Kamrad, J., Pope, S., … Newman, S. (1979). Experimental studies of the etiology of genital exhibitionism. *Archives of Sexual Behavior, 8*, 307–331.

Långström, N. (2010). The DSM diagnostic criteria for exhibitionism, voyeurism, and frotteurism. *Archives of Sexual Behavior, 39*(2), 317–324.

Långström, N., & Seto, M. C. (2006). Exhibitionistic and voyeuristic behavior in a Swedish national population survey. *Archives of Sexual Behavior, 35*(4), 427–435.

Lasègue, C. (1877). *Les exhibitionnistes* (pp. 709–714). Paris: L'union Médicale. [série 3-23].

Lee, J. K. P., Pattison, P., Jackson, H. J., & Ward, T. (2001). The general, common, and specific features of psychopathology for different types of paraphilias. *Criminal Justice and Behavior, 28*, 227–256.

MacPherson, G. J. (2003). Predicting escalation in sexually violent recidivism: Use of the SVR-20 and PCL:SV to predict outcome with noncontact recidivists and contact recidivists. *Journal of Forensic Psychiatry & Psychology, 14*(3), 615–627.

Maletzky, B. M. (1997). Exhibitionism: Assessment and treatment. In D. R. Laws & W. O'Donohue (Eds.), *Sexual deviance: Theory, assessment, and treatment* (pp. 40–74). New York: Guilford.

Marshall, W. L. (2006). Ammonia aversion with an exhibitionist: A case study. *Clinical Case Studies, 5*(1), 15–24.

Marshall, W. L., Anderson, D., & Fernandez, Y. (1999). *Cognitive behavioural treatment of sexual offenders*. New York: John Wiley.

Marshall, W., & Serran, G. (2000). Improving the effectiveness of sexual offender treatment. *Trauma, Violence, and Abuse, 1*, 203–222.

McConaghy, N. (1993). *Sexual behavior: Problems and management*. New York: Plenum.

McGrath, R. J. (1991). Sex-offender risk assessment and disposition planning: A review of empirical and clinical findings. *International Journal of Offender Therapy and Comparative Criminology, 35*, 328–350.

McNally, M. R., & Fremouw, W. J. (2014). Examining risk of escalation: A critical review of the exhibitionistic behavior literature. *Aggression and Violent Behavior, 19*(5), 474–485.

Mohr, J. W., Turner, E. R., & Ball, R. B. (1962). Exhibitionism and pedophilia. *Corrective Psychiatry & Journal of Social Therapy, 8*(4), 172–186.

Monroe, R. R. (1976). Episodic sexual disorders. *Medical Aspects of Human Sexuality, 10*, 55–64.

Morin, J., & Levenson, J. (2008). Exhibitionism: Assessment and treatment. In D. R. Laws & W. T. O'Donohue (Eds.), *Sexual deviance: Theory, assessment, and treatment* (2nd ed., pp. 76–107). New York: Guilford Press.

Murphy, W. D. (1997). Exhibitionism: Psychopathology and theory. In D. R. Laws & W. O'Donohue (Eds.), *Sexual deviance: Theory, assessment, and treatment* (pp. 22–39). New York: Guilford.

Murphy, W., & Page, I. (2008). Exhibitionism: psychopathology and theory. In D. R. Laws & W. T. O'Donohue (Eds.), *Sexual Deviance: Theory, Assessment, and Treatment* (2nd ed., pp. 61–75). Guilford: New York, NY.

Murphy, W. D., & Page, I. J. (2006). Exhibitionism. In McAnulty, R. D. and Burnette,M. M. (Eds.), Sex and sexuality: Sexual deviation and sexual offenses (pp. 1–20). Westport, CT: Praeger Publishers.

O'Donohue, W., Letourneau, E. J., & Dowling, H. (1997). Development and preliminary validation of a paraphilic sexual fantasy questionnaire. *Sexual Abuse: Journal of Research and Treatment, 9*(3), 167–178.

Painter, K. (1996). The influence of street lighting improvements on crime for pedestrian street use, after dark. *Landscape and Urban Planning, 35*, 193–201.

Petri, H. (1969). Exhibitionism: Theoretical and social aspects and treatment with antiandrogens. *Nervenarzt, 40*(5), 220–228.

Plaud, J. J., & Martini, J. R. (1999). The respondent conditioning of male sexual arousal. *Behavior Modification, 23*, 254–268.

Price, M., Gutheil, T. G., Commons, M. L., Kafka, M. P., & Dodd-Kimmey, S. (2001). Telephone scatologia: Comorbidity and theories of etiology. *Psychiatric Annals, 31*, 226–232.

Quinsey, V. L., Skilling, T. A., Lalumi'ere, M. L., & Craig, W. M. (2004). *Juvenile delinquency: Understanding the origins of individual differences*. Washington, DC: American Psychological Association.

Rabinowitz-Greenberg, S. R., Firestone, P., Bradford, J. M., & Greenberg, D. M. (2002). Prediction of recidivism in exhibitionists: Psychological, phallometric, and offense factors. *Sexual Abuse: Journal of Research and Treatment, 14*(4), 329–347.

Rachman, S. (1966). Sexual fetishism: An experimental analogue. *The Psychological Record, 16*, 293–296.

Rachman, S., & Hodgson, R. J. (1968). Experimentally-induced "sexual fetishism": Replication and development. *The Psychological Record, 18*, 25–27.

Raymond, N. C., Coleman, E., Ohlerking, F., Christenson, G. A., & Miner, M. M. (1999). Psychiatric comorbidity in pedophilic sex offenders. *American Journal of Psychiatry, 156*, 786–788.

Rhoads, J., & Borjes, E. (1981). The incident of exhibitionism in Guatemala and the United States. *British Journal of Psychiatry, 139*, 242–244.

Rickles, N. K. (1955). Exhibitionism. *Journal of Social Therapy, 1*, 168–181.

Riordan, S. (1999). Indecent exposure: The impact upon the victim's fear of sexual crime. *Journal of Forensic Psychiatry, 10*, 309–316.

Rooth, F. G. (1971). Indecent exposure and exhibitionism. *British Journal of Psychiatry, 143*, 231–235.

Rooth, F. G. (1973). Exhibitionism, sexual violence, and paedophilia. *British Journal of Psychiatry, 122*(6), 705–710.

Rosen, I. (1964). Exhibitionism, scopophilia and voyeurism. In I. Rosen (Ed.), *The pathology and treatment of sexual deviation*. London: Oxford University Press.

Sadhu, J. M. (2012). Sexting: The impact of a cultural phenomenon on psychiatric practice. *Academic Psychiatry, 36*(1), 76–81.

Schneider, R. D. (1982). Exhibitionism: An exclusively male deviation? *International Journal of Offender Therapy and Comparative Criminology, 26*(2), 173–176.

Serin, R. C., Malcolm, P. B., Khanna, A., & Barbaree, H. E. (1994). Psychopathy and deviant sexual arousal in incarcerated sexual offenders. *Journal of Interpersonal Violence, 9*(1), 3–11.

Seto, M. C., & Barbaree, H. E. (1997). Sexual aggression as antisocial behavior: A developmental model. In D. Stoff, J. Breiling, & J. D. Maser (Eds.), *Handbook of antisocial behavior* (pp. 524–533). New York: Wiley.

Sherman, L. W., & Weisburd, D. (1995). General deterrent effects of police patrol in crime "hot spots": A randomized, controlled trial. *Justice Quarterly, 12*, 625–648.

Stekel, W. (1952). *Patterns of psychosexual infantilism*. New York: Liveright.

Sugarman, P., Dumughn, C., Saad, K., Hinder, S., & Bluglass, R. (1994). Dangerousness in exhibitionists. *Journal of Forensic Psychiatry, 5*, 287–296.

Swindell, S., Stroebel, S. S., O'Keefe, S. L., Beard, K. W., Robinett, S. R., & Kommor, M. J. (2011). Correlates of exhibition-like experiences in childhood and adolescence: A model for development of exhibitionism in heterosexual males. *Sexual Addiction & Compulsivity, 18*(3), 135–156.

Terao, T., & Nakamura, J. (2000). Exhibitionism and low-dose trazodone treatment. *Human Psychopharmacology: Clinical and Experimental, 15*(5), 347–349.

Ullman, S. E., & Filiaps, H. H. (2001). Correlates of formal and informal support seeking in sexual assault victims. *Journal of Interpersonal Violence, 16*, 1028–1047.

von Krafft-Ebing, R. (1965). *Psychopathia sexualis* (12th ed.). New York: Stein & Day. (Original work published 1886).

Venables, N. C., Hall, J. R., & Patrick, C. J. (2013). Differentiating psychopathy from antisocial personality disorder: A triarchic model perspective. *Psychological Medicine, 44*(5), 1005–1013.

World Health Organization. (1992). *The ICD-10 classification of mental and behavioural disorders: Clinical descriptions and diagnostic guidelines*. Geneva: World Health Organization.

Sexual Assault and Female Gang Involvement: A Look at Risk Amplification and Prevention

46

Aubri F. McDonald

Introduction

"There is one aspect of female gang life that does not seem to be changing—the gang as a refuge for young women who have been victimized at home" (Moore & Hagedorn, 2001, p. 3). The purpose of this chapter is to understand the relationship between sexual assault and female gang involvement and to propose a strategy to prevent females from becoming involved with gangs. In particular, the plan is tailored to address the effects of child sexual abuse (CSA) as an underlying risk factor for female gang involvement and an amplifying risk factor for sexual victimization for female gang members. According to Chesney-Lind, Morash, and Irwin (2007), "Evidence of sexual exploitation of female gang members at home and within their gangs is one reason for considering female gang membership a serious social concern" (p. 4).

CSA as a risk factor for gang involvement and sexual revictimization has not been a part of gang involvement prevention strategies. Programs specifically targeted at preventing female gang involvement are underdeveloped. This chapter focuses on girls because of this intervention gap and because, compared to males, the risk for females being victims of CSA is about three times higher (Finkelhor, 2009).[1] Furthermore, children who are victims of sexual abuse are three times more likely to experience sexual victimization again later in life compared to those who have not been sexually abused as children (Boynton-Jarrett, Rich-Edwards, Jun, Hilbert, & Wright, 2011).

Scope of Female Gang Involvement

Females are more involved in gangs than generally acknowledged. Estimates for female gang involvement differ significantly depending on the source. Law enforcement estimates show that of those officially labeled gang offenders, a small percentage is female (Bobrowski, 1988; Spergel, 1995; Thrasher, 1927). A 2004 National Youth Gang Survey gathering data on gangs from a representative sample of police and sheriff departments across the country estimated that 94% of gang members are male (Egley & Ritz, 2006). Research indicates that law enforcement underestimates female gang membership. According to one study, 32% of police jurisdictions surveyed did not, "as a matter of policy," identify females as gang members (Curry & Decker, 1998, p. 98).

A. F. McDonald (✉)
Criminal Justice Department, University of Wisconsin-Parkside, Kenosha, WI, USA

[1]Measuring the prevalence of CSA is problematic. CSA is underreported because many victims never disclose their abuse. It is estimated that the number of cases reported to child protection services is 2.4/1000 or less than one-fourth of 1% (Finkelhor, 1994).

W. T. O'Donohue and P. A. Schewe (eds.), *Handbook of Sexual Assault and Sexual Assault Prevention*,
https://doi.org/10.1007/978-3-030-23645-8_46

Youth surveys reflect substantial female involvement in gangs compared to law enforcement data and show that females constitute as many as one-third of all gang members (Esbensen & Deschenes, 1998; Esbensen, Deschenes, & Winfree Jr, 1999; Esbensen & Huizinga, 1993; Esbensen & Winfree, 1998; Gottfredson & Gottfredson, 2001; Thornberry, Krohn, Lizotte, Smith, & Tobin, 2003). Younger females are more likely to be involved in gangs. Esbensen and Huizinga (1993) found that of gang-involved youth aged 11–15, nearly half were female. Surveying an older group, aged 13–19, they found that a fifth were girls (Esbensen & Huizinga, 1993). Youth surveys may reflect higher estimates of female gang involvement compared to police estimates because survey respondents tend to be younger than youth on police rosters. Females tend to drop out of gang life at earlier ages compared to males. Among Rochester gang members, half of the males and two-thirds of the females stayed in their gangs for a year or less, with very few youth retaining gang membership throughout their adolescent years (Snyder & Sickmund, 2006).

The lack of a standardized definition for what constitutes a gang and what distinguishes a gang member from a "hanger-on" or "wannabe" makes it difficult to accurately determine the scope of youth gang involvement (Snyder & Sickmund, 2006). Female gang members are often characterized as assuming auxiliary roles in gang activities or as assisting male gang members by carrying weapons, providing alibis, or spying for male members (Campbell, 1990; Cohen, 1956; Short & Strodtbeck, 1965; Spergel, 1995).

Female gang involvement varies widely from one location to another. Moore (1991) found that in some US cities, females constitute up to one-third of the members in some gang cliques but are completely absent in others. Female gangs are somewhat more likely to be found in small cities and rural areas than in large cities. Racial or ethnic composition of gangs also varies depending on location. While Latina gangs are predominant in the Southwest, African American gangs are predominant in the Midwest and Northeast (National Youth Gang Center, 2000). National estimates based on survey data show that 50% of all gang members are Hispanic/Latino, 32% are African American, and 11% are Caucasian (National Youth Gang Center, 2010). A 15-city sample found that racial and ethnic proportions of youth reporting gang membership were more evenly distributed among whites (7.3%), blacks (8.3%), and Hispanics (9.0%), but larger (12.9%) for multiracial groups (Esbensen, Brick, Melde, Tusinski, & Taylor, 2008).

Sexualizing Female Gang Members

Research on gangs tends to emphasize the sexuality of female members and their sexual activities with male gang members (see Campbell, 1984, 1990; Taylor, 1993). Male gang researchers traditionally characterized female gang members as maladjusted tomboys or sexual deviants (Joe & Chesney-Lind, 1995). Campbell (1987) noted that early research attributed female gang involvement to "psychological problems and inappropriate gender-role behavior of female gang members" (p. 451). Contemporary perspectives indicate that female gang members are establishing their own ground and taking on an active independent role in crime and violence (Chesney-Lind, 1993; Joe-Laidler & Hunt, 2001).

Female gang members are often stereotyped as "sex objects" for male gang members. Moore and Hagedorn (2001) point out that early research about the "easy sexual availability of female gang members" was based on the male gang members' perspective (p. 3; e.g., Short & Strodtbeck, 1965; Sanchez-Jankowski, 1991). For instance, Decker and Van Winkle (1996) were told by male gang members that female members were initiated into the gang by group sex which the female members dismissed as "ludicrous." In a Mexican American gang in Los Angeles, half the male members said female members were sexually exploited and treated like "possessions," two-thirds of the female members denied they were treated as such, and the other male members said females were treated like family (Moore, 1991).

Sexual exploitation and abuse of female gang members by male gang members is prevalent; however, it does not occur in every gang. Studies involving African American, Mexican American, and Puerto Rican females in gangs reported being sexually victimized by the male members in their gang in Columbus, OH (Miller, 1998), Milwaukee (Hagedorn, 1998), Phoenix, AZ (Portillos, 1999), Chicago (Venkatesh, 1998), and Los Angeles (Moore, 1991). Females from an immigrant Salvadoran gang in San Francisco reported frequent sexual victimization by male gang members, although this rarely happened in a nearby Mexican American gang (Brotherton, 1996). Male gang members of a Mexican American gang in San Antonio, TX, reported that most females who associate with the gang are respected; however, females who frequently partied, used drugs, and were sexually promiscuous were not deemed worthy of respect (Valdez & Cepeda, 1998).

The level and nature of a young women's participation in gang crime may be an indicator of the particular types of victimization risks these young women face. Joe-Laidler and Hunt (1997) found that females in auxiliary gangs were exposed to a greater variety of violence-prone situations tied to their associations with young men. Female gang members who are heavily involved in street crime are at heightened risk for physical violence such as assaults or stabbings. Young women in gangs are also at greater risk for ongoing physical or sexual mistreatment by male gang members (Miller, 2001; Miller & Brunson, 2000).

The experiences of females in gangs suggest a complex relationship with their male counterparts in which the females simultaneously are protected from potentially aggressive situations, but also are open to sexual victimization by their protectors (Joe-Laidler & Hunt, 2001). In Bowker's and colleagues' (1980) study, male gang members in mixed-gender gangs described efforts to protect the females from potentially dangerous situations. The male gang members said that girls were excluded from planning delinquent acts and when girls showed up at the location of a planned incident, it was often postponed or terminated.

Gangs, Delinquency, and Gender

Joe and Chesney-Lind (1995) explain that participating in violence is a stronger normative feature of male gang involvement than it is for females in gangs. Esbensen and Huizinga (1993) found that female gang members are significantly less likely to report high levels of involvement in delinquent activity such as violence, truancy, running away, or using drugs. Female gang members reported an average individual offending rate of 14.0 on a general delinquency scale where the rate for male gang members was nearly triple at 36.9 (Esbensen & Huizinga, 1993).

Youth surveys reflect that female gang members are more delinquent than females and males who are not involved in gangs (Bjerregaard & Smith, 1993; Esbensen & Huizinga, 1993; Fagan, 1990). In the Rochester study, 66% of female gang members and 82% of male gang members reported involvement in at least one serious delinquent act (e.g., car theft, assault with a weapon, breaking and entering) compared with only 7% of non-gang females and 11% of non-gang males (Bjerregaard & Smith, 1993). Fagan (1990) found "prevalence rates for female gang members exceeded rates for non-gang males" for all categories of delinquency.[2]

Fagan's (1990) study surveying gang youth in Chicago, Los Angeles, and San Diego found that compared to male gang members, female gang members were more likely to engage in petty delinquency like theft, vandalism, and selling drugs than serious delinquency such as felony

[2]Categories of delinquency are based off the Denver scale and classified as serious, moderate, and minor delinquency. "Serious delinquency" is an eight-item index that includes car theft, assault with a weapon, and breaking and entering. "Moderate delinquency" is an 11-item index that includes joyriding, fraud, and property destruction. "Minor delinquency" is an eight-item index that includes minor theft, being loud and rowdy in a public place, and lying about one's age (Bjerregaard & Smith, 1993).

assault, robbery, or weapons offenses.[3] The study classified 40% of female gang members and 15% of male gang members as "petty delinquents" while 33% of gang females and 56% gang males were deemed "serious delinquents." Female gang members were also less likely to use hard drugs (33%) compared to male gang members (43%). Hagedorn and Devitt (1999) found that gun use is much more prevalent among male than female gang members.

Research shows that gang-related delinquency for males and females is strongly associated with gender organization of their groups (Joe-Laidler & Hunt, 1997; Miller & Brunson, 2000; Peterson, Miller, & Esbensen, 2001). Peterson et al. (2001) classified youth gangs based on gender composition using data from the G.R.E.A.T. gang prevention project. They found that gangs where all or a majority of the members were female were the least delinquent compared to gangs where members were all male, majority male, or gender-balanced.[4] Studies also show that females are far less likely to be in all female gangs and most often report that their gangs have both male and female members. Miller (2001) found in her comparative study of female gang members in St. Louis and Columbus, Ohio, that 88% were in mixed gender gangs.[5] Curry's (1998) study of female gang members in three cities revealed only about 6% reported membership in autonomous female gangs while 57% described their gangs as mixed gender.[6]

Cultural dynamics and roles related to gender may explain differences between males and females with regard to delinquency and violence. Moore and Hagedorn (1996) suggest that Latina gang members are more bound by "traditional" community patriarchal norms than black female gang members. Joe and Chesney-Lind (1995) indicate that for female gang members, violence "is not celebrated or normative" but rather it is "more directly a consequence of and a response to the abuse, both physical and sexual, that characterizes their lives at home" (p. 428).

Motivations for Gang Involvement

A common public perception is that most youth are coerced into joining a gang (Howell, 2007). Studies show that both young men and women join gangs for many reasons. Bjerregaard and Smith (1993) found that engaging in sexual activity and having delinquent peers were significant factors for why males and females joined gangs. Fifty-four percent of the young men and women in the Rochester study said they had followed the lead of friends or family members, 19% said they joined a gang for protection, and 15% said it was for fun or excitement (Browning, Thornberry, & Porter, 1999; Snyder & Sickmund, 2006). Young people also report joining gangs for a sense of identity and belonging. In Los Angeles, Mexican American gangs were described as "a substitute institution … [providing] meaning and identity" (Quicker, 1983, p. 28) or "their own system in which they [could] belong," in the absence of "clear or satisfactory access to adult status" (Harris, 1988, p. 166). Young men and women may also be drawn to money-making opportunities the gang can provide especially given the economic conditions young men and women at risk for gang involvement often face (i.e., poverty, lack of employment).

[3]"Petty delinquents" reported three or fewer incidents in the past year of minor assault, minor theft, vandalism, or illegal services (buying or selling stolen goods, selling drugs) and no index offenses (felony assault, robbery, or felony theft) in the past year (Fagan, 1990). "Serious delinquents" reported one or two index offenses (felony assault, robbery, or felony theft) within the past year or three or more incidents in the past year of extortion or weapons offenses (Fagan, 1990).

[4]Gender-balanced and majority male gangs were similar in delinquency. Male gang members in gender-balanced gangs differentiated males' and females' participation in delinquent activities. Male gang members in majority-male gangs viewed the few female members in the gang as "one of the guys" and equal partners in delinquent activity.

[5]Many of the young women in the study resisted the label female gang, calling it "stupid," "silly," and "laugh[able]." (Miller, 2001).

[6]36.4% said they were in female gangs affiliated with male gangs.

stood to be related to earlier life experiences" (p. 389).[7]

CSA increases a female's risk for sexual revictimization, and gang involvement amplifies the risk given the prevalence of sexual victimization for female gang members. Both CSA and gang involvement are linked to an increased likelihood to abuse alcohol and drugs, and substance abuse increases the likelihood of sexual revictimization. A study based on a national longitudinal sample of youth makes it clear that gang membership *is* associated with increased drug use as a way to self-medicate in response to that traumatic history (Bjerregaard, 2010). Disinhibition from drugs or alcohol strongly facilitates the occurrence of "reliving" sexual victimization, which then may take the form of acting out violent or sexually traumatic episodes (Pitman, Orr, & Laforque, 1987). In sum, CSA, gang involvement, and substance amplify risk of sexual victimization for females.

Consequences of Gang Involvement

Gang involvement tends to exacerbate problems in a young women's life rather than improve her situation. Gang membership sharply raises a young person's risk of being a victim of violence, not just a perpetrator. Researchers tracking the lives of Rochester gang members to age 22 found evidence of serious adult dysfunction that could not be explained by other factors. Young adults who had been in gangs were more likely to have ended their education prematurely, become pregnant or had children early, and failed to establish stable work lives—all of which were associated with an increased likelihood of being arrested as adults (Snyder & Sickmund, 2006).

Long-term consequences of gang involvement depend on the individual. Some never recover from abuse trauma. Females who were members of gangs reported attempting suicide more than male gang members (Evans et al., 1996). The stigmatization of gang membership can also have long-term consequences. In one study of African American female gang members in Milwaukee, women viewed their gang involvement as an adolescent episode, but for Puerto Ricans in Milwaukee and Mexican Americans in Los Angeles, gang membership constricted their futures (Moore & Hagedorn, 2001). These constrictions included being stigmatized in the community resulting in reduced opportunities for employment. Additionally, most female gang members married male gang members whose careers often involved repeated imprisonments. Most female gang members have children with these male gang members who often abandoned responsibility for their children, leaving the females to be a single parent (Moore & Hagedorn, 2001).

Theoretical Perspectives for Gang Involvement

Robert Sampson (1993) proposed that any theory of crime must begin with the fact that most violent criminals at one time belonged to teenage peer groups, particularly street gangs. There are many theories that may be applied to discuss why females join gangs. Theories addressing delinquency were selected to provide a useful backdrop for understanding the complex interplay of social ecology and female gang involvement. These include social disorganization, social learning model, social control theory, strain theory, and labeling theory.

Social Disorganization

Social disorganization in communities, defined as a breakdown in institutional controls generated by urban change, is one of the oldest explanations of gang membership (Kornhauser, 1978). Examining juvenile delinquency in urban areas, Shaw and McKay (Shaw & McKay, 1942) linked patterns of delinquency to the particular ecological environment in which it occurs.

[7] Survivors of earlier rape and abuse may put themselves at risk of further harm, not because they want to be abused or hurt, but because they may be seeking a different, better outcome, or to have more control (Van der Kolk, 1989).

Frederic Thrasher (Thrasher, 1927) and Irving Spergel (1966) considered gang formation a symptom of underlying disorganization in the community. Forming gangs is also seen as an effort to create order out of disorder (Kornhauser, 1978). Poor, unstable communities often lack the organization and political connections to obtain resources for fighting crime and offering young people an alternative to deviant behavior (Park, Burgess, & McKenzie, 1925). Thrasher (1927) found that most gangs were concentrated in areas with the highest incidence of single-parent families, unemployment, multiple-family dwellings, welfare recipients, and low levels of education. Empirical research has confirmed that measures of social disorganization are useful predictors of gang homicides (Curry & Spergel, 1988).

Social Learning Model

Family and peer groups have a prominent influence on gang involvement. The social learning model posits that youths learn to engage in crime in the same way they learn to engage in conforming behavior, through association with or exposure to others (Burgess & Akers, 1966). Social learning mechanisms include imitation or group pressures to conform. Youths are most at risk for gang involvement in environments where delinquency and/or violence are more likely to be reinforced (and less likely to be punished). Families in a range of settings from the inner city to deindustrialized towns often support girls' violence so that people will not disrespect them, and so girls will learn to "hold their own" and be perceived as such (Brown, 1999; Leitz, 2003; Ness, 2004; Tapper & Boulton, 2000). Gang-involved females are more likely than males to come from a troubled family (Moore, 1991).

Research on female delinquency and gang deviance suggests that peers influence female gang membership (Bowker & Klein, 1983; Campbell, 1990; Giordano, 1978). A study of incarcerated females found that females who identified themselves as being members of either a regular group or a gang were more likely to be delinquent (e.g., running away, fighting, stealing, using drugs, damaging property) than those who had not been part of a group and were receiving support and approval for these behaviors from their girlfriends (Giordano, 1978). Other studies also suggest that the relationships of female adolescents to their girlfriends are strong predictors of both gang membership and delinquency (Bowker & Klein, 1983) and generally support the notion that peers are centrally involved with female gang choices (Campbell, 1984, 1990; Moore, 1991). The "sisterhood" of the gang appears to exert a powerful influence on female as well as male gang membership and behavior (Campbell, 1990).

Social Control

Within inner city areas, a network of interpersonal relationships involving family, gangs, and the neighborhood influences delinquency. If family and relatives offer inadequate supervision or incomplete socialization, children from broken families are more likely to join violent gangs unless others take the parents' place (Shaw & McKay, 1942). Females who do not have positive social controls (e.g., attachment to family, community) within their surroundings are likely to turn to the gang for a surrogate support network (Hirschi, 1969). Community and family in the lives of young female gang members are likely to be fractured and unable to offer sufficient support.

Strain Theory

Cohen (1956) saw gang membership as a solution to the curtailed opportunities for traditional success available to lower-class youth. Poverty and economic marginality are associated with the emergence of youth gangs (Moore & Hagedorn, 2001). Merton's (1968) strain theory posits that an individual looks for ways to satisfy her needs and achieving them may become more important than the means adopted. For instance, females may join gangs for safety, respect, money, empowerment, pride, or self-worth not available through legitimate means. Inadequate social structures or regulation may change an individual's perceptions as to means and opportunities.

Broidy and Agnew (1997) identified gender differences in how males and females perceive and respond to strain. While males are concerned with material success, females are concerned with forming bonds and relationships and may see joining a gang as a way to achieve this. They found that males are likely to take their anger out on others while females tend to internalize anger and blame themselves. Young females living in poverty may find it difficult to meet basic emotional and psychological needs (Tyler, 2002). Overall, young impressionable females living in impoverished areas characterized by narrow opportunities are especially vulnerable to becoming gang-involved.

Labeling Theory

Labeling theory involves negatively labeling those seen as deviating from cultural norms. The labeled individual then self-identifies and operates in accordance to the label (Becker, 1973). That label then triggers processes that increase the likelihood of involvement in deviant groups. Those labeled negatively in a deviant or gang context "are substantially more likely than their peers to become members of a gang in a successive period" (Bernburg, Krohn, & Rivera, 2006, pp. 81–82).

This labeling process can be especially harsh in the context of female gang involvement since being in a gang and delinquency are perceived as being male activities. According to Moore and Hagedorn (2001), "*any* girl who joins a gang is defined as bad" (p. 8). Since most females at risk for gang involvement are African American or Latina, the labeling process for these females is also racialized. For instance, many young black women report that their teachers routinely stereotype them and police often punish them for being "loud" and "insufficiently feminine" (Morris, 2005), while Latinas are ignored and assumed to be headed for dropping out and early motherhood (Kelly, 1993).

Prevention Programs for Female Gang Involvement

Female gangs have received little programmatic attention. In the 1960s, programs for female delinquents were gendered and limited to encouraging females to improve their self-image through cosmetics, dress, and deportment (Moore & Hagedorn, 2001). In the 1970s, "law and order" policies and woman's liberation drew attention to female criminality. By the 1990s, the Federal Government began to recognize that female and male offenders have different programmatic needs. In 1990, the U.S. Department of Health and Human Services (1993) approved funding for gang-prevention programs for adolescent females. The key features of the program included:

- Building support groups for at-risk females
- Promoting cultural awareness
- Empowering youth to succeed
- Expanding community awareness
- Sharing information on conditions that put adolescent females at risk of gang or criminal involvement
- Promoting employment opportunities, building spirituality
- Providing consistency and support

The program lasted 3 years before being discontinued due to "the growing disfavor for non-law-enforcement-based programs in Congress and the non-enthusiastic evaluation results" (U.S. Department of Health and Human Services, 1993, p. 22). In 1992, the Juvenile Justice and Delinquency Prevention Act (JJDPA) of 1974 was reauthorized, mandating that there be more programs focused on female delinquents (Moore & Hagedorn, 2001). JJDPA was reauthorized in 2002 and again in December 2018. However, preventing female gang involvement does not appear to be a priority.

Enduring gang prevention strategies tend to remain male-focused although boys and girls require different approaches in gang prevention. Different approaches are necessary since girls and boys join gangs for different reasons. For instance, a US Department of Justice report on preventing adolescent gang involvement suggests that prevention efforts should be directed at preventing delinquency and that "gangs and gang programs should also be studied within the overall context of juvenile delinquency" (Esbensen, 2000, p. 5). This is problematic because it does not distinguish girls from boys' pathways to gang involvement, nor does it identify major differences in the frequency and types of delinquency. Females in gangs, although more violent than their peers outside of gangs, are not nearly as violent as male gang members (Moore & Hagedorn, 2001). Girls in gangs commit fewer violent crimes than their male counterparts and are more inclined to engage in traditional female offending like status offenses and property offenses (Deschenes & Esbensen, 1999; Moore & Hagedorn, 2001).

Existing Gang Prevention Strategies

CSA as a risk factor for gang involvement has not been a part of gang involvement prevention strategies. Programs specifically targeted at preventing female gang involvement do not exist. Existing gang prevention strategies do not account for the different ways gender can impact a young person's vulnerability for gang involvement. The following are a few examples of prevention strategies for youth at risk for gang involvement.

The G.R.E.A.T. program is school-based and aimed at reducing gang activity and educating about the consequences of gang involvement. Students are provided with "real tools to resist the lure and trap of gangs" including conflict resolution skills, goal setting, communication skills, and information on the negative aspects of gang life (Esbensen, 2000, p. 7). Evaluations of G.R.E.A.T. have reported small but positive effects on students' attitudes and their ability to resist peer pressure (Esbensen & Osgood, 1999; Palumbo & Ferguson, 1995). However, since girls at risk for gang involvement tend to have a low commitment to school compared to boys, a school-based strategy may not be the best approach for preventing female gang involvement (Esbensen & Deschenes, 1998).

The "Gang Prevention Through Targeted Outreach" program through the Boys & Girls Clubs of America aims to reach youth ages 6 to 18 who are at high risk for gang involvement or are already involved with delinquency and gangs. The program uses a network of local community agencies, schools, social service organizations, courts, and police to assess their local gang problem (Esbensen, 2000). The major goal of the program is to satisfy youth interests and their social and physical needs by providing prosocial activities (OJJDP, 2018). The strategy has yielded positive evidence-based results associated with gang involvement and in 2010 was awarded nearly $3 million in grants for initiatives across the USA. Since the program's inception, more than 120 clubs nationwide have been funded, serving more than 6,850 youths (OJJDP, 2018).

The Aggression Replacement Training (ART) program appears equally effective for girls and boys in gangs. It consists of a 10-week, 30-hour cognitive–behavioral program administered to groups of 8–12 adolescents. ART targets and works most effectively with violent gang and non-gang offenders. The program has demonstrated effectiveness with both girls and boys and has showed positive results when tested with gang-involved youth in Brooklyn, New York (Goldstein & Glick, 1994; Goldstein, Glick, & Gibbs, 1998).

Reaffirming Young Sister's Excellence (RYSE) is an intensive community treatment and intervention program designed to provide a continuum of female-specific services to adjudicated females aged 12–17 (Le, Arifuku, & Nunez, 2003). Reducing recidivism is the program's overall goal. Other aims include social, academic, and vocational development of the participants' and interrupting intergenerational family fragmentation by providing services for youths who are pregnant or parenting. Its effectiveness for preventing female gang involvement is unknown.

Risk and Protective Factors for Female Gang Involvement

Rational responses to female gang involvement should include strategies that consider the social, economic and personal contexts that influence females to participate in gangs and young women's victimization within these groups (Miller, 2002). Addressing risk factors for gang involvement can work to cut off pathways to delinquency and prevent female gang involvement. The effectiveness of preventing females from involving themselves with gangs depends on a correct analysis of the pathways to gang involvement and how gangs operate (Fleisher, 2000). CSA is a significant risk factor for gang involvement; however, CSA does not exclusively cause girls to join gangs. CSA and gang involvement are interconnected and are impacted by many of the same factors for the individual and involve their family, peers, and the community in which they live. Protective factors aim to address the risk factors. Table 46.1 is a compiled list of risk factors and corresponding protective factors for female gang involvement across multiple levels of the social ecology.

Individual. Most female gang members are between the ages of 12 and 17 and are African American or Latina (Moore & Hagedorn, 2001). The end of middle school and the transition to high school are considered the riskiest times for adolescent female involvement in delinquent behavior (Acoca & Dedel, 1998). Pertinent to CSA victimization, this transition period in a young girl's life is characterized by a "shift from the relatively asexual gender system of childhood to the overtly sexualized gender systems of adolescence and adulthood" (Thorne, 1993, p. 135). Compared to males, females join and leave gangs earlier. Pregnancy prompts many young women to age out of the gang as they realize they do not want that lifestyle for their child (Moore, 1991). Females involved with gangs tend to be young (i.e., 11–15 years old) and join gangs as young as 11 years old (Esbensen & Huizinga, 1993). Therefore, prevention efforts should target girls ages 8–11, before they enter middle school.

CSA victimization is a significant risk factor as it can have lasting cognitive, psychological, and emotional effects that may render an individual more vulnerable to becoming gang-involved (Tyler, 2002). Cognitive impairment can lead to performing poorly in school and poor decision-making which can lead to dropping out and engaging in risky behavior associated with gang involvement. Psychological effects may include a negative impact on self-esteem rendering an individual susceptible to peer pressure. Victims of CSA may also be suffering from emotional impacts including poor coping skills and the inability to regulate behavioral responses, and CSA victimization may prompt an individual to self-medicate with drugs and alcohol.

Family. Female gang members report that problems within the family, such as sexual victimization, violence, and drug abuse led them to avoid home and join a gang (Chesney-Lind et al., 2007). Both child sexual abuse and gang involvement are linked to deficient parental control, particularly social distance from the maternal figure. The presence of a stepfather doubles the risk for girls, not only for abuse by the stepfather but also by other men before the arrival of the stepfather in the home (Mullen, Martin, Anderson, Romans, & Herbison, 1993). Additionally, parents abusing drugs and alcohol are less able to monitor the activities of their children, thus increasing the likelihood of gang involvement. Families with cultural attitudes that devalue females facilitate abuse and neglect toward females. Living in a household where violence is common and not discouraged effectively socializes youth toward violence. Having a parent or sibling who is a gang member greatly increases the likelihood of being a gang member. Protective measures may

Table 46.1 Risk and protective factors for female gang involvement

Levels	Risk factors	Protective factors
Individual	• Victim of CSA • Ethnic minority—Latina, African American • Age—older less at risk • Academic failure • Poor decision-making/problem solving skills • Poor social skills • Low self-esteem/self-confidence (susceptible to peer pressure) • Aggressive or reactive behavior • Substance, alcohol abuse	• Addressing CSA trauma and other impacts • Support for academic achievement and intellectual abilities • Effective decision-making/problem solving skills • Well-developed interpersonal and social skills • Avenues to enhance sense of worth • High sense of self-esteem, self-efficacy, and personal responsibility • Belief in ability to influence environment in a positive manner • Flexible coping skills • Internal locus of control; reflective vs. impulsive thoughts and behavior • Treatment for substance, alcohol abuse
Family	• Parenting/supervision deficits—especially social distance from mother • Single-parent household • Parental substance, alcohol abuse • Devalued attitude toward females • Approving attitude toward delinquency/violence • Parents/siblings gang members	• Empowerment, respect for females • Reduction of approving attitude toward delinquency/violence • Attentive, balanced parenting • Treatment/avoiding parental substance, alcohol abuse
Peer	• Access to gang-involved peers • Peer approval of violence/delinquency	• Access to non-delinquent peers • Avoidance of delinquent peers • Peer disapproval of violence/delinquency
Community	• Poverty • Gang activity • Approving attitude toward delinquency/violence • Devalued attitude toward females • Damaging portrayals of females in the media • Lack of recreational/employment opportunities • Lack of community support • Racism	• Reduction in gang activity • Community disapproval of delinquency/violence • Respectful attitude toward females • Empowering portrayals of females in the media • Increased opportunities for recreational activities/employment • Increased community support • Addressing racism, finding ways to reduce racist attitudes

involve removing youth from abusive home environments.

Peers. Associating with gang-involved peers is a prominent risk factor for becoming involved in a gang. People tend to trust their friends and become involved in what their friends are doing. This includes joining gangs. Protective factors involve avoiding these peers and making friends with others who are not gang-involved and who frown upon gang activity.

Community. Growing up in segregated and economically disadvantaged neighborhoods and exposure to gang activity are influential determinants in whether girls join gangs. Furthermore, communities with high concentrations of ethnic minorities tend to have cultural attitudes that devalue girls. A study in Phoenix reported a persistent and pervasive double standard among Mexican American gang members—particularly when it came to sexuality (Portillos, 1999). The gender oppression and structural limitations faced by girls in contemporary poverty-stricken neighborhoods play a crucial role in girls' "decisions" to join gangs (Miller, 2001).

Broader societal factors also help create a climate in which violence is encouraged or inhibited. Risks increase when the community fails to provide sufficient youth programs or alternatives to violence.

Proposal for Prevention Plan to Address Female Gang Involvement

A comprehensive strategy is needed to address sexual exploitation and to provide refuge for girls who are victimized by their family, gang, or others. Prevention and intervention programs need to be crafted specifically to meet the needs of teen girls and young women—those on the verge of joining gangs and those already in them (Hong, 2008). As illustrated in Table 46.2, the prevention plan proposed here is a secondary and tertiary strategy for female victims of CSA who are involved in gangs or at risk for gang involvement.

One component of a strategic plan could involve the development of a physical location that operates as a "safe house" for females who have been sexually abused, similar to safe houses for adult victims of domestic violence or adolescent and adult victims of sex trafficking. The safe house would provide the girls with basic needs such as shelter and food but would also include services to prepare them for a more optimistic future (i.e., substance abuse treatment, job training). The services provided at a safe house should be designed around the protective factors for gang involvement.

At the secondary level of prevention, the strategy aims to thwart gang involvement for females by reducing the impact of risk factors that lead to gang involvement. Since CSA serves as a prominent risk factor for gang involvement, a secondary prevention approach would focus on facilitating healing and recovery from CSA. For females who have run away to escape ongoing sexual abuse, the protection of a safe house could both provide a therapeutic environment and meet physical and social needs that gang involvement might otherwise provide. At the tertiary level of prevention, a prevention plan should work to address the impacts of CSA victimization, including gang involvement. This approach would be aimed at females who have already been involved with or joined gangs. For these females, skills training and opportunities for employment, pro-social relationships, and recreation could be provided as an alternative to gang involvement. Such skill-building classes and opportunities could also be offered in a secondary prevention effort for females at risk for gang involvement.

This plan excludes a call for political or legislative action. Gang-involved youths are often not seen as in need of assistance or protection. One gang ethnographer shared that he is "not optimistic about federal or state-level political support necessary to accomplish substantial material change in the lives of impoverished kids let alone gang-affiliated adolescents" (Fleisher, 2000, p. 224). Therefore, the organization, support, and services at the safe house are based on the social ecological model focusing on individual, peer and family, and community-level

Table 46.2 Applying the proximal track for preventing gang involvement for females

	Secondary prevention	Tertiary prevention
Goals	1. Reduce saliency of risk factors 2. Avoid female gang involvement	1. Address impact of CSA victimization on gang involvement 2. Reduce involvement with gangs
Temporal focus	Immediate	Immediate
Target groups	Female victims of CSA at risk for gang involvement	Female victims of CSA involved with gangs
Intervention focus	Provide alternative to abusive situation as a way to prevent victim from becoming gang-involved	1. Address impacts of CSA and gang involvement 2. Provide skills training opportunities for recreation and employment

interventions, with some additional social-marketing recommendations at the societal level of the social ecology.

The "Safe House"

The "safe houses" would need to be in areas with high gang activity, which are likely to have already been identified by law enforcement jurisdictions. The plan should be based on effectiveness. It should be implemented in inner city areas with large populations and in smaller communities with gang activity. Large cities would require a network of interconnected "safe houses" not unlike the very sophisticated and interconnected system of shelters that exists for pets that have been abandoned or abused.

Start-up costs for each safe house would include the property costs related to facility development (i.e., licenses, permits, renovations, security measures, etc.). Additional costs include equipment, materials, and supplies needed to plan and initiate operations at the safe house as well as costs related to staffing (trauma-informed training, team-building, compensation, etc.). Initial operations would include developing a strategy to collect donations and applying for non-profit status so the safe house would be tax-exempt and donor contributions would be tax deductible. Rules would also have to be established to ensure safety of the residents and staff.

Individual. Services should be based on the needs of the individual. Girls who are involved in gangs and who are at risk for gang involvement have unique needs. They require much attention in the way of counseling and trauma-focused cognitive–behavioral therapy to address the effects of trauma and abuse. Counseling is based on the protective factors associated with female gang involvement. The treatment design is especially sensitive to the fact that many of these girls are victims of CSA. Detailed case records including health and criminal background and behavioral conduct would have to be maintained. These records could serve as a reference and could be valuable for reinforcing positive behavior and discouraging negative behavior.

Consequences of gang involvement like delinquency and sexual victimization should also be central to treatment. Conflict resolution and positive coping strategies could be helpful since many of the girls are at risk or engage in aggressive and delinquent behavior. Delinquent females in need of mental health treatment are often incarcerated. It costs less money to treat offenders than to incarcerate them; the money saved from not having to arrest and imprison repeat offenders will save a substantial amount of money (Winkel, 2010).

This population of females could also greatly benefit from sex education, pregnancy prevention, and parenting classes. Another goal of treatment for these girls is the promotion of positive relationships with significant others, sexual partners, family, and peers. These girls need education, training, mentoring, and tutoring to promote positive development. Educational neglect is a common theme among girls who are gang-involved or at risk for gang involvement (Morris, 2005). Links between educational failure and gang membership are clear; compared to better students, low achieving students report greater awareness of gangs, were more often asked to join gangs, reported more friends in gangs, and most importantly were more likely to say they were in gangs (Lopez, Wishard, Gallimore, & Rivera, 2006). Not surprisingly, youths who successfully participate in and complete education have greater opportunities to develop into responsible adults and sever the generational cycle of violence.

Peers and Family. Some of the main reasons girls join gangs are that they come from dysfunctional families or have peers who belong to gangs, and have a family member involved in a gang. Consequently, "ambiguity, mistrust, deception are woven into the fabric of gang members' family lives" (Fleisher, 2000, p. 242). Providing girls with alternatives to dysfunctional or abusive family and peer networks would be the best prevention strategy for girls in gangs and at risk for gang involvement. The safe house could change a girl's social network by adding ties to mainstream social, educational, and economic opportunities. Interaction with college student interns at the safe house could open up opportunities to interact with non-deviant peers and encourage educational attainment. Outreach and counseling could also be carried out by former female gang members who could advise on how to successfully avoid gang membership or remove themselves from the gang. Having former gang members interact with girls could be an important element in treatment since their experiences are likely to be similar.

Community. Female gang members and girls who are at risk for gang involvement are likely to have been raised in a community that lacks support. As mentioned earlier, this deficit extends to other institutions like the educational system and law enforcement. The "safe house" would need to be sustainable; a place where girls can learn responsibility to their community. The girls could be involved in the operation and maintenance of the safe house. The safe house would also require an organized and comprehensive effort from the community which may pose a challenge. Large urban areas often have universities, colleges, and technical schools near the center of the city and not far from areas with high gang activity. This means there are a significant number of students in the area that could function as staff for the safe house. Students within a medical school and within departments like Gender and Women Studies, School of Public Health, Urban Planning and Policy, Latino Studies, and other social sciences departments could be given the opportunity to use their knowledge and skills to volunteer at the safe houses. Instructors could offer course credit in the way of independent studies or internships. Cooperation from university students would also present opportunities for this population to have access to non-delinquent peers as well as ties to mainstream outlets.

Collaborations with local businesses could open up employment opportunities for the girls to acquire workplace skills and a positive work ethic. The safe house would be based on a system where the girls would work for money or in exchange for resources. Businesses where females could express their creativity and gain a sense of accomplishment would be ideal collaborators. For instance, animal shelters could allow opportunities for the girls to train and groom dogs. This collaboration could be modeled after a successful prison program called *Helping Paws* that offers certifications in dog training and grooming.[8]

Local businesses and faith-based organizations could also be commissioned to promote investment in the community. These businesses could sponsor activities that work to clean up the community. For instance, graffiti removal could be made into an event offering incentives like food and games to participants. Creating a garden could be another option where local lawn and garden businesses donate materials. Faith institutions could hold events that promote self-efficacy for girls—like art fairs, theater, or other outlets to express creativity. Networking with other community agencies that offer legal aid, food pantries, soup kitchens, thrift stores, and existing organizations for women who are victims of violence would assist with provisions for volunteers, food, clothing, and other services.

Societal. Factors like poverty, racism, and sexism help to maintain economic or social inequalities between groups in society. It is much more challenging to address societal factors that help create a climate in which violence and delinquency exist. Media portrayals of girls as violent gangbangers create a political climate where the victims of poverty, racism, and sexism can be blamed for their own problems (Chesney-Lind et al., 2007). These media images then influence societal attitudes that promote the demonization of female delinquents. Media frames can then be used as justification for inattention to the actual problems of girls in and around gangs and can facilitate their harsh treatment in the juvenile justice system. As

[8] https://www.pawswithacause.org/what-we-do/pawsprisonpartners.

labeling theory suggests, negative labels can encourage gang involvement as the individual begins to self-identify with the characterization.

Media that counters negative narratives about females could be a possible way to address demonization of delinquent girls. Public awareness through social marketing or social networking could bring attention to female gang involvement. Raising awareness about the connection between child sexual abuse and female gang membership could effectively humanize girls who are in gangs or at risk for gang involvement.

Conclusion

This prevention strategy is not without limitations. Barriers could include local entities not wanting to be affiliated with delinquent youth and problems with trust for employment. Also, there could be issues with dedication to the values of the safe house. Another obstacle could be that the positioning of a "safe house" within a gang area would not provide enough distance between the girls and the dysfunctional relationships and environments that facilitate gang involvement.

Truly understanding the experience of girls in gangs or girls at risk for gang involvement is central to the effectiveness of a prevention plan. While there are a number of shared risk and protective factors for male and female gang involvement, for at risk girls, it is especially important to address the effects that child sexual abuse has on individuals and society as a whole.

References

Acoca, L., & Dedel, K. (1998). *No place to hide: Understanding and meeting the needs of girls in the California Juvenile Justice System*. San Francisco, CA: National Council on Crime and Delinquency.

Bayatpour, M., Wells, R. D., & Holford, S. (1992). Physical and sexual abuse as predictors of substance use and suicide among pregnant teenagers. *Journal of Adolescent Health, 13*(2), 128–132.

Becker, H. (1973). *Outsiders*. New York: Free Press.

Bernburg, J. G., Krohn, M. D., & Rivera, C. J. (2006). Official labeling, criminal embeddedness, and subsequent delinquency: A longitudinal test of labeling theory. *Journal of Research in Crime and Delinquency, 43*(1), 67–88.

Bibring, E. (1943). The conception of the repetition compulsion. *The Psychoanalytic Quarterly, 12*(4), 486–519.

Bjerregaard, B. (2010). Gang membership and drug involvement: Untangling the complex relationship. *Crime & Delinquency, 56*(1), 3–34.

Bjerregaard, B., & Smith, C. (1993). Gender differences in gang participation, delinquency, and substance use. *Journal of Quantitative Criminology, 9*(4), 329–355.

Bobrowski, L. J. (1988). *Collecting, organizing and reporting street gang crime*. Chicago Police Department.

Bowker, L. H., Gross, H. S., & Klein, M. W. (1980). Female participation in delinquent gang activities. *Adolescence, 15*(59), 509.

Bowker, L. H., & Klein, M. W. (1983). The etiology of female juvenile delinquency and gang membership: A test of psychological and social structural explanations. *Adolescence, 18*(72), 739.

Boynton-Jarrett, R., Rich-Edwards, J. W., Jun, H. J., Hilbert, E. N., & Wright, R. J. (2011). Abuse in childhood and risk of uterine leiomyoma: the role of emotional support in biologic resilience. *Epidemiology, 22*(1), 6–14.

Broidy, L., & Agnew, R. (1997). Gender and crime: A general strain theory perspective. *Journal of Research in Crime and Delinquency, 34*(3), 275–306.

Brotherton, D. (1996). "Smartness," "Toughness," and "Autonomy:" Drug use in the context of gang female delinquency. *Journal of Drug Issues, 26*, 261–277.

Brown, L. M. (1999). *Raising their voices: The politics of girls' anger*. Cambridge, MA: Harvard University Press.

Browning, K., Thornberry, T. P., & Porter, P. K. (1999). *Highlights of findings from the Rochester youth development study*. Washington, DC: US Department of Justice, Office of Justice Programs, Office of Juvenile Justice and Delinquency Prevention.

Burgess, E. W., & Akers, R. L. (1966). A differential association-reinforcement theory of criminal behavior. *Social Problems, 14*(2), 128–147.

Campbell, A. (1984). *The Girls in the Gang*. Cambridge, MA: Basil Blackwood.

Campbell, A. (1987). Self-definition by rejection. *Social Problems, 34*, 451–466.

Campbell, A. (1990). Female participation in gangs. In C. R. Huff (Ed.), *Gangs in America* (pp. 163–182). Newbury Park, CA: Sage.

Chesney-Lind, M. (1993). Girls, gangs and violence: Anatomy of a backlash. *Humanity and Society, 17*(3), 321–344.

Chesney-Lind, M., & Hagedorn, J. (Eds.). (1999). *Female gangs in America: Essays on girls, gangs and gender*. Chicago, IL: Lake View Press.

Chesney-Lind, M., Morash, M., & Irwin, K. (2007). Policing girlhood? Relational aggression and violence prevention. *Youth Violence and Juvenile Justice, 5*(3), 328–345.

Cohen, A. K. (1956). *Delinquent boys: The culture of the gang*. NY: Routledge & Kegan Paul.

Curry, D., & Decker, S. (1998). *Confronting gangs*. Los Angeles, CA: Roxbury.

Curry, G. D. (1998). Female gang involvement. *Journal of Research in Crime and Delinquency, 35*(1), 100–118.

Curry, G. D., & Spergel, I. A. (1988). Gang homicide, delinquency, and community. *Criminology, 26*(3), 381–406.

Decker, S., & Van Winkle, B. (1996). *Life in the gang*. New York: Cambridge University Press.

Deschenes, E. P., & Esbensen, F. A. (1999). Violence among girls: Does gang membership make a difference? In M. Chesney-Lind & J. Hagedorn's (Eds.), *Female Gangs in America*. Chicago, IL: Lake View Press.

Egley, A., & Ritz, C. E. (2006). *Highlights of the 2004 National Youth Gang Survey*. Washington, DC: U.S. Department of Justice, Office of Justice Programs, Office of Juvenile Justice and Delinquency Prevention.

Esbensen, F., & Osgood, D. W. (1999). Gang Resistance Education and Training (G.R.E.A.T.): Results from the national evaluation. *Journal of Research in Crime and Delinquency, 36*(2), 194–225.

Esbensen, F. A. (2000). *Preventing adolescent gang involvement*. Washington, DC: U.S. Department of Justice, Office of Justice Programs, Office of Juvenile Justice and Delinquency Prevention, (NCJ 182210).

Esbensen, F. A., Brick, B. T., Melde, C., Tusinski, K., & Taylor, T. J. (2008). The role of race and ethnicity in gang membership. In F. Van Gemert, D. Peterson, & I. L. Lien (Eds.), *Street gangs, migration and ethnicity* (pp. 117–139). Portland, OR: Willan Publishing.

Esbensen, F. A., & Deschenes, E. P. (1998). A multisite examination of youth gang membership: Does gender matter? *Criminology, 36*(4), 799–828.

Esbensen, F. A., Deschenes, E. P., & Winfree, L. T., Jr. (1999). Differences between gang girls and gang boys: Results from a multisite survey. *Youth & Society, 31*(1), 27–53.

Esbensen, F. A., & Huizinga, D. (1993). Gangs, drugs, and delinquency in a survey of urban youth. *Criminology, 31*(4), 565–589.

Esbensen, F. A., & Winfree, L. T. (1998). Race and gender differences between gang and nongang youths: Results from a multisite survey. *Justice Quarterly, 15*(3), 505–526.

Evans, W., Albers, E., Macari, D., & Mason, A. (1996). Suicide ideation, attempts and abuse among incarcerated gang and non-gang delinquents. *Child and Adolescent Social Work Journal, 13*(2), 115–126.

Fagan, J. (1990). Social processes of delinquency and drug use among urban gangs. In C. R. Huff (Ed.), *Gangs in America* (pp. 183–219). Newbury Park, CA: Sage Publications.

Finkelhor, D. (1994). Current information on the scope and nature of child sexual abuse. *The Future of Children, Sexual Abuse of Children, 4*(2), 31–53.

Finkelhor, D. (2009). The prevention of childhood sexual abuse. *The Future of Children, 19*(2), 169–194. https://doi.org/10.1353/foc.0.0035

Fleisher, M. S. (2000). *Dead end kids: Gang girls and the boys they know*. Madison, WI: The University of Wisconsin Press.

Giordano, P. C. (1978). Girls, guys and gangs: The changing social context of female delinquency. *Journal of Criminal Law & Criminology, 69*, 126.

Goldstein, A. P., & Glick, B. (1994). Aggression replacement training: Curriculum and evaluation. *Simulation & Gaming, 25*, 9–26.

Goldstein, A. P., Glick, B., & Gibbs, J. (1998). *Aggression replacement training: A comprehensive intervention for aggressive youth*. Champaign, IL: Research Press.

Gottfredson, G. D., & Gottfredson, D. C. (2001). What schools do to prevent problem behavior and promote safe environments. *Journal of Educational and Psychological Consultation, 12*(4), 313–344.

Hagedorn, J. (1998). *People and folks* (2nd ed.). Chicago, IL: Lakeview Press.

Hagedorn, J., & Devitt, M. (1999). Fighting females: The social construction of the female gang. In M. Chesney-Lind & J. Hagedorn (Eds.), *Female gangs in America*. Chicago, IL: Lakeview Press.

Harris, M. G. (1988). *Cholas: Latino girls and gangs*. New York: AMS Press.

Hill, K. G., Lui, C., & Hawkins, J. D. (2001). *Early precursors of gang membership: A study of Seattle youth*. Washington, DC: US Department of Justice, Office of Justice Programs, Office of Juvenile Justice and Delinquency Prevention.

Hirschi, T. (1969). A control theory of delinquency. In *Criminology theory: Selected classic readings* (pp. 289–305).

Hong, R.S. (2008, December 26). Task force on girl gangs forms. *Pasadena Star-News* (CA).

Howell, J. C. (2007). Menacing or mimicking? Realities of youth gangs. *Juvenile and Family Court Journal, 58*(2), 39–50.

Joe, K. A., & Chesney-Lind, M. (1995). "Just every mother's angel" An analysis of gender and ethnic variations in youth gang membership. *Gender & Society, 9*(4), 408–431.

Joe-Laidler, K., & Hunt, G. (1997). Violence and social organization in female gangs. *Social Justice, 24*(4), 148–169.

Joe-Laidler, K., & Hunt, G. (2001). Accomplishing femininity among the girls in the gang. *British Journal of Criminology, 41*(4), 656–678.

Kaufman, K., Barber, M., Moser, H., & Carter, M. (2002). Reconceptualizing child sexual abuse as a public health concern. In P. Schewe (Ed.), *Preventing violence in relationships* (pp. 27–54). Washington, DC: American Psychological Association.

Kelly, D. (1993). *Last chance high: How girls and boys drop in and out of alternative schools*. New Haven, CT: Yale University Press.

Kilpatrick, D. G., Ruggiero, K. J., Acierno, R., Saunders, B. E., Resnick, H. S., & Best, C. L. (2003). Violence and risk of PTSD, major depression, substance abuse/dependence, and comorbidity: Results from the National Survey of Adolescents. *Journal of Consulting and Clinical Psychology, 1*(4), 692–700.

Kornhauser, R. R. (1978). *Social sources of delinquency: An appraisal of analytic models*. Chicago, IL: University of Chicago Press.

Lauderback, D., Hansen, J., & Waldorf, D. (1992). Sisters are doin' it for themselves: A black female gang in San Francisco. *The Gang Journal, 1*(1), 57–72.

Le, T., Arifuku, I., & Nunez, M. (2003). Girls and culture in delinquency intervention: A case study of RYSE. *Juvenile and Family Court Journal, 54*, 25–34.

Leitz, L. (2003). Girl fights: Exploring females' resistance to educational structures. *International Journal of Sociology and Social Policy, 23*(11), 15–43.

Lopez, E. M., Wishard, A., Gallimore, R., & Rivera, W. (2006). Latino high school students' perceptions of gangs and crews. *Journal of Adolescent Research, 21*(3), 299–318.

Lung, C., & Daro, D. (1996). *Current Trends in Child Abuse Reporting and Fatalities: The Results of the 1995 Annual Fifty State Survey*. Chicago, IL: National Committee to Prevent Child Abuse.

Merton, R. K. (1968). *Social theory and social structure*. New York, NY: Simon and Schuster.

Miller, J. (1998). Gender and victimization risk among young women in gangs. *Journal of Research in Crime and Delinquency, 35*(4), 429–453.

Miller, J. (2001). *One of the guys: Girls, gangs and gender*. New York: Oxford Press.

Miller, J. (2002). The girls in the gang: what we've learned from two decades of research. In C. R. Huff (Ed.), *Gangs in America III* (pp. 175–197). Thousand Oaks, CA: Sage Publications.

Miller, J., & Brunson, R. K. (2000). Gender dynamics in youth gangs: A comparison of males' and females' accounts. *Justice Quarterly, 17*(3), 419–448.

Moore, J. (1991). *Going down to the Barrio: Homeboys and homegirls in change*. Philadelphia, PA: Temple University Press.

Moore, J., & Hagedorn, J. M. (2001, March). *Female gangs: A focus on research*. Washington, DC: U.S. Department of Justice, Office of Justice Programs, Office of Juvenile Justice and Delinquency Prevention, (NCJ 186159).

Moore, J. W., & Hagedorn, J. (1996). What happens to girls in the gang? In C. R. Huff (Ed.), *Gangs in America* (2nd ed.). Thousand Oaks, CA: Sage Publications.

Morris, E. W. (2005). 'Tuck in that shirt!': Race, class, gender, and discipline in an urban school. *Sociological Perspectives, 48*, 25–48.

Mullen, P. E., Martin, J. L., Anderson, J. C., Romans, S. E., & Herbison, G. P. (1993). Childhood sexual abuse and mental health in adult life. *The British Journal of Psychiatry, 163*(6), 721–732.

National Youth Gang Center. (2000). *1998 National Youth Gang Survey*. Washington, DC: U.S. Department of Justice, Office of Justice Programs, Office of Juvenile Justice and Delinquency Prevention.

National Youth Gang Center. (2010). *2008 National Youth Gang Survey*. Washington, DC: U.S. Department of Justice, Office of Justice Programs, Office of Juvenile Justice and Delinquency Prevention.

Ness, C. D. (2004). Why girls fight: Female youth violence in the inner city. *Annals of the American Academy of Political and Social Science, 595*, 32–48.

OJJDP. (2018). *Awards Made for Solicitation, Youth Gang Prevention and Intervention Program*. Retrieved from https://external.ojp.usdoj.gov/SelectorServer/awards/pdf/solicitation/OJJDP%20FY%2010%20Youth%20Gang%20Prevention%20and%20Intervention%20Program.

Palumbo, D. J., & Ferguson, J. L. (1995). Evaluating Gang Resistance Education and Training (GREAT): Is the impact the same as that of Drug Abuse Resistance Education (DARE)? *Evaluation Review, 19*(6), 591–619.

Park, R. E., Burgess, E. W., & McKenzie, R. D. (1925). *The City*. Chicago, IL: University of Chicago Press.

Peterson, D., Miller, J., & Esbensen, F. A. (2001). The impact of sex composition on gangs and gang member delinquency. *Criminology, 39*(2), 411–440.

Peterson, D. (2012). Girlfriends, gun-holders, and ghetto-rats? Moving beyond narrow views of girls in gangs. In Delinquent girls (pp. 71–84). Springer, New York, NY.

Pitman, R., Orr, S., & Laforque, D. (1987). Psychophysiology of PTSD imagery in Vietnam combat veterans. *Archives of General Psychiatry, 44*, 940–976.

Portillos, E. L. (1999). The social construction of gender in the Barrio. In M. Chesney-Lind & J. Hagedorn's (Eds.), *Female gangs in America* (pp. 232–244). Chicago, IL: Lake View Press.

Quicker, J. C. (1983). *Homegirls: Characterizing Chicana gangs*. Madison, CT: International Universities Press.

Sampson, R. J. (1993). The community context of violent crime. In W. J. Wilson (Ed.), *Sociology and the public agenda* (pp. 267–274). Newbury Park, CA: Sage Publications. ISBN 0-8039-5083-7

Sanchez-Jankowski, M. (1991). *Islands in the street*. Berkeley, CA: University of California Press.

Shaw, C. R., & McKay, H. D. (1942). *Juvenile delinquency in urban areas*. Chicago, IL: University of Chicago Press.

Short, J., & Strodtbeck, F. (1965). *Group processes and gang delinquency*. Chicago, IL: University of Chicago Press.

Snyder, H. N., & Sickmund, M. (2006). *Juvenile Offenders And Victims: 2006 National Report*. Washington, DC: Office of Juvenile Justice and Delinquency Prevention.

Spergel, I. (1966). *Street gang work: Theory and practice*. Reading, MA: Addison-Wesley Pub. Co.

Spergel, I. (1995). *The youth gang problem*. New York, NY: Oxford University Press.

Tapper, K., & Boulton, M. (2000). Social representations of physical, verbal and indirect aggression in children:

Sex and age differences. *Aggressive Behavior, 26*, 442–454.

Taylor, C. (1993). *Girls, gangs, women and drugs*. East Lansing, MI: Michigan State University Press.

Thompson, K. M., & Braaten-Antrim, R. (1998). Youth maltreatment and gang involvement. *Journal of Interpersonal Violence, 13*(3), 328–345.

Thornberry, T. P. (1998). Membership in youth gangs and involvement in serious and violent offending. In R. Loeber & D. P. Farrington (Eds.), *Serious & violent juvenile offenders: Risk factors and successful interventions* (pp. 147–166). Thousand Oaks, CA: Sage Publications.

Thornberry, T. P., Krohn, M. D., Lizotte, A. J., Smith, C. A., & Tobin, K. (2003). *Gangs and delinquency in developmental perspective*. Cambridge: Cambridge University Press.

Thorne, B. (1993). *Gender play: Girls and boys in school*. New Brunswick, NJ: Rutgers University Press.

Thrasher, F. (1927). *The gang: A study of 1,313 gangs in Chicago*. Chicago, IL: University of Chicago Press.

Townsend, C. & Rheingold, A. A. (2013). *Estimating a child sexual abuse prevalence rate for practitioners: A review of child sexual abuse prevalence studies*. Charleston, S.C., Darkness to Light Pg 2. Retrieved from www.D2L.org/1in10.

Tyler, K. (2002, November–December). Social and emotional outcomes of childhood sexual abuse: A review of recent research. *Aggression and Violent Behavior, 7*(6), 567–589. https://doi.org/10.1016/S1359-1789(01)00047-7

U.S. Department of Health and Human Services. (1993). *Report to the Congress on the Youth Gang Drug Prevention Program: Fiscal Year1993 Report*. Washington, DC: U.S. Department of Health and Human Services, Administration for Children and Families, Family and Youth Services Bureau.

Valdez, A., & Cepeda, A. (1998). *Homegirls, chicks, and kicking it: Females associated with Mexican American male gangs. Unpublished paper*. San Antonio, TX: University of Texas at San Antonio.

Van der Kolk, B. A. (1989). The compulsion to repeat the trauma: Re-enactment, revictimization, and masochism. *Psychiatric Clinics, 12*(2), 389–411.

Venkatesh, S. A. (1998). Gender and outlaw capitalism: A historical account of the Black Sisters United "girl gang". *Signs, 23*, 683–709.

Vigil, J. D. (1988). Group processes and street identity: Adolescent Chicago gang members. *Ethos, 16*(4), 421–445.

Winkel, B. (2010, July 9). Treating criminals. *Treatment Solutions Network*. Retrieved from http://www.treatmentsolutionsnetwork.com/blog/index.php/2010/07/09/treating-criminals/.

Wurtele, S. K. (2002). School-based child sexual abuse prevention. In P. Schewe (Ed.), *Preventing violence in relationships* (pp. 27–54). Washington, DC: American Psychological Association.

Consistency of Offender Behaviors and Victim Targeting in Serial Sexual Violence: An Overview of the Field

47

C. Gabrielle Salfati

Introduction

Assessing sex offending and understanding the factors that can aid in that process is key in the analysis of crimes such as serial sex offending and serial sexual homicide. Knowledge of the factors, and the empirical backing these factors have, is, therefore, integral to enable more valid and reliable assessments of offending patterns.

Clinical Risk Assessment is a process that aims to determine, based on specific psychological measurements, the likelihood that an offender is going to commit a crime. The field of risk assessment in sexual offending has focused on which offender characteristics are predictive of reoffending, and several tests are employed now in this process. Recent research has, however, shown that the current process involved in risk assessment has had difficulties in reliably assigning offenders to categories of risk that can adequately predict their likelihood of re-offending, and that there is variability in offenders who receive similar "scores" in terms of whether they go on to re-offend or not. One avenue that has been suggested that we may want to explore therefore is a more detailed understanding of an offender's behaviors at the time of the crime and how we can use this information to help refine and increase the reliability of risk predictions (Salfati & Kunkle, 2016).

Offender Profiling, or Behavioral Crime Scene Analysis, is another field that has been developing alongside the field of risk assessment. This process can be seen as the flipside of the risk assessment coin (Salfati, 2015). Instead of predicting unknown future behavior from the characteristics of the offender, it aims to predict characteristics of an unknown offender from the known actions they engaged in at the crime scene (Canter, 2000, 2004). As part of the process, offender profiling aims to examine the actions at the crime scene and categorize these into different behavioral subtypes, which are predictive of separate and distinct sets of offender characteristics. In serial crimes such as sexual homicide and rape, the examination of whether offenders are consistent in their behavior over their series, or whether they change, escalate or whether they engage in predictable trajectories over time, has been added to the profiling process of categorizing offenses into different subtypes (Salfati, 2008a). The overall aim is to use this information to help narrow down and prioritize the most likely characteristics of potential suspects.

Salfati (2015) stressed that both fields bring important pieces to understanding the analysis of sex offending. Adding how an offender shows consistent patterns of behavior across their series to the risk assessment process, may provide a substantial addition to our understanding of the

C. G. Salfati (✉)
John Jay College of Criminal Justice, City University of New York, New York, NY, United States
e-mail: gsalfati@jjay.cuny.edu

W. T. O'Donohue and P. A. Schewe (eds.), *Handbook of Sexual Assault and Sexual Assault Prevention*,
https://doi.org/10.1007/978-3-030-23645-8_47

relationship between psychological assessment of behavior, and ultimately may impact the reliability of predictions and types of re-offending and recidivism.

This chapter aims to give an overview of the field of behavioral crime scene analysis and discuss the advancements that have been made in this field, specifically with reference to understanding consistency patterns across an offender's series in cases of sexual crimes such as rape and homicide. The focus will be on the discussion around understanding the specific components of sexual activity during series, and its different expressions through the behavior itself, the type of crime (rape and sexual homicide), and also how the sexual component may be expressed through the victim targeted, such as in cases of sex workers.

Behavioral Crime Scene Analysis and Investigative Practice

The main aim of behavioral crime scene analysis is to analyze the way an offender commits their crime, to establish discernible patterns and behavioral subtypes, and then link subtypes of crime scene actions to the most likely offender background characteristics, and use this in criminal investigations as a primary tool for the police to narrow their suspect pool down to statistically the most likely type of offender, and identify and link series of crimes.

In the 1970s and 1980s, the early years of what we associate with the beginning of the offender profiling field, most profiling was based on the experiences of investigating officers who had extensive experience investigating cases, as well as clinicians who had been involved in the pre-trial assessment process, treated offenders within the hospital environment, or dealt with them in offender treatment programs within the prison system. Much of this early work was initiated by the FBI and their clinical practitioner colleagues on sexual homicide, specifically with an interest in understanding serial homicide (Douglas, Ressler, Burgess, & Hartman, 1986; Ressler et al., 1986), and although it was meant for criminal investigations, focused on the clinical aspect of violent crimes, notably psychopathology (see reviews by McCann, 1992; Poytheress, Otto, Darkes, & Starr, 1993).

McCann (1992) highlights however that little was done in these early years in the way of published research on the utility, reliability and validity of profiling. As the technique became more and more popular throughout the 1980s onwards, people increasingly began asking questions regarding the validity and the reliability of profiling as a method for analyzing criminal behavior. Specifically, questions arose regarding how accurate these profiles actually were.

In terms of how these issues relate to practice, a number of studies were done early on in the profiling and behavioral crime analysis field. Risinger and Loop (2002) reviewed the history of crime analysis in general, and found that the analysis of criminal behavior was still not based on empirical and scientific evidence. Instead, the field was riddled with people giving their opinions about what they thought an offender's behavior was an indication of, rather than using solidly founded scientific knowledge of human behavior. Alison, Bennell, Mokros, and Ormerod (2002) in another study focusing specifically on profiling also highlighted that much of what was considered standard practice actually fell short of current understandings of various psychological processes and principles and was not based on a long history of research on psychology and the analysis of human behavior. In a subsequent study, Alison, Smith, Eastman, and Rainbow (2003), aiming to further examine the reliability and validity of the practice of profiling, examined 21 actual investigative profiling reports provided by experts, and showed that of the nearly 4000 claims regarding the characteristics of offenders present in the 21 profiles, as much as 80% of the information provided was not supported by empirical evidence. Meyer (2007) additionally did an evaluation of case law internationally to assess the use of criminal behavior methods generally in court. She found that the techniques discussed in the cases reviewed were generally failing the legal test for admissible expert evidence due to the fact they were based on very little valid empirical data. Again, the same picture was coming through: people were giving their opinions, but these opinions were not based on empirical facts.

Behavioral Crime Scene Analysis and Investigative Psychology

Due to the increasing questions being raised in the field relating to the lack of an empirical basis to the practice of behavioral crime scene analysis, the new field of social science of Investigative Psychology emerged in the early 1990s, which aimed to examine the evidence for offender profiling and behavioral crime scene analysis to explore how much we actually knew about what offenders do, how much of our understanding of human behavior we could use to understand criminal behavior specifically, and how we could ultimately use all of this to reliably profile an offender's actions and link that to the type of person they may be, and use this in an investigative context (see Canter, 1994, 2000, 2004).

In the last 30 years, a growing empirical basis to the analysis of criminal behavior has developed under the umbrella of Investigative Psychology, as well as rigorous research methodology associated with this work (Alison, Snook & Stein, 2001; Alison, Smith, & Morgan, 2003; Bateman & Salfati, 2007; Canter, Alison, Alison, & Wentink, 2004; Canter & Wentink, 2004; Salfati, 2008b, 2011; Salfati & Bateman, 2005; Trojan & Salfati, 2008). Investigative Psychology aims to establish an empirical approach to behavioral crime scene analysis and offender profiling (see Salfati, 2011 for an overview of the methodology) and focusses on behavior that can be observed and objectively measured so that the basis for decision-making is based on a scientific method, and not on something that is based on processes fraught with subjectivity and guess work, such as guessing any internal processes like motivation of the offender. The next stage in the profiling process is to empirically (i.e. statistically) categorize behaviors into different subtypes of crime scenes, based on subgroups of observable behaviors, that can be understood by their common psychological meaning. These psychological subgroups will be clearly linked and backed up by validated, and useful, theoretical classification systems. The third step of the profiling process focuses on linking these crime scene types to the types of offender characteristics related to each one of these types. The hypothesis is that a person who commits a particular type of crime scene will be a specific type of person. This is what has been referred to as the A → C equation, or the Actions to Characteristics equation (Canter, 2000, 2004). By using this stepwise system, an empirical basis can be established on each step in the process, which will make the process more valid, and the application of it reliable across practitioners. The last phase of the profiling process can then use this information in practice to help focus a given police inquiry and narrow down the suspect pool to the most likely type of offender, based on an evaluation of the behaviors they engaged in at the crime scene.

Three general interlinked areas have been the focus of this behavioral crime scene analysis and offender profiling research: individual differentiation, behavioral consistency, and inferences about offender characteristics (Canter, 2000; Salfati, 2008a).

1. Individual differentiation aims to establish differences between the behavioral actions of offenders and identify subgroups of crime scene types.
2. Behavioral consistency is a key issue in profiling, specifically for understanding both the development of an offender's criminal career and an individual's consistency across a series of crimes—that is, whether the same subsets of actions are displayed at each crime scene over a series of offenses.
3. Inferences about offender characteristics based on the way an offender acts at the time of the crime are at the core of profiling and use consistency analysis as its main focus.

In the current chapter, we focus specifically on the second component of behavioral consistency.

Behavioral Crime Scene Analysis and Clinical Practice

It is difficult to get a clear estimate of how many mental health professionals are involved in behavioral crime scene analysis and profiling (Torres, Boccaccini, & Miller, 2006). Copson (1995) in an evaluation of profiling in its early years suggests that well over half the operational profiling in the UK was conducted by psychologists and psychiatrists employing a clinical (experience- or judgment-based evaluation rather than database-based) approach. Bartol (1996) conducted a survey of 152 police psychologists working within various policing capacities in 1994, a senior group with an average experience of 11.8 years, most (89%) had PhD's, followed by a variety of other higher degrees. Most obtained their terminal degree in clinical psychology (60.7%) and counseling psychology (17%), and 2% of monthly work time of in-house psychologists and 3.4% of workload by part-time consulting psychologists were directed at profiling. A surprising number Bartol shows, due to the fact that 70% of the survey did not feel comfortable profiling and seriously questioned its validity and usefulness until more research was done to back it as a process. A result which makes sense if we think about the fact that the majority of the respondent had no experience in the method.

However, Torres et al. (2006) state a decade later that this pattern was changing by quoting a 2004 issue of the American Psychological Association's (APA) monthly professional magazine, *Monitoring Psychology*, which highlighted the role of psychologists in criminal profiling (Winerman, 2004a, 2004b). They show that this trend was also evident in the recent publication of profiling research by psychologists, and citing the work by investigative psychologists (e.g., Canter et al., 2004; Canter & Wentink, 2004; Kocsis, 2004; Salfati, 2003; Salfati & Canter, 1999) and in the coverage of profiling in editions of psychology–law textbooks (e.g. Bartol & Bartol, 2004; Constanzo, 2004; Wrightsman & Fulero, 2005).

In a similar study to Bartol's 10 years earlier, Torres et al. (2006) conducted an internet survey of forensic psychologists and psychiatrists and asked questions related to their experiences with and opinions about profiling. Only 9.9% ($N = 161$) of the 1637 forensic mental health professionals (approximately half psychologists and half psychiatrists) who received an e-mail solicitation completed the study. Torres et al. thus caution that the low response rate may make it unlikely that respondents were able to accurately express the amount of variation in beliefs and practices that is present among forensic mental health professionals as a whole. They also highlight that it may be that those who responded were strong proponents or advocates of profiling and that the survey findings represent either an overly positive or an overly negative view of profiling. About 10% of the 161 survey respondents had profiling experience, although more than 25% considered themselves knowledgeable about profiling. Fewer than 25–40% (depending on whether the terms "profiling" or "criminal investigative analysis" was used) believed that the method was reliable profiling was scientifically reliable or valid. Just under a third of forensic mental health professionals reported having knowledge of profiling and criminal investigative analysis (31.5% and 26.1%, respectively) and training in these techniques (16.3% and 20.3%, respectively), only about 10% reported ever having generated a profile or criminal investigative analysis for an actual case. Similarly, only about 10% reported having testified in court about their use of these techniques or their opinion of these techniques in general. Although fewer than half of the forensic mental health professionals questioned the scientific merit of profiling and criminal investigative analysis, the majority responded that these techniques were useful tools for law enforcement. No significant differences between those with and without knowledge were revealed.

When we move from looking at the *opinions* by clinicians, to the *profiling research and work* of clinicians, the picture is however less encouraging, as Canter and Youngs (2009) sum up; *"In a series of studies first published in 1954 and followed up over subsequent decades, it has been found that actuarial decision processes were far more accurate and valid than those based on clinical judgement. In general the scientific approach proves to be far more effective than that based upon personal opinion.*" (Canter & Youngs, 2009, p7).

Snook, Eastwood, Gendreau, Goggin, and Cullen (2007) in their review additionally state that anecdotal arguments were the most frequently endorsed knowledge source in the 130 publications on offender profiling they surveyed. As Douglas et al. (1986) state "*The process used by an investigative profiler in developing a criminal profile is quite similar to that used by clinicians to make a diagnosis and treatment plan... investigators traditionally have learned profiling through brainstorming, intuition, and educated guesswork*" (p. 405). Snook, Cullen, Bennell, Taylor, and Gendreau (2008) discuss how this clinically based process is reminiscent of psychoanalytic approaches to therapy where mental health professionals diagnose their clients through subjective interpretations and unsupported methods (Dawes, 1997; cited in Snook et al., 2008). They go on to discuss how errors such as these, in the profiling realm, may be due to how experience led profilers attain information and use anecdotes. They highlight that empirical research has shown that clinical experience has a limited effect on the accuracy of psychologists' and psychiatrists' judgments across a range of tasks (e.g., Garb, 1998; Garb & Boyle, 2003; Meehl, 1997, cited in Snook et al., 2008), and that there is low intra- and interclinician consistency in judgments of mental health status (Faust & Ziskin, 1988, cited in Snook et al., 2008).

Boon (1997, 1998) in some of the earliest writings discussing clinical perspectives of profiling provides an overview of how personality theory and clinical approaches has been seen to contribute to profiling. West (2000) provides a more integrated approach, and a discussion of how the clinical approach may be integrated with the more behavioral approach that is normally associated with empirical profiling, and by so doing provides the benefit of clinical work to profiling, whilst lending more objective credibility to clinical profiling. He stresses that it is important even for clinical assessment and risk assessment to go beyond the interview and look at what happened during the crime scene and hypothesizes that there might be a link between some behaviors at the scene that relate to key clinical concepts of fantasy and motivation and psychopathology. He proposes many interesting questions about this relationship, the focus however remains on assessment of risk and treatment planning, and thus on motivation and internal psychological processes of the offender, which although the main focus in clinical work, and certainly is of interest to theoretical work, is less applicable to the focus of profiling which aims to elucidate objective behavioral features that can be measured at the crime scene, and more searchable attributes of the offender such as location, criminal records and other factors more often recorded in police files. West (2001) however acknowledges that although clinicians can contribute a great deal based on their experience and contact with patients, "it is important to emphasize that such exposure to offender/patients in a clinical environment is not enough to constitute the knowledge base on which an offender profile can be produced." (p. 101–102), and emphasizes multidisciplinary teams (which is what later happened in the UK profiling practice, see Rainbow, 2008). West (2001, p.103) additionally adds how the American Psychological Association (APA) admonished the FBI for engaging in profiling and making conclusions based on techniques of limited reliability. The British Psychological Society (BPS) in the UK has also admonished psychologists for using profiling in a way for which it was not intended, and based on no actual expertise. The fact that both of the largest organizations regulating psychological practice have at some point commented on the process, further highlights the switch of the focus in the field towards building a valid basis of research, and a reliable process in which to apply it as part of a transparent and regulated process.

Behavioral Crime Scene Analysis and Behavioral Consistency

A key question in the area of Investigative Psychology and a key question in the area of investigating serial crimes is whether we can link crime scenes to each other based on certain consistent actions that the offender engages in at each crime scene, and thereby identify specific series. When we are talking about consistency, we are generally referring to the idea that an offender will display similar actions across crime scenes, which provides the information needed to allow us to link a series together. Alongside being able to identify actions that can be used to link series, we also need to know how to differentiate one series from another series. Key to this process is the question of what offender actions are the most reliable for making these determinations. Central to this question is what is meant by consistency and how this may be displayed at the crime scene in terms of the actions most useful to establish both similarity and differentiation. These questions are the same in risk assessment in clinical practice (Salfati & Kunkle, 2016).

The Problem of Linking in Practice

In 2005, the FBI's National Center for the Analysis of Violent Crime (NCAVC) invited 135 serial murder subject matter experts to discuss the current state of the knowledge of the field since the original work on sexual and serial homicide that was done by the FBI in the 1970s. These experts came from 10 countries and 5 continents, and included law enforcement who had been involved in investigating cases of serial homicide, legal professionals including prosecutors and defense attorneys who had been part of the court process; members of the media and investigative journalists who had reported on these cases, clinicians who had been part of the assessment of serial offenders, and academics who had done research on the topic. One of the conclusions from this meeting (NCAVC, 2005) was that there was a real lack of valid empirical research in the field that could be reliably used. Most of what was known to that point either came from investigative experience, or was based on case studies that were done by clinicians. The report that came out of the meeting specifically highlighted the importance of ensuring that a solid empirical basis exists and concluded that "*the implementation of a tested and reliable case management system...coupled with competent analytical staff, is imperative in serial murder investigations*" (NCAVC, 2008, p.25).

A more recent UK government review of the services needed in crime analysis and investigation of serial crimes also very clearly highlight that; "*Preventing rape and catching perpetrators are activities that are supported by good intelligence material so that the right investigative approach is selected and resources are targeted effectively. Without that material, the risk to the identification of repeat offenders, or perpetrators whose crimes are escalating in seriousness can increase, and opportunities to strengthen prosecutions be lost*" (HMIC, 2012, p. 4).

Empirical Studies on Linking Serial Crimes

A couple of years after the 2005 FBI symposium, Bateman and Salfati (2007) examined the academic literature on linking, confirming that researchers and practitioners until that point, although prolific in the amount of publications, had not explained in detail how they link crimes, so the validity of their statements was left untested. Indeed, much of this early literature was not supported by empirical studies, but instead was a collection of either untested theoretical papers, or practice-led papers that proposed patterns based on clinical judgment or investigative experience. In the same year, Woodhams, Hollin, & Bull (2007) also conducted a review of the literature and concluded that only 11 studies had addressed the actual empirical and methodological issues related to linking (Bennell & Canter, 2002; Bennell & Jones, 2005; Canter et al., 1991; Green, Booth, & Biderman, 1976; Grubin, Kelly, & Brunsdon, 2001; Hammond, 1990; Salfati & Bateman, 2005; Santtila, Fritzon,

& Tamelander, 2005; Santtila, Junkkila, & Sandnabba, 2005; Woodhams & Toye, 2007).

Salfati and Sorochinski (2018) in a more recent review showed that there has been a steady increase in the decade that followed the FBI meeting in the number of studies specifically relating to linking serial crime, with 40 empirical research studies that have been published that directly address the issue of linking serial crimes—including burglary, robbery, rape, arson, and homicide—using behavioral evidence. Most of these studies have specifically focused on resolving the methodological dilemma of how to best use crime scene behaviors to link serial offenses. However, of these 40 studies, only six specifically focused on serial homicide (Bateman & Salfati, 2007; Salfati & Bateman, 2005; Salfati, Horning, Sorochinski, & Labuschagne, 2015; Salo, et al., 2012; Santtila et al., 2008; Sorochinski & Salfati, 2010), and 13 involved series of sexual offenses (Bennell, Jones, & Melnyk, 2009; Grubin et al., 2001; Harbers, Deslauriers-Varin, Beauregard, & van der Kemp, 2012; Hewitt & Beauregard, 2014; Leclerc, Lussier, & Deslauriers-Varin, 2015; Kearns, Salfati, & Jarvis, 2011; Santtila et al., 2005; Slater, Woodhams, & Hamilton-Giachritsis, 2015; Sorochinski & Salfati, 2018; Winter et al., 2013; Woodhams, et al., 2007; Woodhams, Hollin, & Bull, 2008; Woodhams & Labuschagne, 2011).

Sorochinski and Salfati's (2018) review of these linking studies (2018) show that over half of the studies examined the possibilities of behavioral linking using only two crimes from a series, either two consecutive crimes (e.g. Davies, Tonkin, Bull, & Bond, 2012; Tonkin, Grant, & Bond, 2008; Woodhams & Toye, 2007) or a random pair of two crimes (e.g. Bennell & Canter, 2002; Bennell & Jones, 2005) from the series, and determining the predictive validity of various methods in linking the two crimes together. Such an approach may be problematic they state, in that it does not allow for the examination of progression of consistency and change over time, especially since emerging evidence suggests that offenders may become less consistent as their series progress (Kearns et al., 2011; Salfati et al., 2015), highlighting the importance of fully investigating behavioral patterns across a larger number of crimes within series. This is showcased further in the next section, which aims to provide a full review of empirically based consistency studies to date.

Behavioral Consistency

The consistency hypothesis was outlined by Canter (1994) and states that "the way an offender carries out one crime on one occasion will have some characteristic similarities to the way he or she carries out crimes on other occasions" (p. 347).

Studies that examined behavioral consistency in sexual offenses (Canter et al., 1991; Grubin et al., 2001; Santtila, Junkkila, & Sandnabba, 2005) have all provided evidence that offenders are consistent to a degree in their offending behaviors. However, the consistency discussed is far from what is necessary for behavioral linking to be considered empirically validated and useful in practice, which would only be useful if studies could show that offenders are indeed consistent in all, or the vast majority of their crimes, as shown by either individual behaviors they engage in or subtypes. With early studies showing that offenders don't show the consistency patterns hypothesized to exist, where their crimes are similar across their series, recent studies (e.g., Hewitt & Beauregard, 2014; Leclerc et al., 2015; Salfati, 2009; Sorochinski & Salfati, 2010) have suggested that consistency needs to be looked at in a much broader way, and highlight the importance of looking beyond stability of behavior and of additionally incorporating an understanding of consistency in terms of patterns of behavioral change. Salfati (2009) suggests that these patterns may be usefully seen not as consistency in certain behaviors or patterns of behaviors, but instead as the patterns of change, as the offender moved from one crime to the next. The nature of what this change consists of therefore becomes a key area of study in the area of linking.

Of the 6 serial homicide and 13 sexual offense studies on linking mentioned above, only 4 of the studies on serial homicide (Bateman & Salfati,

2007; Salfati et al., 2015; Salfati & Bateman, 2005; Sorochinski & Salfati, 2010) and 2 of the studies on sexual assault (Kearns et al., 2011; Sorochinski & Salfati, 2017) specifically looked at the issue of behavioral consistency.

These studies on behavioral consistency go beyond simply demonstrating the statistical evidence for similarities between random pairs of crimes within series, to more specifically examine the patterns of development, consistency, and change patterns across an offender's full series, so as to start understanding the possible psychology that may underlie an offender's behavioral patterns across time – a much more important and pertinent question when we aim to apply it to both investigations and clinical risk assessment of serial crimes. Although most of these studies did not focus specifically or exclusively on the sexual component, they all discuss the general consistency of these offenders, who often engage in sexual activity during their crimes, and discuss not only the apparent lack of consistency of observable sexual activity but also the issue of overall inconsistency in behavior. All of which is important information for any kind of consistency analysis in practice, whether in an investigative context, or in a clinical context.

In order to further outline the discussion around these issues, the studies will be discussed in date order to show the development of the consistency argument, and the details of the most useful behaviors to focus on and the main psychological theories used in this work, as the research developed over time.

Much of the work in Investigative Psychology has followed two main psychological theories in the work on crime scene classification. Much of the literature on both crime in general and violent crime in particular, has focused on the influence of the interpersonal relationship between the offender and the victim (e.g. Canter, 1994; Wolfgang, 1958). Most studies in the field have therefore focused on this element in classifying crime scenes, and using this as a basis for analysis of an offender's consistency patterns over time. In the work on homicide, originally developed by Salfati (2000), and based on the original work by Fesbach (1964) focusses on two general psychological themes, *Expressive* (Hostile) and *Instrumental* aggression, which are distinguished by their goals or the rewards they offer the perpetrator. The Expressive type of aggression occurs in response to anger-inducing conditions such as insults, physical attack or personal failures, and the goal is to make the victim (the person) suffer. The Instrumental type of aggression comes through the desire for objects or the status possessed by another person, such as jewelry, money or territory, and here the offender tries to obtain the desired object regardless of the cost. In the work on rape and sexual assaults, and later also serial homicides, the field of Investigative Psychology has focused on the Interpersonal model outlined by Canter (1994) relating to how an offender may interact with the victim based on the psychological meaning they may assign to the victim, which includes the sexual element of the crime - notably *Person* (the victim has a personal meaning to the offender, or is selected for specific characteristics of emotional meaning); *Object* (the victim is not individually important, but instead is acted upon in an objectifying way where the victim themselves, or the body of the victim are mere objects to be acted upon, or used by the offender; or *Vehicle* (where the offender picks a victim that they use as a vehicle for an ulterior gain, such as a victim that may represents a category or type of person of some importance to the offender, or a victim that will be used as a vehicle to reach the offender's ulterior aim such as theft or a psychological need). Although individual studies on both homicide and rape have adapted and modified the specifics of these theories, the overall ideas behind the works have remained present.

Salfati and Bateman (2005) in a study of the first three crime scenes in 23 serial homicide series, provided the first empirical study focusing on developing methodological benchmarks for classification of crime scenes in serial homicide offenses. The authors based their work on a framework (e.g., Salfati, 2000; Salfati & Canter, 1999) originally developed to classify single homicides into two types of interpersonal interaction with the victim, notably expressive and instrumental. Although sexual behaviors were included in this model, it was not an individual focus since the model was based on the display of the percent of behaviors in each theme, rather than what specific behaviors were present. They classified each crime scene based on its dominant theme and then went on to test the consistency with which offenders offended according to the same theme across their series - the idea being that by focusing on overall themes, rather than specific individual behaviors, more of the situational factors affecting individual behaviors could be factored out. Results from this study showed that although a thematically based homicide classification was more productive in analyzing consistency than single behaviors, consistency levels were still not high. In addition, they showed that the differences in results depended on which criterion of stringency they employed for testing consistency, something that previous literature had not dealt with. Their study highlighted the importance of providing clear guidelines for how cases are allocated to theme, and how cases are linked, and the guidelines that they provided have since been used in numerous studies to date (see Trojan & Salfati, 2008, for a full discussion). Prior to the publication of this study, any studies that discussed "allocating" an offender to a subtype, did not provide any guidelines, or clear methodologically thought-out criteria, which led to too much unreliability in the process, with individual decision makers using their own judgement versus a reliable consistent method. Using a moderately stringent criteria (where a case was allocated to a theme if it had a minimum of 1.5 times as many behaviors in one theme than in the alternative theme), 26% of the 23 series remained consistent across the first three crime scenes in the series. Using a stringent classification criterion (where a case was allocated to a theme if it had a minimum of 2 times as many behaviors in one theme than in the alternative theme), only 13% of the 23 series were completely consistent in the theme (subtype) displayed across the first three crimes in the series. This was the first time any study had provided any quantification to illustrate how consistent offenders actually are, and with the numbers showed that the numbers were much lower than what the theoretical literature has postulated. However, what must also be kept in mind is that this was the first study to look at consistency, and that the specific actions used may not have been the strongest for the analysis. As Canter (2000) discusses when he outlines the idea of the Canonical equation, each behavior or action that goes in to a theme, may individually have more or less weight depending on their salience (i.e. theoretical importance), as well as having a weight related to their statistical impact (i.e. how frequent or rare the behavior is, i.e. how common to the sample or how specific to the individual case it may be). One of the issues the study highlighted was that the individual behaviors that make up each theme still need to be refined to factor out behaviors that are more dependent on the situation than on the offender's psychology. The study therefore highlighted the importance of further investigating the nature of individual behaviors themselves so that the understanding of the consistency and stability of these can be fed back into a more thematic model.

Bateman and Salfati (2007) did a similar study on 90 serial homicide offenses, looking at individual behaviors instead of themes. They identified six key behavioral categories discussed in the literature on signatures and serial homicide: body disposal behaviors; forensic awareness behaviors; mutilation behaviors; weapons used; theft behaviors; and sexual behaviors. Each one of these categories in turn contained a diverse number of objectively defined and physically observable behaviors from the crime scene adhering to the description of the category. An 80% consistency criterion was used, meaning that an offender was only deemed consistent if he employed an individual behavior in four out of his first five crime scenes in the series. The results showed that there were inherent difficulties in using individual behaviors to identify consistency patterns across a series, and consequently to link cases. Serial homicide offenders did not show consistency in their use of the same crime scene behaviors, nor did this consistency increase when behaviors were looked at as general groups—i.e., the offenders showing the use of any kind of sexual behavior, any kind of body disposal behavior, etc. This study provided the first empirical study in a wave of empirical testing that questioned early theories in the literature on serial homicide, which have suggested that specific behaviors are key in understanding the consistency in an offender's behavior across their crimes. Indeed, the sexual component which had been the focus of much of the literature showed the least amount of consistency of all the subgroups of behaviors in the study. Instead, the behaviors that did show any level of consistency, were all reflective of an underlying psychological issue of control.

Sorochinski and Salfati (2010) in their study aimed to bring together the basis for classification used in both the previous two studies on serial homicide and specifically constructed subtypes by selecting specific individual behaviors to include into their analysis that showed a greater potential for consistency. They included the level pre or post offense planning (as a more detailed examination of how the offender may control the crime scene), the type of violence in terms of whether it was goal or process oriented (to examine different ways in which the offender may use violence, notably to control or to simply cause harm), and also used the Interpersonal model outlined by Canter (1994) relating to how an offender may interact with the victim based on the psychological meaning they may assign to the victim (Person, Object, Vehicle), which includes the sexual element of the crime. Using these factors, their study examined behavioral consistency and behavioral change patterns across the first three offenses, and showed a higher level of consistency than previous studies. Of the 19 series examined, eight (42.1%) were found to consistently exhibit behaviors from the same planning strategy theme across all three offenses. Of these, four offenders consistently fell within the pre-planning theme, three offenders consistently used post-planning and one offender did not present any of the behaviors within this theme in any of his crime scenes (this was still determined to represent consistency as consistent lack of planning behaviors may be nonetheless telling for the purposes of linking offenses). Thematic consistency of wounding was found in six (31.5%) of the series. Of those, half were consistently process-oriented in the way they killed the victim and half were goal-oriented. Consistency in Victim-offender interaction was found in 11 (57.9%) of the series, seven of which were consistent using the vehicle theme.

Sorochinski and Salfati (2010) also analyzed the consistency and change patterns within each of the three behavioral subgroups (planning, wounding, and victim-offender interaction) revealed that offenders are most consistent in the way they interact with the victim. Within the planning behavioral subgroup, offenders changed most from their first to second offense while for their third offense they often came back to their initial planning style, which may be evidence of experimentation and learning the best strategy for the successful accomplishment of their goal. Patterns relating to the wounding subgroup were the least consistent, which is likely due to the situational factors (such as victim resistance) affecting this behavioral subgroup. The study also looked at whether offenders who were found to be consistent within one behavioral subgroup were also consistent across other subgroups. Only two offenders (10.5%) were consistent across the three subgroups. Five (26.3%) offenders were consistent in two out of three behavioral subgroups, eight (42.1%) offenders consistently employed the same cognitive strategy throughout their series in only one of the behavioral subgroups, and four (21.1%) offenders were inconsistent across all behavioral subgroups. Thus, while overall consistency across all subgroups is low, the majority of offenders are consistent in at least one aspect of their homicide behavior (i.e. planning, wounding, or interaction with the victim). Although no specific conclusions were made regarding the sexual activity in the crimes as this was not the focus of the study, the study did highlight the usefulness of looking for behavioral consistency in terms of behavioral trajectories, i.e. escalating in degree or switching from one behavioral subtype to another, thus starting to show that consistency may not be as liner or simple as previously defined.

Kearns et al. (2011) in a study of the first 4 offenses in 23 serial rape series (92 offenses) also examined behavioral consistency and patterns of change in rape series, by focusing on themes based on the previously outline 3 interpersonal interaction styles with the victim (victim as Person, Vehicle, or Object, see Canter, 1994 for details of this model). Results from the study indicated that most of the 92 individual crime scenes showed a dominant interactional style. However, when the offenses were looked at as series, i.e. when the first 4 offenses in each series was examined for their consistency patterns, only 9 series were classified as showing consistency. However, even within these 9 series, 5 had one offense within the series that did not exhibit the dominant theme of the rest of the offenses. In 4 out of these 5 series, it was the fourth offense in the series that displayed an inconsistent theme, which suggests that thematic behavioral consistency decreased as the series progressed. When looked at further, results showed that the vast majority of the offenders exhibited behaviors from multiple themes. The finding that serial rape offenders do not exemplify behaviors that are strictly within one behavior theme highlights the difference between examining behavioral consistency in theory and in practice. Theoretically, an offender's individual behaviors may change from crime to crime due to contextual issues, but would always be part of the same theme "pool" of behaviors over the course of the series. However, the results from the study shows that in practice almost all offenders utilized behaviors in multiple themes and changed their patterns of offending throughout a series. As highlighted by Sorochinski and Salfati (2010), these patterns of change again highlight the importance of examining behavioral consistency over the course of a series, and not simply as random pair-wise linkage analyses, which has been done by other studies in the linking field.

Salfati et al. (2015) in a study of 30 serial homicides with a total of 283 victims and 235 crime scenes in South Africa, also examined the role of the victim by using a similar definition as that outlined by Canter (1994) and also modified and used as a guide the examination of offending styles in the previous studies above. When looking at the consistency levels with which offenders engaged in a dominant interaction style, these were much higher (50%) than those previously reported by Salfati and Bateman (2005) due to both refinements in the data collection and selection of more reliable behaviors. The analysis showed that using this model, almost two-thirds of the cases showed a dominant Victim as Vehicle theme. A lower percentage of offenders used the Victim as Object theme. However, many of those that began with this theme remained consistent. Conversely, offenders who engaged in the Victim as Vehicle theme remained less consistent as the series progressed. These results, they suggest, may indicate that an offender's focus and involvement with the victim may be influential in consistency patterns. This lends an additional level of complexity to the analysis and definition of consistency, by incorporating change as possibly being part of a consistency pattern (Salfati, 2008a). When the stability of individual victim features were looked at as a whole in relation to consistency level as the series progressed, the decrease in consistency was even more marked, from 60% when looking at the first two crime scenes in a series, to 25% when looking at the first four crime scenes in a series. Most of the individual victim features (couples, live victims, vulnerable victims) which were key in defining each of the victim-based types (Object/Vehicle) were also in and of themselves not stable as the series progressed. Offenders tended to consistently target vulnerable victims in the beginning of the series; however, as the series progressed, offenders changed pattern and there was a substantial decrease in procuring vulnerable victims. The authors concluded that it may be in the beginning that offenders are operating in their comfort zone and target these types of victims because they are easily accessible, and then offenders may become bolder or more experimental in their victim selection as the series continues. These are all patterns they recommend need to be explored further as we move forwards in elucidating victim-focused consistency patterns in serial homicide. These results from the analysis of individual components of each theme, however, support the original conclusions made by Bateman and Salfati (2007), who also found very low levels of consistency when focusing on individual isolated features, and who recommended that moving from an individual behavior focus to a theme- or type-based focus, would be more useful as it would be able to factor in behavioral change due to the situation or interaction with the victim. Another possible explanation to change patterns as the series moved forward, the authors suggest, may be that offenders changed interaction patterns (both thematically and in terms of length of offense) in response to the type of victim selected, and this should also be explored in more depth. Results therefore suggest again that thematic stability or instability across the series may be due to the type of victim targeted, and the question remains whether identifiable patterns may be determined based on these changing features as the series develops.

Sorochinski and Salfati (2017) in an analysis of 30 series of sexual assault and rape showed that the control (including verbal control, control by using constraints such as binding and gagging, and control through using a weapon, and control through physical violence) and violent (at the start, during the offense, and at the end, and using manual violence and/or using a weapon) behavior subtypes could best understood quantitatively (i.e. in terms of the degree of the behavior employed), whilst the sexual activity (ranging from foreplay, to penetration, to demanding victim participation, and verbal sexual activity) was most usefully understood qualitatively in terms of the specific subtype exhibited. The analysis of consistency and behavioral trajectories showed that whilst none of the offenders exhibited complete consistency across the 3 behavioral subtypes, a subsample of offenders remained fully consistent in at least one. Furthermore, of those who were not consistent, the vast majority followed an identifiable trajectory of change. This finding is in line with Sorochinski and Salfati's (2010) study of behavioral patterns of serial homicide offenders and suggests that searching for consistency in specific behavioral domains is more productive than looking for consistency across a large number of offending behaviors together. The study additionally showed that by combining specific subtypes and degree of presence together in the analysis of behavior, allows for more flexibility in individually differentiating crime scenes, and confirming that the search for consistency in serial crime should not stop at exact matching, but rather should go into more depth in the analysis of the trajectories of behavioral change.

Moving Towards Understanding Consistency in Inconsistency

Salfati (2008a) highlighted the need to expand the framework for looking at consistency to not simply restricting it to series within one crime type, such as homicide or rape, but instead look at how many series included both types of legally defined crimes, but from a psychological perspective included different varying levels of lethal violence in their series, and exhibited sexual activity towards some of their victims, and not to others. The focus was again on expanding the understanding of how we define consistency not only in the exact pattern matching of individual behaviors, but instead take a more global look at understanding the trajectory of the behaviors of the offender over time.

Fleeson and Noftle (2008) also in their theoretical work on the consistency of human behavior argued that "the question is not whether behavior is consistent or not, rather the question is which ways behavior is more consistent and which ways it is less consistent" (p. 1357). Fleeson and Noftle further suggested that consistency does not have to be manifested through the identical repetition of a given behavior, but rather can manifest itself in complex patterns. Other recent studies (e.g., Hewitt & Beauregard, 2014; Leclerc et al., 2015) have also started to highlight the importance of looking beyond stability of behavior and of understanding consistency in terms of patterns of behavioral change.

Exploring Behavioral Consistency Though Victimology

Proulx (2007), in his comprehensive report on the current understanding of sexual homicide, highlights the importance of focusing not only on what offenders do during their crimes but also on how these offenders differ depending on the victim group they target. Furthermore, Chan, Beauregard, and Meyers (2015), in their study of Canadian serial and single sexual homicides, found that serial offenders are significantly more likely to have specific victim-type preferences.

In much of the above literature on consistency, although it focuses on behavior, the underlying psychological focus has been on how these behaviors may reflect something about how the offender interacts with the victim. At the heart of the behavioral crime scene analysis work therefore, has been the question of the role of the victim.

Another body of research in the literature on behavioral consistency has therefore been to focus on the type of victim that the offender targets, in a more direct way. This body of work has also aimed to take on board the more expanded view of how we may define a series, and has included an exploration of consistency in series that include both sexual assaults of live victims and homicides and sexual homicides.

One of the groups of victims of particular focus in this work has been that of vulnerable victims, and subgroups of highly targeted women such as sex workers (e.g., Abrams, Palmer, & Salfati, 2016; Salfati, 2013; Salfati, Horning, Sorochinski, & Labuschagne, 2014; Salfati, James, & Ferguson, 2008; Salfati & Sorochinski, 2018; Sorochinski & Salfati, 2010). This body of work provides a further expansion of the discussion on how we should look at consistency, and includes the factor of victim targeting.

Egger (1984) in one of the earliest writings on serial homicide, wrote that the key challenge for investigators is what he terms "linkage blindness." Linkage blindness is a situation whereby crime scenes that are part of the same series are not identified as such due to overt factors (such as type of victim) looking dissimilar, and as such conclusions are made that they are unlinked. In the case of offenders who target different types of victims, and victimology being a key salient feature of linkage analysis, this poses a very real problem. It is therefore of utmost importance that the issue underlying victim targeting is more fully understood.

Egger (2003) points out that 65% of serial homicide victims are female, and nearly 78% of female victims of serial homicide offenders are sex workers. As a subgroup of vulnerable victims, they therefore present a specifically highly targeted group. Recent figures have also suggested that 32% of serial homicides involve sex workers (Quinet, 2011). Potterat et al., 2004 further suggest that being a sex worker makes a woman 18 times more likely to be killed than non-sex worker women of similar demographics. When sex workers as a group are looked at the context of a national health issue, figures show that homicide is the second-leading cause of death amongst sex workers (Lowman & Fraser, 1995). In addition, despite the overall general decline in serial homicide cases between the 1980s and 2000s, research indicates that serial homicide cases involving sex worker victims has dramatically increased by decade (Quinet, 2011). Quinet also found that the average length of time that offenders were active was longer for cases involving sex worker victims. This undoubtedly relates to the fact that sex worker homicides are some of the most difficult to solve, which is supported by some statistics that show that 10 years on, 69% of sex worker homicides are still unsolved (Kinnell, 2001).

Offenders Who Target Sex Workers

In terms of the offenders who target sex workers, Salfati et al. (2008) in their study on homicides of sex workers also show that almost half of offenders who had previous violent convictions, had a pre-conviction for at least one homicide, and that with figures as high as these, they suggest that it is likely that a sex worker will come into contact with clients with violent pre-convictions on a relatively regular basis. Brooks-Gordon, 2006 further concludes from her study that the majority of violence on sex workers is committed by a small proportion of offenders, and concludes that this suggest that many are serial offenders. Kinnell, 2006, in a study of 84 homicides against street workers, additionally discusses the vulnerability of sex workers to serial killers. Research in the US has shown that when sex worker victims are killed, in at least 35% of cases, a serial offender will be involved (Brewer et al., 2006).

Additional research shows that offenders who target sex workers often show a pattern of generalized violence against women. In an analysis of the criminal records of 77 clients stopped by the police, Brooks-Gordon (2006) found that 63 had a previous criminal record. The type most frequent previous conviction was for violence (21%), and 7% had previous convictions for sex offenses. Brooks-Gordon followed these men up, and found that 11 of them were re-convicted within 23 months after their arrest for approaching sex workers. Of these 11 men, six of them were convicted of a violent offense against the person, and one was convicted for a sexual offense. She therefore tentatively concludes that, with keeping in mind the small numbers, the research suggests a link between soliciting sex workers and more serious crimes committed by only a small number of these men, who are likely to be repeat offenders. Looking at previous convictions of offenders who killed women in different offense groups, Salfati et al. (2008) report that offenders who kill sex workers were the least likely to have previous nonviolent offenses (20%) when compared to offenders who killed non-sex worker women (offenders who killed and sexually assaulted, 41%; offenders who killed but did not sexual assault, 81%). Conversely, offenders who killed sex workers had significantly more pre-convictions for sexual offenses compared to offenders who killed non-sex workers. They also reported that significantly more sex worker homicide offenders (69%) had spent time in prison than offenders who killed non-sex workers (nonsexual, 27% and sexual, 29%). In accord with the general literature on violence against sex workers, a study by Salfati et al. (2008) shows that in a large proportion (14 out of 19) of offenders who had previous violent convictions, 6 involved a pre-conviction for at least one murder. With figures as high as these they suggest that it is likely that a prostitute will come into contact with clients with violent pre-convictions on a relatively regular basis. Indeed, in one sex worker homicide case in their study, the victim had had sex with a client who had previous convictions for attempted murder and serious sexual assaults on women, in the same night as she was killed by another client who also had previous convictions for attempted murder.

Salfati (2009) in a comprehensive review of the literature on men who target sex workers, also showed that men who assault sex workers often have convictions for assaulting other women as well, which supports some of the general literature suggesting that violence against sex workers may be considered as part of a continuum of violence against women more generally, and not just against sex workers specifically. Salfati (2009) therefore goes on to suggests that violence against sex workers may be considered as part of a continuum of violence against women more generally, and not just against sex workers specifically. This additional cross-over between groups of women, as well as cross-over of crime types (rape and sexual homicide), however, adds an additional level of complexity to issues of understanding consistency.

Recent studies have shown that serial offenders who target sex workers also target non-sex workers. Salfati (2007, 2013) looked at 19 series of 106 victims involving at least one sex worker victim. Of these, she showed that 42% of series were composed of sex worker victims only, and 58% were mixed, i.e. the series included both sex worker victims and non-sex worker victims. These initial results go against much of the belief in the field that offenders are behaviorally consistent and display victim preferences. In order to gain an understanding of what factors may link these victims to each other, other than overt victim type, specifically the sexual part of the crime, either as victim type (sex workers) or as behavior (sexual assault), the study compared the sex worker victims ($N = 16$) and non-sex worker victims ($N = 90$) on sexual assault, and the study estimated that 43% of sex workers and 44% of non-sex workers were sexually assaulted. When the sexual element was looked at to determine whether it provided the element of consistency that ties the different types of victims together, the analysis further showed that, of the 19 series, 2 series included sex worker victims who were all sexually assaulted, 5 series included sex worker victims who were not sexually assaulted, and 11 series included mixed victim types (sex workers and non-sex workers) and a mix of sexual assaults and no sexual assaults. The results thus indicate that overt sexual assault is not a simple distinguishing factor between victim types, thus again showing that the sexual element in sexual homicides may not be the most reliable focus to understand consistency.

Abrams, Palmer and Salfati (2016) using a different dataset of 21 offenders that encompassed 9 single series (43%), 7 sex-worker only series (33%), and 5 mixed series (24%) found that single and serial sex worker offenders had a dominant noncriminal lifestyle (living with someone, being employed, and being in a relationship with someone) compared to the mixed series offenders who had a dominant criminal lifestyle (history of drug use, history of property offense, history of violent offense and history of sex offense). In addition, mixed victim series were longer and more victims when compared to sex worker only series, but their analysis found no discernible victim patterns that could elucidate what may be happening.

Salfati and Sorochinski (2015, 2018) aimed to look at the victim patterns in more detail, through looking at the interplay between sexual activity and victim type (sex workers and non-sex workers), to investigate how the overt and covert sexual nature of the crimes may affect our understanding of consistency patterns in series of sexual offenses. Their study included 67 international solved homicide series (with 474 victims) that included at least one sex worker victim in each series. Their results were similar to previous studies, showing that 30 series (45%) included only sex worker victims, 28 series (42%) were mixed (i.e., had at least one known sex worker victim and at least one known non-sex worker victim), and 9 series (13%) included at least one sex worker victim, but also at least one victim whose occupation was not known. Their study looked further at the interchange between lethal violence and sexual violence, particularly with non-sex worker victims, and found that non-sex worker victims were significantly more likely to have been left alive by the offender, and commonly sexually assaulted. Furthermore, of the non-sex worker victims who survived the attack, 81.1% were sexually assaulted, and of those that were killed, 32.4% were known to have been sexually assaulted. As has been theorized by Sorochinski and Salfati (2010), it is possible that the consistency of actions for these offenders is victim-specific: in other words, rather than having one overall behavioral pattern, these offenders exhibit different (consistent) patterns of behavior that is specific to each type of victim. The meaning of the overt sexual activity therefore becomes an intricate one, with some victims perhaps representing sex, whilst others became sexual victims through the sexual assault itself.

Overall, Salfati and Sorochinski identified 3 main victim-targeting patterns: sex worker-only series, mixed-crossover series, and mixed-homicide series. In the 30 series composed only of sex workers, offenders could be seen to target their violence specifically at only this victim type. The authors hypothesized that offenders may have either a psychotic disorder (e.g., a fixated conviction that they must rid the world of sex workers), or may have focused on sex workers due to their potential to satisfy sexually violent fantasies, or their status as easy targets. In the 28 mixed victim series, in order to further look at the interplay between whether the victim was a sex worker or not, whether the victim was killed or left alive, and whether there was evidence of a sexual assault, results showed that sex workers still made up the majority of victims (56.8% sex workers vs. 27.8% non-sex workers and 15.4% unknown). Further examination of the mixed series also indicated two separate types of trajectories, the crossover type, and the homicide type. In the crossover trajectory, the series usually started with a non-sex worker, the victims were often known to the offender (e.g., ex-girlfriend, relative), and were often left alive. As the series progressed, however, many of these offenders would go on to target and kill sex workers who were strangers. There was an overall lack of consistency in the types of crimes that were committed (sexual assault, sexual homicide, homicide), the type of victim (non-sex workers and sex workers), as well as the type of relationship with the victim prior to the attack (intimate partner, acquaintance, stranger), with most of the known victims being left alive (but sexually assaulted), and most stranger victims killed. The crossover trajectory can be seen to be particularly problematic for the investigation, as victimology and crime type consistency are among the most common elements that the investigators rely on for linking series. In the homicide trajectory, the series usually started with a sex worker. In the opposite pattern from the crossover trajectory, the first victim was often a stranger to the offender, and was killed. As the series progressed, these offenders would continue to kill sex workers strangers victims, but many of these offenders would also have an additional one or two non-sex worker non-stranger victims. However, in this type of series, all victims were killed. No consistency pattern for presence of sexual assault was observed in this trajectory. However, the authors stressed it is often impossible to determine the presence of sexual assault in homicides of sex workers. In the homicide trajectory, offenders were observed to be consistent in the type of crime (homicide), with the victims predominantly sex workers. In many cases, non-sex worker victims occurred toward the end of their series, suggesting that these victims may in some cases be the factor that led to the case being solved.

Salfati and Sorochinski concluded by stating that the presence of several distinct patterns that, while not all consistent, showed that behavioral trajectories in the actions by offenders could be identified, and are in line with current trends in the violent serial crime literature (e.g., Hewitt & Beauregard, 2014; Leclerc et al., 2015; Salfati, 2008a; Sorochinski & Salfati, 2010, 2018), which highlights the importance of looking beyond complete consistency and into the ways that offenders may change their behavioral patterns across series. The issue of sex may interplay with victim type, and either be implicit in terms of who the victim is (e.g., sex worker), or explicit, in terms of the assault itself (e.g. behavior).

Conclusion

Assessing sex offending and understanding the factors that can aid in that process is key in the analysis of crimes such as serial sex offending and serial sexual homicide. Knowledge of the factors, and the empirical backing these factors have, is, therefore, integral to enable more valid and reliable assessments of offending patterns.

Salfati (2015) and Salfati and Kunkle (2016) stressed that adding how an offender shows consistent patterns of behavior across their series to both crime scene analysis as well as clinical assessment, may provide a substantial addition to our understanding of the factors that are at play when assessing a serial offender's behavior, and provides the empirical basis for future research and investigative and clinical assessment and practice.

This chapter has aimed to give a detailed overview of what empirical studies have been done to back up our understanding of behavioral consistency, specifically as it applies to serial sexual violence such as sexual assaults and serial homicides. The specific focus has been on understanding the specific components of sexual activity during series, its different expressions through the behavior itself, the type of crime (rape and sexual homicide), and also how the sexual component may be expressed through the victim targeted, such as in cases of sex workers. The review has aimed to outline what we know, what some of the constructs are that have been used in understanding behavioral consistency, and has provided a historical overview of the empirical development of the field of behavioral crime scene analysis as it pertains to linking and behavioral consistency.

To date a substantial amount of empirical research has been done in the area of linking serial crimes; however, the subset of studies that have empirically examined linking issues in serial sexual assaults and homicide is small, and smaller still when we specifically look for studies that has aimed to understand the patterns of consistency in the trajectory of behavior across an offender's full series.

Overall, however, the research has highlighted that we have come a long way in our understanding of how offenders display consistency, and how we may go beyond simply looking for exact behavioral similarities, to taking a more complex approach to assessing consistency.

References

Abrams, M. M., Palmer, B., & Salfati, C. G. (2016). *Patterns of sex worker and non-sex worker victim selection: Relationship to offender characteristics*. New Orleans, LA: American Society of Criminology.

Alison, L., Smith, M. D., Eastman, O., & Rainbow, L. (2003). Toulmin's philosophy of argument and its relevance to offender profiling. *Psychology, Crime & Law, 9*(2), 173–183.

Alison, L., Smith, M. D., & Morgan, K. (2003). Interpreting the accuracy of offender profiles. *Psychology, Crime & Law, 9*(2), 185–195.

Alison, L. J., Bennell, C., Mokros, A., & Ormerod, D. (2002). Ten years after the personality paradox in offender profiling: A theoretical review of the processes involved in deriving background characteristics from crime scene actions. *Psychology, Public Policy, and Law, 8*, 115–135.

Alison, L., Snook, B., & L. Stein, K. (2001). Unobtrusive measurement: Using police information for forensic research. *Qualitative Research, 1*, 241–254. https://doi.org/10.1177/146879410100100208

Bartol, C. R. (1996). Police psychology: Then, now, and beyond. *Criminal Justice and Behavior, 23*, 70–89.

Bartol, C. R., & Bartol, A. M. (2004). *Psychology and law* (3rd ed.). Belmont, CA: Wadsworth.

Bateman, A., & Salfati, G. (2007). An examination of behavioral consistency using individual behaviors or groups of behaviors in serial homicide. *Behavioral Sciences & the Law, 25*, 527–544.

Bennell, C., & Canter, D. (2002). Linking commercial burglaries by modus operandi: Tests using regression and ROC analysis. *Science & Justice, 42*, 153–164.

Bennell, C., & Jones, N. J. (2005). Between a ROC and a hard place: A method for linking serial burglaries by modus operandi. *Journal of Investigative Psychology and Offender Profiling, 2*, 23–41.

Bennell, C., Jones, N. J., & Melnyk, T. (2009). Addressing problems with traditional crime linking methods using receiver operating characteristic analysis. *Legal and Criminological Psychology, 14*, 293–310. https://doi.org/10.1348/135532508X349336

Boon, J. C. W. (1997). The contribution of personality theories to psychological profiling. In J. L. Jackson & D. A. Bekerian (Eds.), *Offender profiling: Theory, research, and practice* (pp. 43–59). Chichester: Wiley.

Boon, J. C. W. (1998). Science, psychology and psychological profiling. In C. A. Unit (Ed.), *Case analysis Unit (BKA), method of case analysis: An international symposium* (pp. 143–154). Bundeskriminalamt Kriminalistisches Institut: Wiesbaden.

Brewer, D. D., Dudek, J. A., Potterat, J. J., Muth, S. Q., Roberts, J. M., & Woodhouse, D. E. (2006). Extents, trends, and perpetrators of prostitution related homicide in the United States. *Journal of Forensic Science, 51*(5), 1101–1108.

Brooks-Gordon, B. (2006). *The price of sex: Prostitution, policy and society*. Cullumpton, Devon: Willan Publishing.

Canter, D., & Youngs, D. (2009). *Investigative psychology: Offender profiling and the analysis of criminal action*. Chichester: Wiley.

Canter, D. V. (1994). *Criminal shadows*. London: Harper Collins.

Canter, D. V. (2000). Offender profiling and criminal differentiation. *Legal and Criminological Psychology, 5*, 23–46.

Canter, D. V. (2004). Offender profiling and investigative psychology. *Journal of Investigative Psychology and Offender Profiling., 1*(1), 1–15. https://doi.org/10.1002/jip.7

Canter, D. V., Alison, L. J., Alison, E., & Wentink, N. (2004). The organized/disorganized typology of serial murder: Myth or model? *Psychology, Public Policy Law, 10*, 293–320.

Canter, D. V., Heritage, R., Wilson, M., Davies, A., Kirby, S, Holden, R., McGinley, J., Hughes, H., Larkin, P., Martin, L., Tsang, E., Vaughan, G, and Doanld, I. (1991) A facet approach to offender profiling, volume 1. Final Report to the Home Office

Canter, D. V., & Wentink, N. (2004). An empirical test of Holmes and Holmes's serial murder typology. *Criminal Justice and Behaviour, 31*, 489–515.

Chan, H. C., Beauregard, E., & Myers, W. C. (2015). Single-victim and serial sexual homicide offenders: Differences in crime, paraphilias and personality traits. *Criminal Behaviour and Mental Health, 25*(1), 66–78.

Constanzo, M. (2004). *Psychology applied to law*. Belmont, CA: Wadsworth.

Copson, G. (1995). *Coals to Newcastle? Part 1: A study of offender profiling*. London: Home Office Police Research Group. Special Interest Series.

Davies, K., Tonkin, M., Bull, R., & Bond, J. W. (2012). The course of case linkage never did run smooth: A new investigation to tackle the behavioural changes in serial car theft. *Journal of Investigative Psychology Offender Profiling, 9*, 274–295.

Dawes, R. M. (1997). *House of cards: Psychology and psychotherapy built on myth*. New York: Free Press.

Douglas, J. E., Ressler, R. K., Burgess, A. W., & Hartman, C. R. (1986). Criminal profiling from crime scene analysis. *Behavioral Sciences & the Law, 4*(4), 401–421.

Egger, S. A. (1984). Working definition of serial murder and the reduction of linkage blindness. *Journal of Police Science and Administration, 12*(3), 348–357.

Egger, S. A. (2003). *The need to kill*. Upper Saddle River, NJ: Prentice Hall.

Faust, D., & Ziskin, J. (1988). The expert witness in psychology and psychiatry. *Science, 241*, 31–35.

Fesbach, S. (1964). The function of aggression and the regulation of aggressive drive. *Psychological Review, 71*, 257–272.

Fleeson, W., & Noftle, E. E. (2008). Where does personality have its influence? A supermatrix of consistency concepts. *Journal of Personality, 76*, 1355–1386. https://doi.org/10.1111/j.1467-6494.2008.00525.x

Garb, H. N. (1998). *Studying the clinician: Judgment research and psychological assessment*. Washington, DC: American Psychological Association.

Garb, H. N., & Boyle, P. A. (2003). Understanding why some clinicians use pseudoscientific methods: Findings from research on clinical judgment. In S. O. Lilienfeld, S. J. Lynn, & J. M. Lohr (Eds.), *Science and pseudoscience in clinical psychology* (pp. 17–38). New York: Guilford.

Green, E. J., Booth, C. E., & Biderman, M. D. (1976). Cluster analysis of burglary MO's. *Journal of Police Science and Administration, 4*, 382–387.

Grubin, D., Kelly, P., & Brunsdon, C. (2001). *Linking serious sexual assaults through behavior*. London: Home Office, Research, Development and Statistics Directorate.

Hammond, K. J. (1990). Case-based planning: A framework for planning from experience. *Cognitive Science, 14*(3), 385–443. https://doi.org/10.1016/0364-0213(90)90018-R

Harbers, E., Deslauriers-Varin, N., Beauregard, E., & van der Kemp., J. J. (2012). Testing the behavioural and environmental consistency of serial sex offenders: A signature approach. *Journal of Investigative Psychology & Offender Profiling, 9*, 259–273. https://doi.org/10.1002/jip.1368

Her Majesty's Inspectorate of Constabulary (HMIC) and Her Majesty's Inspectorate of the Crown Prosecution Service (HMICPS) (2012). *Forging the links: Rape investigation and prosecution*. Retrieved from http://www.hmic.gov.uk/media/forging-the-links-rape-investigation-and-prosecution-20120228.pdf

Hewitt, A., & Beauregard, E. (2014). Offending patterns of serial sexual offenders: Escalation, de-escalation, and consistency of sexually intrusive and violent behaviours. *Journal of Investigative Psychology & Offender Profiling, 11*, 57–80. https://doi.org/10.1002/jip.1407

Kearns, E., Salfati, C. G., & Jarvis, J. (2011). *Serial rape: The relationship between geographic patterns, crime locations and offender demographics*. Washington, DC: Poster at Annual American Society of Criminology Conference.

Kinnell, H. (2001). Violence against sex workers. Response to Church et al. (2001). *British Medical Journal, 322*, 524.

Kinnell, H. (2006). Murder made easy: The final solution to prostitution? In R. Campbell & M. O'Neill (Eds.), *Sex work now* (pp. 141–168). Cullompton, Devon: Willan Publishing.

Kocsis, R. N. (2004). Profiling the criminal mind: Does it actually work? *The Lancet, 364*, 14–15.

Leclerc, B., Lussier, P., & Deslauriers-Varin, N. (2015). Offending patterns over time: An examination of specialization, escalation and de-escalation in the commission of sexual offences. In A. Blokland & P. Lussier (Eds.), *Sex offenders: A criminal career approach*. Oxford: Wiley.

Lowman, J., & Fraser, L. (1995) *Violence against persons who sex worker: The experience in British Columbia*. Retrieved from http://mypage.uniserve.ca/~lowman/.

McCann, J. T. (1992). Criminal personality profiling in the investigation of violent crime: Recent advances and future directions. *Behavioral Sciences & the Law, 10*(4), 475–481.

Meehl, P. E. (1997). Credentialed persons, credentialed knowledge. *Clinical Psychology: Science and Practice, 4*, 91–98.

Meyer, C. B. (2007). Criminal profiling as expert evidence? An international case law perspective. In R. N. Kocsis (Ed.), *Criminal profiling: International theory, research and practice* (pp. 207–247). Totowa, NJ: Humana Press.

NCAVC. (2005). Serial murder multi-disciplinary perspectives for investigators. Beavioral analysis unit, National Center for the Analysis of Violent Crime. Retrived from https://www.fbi.gov/stats-services/publications/serial-murder

NCAVC. (2008). In R. J. Morton & M. A. Hilts (Eds.), *Serial murder: Multidisciplinary perspective for investigators*. Quantico, VA: Federal Bureau of Investigation, National Center for the Analysis of Violent Crime (NCAVC).

Potterat, J. J., Brewer, D. D., Muth, S. Q., Rothberg, R. B., Woodhouse, D. E., Muth, J. B., … Brody, S. (2004). Mortality in a long-term open cohort of sex worker women. *American Journal of Epidemiology., 159*(8), 778–785.

Poytheress, N., Otto, R. K., Darkes, J., & Starr, L. (1993). APA's expert panel in the congressional hearing review of the USS Iowa incident. *American Psychologist, 48*, 8–15.

Proulx, J. (2007). Sexual murderers: Theories, assessment and treatment. In *Sexual homicide and paraphilias: The correctional Service of Canada's experts forum* (pp. 215–233). Ottawa, ON: Canadian Government Publishing. Retrieved from http://www.csc-scc.gc.ca/research/shp2007-paraphil12-eng.shtml

Quinet, K. (2011). Prostitutes as victims of serial homicide: Trends and case characteristics from 1970–2009. *Homicide Studies, 15*(1), 74–100.

Rainbow, L. (2008). Taming the beast: The UK approach to the management of behavioral investigative advice.

Journal of Police and Criminal Psychology, 23(2), 90–97.

Ressler, R. K., Burgess, A. W., Douglas, J. E., Hartman, C. R., d'Agostino, R. B. (1986). Sexual killers and their victims: Identifying patterns through crime scene analysis. *Journal of Interpesonal Violence, 1*(3), 288–308.

Risinger, D. M., & Loop, J. L. (2002). Three card Monte, Monty hall, modus operandi, and "offender profiling": Some lessons of modern cognitive science for the law of evidence. *Cardozo Law Review, 24*, 193–285.

Salfati, C. G. (2000). The nature of expressiveness and instrumentality in homicide. *Homicide Studies, 3*(4), 265–293.

Salfati, C. G. (2003). Offender interaction with victims in homicide: A multidimensional analysis of frequencies in crime scene behaviors. *Journal of Interpersonal Violence, 18*(5), 490–512.

Salfati, C. G. (2007). *Prostitutes: Vulnerable or sexual targets of serial homicide*? Presented at the Annual American Society of Criminology Conference, Atlanta, GA.

Salfati, C. G. (2008a). Linking serial crimes. In J. Fossi & L. Falshaw (Eds.), *Issues in forensic psychology* (Vol. 8). London: British Psychological Society, Division of Forensic Psychology Publications.

Salfati, C. G. (2008b). *Prostitute victims of serial homicide: Investigative concerns*. Paper presented at the Academy of Criminal Justice Sciences, Cincinnati, OH.

Salfati, C. G. (2009). Prostitute homicide: An overview of the literature and comparison to sexual and non-sexual female victim homicide. In D. Canter, M. Ioannou, & D. Youngs (Eds.), *Safer sex in the city: The experience and management of street prostitution* (The psychology, crime and law series) (pp. 51–68). Aldershot: Ashgate.

Salfati, C. G. (2011). Research methods in offender profiling research. In B. Rosenfeld & S. Penrod (Eds.), *Research methods in forensic psychology* (pp. 122–135). Hoboken, NJ: Wiley.

Salfati, C. G. (2013). Linkage analysis of serial murder cases involving prostitute victims. In J. Helfgott (Ed.), *Criminal psychology reference set* (Vol. 3, pp. 211–228). Westport, CT: Praeger Publishers.

Salfati, C. G., & Bateman, A. (2005). Serial homicide: An investigation of behavioral consistency. *Journal of Investigative Psychology and Offender Profiling, 2*(2), 121–144.

Salfati, C. G., & Canter, D. V. (1999). Differentiating stranger murders: Profiling offender characteristics from behavioral styles. *Behavioral Sciences & the Law, 17*, 391–406.

Salfati, C. G., Horning, A., Sorochinski, M., & Labuschagne, G. (2014). South African serial homicide: Consistency in victim target and behaviors across series. *Journal of Investigative Psychology and Offender Profiling*.

Salfati, C. G., Horning, A., Sorochinski, M., & Labuschagne, G. (2015). South African serial homicide: Consistency in victim types and crime scene actions across series. *Journal of Investigative Psychology and Offender Profiling, 12*(1), 83–106.

Salfati, C. G. (2015, October 26). Offender profiling & risk assessment – opposite sides of the same coin. Retrieved from https://drexel.edu/cnhp/news/current/archive/2015/October/2015-10-26-offender-profiling-and-risk-assessment-opposite-sides-of-the-same-coin/

Salfati, C. G., James, A. R., & Ferguson, L. (2008). Prostitution homicides: A descriptive study. *Journal of Interpersonal Violence., 23*, 3.

Salfati, C. G. and Kunkle, C. (2016) *Offender profiling & risk assessment: Combining forces to strengthen the validity of behavioral analysis of serial sexual offending*. Presentation at the International Academy of Investigative Psychology 17th Conference. New York.

Salfati, C. G. & Sorochinski, M. (2015) *Sex worker victims: A specific target for serial homicide offenders or part of a generalized violence pattern*? Presentation at the Annual Meeting of the American Society of Criminology, Washington, DC.

Salfati, C. G., & Sorochinski, M. (2018). Sex worker victims: Consistency vs inconsistency in victimization patterns by serial sexual homicide offenders. In J. Proulx, A. Carter, É. Beauregard, A. Mokros, R. Darjee, & J. James (Eds.), *International handbook of sexual homicide*. New York: Routledge.

Salo, B., Sirén, J., Corander, J., Zappalà, A., Bosco, D., Mokros, A., & Santtila, P. (2012). Using Bayes' theorem in behavioural crime linking in serial homicide. *Legal and Criminological Psychology, 18*(2), 356–370. https://doi.org/10.1111/j.2044-8333.2011.02043.x

Santtila, P., Fritzon, K., & Tamelander, A. L. (2005). Linking arson incidents on the basis of crime scene behaviour. *Journal of Police and Criminal Psychology, 19*, 1–16. https://doi.org/10.1007/BF02802570

Santtila, P., Junkkila, J., & Sandnabba, N. K. (2005). Behavioural linking of stranger rapes. *Journal of Investigative Psychology and Offender Profiling, 2*, 87–103. https://doi.org/10.1002/jip.26

Santtila, P., Pakkanen, T., Zappala, A., Bosco, D., Valkama, M., & Mokros, A. (2008). Behavioural crime linking in serial homicide. *Psychology, Crime & Law, 14*, 245–265. https://doi.org/10.1080/10683160701739679

Slater, C., Woodhams, J., & Hamilton-Giachritsis, C. (2015). Testing the assumptions of crime linkage with stranger sex offenses: A more ecologically-valid study. *Journal of Police and Criminal Psychology, 30*(4), 261–273.

Snook, B., Cullen, R. M., Bennell, C., Taylor, P. J., & Gendreau, P. (2008). The criminal profiling illusion: What's behind the smoke and mirrors? *Criminal Justice and Behavior, 35*(10), 1257–1276.

Snook, B., Eastwood, J., Gendreau, P., Goggin, C., & Cullen, R. M. (2007). Taking stock of criminal profiling: A narrative review and meta-analysis. *Criminal Justice and Behavior, 34*(4), 437–453.

Sorochinski, M., & Salfati, C. G. (2010). The consistency of inconsistency in serial homicide: Patterns of behavioral change across series. *Journal of Investigative*

Psychology and Offender Profiling, 7(2), 109–136. https://doi.org/10.1002/jip.118
Sorochinski, M., & Salfati, C. G. (2017). Assumptions underlying behavioral linkage revisited: A revised approach to ascertaining individual differentiation and consistency in serial rape. In P. A. Granhag, R. Bull, A. Shaboltas, & E. Dozortseva (Eds.), *Psychology & law in Europe: When West meets east* (pp. 51–78). Boca Raton, FL: Taylor & Francis/CRC Press. ISBN 9781498780988.
Sorochinski, M., & Salfati, C. G. (2018). A multidimensional approach to ascertaining individual differentiation and consistency in serial sexual assault: Is it time to redefine and refine? *Journal of Police and Criminal Psychology, 33*(1), 63–83. https://doi.org/10.1007/s11896-017-9235-z
Tonkin, M., Grant, T. D., & Bond, J. W. (2008). To link or not to link: A test of the case linkage principles using serial car theft data. *Journal of Investigative Psychology and Offender Profiling, 5*, 59–77.
Torres, A., Boccaccini, M., & Miller, H. (2006). Perceptions of the validity and utility of criminal profiling among forensic psychologists and psychiatrists. *Professional Psychology: Research and Practice, 37*(1), 51–58.
Trojan, C., & Salfati, C. G. (2008). Methodological considerations of determining dominance in multidimensional analyses of crime scene behaviors and offender characteristics. *Journal of Investigative Psychology & Offender Profiling, 5*(3), 125–146.
West, A. (2000). Clinical assessment of homicide offenders: The significance of crime scene in offense and offender analysis clinical assessment of homicide offenders: The significance of crime. *Homicide Studies, 4*, 219–233.
West, A.(2001). Current approaches to sex-offender risk assessment: A critical review. *The British Journal of Forensic Practice, 3*(3), 31–41.
Winerman, L. (2004a). Criminal profiling: The reality behind the myth. *Monitor on Psychology, 35*(7), 66.
Winerman, L. (2004b). Does profiling really work? *Monitor on Psychology, 35*(7), 67.
Winter, J., Lemeire, J., Meganck, S., Geboers, J., Rossi, G., & Mokros, A. (2013). Comparing the predictive accuracy of case linkage methods in serious sexual assaults. *Journal of Investigative Psychology & Offender Profiling, 10*, 28–56. https://doi.org/10.1002/jip.1372
Wolfgang, M. E. (1958). Patterns in criminal homicide. Oxford, UK: University of Pennsylvania Press.
Woodhams, J., Hollin, C. R., & Bull, R. (2007). The psychology of linking crimes: A review of the evidence. *Legal and Criminological Psychology, 12*, 233–249.
Woodhams, J., Hollin, C. R., & Bull, R. (2008). Incorporating context in linking crimes: An exploratory study of situational similarity and if-then contingencies. *Journal of Investigative Psychology & Offender Profiling, 5*, 1–23. https://doi.org/10.1002/jip.75
Woodhams, J., & Labuschagne, G. (2011). A test of case linage principles with solved and unsolved serial rapes. *Journal of Police and Criminal Psychology, 27*(1), 85–98. https://doi.org/10.1007/s11896-011-9091-1
Woodhams, J., & Toye, K. (2007). An empirical test of the assumptions of case linkage and offender profiling with serial commercial robberies. *Psychology, Public Policy, and Law, 13*, 59–85.
Wrightsman, L. S., & Fulero, S. M. (2005). *Forensic psychology* (2nd ed.). Belmont, CA: Wadsworth.

Intimate Partner Sexual Violence and Gender Asymmetry

48

Du Nguyen and Amy E. Naugle

Intimate Partner Violence

Intimate partner violence (IPV) is a significant concern that can be observed on many system levels. IPV is often synonymously referred to as domestic violence in research literature and in legal proceedings. Though domestic violence may also broadly encompass abuse observed in the family structure by any household member, IPV more precisely refers to violence by current or former intimate partners (i.e., spouse, boyfriend/girlfriend, dating partner, or ongoing sexual partner; Breiding, Basile, Smith, Black, & Mahendra, 2015). The National Intimate Partner and Sexual Violence Survey (NISVS) reported that 1 in 4 adult women and 1 in 9 adult men have experienced some form of IPV in their lifetime (Smith et al., 2017). Data collected from the WHO multicountry study on women's health and domestic violence against women (Garcia-Moreno, Jansen, Ellsberg, Heise, & Watts, 2005) indicate that IPV is a global problem, with wide lifetime prevalence rates across countries ranging from 6–59% for sexual violence and 23–62% for physical violence.

In the United States, IPV against women is recognized as an economic burden with total estimates exceeding $5 billion in direct costs (e.g., health care) and indirect costs (e.g., lost productivity and present value of lifetime earnings; National Center for Injury Prevention and Control, 2003). Compared to women who did not report a history of IPV, women with a history of IPV were more likely to utilize mental health services, alcohol/drug services, and both inpatient and outpatient care during and after their IPV experience, with a 19% higher annual cost of care than women without a history of IPV (Rivara et al., 2007). This pattern persisted for upwards of 5 years after the experience. On an individual level, IPV has been associated with a number of immediate and long-term negative health consequences, including higher rates of depression, substance abuse, PTSD, and suicidality in women (Golding, 1999) with a similar pattern of outcomes shown in men (Coker et al., 2002). Smith et al. (2017) reported that IPV victims were more likely to experience health conditions such as chronic pain, difficulSties with sleeping, activity limitations, and overall poor physical and mental health.

While IPV has been represented in the literature for the past several decades, it has not been comprehensively defined. A number of theoretical frameworks for IPV have been offered, including psychological (e.g., social learning theory), biobehavioral (e.g., genetics), feminist, and sociological (e.g., Goode's resource theory) approaches, as well as an attempt at an integrative multidimensional approach adapted from

D. Nguyen · A. E. Naugle (✉)
Department of Psychology, Western Michigan University, Kalamazoo, MI, USA
e-mail: amy.naugle@wmich.edu

W. T. O'Donohue and P. A. Schewe (eds.), *Handbook of Sexual Assault and Sexual Assault Prevention*,
https://doi.org/10.1007/978-3-030-23645-8_48

Bronfenbrenner's Social Ecological Model (Mitchell & Vanya, 2009). Though Heise (2012) has questioned whether IPV should be considered dimensionally based on severity of violence rather than by type or form, by and large the majority of research continues to conceptualize IPV based on types. Johnson (2006) presents a categorization of IPV types based on the control motives of the perpetrator. He presents four distinctions (i.e., situational couple violence, intimate terrorism, violent resistance, and mutual violent control) due to fundamental differences in their causes, trajectories, and subsequent treatment needs. The CDC also conceptualizes topographically different forms of IPV: physical violence, sexual violence, stalking, and psychological aggression (Breiding et al., 2015). The World Health Organization (WHO; Heise & Garcia-Moreno, 2002) and Hart and Klein (2013) offer similar definitions as the CDC, with the inclusion of controlling behaviors and economic abuse, respectively.

One crucial argument for viewing IPV types separately and not as a singular construct is to better understand issues of gender differences in the rate and severity of perpetrated violence (i.e., gender asymmetry) or the degree of bidirectional/reciprocal violence within an intimate relationship (Archer, 2000), particularly if there are discrepancies across the types. There have been mixed findings regarding gender symmetry in IPV perpetration, with some researchers reporting evidence for a disproportionate pattern of perpetration in heterosexual partners in which men act as the perpetrators and women as the victims (Jacobson & Gottman, 1998), while others have found gender symmetry in perpetration (Chan, 2012; Teten, Sherman, & Han, 2008). In his review, Chan (2011) reported comparable rates of perpetration in both men and women, supporting gender symmetry in IPV. However, he also notes when the severity of the violence and resulting consequences were taken into account, it appears that men more often acted as the perpetrators. Overall, conceptualizing IPV as an overarching umbrella term for separate violence types has been advantageous for parsing out and comparing gender symmetry across types.

Intimate Partner Sexual Violence

Perhaps one of the more evident examples for gender asymmetry represented in the present literature on IPV prevalence and reporting is in the realm of sexual violence. Intimate partner sexual violence (IPSV) describes any form of nonconsensual sexual violence by a current or former intimate partner, which may include noncontact sexual experiences (e.g., verbal or behavioral sexual harassment and threats of sexual violence), sexual contact (e.g., intentional touching), penetration (e.g., sexual assault), and sexual coercion (e.g., pressured to concede to sexual activity; Breiding et al., 2015). As with the broader IPV, IPSV is associated with similar negative health consequences and several unique health outcomes, particularly in the areas of sexual health and reproduction (e.g., sexually transmitted infections, unwanted pregnancy; Campbell, Dworkin, & Cabral, 2009).

For both men and women who have experienced some form of sexual violence, the perpetrator was often known to them, with a large portion represented by a former or current intimate partner (Smith et al., 2017). In terms of gender asymmetry, a higher prevalence rate has consistently been found for male sexual perpetration and female victimization in heterosexual couples (Chan, 2012; Kar & O'Leary, 2010). Perpetration by men also proves to result in both more severe short-term and long-term injurious consequences (Tjaden & Thoennes, 2000). However, consideration needs to be given to sampling techniques (e.g., general population versus emergency room recruitment). Researchers have acknowledged that the majority of sexual violence research has approached the issue from the lens of gender-based violence and may have inadvertently led to skewed estimates of the asymmetrical or symmetrical nature of IPSV (Straus, 2011).

Male Sexual Assault

The unfortunate result is that the area of male sexual assault (MSA) victimization has largely been ignored, disregarded, or simply has not kept pace with more mainstream IPSV research and practice. False beliefs and stigmatizations regarding male victims pervades not only the interpersonal level but can also be observed on higher institutional levels, evident from the gendering of sexual assault, specifically penetrative rape, which has had significant long-term implications in the acceptance and understanding of MSA (Capers, 2011). Over the past few decades, rape law reform movements have advocated for alterations to judicial laws across the country based on the growing knowledge of sexual assault, with notable successful reforms including the use of gender-neutral language, the abolishment of the marriage exemption in sexual assault, and an expanded definition of forcible rape that goes beyond penile–vaginal penetration to include other forms of sexual contact (Cocca, 2004; Rumney, 2007). The FBI's Uniform Crime Reporting (UCR) Program continued to recognize forcible rape as "the carnal knowledge of a female forcibly and against her will" up until 2013, resulting in the explicit exclusion of MSA in their data collection and reporting (U.S. Department of Justice, 2013). The 2013 revision expanded the definition of rape to include "penetration, no matter how slight, of the vagina or anus with any body part or object, or oral penetration by a sex organ of another person, without the consent of the victim" (U.S. Department of Justice, 2014) in order to increase gender neutrality. However, Capers (2011) reports that the entrenched judicial establishment has persisted largely unchanged, with the enforcement of rape statues remaining gendered, despite reforms in the vast majority of states.

An example of this ongoing issue can be seen in sexual assault reporting rates. Although underreporting of sexual assault incidents by female victims has consistently been a pressing matter, with official reports sought for only one-third of cases, it has been suggested that underreporting and low help-seeking behaviors may be an even greater issue in the general male population (Archer, 2000; Clayton & Beckson, 2011; Truman & Morgan, 2016). This issue is further amplified in certain groups, such as within the prison system and in the military, where an estimated 17–22% male victims made an official report to administrative personnel (Miller, 2010; United States Department of Defense, 2014).

The historical disregard for MSA is due in part to culturally held beliefs regarding traditional masculinity and gender-role socialization, particularly role norms that are associated with dominance and dictate the ability to protect oneself (Kassing, Beesley, & Frey, 2005). Several false rape myths have been identified, including "men cannot be overpowered and assaulted," "men are less affected by sexual assault," "male victims who were assaulted by men are gay and were more culpable" (Coxell & King, 2010; Struckman-Johnson & Struckman-Johnson, 1992). Rape myths may be especially problematic for male victims as men tend to report more acceptance of both male and female rape myths than women (Davies, Gilston, & Rogers, 2012).

Intersectional Considerations

What must not be overlooked is the need for an intersectional framework in examining male sexual assault. Breiding, Chen, and Black (2014), as part of the NISVS data, reported that a significantly higher number of American Indian or Alaska Native, Black, and multiracial men experienced lifetime IPV compared to white men. Male victims were more likely than not to report housing and food insecurity, have a combined household income of less than $50,000, be physically disabled, and experience their first rape before the age of 18 (Breiding et al., 2014; Haydon, McRee, & Halpern, 2011; Tjaden & Thoennes, 2006).

In regards to sexual victimization within the LGBTQ+ community, transgender individuals experience significantly higher rates of IPV than their cisgender counterparts (Langenderfer-Magruder, Whitfield, Walls, Kattari, & Ramos, 2016; Turell, 2000). Both gay and bisexual men experienced more lifetime nonrape sexual assaults compared to heterosexual men (Breiding et al., 2014). Sexual minority individuals may be distinctively vulnerable due to the usage of IPV tactics specific to this population (e.g., coercive threats of outing a partner; Badenes-Ribera, Bonilla-Campos, Frias-Navarro, Pons-Salvador, & Monterde-i-Bort, 2016). A consistent result that has been established within the literature is a high degree of victim blaming and negative attitudes shown towards gay victims by heterosexual men (Davies & Boden, 2012; Davies & Hudson, 2011), which has been suggested to be, in part, motivated by the endorsement of rigid gender-role distinctions (Whitley, 2001). Homonegativity (or homophobia), particularly for men, was related to greater acceptance of male rape myths and predicted more negative perceptions of not only sexual minority men but also all male victims (Anderson, 2004; Kassing et al., 2005).

Response to Male Sexual Assault

Pervading rape myths and negative attitudes towards sexual assault is evident even within professional fields that encounter the aftermath of sexual violence at high rates. Jamel, Bull, and Sheridan (2008) found that some key reasons male victims did not report their assault to the police were their expectations of not being believed or treated poorly, and their fear of assumptions that may be made about their sexuality. Their fears are not baseless; Struckman-Johnson and Struckman-Johnson (1992) reported that greater acceptance of rape myths was related to an increased likelihood of an inappropriate response directed at the victim. The concern for inappropriate responding may be exacerbated even further as some researchers have found that police officers may hold "real rape" stereotypes (e.g., victim physically resisted; Estrich, 1987) when deciding the credibility of a rape scenario, despite many rape cases not realistically meeting these standards (Krahe, 1991).

Furthermore, men may not seek medical attention unless they had suffered a serious injury (Tjaden & Thoennes, 2006). When male IPSV victims do exhibit help-seeking behaviors, they often run into significant barriers. Several victims reported that there was a lack of therapeutic treatments available that adequately addressed specific concerns of male victims (Washington, 1999). Victims faced obstacles with available services such as perceived discriminatory practices when seeking medical services (Tsui, 2014), encountering health care professionals early on in care (e.g., nurses) who lack training and competency in treatment of male victims (Barber, 2013), and experiencing incidences of secondary victimization (i.e., insensitive behaviors that may exacerbate distress; Machado, Santos, Graham-Kevan, & Matos, 2017). For men in the LGBTQ+ community, there are additional hurdles. In their qualitative study, Bornstein, Fawcett, Sullivan, Senturia, and Shiu-Thornton (2006) concluded that comprehensive research and services continues to be hampered by a lack of attention to the specific needs of LGBTQ individuals. The researchers point to a number of limitations: difficulty identifying instances of domestic violence due to a paucity of resources for queer relationships or resources that define domestic violence from a gendered heteronormative perspective; limited community awareness of domestic violence in queer relationships; and lower rates of reporting and non-queer-specific support seeking due to a fear of systemic discrimination.

Consequences of Male Sexual Assault

The majority of outcome research in regards to sexual victimization was compiled primarily on the basis of research on female sexual assault. Though sexual victimization overall has been associated with a number of negative mental and physical health consequences, there are some notable gender differences in the aftermath of sexual assault. Male victims are more likely to experience adverse externalizing behaviors (e.g., everyday smoking), while female victims are more likely to report internalizing behaviors (e.g., depression; Choudhary, Coben, & Bossarte, 2008). In a descriptive analysis regarding the effects of male rape, a majority of the participants reported long-term concerns with anger and revenge fantasies, a loss of masculinity (e.g., inability to prevent the assault), changes in their sexual attitude or behaviors (e.g., increased promiscuity), and feelings of guilt and disgust (Walker, Archer, & Davies, 2005). Male victims who reported more rape myth acceptance were also more likely to demonstrate greater levels of self-blame for their victimization, with some evidence pointing to rape myths operating more strongly when the perpetrator was a woman (Struckman-Johnson & Struckman-Johnson, 1992). The issue of homonegativity may also influence male victims themselves. Gay men endorsing strong internalized homophobia may view their assault as punishment for their sexuality (Garnets, Herek, & Levy, 1990), while heterosexual men report confusion about their sexuality in the aftermath of a sexual assault by a female perpetrator (Davies, 2002), perhaps due to the rape myth that men should encourage all opportunities for sex with a willing woman (Smith, Pine, & Hawley, 1988).

Female Perpetration

Female-perpetrated MSA is a subset of IPSV that is often overlooked in favor of the more prevalent male-perpetrated female sexual assault and, to a lesser extent, male-perpetrated MSA. While men, at much higher frequencies, face sexual violence at the hands of other men (Tjaden & Thoennes, 2006), Krahe, Waizenhofer, and Moller (2003) argue for the relevance of the topic in forming a comprehensive understanding of aggression that is not engrossed in the myth of passive women and aggression as a male trait. The researchers also argue that the disregard for the heterogeneity of sexual violence leads to an overemphasis on physical violence and less attention paid to verbal sexual coercion. Sexual coercion perpetrated by women was associated with psychological aggression and the women tended towards subtle, nonphysical means, such as with seduction (e.g., deceptive flirting that leads to high ambiguity) and manipulation (e.g., threatening to end the relationship) tactics, rather than other forms of aggression (Fontaine, Parent, & Guay, 2018).

Motivations and Risk Factors for IPSV Perpetration

There have been a number of motivators proposed as antecedents for the initiation of IPV. These motivators can be grouped into prominent themes. For the most part, violence motivators span across genders, with some themes predominately expressed by men or women (Malloy, McCloskey, Grigsby, & Gardner, 2003). The majority of research has viewed IPV perpetration unitarily when exploring motives for the violence, with evidence pointing to the presence of multiple motivations and bidirectional patterns of violence (Straus, 2007), as well as a contextually informed framework from which to understand the dynamics of IPV (Bell & Naugle, 2008).

Historically, self-defense has been viewed as the most prevalent, if not the only, reason for IPV perpetration in women, though there is greater evidence challenging this notion by reporting similar rates of perpetration due to retaliation, particularly against previous violence (Hamberger, 2005) and low rates of reporting for self-defense as compared to other proximal motivations (Leisring, 2013; Olson & Lloyd, 2005). Miron, Brummet, Ruggles, and Brehm (2008) suggested that retaliation is an anger-motivated behavior and that a goal of anger may be to sustain retaliation. Anger may be internally suppressed or expressed externally, likely in the form of aggression (Daniel, Goldston, Erkanli, Franklin, & Mayfield, 2009), and more specifically, has been related to sexual offending (Ahmed, 2014). Olson and Lloyd (2005) identified 12 categories of motives in a sample of women perpetrators, most notably psychological factors (e.g., personality traits, anger), rule violations (e.g., dissatisfaction with partner behavior), gain attention and compliance (e.g., demanding for attention due to partner's avoidance/withdrawal), and restoration of face threat (e.g., use of aggression to restore face/self-image).

The Social Ecological Model (Bronfenbrenner, 1979) provides a framework by which to understand the complex interplay of factors that may influence violence. Typically, the model includes four levels: individual (i.e., biological factors, personal history, and beliefs and attitudes), relationship (i.e., close social relationships), community (i.e., environments that the individual and relationship resides), and societal (i.e., social norms, institutional structures). The majority of studies focus on individual-level factors and less on macro-level risk factors (Kovacs, 2017). As part of their systematic qualitative review, Tharp et al. (2012) identified 67 risk and protective factors for IPSV within the four levels and subdomains, several of which had predominately significant findings in the extant literature. Besides compiling a comprehensive list of influential factors for IPSV, the researchers make two important points: firstly, multiple interactions among the factors imply that risk factors interact to increase the overall risk for IPSV; secondly, both risk factors and protective factors are context dependent and become activated under certain circumstances. Additionally, IPSV and sexual violence share a number of risk factors, including adherence to traditional gender roles, poverty, substance misuse, and exposure to violence in childhood (Harvey, Garcia-Moreno, & Butchart, 2007). The significance of this is the acknowledgment that IPSV does not exist in a vacuum and research into sexual victimization should not be arbitrarily isolated based solely on the relationship of the perpetrator to the victim.

Primary, Secondary, and Tertiary Interventions

Although there has been a growth in IPSV research, there is room for significant improvement in the understanding and implementation of both preventative and responsive interventions, particularly for groups who may experience elevated risk for IPV. For example, even though IPV has been observed across demographic characteristics, racial minority status, low socioeconomic status (SES), and low formal education attainment continue to be associated with an increased likelihood of experiencing IPV (Breiding et al., 2014; Cox, Kotch, & Everson, 2003). Despite this, rape victims may find themselves in the position of needing costly long-term medical and mental health services (National Center for Injury Prevention and Control, 2003). There is also concern that current wide-spread interventions lack the cultural sensitivity needed to address the nuanced needs of minority individuals (Waller, 2016).

When evaluating interventions for IPV, it is important to identify the three different levels (Coker, 2004), an approach that is complementary to the Social Ecological Model for understanding the factors of IPV. The tertiary level describes response efforts to current violence to prevent future violence, disability, or mortality, including resources such as shelters for the victims, support groups, and treatment programs for the perpetrators. The secondary level describes early detection, or screening, to reduce the progression of negative health consequences with existing treatments (e.g., treatment for HIV). Finally, the primary level addresses public health efforts to reduce the risk of IPV, including antiviolence media campaigns.

In the tertiary level, most treatment programs are dichotomous and are either focused on perpetrators or victims. Intervention research for victims is limited and has been restricted by its focus on revictimization alone as an intervention outcome, without consideration for other outcome variables such as safety behaviors, reduction in negative consequences, and enhancement of quality of life (Eckhardt et al., 2013). Davies (2002) further argues that intervention services for men lag behind those for women, calling for more inclusion of resources that are gender-neutral or male-specific to be available for male victims. At this point in time, there is little progress on addressing specific issues that may arise in the aftermath of MSA and the majority of treatments focus on the common symptomology observed with other forms of IPV (Wall & Quadara, 2014).

The most common program designed for perpetrators is the "Batterer Intervention Programs" (BIPs). A review of IPV interventions found that most studies of BIPs typically used a group format and run for approximately 22 sessions (Eckhardt et al., 2013). They often follow one of two main approaches. The first approach is based in large part on the traditional gendered feminist framework and emphasizes patriarchal socialization and male power and control as the true culprits of IPV (e.g., the Duluth model; Maiuro & Eberle, 2008; Pence & Paymar, 1993). In US states that have adopted standards of treatment for IPV perpetrators, Maiuro and Eberle (2008) reported that 95% include the conceptualization of power and control as the main, and sometimes only, framework for IPV. The second BIP approach has a more therapeutic leaning based on Cognitive Behavioral Therapy (CBT) and is more relevant for female perpetrators. This approach widens the scope of interest and acknowledges other associated factors beyond power and control, such as social skills deficit and emotion dysregulation (Shorey, Brasfield, Febres, & Stuart, 2011; Tharp et al., 2012), with a similar goal of behavior change as with CBT for psychopathology (Beck, 1976). Buttell, Powers, and Wong (2012) found that women were more likely to complete the program if they had supportive services and had adequate supervision of their participation within the program. Unfortunately, there is lackluster support for the efficacy of BIPs in regards to recidivism rates at best (Arias, Arce, & Vilariño, 2013; Babcock, Green, & Robie, 2004), with many problematic issues found, including lack of outcome data for BIPSs, the singular usage of English in many programs, and à "one size fit all" approach despite the heterogeneity of perpetrators (Price & Rosenbaum, 2009). Therefore, BIPs may benefit from matching to the type of violence, type of abuser (e.g., IPV only perpetrator vs. perpetrator of general violence), and certain personality traits (e.g., violent antisocial) in order to better address risk severity of the perpetrators (Aaron & Beaulaurier, 2017).

Alternative interventions to BIPs for IPSV have been limited by the predominant focus on physical and psychological aggression, often to the exclusion of sexual violence. Of the available research that includes sexual violence within their purview, many focus on enhancing current BIP interventions for IPV perpetration. Buttell et al. (2012) suggest that early drop outs observed with BIPs are due to the perpetrators still remaining in the pre-contemplative stage when BIPs often require active participation. Providing evidence for the utility of motivational interviewing (MI; Miller & Rollnick, 2013) to resolve ambivalence to change prior to court-mandated BIP, a study evaluating the efficacy of a one-session brief motivational enhancement treatment (BME) found similar results of increased compliance to BIP and no difference in recidivism rates compared to the control group (Crane & Eckhardt, 2013). Some have responded to the weak support for the Duluth/CBT model by proposing better integration of existing models. One such example is the integration of cognitive-behavioral therapy and psychodynamic psychotherapy (CBT/PT) proposed by Lawson, Kellam, Quinn, and Malnar (2012). This model contains elements of MI and a psychodynamic analysis of interpersonal relationship issues in addition to the standard Duluth/CBT components. Additionally, there is initial support for an Acceptance and Commitment Therapy (ACT)-based program labeled Achieving Change Through Values-Based Behavior (ACTV) that emphasizes acting on values-consistent behaviors in the presence of challenging thoughts when compared to the traditional Duluth/CBT program (Zarling, Bannon, & Berta, 2017). There was a reduction in recidivism rates, including domestic assault charges, for ACTV participants during a 12-month postintervention time period.

While the tertiary level focuses on interventions in response to ongoing or past IPV, the secondary and primary levels are more concerned with prevention. The literature on rape myths in regards to sexual violence response suggests that reducing rape myth acceptance may be a common goal in prevention services. In a study involving two incoming cohorts at the United States Naval Academy, Rosenstein (2015) suggests that additional gender-neutral training sessions were associated with decreases in rape myth acceptance for both men and women, suggesting that preventative intervention tools for civilians should also consider implementing more gender-neutral language in order to better reach male victims and possibly promote their audience's awareness of prevention and response to IPSV. Future research is still needed to evaluate whether the reduction of rape myth acceptance is successful in addressing perpetration of sexual violence.

Finally, primary prevention is the interplay between several system levels to reduce IPSV in the population and foster a healthier environment. Parks, Cohen, and Kravitz-Wirtz (2007) offer a useful framework by which to evaluate primary prevention approaches. The Spectrum of Prevention of IPV covers several facets: strengthening individual knowledge and skills, promoting community education, educating providers, fostering coalitions and networks, changing organizational practices, and influencing policy and legislation. This framework allows for evaluation of primary prevention across the lifespan and in the broader societal scope. Of the six facets of the Spectrum, the first three sublevels in the Spectrum represent more immediate processes for positive change. Strengthening individual knowledge and skills can be addressed across the lifespan. For example, it has been well documented that dating violence and sexual violence victimization during adolescence is a risk factor for later adult IPV (Tharp et al., 2012). A review examining interventions for adolescent IPV and SV found promising evidence for school-based violence interventions (e.g., targeting nonviolent conflict resolution) and community-based interventions to promote gender-equitable attitudes for adolescent boys and girls (Lundgren & Amin, 2014). As for provider education, secondary victimization by providers frequently occurs for IPSV victims and while there has been a call for increased educational interventions, the establishment of such interventions is still restricted. However, there is some evidence that family doctors in primary care settings reported feeling more prepared after the implementation of a 1.5 day educational training containing both theoretical discussions and role-plays (Lo Fo Wong, Wester, Mol, & Lagro-Janssen, 2007).

The latter three have the most potential impact on systematic change. IPV prevention media campaigns are a popular method of raising awareness and distributing public information. Outside of multiple-intervention type campaigns, media campaigns are not usually enough to lead to behavior change (National Cancer Institute, 2002). Some researchers have also raised the question of the effectiveness of these campaigns for men. Women tend to view IPV as being a more serious issue and men were found to be resistant to campaigns portraying a gender-specific message of male perpetration (Keller & Honea, 2015), which raises the question of how to best address IPV for women without alienating men.

Based on what is currently known about IPSV, there is both much to be enthusiastic about and a great number of areas of needed growth. When compared to physical or psychological abuse by intimate partners, sexual violence is still often overlooked in research and intervention. Therefore, it is essential to better understand the course of IPSV, from motivators and risk factors to the intervention response in diverse socioeconomic and cultural contexts. Additionally, evaluation for any gender asymmetric aspect of IPSV should not take precedence over a more expansive gender-informed approach to IPV beyond a traditional feminist perspective that exclusively frames men as the perpetrators and women as the victims (McCarrick, Davis-McCabe, & Hirst-Winthrop, 2016). Future research must also assess the efficacy of primary, secondary, and tertiary preventative approaches and the best strategy by which to disseminate knowledge about IPSV, especially to populations at increased risk and/or with limited available resources that have too often been neglected in intervention literature, such as female perpetrators and male victims. Systematic multilevel preventative efforts that address the individual, relationship, community, and societal levels need to be promoted. Future intervention research should also broaden the scope of evaluation in regards to outcome variables, particularly being attentive to potentially overlooked positive family and parenting outcomes that may be especially potent motivators for change to both victims and perpetrators engaged in intervention programs. Finally, integration of theoretical frameworks informing research is essential to better encapsulate the complexity and extent of IPSV.

References

Aaron, S. M., & Beaulaurier, R. L. (2017). The need for new emphasis on batterers intervention programs. *Trauma, Violence, & Abuse, 18*(4), 425–432. https://doi.org/10.1177/1524838015622440

Ahmed, A. G. (2014). Dysfunctional anger and sexual violence. *Psychiatric Clinics of North America, 37*(2), 231–238.

Anderson, I. (2004). Explaining negative rape victim perception: Homophobia and the male rape victim. *Current Research in Social Psychology, 10*(4), 43–57.

Archer, J. (2000). Sex differences in aggression between heterosexual partners: A meta-analytic review. *Psychological Bulletin, 126*(5), 651–680.

Arias, E., Arce, R., & Vilariño, M. (2013). Batterer intervention programmes: A meta-analytic review of effectiveness. *Psychosocial Intervention, 22*, 153–160.

Babcock, J. C., Green, C. E., & Robie, C. (2004). Does batterers' treatment work? A meta-analytic review of domestic violence treatment. *Clinical Psychology Review, 23*(8), 1023–1053.

Badenes-Ribera, L., Bonilla-Campos, A., Frias-Navarro, D., Pons-Salvador, G., & Monterde-i-Bort, H. (2016). Intimate partner violence in self-identified lesbians: A systematic review of its prevalence and correlates. *Trauma, Violence, & Abuse, 17*(3), 284–297. https://doi.org/10.1177/1524838015584363

Barber, C. F. (2013). Domestic violence against men. *Nursing Standard, 22*(51), 35–39.

Beck, A. T. (1976). *Cognitive therapy and the emotional disorders*. New York, NY: International Universities Press.

Bell, K. M., & Naugle, A. E. (2008). Intimate partner violence theoretical considerations: Moving towards a contextual framework. *Clinical Psychology Review, 28*(7), 1096–1107.

Bornstein, D. R., Fawcett, J., Sullivan, M., Senturia, K. D., & Shiu-Thornton, S. (2006). Understanding the experiences of lesbian, bisexual and trans survivors of domestic violence: A qualitative study. *Journal of Homosexuality, 51*(1), 159–181. https://doi.org/10.1300/J082v51n01_08

Breiding, M. J., Basile, K. C., Smith, S. G., Black, M. C., & Mahendra, R. R. (2015). *Intimate partner violence surveillance: Uniform definitions and recommended data elements, version 2.0*. Atlanta, GA: National Center for Injury Prevention and Control, Centers for Disease Control and Prevention.

Breiding, M. J., Chen, J., & Black, M. C. (2014). *Intimate partner violence in the United States – 2010*. Atlanta, GA: National Center for Injury Prevention and Control, Centers for Disease Control and Prevention.

Bronfenbrenner, U. (1979). *The ecology of human development*. Cambridge, MA: Harvard University Press.

Buttell, F. P., Powers, D., & Wong, A. (2012). Evaluating the predictors of program attrition among women mandated into Batterer Intervention Treatment. *Research on Social Work Practices, 22*(1), 20–28. https://doi.org/10.1177/1049731511413473

Campbell, R., Dworkin, E., & Cabral, G. (2009). An ecological model of the impact of sexual assault on women's mental health. *Trauma, Violence, & Abuse, 10*(3), 225–246. https://doi.org/10.1177/1524838009334456

Capers, B. (2011). Real rape too. *California Law Review, 99*(5), 1259–1307.

Chan, K. L. (2011). Gender differences in self-reports of intimate partner violence: A review. *Aggression and Violent Behavior, 16*(2), 167–175.

Chan, K. L. (2012). Gender symmetry in the self-reporting of intimate partner violence. *Journal of Interpersonal Violence, 27*(2), 263–286. https://doi.org/10.1177/0886260511416463

Choudhary, E., Coben, J. H., & Bossarte, R. M. (2008). Gender and time differences in the associations between sexual violence victimization, health outcomes, and risk behaviors. *American Journal of Men's Health, 2*(3), 254–259. https://doi.org/10.1177/1557988307313819

Clayton, M. B., & Beckson, M. (2011). Male victims of sexual assault: Phenomenology, psychology, physiology. *Journal of the American Academy of Psychiatry and the Law, 39*(2), 197–205.

Cocca, C. (2004). *Statutory rape laws in historical context. Jailbait: The politics of statutory rape laws in the United States* (pp. 9–28). Albany, NY: SUNY Press.

Coker, A. L. (2004). Primary prevention of intimate partner violence for women's health: A response to Plichta. *Journal of Interpersonal Violence, 19*(11), 1324–1334. https://doi.org/10.1177/0886260504269686

Coker, A. L., Davis, K. E., Arias, I., Desai, S., Sanderson, M., Brandt, H. M., & Smith, P. H. (2002). Physical and mental health effects of intimate partner violence for men and women. *American Journal of Preventative Medicine, 23*(4), 260–268.

Cox, C. E., Kotch, J. B., & Everson, M. D. (2003). A longitudinal study of modifying influences in the relationship between domestic violence and child maltreatment. *Journal of Family Violence, 18*(1), 5–17.

Coxell, A. W., & King, M. B. (2010). Male victims of rape and sexual abuse. *Sexual and Relationship Therapy, 25*(4), 380–391.

Crane, C. A., & Eckhardt, C. I. (2013). Evaluation of a single-session brief motivational enhancement intervention for partner abusive men. *Journal of Counseling Psychology, 60*(2), 180–187. https://doi.org/10.1037/a0032178

Daniel, S. S., Goldston, D. B., Erkanli, A., Franklin, J. C., & Mayfield, A. M. (2009). Trait anger, anger expression, and suicide attempts among adolescents and young adults: A prospective study. *Journal of Clinical Child & Adolescent Psychology, 38*(5), 661–671. https://doi.org/10.1080/15374410903103494

Davies, M. (2002). Male sexual assault victims: A selective review of the literature and implications for support services. *Aggression and Violent Behavior, 7*, 203–214.

Davies, M., & Boden, S. J. (2012). Examining the sexual preference effect in depicting male sexual assault. *Journal of Aggression, Conflict and Peace Research, 4*(3), 136–143.

Davies, M., Gilston, J., & Rogers, P. (2012). Examining the relationship between male rape myth acceptance, female rape myth acceptance, victim blame, homophobia, gender roles, and ambivalent sexism. *Journal of Interpersonal Violence, 27*(14), 2807–2823. https://doi.org/10.1177/0886260512438281

Davies, M., & Hudson, J. (2011). Judgments towards male and transgendered victims in a depicted stranger rape. *Journal of Homosexuality, 58*, 237–247. https://doi.org/10.1080/00918369.2011.540179

Eckhardt, C. I., Murphy, C. M., Whitaker, D. J., Sprunger, J., Dykstra, R., & Woodard, K. (2013). The effectiveness of intervention programs for perpetrators and victims of intimate partner violence. *Partner Abuse, 4*(2), 196–231.

Estrich, S. (1987). *Real rape*. Cambridge, MA: Harvard University Press.

Fontaine, N. M. G., Parent, G., & Guay, J.-P. (2018). Female sexual coercion examined from a developmental criminology perspective. *Sexologies, 27*(2), e45–e50.

Garcia-Moreno, C., Jansen, H. A., Ellsberg, M., Heise, L., & Watts, C. (2005). *WHO multi-country study on women's health and domestic violence against women: Initial results on prevalence, health outcomes and women's responses*. Geneva: World Health Organization.

Garnets, L., Herek, G. M., & Levy, B. (1990). Violence and victimization of lesbians and gay men. *Journal of Interpersonal Violence, 5*(3), 366–383.

Golding, J. M. (1999). Intimate partner violence as a risk factor for mental disorders: A meta-analysis. *Journal of Family Violence, 14*(2), 99–132.

Hamberger, L. K. (2005). Men's and women's use of intimate partner violence in clinical samples: Toward a gender-sensitive analysis. *Violence and Victims, 20*(2), 131–151.

Hart, B. J., & Klein, A. R. (2013). Practical implications of current intimate partner violence research for victim advocates and service providers (NJC 244348). National Criminal Justice Reference Service. Retrieved from https://www.ncjrs.gov/pdffiles1/nij/grants/244348.pdf

Harvey, A., Garcia-Moreno, C., & Butchart, A. (2007). *Primary prevention of intimate-partner violence and sexual violence: Background paper for WHO expert meeting May 2–3, 2007*. New York: WHO. Retrieved from http://www.who.int/violence_injury_prevention/publications/violence/IPV-SV.pdf

Haydon, A. A., McRee, A.-L., & Halpern, C. T. (2011). Unwanted sex among young adults in the United States: The role of physical disability and cognitive performance. *Journal of Interpersonal Violence, 26*(17), 3476–3493. https://doi.org/10.1177/0886260511403756

Heise, L. (2012). *Determinants of partner violence in low and middle-income countries: Exploring variation in individual and population level risk*. London: London School of Hygiene Tropical Medicine.

Heise, L., & Garcia-Moreno, C. (2002). Violence by intimate partners. In E. G. Krug et al. (Eds.), *World report on violence and health* (pp. 87–121). World Health Organization: Geneva.

Jacobson, N. S., & Gottman, J. M. (1998). *When men batter women: New insights into ending abusive relationships*. New York: Simon & Schuster.

Jamel, J., Bull, R., & Sheridan, L. (2008). An investigation of the specialist police service provided to male rape survivors. *International Journal of Police Science & Management, 10*(4), 486–508. https://doi.org/10.1350/ijps.2008.10.4.101

Johnson, M. P. (2006). Conflict and control: Gender symmetry and asymmetry in domestic violence. *Violence Against Women, 12*(11), 1003–1018. https://doi.org/10.1177/1077801206293328

Kar, H. L., & O'Leary, K. D. (2010). Gender symmetry or asymmetry in intimate partner victimization? Not an either/or answer. *Partner Abuse, 1*(2), 152–168. https://doi.org/10.1891/1946-6560.1.2.152

Kassing, L. R., Beesley, D., & Frey, L. L. (2005). Gender role conflict, homophobia, age, and education as predictors of male rape myth acceptance. *Journal of Mental Health Counseling, 27*(4), 311–328.

Keller, S. N., & Honea, J. C. (2015). Navigating the gender minefield: An IPV prevention campaign sheds light on the gender gap. *Global Public Health, 11*(1–2), 184–197. https://doi.org/10.1080/17441692.2015.1036765

Kovacs, R. J. (2017). The macro-level drivers of intimate partner violence: New evidence from a multilevel dataset. *Global Public Health, 13*(7), 944–956. https://doi.org/10.1080/17441692.2017.1317010

Krahe, B. (1991). Police officers' definitions of rape: A prototype study. *Journal of Community and Applied Social Psychology, 1*, 223–244.

Krahe, B., Waizenhofer, E., & Moller, I. (2003). Women's sexual aggression against men: Prevalence and predictors. *Sex Roles, 49*(5/6), 219–232.

Langenderfer-Magruder, L., Whitfield, D. L., Walls, N. E., Kattari, S. K., & Ramos, D. (2016). Experiences of intimate partner violence and subsequent police reporting among lesbian, gay, bisexual, transgender, and queer adults in Colorado: Comparing rates of cisgender and transgender victimization. *Journal of Interpersonal Violence, 31*(5), 855–871. https://doi.org/10.1177/0886260514556767

Lawson, D. M., Kellam, M., Quinn, J., & Malnar, S. G. (2012). Integrated cognitive-behavioral and psychodynamic psychotherapy for intimate partner violent men. *Psychotherapy, 49*(2), 190–201. https://doi.org/10.1037/a0028255

Leisring, P. A. (2013). Physical and emotional abuse in romantic relationships: Motivation for perpetration among college women. *Journal of Interpersonal Violence, 28*(7), 1437–1454. https://doi.org/10.1177/0886260512468236

Lo Fo Wong, S., Wester, F., Mol, S., & Lagro-Janssen, T. (2007). "I am not frustrated anymore": Family doctors' evaluation of a comprehensive training on partner abuse. *Patient Education and Counseling, 66*(2), 129–137.

Lundgren, R., & Amin, A. (2014). Addressing intimate partner violence and sexual violence among adolescents: Emerging evidence of effectiveness. *Journal of Adolescent Health, 56*, 542–550.

Machado, A., Santos, A., Graham-Kevan, N., & Matos, M. (2017). Exploring help seeking experiences of male victims of female perpetrators of IPV. *Journal of Family Violence, 32*(5), 513–523.

Maiuro, R. D., & Eberle, J. A. (2008). State standards for domestic violence perpetrator treatment: Current status, trends, and recommendations. *Violence and Victims, 23*(2), 133–155. https://doi.org/10.1891/0886-6708.23.2.133

Malloy, K. A., McCloskey, K. A., Grigsby, N., & Gardner, D. (2003). Women's use of violence within intimate relationships. *Journal of Aggression, Maltreatment & Trauma, 6*(2), 37–59. https://doi.org/10.1300/J146v06n02_03

McCarrick, J., Davis-McCabe, C., & Hirst-Winthrop, S. (2016). Men's experience of the criminal justice system following female perpetrated intimate partner violence. *Journal of Family Violence, 31*(2), 203–213.

Miller, K. L. (2010). The darkest figure of crime: Perceptions of reasons for male inmates to not report sexual assault. *Justice Quarterly, 27*(5), 692–712. https://doi.org/10.1080/07418820903292284

Miller, W. R., & Rollnick, S. (2013). *Motivational interviewing: Helping people change*. New York, NY: Guilford Press.

Miron, A. M., Brummett, B., Ruggles, B., & Brehm, J. W. (2008). Deterring anger and anger-motivated behaviors. *Basic and Applied Social Psychology, 30*(4), 326–338. https://doi.org/10.1080/01973530802502259

Mitchell, C., & Vanya, M. (2009). Explanatory frameworks of intimate partner violence. In C. Mitchell & D. Anglin (Eds.), *Intimate partner violence: A health-based perspective* (pp. 39–52). New York, NY: Oxford University Press.

National Cancer Institute (NCI). (2002). *Making health communications programs work*. Washington, DC: National Cancer Institute (USDHHS/NIH/NCI).

National Center for Injury Prevention and Control. (2003). *Costs of intimate partner violence against women in the United States*. Atlanta, GA: Centers for Disease Control and Prevention.

Olson, L. N., & Lloyd, S. A. (2005). "It depends on what you mean by starting": An exploration of how women define initiation of aggression and their motives for behaving aggressively. *Sex Roles, 53*(7–8), 603–617. https://doi.org/10.1007/s11199-005-7145-5

Parks, L., Cohen, L., & Kravitz-Writz, N. (2007). *Poised for prevention: Advancing promising approaches to primary prevention of intimate partner violence*. Oakland: Robert Wood Johnson Foundation.

Pence, E., & Paymar, M. (1993). *Education groups for men who batter: The Duluth model*. New York: Springer.

Price, B. J., & Rosenbaum, A. (2009). Batterer intervention programs: A report from the field. *Violence and Victims, 24*(6), 757–770. https://doi.org/10.1891/0886-6708.24.6.757

Rivara, F. P., Anderson, M. L., Fishman, P., Bonomi, A., Reid, R. J., Carrell, D., & Thompson, R. S. (2007). Healthcare utilization and costs for women with a history of intimate partner violence. *American Journal of Preventive Medicine, 32*(2), 89–96.

Rosenstein, J. E. (2015). Military sexual assault prevention and male rape myth acceptance. *Military Behavioral Health, 3*(4), 207–211. https://doi.org/10.1080/21635781.2015.1038404

Rumney, P. N. S. (2007). In defense of gender neutrality within rape. *Seattle Journal for Social Justice, 6*(1), 481–526.

Shorey, R. C., Brasfield, H., Febres, J., & Stuart, G. L. (2011). An examination of the association between difficulties with emotion regulation and dating violence perpetration. *Journal of Aggression, Maltreatment, & Trauma, 20*(8), 870–885. https://doi.org/10.1080/10926771.2011.629342

Smith, R. E., Pine, C. J., & Hawley, M. E. (1988). Social cognition about adult male victims of female sexual assault. *Journal of Sex Research, 25*, 101–112.

Smith, S. G., Chen, J., Basile, K. C., Gilbert, L. K., Merrick, M. T., Patel, N., … Jain, A. (2017). *The National Intimate Partner and Sexual Violence Survey*

(NISVS): 2010–2012 State Report. Atlanta, GA: National Center for Injury Prevention and Control, Centers for Disease Control and Prevention.

Straus, M. A. (2007). Dominance and symmetry in partner violence by male and female university students in 32 nations. *Children and Youth Services Review, 30*(3), 252–275.

Straus, M. A. (2011). Gender symmetry and mutuality in perpetration of clinical-level partner violence: Empirical evidence and implications for prevention and treatment. *Aggression and Violent Behavior, 16*(4), 279–288.

Struckman-Johnson, C., & Struckman-Johnson, D. (1992). Acceptance of male rape myths among college men and women. *Sex Roles, 27*, 85–100.

Teten, A. L., Sherman, M. D., & Han, X. (2008). Violence between therapy-seeking veterans and their partners: Prevalence and characteristics of nonviolent, mutually violent, and one-sided violent couples. *Journal of Interpersonal Violence, 24*(1), 111–127.

Tharp, A. T., DeGue, S., Valle, L. A., Brookmeyer, K. A., Massetti, G. M., & Matjasko, J. L. (2012). A systematic qualitative review of risk and protective factors for sexual violence perpetration. *Trauma, Violence, & Abuse, 14*(2), 133–167. https://doi.org/10.1177/1524838012470031

Tjaden, P., & Thoennes, N. (2000). *Full report of the prevalence, incidence, and consequences of violence against women: Findings from the national violence against women survey*. Washington, DC: National Institute of Justice.

Tjaden, P., & Thoennes, N. (2006). *Extent, nature, and consequences of rape victimization: Findings from the National Violence Against Women Survey (NCJ 210346)*. Washingon, DC: U.S. Department of Justice, National Institute of Justice.

Truman, J. L., & Morgan, R. E. (2016). *Criminal victimization, 2015*. Bureau of Justice Statistics: U.S. Department of Justice.

Tsui, V. (2014). Male victims of intimate partner abuse: Use and helpfulness of services. *Social Work, 59*(2), 121–130.

Turell, S. C. (2000). A descriptive analysis of same-sex relationship violence for a diverse sample. *Journal of Family Violence, 15*(3), 281–293.

United States Department of Defense, Sexual Assault Prevention and Response Office. (2014). *Annual Report on Sexual Assault in the Military*. Retrieved from http://sapr.mil/public/docs/reports/FY14_Annual/FY14_DoD_SAPRO_Annual_Report_on_Sexual_Assault.pdf.

United States Department of Justice, Federal Bureau of Investigation. (2013). *Uniform Crime Report: Crime in the United States, 2012*. Retrieved from https://ucr.fbi.gov/crime-in-the-u.s/2012/crime-in-the-u.s.-2012/violent-crime/rape/rapemain.pdf.

United States Department of Justice, Federal Bureau of Investigation. (2014). *Uniform Crime Report: Crime in the United States, 2013*. Retrieved from https://ucr.fbi.gov/crime-in-the-u.s/2013/crime-in-the-u.s.-2013/violent-crime/rape/rapemain_final.pdf.

Walker, J., Archer, J., & Davies, M. (2005). Effects of male rape on psychological functioning. *British Journal of Clinical Psychology, 44*(3), 445–451. https://doi.org/10.1348/014466505X52750

Wall, L., & Quadara, A. (2014). Acknowledging complexity in the impacts of sexual victimization trauma. *ACSSA Issues: Australian Centre for the Study of Sexual Assault, 16*, 1–123.

Waller, B. (2016). Broken fixes: A systematic analysis of the effectiveness of modern and postmodern interventions utilized to decrease IPV perpetration among Black males remanded to treatment. *Aggression and Violent Behavior, 27*, 42–49.

Washington, P. A. (1999). Second assault of male survivors of sexual violence. *Journal of Interpersonal Violence, 14*(7), 713–730.

Whitley, B. E. (2001). Gender-role variables and attitudes towards homosexuality. *Sex Roles, 45*(11/12), 691–721.

Zarling, A., Bannon, S., & Berta, M. (2017). Evaluation of acceptance and commitment therapy for domestic violence offenders. *Psychology of Violence, 9*(3), 257–266.

Exploring the Relationship Between Intimate Partner Sexual Assault, Severe Abuse, and Coercive Control

49

Shannon B. Harper

And they say marital rape is not as bad as stranger rape. I don't know. I have never been raped by a stranger. But I think being raped by your husband in your own home must be worse in some ways. At least if you're attacked by a perfect stranger it is not so personal. Your husband is the person whom you should be able to turn to for comfort, who should protect you. When it is the person you have entrusted your life to who abuses you, it isn't just physical or sexual assault, it is a betrayal of the very core of your marriage or your person, your trust. If you're not safe in your own home, next to your husband, where are you safe?

(Linda, Intimate partner sexual assault survivor, (Esteal & McOrmond-Plummer, 2005, p. 116)

Introduction

It is estimated that more than 7 million women in the United States have been sexually assaulted by an intimate partner (current or former spouse, girlfriend, or boyfriend; Bergen & Barnhill, 2006). Intimate partner sexual assault (IPSA) is the most common form of sexual assault (Tjaden & Thoennes, 2000), and can be defined as any unwanted oral, vaginal, or anal intercourse or penetration (with fingers, tongue, penis, or objects) obtained by force, by threat of force, or when a partner is unable to consent (i.e., due to drug or alcohol intoxication or being asleep or unconscious; Bagwell-Gray, Messing, & Baldwin-White, 2015). Lifetime rates of IPSA range between 7.7% and 14% (Basile, 2002; Tjaden & Thoennes, 2000). Among women who have been physically abused by an intimate partner, the rates of IPSA are even higher, ranging from 28% (Eby, Campbell, Sullivan, & Davidson, 1995) to 68%[1] (McFarlane, Malecha, Watson, et al., 2005).

Current research has identified, defined, and measured IPSA using inconsistent terminology and measurement. Sexual assault has been defined in the literature using several terms, including intimate partner sexual violence, forced sex,[2] rape, sexual coercion, sexual aggression, and sexual victimization (Bagwell-Gray et al.,

S. B. Harper (✉)
Sociology Department, Iowa State University, Ames, IA, USA
e-mail: sharper@iastate.edu

[1]This prevalence range is very wide and provides very little specificity about the scope and nature of IPSA. This expansive range may speak to issues associated with measuring IPSA across studies and the necessity for future and replicative research.

[2]Forced sex is a problematic term due to its association with consensual sex; however, some scholars (e.g., Campbell & Soeken, 1999) use this term because women who are sexually assaulted by their intimate partners often do not want to define what they experienced as sexual assault or rape because the act was committed by someone they love and/or care for.

W. T. O'Donohue and P. A. Schewe (eds.), *Handbook of Sexual Assault and Sexual Assault Prevention*,
https://doi.org/10.1007/978-3-030-23645-8_49

2015). I use the term "sexual assault" as opposed to the term "rape" because the latter commonly conveys the message that the perpetrator is a stranger to or acquaintance of the survivor rather than their intimate partner (Bagwell-Gray et al., 2015). Additionally, some survivors may not feel comfortable referring to their victimization as rape because an intimate partner committed the offense (Bagwell-Gray et al., 2015). Due to overwhelming evidence indicating that the majority of sexual assaults are perpetrated by men against women (e.g., Breiding et al., 2014; Davis et al., 2012), as well as the limited research on IPSA in same-sex relationships, this chapter uses the term IPSA to primarily examine sexual assault in opposite-sex (heterosexual) intimate relationships wherein males victimize their female intimate partners. We know very little about sexual assault in lesbian, gay, bisexual, and transgender (LGBT) people's intimate relationships; however, some studies suggest that bisexual women and transgender people experience higher levels of IPSA than heterosexual/cisgender (i.e., personal identity and gender correspond with birth sex) women (see Brown & Herman, 2015). Bisexual women are 2.6 times more likely to have experienced IPSA when compared to heterosexual women (Walters, Chen, & Breiding, 2013); and the prevalence of IPSA among transgender people ranges from 25% to 47% (Risser et al., 2005; Roch, Morton, & Ritchie, 2010; Turrell, 2000), which are rates approximately 3 times higher than cisgender women (Tjaden & Thoennes, 2000). While there is minimal research on IPSA among women overall, far less research exists on IPSA among women/people of color. Available literature suggests that White women are more likely than Black and Hispanic/Latina women to experience IPSA (McFarlane, Malecha, Watson, et al., 2005).

Although IPSA does not exclusively occur within relationships involving intimate partner violence (IPV; i.e., physical, sexual, psychological, and/or emotional abuse, threats of abuse, and/or stalking by a current or former intimate partner; Saltzman, Fanslow, McMahon, & Shelley, 2002), there is a small likelihood of finding research that documents IPSA occurring absent the presence of physical IPV (Bagwell-Gray et al., 2015). Consequently, this chapter examines IPSA as one component of IPV,[3] which often coexists with emotional, physical, and other forms of abuse (Hall, Walters, & Basile, 2012; Tjaden & Thoennes, 2000) and occurs across age, race, ethnicity, and social class. Approximately 34–59%[4] of women who experience IPSA are also physically assaulted by an intimate partner (McFarlane, Malecha, Watson, et al., 2005). Nineteen percent of women experience both physical violence (minor or severe) and severe sexual violence (Parker, Gielen, Castillo, & Webster, 2015). Intimate partner sexual assault has been overlooked in empirical research on both IPV and sexual violence despite its widespread prevalence. Researchers frequently fail to analyze IPSA as a distinctive subtype of IPV and its unique consequences and correlates apart from other forms of IPV (Bagwell-Gray et al., 2015).

Women who have experienced IPSA report physical violence (that may occur during episodes of IPSA or separate from physical violence in intimate relationships) that is twice as severe when compared to women who have not experienced IPSA (Weaver et al., 2007). There is a strong relationship between severe physical IPV, IPSA, and intimate terrorism (Johnson, 1995)/coercive control (Stark, 2007), which will be explored throughout this chapter. It is important to note that this relationship has not yet been firmly established in the literature, so this chapter utilizes available research on IPSA as a mechanism of severe IPV and applies the theoretical construct of and research findings specific to coercive control to make a conceptual argument.[5] Specifically—in situations of severe abuse, abusive men may perpetrate IPSA as a mechanism of intimate terrorism (Johnson, 1995, 2008) and coercive control. Intimate terrorism was conceptualized by Johnson (1995) and involves a pattern

[3] IPV affects more than one in three women experiencing sexual or physical abuse by an intimate partner in their lifetime (Bagwell-Gray et al., 2015).

[4] See endnote 1 above.

[5] Future research is needed.

of abusive tactics employed to control and manipulate the survivor's actions, relationships, and activities. Abusive men may exact intimate terrorism through a combination of physical, sexual, emotional/psychological violence or individual forms of violence to establish/maintain control over/of the victim. Using intimate terrorism (Johnson, 1995) as a framework, Stark (2007) developed the concept of coercive control to describe a pattern of violence, intimidation, isolation, and control where the main goal is to degrade, isolate, and deprive women of their rights to physical security, dignity, and respect (Stark, 2007).

This chapter begins by situating a discussion of IPSA in relation to severe IPV and coercive control. Next, the detrimental emotional and physical health and behavioral consequences of IPSA, including posttraumatic stress disorder (PTSD), depression, suicide ideation, and substance use and abuse within the context of coercive control are examined. These consequences minimize survivors' capacity to live full, autonomous lives, and help to perpetuate abusive men's domination. This discussion is followed by an analysis of how diminished help-seeking among IPSA survivors exacerbates coercive control limiting survivors' ability to keep themselves safe from harm. Finally, important considerations when examining consent and sexual assault within intimate relationships are discussed.

Severe IPV, Coercive Control, and IPSA

Feminist theory addresses the link between patriarchy and sexual assault wherein men commit the offense to maintain and perform hegemonic masculinity (i.e., the male sexual assault offender seeks power and control over their powerless woman subordinate; Javaid, 2016). Feminists argue that sexual assault operates to enable men to exercise power and control over women due to the crime being entrenched in an extensive social structure supported by a hierarchy of patriarchal relations (Javaid, 2016; MacKinnon, 1991). Sexual assault thus can be understood "as an extension of male power and control over women where male offenders regard their female victims as inferior, weak and subordinate, revealing the intrinsic issue of domination that accompanies the hegemony" (Javaid, 2016, p. 284; Stanko, 1990). Within this context, abusive men may sexually assault their female intimate partner to degrade them and make them feel inferior so as to reinforce socially supported male superiority (Javaid, 2016). Research suggests that IPSA survivors often feel that their partners inflict sexual violence to obtain or maintain power and control over them (Temple, Weston, Rodriguez, & Marshall, 2007). One study found that 78% of IPSA survivors believed that their partners assaulted them to prove their manhood (Frieze, 1983). Sexual degradation and humiliation are coercive control tactics and may occur in intimate relationships involving and not involving sexual assault (see Important Considerations concluding section). What is sexually degrading for one woman may not be sexually degrading for another; however, research suggests that a significant number of women find specific types of tactics especially degrading, including being forced to watch pornography, insulting sexual performance, violence inflicted during consensual sex, and continuing sex despite it causing the victim pain (Logan, Cole, & Shannon, 2007). Among women who had experienced IPSA, 80.6–90% had been sexually demeaned by their intimate partners before, during, or after sex (compared to 21.3–29% who had not experienced IPSA); 61.3–81.8% had been pressured to watch pornography when they did not want to (compared to 16–23.4% of women who had not experienced IPSA); and 90.9% reported that their intimate partners had used sex as a way to control them (compared to 46.8% of women who had not experienced IPSA; Logan, 2011; Logan et al., 2007).

Historically, if a husband sexually assaulted his wife, he would be exempt from arrest and punishment (Temple et al., 2007) as marital rape did not become a crime in the U.S. until the early 1990s. Sexual assault within married relationships is often socially considered a contradiction in terms as it is not "necessary" for a man to sexually assault his wife (Bennice & Resick, 2003). Such beliefs are embedded in notions that the woman's sexuality is a commodity; women's bodies are the property of their fathers and husbands; that only husband and wife are privy to what occurs sexually in the bedroom; a husband is entitled to have sex with his wife whenever he pleases; and the wife should consent to her husband's wishes regardless of her own (Temple et al., 2007). While the aforementioned refers to martial relationships specifically, patriarchal notions of power and control extend beyond marital relationships to nonmarital relationships and infiltrate all areas of the social sphere (e.g., families, social relations, religions, laws, schools, textbooks, media, offices). When IPSA survivors report their victimization, they are often met with skepticism because of socially prevalent beliefs that their prior consensual sexual relations with their intimate partners implies their willingness to engage in sex at any time (Monson, Langhinrichsen-Rohling, & Binderup, 2000; see Important Considerations concluding section). Sexual assault/rape myths become stronger as the relational distance between the sexual assault survivor and perpetrator decreases where women who are sexually assaulted by an intimate partner are stereotyped more harshly than women who are sexually assaulted by a stranger (Basile, 2002).

Intimate partner sexual assault and intimate terrorism/coercive control are part of continuum of power and control within this patriarchal framework (Stark, 2009). Wilson and Daly (1992) have argued that abusive men may exact sexual violence as an aggressive mechanism of coercive control so as to enforce control of and ownership over their partners' sexuality. The abuser may exert control through acts of sexual violence as well as physical, emotional, psychological, verbal threats, financial abuse, and/or other types of violence that may occur in multiple variations (e.g., physical violence and sexual assault; emotional violence and sexual assault; emotional violence, physical violence, and sexual assault; verbal threats and sexual assault) concurrently or individually in a patterned fashion. Sexual assault in intimate relationships is associated with increased frequency and severity of violence (Campbell et al., 2002), and increased frequency and severity of violence is strongly associated with intimate terrorism/coercive control (although severe violence is not exclusive to intimate terrorism; Johnson & Leone, 2005). Intimate terrorism/coercive control is typically associated with IPV that accounts for the most serious injury and death (Johnson, 1995; Ogle, Maier-Katkin, & Bernard, 1995). More than 40% of women who have been sexually and physically assaulted by an intimate partner at some point in their lives sustain a physical injury (Graffunder, Noonan, Cox, & Wheaton, 2004), and IPSA/severe IPV is a significant predictor of intimate partner homicide (IPH; Bagwell-Gray, 2016; McFarlane, Campbell, Sharps, & Watson, 2002; McFarlane, Malecha, Watson, et al., 2005; McFarlane, Malecha, Gist, et al., 2005). Because Stark's (2007) coercive control concept incorporates intimate terrorism, this chapter specifically explores coercive control in relation to IPSA and severe physical violence.

Multiple studies indicate that intimate relationships that involve sexual assault tend to involve higher frequencies and levels of severe physical injury (Bagwell-Gray, 2016; Campbell et al., 2003; Dutton, Kaltman, Goodman, Weinfurt, & Vankos, 2005). Severe abuse is often associated with intimate terrorism where abusive men use sexual assault as a mechanism of coercive control to dominate their intimate partners and deprive them of their dignity, autonomy, and social supports in ways that compromise their capacity to seek help, escape the relationship, or perform and maintain self-care (Stark, 2012). Coercive control is an ongoing pattern of domination by which male abusive partners exact repetitive sexual, emotional, and/or physical violence and employ tactics of intimidation, sexual degradation, isolation, and control to entrap their intimate partners within the relationship (Stark, 2012). Entrapment denotes a hostage-like situation wherein sexual assault operates to enforce gender control and inflict serious harm to the survivor's dignity, liberty, and personhood, as well as to physical and psychological integrity (Stark, 2007). Coercive control is a deliberate and calculated pattern of behavior designed to isolate, manipulate, and terrorize a victim into obedience (Stark, 2007). In coercively controlling relationships, abused women often experience a spectrum of abuse where sexual assault victimization coexists with other forms of abuse. Relationships involving high levels of sexual assault also involve high levels of physical violence, psychological abuse, and stalking (Dutton et al., 2005). Research suggests that severe psychological abuse in which the abuser dominates and isolates his intimate partner through behaviors such as acting jealous or possessive, restricting access to the telephone, use of vehicles, or access to money/finances cooccurs with sexual assault (Hall et al., 2012). These findings imply a pattern of violence and behaviors intended to control the intimate partner and deny her autonomy.

Power and control are commonly associated with IPV generally (Johnson, 1995) and IPSA specifically (Wilson & Daly, 1992). Wilson and Daly (1992) coined the term "sexual proprietariness" to describe men who respond to their feelings of jealousy by using violence, including sexual assault, to declare ownership over their intimate partner's sexuality. Research indicates that jealousy is a major trigger for violence in intimate relationships where men who fear their intimate partners will leave them or sleep with another man are more likely to abuse their partners in an effort to stop them from leaving the relationship (Sugihara & Warner, 2002). The risk of IPSA significantly increases when abusive men exhibit jealous behavior (Gage & Hutchinson, 2006). Intimate partner sexual assault survivors are more likely than women who have not experienced IPSA to state that their abusive partners display jealousy (Messing, Amanor-Boadu, Cavanaugh, Glass, & Campbell, 2013). Abusive men may sexually assault their intimate partners when they are denied sex, which reestablishes the power they feel they have lost and reinstates feelings of control over their significant others (Finkelhor & Yllo, 1985). Bergen's (1996) research suggests that men who sexually assault their wives are motivated by a desire to control their behaviors and a sense of entitlement to sexual gratification (see also Finkelhor & Yllo, 1985). Russell (1990) argued that men who sexually assault their wives feel a patriarchal sense of ownership of them. As one abusive man who sexually assaulted his wife explained: "When she would not give it freely … I would take it. That's as honest as I can get … [He felt] You can't deny me. I have a right to this. You're not satisfying my needs" (Finkelhor & Yllo, 1985, p. 72). The man in this study and men like him may perpetrate sexual assault to dominate their intimate partners, which inflicts harm on the survivor's ability to make self-interested decisions (Stark, 2012). Sexual assault violently denies survivors the ability to make decisions about their sexuality and protect their physical and emotional well-being, placing them at the mercy of their abusers and exacerbating the risk of future and more severe harm. Several studies have found that the primary motive for male-perpetrated IPH is sexual proprietariness (e.g., Campbell, 1992; Daly, Wiseman, & Wilson, 1997), so it is not surprising that IPSA is similarly a significant predictor of IPH (Bagwell-Gray, 2016; McFarlane et al., 2002; McFarlane, Malecha, Gist, et al., 2005).

This form of coercively controlling violence is not limited to marital relationships. In a study involving interviews with severely abused women who were at risk for IPH, one woman indicated that her boyfriend sexually assaulted her while refusing to wear a condom (compelling her to get a tubal ligation in secret; Bagwell-Gray, 2016). These forms of sexual assault are indicators of coercive control where abusers deny their intimate partners the right to make decisions about their reproductive and sexual health. Coercively controlling men may forbid their intimate partners access to contraceptives because they do not accept or approve of them (Rickert, Wiemann, Harrykissoon, Berenson, & Kolb, 2002). Abusers may also use sexual and physical violence or the threat of violence to force their intimate partners into undergoing tubal ligations or hysterectomies (Akyuz, Şahiner, & Bakır, 2008). One study found that 8.7% of women were forced by their intimate partners to undergo these procedures

(Raj, Liu, McCleary, & Silverman, 2005). Sexual assault as a mechanism of coercive control serves to forcefully remove women's options to make self-interested decisions about their bodies not to mention the high likelihood of emotional devastation associated with being forced to endure such procedures. Another woman reported that her ex-husband would deprive her of sleep until she was so exhausted she could no longer fight off his unwanted sexual advances (Bagwell-Gray, 2016). This control tactic can be likened to torture tactics used against prisoners of war to annihilate their will and deny their humanity (Stark, 2009).

Survivors of IPSA also suffer the highest frequency of multiple sexual assaults (McFarlane, Malecha, Watson, et al., 2005; Tjaden & Thoennes, 2000). Married women who are sexually assaulted by their husbands are 10 times more likely to experience multiple sexual assaults than are women sexually assaulted by a stranger (Russell, 1990). Bergen (1995) found that married women in relationships involving sexual violence reported being sexually assaulted more than 20 times before they were able to end the abuse. Prior IPSA victimization may be a risk factor for repetitive IPSA victimization within intimate relationships because the violence occurs within ongoing intimate relationships where sex is often expected and/or customary. Another study revealed that IPSA survivors experienced nonfatal strangulation while being sexually assaulted at a rate 4–7 times greater ($n = 46$, 22.5%) than women who were sexually assaulted by other types of perpetrators (acquaintance/friend, $n = 20$, 3.3%; stranger, $n = 11$, 5.6%; and other, $n = 2$, 2.9%; Zilkens et al., 2016). Collectively, these findings suggest that abusive men may use these forms of sexual violence specifically to humiliate, punish, demoralize, and establish ownership of their intimate partners. Intimate partner sexual assault that involves degrading behavior may exacerbate the risk of self-esteem problems, depression, and other mental health problems among survivors (see Detrimental Health Effects of IPSA section), which may make them more vulnerable to the power and control tactics of their abusers and reduce their ability and motivation to seek help for the violence they are experiencing (see IPSA and Help-Seeking section).

In situations of severe IPV or battering, abusive men may also sexually assault their intimate partners while they are under the influence of drugs or alcohol or after beating them (Finkelhor & Yllo, 1985; Russell, 1990), and/or when they are asleep, sick, or incapacitated in some way (e.g., Abbey, Parkhill, BeShears, Clinton-Sherrod, & Zawacki, 2006). One could posit that IPSA within these contexts also suggests coercive control where abusers inflict sexual assault to subjugate their intimate partners who are disproportionately more vulnerable due to intoxication and/or incapacitation. The consequence of IPSA in these circumstances (in addition to IPSA in any set of circumstances) may be increased PTSD symptomology and depression, which have been found to be significantly associated with IPSA (Bennice, Resick, Mechanic, & Astin, 2003), thus potentially resulting in survivors' increased isolation due to shame and inability to reconcile what they experienced.[6] When compared to stranger sexual assault survivors, IPSA survivors may be less likely to seek help after realizing they have been assaulted because they have been victimized by someone they care for, love, and trust (Bergen, 2006), which may lead to more severe, detrimental, and long-lasting mental health consequences (see Detrimental Health Effects of IPSA section).

Pregnancies following sexual assault are unintended and unintended pregnancies account for about one half of all pregnancies in the U.S. (Henshaw, 1998). One study found that 26% ($n = 20$) of the sexually assaulted women who had been pregnant ($N = 77$) experienced a sexual assault-induced pregnancy (5 times the national average of unintended pregnancies), and the number of sexual assault-induced pregnancies per woman ranged from one to four (McFarlane, Malecha, Watson, et al., 2005). Abusive men may

[6]There is a strong relationship between IPSA and survivors' feelings of fear, guilt, humiliation, and self-blame (not accounting for degrading sexual violence specifically; Finkelhor & Yllo, 1985).

control their partner's contraceptive use leading to unintended pregnancies (Campbell, Pugh, Campbell, & Visscher, 1995; Gazmararian et al., 1995). Sexual assault induced pregnancies eliminate women's ability to plan for pregnancy, which may increase the likelihood of detrimental health outcomes and elective abortions. McFarlane, Malecha, Watson, et al. (2005) found that women who were sexually assaulted during conception reported fewer live births and more elective abortions when compared to abused women who were not sexually assaulted at conception. Women who experience sexual assault induced pregnancies may elect to obtain abortions because their abusers have violated their bodies and stripped them of their rights to make decisions about their reproduction, limiting their ability to continue their pregnancies in their own self-interests and enjoy the prospect of a child. Moreover, because women may associate love with conception more so than men (Swayne, 2014), and develop deep feelings of love for their developing babies, the bodily degradation and violence associated with IPSA may dissuade women from wanting to continue their pregnancies.

Sexual assault as a mechanism of coercive control sometimes continues during pregnancy. Approximately 13% of women in abusive relationships have been sexually assaulted during pregnancy (McFarlane, 2007; McFarlane, Malecha, Gist, et al., 2005). Women who are physically or sexually abused while pregnant report more frequent and severe physical or sexual abuse when compared with women physically or sexually abused before pregnancy, but not during pregnancy (McFarlane, Campbell, & Soeken, 1995). Between 4% and 8% of pregnant women are physically abused at least once during pregnancy (Gazmararian et al., 2000). Some research suggests that physical and sexual assault increases during pregnancy (Helton, McFarlane, & Anderson, 1987; although other research reveals opposite or mixed findings). Adverse pregnancy outcomes associated with sexual and physical assault during pregnancy include preterm delivery (Coker, Sanderson, & Dong, 2004), maternal death (Horon & Cheng, 2001), sexually transmitted infections (STIs; McFarlane, Malecha, Watson, et al., 2005), and additional complications for the mother during pregnancy and after the baby is born (King, 2003). Additionally, women who are sexually assaulted and physically abused during pregnancy are more likely to terminate their pregnancies. One study revealed that in the past year, 19.5% of women seeking an abortion (N = 312) had been physically assaulted and 3.7% reported sexual abuse, including sexual assault (Keeling, Birch, & Green, 2004; McFarlane, 2007). More than half of the women who reported sexual abuse indicated that sexual assault caused the pregnancy for which they were seeking an abortion (Keeling et al., 2004). Another study found that 16% of women (n = 32) who were sexually assaulted during pregnancy had an elective abortion (McFarlane, Malecha, Watson, et al., 2005).

As tools of coercive control, sexual assault and other forms of violence within intimate relationships may deny women the capacity to control their own environments well enough to ensure infant/child safety thus eliminating full-term pregnancy as a viable alternative to abortion. Indeed, women who have been sexually assaulted by their intimate partners may lack confidence that they can keep their children safe given they cannot protect themselves from sexual violence. Intimate partner sexual assault survivors may terminate their pregnancies to remove them as a source of power and control for their abuser in the relationship (McFarlane, Malecha, Watson, et al., 2005). Similarly, due to women's increased vulnerability during pregnancy, abusive men may find it easier to force their intimate partners to fulfill their sexual wants. An abusive man may sexually assault his intimate partner—as well as employ a variety of other coercive control mechanisms such as emotional, physical, and financial abuse—during pregnancy to force her to refocus her attention away from her unborn child and back toward him. One study found that abusive men often feel jealous of their unborn children, with one study subject indicating that her abusive partner told her he wanted to remain at the center of her attention and could not handle being a secondary priority (Stockl & Gardner,

2013). This same man strangled the woman after her daughter was born when she said that her daughter was "her life." Thus, it is not surprising that women abused during pregnancy are at a three-fold risk of becoming an attempted or completed femicide victim (i.e., the killing of a woman; McFarlane et al., 2002).

Research reveals a strong link between sexual assault and femicide (see Bagwell-Gray, 2016). Women who are sexually assaulted in intimate relationships have higher scores on homicide risk assessments even after controlling for physical and nonphysical abuse (Bagwell-Gray, 2016; Campbell & Soeken, 1999). In cases of femicide, victims were 1.87 times more likely to have been sexually assaulted by their intimate partners compared to women who were IPV survivors but not killed by their significant others (Campbell & Soeken, 1999). Threats to kill and strangulation are two significant homicide indicators that are associated with IPSA (Messing, Thaller, & Bagwell, 2014).

Additionally, abused women may file for protection orders to protect themselves from IPSA and homicide victimization. Approximately 16.4% of IPSA survivors obtain protection orders to address the sexual violence they are experiencing (Tjaden & Thoennes, 2000). Women who obtain protection orders against their intimate partners are at a higher risk of IPH as abusive men may use deadly force to retaliate against their intimate partners when they seek this form or other types of assistance or attempt to leave the relationship (Maddoux, McFarlane, Liu, & Liu, 2015). One study found that women experienced higher levels of threats, physical violence, and sexual assault after their abusers violated the terms of their protection orders (Maddoux et al., 2015). This violent retaliation may be in response to the woman attempting to live independently of her abuser and reduce her abuser's ability to impose power and control over her life.

As discussed previously, sexual proprietariness is positively associated with IPSA and IPH. Men who are possessive of their intimate partners are more likely than those who are not to use deadly force against their partners, and women are at the greatest risk of homicide when they leave or attempt to leave their abusive relationships (Dichter & Gelles, 2012). Campbell et al. (2003) conducted a study on risk factors for femicide using sexual assault, stalking, strangulation, and abuse during pregnancy as variables, which are typically associated with increased and escalating frequency and severity of violence in intimate relationships. Interestingly, the only variable in the full predictive model that achieved significance was sexual assault, suggesting that sexual assault has more dangerous implications for women when compared to other forms of IPV that have typically been found to be associated with femicide (i.e., the full prediction model combined the aforementioned variables and other risk factors for IPH) (Bagwell-Gray, 2016).

Detrimental Health Effects of IPSA

Evidence from several studies suggests that as the severity and frequency of violence in an intimate relationship increases, so too does the severity of detrimental health effects associated with that violence (e.g., Cox et al., 2006). In relation to post-assault mental health symptomology, IPSA survivors are at a higher risk of PTSD, anxiety, depression, attempted and actual suicide, and psychological distress than survivors of other forms of IPV (Weaver et al., 2007). Similarly, IPSA survivors are 4–5 times more likely to suffer from depression or anxiety than women who did not experience any violence, and 3 times more likely than physical abuse survivors and 2 times more likely than stranger sexual assault survivors to be diagnosed with depression and anxiety (Plichta & Falik, 2001). When compared to survivors of stranger sexual assault, IPSA survivors may experience more emotional harm and trauma because the violence occurs within the context of an ongoing intimate relationship (Campbell & Soeken, 1999).

Literature has documented a strong positive relationship between PTSD and IPSA (Barnawi, 2017; Dutton et al., 2005; Temple et al., 2007). The severity of a partner's sexual assault significantly predicts women's level of PTSD symptoms even after controlling for physical violence and associated consequences (Bennice et al., 2003). The severity of PTSD symptoms is directly related to the level of physical violence (Kemp, Green, Hovanitz, & Rawlings, 1995), and relationships involving sexual assault tend to also involve more severe physical violence (Weaver et al., 2007). For example, one study found a significant and positive relationship between physical and sexual assault severity and sexual assault severity and PTSD severity (Bennice et al., 2003). The strong relationship between severe abuse and IPSA may imply a strong relationship between IPSA and coercive control, and women in relationships involving coercive control experience more severe PTSD and depression symptomology than women who are in relationships involving only situational couple violence (i.e., IPV arising out of particular conflicts, Johnson & Leone, 2005). This may be because the persistence and severity of abuse (physical, sexual, and/or emotional) combined with nonviolent coercive control tactics (e.g., emotional abuse, isolation, using children, using male privilege, economic abuse, threats, intimidation, and blaming; Stark, 2009) may cause survivors to feel entrapped and bereft of hope that their lives will improve leading to increased mental health problems and symptomology. Posttraumatic stress disorder symptoms such as flashbacks, nightmares, emotional numbness, and hypervigilance may occur persistently and relentlessly in these circumstances. As Johnson and Leone (2005) suggested, a core idea of coercive control is that even the nonviolent control tactics take on a violent meaning that they would not have in the absence of their connection with violence. Imagine, for example, the different meaning and emotional impact of an intimidating look from a nonviolent partner and a similar gesture from a partner who has already demonstrated his willingness to be violent. As the victims of intimate terrorism often report, 'all he had to do was look at me that way and I would do whatever he wanted.' (p. 324).

Similarly, sexual assault committed by an intimate partner results in suicide ideation at levels equal to or greater than other forms of IPV and sexual assault committed by strangers or acquaintances (McFarlane, Malecha, Gist, et al., 2005; Weaver et al., 2007). One study found that 34% of women (17 out of 50) living in a battered women's shelter had thought about killing themselves and severe symptoms of PTSD and moderately severe symptoms of depression (Weaver et al., 2007). McFarlane, Malecha, Gist, et al.'s (2005) study similarly revealed that women reporting IPSA were significantly more likely to report threatening or attempting suicide within 90 days of the report compared to women who only experienced physical abuse. Sexual assault within intimate relationships may be a stronger predictor of suicide ideation than other psychological maladies because this form of assault is often chronic in nature and associated with more severe levels of physical violence (Weaver et al., 2007). However, more research examining the relationship between suicidality and sexual assault within intimate relationships is needed.

One could argue that as a mechanism of coercive control in severely abusive relationships, an abusive man may perpetrate sexual assault to degrade and humiliate his intimate partner so as to force her compliance with his wishes and demands, or reduce her capacity, energy, and strength to physically resist or aggressively fight back against sexual assault (and other abuse) victimization. Such circumstances epitomize emotional devastation where suicide may appear the only recourse. Research has found that the cumulative effects of sexual and physical assault in intimate relationships are more severe, and in some ways different from, the consequences of physical abuse alone (McFarlane, 2007; McFarlane, Malecha, Watson, et al., 2005). Women who have been sexually and physically assaulted by their intimate partners experience more severe health problems, lower self-esteem, more distorted body image, greater levels anxiety, and feel less in control of their lives (Howard, Riger, Campbell, & Wasco, 2003). This symptomology among women who are abused may make it easier for men who are abusive to manipulate their partners' feelings and control their behaviors leading to not only increased suicide ideation, but also diminished ability/effectiveness to defend themselves, resist violence, seek help, or leave their relationships.

Women who have been sexually assaulted by an intimate partner are also affected by detrimental physical health outcomes. Between 6.5% (Campbell & Alford, 1989) and 15% (McFarlane, Malecha, Watson, et al., 2005) of women sexually assaulted by an intimate partner report contracting a STI due to IPSA. Fifteen percent of women reported one or more STIs after being sexually assaulted by their intimate partners repetitively (McFarlane, Malecha, Watson, et al., 2005). Multiple studies report a link between IPSA and increased risk of HIV infection (e.g., Dunkle, Jewkes, Brown, & Gray, 2004; Raj, Silverman, & Amaro, 2004). Research employing qualitative methods has demonstrated the relationship between HIV/AIDS, inequality between men and women, and IPV, which is rooted in socialized patriarchal gender ideals and expectations for men to control and dominate their intimate partners (Jewkes, Dunkle, Nduna, & Shai, 2010). These patriarchal ideals and expectations translate into risky sexual behavior and predatory sexual practices (Garcia-Moreno & Watts, 2000) that allow men to have multiple partners and control how they interact with women sexually (Jewkes et al., 2010). Abusive men commonly engage in behaviors that put their partners at greater risk for HIV infection. Global studies have found that men who abuse their intimate partners are more likely to have multiple sex partners than men who are not abusive (Garcia-Moreno, Jansen, Ellsberg, Heise, & Watts, 2006). Additionally, physical IPV has been found to be associated with higher numbers of sexual partners within the past year, lifetime sexual partners, more frequent intercourse in the recent past, and increased number of casual sexual partners (Dunkle et al., 2006).

As a mechanism of coercive control, abusive men engaging in sex with multiple partners coupled with perpetrating IPSA may suggest they feel superior to their intimate partners and as if they are sexually entitled to receive sexual gratification whenever they please regardless of the emotional and physical health consequences of their behaviors (Bancroft, 2002). Pitman (2017) explained that men's sense of superiority and entitlement infiltrates the relationships they have with their intimate partners and establishes the acceptability of double standards. That is—abusive men can control the sexual behaviors of their intimate partners and inflict abuse to ensure they do not have sex with other men while engaging in reckless sexual behavior without penalty. Abusive men may refuse to wear condoms and insist on controlling their partners' use of contraceptives, which is associated with increased risk of STIs among women who are abused (rather than risky behavior on the woman's part; e.g., multiple casual sexual partners or IV drug use; Eby & Campbell, 1995). Men who reported sexually assaulting their intimate partners during the past year also reported higher rates of inconsistent or no condom use, perpetrating sexual assault without a condom, and having fathered more than three children (Raj et al., 2006). Intimate partner sexual assault survivors are often less able to protect themselves from HIV due to lack of control and fear of their intimate partners (Jewkes et al., 2010). Indeed, women sexually assaulted by their intimate partners often feel as if they have a lack of control over their sexuality (Wingood, DiClemente, McCree, Harrington, & Davies, 2001).

Additionally, research suggests that IPSA survivors report significantly more substance use as compared with women who were physically abused only (McFarlane, 2007; McFarlane, Malecha, Gist, et al., 2005). One study found that IPSA survivors who experienced more than one sexual assault were 3 times more likely to report beginning or increasing their use of substances compared to IPSA survivors who experienced only one sexual assault, and alcohol was the substance most frequently reported (McFarlane, Malecha, Gist, et al., 2005). The former group of survivors was also most likely to report illegal drug use when compared to the latter group of survivors. Other research indicates that among women who were severely abused and had filed for a protection order (N = 676), significantly more women who abused or were dependent on alcohol (33.8%) reported sexual assault within the last year of their abusive relationships compared with women who did not use alcohol (21.9%) and women who drank alcohol infrequently (20.4%; Shannon, Logan, Cole, & Walker, 2008). Intimate partner violence generally is associated with higher rates of drug abuse, heavy drinking, and general substance use (Zweig, Yahner, & Rossman, 2012), and women may use and abuse substances as a coping mechanism (Kayson et al., 2007). However, the cumulative traumatic effects of IPSA combined with severe abuse and other coercively controlling behaviors within relationships where the perpetrator is a loved intimate partner may increase the perceived necessity of substance use among survivors to self-medicate emotional trauma when compared to women who are sexually assaulted by strangers or who have not been sexually victimized by an intimate partner.[7]

IPSA and Help-Seeking

As the level of severe violence in a relationship escalates, so too do women's help-seeking behaviors (Gondolf & Fisher, 1988). Cattaneo, DeLoveh, and Zweig (2008) found that survivors of IPSA and physical IPV (n = 470; 44% of the sample) sought significantly more help from varying resources and were more likely to seek out legal help than survivors of physical IPV alone. Women who are experiencing both physical and sexual assault may have greater need for legal protection than women who are experiencing only physical assault due to the cumulative effects and associated negative outcomes associated with experiencing both forms of violence. One study found that 78% of women seeking protection orders (N = 197) experienced severe physical violence and 19% experienced both severe physical violence and severe sexual violence, including sexual assault (Parker, Gielen, Castillo, & Webster, 2015). Survivors of IPSA may seek out protection orders because they need emergency help to stop their abusers from inflicting additional violence. For instance, research has found that 77% of women seeking protection orders for severe physical and sexual assault (N = 197) experienced severe injury from IPV (Parker et al., 2015).

While IPSA survivors may seek help more often as the severity of violence increases, they may not have access to or seek help from all available formal and informal supports. For example, women with lower incomes experiencing IPSA are less likely than women with higher incomes experiencing IPSA to seek out legal or other forms of assistance despite needing the help (Parker et al., 2015). Coercively controlling men may isolate their intimate partners, severing their access to resources that may be desperately needed to address the severity of violence they are experiencing. Limited access to IPV resources is exacerbated among women who are poor as they may depend on their abuser's income to survive (as well as to ensure the survival of their children; Bornstein, 2006), and/or their abusers may forbid them from working (i.e., coercive control) resulting in reduced help-seeking behaviors. Women who are sexually assaulted by their intimate partners are also less likely than women who experience exclusively physical violence to reach out to tell someone about the violence (Fanslow & Robinson, 2010). This finding may be due to the emotional toll of IPSA and feelings of low self-esteem and shame (Shields & Hanneke, 1983)—which are exacerbated by coercive control (Stark, 2012)—the consequence of which may be diminished ability to identify, access, and use community and social support, lower self-efficacy, and increased self-blame (Howard et al., 2003).

Cattaneo et al. (2008) study revealed that while IPSA survivors were more likely to report a greater degree of help-seeking than women who had not experienced IPSA, they were also more likely to report that they did not seek help when they needed it, which may be because they feared their abusers would inflict more repetitive and severe sexual violence. Indeed, fear was the greatest obstacle for reaching out for help. Forty-six percent of IPSA and physical IPV survivors reported that they needed access to a hotline but did not seek this assistance. These results are troubling as one could argue that women who are

[7] More research is needed to examine this contention.

being severely sexually and physically assaulted by an intimate partner have a greater need for outside assistance when compared to those who are not experiencing both forms of violence or severe violence. As examined throughout this chapter, IPSA survivors are at an increased risk of IPH victimization (Bagwell-Gray, 2016; McFarlane et al., 2002; McFarlane, Malecha, Watson, et al., 2005; McFarlane, Malecha, Gist, et al., 2005).

The studies above point to a lack of survival strategies available to IPSA survivors despite the significant need for such assistance. Rather than rely on outside services such as police or IPV advocacy organizations, IPSA survivors are significantly more likely to use placation strategies (Meyer, Wagner, & Dutton, 2010; Parker et al., 2015). However, although IPSA survivors prefer placation over these other resources, they also perceive placation to be less effective than these other services (Parker et al., 2015). Why might IPSA survivors choose to placate their abusers rather than seek these services if in fact they are perceived as more effective? Although the specified study did not specifically examine the dimensions and context of women's perceptions, the answer to this question may lie in how women perceive short and long-term effectiveness of IPV resources. Research suggests that when women leave their intimate relationships or seek help, the severity and frequency of violence escalates, as does the risk of lethal violence (Websdale, 1999). Additionally, women are often unable to defend themselves against men's violence, and friends, family, and other resources cannot be present all the time to ensure that the survivor has protection. Intimate partner sexual assault survivors may perceive outside services such as police as effective in reducing violence in the short-term, but entirely ineffective at reducing repetitive, increasingly severe, and long-term violence. When short-term options fail to provide long-term reprieve, IPSA survivors may feel like placation is the best option available, which is a troubling contention as the effectiveness of placation in reducing violence depends on the efficacy of the survivor in calming her abuser, which is unlikely to be reliable or consistently effective especially during times of escalating and increasingly dangerous violence. Thus, in the absence of viable alternatives, IPSA survivors may feel as if they are "grasping at straws" (i.e., placation) to ensure they survive coercively controlling violence that has denied them the opportunity and capacity to use and benefit from services that may help them to thrive and ultimately, stay alive.[8] The consequence is increased entrapment within their abusive relationships wherein abusive men exact IPSA and/or physical violence as part of a life-threatening "regime of domination" (Stark, 2012, p. 8).

As the level of coercive control escalates in a relationship, so too does IPSA and the risk of severe and fatal violence (Stark, 2012). A study conducted across several cities found that the level of control in an abusive relationship increased the risk of homicide victimization by a factor of nine (Glass, Manganello, & Campbell, 2004; Stark, 2012). Other research has demonstrated that coercive control was a stronger indicator than physical IPV (by four times) of escalated violence (81% vs. 20%), death threats (80% vs. 17%), and IPSA (76% vs. 24%) after both partners had separated (Beck & Raghavan, 2010; Stark, 2012). These findings suggest that "women's vulnerability to physical and sexual abuse is typically a byproduct of an already established pattern of domination that has disabled their capacity to mobilize personal, material and social resources to resist or escape" (Stark, 2012, pp. 13–14).

Important Considerations

The conceptual argument presented above is premised upon a liberal/radical feminist theoretical framework that considers sexual assault offending to be specifically motivated by power and control rather than other sexual assault causal factors that have also been empirically supported such as opportunity, pervasive anger, sexual grat-

[8] At the same time, research also suggests that increased IPV resource use may increase the risk of IPH in some cases (Reckdenwald & Parker, 2012).

ification, and/or vindictiveness (Cossins, 2000; Knight, 1999; McPhail, 2015; Scully & Marolla, 1985; White & Post, 2003). Feminist theories of sexual assault have been critiqued for being essentialist in nature and focusing primarily on power and control as the single factor motivating offending (Ward, Polaschek, & Beech, 2006) without accounting for other causal multifactor mechanisms, including those that are developmental (e.g., attachment disorders, early sexual initiation, intimacy deficits, and peer pressure), biological (e.g., genetic factors, androgens, neurological deficits), environmental (e.g., child abuse [sexual and physical] and parental IPV), situational (e.g., alcohol and drug use and misuse, firearms, gang membership, juvenile delinquency), and/or psychological (e.g., low self-esteem, low empathy, poor mental health). All of these multifactor mechanisms/theories are supported in the literature in relation to sexual assault perpetration generally (i.e., not IPSA specifically; Abbey & McAuslan, 2004; Abbey, Parkhill, Clinton-Sherrod, & Zawacki, 2007; Beech & Mitchell, 2005; Beech & Ward, 2004; Brown & Forth, 1997; Burk & Burkhart, 2003; Chesire, 2004; Jewkes, Sikweyiya, Morrell, & Dunkle, 2011; Johansson et al., 2008; Malamuth, Linz, Heavey, Barnes, & Acker, 1995; Maniglio, 2010; Prentky et al., 1989; Siegert & Ward, 2003; Thornton, 2002; Ward & Beech, 2006), however, we know very little about their effects on IPSA specifically. More research is definitively needed as feminist-oriented perspectives are not the only conceptual lenses with which to examine IPSA, and coercive control is not the only motivation for IPSA offending.

Scholars have argued that it is difficult to measure and understand consent in intimate relationships due to the unique nature of sexual intimacy within those relationships (see Logan, Walker, & Cole, 2015), where there is often a presumption of continuous consent for intercourse and other sexual relations (Lazar, 2010; Logan et al., 2015; Monson et al., 2000; Shotland & Goodstein, 1992; Yllo, 1999). For example, when intimate partners initially engage in consensual sex, they may believe this establishes an unspoken "contract" for sex with one another (Logan et al., 2015). As the relationship progresses and becomes more permanent, consent may then become more implicit and assumed (Logan et al., 2015). While consent for sexual activity is perceived legally and socially as a singular, discrete event that can be revoked, it may actually be more fluid within intimate relationships and thus conceptualized as something that can be continually negotiated (Logan et al., 2015). That is, because a woman has consented to sexual activity in the past, her intimate partner may treat this as evidence of consent for current and future sexual relations relieving him of the legal obligation to ask for consent (Lazar, 2010). Lazar (2010) explained that when a woman's consent is perceived as continual, her actual wants and needs in relation to any specific sex act are removed, thus denying her the agency and freedom to make choices about the sexual acts to which she engages.

The line between sexual assault and consensual sex may also become blurred in intimate relationships when women acquiesce to unwanted sex with their spouse/intimate partners due to perceptions of personal sexual duty or obligation based in part on socialized and antiquated gender role expectations (e.g., belief that women must satisfy their husbands and remain submissive in intimate relationships), the historical failure of the law to recognize sexual assault within marital relationships, and/or religious beliefs (Basile, 1999). Feelings of sexual obligation are often reinforced by socialization, the legal system, religion, and the institution of marriage that defines what it means to be a good wife and/or girlfriend (Finkelhor & Yllo, 1985; Logan et al., 2015). Women may be coerced, tricked, pressured, manipulated, or bullied to have sex and give in despite not wanting to participate, the absence of violence, and not being physically forced or threatened to do so (Basile, 1999; McPhail, 2015). This behavior falls into the subtle realm of sexual coercion without necessarily qualifying as sexual assault (Basile, 1999). Scholars have documented types of coerced sex between married or other intimate partners that may or may not legally qualify as sexual assault (Basile, 1999, 2002; Campbell & Soeken, 1999;

Finkelhor & Yllo, 1985). Research suggests that women are sometimes confused about whether what they experienced was sexual assault due to not explicitly saying "no" to sex with their intimate partners, yet still expressing discontent with participating; or giving in to sex so as to avoid negative consequences (e.g., violence, disappointment, emotional manipulation, arguments) if they refuse (Basile, 1999). As Basile (1999) explained:

> If they do not define their experiences as rape, women who give in to unwanted sex with their husbands have no shared language with which to describe the incidents. It is as if the only available cultural labels are "rape" or "not rape," and this dichotomy leaves no room to acknowledge or label undesired sex of a less violent and physically coerced nature. (p. 1053)

Consistent with the theoretical framework of this paper, feminists may argue that this confusion is the result of a power imbalance between men and women in intimate relationships. Specifically—the definition of sexual assault becomes ambiguous when women provide consent within a patriarchal society that serves to maintain their second-class status (Basile, 1999; MacKinnon, 1983). Within a society that socializes men to believe that "no" means "yes" or "maybe" or "keep trying" (Basile, 1999; Searles & Berger, 1995), the distinction between acquiescence and consent is continuously unclear, and this ambiguity is more pronounced within marital/intimate relationships (Basile, 1999). Defining clear consent boundaries may be dependent on the context of the intimate relationship at the time thus complicating scholars' ability to measure sexual assault and violence within intimate relationships (Logan et al., 2015) and raising concerns and questions about women's autonomy and control in intimate relationships (Basile, 1999).

Conclusion

This chapter has examined how IPSA may operate as a mechanism of coercive control within severely abusive relationships. When IPSA and IPV coexist, they may occur as part of a pattern of escalating frequency and severity of control and violence leading to higher rates of injury and psychological, physical, and behavioral health problems as well as increased risk of femicide. The severe nature of this context of abuse coupled with the emotional devastation associated with being sexually assaulted by a loved one may operate to control survivors' behaviors, reduce their capacity to care for themselves and control their environments, and prevent them from developing socially and economically (Stark, 2012). Intimate partner sexual assault as part of a pattern of domination may target the survivor's autonomy, equality, liberty, social supports, and dignity, subjugating their ability to make autonomous, self-interested decisions fundamental to seeking and accessing help and/or escaping the violence (Stark, 2012). The consequence can be compared to a hostage-like situation wherein survivors are entrapped within their relationships (Stark, 2012).

Additional research is necessary to further explore IPSA and its correlates and consequences separate from physical IPV, as well as how coercive control operates within relationships involving IPSA. Furthermore, while we know that women who are severely abused and experience IPSA are more likely to reach out for help from varying resources (presumably on multiple occasions), research suggests that assistance has not been entirely effective in reducing the violence (Parker et al., 2015) or minimizing the risk of homicide (Maddoux et al., 2015). It goes without saying that IPV organizations need more funding to target their services to the women most in need of their assistance and more research may be needed to assess how these organizations can better enhance safety and address the needs of these marginalized survivors.

References

Abbey, A., & McAuslan, P. (2004). A longitudinal examination of male college student's perpetration of sexual assault. *Journal of Consulting and Clinical Psychology, 72*, 747–756.

Abbey, A., Parkhill, M. R., BeShears, R., Clinton-Sherrod, A. M., & Zawacki, T. (2006). Cross-sectional predictors of sexual assault perpetration in a community sample of single African American and Caucasian men. *Aggressive Behavior, 32*(1), 54–67.

Abbey, A., Parkhill, M. R., Clinton-Sherrod, A. M., & Zawacki, T. (2007). A comparison on men who committed different types of sexual assault in a community sample. *Journal of Interpersonal Violence, 22*, 1567–1580.

Akyuz, A., Şahiner, G., & Bakır, B. (2008). Marital violence: Is it a factor affecting the reproductive health status of women? *Journal of Family Violence, 23*(6), 437–445.

Bagwell-Gray, M. (2016). Intimate partner sexual violence poses risk factor for homicide. *Family & Intimate Partner Violence Quarterly, 9*(1), 41–51.

Bagwell-Gray, M. E., Messing, J. T., & Baldwin-White, A. (2015). Intimate partner sexual violence: A review of terms, definitions, and prevalence. *Trauma, Violence, & Abuse, 16*(3), 316–335.

Bancroft, L. (2002). *Why does he do that? Inside the minds of abusive and angry men*. New York: The Berkeley Publishing Group.

Barnawi, F. H. (2017). Prevalence and risk factors of domestic violence against women attending a primary care center in Riyadh, Saudi Arabia. *Journal of Interpersonal Violence, 32*(8), 1171–1186.

Basile, K. C. (1999). Rape by acquiescence: The ways in which women "give in" to unwanted sex with their husbands. *Violence Against Women, 5*, 1036–1058.

Basile, K. C. (2002). Prevalence of wife rape and other intimate partner sexual coercion in a nationally representative sample of women. *Violence and Victims, 17*, 511–524.

Beck, C. J. A., & Raghavan, C. (2010). Intimate partner abuse screening in custody mediation: The importance of assessing coercive control. *Family Court Review, 48*(3), 555–565.

Beech, A. R., & Mitchell, I. J. (2005). A neurobiological perspective on attachment problems in sexual offenders and the role of selective serotonin re-uptake inhibitors in treatment of such problems. *Clinical Psychology Review, 25*, 153–182.

Beech, A. R., & Ward, T. (2004). The integration of etiology and risk in sex offenders: A theoretical model. *Aggression and Violent Behavior, 10*, 31–63.

Bennice, J. A., & Resick, P. A. (2003). Marital rape: History, research, and practice. *Trauma, Violence, & Abuse, 4*, 228–246.

Bennice, J. A., Resick, P. A., Mechanic, M., & Astin, M. (2003). The relative effects of intimate partner physical and sexual violence on post-traumatic stress disorder. *Violence and Victims, 18*, 87–94.

Bergen, R. K. (1995). Surviving wife rape: How women define and cope with the violence. *Violence Against Women, 1*(2), 117–138.

Bergen, R. K. (1996). *Wife rape: Understanding the responses of survivors and service providers*. Thousand Oaks, CA: Sage.

Bergen, R. K. (2006). *Marital rape: New research and directions*. VAWnet: The National Online Resource Center on Violence Against Women. Retrieved from https://vawnet.org/material/marital-rape-new-research-and-directions

Bergen, R. K., & Barnhill, E. (2006). *Marital rape: New research and directions*. VAWnet: National Resource Center on Domestic Violence. Retrieved from https://www.nycourts.gov/ip/womeninthecourts/pdfs/MARITAL%20RAPE_1_d_1.pdf

Bornstein, R. F. (2006). The complex relationship between dependency and domestic violence: Converging psychological factors and social forces. *American Psychologist, 61*(6), 595–606.

Breiding, M. J., Smith, S. G., Basile, K. C., Walters, M. L., Chen, J., & Merrick, M. T. (2014). Prevalence and characteristics of sexual violence, stalking, and intimate partner violence victimization—National Intimate Partner and Sexual Violence Survey, United States, 2011. Centers for Disease Control and Prevention, Surveillance Summaries, 63(SS08), 1–18.

Brown, S. L., & Forth, A. E. (1997). Psychopathy and sexual assault: Static risk factors, emotional precursors, and rapist subtypes. *Journal of Consulting and Clinical Psychology, 65*, 848–857.

Brown, T. N. T., & Herman, J. L. (2015). *Intimate partner violence and sexual abuse among LGBT people*. The Williams Institute. Retrieved from https://williamsinstitute.law.ucla.edu/wp-content/uploads/Intimate-Partner-Violence-and-Sexual-Abuse-among-LGBT-People.pdf.

Burk, L. R., & Burkhart, B. R. (2003). Disorganized attachment as a diathesis for sexual deviance developmental experience and the motivation for sexual offending. *Aggression and Violent Behavior, 8*, 487–511.

Campbell, J. C. (1992). "If I can't have you, no one can": Power and control in homicide of female partners. In J. Radford & D. E. H. Russell (Eds.), *Femicide: The politics of woman killing* (pp. 99–113). New York: Twayne.

Campbell, J. C., & Alford, P. (1989). The dark consequences of marital rape. *American Journal of Nursing, 89*, 946–949.

Campbell, J. C., Jones, A. S., Dienemann, J., Kub, J., Schollenberger, J., O'Campo, P., … Wynne, C. (2002). Intimate partner violence and physical health consequences. *Archives of Internal Medicine, 167*, 1157–1163.

Campbell, J. C., Pugh, L. C., Campbell, D., & Visscher, M. (1995). The influence of abuse on pregnancy intention. *Women's Health Issues, 5*, 214–223.

Campbell, J. C., & Soeken, K. (1999). Forced sex and intimate partner violence: Effects on women's health. *Violence Against Women, 5*, 1017–1035.

Campbell, J. C., Webster, D., Koziol-McLain, J., Block, C., Campbell, D., Curry, M. A., … Laughon, K. (2003). Risk factors for femicide in abusive relationships: Results from a multisite case control study. *American Journal of Public Health, 93*(7), 1089–1097.

Cattaneo, L. B., DeLoveh, H. L. M., & Zweig, J. M. (2008). Sexual assault within intimate partner violence:

Impact on helpseeking in a national sample. *Journal of Prevention & Intervention in the Community, 36*(1–2), 137–153.

Chesire, J. D. (2004). Review, critique, and synthesis of personality theory in motivation to sexually assault. *Aggression and Violent Behavior, 9*, 633–644.

Coker, A. L., Sanderson, M., & Dong, B. (2004). Partner violence during pregnancy and risk of adverse pregnancy outcomes. *Pediatric and Perinatal Epidemiology, 18*, 260–269.

Cossins, A. (2000). *Masculinities, sexualities, and child sexual abuse*. The Hague: Kluwer Law International.

Cox, A. L., Coles, A. J., Nortje, J., Bradley, P. G., Chatfield, D. A., Thompson, S. J., & Menon, D. K. (2006). An investigation of auto-reactivity after head-injury. *Journal of Neuroimmunology, 174*, 180–186.

Daly, M., Wiseman, K. A., & Wilson, M. (1997). Women with children sired by previous partners incur excess risk of uxoricide. *Homicide Studies, 1*, 61–71.

Davis, K. C., Kiekel, P. A., Schraufnagel, T. J., Norris, J., George, W. H., & Kajumulo, K. F. (2012). Men's alcohol intoxication and condom use during sexual assault perpetration. *Journal of Interpersonal Violence, 27*(14), 2790–2806.

Dichter, M. E., & Gelles, R. J. (2012). Women's perceptions of safety and risk following police intervention for intimate partner violence. *Violence Against Women, 18*(1), 44–63.

Dunkle, K. L., Jewkes, R. K., Brown, H. C., & Gray, G. E. (2004). Gender-based violence, relationship power, and risk of HIV infection in women attending antenatal clinics in South Africa. *The Lancet, 363*(9419), 1415–1421.

Dunkle, K. L., Jewkes, R. K., Nduna, M., Levin, J., Jama, N., Khuzwayo, N., … Duvvury, N. (2006). Perpetration of partner violence and HIV risk behaviour among young men in the rural Eastern Cape, South Africa. *AIDS, 20*, 2107–2114.

Dutton, M. A., Kaltman, S., Goodman, L. A., Weinfurt, K., & Vankos, N. (2005). Patterns of intimate partner violence: Correlates and outcomes. *Violence and Victims, 20*(5), 483–497.

Eby, K. K., & Campbell, J. C. (1995). Health effects of experiences of sexual violence for women with abusive partners. *Women's Health Care International, 14*, 563–576.

Eby, K. K., Campbell, J. C., Sullivan, C. M., & Davidson, W. S., II. (1995). Health effects of experiences of sexual violence for women with abusive partners. *Health Care for Women International, 16*, 563–576.

Esteal, P., & McOrmond-Plummer, L. (2005). *Real rape, real pain: Help for women sexually assaulted by male partners*. Melbourne: Hybrid Publishers.

Fanslow, J. L., & Robinson, E. M. (2010). Help-Seeking behaviors and reasons for help seeking reported by a representative sample of women victims of intimate partner violence in New Zealand. *Journal of Interpersonal Violence, 25*(5), 929–951.

Finkelhor, D., & Yllo, K. (1985). *License to rape: Sexual abuse of wives*. New York: Holt, Rinehart, & Winston.

Frieze, I. (1983). Investigating the causes and consequences of marital rape. *Signs, 8*, 532–553.

Gage, A. J., & Hutchinson, P. L. (2006). Power, control, and intimate partner sexual violence in Haiti. *Archives of Sexual Behavior, 35*(1), 11–24.

Garcia-Moreno, C., Jansen, H. A. F. M., Ellsberg, M., Heise, L., & Watts, C. H. (2006). Prevalence of intimate partner violence: Findings from the WHO multicountry study on women's health and domestic violence. *The Lancet, 368*, 1260–1269.

Garcia-Moreno, C., & Watts, C. (2000). Violence against women: Its importance for HIV/AIDS. *AIDS, 14*(suppl 3), 253–265.

Gazmararian, J. A., Adams, M. M., Saltzman, L. E., Johnson, C. H., Bruce, F. C., Marks, J. S., & Zahniser, S. C. (1995). The relationship between intendedness and physical violence in mothers of newborns. *Obstetrics and Gynecology, 85*, 131–138.

Gazmararian, J. A., Petersen, R., Spitz, A. M., Goodwin, M. M., Saltzman, L. E., & Marks, J. S. (2000). Violence and reproductive health: Current knowledge and future research directions. *Maternal and Child Health Journal, 4*(2), 79–84.

Glass, N., Manganello, J., & Campbell, J. C. (2004). Risk for intimate partner femicide in violent relationships. *DV Report, 9*(2), 30–33.

Gondolf, E. W., & Fisher, E. R. (1988). *Battered women as survivors*. New York: Lexington.

Graffunder, D. M., Noonan, R. K., Cox, P., & Wheaton, J. (2004). Through a public health lens. Preventing violence against women: An update from the U.S. Centers for Disease Control and Prevention. *Journal of Women's Health, 3*, 5–14.

Hall, J. E., Walters, M. L., & Basile, K. C. (2012). Intimate partner violence perpetration by court-ordered men: Distinctions among subtypes of physical violence, sexual violence, psychological abuse, and stalking. *Journal of Interpersonal Violence, 27*(7), 1374–1395.

Helton, A. S., McFarlane, J., & Anderson, E. T. (1987). Battered and pregnant: A prevalence study. *American Journal of Public Health, 77*, 1337–1339.

Henshaw, S. K. (1998). Unintended pregnancy in the United States. *Family Planning Perspectives, 30*, 24–29.

Horon, I. L., & Cheng, D. (2001). Enhanced surveillance for pregnancy associated mortality in Maryland, 1993-1998. *Journal of the American Medical Association, 285*, 1455–1459.

Howard, A., Riger, S., Campbell, R., & Wasco, S. (2003). Counseling services for battered women: A comparison for physical and sexual assault survivors. *Journal of Interpersonal Violence, 18*(7), 717–734.

Javaid, A. (2016). Feminism, masculinity and male rape: Bringing male rape 'out of the closet'. *Journal of Gender Studies, 25*(3), 283–293.

Jewkes, R., Sikweyiya, Y., Morrell, R., & Dunkle, K. (2011). Gender inequitable masculinity and sexual entitlement in rape perpetration South Africa: Findings of a cross-sectional study. *PLoS One, 6*, e29590.

Jewkes, R. K., Dunkle, K., Nduna, M., & Shai, N. (2010). Intimate partner violence, relationship power inequity, and incidence of HIV infection in young women in South Africa: A cohort study. *Lancet, 376*, 41–48.

Johansson, A., Santtila, P., Harlaar, N., von der Pahlen, B., Witting, K., Algars, M., … Sandnabba, N. K. (2008). Genetic effects on male sexual coercion. *Aggressive Behavior, 34*, 190–202.

Johnson, M. P. (1995). Patriarchal terrorism and common couple violence: Two forms of violence against women. *Journal of Marriage and the Family, 57*, 283-294.

Johnson, M. P. (2008). *A typology of domestic violence: Intimate terrorism, violent resistance, and situational couple violence*. Lebanon, NH: Northeastern University Press.

Johnson, M. P., & Leone, J. M. (2005). The differential effects of intimate terrorism and situational couple violence. *Journal of Family Issues, 26*(3), 322–349.

Kayson, D., Dillworth, T. M., Simpson, T., Waldrop, A., Larimer, M. E., & Resick, P. A. (2007). Domestic violence and alcohol use: Trauma-related symptoms and motives for drinking. *Addictive Behaviors, 32*, 1272–1283.

Keeling, J., Birch, L., & Green, P. (2004). Pregnancy counseling clinic: A questionnaire survey of intimate partner abuse. *The Journal of Family Planning and Reproductive Health Care, 30*(3), 165–168.

Kemp, A., Green, B. L., Hovanitz, C., & Rawlings, E. I. (1995). Incidence and correlates of posttraumatic stress disorder in battered women: Shelter and community samples. *Journal of Interpersonal Violence, 10*, 43–55.

King, J. C. (2003). The risk of maternal nutritional depletion and poor outcomes increases in early or closely spaced pregnancies. *Journal of Nutrition, 133*, 1732S–1736S.

Knight, R. A. (1999). Validation of a typology for rapists. *Journal of Interpersonal Violence, 14*, 303–330.

Lazar, R. (2010). Negotiating sex: The legal construct of consent in cases of wife rape in Ontario, Canada. *Canadian Journal of Women and the Law, 22*, 329–363.

Logan, T. (2011). *The pilot study data results*. Unpublished data.

Logan, T., Cole, J., & Shannon, L. (2007). A mixed-methods examination of sexual coercion and degradation among women in violent relationships who do and do not report forced sex. *Violence and Victims, 22*, 71–94.

Logan, T. K., Walker, R., & Cole, J. (2015). Silenced suffering: The need for a better understanding of partner sexual violence. *Trauma, Violence, & Abuse, 16*(2), 111–135.

MacKinnon, C. (1983). Feminism, marxism, method, and the state: Toward feminist jurisprudence. *Signs, 8*(4), 635–658.

MacKinnon, C. (1991). Reflections on sex equality under law. *The Yale Law Journal, 100*, 1281–1328.

Maddoux, J., McFarlane, J., Liu, F., & Liu, F. (2015). Risks for women from abusers violating protection orders. *American Journal of Family Law, 29*(1), 32–40.

Malamuth, N. M., Linz, D., Heavey, C. L., Barnes, G., & Acker, M. (1995). Using the confluence model of sexual aggression to predict men's conflict with women: A 10 year follow up study. *Journal of Personality & Social Psychology, 69*, 353–369.

Maniglio, R. (2010). The role of deviant sexual fantasy in the etiopathogenesis of sexual homicide: A systemic review. *Aggression and Violent Behavior, 15*, 294–302.

McFarlane, J. (2007). Pregnancy following partner rape: What we know and what we need to know. *Trauma, Violence, & Abuse, 8*, 127–134.

McFarlane, J., Campbell, J. C., Sharps, P., & Watson, K. (2002). Abuse during pregnancy and femicide: urgent implications for women's health. *Obstetrics and Gynecology, 100*(1), 27–36.

McFarlane, J., Campbell, J. C., & Soeken, K. (1995). Abuse during pregnancy: Frequency, severity, perpetrator, and risk factors of homicide. *Public Health Nursing, 12*(5), 284–289.

McFarlane, J., Malecha, A., Gist, J., Watson, K., Batten, E., Hall, I., & Smith, S. (2005). Intimate partner sexual assault against women and associated victim substance use, suicidality, and risk factors for femicide. *Issues in Mental Health Nursing, 26*, 953–967.

McFarlane, J., Malecha, A., Watson, K., Gist, J., Batten, E., Hall, I., & Smith, S. (2005). Intimate partner sexual assault against women: Frequency, health consequences, and treatment outcomes. *Obstetrics and Gynecology, 105*, 99–108.

McPhail, B. A. (2015). Feminist framework plus: Knitting feminist theories of rape etiology into a comprehensive model. *Trauma, Violence, & Abuse, 17*(3), 314–329.

Messing, J. T., Amanor-Boadu, Y., Cavanaugh, C. E., Glass, N. E., & Campbell, J. C. (2013). Culturally competent intimate partner violence risk assessment: Adapting the danger assessment for immigrant women. *Social Work Research, 37*(3), 263–275.

Messing, J. T., Thaller, J., & Bagwell, M. (2014). Factors related to sexual abuse and forced sex in a sample of women experiencing police-involved intimate partner violence. *Health & Social Work, 39*, 181–191.

Meyer, A., Wagner, B., & Dutton, M. A. (2010). The relationship between battered women's causal attributions for violence and coping efforts. *Journal of Interpersonal Violence, 25*(5), 900–918.

Monson, C. M., Langhinrichsen-Rohling, J., & Binderup, T. (2000). Does "no" really mean "no" after you say "yes"? Attributions about date and marital rape. *Journal of Interpersonal Violence, 15*(11), 1156–1174.

Ogle, R. S., Maier-Katkin, D., & Bernard, T. J. (1995). A theory of homicidal behavior among women. *Criminology, 33*, 173–194.

Parker, E. M., Gielen, A. C., Castillo, R., & Webster, D. (2015). Safety strategy use among women seeking temporary protective orders: The relationship between violence experienced, strategy effectiveness, and risk perception. *Violence and Victims, 30*(4), 615–635.

Pitman, T. (2017). Living with coercive control: Trapped within a complex web of double standards, double binds and boundary violations. *The British Journal of Social Work, 47*(1), 143–161.

Plichta, S. B., & Falik, M. (2001). Prevalence of violence and its implications for women's health. *Women's Health Issues, 11*, 244–258.

Prentky, R. A., Knight, R. A., Sims-Knight, J. E., Straus, H., Rokous, F., & Cerce, D. (1989). Developmental antecedents of sexual aggression. *Development and Psychopathology, 1*, 153–169.

Raj, A., Liu, R., McCleary, J., & Silverman, J. G. (2005). South Asian victims of intimate partner violence more likely than non-victims to report sexual health concerns. *Journal of Immigrant Health, 7*(2), 85–91.

Raj, A., Santana, M. C., La Marche, A., Amaro, H., Cranston, K., & Silverman, J. G. (2006). Perpetration of intimate partner violence associated with sexual risk behaviors among young adult men. *American Journal of Public Health, 96*, 1873–1878.

Raj, A., Silverman, J. G., & Amaro, H. (2004). Abused women report greater male partner risk and gender-based risk for HIV: Findings from a community-based study with Hispanic women. *AIDS Care, 16*, 519–529.

Reckdenwald, A., & Parker, K. F. (2012). Understanding the change in male and female intimate partner homicide over time: A policy-and-theory-relevant investigation. *Feminist Criminology, 7*(3), 167–195.

Rickert, V. I., Wiemann, C. M., Harrykissoon, S. D., Berenson, A. B., & Kolb, E. (2002). The relationship among demographics, reproductive characteristics, and intimate partner violence. *American Journal of Obstetrics and Gynecology, 187*, 1002–1007.

Risser, J. M. H., Shelton, A., McCurdy, S., Atkinson, J., Padgett, P., Useche, B., … Williams, M. (2005). Sex, drugs, violence, and HIV status among male-to- female transgender persons in Houston, Texas. *International Journal of Transgenderism, 8*(2–3), 67–74.

Roch, A., Morton, J., & Ritchie, G. (2010). *Out of sight, out of mind? Transgender people's experiences of domestic abuse*. LGBTYouth Scotland & Equality Network

Russell, D. E. H. (1990). *Rape in marriage*. Bloomington, IN: Indiana University Press.

Saltzman, L. E., Fanslow, J. L., McMahon, P. M., & Shelley, G. A. (2002). *Intimate partner violence surveillance: Uniform definitions and recommended data elements (version 1.0)*. Atlanta, GA: Centers for Disease Control and Prevention, National Center for Injury Prevention and Control.

Scully, D., & Marolla, J. (1985). Riding the bull at Gilley's: Convicted rapists describe the rewards of rape. *Social Problems, 32*, 251–263.

Searles, P., & Berger, R. J. (Eds.). (1995). *Rape and society: Readings on the problem of sexual assault*. Boulder, CO: Westview.

Shannon, L., Logan, T. K., Cole, J., & Walker, R. W. (2008). An examination of women's alcohol use and partner victimization experiences among women with protective orders. *Substance Use & Misuse, 43*, 1110–1128.

Shields, N., & Hanneke, C. (1983). Battered wives reactions to marital rape. In D. Finkelhor, R. Gelles, et al. (Eds.), *The dark side of families: Current family violence research* (pp. 131–148). Thousand Oaks, CA: Sage Publications.

Shotland, R. L., & Goodstein, L. (1992). Sexual precedence reduces the perceived legitimacy of sexual refusal: An examination of attributions concerning date rape and consensual sex. *Personality and Social Psychology Bulletin, 18*, 756–764.

Siegert, R. J., & Ward, T. (2003). Back to the future: Evolutionary explanations of rape. In T. Ward, D. R. Laws, & S. M. Hudson (Eds.), *Sexual deviance: Issues and controversies* (pp. 45–64). Thousand Oaks, CA: Sage.

Stanko, E. A. (1990). *Everyday violence: How women and men experience sexual and physical danger*. London: Harper Collins.

Stark, E. (2007). *Coercive control: How men entrap women in personal life*. New York: Oxford University Press.

Stark, E. (2009). *Coercive control: How men entrap women in personal life*. New York: Oxford University Press.

Stark, E. (2012). Re-presenting battered women: Coercive control and the defense of liberty. Violence Against Women: Complex Realities and New Issues in a Changing World. Les Presses de l'Université du Québec, 3–19. Retrieved from http://www.stopvaw.org/uploads/evan_stark_article_final_100812.pdf.

Stockl, H., & Gardner, F. (2013). Women's perceptions on how pregnancy influences the context of intimate partner violence. *Culture, Health, & Sexuality, 15*(10), 1206–1220.

Sugihara, Y., & Warner, J. A. (2002). Dominance and domestic abuse among Mexican Americans: Gender differences in the etiology of violence in intimate relationships. *Journal of Family Violence, 17*(4), 315–340.

Swayne, M. (2014, August 19). Love makes sex better for most women. *Penn State News*. Retrieved from https://news.psu.edu/story/323224/2014/08/19/research/love-makes-sex-better-most-women.

Temple, J. R., Weston, R., Rodriguez, B. F., & Marshall, L. L. (2007). Differing effects of partner and nonpartner sexual assault on women's mental health. *Violence Against Women, 13*(3), 285–297.

Thornton, D. (2002). Constructing and testing a framework for dynamic risk assessment. *Sexual Abuse, 14*, 139–154.

Tjaden, P., & Thoennes, N. (2000). *Full report of prevalence, incidence, and consequences of violence against women: Findings from the national violence against women survey (NCJ 183781)*. Washington, DC: U.S. Department of Justice, National Institute of Justice.

Turrell, S. C. (2000). A descriptive analysis of same-sex relationship violence for a diverse sample. *Journal of Family Violence, 15*(3), 281–293.

Walters, M. L., Chen, J., & Breiding, M. J. (2013). *The National Intimate Partner and Sexual Violence Survey (NISVS): 2010 findings on victimization by sexual orientation*. Atlanta, GA: National Center for Injury Prevention and Control, Centers for Disease Control and Prevention. Retrieved from https://www.cdc.gov/violenceprevention/pdf/nisvs_sofindings.pdf

Ward, T., & Beech, A. (2006). An integrated theory of sexual offending. *Aggression and Violent Behavior, 11*, 44–63.

Ward, T., Polaschek, D. L. L., & Beech, A. R. (2006). *Theories of sexual offending*. West Sussex: John Wiley & Sons.

Weaver, T. L., Allen, J. A., Hopper, E., Maglione, M. L., McLaughlin, D., McCullough, M. A., ... Brewer, T. (2007). Mediators of suicidal ideation within a sheltered sample of raped and battered women. *Health Care for Women International, 28*, 478–448.

Websdale, N. (1999). *Understanding domestic homicide*. Lebanon, NH: Northeastern University Press.

White, J. W., & Post, L. A. (2003). Understanding rape: A metatheoretical framework. In C. B. Travis (Ed.), *Evolution, gender, and rape* (pp. 383–411). Cambridge, MA: MIT Press.

Wilson, M. I., & Daly, M. (1992). Who kills whom in spouse killings? On the exceptional sex ratio of spousal homicides in the United States. *Criminology, 30*, 189–215.

Wingood, G. M., DiClemente, R. J., McCree, D. H., Harrington, K., & Davies, S. L. (2001). Dating violence and the sexual health of black adolescent females. *Pediatrics, 107*, E72.

Yllo, K. (1999). The silence surrounding sexual violence: The issue of marital rape and the challenges it poses for the Duluth model. In M. Shepard & E. Pence (Eds.), *Coordinating community responses to domestic violence: Lessons from the Duluth model* (pp. 223–238). Thousand Oaks, CA: Sage.

Zilkens, R. R., Phillips, M. A., Kelly, M. C., Mukhtar, S. A., Semmens, J. B., & Smith, D. A. (2016). Non-fatal strangulation in sexual assault: A study of clinical and assault characteristics highlighting the role of intimate partner violence. *Journal of Forensic and Legal Medicine, 43*, 1–7.

Zweig, J. M., Yahner, J., & Rossman, S. B. (2012). Does recent physical and sexual victimization affect further substance use for adult drug-involved offenders? *Journal of Interpersonal Violence, 27*, 2348–2372.

Shannon B. Harper, Ph.D. is an Assistant Professor of criminal justice studies in the Sociology Department at Iowa State University. Shannon's current research examines how domestic violence resources affect neighborhood intimate partner homicide (IPH) trajectories and how severely abused women (i.e., women at risk of homicide) construct the relevance and accessibility of those resources. Shannon's published works can be found in *Feminist Criminology*, *Sociology Compass*, and the *Journal of School Violence*.

Index

W. T. O'Donohue and P. A. Schewe (eds.), *Handbook of Sexual Assault and Sexual Assault Prevention*,
https://doi.org/10.1007/978-3-030-23645-8

I

J

Q

R

T

U